AF548695

Atlas of limb prosthetics

SURGICAL AND PROSTHETIC PRINCIPLES

American Academy of Orthopaedic Surgeons

Atlas of limb prosthetics

SURGICAL AND PROSTHETIC PRINCIPLES

American Academy of Orthopaedic Surgeons

with 1168 *illustrations*

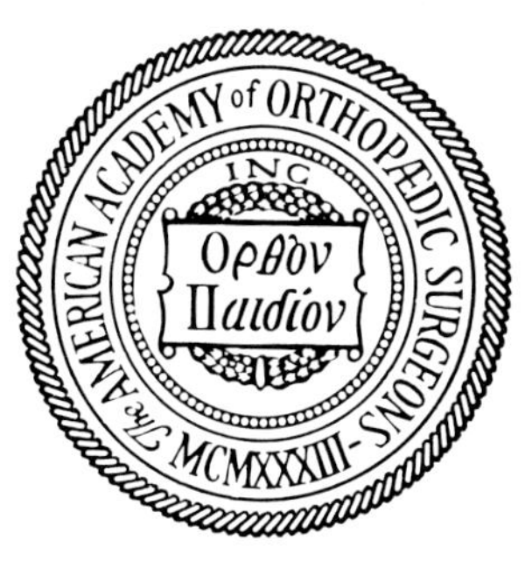

The C. V. Mosby Company

ST. LOUIS • TORONTO • LONDON 1981

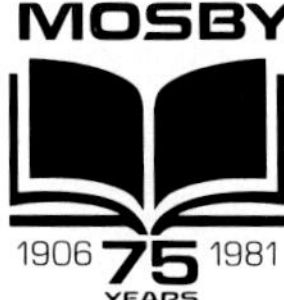

A TRADITION OF PUBLISHING EXCELLENCE

Printed in the United States of America

The C. V. Mosby Company
11830 Westline Industrial Drive, St. Louis, Missouri 63141

Library of Congress Cataloging in Publication Data

American Academy of Orthopaedic Surgeons.
Atlas of limb prosthetics.

Bibliography: p.
Includes index.
1. Artificial limbs. 2. Amputation. I. Title.
[DNLM: 1. Amputation—Atlases. 2. Amputees—Atlases. 3. Artificial limbs—Atlases. WE17 A512a]
RD756.A38 1980 617′.58 80-16572
ISBN 0-8016-0058-8

C/U/B 9 8 7 6 5 4 3 2 1 05/B/597

Contributors

GEORGE T. AITKEN, M.D.

Former Medical Director, Area Child Amputee Program; Clinical Professor, Department of Surgery, Michigan State University College of Human Medicine, Grand Rapids, Michigan

NORMAN BERGER, B.S., M.S.

Senior Research Scientist, Orthopedic Surgery, New York University Medical Center, New York, New York

SIDNEY J. BLAIR, M.D.

Chief, Section of Hand Surgery; Associate Professor, Orthopedic Surgery, Loyola University Stritch School of Medicine, Maywood, Illinois

JOHN H. BOWKER, M.D.

Professor, Department of Orthopaedic Surgery, University of Arkansas College of Medicine, Little Rock, Arkansas; Medical Director, Arkansas Rehabilitation Institute, Little Rock, Arkansas

MARTIN L. BUCKNER, C.P.O.

Director of Prosthetics and Orthotics, Mississippi Methodist Rehabilitation Center, Jackson, Mississippi

WILTON H. BUNCH, M.D., Ph.D.

Professor and Chairman, Department of Orthopedics, Loyola University Medical Center, Maywood, Illinois

ERNEST M. BURGESS, M.D.

Principal Investigator, Prosthetics Research Study, Seattle, Washington; Clinical Professor, Department of Orthopedics, University of Washington, Seattle, Washington

WILLIAM E. BURKHALTER, M.D.

Professor of Orthopaedics and Chief, Division of Hand Surgery, Department of Orthopaedics and Rehabilitation, University of Miami School of Medicine, Miami, Florida

JAMES M. CARY, M.D.

Assistant Clinical Professor of Orthopaedic Surgery, Yale University School of Medicine, New Haven, Connecticut

DUDLEY S. CHILDRESS, Ph.D.

Professor (Dual Appointment), Orthopaedic Surgery and Electrical Engineering and Computer Science, Northwestern University, Chicago, Illinois

RUTH DICKEY, B.S., O.T.R.

Occupational Therapist, Rehabilitation Engineering Center, Institute of Rehabilitation Medicine, New York University Medical Center, New York, New York

CHARLES M. FRYER, B.S., M.S.

Assistant Professor, Orthopaedic Surgery, Northwestern University Medical School, Chicago, Illinois

BERT GORALNIK, C.P., M.S.

Technical Assistant to the Director, Veterans Administration Rehabilitation Engineering Center, New York, New York

FREDERICK L. HAMPTON, C.P.

Director, Prosthetic and Orthotic Education, Department of Orthopaedics and Rehabilitation, University of Miami School of Medicine, Miami, Florida

ANNE R. HARRIS, R.P.T.

Assistant Chief Physical Therapist, Supervisor of Amputees, Department of Orthopaedics and Rehabilitation, Physical Therapy Department, University of Miami School of Medicine, Jackson Memorial Hospital, Miami, Florida

ROBERT HAYES, C.P.

President, Hayes Prosthetics, Inc., West Springfield, Massachusetts

CHARLES A. HOFMANN, S.J., Ph.D.

Archdiocesan Consultation Service, Archdiocese of Cincinnati, 29 East Eighth Street, Cincinnati, Ohio

†HECTOR W. KAY

Assistant Executive Director, Committee on Prosthetics Research and Development, National Academy of Sciences—National Research Council, Washington, D.C.

BERNICE KEGEL, R.P.T.

Chief of Rehabilitation, Prosthetics Research Study, Seattle, Washington

JOANNE SIMON KESTNBAUM, B.S., M.A., A.C.S.W.

Evanston, Illinois

STEPHEN KRAMER, C.P.O.

President, Universal Orthopedic Laboratories, Inc., Chicago, Illinois

ALFRED E. KRITTER, M.D.

Associate Clinical Professor of Orthopaedics, Orthopaedics, Medical College of Wisconsin, Milwaukee, Wisconsin

LEON M. KRUGER, M.D.

Chief of Staff, Shriners Hospital for Crippled Children, Springfield, Massachusetts; Clinical Professor of Orthopaedic Surgery, Department of Orthopaedic Surgery, New York University School of Medicine, Postgraduate Medical School, New York, New York; Clinical Professor of Orthopedic Surgery, Boston University Medical Center, Boston, Massachusetts

MADELYN M. LABORIEL, M.D.

Department of Pediatrics, University of California Los Angeles School of Medicine, Los Angeles, California

CLAUDE N. LAMBERT, M.D.

Emeritus Professor and former Chairman, Department of Orthopaedic Surgery, University of Illinois College of Medicine, Chicago, Illinois

H. RICHARD LEHNEIS, Ph.D., C.P.O.

Research Assistant Professor of Rehabilitation Medicine; Director, Orthotics and Prosthetics, Institute of Rehabilitation Medicine, New York University Medical Center, New York, New York

FRED LEVIT, M.D.

Professor of Clinical Dermatology, Department of Dermatology, Northwestern University, Chicago, Illinois

THOMAS LUNSFORD, M.S.E., C.O.

Chief, Orthotics Department; Director, Orthotic Education, Rancho Los Amigos Hospital, Downey, California

ERNST MARQUARDT, M.D.

Professor Doctor of Medicine, Head of Dysmelia Department and Technical Orthopaedics, Orthopaedic Hospital, University of Heidelberg, Heidelberg, Germany

NEWTON C. McCOLLOUGH, III, M.D.

Professor and Chairman, Department of Orthopaedics and Rehabilitation, Director of Rehabilitation Center, Jackson Memorial Hospital, University of Miami School of Medicine, Miami, Florida

VERT MOONEY, M.D.

Professor and Chairman, Division of Orthopedic Surgery, The University of Texas Health Science Center at Dallas, Dallas, Texas

EDWARD PEIZER, Ph.D.

Assistant Director, Veterans Administration Rehabilitation Engineering Center, New York, New York

†Deceased.

RAYMOND J. PELLICORE, M.D.

Assistant Clinical Professor, Abraham Lincoln School of Medicine, and Chairman, Department of Orthopaedics, Illinois Central Hospital and St. Mary of Nazareth Hospital, Chicago, Illinois

JACQUELIN PERRY, M.D.

Chief of Pathokinesiology, Rancho Los Amigos Hospital, Downey, California; Professor of Orthopaedics, University of Southern California, Los Angeles, California

MICHAEL J. QUIGLEY

President, Amerimed, Inc., River Forest, Illinois

GUSTAV RUBIN, M.D.

Orthopaedic Consultant, Veterans Administration Rehabilitation Engineering Center, New York, New York

SHAHAN K. SARRAFIAN, M.D.

Assistant Professor, Orthopedic Surgery, Northwestern University Medical School, Chicago, Illinois

MAURICE D. SCHNELL, M.D.

Associate Professor, Department of Orthopedics, University of Virginia Medical School, Charlottesville, Virginia

YOSHIO SETOGUCHI, M.D.

Adjunct Professor of Pediatrics, Department of Pediatrics, University of California Los Angeles School of Medicine, Los Angeles, California

JAY D. SHEARER, M.Ed., M.T.R.S.

Therapeutic Recreation Specialist, Arkansas Rehabilitation Institute, Little Rock, Arkansas

JANET S. SMELTZER, O.T.R.

Assistant Chief, Occupational Therapy, Occupational Therapy—Rehabilitation, Jackson Memorial Hospital, Miami, Florida

ANTHONY STAROS, M.S., P.E.

Director, Veterans Administration Rehabilitation Engineering Center, New York, New York

ROBERT G. THOMPSON, M.D.

Clinical Professor of Orthopaedic Surgery, Department of Orthopaedic Surgery, Northwestern University Medical School, Chicago, Illinois

ROBERT E. TOOMS, M.D.

Clinical Professor, Department of Orthopedic Surgery, University of Tennessee Center for the Health Sciences, Memphis, Tennessee; Active Staff, Campbell Clinic, Memphis, Tennessee

RICHARD VONER, C.P.O.

Orthomedics, Inc., Chief Clinical Prosthetist, Rancho Los Amigos Hospital, Downey, California

F. WILLIAM WAGNER, Jr., M.D.

Clinical Professor, Orthopedic Surgery, University of Southern California, Los Angeles, California; Chief, Ortho-Diabetes Service, Rancho Los Amigos Hospital, Downey, California

ROBERT L. WATERS, M.D.

Chief of Surgery, Rancho Los Amigos Hospital, Downey, California

HUGH G. WATTS, M.D.

Professor, Department of Orthopaedics, University of Pennsylvania School of Medicine, Philadelphia, Pennsylvania

A. BENNETT WILSON, Jr., B.S.M.E.

Director, Rehabilitation Engineering, Division of Orthopedics, The University of Texas Health Science Center at Dallas, Dallas, Texas

Preface

The wars of the past 40 years have yielded untold numbers of young men in their prime whose limb loss has stimulated extensive research in the management of the amputee. Progress has been made in many areas of amputee rehabilitation, including new surgical techniques, better understanding of the biomechanical principles involved in normal and abnormal human locomotion, and improved design of artificial limbs using new materials and components.

In the lower limb, appreciation of biomechanical principles and energy costs, combined with the capability for more versatile prosthetic design, have altered many of our old concepts regarding "site of election" for amputation. Although the stimulus to improvement in care of the lower limb amputee can be traced to the tragedy of war, the cobeneficiary of such endeavors has been the patient with circulatory insufficiency, which commonly necessitates amputation of one or both lower limbs. In current practice, lower limb amputation accounts for over 80% of all amputations performed.

Upper limb amputation, by contrast, is far less frequent and presents a far greater challenge in prosthetic replacement. As in the lower limb, the success of rehabilitation can be correlated closely with the level of amputation. Nevertheless, immense problems remain in prosthetically restoring sensory capacity and manipulation of objects within the grasp, both of which are essential to optimum upper limb function. Major advances have been made in the areas of myoelectric control and powered components, but much remains to be accomplished.

In 1962, the Committee to Study Braces and Prostheses of the American Academy of Orthopaedic Surgeons published volume II of the *Orthopaedic Appliance Atlas,* a monumental work on limb prosthetics. This volume provided much needed information on the technical aspects of prosthetic substitution.

It is the purpose of this book to relate the surgical procedure of amputation to the rehabilitation of the amputee. Surgical procedures are presented primarily in the context of restoring maximum function to the patient following limb ablation. The text is organized to provide general information as an overview and specific information regarding surgical considerations, prosthetic replacement, and prosthetic rehabilitation for each level of amputation. The final part is devoted to the juvenile amputee, covering both acquired amputations and congenital limb deficiency. Outstanding authorities from the fields of amputation surgery, prosthetics, physical and occupational therapy, engineering, and numerous other allied professions have contributed material for this atlas. Thus a spectrum of information is provided to the reader regarding the amputee from the initial surgical decision to the completion of rehabilitation.

The material presented in this book has been made available by the American Academy of Orthopaedic Surgeons for educational purposes only. This material is not intended to represent the only, or necessarily best, methods or procedures appropriate for the medical situations discussed, but rather is intended to present an approach, view, statement, or opinion of the authors, which may be helpful to others who face similar situations.

It is hoped that all professionals involved with the care of the amputee will benefit from the contents of this text, perhaps more from parts that are written by persons from disciplines other than their own. The ultimate beneficiaries of this work will undoubtedly be the amputee and the congenital limb-deficient individual. It is to this segment of our handicapped population that we have dedicated our effort.

The Committee on Prosthetics and Orthotics wishes to gratefully acknowledge the extensive financial and technical assistance provided by the Veterans Administration without which the publication of this book would not have been possible. To the many authors who have contributed material for this atlas, the Committee is indeed most appreciative and indebted.

The Committee on Prosthetics and Orthotics,
American Academy of Orthopaedic Surgeons

Newton C. McCollough, III, *Chairman*
Wilton H. Bunch, *Secretary*
Ernest M. Burgess, *Advisor*
Frank W. Clippinger
Alfred E. Kritter
Leon M. Kruger
Joseph G. Matthews
Paul R. Meyer
Maurice D. Schnell
Anthony Staros

Prior contributing members

John H. Bowker
James M. Cary
Raymond J. Pellicore
Jacquelin Perry
Robert G. Thompson *(ex officio)*

Contents

PART ONE

Introduction

CHAPTER 1

History of amputation surgery and prosthetics

A. BENNETT WILSON, Jr.

No doubt artificial limbs of some type, such as a forked stick, have been used since the beginning of mankind, but the earliest recorded use of a limb prosthesis is that of a Persian soldier, Hegesistratus, who Herodotus[49] reported escaped about 484 BC from stocks by cutting off his foot and replacing it with a wooden one. The oldest known artificial limb in existence was a copper and wood leg unearthed at Capri, Italy, in 1858, which was supposedly made about 300 BC. Unfortunately, it was destroyed during a bombing of London in World War II.

Artificial hands made of iron were used by knights in the fifteenth century. The Alt-Ruppin hand, shown along with other hands from the fifteenth century in the Stibbert Museum, Florence, Italy, is a good example of the work of that age.

With respect to surgery, Hippocrates described the use of ligatures, but this technique was lost during the Dark Ages. It was reintroduced in 1529 by Ambroise Pare,[44] a French military surgeon. As a result, amputations came to be used more and more as a lifesaving measure, since the rate of survival was much higher when ligatures were used.

Morel[24] introduced the tourniquet in 1674, which gave another impetus to amputation surgery. Pare[44] carried out the first elbow disarticulation procedure in 1536. Sir James Syme[39] reported the Syme procedure for amputation at the ankle in 1843.

The introduction of antiseptic techniques by Lord Lister[25] (1867), a student and son-in-law of Syme, contributed greatly to the overall success of amputation surgery, as did the use of chloroform and ether about the same time.

The concept of kineplasty to power upper limb prostheses directly by muscle contraction was introduced by Vanghetti[55] in 1898 while trying to improve the function of Italian soldiers who had had their hands amputated by the Abyssinians. Vanghetti's associate, Ceci,[12] performed the first operation of this type on humans in 1900. Sauerbruch[48] (1916), in Germany, developed the skin-lined muscle tunnel, and Bosch Arana,[8] in Argentina, carried out clinical studies of this procedure in the 1920s.

Ertl in Germany (1949) developed the technique known as "myodesis," which consists of tying the distal ends of the cut muscle of the stump to the bone in such a way that reattachment is encouraged.[20] This idea seems to have been abandoned until much later, when it was revived by Dederich in the 1950s.[16]

Each major war seems to have been the stimulus not only for improvement of amputation surgical techniques, but also for the development of improved prostheses. World War II was no exception. Toward the end of World War II, amputees in military hospitals in the United States began voicing their disappointment about the performance afforded by their artificial limbs. To ensure that they received the best care possible, the Surgeon General of the Army, Norman T. Kirk, an orthopaedic surgeon by training, turned to the National Academy of Sciences (NAS) for advice.

A COORDINATED PROGRAM FOR AMPUTEES

A conference of surgeons, prosthetists, and scientists organized by the NAS early in 1945 revealed that little modern scientific effort had gone into the development of artificial limbs, and a "crash" research program was launched later in 1945 through the NAS.[14] This effort was initially funded by the Office of Scientific Research and Development (OSRD). At the end of the war, when OSRD was disbanded, the Office of the Surgeon General of the Army continued support that was later assumed by the Veterans Administration, which had also inherited the responsibility for the care of amputees after discharge from the armed services.

For the first 2 years the NAS, through the Committee on Artificial Limbs (CAL), actually operated the program through subcontracts with several universities and industrial laboratories. On June 30, 1947, the CAL disbanded, and the role of the NAS became an advisory one to the Veterans Administration, which contracted directly with various research groups. In 1947, the Veterans Administration also established its own testing and development laboratory in New York City. The army and navy cooperated by supporting prosthetics research laboratories within their own organizations. From July 1, 1947, to December 1, 1955, the group within the NAS was known as the Advisory Committee on Artificial Limbs. The Prosthetics Research Board was created to carry out the NAS responsibility from December 1, 1955, to June 30, 1959. In July, 1959, the Committee on Prosthetics Research and Development and the Committee on Prosthetics Education and Information (later called the Committee on Prosthetics-Orthotics Education), both subgroups of the board, assumed this role until their dissolution by the parent NAS in 1976, the reason for which has never been made completely clear.

The Artificial Limb Program, as it came to be known, was started initially with the idea that physicians and surgeons could provide engineers with design criteria for components such as ankle and knee joints and that good engineering design based on these criteria and coupled with modern materials would result in devices that could solve many of the problems of the amputee. Although some progress by this approach was made early in the program, it soon became apparent that fundamental information on how human limbs function was needed before adequate design criteria could be formulated. To provide such information on lower limb function, a project was established at the University of California, Berkeley, as a joint responsibility of the Engineering and Medical Schools. Eberhart et al.,[18] who had collaborated previously in a biomechanical analysis of the shoulder, directed this program, which began by using the latest technology to refine and add to the existing knowledge of human locomotion. A concurrent program was initiated under Taylor in the Engineering School at the University of California, Los Angeles, on the function of the upper limbs.[14]

At the same time design and development projects were being carried out at Northrop Aviation, Inc.; Catranis, Inc.; the Army Prosthetics Research Laboratory; the U.S. Naval Hospital, Mare Island (which later became the Navy Prosthetics Research Laboratory, Oakland Naval Hospital); and a U.S. Army Air Force unit at Wright Field. New York University was engaged in 1947 to evaluate the devices that resulted from the research and development program. The Veterans Administration's laboratory in New York also performed evaluations primarily by means of mechanical and chemical testing projects; later this laboratory became part of the Veterans Administration Prosthetics Center (VAPC),* which contributed heavily to development and evaluation projects established within the program. Although progress was made with new devices and substitutions of materials, more significant advances were in the areas of socket design and alignment of the various types of prostheses.

As a result of a visit by a commission to Europe in 1946[54] a study of the suction socket for above-knee prostheses was made by the University of California.[19] The results of this study, coupled with information derived from the locomotion studies at the University of California, Berkeley, led to a biomechanical rationale for the design and fabrication of the socket and the alignment of above-knee prostheses.[3]

Innovative techniques for providing improved prostheses for Syme[60] and hip disarticulation[39] amputees were developed by McLaurin and his associates while working at Sunnybrook Hospi-

*As of July 1, 1980, the name Veterans Administration Prosthetics Center was changed to Veterans Administration Rehabilitation Engineering Center (VAREC).

tal, Toronto, under the auspices of the Department of Veterans Affairs of Canada. Much of this work was carried to fruition at the University of California, Berkeley, after Foort transferred there in 1955 from Toronto.[60] Variations on the early designs of Syme prostheses were made by VAPC prosthetists.[60] Thus a body of knowledge of management of Syme and hip disarticulation (and hemipelvectomy) amputees was developed and then disseminated to clinicians through a formal education program.

Concurrently, on the basis of a number of innovations in below-knee socket designs made by practitioners in various parts of the country, Radcliffe and Foort[46] developed the rationale and techniques of fabrication for what is now known as the "patellar-tendon-bearing (PTB)" prosthesis. Education in fabrication and application was first offered through university education programs in 1960. A number of variations in technique are now used successfully in practice, but the principles set forth originally by Radcliffe and Foort have stood the test of time.

In 1963 Weiss, an orthopaedic surgeon from Poland,[59] visited the United States under the auspices of the Office of Vocational Rehabilitation at which time he described techniques he was using in management of lower limb amputees. These included fitting of temporary prostheses immediately after surgery, adapted from Berlemont[6] and osteoplasty and myoplasty techniques adapted from Ertl[20] and Dederich.[16,35]

Weiss' presentations prompted the Veterans Administration in Seattle to initiate in 1964 under Burgess[10] a study to determine the feasibility of immediate postsurgical fitting, osteoplasty, and myoplasty. Projects were also started at the Navy Prosthetics Research Laboratory[26] and the University of Miami.[15] Just prior to this a team at Duke University[27] had been studying the effects of early fitting, that is, providing the patient with temporary prostheses with well-defined sockets within a month of the amputation.

As a result of these efforts many amputees are now being fitted with rigid dressings immediately after surgery and with definitive prostheses much earlier than was previously considered possible. Hospital and training costs for amputees thereby have been reduced considerably.

Pedersen[45] and others began, about 1958, to promote the idea that knee joints in many elderly patients with vascular disease could be saved if proper care were given postsurgically, although the classic instruction until then was to amputate above the knee when circulation was impaired, so that healing could be ensured. Weiss agreed with the view that knees could be saved and pointed out that the use of a rigid dressing should improve healing by reducing edema. Consequently, the ratio of above-knee to below-knee amputations since 1965 in the United States has almost been reversed from 70:30 to 30:70.[32] This has had a profound effect on the rehabilitation potential of dysvascular and geriatric amputees.

Although the Veterans Administration had no direct responsibility for children, it did provide indirect support to the Children's Bureau in adapting some of the devices and techniques developed for adults. Frantz[23] and Aitken[1] and the Michigan Crippled Children's Commission initiated a project to develop methods of management for child amputees in Grand Rapids in 1952. A similar project was launched at University of California, Los Angeles, in 1955, and New York University was funded to evaluate further the devices and techniques emanating from these projects. The Children's Bureau also provided the NAS with some funds for coordination of activities in child prosthetics. From this emerged the Child Amputee Clinic Chiefs Program, which has held meetings nearly every year since 1958, and the Inter-Clinic Information Bulletin, a small monthly that has proven to be useful for the dissemination of results of research and development.

AMPUTEE PROGRAMS IN OTHER COUNTRIES

In Great Britain, the Limb Fitting Centre at Queen Mary's Hospital, Roehampton, expanded its research effort shortly after the end of World War II and became known as the Biomechanical Research and Development Unit. The Scottish Department of Home and Health Services has sponsored research and development at the Limb Fitting Centre, Dundee; University of Strathclyde; and Princess Margaret Rose Hospital, Edinburgh. The work in Edinburgh is devoted mainly to children. At the University of Strathclyde, there has been established a 3-year education program in prosthetics and orthotics.

Work concerning children's problems is also being carried out in other places in Great Britain, namely at Chailey Heritage and the Nuffield Clinic, Oxford. Suppliers of artificial limbs in Great Britain also support research and development within their own organizations.

A number of research and development efforts were started in Germany after World War II, but there appears to have been little coordination of this effort. The work at the University of Munster in body-powered upper limb prosthetics has influenced practice elsewhere, as has the work at the University of Heidelberg with severely involved child amputees. A formal education program for prosthetists has been in operation in Frankfort for many years.

The thalidomide tragedy prompted the Swedish government to expand its research and development work in technical aids for the handicapped to include artificial limbs in 1962. This program continues today.

The French government in recent years has expanded its support of artificial limb research mainly through the Ministre des Anciens Combattants et Victimes de Guerre.

Research and development in artificial limbs in Italy have a long history. A research unit has been in operation at the University of Bologna for many years, and a group at the Prosthetic Centre in Budrio is very active in the development of externally powered upper limb prostheses.

Two projects in Poland that have made significant contributions to limb prosthetics are the Rehabilitation Center at Konstancin and the University of Poznan.

Not a great deal is known about activities in Russia but research units are located in Leningrad and Moscow. Their contribution has been the first clinically useful myoelectrically controlled hand.

The United States government, through the Surplus Agricultural Commodity Act (P.L. 480), has supported work in Poland, Yugoslavia, Israel, Egypt, India, and Pakistan.

Some prosthetic research has been carried out in Japan but as yet has had little effect on practices in the United States.

RELATED ORGANIZATIONS

The American Orthotics and Prosthetics Association (AOPA) is an organization of privately operated prosthetics and orthotics facilities in the United States and Canada to assist facilities in providing the best possible services. The parent group was organized in 1917 as the Artificial Limb Manufacturers' Association. The name was changed shortly afterward to the Orthopedic Appliance and Limb Manufacturers' Association when orthotists joined, and the present name was adopted in 1958. AOPA publishes quarterly *Orthotics and Prosthetics* for the purpose of reporting on the latest clinical practices.

The American Board for Certification in Prosthetics and Orthotics was established in 1948 as an accreditation body to certify the professional competence of practitioners and facilities in these disciplines. In addition to its accreditation activities, the board also seeks to advance the highest levels of competency and ethics in the prosthetic/orthotic profession.

In 1952 the International Society for the Rehabilitation of the Disabled (now called Rehabilitation International) appointed an International Committee on Prosthetics and Orthotics to promote the dissemination of knowledge of prosthetics and orthotics throughout the world. The chairman was Knud Jansen, and headquarters for the committee were established in Copenhagen, where a number of very successful international seminars were conducted in the late 1950s and 1960s. The committee also sponsored courses and conferences at other locations during this period and, in 1971, with the concurrence of Rehabilitation International, the members of the committee and others, formed the International Society for Prosthetics and Orthotics (ISPO) "to promote high quality prosthetics and orthotics care to all people with neuromuscular and skeletal disabilities." ISPO, an organization of all professionals associated with prosthetics and orthotics, conducts an International Congress at 3-year intervals to bring together clinicians, educators, research personnel, and administrators to exchange information and ideas and to make plans for cooperative programs. ISPO publishes three times a year *Prosthetics and Orthotics International,* which contains research reports and results of clinical evaluation of new devices and techniques.

The American Academy of Orthotists and Prosthetists (AAOP) was founded in 1970 by practicing prosthetists and orthotists as a professional society to promote the advancement of knowledge in the field of prosthetics and orthotics. Its goals and organization relate primarily to education. The AAOP publishes quarterly *Newsletter—Prosthetics and Orthotics Clinic.*

The Veterans Administration publishes the *Bulletin of Prosthetics Research* biannually, which summarizes current research in the field.

DEVELOPMENTS IN LOWER LIMB PROSTHETICS

Sockets and suspension

Prior to the United States' research program, the most common approach to the design of the above-knee socket was the carved "plug fit" wooden socket with a conical interior shape. The weight of the amputee during the stance phase of walking and during standing was transferred to the skeletal system through the muscles about the thigh.

The above-knee socket design introduced by the University of California about 1950 was shaped to permit use of the remaining musculature. It contained well-defined walls and became known as the "quadrilateral socket."[3] The posterior wall was shaped to provide ischial-gluteal weight bearing. Following the German practice an air space was left at the distal end of the stump, and an air valve was installed in one of the walls, usually the medial one. Most of the patients used this system successfully but a significant number experienced edema and dermatological problems that warranted further study.

Concurrently at the University of California, Berkeley, and San Francisco, studies of the problems of the below-knee amputee resulted in the PTB prosthesis, which involved total contact between the stump and socket. Further analysis of problems with above-knee amputation and experience with the PTB prosthesis resulted in the total-contact quadrilateral above-knee socket, which minimized the problems of terminal edema.

Immediately after World War II the vast majority of lower limb prostheses were constructed of a combination of wood and leather. These materials, alone and together, have many properties desirable for the construction of artificial limbs but they also possess properties that make them a good deal less than perfect. Wood requires the skill of carving and shaping, and leather absorbs perspiration and is difficult to keep clean.

To overcome some of the deficiencies of wood and leather, Northrop Aviation, Inc., introduced the use of thermosetting resins for laminating tubular stockinette-over-plastic replicas of the stump to form sockets and structural components of upper limb prostheses. The Veterans Administration Prosthetics Center conducted extensive demonstrations to get prosthetists to start using plastic laminates over wood, furthering the trend toward the use of plastics.

McLaurin[60] and his co-workers in Toronto coupled the plastic laminating technique with a good engineering analysis of the problem to produce the Canadian Syme prosthesis, which was a significant improvement over former practice. This design and variations developed by the Veterans Administration Prosthetics Center were adopted worldwide as prosthetists learned to use plastic laminates. (This design also incorporated a foot section that led to the SACH foot.) The same group also conceived and developed the plastic-socket Canadian hip disarticulation prosthesis about 1955, which also was soon adopted worldwide.[5,38]

The plastic laminating techniques made total-contact sockets practical; most of the prostheses used throughout the world are total-contact sockets made essentially of a plastic laminate.

The search for a practical method of making transparent sockets was highlighted in 1972 when Snelson and Mooney developed a method for vacuum-forming polycarbonate over a positive model of the stump. Although not suitable for definitive prostheses because of brittleness, polycarbonate sockets are useful as check sockets and as an aid in teaching. Vacuum-forming polypropylene, the properties of which seem to make it appropriate for definitive use, was introduced in 1975 by Moss Rehabilitation Hospital in Philadelphia.

The introduction of socket designs that take full advantage of the functions and properties of the stump in conjunction with a rationale for alignment probably represents the greatest achievement in prosthetics since World War II.

Prior to the development of socket designs based on biomechanics, suspension of most lower limb prostheses presented formidable problems. Until the introduction of the pelvic band about the time of World War I, over-the-shoulder suspenders were used almost universally for keeping above-knee prostheses in place. Until the development of the PTB prosthesis the side bars of the thigh lacers, or corset, of the below-knee prosthesis were bent to conform to the medial and lateral surfaces of the thigh to provide suspension. This arrangement was often supplemented by a waist belt.

The quadrilateral design not only permits the use of suction for suspension but makes the suspension problem easier because the muscle action of the stump within the intimately fitting socket also helps hold the prosthesis in place. Suction is seldom used in the below-knee socket. The intimate fit makes it possible in most cases to achieve adequate suspension by a supracondylar strap. Variations of the original PTB prosthesis design (supracondylar or supracondylar-suprapatellar) employ more proximal brims that are contoured to make the supracondylar straps unnecessary.

The goal for many years to achieve a practical transparent socket was reached by Mooney and

Snelson in 1971 by using a vacuum-forming polycarbonate sheet.[41] This technique has proven extremely valuable in teaching and in use as a check socket in difficult cases. Wilson and Stills[63] have demonstrated that it is possible to provide below-knee prostheses that weigh only one third as much as the conventional PTB prosthesis design by thermoforming polypropylene.

The ultimate arrangement for achieving suspension would seem to be attaching the prosthesis directly to the bone. The first recorded efforts in what is often called "skeletal attachment" seem to have been made in Germany in the 1940s. Some work was considered at the University of California, but the first experimental work in the United States was probably that of Esslinger[21] in Birmingham, Michigan, during the 1960s, which was undertaken on a small scale with support from the Veterans Administration. Results with dogs were encouraging. Hall[30] of Southwest Research Institute continued this work for a while as a result of some experiences he had had with horses, and Mooney[40] has been investigating the problem at Rancho Los Amigos Hospital, Downey, California, as time and circumstances permit.

Prosthetic knees

Locomotion studies at the University of California showed that swing-phase control of the shank is as important as stance-phase control in lower limb prosthetics. Until that time, control of the shank during swing phase in most above-knee prostheses was provided by introducing friction about the knee bolt, the so-called constant friction knee, an arrangement that provides a smooth gait at only one cadence for a given amount of friction.

The Navy Variable Cadence Knee Unit[43] was designed to overcome, to some degree, the shortcoming of the constant friction unit by increasing the friction toward the end of the swing phase. The Navy design, introduced about 1950, did indeed permit improvement in the gait pattern but the materials available at that time soon failed as a result of wear, and maintenance became a problem. The same principle is employed in the Northwestern University variable cadence knee,[52] which is presently available commercially.

In 1949 the Vickers Corporation in Detroit requested assistance from the government through the NAS in perfecting the Stewart-Vickers Hydraulic Above-Knee Leg, a design by Jack Stewart, who was an above-knee amputee. This system used hydraulic principles to lock the knee on heel contact and to provide coordinated motion between the knee and ankle during swing phase.[43] Laboratory and clinical trials at New York University with a dozen units showed that the prosthesis was well accepted by a good proportion of amputees, apparently because of the swing-phase control resulting from the hydraulic system that had been provided primarily for stance-phase control and not because of the stance-phase control itself. It was learned later that the ease of plantar flexion of the ankle during the early stages of stance phase was beneficial in providing stability during stance phase.

Results of the New York University evaluation program and other efforts prompted the United States Manufacturing Company to make a version of the Stewart-Vickers design available commercially. Known as the Hydra-Cadence, this unit retained the swing phase and hydraulic ankle features but, because of the high cost, the stance-phase control feature was not included.[58]

Mauch, who along with Henschke had been developing a hydraulically actuated stance-phase control unit under the auspices of the U.S. Air Force since 1946, was persuaded in 1951 to concentrate his efforts on the use of hydraulic principles for control of the shank during swing phase.[57] The result was the model "B" Henschke-Mauch Knee Unit. The swing-phase feature was later incorporated into the stance-phase system (model A) and called the Mauch S' n 'S System, which is the unit available today. Other hydraulic swing-phase units now available as a result of the research program are the Dupaco Hermes[56] and the Dynaplex.[6,61]

To overcome the high costs involved in manufacturing hydraulic units and yet retain the advantages, a pneumatically controlled system was designed at the University of California, which is now available and known as the UC-BL Pneumatic Swing Control.[61]

To eliminate the bulk usually associated with knee disarticulation prostheses Lyquist[36] designed in 1973 the OHC (Orthopaedic Hospital, Copenhagen) knee unit, which uses a four-bar linkage within the shank to provide an effective knee axis that approximately matches the normal knee axis. The OHC unit, by virtue of the four-bar linkage, is quite stable during stance phase, and it is available with a hydraulically controlled swing-phase system.

Other stance-phase controls have been developed by commercial organizations (Otto Bock, Orthopedic Industries, Inc., U.S. Manufacturing Co.). These are essentially mechanical systems with an incremental resistance added on weight bearing. These stance-phase controls (Bock Safety Knee, USMC Kolman Knee) are also commercially available.

Prosthetic feet

Through the years great attention was devoted to the design of artificial feet to provide better function than allowed by the standard single-axis wood foot. Considerable effort in the early years of the program was given to the design of articulated feet with the expectation that such designs would enhance the amputee's ability to walk. An outstanding achievement of the early years was the "Navy ankle" developed by the Naval Prosthetic Research Laboratory in Oakland, California. This ankle contained a block of rubber with variable stiffness to control motions in all three planes. However, excessive maintenance prevented it from being a commercial success. The Greissinger foot, developed in Germany to offer the kind of function provided by the navy unit, has commonly been used to provide "three-way action." Meanwhile the introduction of the solid ankle cushion heel (SACH) foot with the PTB prosthesis represented the ultimate in simplicity, while providing adequate function for most patients. The SACH foot has had outstanding success in the marketplace primarily because of its simplicity.

Endoskeletal prostheses

The first endoskeletal designs were used as temporary prostheses. In the first 10 years or so of the research program the use of temporary prostheses was discouraged because it was believed that more harm than good would result from the use of crudely made, poorly fitting sockets mounted on peg legs. However, after the rationale for socket configuration was fully developed and plastics had proven to require less time but resulted in better fit than earlier methods of fabrication, the idea of temporary prostheses was revived.

Pylons, or endoskeletal prostheses, with adjustment features began to appear about 1960. Staros[51] established the criteria for their use as temporary limbs. Their use was then accelerated by immediate postsurgical fitting studies, and various designs began to appear on both sides of the North Atlantic, the ultimate concept being an adjustable endoskeletal structure that could be carried over into the definitive prosthesis, the "pylon" being covered with a resilient foam shaped to match the contralateral leg.

These designs, usually referred to as modular endoskeletal limbs, have gradually had more and more success despite the difficulty in shaping and maintaining their foam covers.[62]

DEVELOPMENTS IN UPPER LIMB PROSTHETICS

Early in the Artificial Limb Program it was decided that the best approach to take at that time for upper limb replacement was to develop a variety of components, socket designs, and harnessing methods that could be assembled to best meet the needs of individual patients, rather than trying to develop special systems for each level of amputation.

The primary assignment to the Army Prosthetics Research Laboratory (APRL) was the development of artificial arms with emphasis on artificial hands. Out of this effort came the voluntary-closing APRL hand and the APRL hook.[22] These devices were well received by a significant proportion of the amputee population, but it was difficult for the manufacturer to produce quality devices at a competitive price because of the close mechanical tolerances required. These devices are still available today but the high costs preclude widespread use.

Although the APRL hand and hook are not used widely, the basic research required led to the development of the sizes and configurations[17] that are now standard for most artificial hands produced today. The manufacturer of nearly all of the cosmetic gloves provided for artificial hands is based on techniques[11] developed at the APRL.

Northrop Aviation, Inc., produced many ingenious designs for artificial arms in addition to introducing plastic laminating techniques.[42] The alternating-lock elbow unit operated from the harness for above-elbow amputees was first developed by Northrop in 1947. After becoming available commercially, it soon replaced other available units, all of which required use of the contralateral hand or motion against a fixed object to activate the lock. This basic design is in use throughout the world.

Northrop also initiated a study in harness design that was later taken over by the University of California, Los Angeles. UCLA also developed socket designs for all levels of upper limb amputation based on anatomical and physiological principles. Refinements of these basic socket and harness designs are still the standard for body-powered upper limb prosthetics.

The hardware, socket, and harness designs produced by Northrop, APRL, UCLA, and others between 1946 and 1950 made it practical and desirable for the surgeon to save all length possible in amputation through the upper limb.[29] Unfortunately, except for external power systems, no major advances that have found widespread use have been made in upper limb prosthetics since the 1950s.

External power

Although some work was done in Germany earlier,[7] it was Alderson[2] who, with support from the United States government and International Business Machines, developed the first working model of an electrically powered artificial arm, which appeared about 1949. Demonstrations were impressive but evaluations at New York University and UCLA in 1953 revealed that amputees could not operate any of the designs without conscious thought, primarily because the sensory feedback so necessary for automatic or semiautomatic operation was not adequate. For this reason, the development of devices was discontinued at that time, and some effort was put into a study of sensory feedback.

In 1958 Russian workers[34] announced that a "thought-controlled" artificial arm had been perfected, which proved to be an electric hand controlled by myoelectric signals from the flexors and extensors of the wrist, and was suitable for below-elbow amputees. Again, adequate feedback signals were lacking.

Rights to manufacture these devices were purchased by groups in Canada and Great Britain, but these units were never widely accepted. However, Otto Bock Orthopedic Industry, Inc., in Germany and Viennatone in Austria made available versions of the Russian design that they presently market. An interesting design was proposed in Yugoslavia[48] but was never carried to fruition. Mason of the Veterans Administration Prosthetics Center and Childress[13] at Northwestern University provided refined designs, in which the batteries are within the hand or wrist unit. New socket designs for below-elbow amputees, which provide self-suspension, were developed, thus eliminating the need for any wiring or harness above the elbow. These components are available commercially in the United States from the Fidelity Electronics Co.

The thalidomide tragedy[1,23] created a great deal of interest in externally powered prostheses, especially in Germany,[37] Sweden, England, and Canada, beginning about 1960. Initial efforts in Germany centered around pneumatically operated prostheses and by arrangement with the University of Heidelberg, Kessler and Kiessling[33] in the United States undertook complementary development work. Results on some severely disabled adults and children were impressive but lack of funds curtailed this effort in 1968. Simpson,[50] in Edinburgh, is using pneumatic prostheses of his own design quite successfully for severely disabled children, but the design is not available outside the United Kingdom.

A great deal of effort has been expended on the development of electric elbows by the Veterans Administration and others. To date in the United States only the VAPC electric elbow is commercially available. Reports from Italy claim that electric elbows are used widely there, but they do not seem to be accepted in other places in Europe. A child-size electric elbow is available from Variety Village in Toronto, Canada.

Some work has been carried out by the Veterans Administration Prosthetics Center and Northwestern University in the development of electrically powered hooks, but to date the only externally powered terminal devices available in the United States are electric hands.

Special procedures

The idea of harnessing a muscle directly to power an arm prosthesis (Vanghetti[55] in Italy, Sauerbruch[48] in Germany, and Bosch Arana[8] in Argentina) appealed to a number of investigators in the United States immediately after World War II. The only practical system that could be devised after extensive investigation of use of muscle tunnels through the wrist flexors and extensors in below-elbow amputees, biceps and triceps in below-elbow and above-elbow amputees, and pectoral muscles in above-elbow and shoulder disarticulation cases was one involving the biceps tunnel for the below-elbow amputee.[4,9] Although many kineplasty procedures were performed, the technique has been abandoned largely because of the extra surgery involved and the considerable care that must be used in keeping the tunnel clean if complications are to be avoided. One positive result of the kineplasty program was that it provided for the first time the opportunity to study the biomechanical characteristics of an intact human muscle.[31]

The Krukenberg[64] procedure, in which the forearm stump is split between the ulna and radius and the forearm muscles are attached to them in such a way as to provide a functional pincer grasp, was originated in Germany and is used there today, especially for blind amputees because of the sensory feedback provided. Because of its grotesque appearance, the Krukenberg procedure is seldom used in the United States despite the success reported by Swanson.[53]

EARLY EDUCATION AND TRAINING

Pilot courses sponsored by the University of California, Berkeley, in 1949 in prescription, fabrication, and alignment of the suction-socket above-knee prosthesis were followed by local courses presented in key areas of the country by the Veterans Administration Prosthetics and Sensory Aids Service (PSAS) and the Orthopaedic Appliance and Limb Manufacturers Association (now American Orthotic and Prosthetic Association).[28] In these courses orthopaedic surgeons and prosthetists received instructions together. Prior to this, the education of a prosthetist consisted of an informal apprenticeship program in which very little formal instruction was available.

Although a number of prosthetists and surgeons had advocated through the years that teamwork between the two disciplines would result in improved service, little was done until 1949 when the Veterans Administration PSAS organized thirty amputee clinic teams, consisting of a surgeon, prosthetist, physical therapist, occupational therapist, and prosthetics representative.

While this experimental teaching program on the suction socket was being carried out and the clinic teams were being formed, a body of knowledge in upper limb prosthetics was being accumulated at UCLA. A rationale for socket and harness design was developed for every level of amputation in the upper limb, including shoulder disarticulation and the forequarter amputation. Components that could be selected and assembled to meet the individual needs of upper limb amputees were designed and tested and most had been made available through regular commercial channels. Thus it was possible for surgeons to save all length possible in upper limb amputations.

With financial assistance from the Veterans Administration, UCLA initiated a series of formal 6-week courses in upper limb prosthetics for the amputee clinic teams in 1952. Twelve of these courses were offered to clinicians in the United States on a regional basis during 1953 and 1954 with tremendous success. Civilian as well as Veterans Administration teams attended. Approximately 140 Veterans Administration and civilian teams were trained. Because the Veterans Administration teams, almost without exception, consisted of surgeons and prosthetists in private practice, the results of the training program reached the nonveteran population as well, and civilian clinics were established throughout the United States and Canada.

The material presented in the original series of suction-socket courses was refined and supplemented with new material on alignment by the University of California, Berkeley, Biomechanics Laboratory. A pilot school based on this material presented to leading prosthetists, surgeons, and therapists in Berkeley in 1955 led the way to establishing formal courses in 1956 at UCLA in above-knee prosthetics for practicing clinic teams.

Because UCLA could not meet the needs of the country with respect to the number of teams that desired training, the Veterans Administration sponsored the establishment of a Prosthetics Education Program at New York University in the Post-Graduate Medical School in 1956. To provide a similar facility in the Midwest the Office of Vocational Rehabilitation (now Rehabilitation Services Administration) of the Department of Health, Education, and Welfare sponsored the establishment of the prosthetic Education Program at Northwestern University in 1959. Since 1960, these three universities have continued to provide ongoing educational programs in all aspects of prosthetics. Other formal programs have been added through the years.

REFERENCES

1. Aitken, G. T.: Hazards to health, etiology of traumatic amputations in children, N. Engl. J. Med. **265:**133-134, July 20, 1961.
2. Alderson, S. W.: The electric arm. In Klopsteg, P. E., and Wilson, P. D.: Human limbs and their substitutes, New York, 1954, McGraw-Hill, Inc. Reprinted by Hafner Press, New York, 1960.
3. Anderson, M. H., et al.: Prosthetic principles, above-knee amputations, Springfield, Ill., 1960, Charles C thomas, Publisher.
4. Bechtol, C. D., and Aitken, G. T.: Cineplasty. In American Academy of Orthopaedic Surgeons: Orthopaedic appliances atlas, vol. 2, Ann Arbor, Mich., 1960, Edwards Brothers.
5. Bell, C. A.: Canadian hip disarticulation prosthesis, Orthop. Prosthet. Appliance J. **10**(1):35-39, March, 1956.
6. Berlemont, M., Weber, R., and Willot, J. P.: Ten years of experience with the immediate application of prosthetic devices to amputees of the lower extremities on the operating table, Prosthet. Orthot. Int. **3:**8-18, 1969.
7. Borchardt, M., et al., editors: Ersatzglieder and arbeitshilfen, Berlin, 1919, Springer.
8. Bosch Arana, G.: Kineplastic amputations: arm bimotor and a prosthesis, Surg. Gynecol. Obstet. **42:**416-420, 1926.

9. Brav, E. A., et al.: Cineplasty, an end-result study, J. Bone Joint Surg. **46A**(1):59-76, Jan., 1957.
10. Burgess, E., Traub, J. E., and Wilson, A. B., Jr.: Immediate postsurgical prosthetics in the management of lower extremity amputees, Washington, D.C. 1967, Veterans Administration.
11. Carnelli, W. A., DeFries, M. G., and Leonard, J.: Color realism in the cosmetic glove, Artif. Limbs **2**(2):57-65, May, 1955.
12. Ceci, A.: Amputations cineplastiques des membres superieurs (Cineplastic amputations of the upper extremity), Presse Med. **14:**745-747, 1906.
13. Childress, D., Billock, J. N.: Self-containment and self-suspension of externally powered prostheses for the forearm, Bull. Prosthet. Res., 10-14, Fall, 1970.
14. Committee on Artificial Limbs, National Research Council: Terminal Research Reports on Artificial Limbs (covering the period from April 1, 1945, through June 30, 1947), Washington, D.C., 1947.
15. Committee on Prosthetic Research and Development: Immediate postsurgical fitting of prostheses – report of a workshop, Washington D.C. 1968, National Academy of Sciences.
16. Dederich, R.: Amputationsstumpf knankheiten und ihre chirurgische Behandlung, Mschr. Unfallheilk, **63:**101, 1960.
17. DeFries, M. G.: Sizing of cosmetic hands to fit the child and adult population, Technical Report No. 5441, Sept., 1954, Washington, D.C., Sept., 1954, U.S. Army Medical Biomechanical Research Laboratory, Walter Reed Army Medical Center.
18. Eberhart, H. D., Inman, V. T., Dec, J. B., Saunders, M., Levens, A. S., Bresler, B., and McCowan, T. D.: Fundamental studies of human locomotion and other information relating to the design of artificial limbs, a report to the National Research Council, Committee on Artificial Limbs, Berkeley, Calif., 1947, University of California.
19. Eberhart, H. D., and McKennon, J. C.: Suction-socket suspension of the above-knee prosthesis. In Klopsteg, P. E., and Wilson, P. D.: Human limbs and their substitutes, New York, 1954, McGraw-Hill, Inc. Reprinted by Hafner Press, New York, 1960.
20. Ertl, J.: Über amputationsstümpfe, Chirurg. **20:**218-224, 1949.
21. Esslinger, J. O.: A basic study in semiburied implants and osseous attachments for application in amputation prostheses, Bull. Prosthet. Res., 10-13, Spring, 1970.
22. Fletcher, M. J.: Problems in designing of artificial hands, Orthop. Prosthet. Appliance J. **9**(2):59-68, June, 1955.
23. Frantz, C. H.: An evolution in the care of the child amputee, Artif. Limbs **10**(1):1-4, Spring, 1966.
24. Garrison, F. H.: An introduction to the history of medicine, Philadelphia, 1963, W. B. Saunders Co.
25. Garrison, F. H.: An introduction to the history of medicine, Philadelphia, 1963, W. B. Saunders Co.
26. Golbranson, F. L., Asbelle, C., and Strand, D.: Immediate postsurgical fitting and early ambulation, Clin. Orthop. **56:**119-131, 1968.
27. Goldner, J. L., Clippinger, F. W., Jr., and Titus, B. R.: Use of temporary plaster or plastic pylons preparatory to fitting a permanent above knee or below knee prosthesis. Final Report of Project No. 1363 to (U.S.) Vocational Rehabilitation Administration by Duke University Medical Center, Durham, N.C., 1967.
28. Haddan, C. C., and Thomas, A.: Status of the above-knee suction socket in the United States, Artif. Limbs **4**(2): 29-39, May, 1954.
29. Hall, C. B., and Bechtol, C. O.: Modern amputation technique in the upper extremity, J. Bone Joint Surg. **45A:** 1717-1722, 1963.
30. Hall, C. W., Cox, P. H., and Mallow, W. A.: Skeletal extension development: criteria for future designs, BPR-10-25.
31. Inman, V. T., and Ralston, H. J.: The mechanics of voluntary muscle. In Klopsteg, P. E., and Wilson, P. D.: Human limbs and their substitutes, New York, 1954, McGraw-Hill, Inc. Reprinted by Hafner Press, New York, 1960.
32. Kay, H. W., and Newman, J. D.: Relative incidences of new amputations, Orthop. Prosthet. **29:**3-16, June, 1975.
33. Kessler, H. H., and Kiessling, E. A.: Pneumatic arm prosthesis, Am. J. Nurs. **65**(6), June, 1965.
34. Kobrinski, A. E., Bolhovitin, S. V., Voskoboinikova, L. M., Ioffe, D. M., Polyan, E. P., Popov, B. P., Slavutski, Y. L., Sysin, A. Y., and Yakobson, Y. S.: Problems of bioelectric control in automatic and remote control. Proceedings of the First International Congress of the International Federation of Automatic Control, Moscow, 1960, vol. 2, London, Butterworth & Co. (Publishers) Ltd.
35. Loon, H. E.: Below-knee amputation surgery, Artif. Limbs **6**(6):86-99, June, 1962.
36. Lyquist, E.: The OHC knee-disarticulation prosthesis, Orthop. Prosthet. **30:**27-28, June, 1976.
37. Marquardt, E.: Heidelburg pneumatic arm prosthesis, J. Bone Joint Surg. **47B**(3):425-434, Aug., 1965.
38. McLaurin, C. A.: The evolution of the Canadian-type hip-disarticulation prosthesis, Artif. Limbs **4**(2):22-28, Autumn, 1957.
39. Mercer, W.: Syme's amputation, J. Bone Joint Surg. **37-B**(3):611-612, Aug., 1956.
40. Mooney, V.: Personal communication, 1978.
41. Mooney, V., and Snelson, R.: Fabrication and application of transparent sockets, Orthop. Prosthet. **26:**1-13, March, 1972.
42. Motis, G. M.: Final report on artificial arm and leg research and development, Northrop Aircraft, Inc., Hawthorne, Calif. Final Report to the National Research Council Advisory Committee on Artificial Limbs, Feb., 1951.
43. Murphy, E. R.: Lower-extremity components. In American Academy of Orthopaedic Surgeons: Orthopaedic appliance atlas, vol. 2, Ann Arbor, Mich., 1960, Edwards Brothers.
44. Pare, A.: Oeuvres completes, Edition Malgaigne, Paris **1:** 616-621, 1840.
45. Pederson, H. E.: The problem of the geriatric amputee, Artif. Limbs **12**(1):i-iii, 1968.
46. Radcliffe, C. W., and Foort, J.: Patellar-tendon-bearing below-knee prosthesis, Bioengineering Laboratory, Berkeley, Calif., 1961, University of California.
47. Rakic, M.: Practical design of a hand prosthesis with sensory elements. Proceedings of the International Symposium of the Application of Automatic Control in Prosthetics Design, Aug. 27-31, 1962, Belgrade, Yugoslavia.
48. Sauerbruch, F., and ten Horn, C.: Die willkurlich bewegbare kunstliche hand (artificial hand capable of voluntary movement), Berlin, 1923, Springer Verlag.
49. Selincourt, A., editor: Herodotus, the histories, New York, 1954, Penguin Books.
50. Simpson, D. C.: Powered upper arm prostheses for young

children. Digest, Sixth International Conference on Medical Electronics and Biological Engineering, 1965, Tokyo, Japan.
51. Staros, A.: The temporary prosthesis for the above-knee amputee in geriatric amputee, Publication 919, Washington, D.C., 1961, National Academy of Sciences.
52. Staros, A., and Peizer, E.: Northwestern University intermittent mechanical friction system (disk-type), Artif. Limbs **9**(1):45-52, Spring, 1965.
53. Swanson, A. B.: The Krukenberg procedure in the juvenile amputee, J. Bone Joint Surg. **46A:**1540-1548, Oct., 1964.
54. United States Army, Surgeon General's Office, Commission on Amputations and Prostheses: Report on European Observations, Washington, D.C. 1946.
55. Vanghetti, G.: Plastica dei monconi a scopo di protesi cinematica (plastic surgery of stumps for cinematic prostheses), Arch. de Ortop. **XVI:** 305, 385, 1899.
56. Veterans Administration, Prosthetic and Sensory Aids Service, Clinical application study of the Dupaco "Hermes" hydraulic control unit, TR-4, New York, Jan. 4, 1965.
57. Veterans Administration, Prosthetic and Sensory Aids Service, Clinical application study of the Henschke-Mauch "Hydraulik" swing control system, New York, TR-3, Dec. 1, 1964.
58. Veterans Administration, Prosthetic and Sensory Aids Service, Clinical application study of the Hydra-Cadence above-knee prosthesis, New York, TR-2, Nov. 1, 1963.
59. Weiss, M., Gielzynski, A., and Wirski, J.: Myoplasty immediate fitting ambulation, New York, International Society for Rehabilitation of the Disabled (Reprint of paper presented at the sessions of the World Commission on Research in Rehabilitation, Tenth World Congress of the International Society for Rehabilitation of the Disabled, Wiesbaden, Germany, Sept., 1966).
60. Wilson, A. B., Jr.: Prostheses for Syme's amputation, Artif. Limbs **6**(1):52-75, April, 1961.
61. Wilson, A. B., Jr.: Recent advances in above-knee prosthetics, Artif. Limbs **12:**1-27, Autumn, 1968.
62. Wilson, A. B., Jr.: Lower-limb modular prostheses: a status report, Orthop. Prosthet. **29:**23-32, March, 1975.
63. Wilson, A. B., Jr., and Stills, M.: Ultra-light prostheses for below-knee amputees, Orthop. Prosthet. **30:**43-47, March, 1976.
64. Zanoli, R.: Krukenberg-Putti amputation-plasty, J. Bone Joint Surg. **39-B**(2):230-232, May, 1957.

CHAPTER 2

General principles of amputation surgery

ERNEST M. BURGESS

Our limbs provide a major and primary contact with the physical environment. Loss of part or all of a limb progressively circumscribes our ability to move, work, and play, and even to survive in the world about us. The amputee must depend on remaining organ systems and mechanical substitutes to replace lost function. Amputation transversely severs all of the varied tissues of the limb. Each must heal in its own particular manner under the broad canopy of cell regeneration and repair.

Not only does amputation cause physical and functional loss, it also presents a unique psychological circumstance. The body image is altered and distorted by the absent part. No amount of psychological testing and evaluation can completely measure this effect. Only the amputee can define these feelings.

Amputation surgery has two goals: ablation and reconstruction. The surgery must remove all or that portion of the limb necessary to eliminate the pathological state and provide primary or secondary wound healing. The reconstruction must create the optimum motor and sensory end organ for prosthetic substitution and restoration of function. The success of every primary amputation or revision depends on adherence to these two principles. To be effective, the surgeon must understand functional limb physiology and the nature of prosthetic substitutes.

LEVELS OF AMPUTATION

For many years, the level of amputation was determined not only by surgical adjustment and necessity, but also by the type of prosthetic substitute available. In the lower limb, for example, the Syme amputation and knee disarticulation have been regarded as relatively unsatisfactory because available prostheses were inadequate. Improvements in design and engineering of prostheses have, with a few exceptions, eliminated these considerations as the determinant for level selection. The prosthesis interfaces with the residual limb as a glove fits the hand. Except those few levels which will be specifically discussed in later chapters, the surgeon will select the most distal level of amputation consistent with the disease state and a well-healed, nontender, physiological residual limb. Conservation of residual limb length is a basic principle of modern amputation surgery. This principle is balanced against the requirement for uneventful wound healing. Since levels of amputation are no longer as rigidly defined as in the past, the surgeon will have considerable latitude of judgment in each case. The less the limb loss, the less the functional replacement needed. Selecting the appropriate level of amputation is the first of many decisions needed not only to remove the limb but also to reconstruct a physiological remaining structure.

THE SKIN

The general principles of plastic and reconstructive surgery apply to scar placement in amputations. A pliable, painless, nonadherent, well-healed scar is desired. Location of the scar is of secondary importance in the modern total-contact socket. The amputation site in the upper limb becomes, in essence, the patient's hand. The skin should therefore be managed as carefully as in hand surgery. The amputation site in the lower limb now functions as the patient's foot and requires similar attention to careful skin management.

Skin flaps should be made as broad-based as possible to avoid compromising blood supply. The skin closure should be without tension, but not redundant. In the dysvascular limb, attention should be taken to avoid elevation of skin flaps. Care should also be taken to avoid pressure-sensitive areas and scar adherence where skin lies directly over bone. Skin tolerance to socket pressures can often be gradually increased. The larger the amount of skin surface available for contact with the socket, the less pressure will be applied to each unit area of skin surface. A cylindrical, muscular residual limb presents fewer skin problems than the bony, atrophic, tapered one.

With modern prostheses, skin grafts over or near the amputation site are permissible. Depending on their location, split-thickness and full-thickness free grafts can be useful and need not necessarily be replaced by pedicle grafts. When preservation of limb length is critical, skin grafts are accommodated by prosthetic innovation. Amputations in burned limbs are an example of these circumstances. Gradual improvement in pressure tolerance of grafted skin can be expected if the pressures, shear and skin stretch, are moderated by careful prosthetic fit with the time of limb wearing and the amount of forces gradually increased. Over a period of months, a badly burned limb with amputation and free graft coverage may develop a tolerance approaching normal. In such cases, patients using innovative prostheses may avoid extensive plastic surgery or amputation at a higher level. Complicated skin problems in the amputee should be handled by a team that includes the various relevant disciplines.

THE MUSCLE

Muscles make up the bulk of limb soft tissues. Maximum retention of functioning muscle is essential to provide the residual limb with effective strength, size, shape, circulation, metabolic exchange, and proprioception. The muscular limb seems to be less prone to develop pain syndromes.

Muscle function depends on fixed origin and attachment. Without fixed resistance against which muscle tissue can forcefully contract, progressive weakness and atrophy develop. Whenever possible, then, the sectioned muscles and their extensions (i.e., tendon, aponeurosis, and fascia) should be stabilized. Distal muscle stabilization is a primary principle of amputation surgery.

Muscle stabilization can be surgically accomplished with varying degrees of efficiency by myofascial closure, myoplasty, myodesis, and tenodesis. Myofascial closure simply encases the muscles in a closed fascial envelope and to some degree provides distal fixation for those muscles with fascial attachment. It is by itself an ineffective means of muscle stabilization. It is used primarily when ischemia prevents more efficient means of distal muscle fixation as in the dysvascular amputee. Tenodesis, the firm distal attachment of the severed tendon, is the most physiological and effective means of stabilization. Attachment of the patellar tendon to the cruciate ligaments or to the femur in knee disarticulation exemplifies this technique. Where anatomical circumstances permit, distal attachment of tendons and aponeuroses to the periosteum and/or bone should be performed. When the amputation transects muscles, as in most diaphyseal areas, attachment of the severed muscles becomes more difficult. This is particularly true in areas such as the midportion of the femur where muscle bulk is great and bone surface is small. The muscles may be sewn over the end of the bone to opposing muscle groups. Unless stabilized by scar tissue, however, muscles attached in this manner may work as a sling, sliding back and forth over the end of the bone. This movement often causes bursa formation, crepitus, and discomfort. Therefore, in addition to muscle-to-muscle suture, the muscle groups must be attached to the periosteum or to the bone itself as well as to each other. Suture of muscle to the periosteum and/or bone (myodesis) is effective alone or can be combined with muscle-to-muscle and myofascial closure. The specific techniques of myofascial closure, tenodesis, myoplasty, and myodesis will be described under individual sections.

For most effective residual limb muscle activity, the muscles should be stabilized under physiological tension. The use of spring tensiometers and other devices in surgery to establish proper muscle tension for suture is not practical at this time. The general principles used in muscle and tendon transfer surgery apply. A review of muscle-stabilized amputations indicates that, in general, the muscles tend to be too lax rather than too tight. It is possible, of course, to stabilize muscle groups with excessive or unbalanced tension, as with the quadriceps in thigh amputations. Hip flexion deformity may occur when the quadriceps is tight, overbalancing hamstring function. Excessive muscle tension may produce long-standing pain. Research on effective means of muscle stabilization at the various levels of amputation continues. The principles of muscle stabilization are unquestioned. Application of these principles requires considerable surgical ingenuity.

THE NERVES

Management of sectioned nerves has been troublesome and controversial. The free end of a divided nerve heals by neuroma formation. This intertwined mass of scar and nerve tissue can be painful to pressure, stretching, and other types of physical manipulation. Even when completely undisturbed, electrical potentials may arise within it, causing local and distant sensory and motor phenomena, often disagreeable and painful. Numerous techniques have been devised in an attempt to minimize neuroma formation. Nerve ends have been cauterized by chemicals or heat, buried in bone, enclosed in impervious material, injected with a variety of chemicals, sewn to other nerves or to a more proximal portion of the sectioned nerve itself, ligated, or simply divided and allowed to retract. Since neuroma formation is inevitable, the generally accepted procedure is to section the nerve in such a manner that the subsequent neuroma will lie well cushioned in soft tissues at a site away from the incision scar and not subject to irritation by traction or pressure from the wall of the prosthesis or other sources of contact.

Neuromas in scarred areas tend to be symptomatic. Most surgeons prefer to ligate the nerve under moderate tension, then section it cleanly, just distal to the ligation, allowing retraction away from the site of amputation into proximal soft tissues. In this way, hemostasis is controlled, the size of a neuroma tends to be smaller than when the cut nerve end is not ligated, and there is less chance in the healing process for adhesion formation about the neuroma. Traction on the nerve at the time of sectioning should not be excessive, thus avoiding proximal painful traction neuropathy.

As with muscle tissue in the residual limb, the surgeon's goal is to retain and usefully employ nerve function. Care should be exercised to avoid disturbing nerve fibers innervating remaining limb structures, especially muscles and skin.

BLOOD VESSELS

Adequate hemostasis applies to amputation surgery as in any operative procedure. Arteries and veins are isolated and securely ligated. Cautery is used sparingly and is reserved for small bleeding points only. Double ligation of large arteries may be required when the amputation is carried out in the presence of normal blood supply. The central artery of large nerves can be a source of troublesome bleeding. This is avoided by nerve ligation as described. Bleeding from a sectioned bone end is best controlled by pressure. Occasionally, a cortical artery will require cautery. Bone wax is rarely, if ever, used, and hemostatics are seldom required.

Adequate blood supply must be preserved to allow wound healing. Dissection should avoid proximal damage to blood vessels supplying distal tissue, particularly skin. Skin flaps, even when broad based, should be developed with attention to blood supply. When amputating for ischemia, it is particularly important not to dissect the soft tissues in layers and to preserve all available tissue nutrition. Attention to detail in securing hemostasis may make the difference between healing and failure when blood supply is marginal.

The amputation site should usually be drained because sectioned muscles and bone often bleed from small vessels that are difficult to completely control. Suction drainage and/or through-and-through drainage may be used as indicated. A hematoma is a major complication, predisposing to infection, which may delay wound healing or fail completely. Revision surgery and even higher amputation have been the result of hematoma formation. The inconvenience of a postoperative drain system with possible minor attendant complications is preferred to the major disaster caused by development of a hematoma.

BONE

Complications caused by improper management of the bone are common. Force transmitted between the limb and the prosthesis is in large part transmitted through the retained skeleton within the residual limb. Diaphyseal bone should be sectioned at the appropriate length consistent with soft tissue closure. A fine-tooth reciprocating saw or a sharp handsaw or Gigli saw may be used. Sharp cortical bone edges and irregularities are carefully rounded. Applying the surgical concept of constructing a terminal motor and sensory end organ dictates smooth distal bone surfaces. Areas of high pressure at the bone-socket interface should be avoided by proper attention to detail in bone preparation.

Amputations through diaphyseal bone and joints should take into account the available prostheses at the level of amputation. Residual limbs that are large distally and bulbous cause problems in donning the prosthesis. Some variation in residual limb contour can assist in prosthetic suspension but must be weighed against cosmesis, pressure against the adjacent limb, and awkwardness. These principles apply particularly to disarticulation. Bone ends are rarely just beveled; they are rounded. There are no sharp, angular bone surfaces in the palm of the normal hand or sole of the normal foot. Retained distal bone in the amputation should mirror this natural state.

Management of the periosteum is less clearly defined. Decisions regarding treatment of the periosteum apply primarily to diaphyseal amputation. Diaphyseal bone does not exist open in the natural state. It appears physiological to seal the bone end, if possible, at the time of surgery; however, this will inevitably occur slowly by scar during the course of healing. When a cuff of periosteum is available, it may be sutured over the end of the bone or resected circularly from the distal diaphyseal bone in the immature skeleton.

Children tend to form new bone with periosteal and endosteal bone overgrowth at the diaphyseal amputation site. Intramedullary bone plugs and caps of inert material have been used to circumvent this problem. In general, they have been unsuccessful. Specific techniques as they relate to diaphyseal amputation in children will be covered later in the book.

CLOSURE

General surgical principles apply to wound closure. Dead spaces are eliminated. Drainage systems are used when needed. Opposing tissue layers are sewn under physiological tension, and the closure should be neither too tight nor too loose. As with all surgery, good surgical judgment applies to closure and suture selections in amputations.

STAGED AMPUTATIONS

Amputations are carried out in two or more stages when primary closure is inadvisable. The initial amputation may be for the purpose of providing adequate drainage as in the case of a preliminary open ankle disarticulation in the presence of a septic, ischemic diabetic foot. When the infection has been controlled by the first definitive amputation and other appropriate measures, a procedure at a higher level can then be carried out. If the infection is locally controlled and the amputation is to be performed through and immediately adjacent to a contaminated or infected area, the deep soft tissues and skin flaps are prepared for closure at the definitive bone length, leaving adequate viable skin. The bone is also divided and prepared at its definitive level. The wound is then left open. A secondary closure is performed subsequently; the time interval depends on tissue response. Contaminated amputations, usually a result of trauma, are treated in a similar manner by open flap preparation and delayed closure.

For centuries, open and infected amputations, often guillotine, have been treated by continuous traction, secondary closure, and, if necessary, later revision. There is still a useful place for this technique. When skin and soft tissue loss has been extensive and residual limb length critical, traction is the method of choice to prevent soft tissue retraction with ultimate loss of needed limb length. Traction-revision techniques, time-honored in war, should not be discarded as obsolete. They can be the most conservative and appropriate way to achieve the two basic principles of all amputation surgery, ablation and reconstruction.

REVISION AMPUTATION

The general principles of primary amputation apply to revision surgery. Revision is necessitated because the primary amputation failed to heal or because the healed residual limb is unsatisfactory for prosthetic fit and the patient's functional requirements. As prosthetic engineering has improved, revision surgery is practiced more often. This position is contrary to generally accepted views that improved modern prostheses can fit an undesirable residual limb. However, it is important to remember that prosthetic excellence can also restore function at a higher level amputation; there is a greater functional compromise when attempting to fit a longer but unsatisfactory residual limb.

When most traumatic amputations were treated by guillotine-type surgery and prolonged traction, the scarred residual limbs were routinely revised. Modern amputation techniques have, to a large degree, eliminated revision surgery in this situation. Today, revisions are required more often following wound breakdown when low levels of amputation have failed in the ischemic limb. As our understanding of dynamic limb blood flow increases, there will be less error in level determination. Revision amputation for ischemia will be needed less frequently.

When revising an amputation, the surgeon manages each tissue in the same manner and with the same goals as with primary amputation. Muscles may be scarred and atrophic so that muscle stabilization is usually less than effective. Nonetheless, it should be used, if possible, in the reconstruction. Some muscle stabilization is better than none. Revision for pain alone will fail unless the revision is related to demonstrable local abnormality.

The surgeon is but one member of the amputee rehabilitation team. The team approach to enlightened amputee rehabilitation requires more than postoperative evaluation in the amputee clinic. The surgeon as leader of the team will benefit by the wisdom and judgment of other team members in preoperative evaluation. Established rehabilitation goals are best achieved in this setting.

BIBLIOGRAPHY

Burgess, E. M., Romano, R. L., and Zettl, J. H.: The management of lower extremity amputations, TR 10-6, Aug. 1969, Washington, D.C., 1969, U.S. Government Printing Office.

Dale, W. A., editor: Management of arterial occlusive disease, Chicago, 1971, Year Book Medical Publishers, Inc.

Edmondson, A. S., and Crenshaw, A. H., editors: Campbell's operative orthopaedics, ed. 6, St. Louis, 1980, The C. V. Mosby Co.

Lindholm, R.: Features of amputation surgery among civilians during the period 1930-1960, Acta Orthop. Scan. **8**:74-89, 1964.

Little, J. M.: Amputation of the leg—a dull topic revisited, Med. J. Australia **2**:442-445, Sept., 1973.

Murdoch, G.: Amputation surgery in the lower extremity, Prosthet. Orthot. Int. **1**:72-83, Aug., 1977.

Pedersen, H. E.: The problem of the geriatric amputee, Artif. Limbs **12**(2):i-iii, 1968.

Slocum, D. B.: An atlas of amputations, St. Louis, 1959, The C. V. Mosby Co.

Weiss, M.: Myoplastic amputation, immediate prosthesis and early ambulation, Department of Health, Education, and Welfare, 1964, U.S. Government Printing Office.

Wilson, P. D.: Early weightbearing in the treatment of amputations of the lower limbs, J. Bone Joint Surg. **4**(2):224-247, April, 1922.

CHAPTER 3

Postoperative management

ERNEST M. BURGESS

The primary goal of postsurgical amputation management is prompt, uncomplicated healing. With many surgical procedures, treatment is then considered finished; however, this does not apply to the amputation. Unless the healed residual limb is fit with an appropriate limb substitute, no functional restoration is possible. The empty sleeve or the empty trouser leg starkly portrays incomplete postoperative management. Since postoperative care requires the residual limb to interface and direct the prosthesis, surgical responsibility ends only when maximum functional restoration has been gained.

Until recently, it has been a generally accepted practice to bandage the limb postoperatively with soft supportive dressings and then begin early progressive conditioning by exercise, stretching, and other physical methods. Physical therapists and others have for many years been carefully instructed in the techniques of residual limb bandaging and wrapping. The need for compressive wound dressings has long been recognized as essential to control swelling and promote stable limb volume. This so-called limb shrinkage or maturation permits prosthetic fit without requiring frequent changes in the size and configuration of the prosthetic socket. More recently, a number of techniques have been advocated using an immediate postsurgical rigid dressing that incorporates pressure and support as well as, under certain circumstances, some immediate substitute limb function early in the postsurgical period. The general principles of these systems of management will be considered.

SOFT DRESSINGS

Following surgery, the wound is covered with sterile, compressible soft dressings such as fluff gauze, mechanic's waste, natural sponges, or other materials. The limb is then carefully wrapped with elastic bandages, which are applied to support the amputation site itself under pressure, yet avoid proximal constriction. The supportive elastic bandages are changed frequently, often several times a day, in an attempt to maintain appropriate wound support and pressure. As healing progresses, the patient or relatives of the patient are instructed in bandage application. An elasticized, tapered, closed-end stocking is alternatively used. When, on the basis of the experience and the judgment of the supervising personnel, wound maturity has proceeded to a degree permitting provisional or definitive limb fitting, then the prosthesis is applied and progressively used. Under this system of management, the time interval from amputation to limb fit may take many months. Joint contractures frequently develop, and muscle conditioning is difficult, especially if the limb is painful.

Investigations have shown that pressure under soft "pressure support dressings" is unpredictable, often poorly localized, and can frequently have a tourniquet effect. Moisture, humidity, wound surface, temperature, and sterility under soft conventional dressings are difficult to monitor and control. The frequent movement and manipulation of the tender, healing tissue not only may promote prolonged and deep-seated pain patterns, but also may serve as a source of continuing apprehension and discomfort during the healing period. Patients, especially older peripheral vascular disease amputees, hesitate to move about actively. The need for analgesics and sedatives complicates this immobility. The patient is then placed at increased risk for postoperative complications both local and general.

The advantages of soft dressing management are the ease of application and an opportunity to frequently inspect the healing wound site and quickly change the physical wound environment by replacing and altering the dressings. Even though the system is being outdated by more physiological semirigid and rigid dressing techniques, older teaching and tradition tend to prevail. The soft tissue residual limb wrapping system of management is still used by a majority of surgeons.

SEMIRIGID AND RIGID DRESSINGS

Injured tissues heal best when initially supported and placed at rest. This applies to all tissues of the extremity from skin through bone. This fact is demonstrated in animals and humans by physiological tissue splinting after trauma. Where initial immobilization is combined with appropriate local pressure and elevation of the injured limb, the inflammatory response of early healing is minimized and is beneficially modified by edema control. This practice of immobilization, pressure, and infrequent dressing changes is an axiom of good surgery, yet it seems to be periodically forgotten and has to be relearned by each new generation of surgeons. Curiosity prompts frequent dressings and inspections of early healing wounds. This practice, together with the application of a variety of chemicals that are often oily, irritating, and air occlusive, in general does more harm than good. Nowhere are these principles more impressively demonstrated than in extensive war wounds, open fractures, burns, infected fractures with nonunion, and amputations.

Orr, Trueta, and many other observers, both before and after them, have accumulated overwhelming evidence of the value of closed, rigid dressing techniques. It is unfortunate that these principles, like many others in surgery, are overlooked or forgotten in a day of "miracle" drugs and chemically treated dressings.

Both open and closed amputations have for many years, been treated by early application of rigid dressings. During the latter years of World War I, this experience was well documented both with clean and infected lower limb amputations. Simple functional prosthetic units were applied to the rigid dressings, allowing ambulation and some degree of weight bearing. The method was revived again after World War II, primarily in France and Poland. At the end of the European phase of the war, many thousands of individuals throughout Central and Western Europe were left with poorly healed or unhealed amputations. Working with them, Berlemont in France and Weiss in Poland revived interest in the rigid dressing technique. Their experience has been enlarged and new methods developed throughout much of the world today.

Semirigid and rigid dressings can be fabricated of a variety of materials including Unna paste, conventional plaster of Paris, elastic plaster of Paris, thermolabile polymers, and a number of other splinting materials. The simple encasing of the limb in a plaster cast or similar immobilizing dressing does not fulfill all the requirements of the rigid dressing. The rigid dressing wound environment is designed to achieve a therapeutic degree of terminal pressure and a relatively sterile, dry wound surface, with no restriction to tissue fluid exchange. This implies no proximal constriction as well as adequate suspension of the dressing, that is, the cast. Contour suspension by molding the cast while setting should be reinforced by additional suspension devices such as a waist belt or shoulder harness to straps incorporated in the rigid dressing. Careful attention to suspension will minimize "falling away" of the cast distally, thus allowing terminal edema.

The maintenance of gentle pressure distally is also accomplished by means of compressible materials placed between the site of surgery and the adjacent rigid support. Among the many materials used, sterile polyurethane foam provides an excellent pressure interface material. It does not retain heat, liquids flow through it freely, maceration does not occur, and it is inexpensive and easily contoured. The rigid dressing is applied at the conclusion of surgery and changed as indicated throughout the postoperative period to definitive limb fit.

The primary objection to this form of postsurgical management is the inability to inspect the operative site easily and at will. In terms of the effect on wound healing, this objection actually describes one of the advantages of the closed, rigid dressing system, an undisturbed operative site that is properly supported. Unusual pain, fever, or other clinical evidence of possible complications requires cast removal and wound inspection.

Skill is required in the proper application of a

rigid postamputation dressing. In truth, application of the rigid dressing requires neither more nor less skill than proper application of soft tissue supportive wrappings. The rigid dressing, however, incorporates advantages of comfort, improved wound environment, and easier mobility of the patient. Surgeons performing amputations are obligated in the name of modern amputation management to understand and properly use the postsurgical rigid dressing technique.

Infected and staged amputations are also managed with advantage by a rigid postoperative dressing. In fact, the closed cast techniques successfully popularized by Orr, Trueta, and others were directed toward the treatment of infected and open wounds. Staged amputations are handled in a similar manner with equal success.

IMMEDIATE POSTSURGICAL PROSTHESES

The immediate postsurgical rigid dressing can serve as a socket for a temporary prosthetic device in both the upper and lower limbs. Physical and psychological advantages are attributed to this functional immediate prosthetic system. The patient does not undergo a limbless time interval. Some degree of functional restoration begins immediately. Established pathways of neuromuscular control are less likely to fade with early limb use. Residual limb pain is described as being seen far less in the patient who has a rigid dressing immediately after surgery than with conventional soft tissue management. The time for limb maturation and overall amputee rehabilitation, including hospitalization, is reported to be considerably shorter with this system. The general physical and mental state of the patient is benefited by early general physical activities as well as physiological limb function.

Although some of the described benefits have not been statistically documented, the worldwide experience in immediate postsurgical prosthetic fitting certainly supports many of its advocates' assertions. Areas of disagreement regarding immediate postsurgical prosthetic fitting have centered about the injurious effects of early function, particularly limited weight bearing in lower extremity amputations, inability to easily inspect the operative site, thus anticipating complications early, and technical difficulties in the proper application of the rigid dressing and prosthesis. Of these, the major concern is local tissue damage with wound breakdown when excessive stresses have been applied. This hazard is both significant and real. Early publicity dramatized the spectacular situation in which a patient underwent an amputation and was walking on the day of surgery or the following day. The emphasis on early weight bearing in the lower limb distorted the more significant real value of the rigid dressing–immediate fit system. Experience has demonstrated the fact that early weight bearing must be individualized. In general, little or no weight bearing is allowed other than prosthetic touchdown until the wound has sufficiently healed to permit the gradually increasing wound stress associated with tissue loading. Wound healing potential is marginal with the ischemic amputee. The additional stress of early weight bearing through the rigid dressing can delay wound healing or even cause wound disruption. The amount of wound stress produced by terminal device function must be carefully controlled. Uneventful, quiet wound healing is the primary goal for both the amputation surgery and postsurgical management. Terminal device function can be beneficial but must in no way compromise this benign course.

Immediate postsurgical prosthetic fitting has made surgeons aware of early functional restoration in the amputee. Emphasis is diverted from the surgery as the central fact of treatment. Return of function to an attainable rehabilitation level now becomes the primary goal of treatment. As a result of this constructive and expanded concept, surgeons are modifying and improvising a variety of postsurgical regimens toward early residual limb maturation and definitive limb fit. A variety of simple and inexpensive provisional limbs are fitted early, regardless as to whether the patient has had an immediate prosthetic fitting or not. In keeping with this attitude, some surgeons have been incorporating electrodes, both implant and surface types, to allow voluntary myoelectric terminal device control immediately or early in the postoperative course. This application is of primary use in the upper limb but has also been tried on an experimental basis with lower extremity amputations.

CONTROLLED POSTOPERATIVE ENVIRONMENT TREATMENT WITH AIR SPLINTS AND RELATED DEVICES

Compressed gas can be used as a dressing medium following amputation. The importance of terminal pressure for edema control has stimulated the development of a variety of compressed air dressing bags incorporating the residual limb. The wound need have no other dressings, and if the bag or container is transparent, the limb, including the operative site, can be visually inspected or even palpated through the bag wall without disturbing sterility. The drawbacks to an air bag system are a rapid accumulation of moisture within the bag, creating undesirable humidity and heat with accompanying increased chance of wound maceration and infection. It is necessary to provide a flow-through gas system rather than a sealed static air pressure device if wound pressure, humidity, temperature, and sterility are optimally controlled. Equipment of this type is commercially available today and has been used successfully by the British Research and Development Unit, Roehampton, England, as well as by the Veterans Administration's Prosthetics Research Study, who have coinvestigated the Controlled Environment Treatment in the Western hemisphere. With this system, the physical parameters applied to the amputation are scientifically controlled and monitored by a console to which the bag is attached by means of a flexible tube. The pressure may be intermittent or continuous. Gas composition can be varied should the surgeon so desire. The air flows through the dressing bag, venting proximally through a leaf-flutter system that absolutely prevents proximal constriction. The disposable equipment necessary for this form of management is only slightly more expensive than conventional dressings. The console is permanent equipment. After surgery, patients may be up and about in a chair and on crutches as soon as their general physical condition permits.

Attachment of temporary prosthetic components to the bag is used by some surgeons. Lack of firm support as provided by the rigid dressing technique is at this time a drawback to full effectiveness of the air splint system; however, it is not difficult to incorporate the best features of both the immediate rigid dressing and the air bag control system.

Developments in controlling the physical environment of the amputation wound are progressing rapidly at this time. Innovations and improvements can be expected. All are directed toward the same goal of prompt, uneventful wound healing with early functional restoration, minimized complications, and a positive psychological attitude on the part of the patient.

It has long been recognized that postoperative amputee care directed only toward a healed operative site is inadequate. The complete interdependence of all aspects of amputee management will be repeatedly stressed throughout this atlas. Interdisciplinary cooperation demonstrated by the amputee team is more critical and essential than with most areas of surgery involving functional loss. Physical rehabilitation of the patient, and more specifically the involved limb or limbs, proceeds within obtainable rehabilitation goals from the date of surgery. Exercises, joint contracture prevention, and supportive compression dressings all are part of well-established postsurgical rehabilitation regimens designed to achieve rehabilitation goals and accomplish early restoration of function.

The immediate postsurgical prosthetic concept, including immediate and early substitute limb function through temporary prostheses, is an ideal mechanism both physically and psychologically to advance prompt recovery. With improved amputation surgery designed to retain residual limb function, specifically voluntary muscle strength and control as well as sense of position and movement, it is necessary to attempt to retain and enhance these vital physical characteristics of the residual limb early after surgery. This is in contrast to past conventional thinking. Limb conditioning was and still is in many places designed to "shrink and mature" the limb to provide stability for socket fit. Physical stability is desirable, but even more important is the retention of the functional potential of the limb as a neuromuscular end organ.

As a result of this, modern surgery and postsurgical methods are now used and are being further developed to enhance limb strength and sensibility, with voluntary and reflex control of the prosthesis in a more normal, physiological manner. Stump muscle training, biofeedback techniques, gait pattern education, and skill acquisition beyond the basic requirement of stance and gait are all emerging as elements of increasing importance in postoperative care. Acquiring and developing these residual limb qualities parallel physical wound healing and are an integral part of the postsurgical management. They should begin either immediately or early after surgery.

The entire field of amputation surgery, postsurgical management, and early rehabilitation is exciting and rewarding both to the patient and professional. There are few areas where the surgeon has the unique opportunity to work so closely with other health care disciplines, primarily engineering. Civilian amputations throughout the world continue to increase rapidly in number, mostly the result of degenerative and occlusive arterial disease. Surgeons performing amputations today are committed to a current working knowledge of the rapid developments taking place in this field. Patients are entitled to the improved clinical benefit inherent in modern amputation surgery and aftercare.

BIBLIOGRAPHY

Berlemont, M., et al.: Ten years of experience with immediate application of prosthetic devices to amputations of the lower extremities on the operating table, Prosthet. Orthot. Int. vol. 3, issue no. 8, 1969.

Burgess, E. M.: Wound healing after amputation: effect of controlled environment treatment, J. Bone Joint Surg. **60A**(2): 245-246, 1978.

Burgess, E. M., and Romano, R. L.: The management of lower extremity amputees using immediate postsurgical prostheses, Clin. Orthop. **57**:137-146, March-April, 1968.

Burgess, E. M., Romano, R. L., and Zettl, J. H.: The management of lower extremity amputations, TR 10-6, Aug., 1969, U.S. Government Printing Office.

Ghiulamila, R. I.: Semi-rigid dressing for postoperative fitting of below knee prosthesis, Arch. Phys. Med. Rehabil. **53**:186-190, April, 1972.

Golbranson, F.: Immediate postsurgical fitting and early ambulation, Clin. Orthop. **56**:119-131, 1968.

Sarmiento, A., et al.: Lower extremity amputation: the impact of immediate postsurgical prosthetic fitting, Clin. Orthop. **68**:22-31, Jan-Feb., 1970.

Vitali, M., et al.: Amputations and prostheses, New York, 1978, Macmillan Publishing Co., Inc.

Weiss, M.: Myoplastic amputation, immediate prosthesis and early ambulation, Washington, D.C., Department of Health, Education, and Welfare, U.S. Government Printing Office.

Wilson, P. D.: Early weightbearing in the treatment of amputations of the lower limbs, J. Bone Joint Surg. **4**(2):224-247, April, 1922.

CHAPTER 4

Planning for optimum function in amputation surgery

JAMES M. CARY
ROBERT G. THOMPSON

AMPUTATION SURGERY AS CONSTRUCTIVE SURGERY

Amputation surgery is most frequently performed to rid the patient of a painful, life-threatening, troublesome, or cumbersome part. Emphasis on ablation of a lesion may obscure the concept that successful amputation surgery must also be a constructive treatment program, carefully planned to leave the patient with the least amount of residual disability.

Function does not depend only on the substitution of a prosthesis for the ablated part and is not the responsibility of a limb maker alone. Optimum function is attained only when a prosthesis of excellent design and fabrication is applied, with intelligent selection, to the most durable and effective stump that circumstances allow. Optimum function can be achieved only in a patient with optimistic motivation whose physical strength and skill have been developed by adequate rehabilitation.

PROGRAM PLANNING AS THE PHYSICIAN'S RESPONSIBILITY

This goal of optimum function is a major challenge. Although its implementation will require the efforts of a number of team workers, the planning, coordination, and supervision of the program is the obligation of the physician to the patient. This requires a thorough knowledge and realistic appreciation of amputee function. Following are a number of factors that make program planning the responsibility of the physician:

1. *The surgical procedure itself is part of the overall plan.* The level of function to be attained is dictated, in major part, by the level and effective construction of the amputation stump. The surgeon must have the eventual function in mind when planning the operative procedure.

2. *A realistic and attainable goal of function must be set.* The entire treatment team should be made aware of the extent and limits of this goal so that each member can work effectively and efficiently with consistent expectations. The input of other team members into planning is important, but the physician's experience and knowledge of the individual patient's physical abilities and limitations should allow direction of a functional goal toward attainable reality.

3. *Priorities of function should be established and placed in perspective.* These priorities may differ between individual patients or groups of patients. A young, athletic, traumatic amputee, for example, will have a high priority for durability and comfort of the stump for hard usage. This might, in some instances, not be afforded by a

short, painful, scarred, or poorly muscled below-knee amputation. A geriatric amputee, on the other hand, may have an overriding priority for balance, limb control and proprioception and might require the below-knee level amputation, even though it is defective from a durability standpoint, in order to walk at all.

As another example, a powered prosthetic elbow unit might be essential to the strength and stability function of a bilateral above-elbow amputee, but of little value to a unilateral amputee whose major priority is rapidity of action and proprioceptive feedback for the prosthetic "helping hand."

Priority determinations require thought and clinical judgment, as well as some experience, but they are decisions that have to be made if optimum function is to be attained.

4. *Future problems should be anticipated.* Measures to prevent or correct future problems should be incorporated into the planning from the start. The juvenile amputee presents an obvious example of problems to be anticipated with growth. Eventual prosthetic use requires long-term planning, for the adult, and not simply for the immediate needs of the youngster.[6] Identification of problems will require analysis of growth and consideration of alternatives for an optimum plan of management through life.[17]

Other future problems may be less obvious. An upper limb amputee, for example, with fairly dextrous use of a prosthesis by the therapist's standards, may reject it.[34] Often the precipitating event is frustration by some simple, but necessary, task at home or work that was not included in the instruction. Periodic check on function and usage, with emphasis on specific problem solution, might have helped to maintain useful function. In planning, the physician must ensure that rehabilitation is adequate and relevant to the patient's needs.

Although each patient presents an individual problem and has individual needs and priorities for function, several groupings of patients can be identified in which these priorities and goals for optimum function may differ significantly. We have selected as examples for special comment the traumatic amputee, limb-deficient child, and dysvascular or geriatric amputee. Constructive surgical planning may have a different emphasis in each. The pitfalls to be avoided, as well as the prerequisites for attainment of optimum function, can serve as a general framework for modeling individual treatment programs.

THE TRAUMATIC AMPUTEE

Primary management

The extent to which optimal function can be provided for the patient who is a victim of traumatic limb loss is often determined by the primary management of the injury. In the severely traumatized and contaminated wound, avoidance of further infection and increased vascular compromise is essential. Constructive planning, with its major consideration eventual optimal stump condition, may dictate the need for staging in the management of the amputation.

Military surgeons have long recognized that the avoidance of complication and, in fact, the functional outcome in traumatic amputations, as well as in other types of limb trauma, is in the hands of physicians providing definitive primary care. Experience with thousands of cases in several major wars has provided guidelines for this primary management. In time of war these guidelines were not offered as suggestions, but as firm directives.[18,25,29] For limb amputations directives for primary surgical treatment can be summarized as follows:

1. Ablation will be at the most distal viable level.
2. Viable skin will be preserved.
3. No wound closure of any type will be attempted.
4. Skin traction will be employed.
5. The proximal joint will be immobilized in a functional position.
6. Plaster will be split to avoid constriction.

This regimen is based on the following five principles of wound management, which are so well established by empirical military experience that they are considered axiomatic:

1. Any wound that could be closed at the time of initial debridement can be repaired with equal facility and far greater safety 5 to 9 days later.

2. Invasive infection does not occur in a completely debrided open wound with viable tissue.

3. Increasing vascular embarrassment due to closed space edema does not occur in a completely debrided, fasciotomized, open wound.

4. Inevitable errors in the estimation of tissue viability and wound contamination can be corrected by secondary debridement at the time of delayed closure.

5. In a severely traumatized and potentially contaminated limb wound there is no real justification for immediate closure.

Fig. 4-1 illustrates the complication of tissue necrosis and infection occurring in a patient with

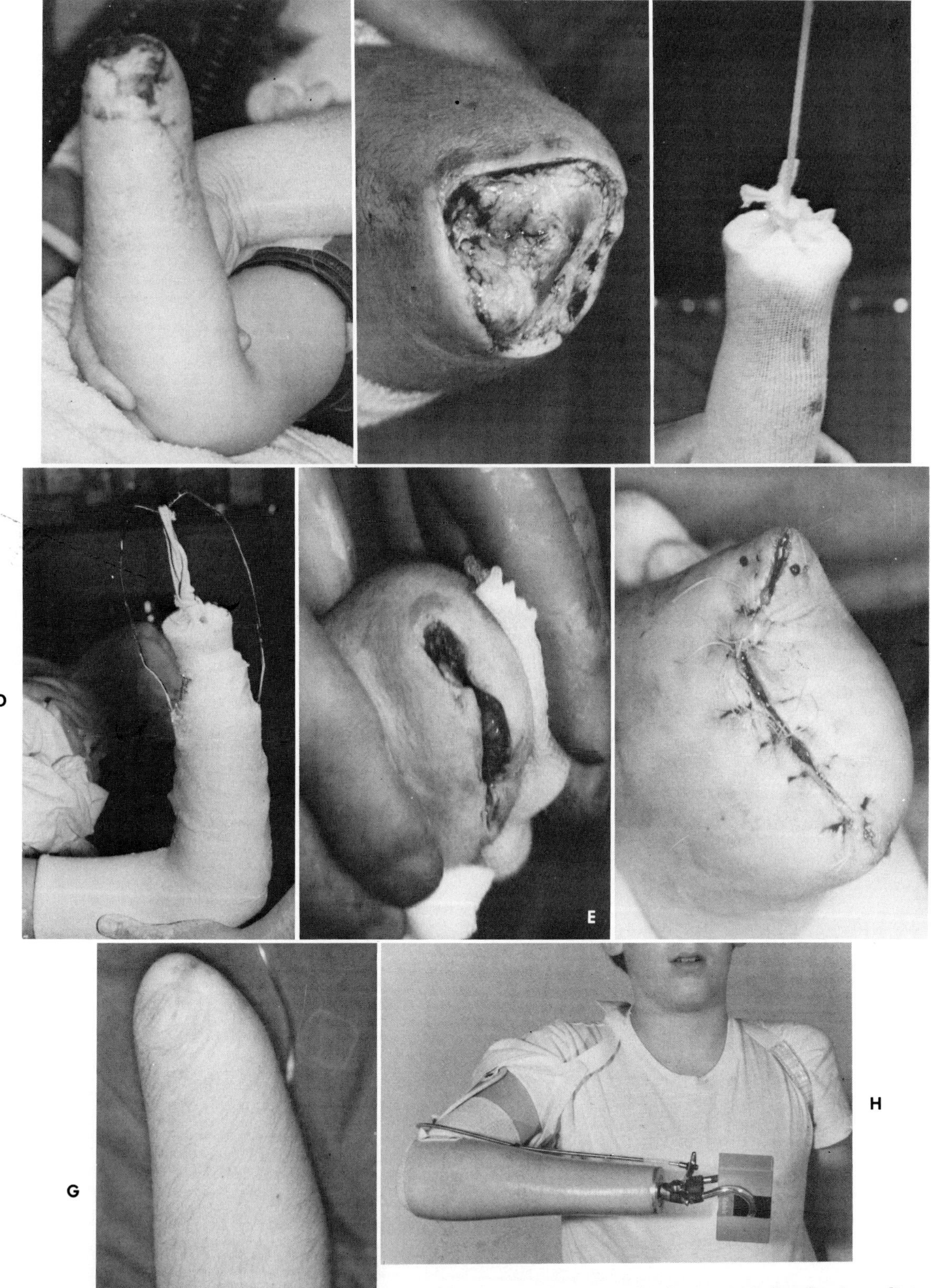

Fig. 4-1. A, Necrosis and infection 3 weeks after immediate skin closure of traumatic amputation of hand and wrist. **B,** Stump completely redebrided. **C,** Stockinette skin traction applied. **D,** Traction cast with elastic bands and outrigger. **E,** Skin mobility after undermining edges on ninth postoperative day. **F,** Delayed closure, ninth day. **G,** Uncomplicated healing. **H,** Length and pronation-supination motion retained.

traumatic wrist disarticulation, which was subjected to immediate primary closure. The techniques employed in the *secondary* treatment of the complication would have been suitable for the *primary* management of the original severely traumatized and potentially contaminated amputation. Fortunately, infection was neither invasive nor advanced so that adequate debridement and skin traction made possible the retrieval of skin cover for delayed closure without loss of optimum stump length and mobility.

Staging for optimal function

In dealing with a traumatic amputation constructive planning is required to salvage the best possible function. Once amputation of the traumatized limb is seen to be inevitable, this planning for function in prosthetic use should be the obvious next step.

At this point it might be wise for the surgeon to stop and consider his own frame of mind. Considerable mental effort has been exerted in an attempt to save the injured part. This effort has failed. Loss of a limb has a considerable emotional impact, not only on the patient and family, but on the surgeon as well. This factor, in itself, may inhibit resumption of the mental effort necessary to think constructively about the amputation.

Good amputee function requires an optimal conversion site, pliable skin cover with sensation, uncomplicated healing, freedom from infection, good vascular stump nutrition, and, if possible, a well-muscled stump. Reasonably prompt prosthetic fitting and rapid rehabilitation are desirable to avoid serious psychological problems.[15,32]

Staging of treatment may be necessary to provide these objectives safely and with assurance. A lower limb amputation must bear weight. If the length and level of the amputation is dictated by the skin available for immediate closure, not only bone length, but the opportunity for revision to an optimal functional stump may well be lost. If a compromise with skin tension in closure is accepted, wound breakdown, infection, or a tender adherent scar are almost inevitable. Patients with persistent sinuses overlying necrotic tissues in primarily closed below-knee stumps are seen all too frequently in civilian practice. Open revisions result in further shortening, often with tender, poorly muscled stumps. During the Korean War and throughout the Vietnam conflict, the practice of lower leg guillotine amputation at optimal bone length was abandoned in favor of open amputation at the most distal viable level. Skin traction was employed, and late revision to optimal stump length was performed, using myodesis where possible. Improved functional results and the lowered incidence of wound complication have been convincing.[18]

The trauma necessitating amputation in civilian practice is not far different from that of the wounds of war. The incidence of complication in immediate wound closure in civilian traumatic amputations strongly suggests that the military experience and recommendation in the treatment of such injuries should be accepted.[16]

Management of specific lower limb traumatic amputations

Specific programs for management of several levels of severe trauma may serve as examples of staged management for optimum function.

The Syme amputation. Severely traumatized or crushing injuries to the foot are not uncommon in civilian practice. Forefoot vascularity and nutrition are easily compromised, and infection is a frequent complication. In these severe foot injuries, however, the functional advantages of Syme amputation make it far superior to higher level amputation. Attempts to retrieve a viable end-bearing heel pad, if they can be done safely and without invasive infection, are fully justified.[7,26]

On occasion diaphyseal tibial amputation cannot be avoided, but the massive injury is often restricted to the forefoot. The skin over the heel, although traumatized, may be salvageable. In these instances the Syme amputation is elected. The Chopart and Lisfranc amputations can be fit with prostheses, which are occasionally tolerated, but they usually give less than adequate functional prosthetic use.

In World War II the Syme amputation was used freely and frequently by the Canadian and British Medical Corps, but was not favored by American military surgeons, who cited the high rate of complication and the number of below-knee revisions required. Understanding of the procedure has improved, and it is now more widely favored. The complications, however, that prompted the procedure's original unpopularity should be considered to see how they can be best avoided.

In the traumatized foot there are several possibilities for Syme conversion. Where the tissues about the heel and plantar skin are not traumatized, a primary loose, well-drained closure of the Syme amputation might be considered. Where these tissues are traumatized, although viable, as is frequently the case in severe foot injuries, it would seem unwise to subject the heel pad to the further trauma of surgical dissection, as in the Canadian military practice of open-flap Syme amputation. These heel pads, after open-flap treatment, are often scarred, tender, and perhaps poorly adapted for end-bearing function after delayed closure. In children there is further reason for rejection of the open-flap techniuqe. The operation is not performed, as it is in adults, with resection of the cartilage surfaces of the ankle, but is a true disarticulation that leaves the distal epiphyses of the tibia and fibula undisturbed.[5] Open disarticulations are troublesome. Cartilage deprived of nutrition undergoes necrosis and desquamation. The recesses of the joint invite persistent bacterial invasion. In a severe foot injury, where the heel pad is believed to be viable, an open forefoot amputation may be performed as a first stage. Surface cartilage is debrided. After edema has been resolved and nutrition of the tissues is established, a delayed formal revision to Syme amputation can be performed with relative safety. In those cases in which there is persistent wound edema or surface infection or where restoration of tissue nutrition is delayed, the application of a very thin split-thickness skin graft as temporary wound cover will usually result in a clean, dry, closed wound. This can subsequently be revised with safety.

The below-knee amputation. The below-knee amputation cannot match the functional ability of the Syme amputation. Only if the stump is well constructed, firm, and muscular and has a pliable skin cover can the younger, active amputee gain the degree of functional ambulation desired and needed.

In 1941, Gallie commented on the poor function and multiple problems encountered in below-knee amputations of 2448 Canadian war veterans.[23] Norman T. Kirk, later to become Surgeon General of the United States Army, did not agree with this unfavorable report, but did emphasize the importance of below-knee stumps "properly fashioned at the site of election."[29]

Since that time, there has been a remarkable increase in the sophistication and versatility of design and fabrication of lower limb prostheses, so much so that the concept of "site of election" and the ideal stump has all but disappeared. It might be hoped that this prosthetic improvement would solve all the problems of the below-knee amputee but this, unfortunately, has not occurred. Many patients with traumatic below-knee amputations continue to have problems in adequate limb fitting, durability, comfort, and endurance.

Planning for optimum function should include the construction of a well-muscled, durable stump of effective length, with a pliable skin cover that has adequate sensation. A prosthesis of sound biomechanical design must be available, and the prosthetist must be aware of any special attributes or limitations of the stump so that these may be incorporated into the selection and design of the artificial limb. When treating a patient with traumatic limb loss these should be the goals of the responsible surgeon. Again, staging for avoidance of complication is often necessary for their assured accomplishment.[19,21]

Fig. 4-2 demonstrates the staged construction of an effective below-knee stump in a patient in whom vascular trauma had resulted in necrosis and chronic infection.

Although an adequate stump was retrieved in this patient, 6 months elapsed from the date of primary injury, and morbidity was excessive. A realistic goal of below-knee amputation could have been determined near the outset. Recognition that the skin of the heel was insensate might have suggested a primary open procedure at distal calf level, avoiding continued necrosis and infection of tissues. The constructive revision might then have been accomplished sooner and with greater safety.

Salvaging an effective above-knee stump. The above-knee amputation, at best, results in much greater disability than one performed below the knee. Only with an ideal muscular stump of effective length can the above-knee amputee function without significant impairment.[37]

In the young child the importance of preservation of the distal femoral epiphysis cannot be overemphasized. About 75% to 80% of the increment in femoral growth is from the distal growth plate. Loss of this growth center may result in progressive and excessive relative shortening of the stump.[5]

The ability to salvage an effective above-knee stump in either the adult or the child with severe proximal lower leg trauma and popliteal artery damage has, again, resulted from military experience. In this instance the ability to salvage an effective above-knee stump was the by-product of failure. The special vascular research team assigned to emergency treatment of arterial injuries during the Korean War had notable successes with femoral artery injuries, but failures of popliteal and trifurcation repairs, particularly

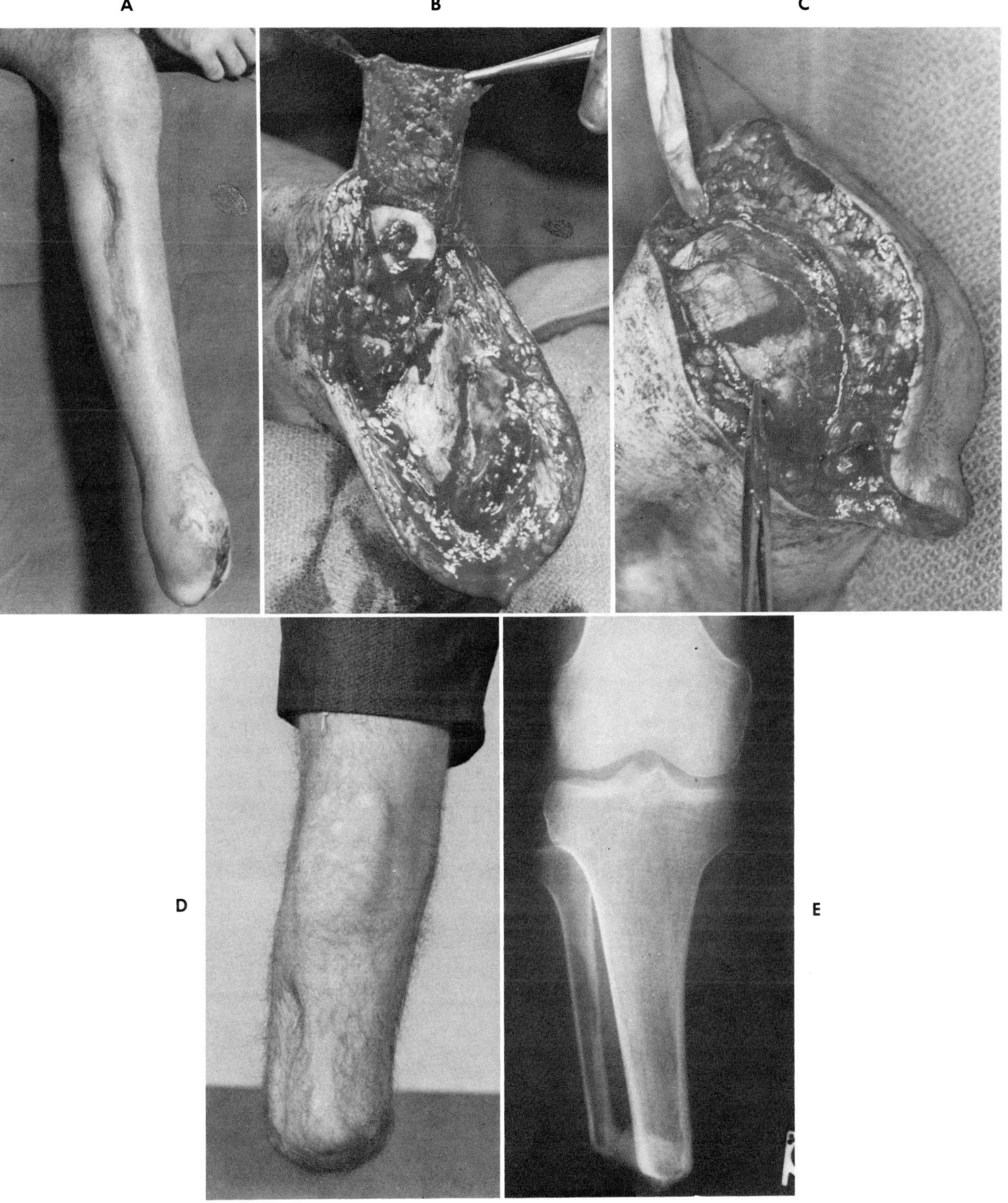

Fig. 4-2. A, Limb of 17-year-old male 6 months after penetrating wound of anterior calf in which trifurcation of popliteal artery was severed. Vascular repair failed, with necrosis of foot and persistent infection of tissues. **B,** After first-stage open amputation in distal tibia with skin traction had controlled infection, definitive revision with Ertl osteoplastic technique was performed. Osteoperiosteal flap used to bridge distal tibia and fibula is shown. **C,** Firmly anchored myodesis under normal muscle tension overlies osteoperiosteal bridge. **D,** Stump is firm, muscular, and capable of partial end bearing in total-contact soft-socket PTB prosthesis. It has provided excellent function. **E,** X-ray film after 1 year of use. Bone bridge and osseous structure of tibia and fibula show hypertrophy rather than usual demineralization seen with less functional stumps.

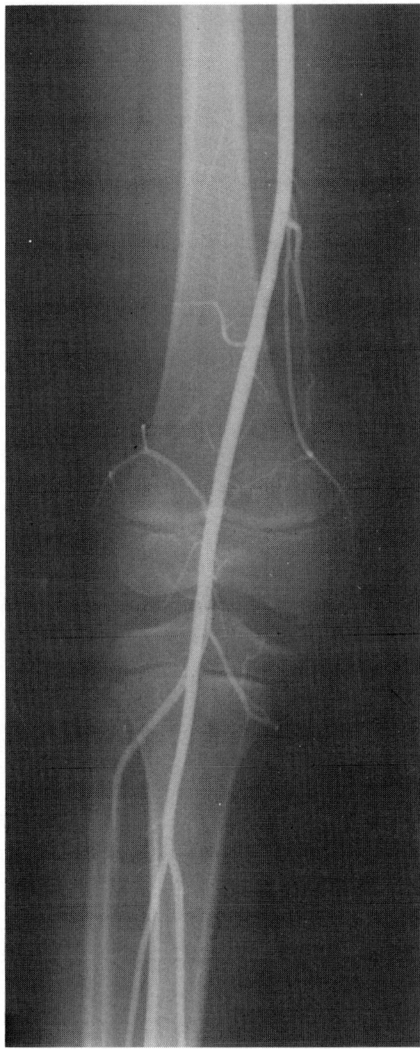

Fig. 4-3. Arteriogram demonstrating geniculate arterial distribution.

when associated with severe lower leg trauma, were frequent.[27]

The key to amputation salvage in these cases is the geniculate circulation (Fig. 4-3). This can provide nutrition and viability to a very short, open below-knee amputation performed as a first-stage temporary procedure, if devitalized calf muscle tissue is removed. Observation of the demarcation of necrosis after popliteal repair failure established the feasibility of this level. This technique of open amputation with skin traction was started late in the Korean War and became standard practice in Vietnam. There is, of course, insufficient soft tissue for an effective below-knee stump, nor should the surgeon consider below-knee prosthetic use at this level in the younger patient (Fig. 4-4). With skin healing and freedom

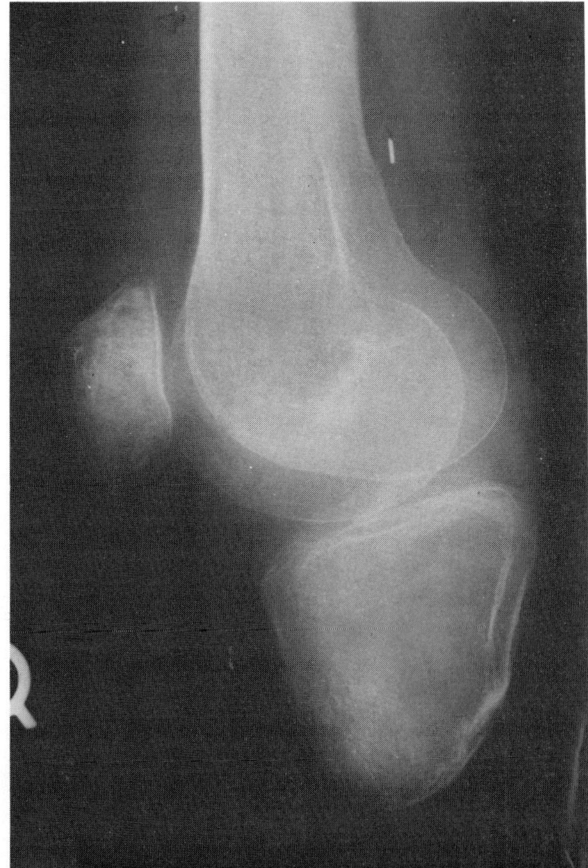

Fig. 4-4. Viable level of first-stage amputation after popliteal artery damage associated with severe lower leg trauma.

from infection and further vascular embarrassment, however, revision to an above-knee transcondylar level in the adult or a knee disarticulation in the younger child with open epiphyses can be readily accomplished as a secondary staged procedure.

Summary

When faced with an injury in which severe trauma and vascular compromise will necessitate limb loss, the surgeon must make a realistic assessment of the amputation level that can be provided the patient under the circumstances. The measures needed to construct the most effective stump for this level must be planned. The surgeon must avoid complications that may jeopardize the planned outcome. Staging of treatment, for avoidance of complication and retention of maximum tissue viability, will usually lead to the desired result.[13]

The mass casualties of wartime have given military surgeons an opportunity to objectively evaluate treatment results in a statistically significant number of severe injuries, which, for the civilian surgeon, are but an occasional experience. Familiarity with and a respect for the principles of treatment that evolved from this experience can be of great value in the primary management and constructive planning of treatment for the patient with an injury that necessitates amputation.

THE LIMB-DEFICIENT CHILD

Selection for treatment

The effective treatment of the child with a serious limb deficiency, either congenital or acquired, will require careful planning and clinical judgment to provide optimum function. Five principles of pediatric orthopaedic surgery can serve as a general outline for this planning:

1. The end product should be defined in terms of eventual adult function, not simply in terms of temporary gains for the youngster. Small children may be transiently improved by some procedures or reconstructions and yet not retain these functional gains into adult life.
2. Problems, therefore, should be identified in terms of adult function. Future problems that will occur as the child grows must be anticipated, and the treatment plan must incorporate solutions.
3. It is necessary to analyze growth, not only in its effect on the disorder, but also for its effect on the proposed treatment.
4. Valid alternatives of treatment should be considered so that the optimum plan may be selected.
5. The whole child, not just the motor-skeletal parts, must function in society. Social, educational, and developmental priorities, which may be even more important to total function, must be considered in the treatment plan.

Congenital limb deficiencies may be divided into an anatomical classification.[22,28] Those deficiencies classified as transverse and terminal are obvious and are accepted for prosthetic treatment. It is in the longitudinal deficiencies that planning is more difficult. Objective decision and clinical judgment are necessary. It can be postulated from experience that some limb anomalies are more effectively treated with prosthetic fitting as amputees than by attempts at limb reconstructions which fail to retain functional improvement through the growth period (Fig. 4-5).[2,31]

This decision, however, is not an easy one. The conditioned attitudes of society, and perhaps even of the surgeon, consider amputation an unmitigated disaster. When seen in the infant or small child these deformities may not seem severe to the parents or family. A critical assessment of the problems involved is necessary to arrive at competent clinical judgment. The biomechanical losses in the limb deficiency must be accurately identified. The major defect is usually a notable inequality of limb length. This is often combined with malalignment or malrotation of the limb and may be associated with absence of adequate proximal musculature or functional instability of proximal joints. The prosthetic alternative of treatment allows for immediate and continuing

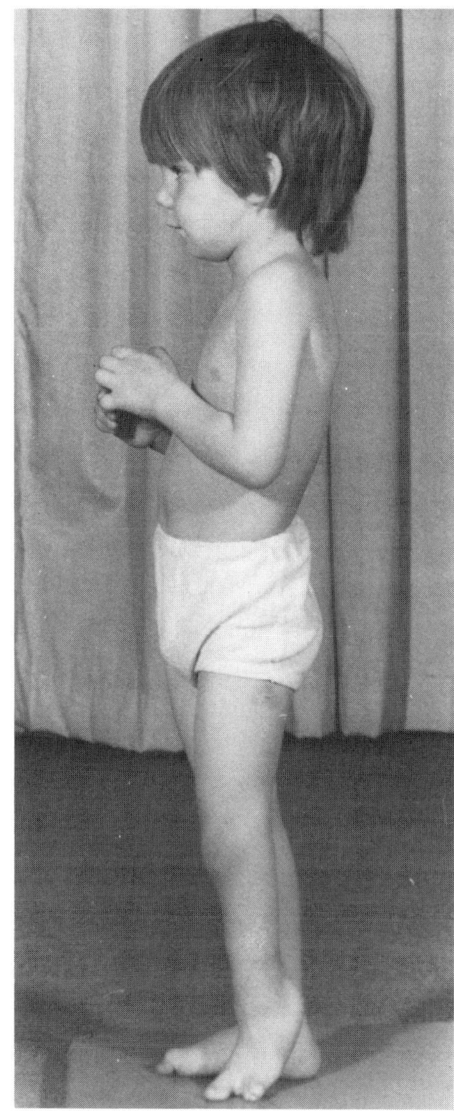

Fig. 4-5. Patient with paraxial (longitudinal) fibular hemimelia. Limb deficiency appropriately treated by conversion and prosthetic fitting.

length equalization. In the lower limb, realignment and proper foot placement can be provided by the prosthesis. Stabilization of joints can be attained by prosthetic mechanisms.

The severity of the biomechanical losses present can be more accurately projected in terms of adult function if certain physical laws are appreciated. The law of magnitude has been known to architects and engineers for centuries, but its application to medical and biological sciences may still not be fully appreciated.[24] Briefly stated, mass, and therefore weight and force, increases as the cube, strength only as the square, of an increasing linear dimension such as height or length. Parameters of mass in the human body can be recognized as weight, reactive joint force, and demand for muscle strength. With growth these increase disproportionately to the squared area parameters such as tissue strength, joint surface area for reception of force, and available muscle strength. Deterioration of functions that are marginal may occur as a child grows. The scale model fallacy—the expectation that initial function in the small child will be retained unimpaired into adult life—has in the past led to errors in judgment in planning reconstructive surgery.

The effect of amputation on the child is quite different than it is in the adult. In the adult, loss of a limb effects a radical and often disastrous change in the life-style and adjustment of the patient. In the young child the limb loss can be amalgamated into a developing life-style without major disruption to the individual's adjustment. The parents, of course, require continuing education in acceptance to avoid imparting a psychological burden to the child.

The decision for amputation and prosthetic management must be based on study of the individual case. It is important to total the whole deficit, since most cases of longitudinal limb deficiency have other implications. One should not concentrate only on the major anomaly. Hypoplasia of the whole limb is common. The effect on continued growth of the limb should be assessed. It is enough to suggest that prosthetic treatment may be considered, without prejudice, as one of the alternatives of management. A knowledge of prosthetic principles, growth, and functional kinesiology of gait is required for objective decision making.

Decision making may be made easier if it is recognized that immediate conversion of the defective limb is rarely necessary. Initially orthotic fitting around the anomaly to allow developing function may be employed. Parents' acceptance is usually attained as they observe function and recognize the cosmetic and functional advantages of prosthetic substitution.

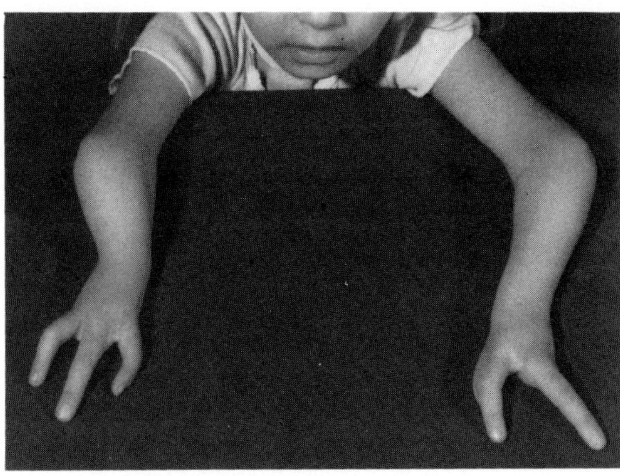

Fig. 4-6. Patient with bilateral ulnar hemimelia. Despite deficiencies in motion and strength, surgical reconstruction of limbs is superior to prosthetic function.

The initial decision in constructive planning is either surgical reconstruction for an intact limb or conversion to an amputation homologue for prosthetic usage. The judgmental criteria on which this decision is based differ significantly between upper and lower limb deficiencies. In each case there are trade-offs for optimization of total function to be made.

In the upper limb, the major prosthetic deficit is lack of sensory feedback, both tactile and proprioceptive. This may serve as a major indication for constructive surgery, despite other deficits in adapted limb prehension, such as reach, prepositioning, strength, and span. In the upper limb, the goal of reconstruction is useful prehensile function, not cosmesis. A key prerequisite for reconstruction is that at least rudimentary grasping action and grasp reflex be present. Quantitative criteria to be assessed are available strength, both prehensile and proximal, limb length that allows useful reach, and proximal joint mobility for needed prepositioning.[1,20,38,43] Bilaterality of the defect may be a relative indication for reconstructive surgery (Fig. 4-6).[30] The surgeon must be assured of the retention of the initial gain through the growth period. Competent clinical judgment requires that a quantitative assessment of these criteria, plus the value of sensory feedback, be compared with the potential function to be expected with prosthetic use.[3,39]

In the lower limb the value of sensory feedback

CONTRIBUTION TO GROWTH OF INDIVIDUAL EPIPHYSES

Distal femur	40%
Proximal tibia	27%
Distal tibia	21%
Proximal humerus	40%
Distal humerus	10%
Proximal ulna	10%
Distal ulna	40%
Proximal radius	13%
Distal radius	37%

takes a lower priority when compared with the necessity for equalization of leg length and stability of the limb for weight-bearing function. Before advising reconstructive surgery for the limb the surgeon must be assured of solving these major problems.

Surgical guidelines for conversion

If prosthetic management is determined to be the best alternative for treatment, it should be noted that approximately 50% of congenital lower limb deficiencies require some type of surgical conversion for optimum prosthetic usage. This may be contrasted with a less than 10% necessity for surgical conversion in upper limb deficiencies. The goal of conversion surgery is to fashion an amputation stump that provides satisfactory function, not only immediately, but throughout the course of proportionate longitudinal bone growth. Following are five general guidelines for planning optimum function for prosthetic use:

1. *Unnecessary procedure should be avoided.* It should be obvious that if prosthetic management is ultimately the best alternative, attempts at reconstructive surgery of the limb for temporary improvement are not indicated. Ineffective surgery is unnecessary surgery, no matter how well intentioned. If good prosthetic function is the ultimate priority, the skin scarring and potential epiphyseal damage that may be incurred in temporary reconstructions should be avoided. Emphasis and priority should be on the eventual integrity and effectiveness of the converted amputation stump.

2. *Epiphyseal growth should be preserved.* Contributions to the increment in limb length from each epiphysis should be kept in mind (see above).

The average increment in length of a lower limb from ages 4 to 16 is 37 cm. Loss of a distal epiphysis, such as that of the femur, with resulting sacrifice of 15 cm of length can be appreciated as a significant future problem.

3. *It is necessary to identify the key joint for prosthetic function.* This can be defined as the most distal stable joint beyond which there is enough tissue to act as a stump. Its requirements, in both the upper and lower limbs, are stability for positioning the prosthesis, sufficient mobility to provide necessary prosthetic excursion, and effective power to control the action of the prosthesis. This key joint concept seems obvious, but is, in fact, a common error in judgment that may result in failure to obtain and maintain optimum function in the growing child.

Fibular transposition at the knee has been advocated for attaining a below-knee amputation level in tibial hemimelia.[11,12] Acceptable use has been attained initially on occasion, but as growth continues, lack of stability, muscle power, and motion in the defective knee joint usually become manifest, and prosthetic function inadequate. Initial acceptance of a knee disarticulation might have resulted in better, more comfortable and durable function, without additional surgical procedures (Fig. 4-7).

4. *Diaphyseal amputation should be avoided when at all possible.* Not only is there a loss of the distal epiphysis, but in the growing child there is progressive loss in the lower limb of end-bearing capacity, firmness, and muscularity of the stump. In the young child, particularly if younger than 8 years old, the phenomenon of overgrowth, a proliferation of bone that results in a sharp, pointed stump, occurs with great frequency (Fig. 4-8). In the absence of firm musculature the skin of the stump is lax, and a hammocking effect induces areas of internal pressure and skin breakdown over the prominent bone end (Fig. 4-9). This necessitates revision with further shortening of the stump. Overgrowth is not epiphyseal in origin but is due to appositional proliferation of growing bone. It is not corrected or prevented by proximal epiphysiodesis, and this procedure should not be performed.

A special note should be made of the congenital band disorder, which is the true congenital amputation. Usually the band occurs in a diaphyseal location. Sometimes, because of intrauterine necrosis, diaphyseal amputation cannot be avoided, but where there is distal viability, even though the part may seem grotesquely deformed or unsalvageable, the problems with diaphyseal amputation should serve as an indication for staged Z-plasty revisions of the congenital band. Even where the distal part cannot be totally salvaged, the distal epiphysis may be saved and an effective amputation stump constructed (Fig. 4-10).

5. *Length should, in general, be preserved.* Skin grafting and scarring that might be unacceptable in the adult amputee may be tolerated and may give good continued function in the child.[40] This is particularly pertinent to the traumatic amputation in childhood. Even if the defective skin does not maintain prosthetic tolerance into adult life, later revisions to an optimum stump may be possible.

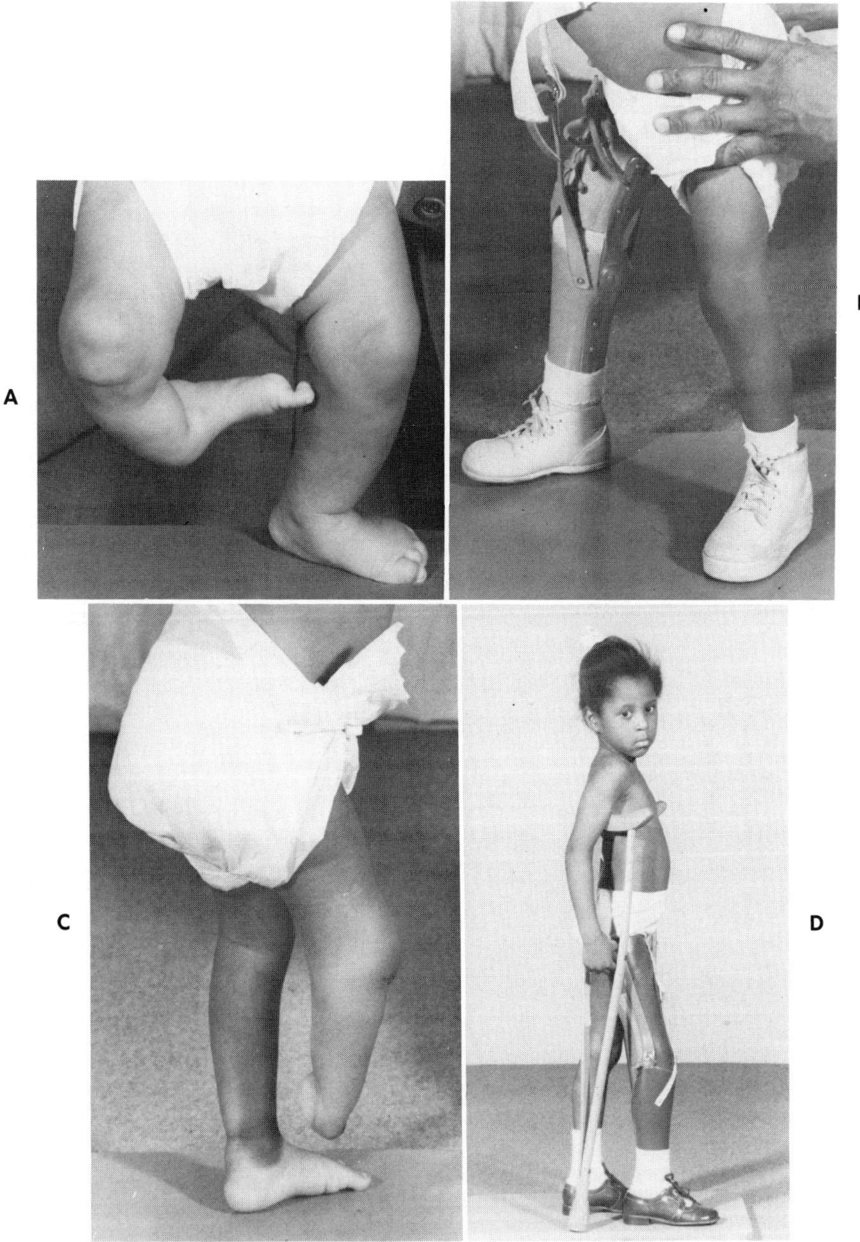

Fig. 4-7. A, Tibial hemimelia. **B,** After Putti-Brown fibular transposition, prosthesis gives early toddler function only. **C,** Reconstructed knee joint lacks stability, muscle power, and motion necessary to key joint for prosthetic use. **D,** Knee disarticulation has provided better prosthetic function.

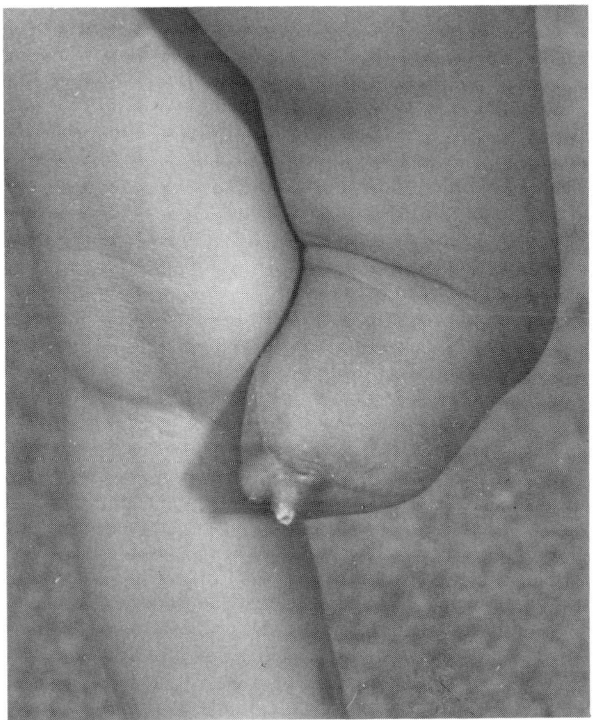

Fig. 4-8. Overgrowth of tibia and fibula in diaphyseal amputation in young child.

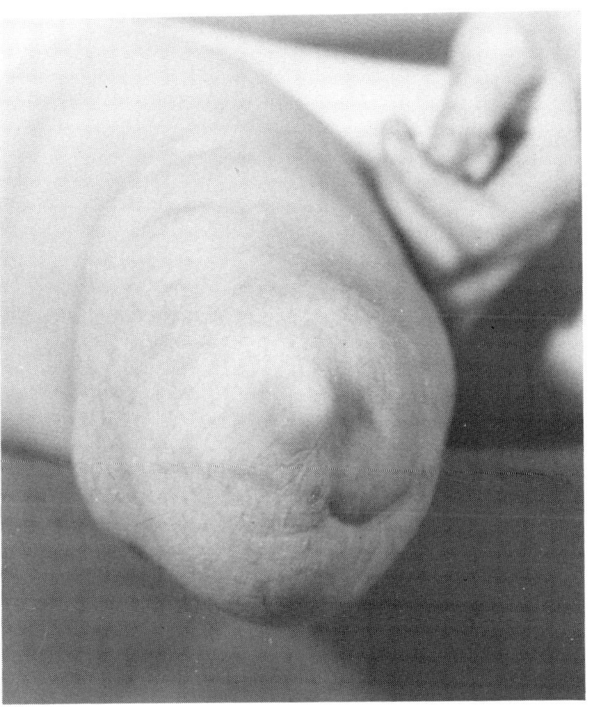

Fig. 4-9. Hammocking of skin and functional prominence of bone end in flabby stump in older child.

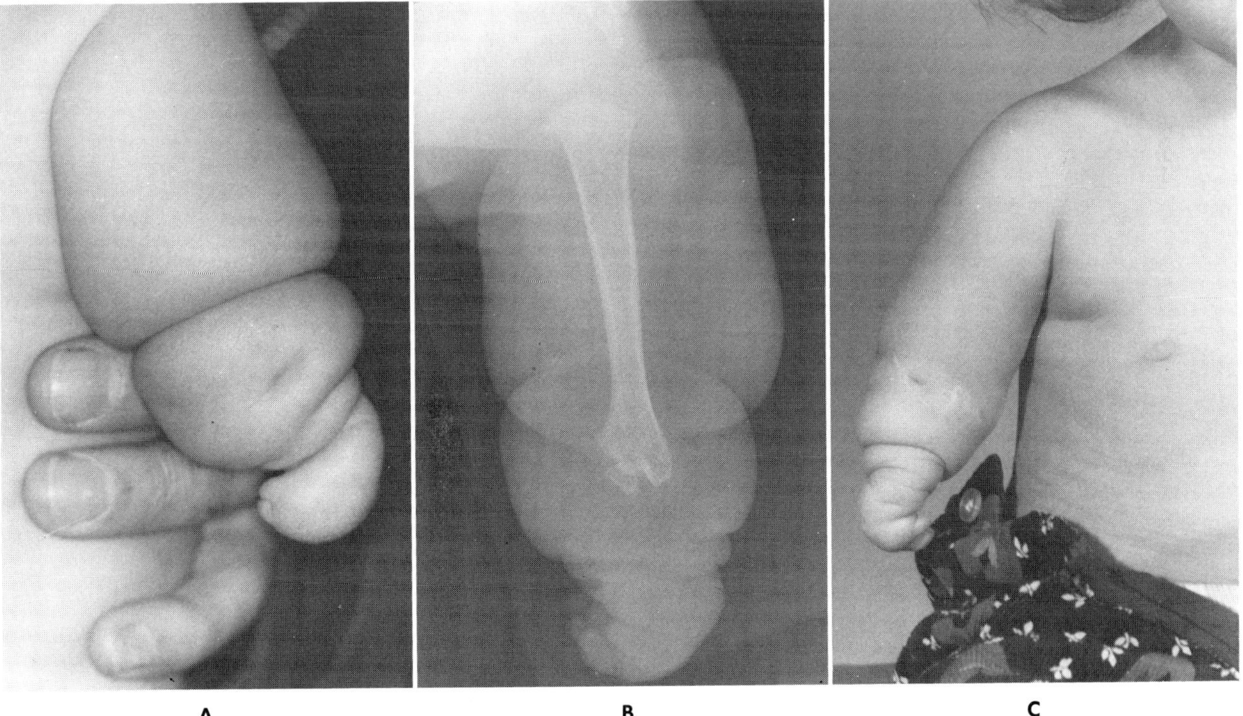

A B C

Fig. 4-10. A, Congenital band with deep cleft about distal humerus. **B,** Distal epiphysis is isolated by circumferential band. **C,** Staged Z-plasties have been completed to ensure nutrition and growth of distal humeral epiphysis and improve prosthetic fitting.

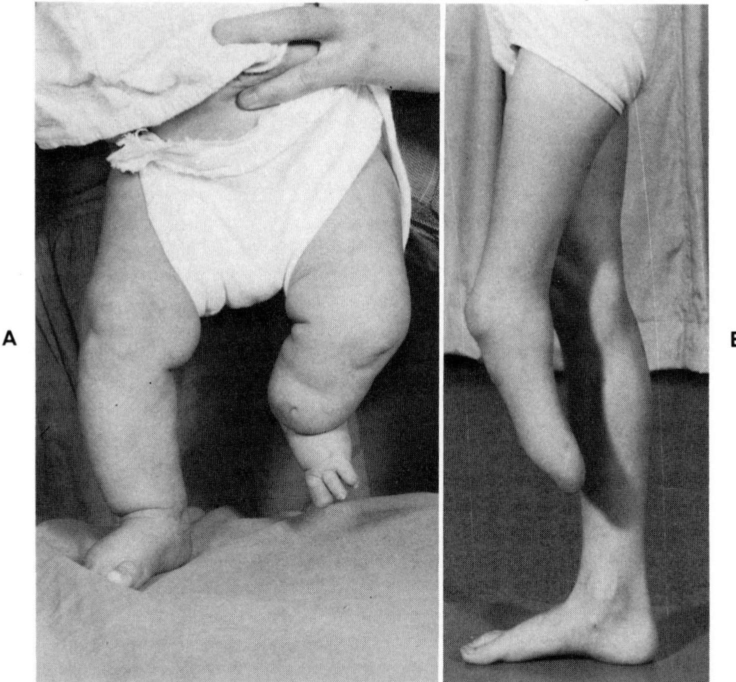

Fig. 4-11. A, Fibular hemimelia (type II) with severe anterior tibial bowing. **B,** With growth, bowing presents prosthetic fitting problems.

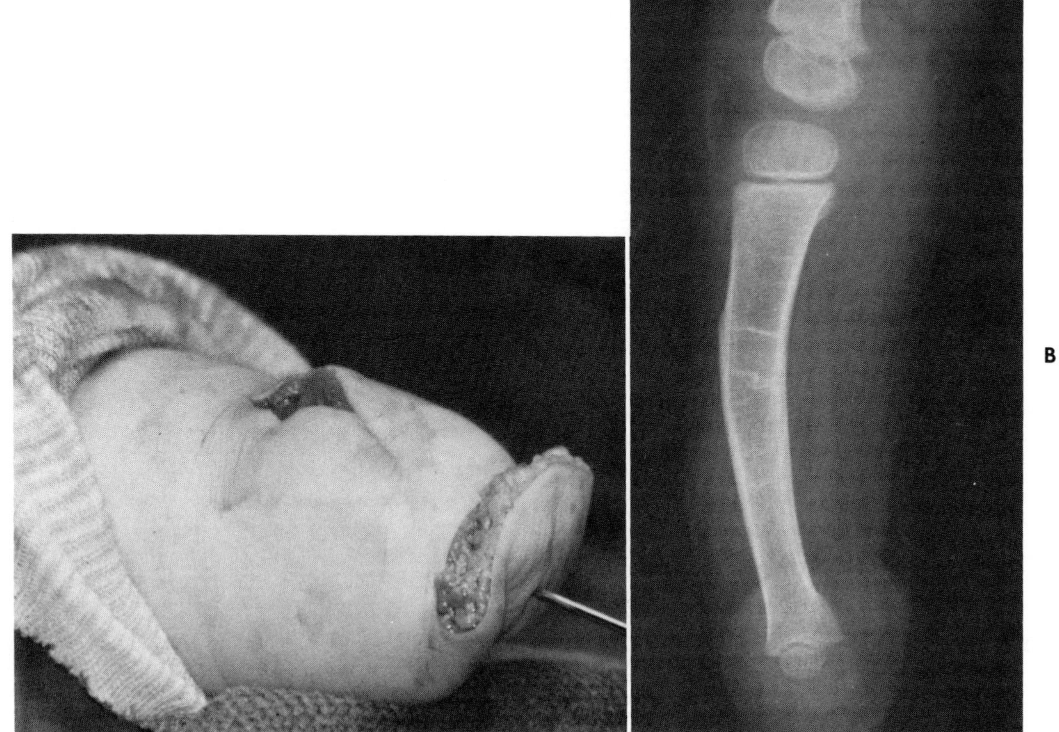

Fig. 4-12. A, Osteotomy at time of initial conversion in another patient. **B,** Straighter stump, with better prosthetic function, has resulted.

Reconstructive procedures for optimum amputee function

Planning for optimum adult function in the limb-deficient child may require more than simple conversion. Procedures to optimize the amputation stump and its prosthetic control may need to be incorporated into the treatment program. If so, the timing of these procedures must be considered in light of the growth and development of the child.

Partial foot absences of the transverse tarsal type require clinical judgment to determine whether they should be accepted or converted to a Syme or Boyd stump for improved adult function. Most small children with partial foot deficiencies, either congenital or acquired, do quite well with simple prosthetic fittings. As weight and force increase, however, gait and prosthetic comfort may deteriorate and provide less than optimum usage for the adult. Certain prerequisites for satisfactory function in the partial foot that can serve as judgmental criteria are as follows:

1. An adequate weight-bearing area for distribution of force should be present in the remaining plantar skin pad.
2. Sensation should be normal.
3. There should be sufficient muscle balance in the hindfoot to provide lateral stability and to prevent progressive deformity with growth.
4. There should be enough tissue anterior to the ankle joint axis to provide a translatable plantar flexion–knee extension couple. If this is absent, pressure and friction transmitted to the skin of the stump and shin may be excessive in the distally unstable fittings provided, for instance, for deficiencies at the Lisfranc or Chopart amputation levels. A shortened stride length and halting gait is observed in the adult patient. These gait defects are not seen with the enclosed, stable end bearing of the Syme stump, and transmission of dorsiflexion moment from the SACH foot to a PTB prosthesis contour of the proximal socket allows comfortable acceptance of pressure in stance.

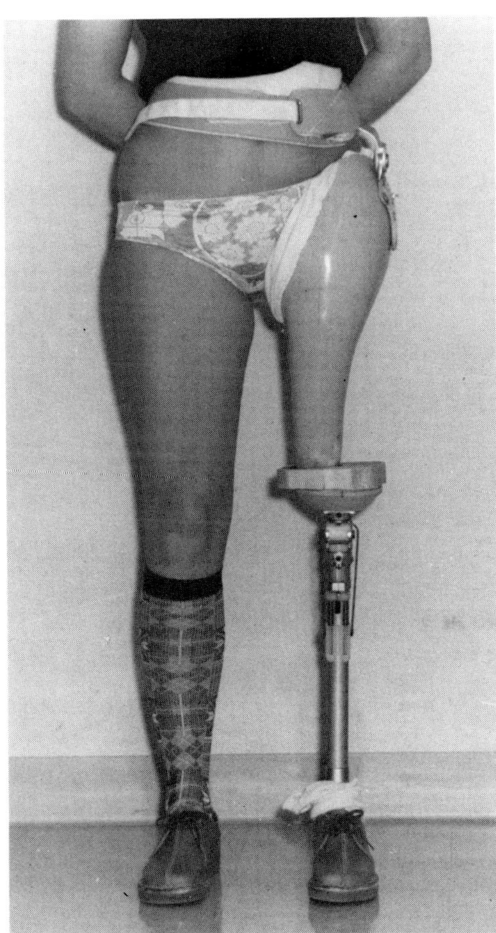

Fig. 4-13. Dynamic alignment of endoskeletal prosthesis for adult with proximal femoral focal deficiency. Above-knee level of fitting, alignment, and accessory components are shown.

Other stump deformities and mechanical malalignments, tolerated in the young child, may give unacceptable functional alignment and prosthetic fitting in the adult. Fibular deficiencies associated with significant anterior and medial bowing of the tibia can be fitted and tolerated in a small child after simple ankle disarticulation has been accomplished. As the child grows, however, the persistent angulation of the stump makes it increasingly difficult to align the prosthesis to provide appropriate gait mechanics. Poor distribution of pressure from prosthesis to skin may result in problems. In certain cases with this deformity, osteotomy at the time of conversion can be expected to maintain a well-aligned amputation stump and ease of prosthetic fitting into adult life (Figs. 4-11 and 4-12).

In certain limb deficiencies the planning of procedures that are not specifically directed toward the amputation stump itself may be needed to optimize adult function. These require careful individual analysis. Unilateral proximal femoral focal deficiency may serve as an example. There seems to be no general agreement on a single treatment program for this condition. Many procedures and approaches have been advocated in attempts to gain optimal function.[42] Experience indicates that the majority of these patients, will, at full growth, walk with an above-knee amputee gait and prosthetic fitting (Fig. 4-13).[4,8,36] If this is

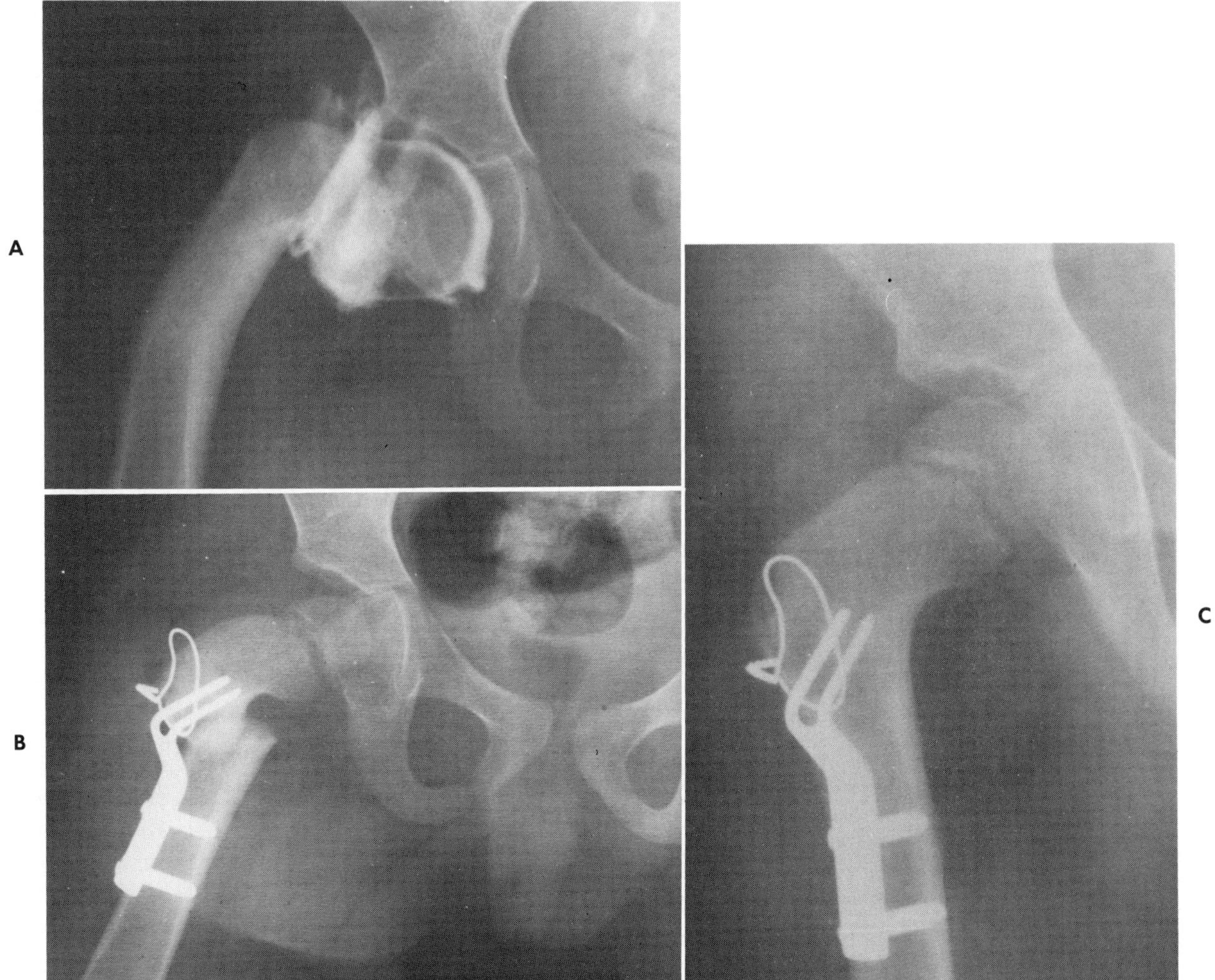

Fig. 4-14. A, Arthrogram showing prerequisites for hip realignment in proximal femoral focal deficiency. **B,** Pauwel Y-type subtrochanteric osteotomy type is combined with transfer of greater trochanteric insertion of gluteal musculature. **C,** Continued development of hip joint follows restoration of muscle function and gluteal moment.

the eventual adult prognosis, it would seem reasonable that planning for optimum function should incorporate the solution, if possible, of those specific biomechanical deficits in the anomaly which interfere with optimal function as an above-knee amputee.

From observation of the older patient with the disorder, a major deficit would seem to be the hip instability and abductor insufficiency present in untreated cases. Selected patients may be candidates for hip reconstruction in an attempt to afford a stable fulcrum for weight bearing at the hip, as well as to provide an appropriate mechanical advantage for the hip abductor muscles. Satisfactory accomplishment of this goal must include not only osteotomy to correct the deformity, but reproduction of normal hip mechanics by transfer of the greater trochanter and abductor muscle insertion. Adequate femoral neck length and abductor moment arm must be achieved. This suggests stringent prerequisites for success. A spherical femoral head must be present in a competent acetabulum. Abductor musculature must be demonstrably functional. Epiphyseal growth damage, either directly through encroachment by a fixation device or by excessive muscle tension spanning the hip, must be avoided. Femoral shortening through the defective subtrochanteric region to avoid excessive muscle tension, as well as to promote good bony healing, is essential. Attempted reconstruction of a hip that will be defective or at risk for subluxation will result in early degenerative change, pain, and stiffness, which are probably more disabling than the original

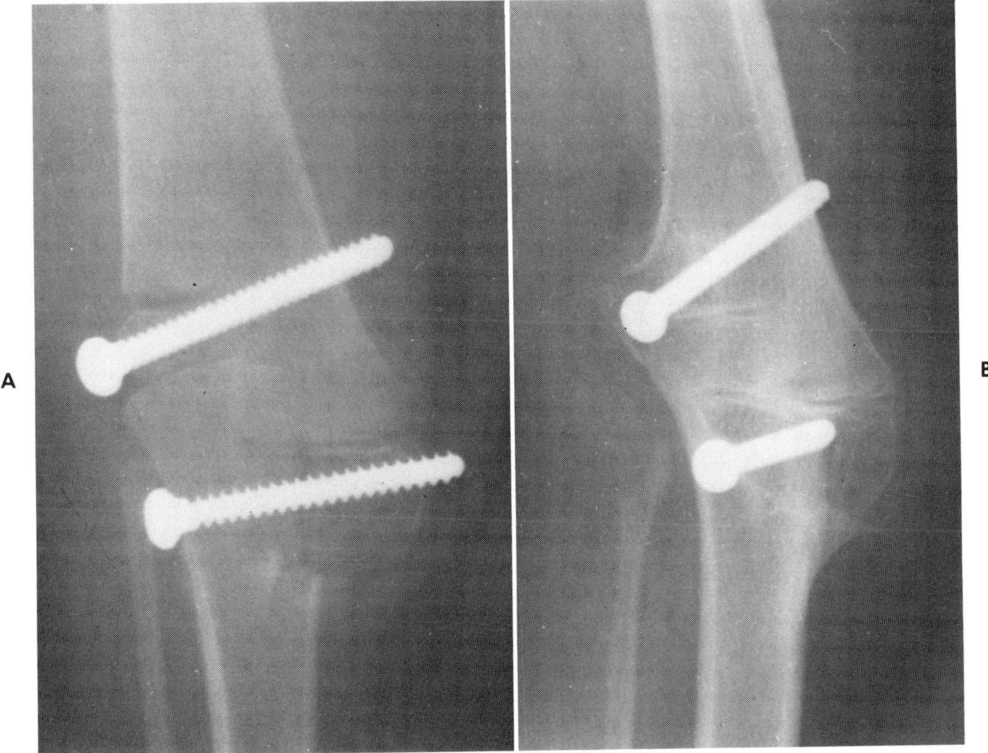

Fig. 4-15. A, "Step-cut" knee arthrodesis designed to combine epiphysiodesis to control stump length in proximal femoral focal deficiency. **B,** Healed arthrodesis has accomplished epiphyseal arrest.

instability. However, cases in the type A group[4] of this anomaly are suitable for hip realignment (Fig. 4-14).

A second biomechanical problem in this condition is that the stump-socket instability which occurs when the level of the knee, situated proximally near the brim of the prosthesis, combines with the malrotation of the leg to hamper active control of prosthetic swing and placement. In those patients who must function as above-knee amputees, a knee arthrodesis can relieve this particular problem. The arthrodesis is more easily performed in the child before hip and knee flexion contractures become severe or fixed.

For above-knee prosthetic usage the stump length and level of the prosthetic knee-hinge is important to an even gait. Careful growth analysis and prediction is important to time control of this length by appropriate epiphysiodesis if needed. This length control can be considered in planning the timing for knee arthrodesis as a combined procedure (Fig. 4-15).

It should be noted that in *bilateral* proximal femoral focal deficiency (PFFD), prosthetic use is not sufficiently good to permit the sacrifice of adapted use, out of prostheses, of the anomalous limbs. It is unwise in the bilateral PFFD to ablate weight-bearing feet. Prosthetic fitting around the anomalies, without conversion, is the best alternative for overall function in most, if not all, bilateral cases.

Summary

In planning for optimum function for the limb-deficient child a treatment program should be established with its ultimate goal the function of the fully grown adult. It is necessary for the surgeon to identify those problems which may interfere with this optimal adult function. Analysis of growth and the implications of the law of magnitude should be appreciated so that the surgeon is not deceived by temporary acceptable function in the small child. Congenital limb deficiencies, in particular, require the combined effort of surgeon and prosthetist to attain optimum adult function. Planning is necessary, and compromise with future function accepted only with reluctance. The family should be a party to the treatment planning so that full cooperation and support with each step is obtained. Valid alternatives should be considered so that an optimum plan can be selected. The development of the whole child, including physical growth and muscular coordination, as well as social and educational obligations, must be fully considered in this treatment program.

THE DYSVASCULAR AMPUTEE

Although some of the techniques and, particularly, the priorities may differ in the dysvascular or geriatric amputee from the younger patients previously discussed, the goal of treatment remains the same. The essential objective is rehabilitation of the patient to the maximum function possible, rather than simply the ablation of an impaired limb and attainment of primary wound healing. Planning for this goal is required in all three phases of treatment of the dysvascular limb: preoperative, operative, and postoperative.

Preoperative considerations

Since the majority of geriatric patients who require amputations will have vascular disease, it is important that the vascular or general surgeons who care for these patients be aware of conditions that may interfere with patient function in the postamputation period. Many of these patients will have had explorations of their arterial system. Some may have had arterial grafts, either synthetic or autogenous, placed to improve circulatory status. It is important to emphasize satisfactory locations for exploratory incisions in the lower limb. If the incision in the femoral area must cross the inguinal crease, the incision should parallel the inguinal ligament, rather than cross it at a perpendicular angle (Fig. 4-16).

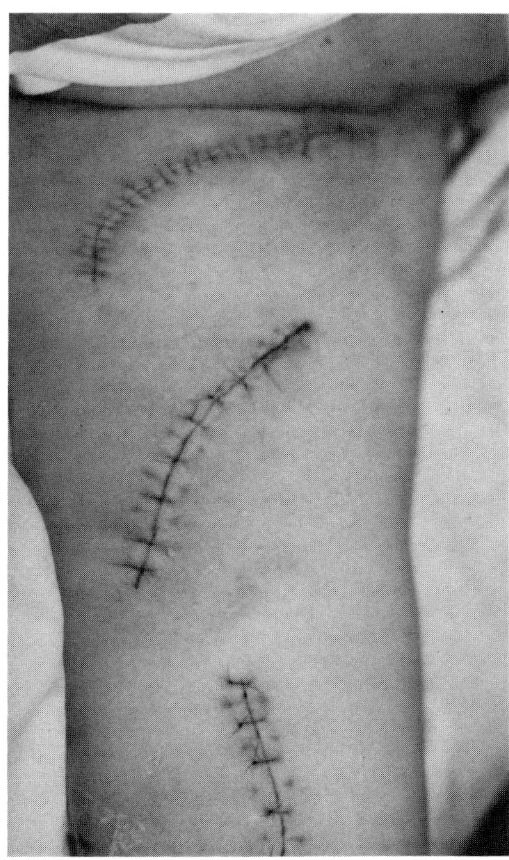

Fig. 4-16. Incisions for vascular explorations, which will not interfere with subsequent amputation surgery or prosthetic usage.

If the patient should subsequently require an above-knee amputation, the quadrilateral socket generally used is carried high onto the anterior aspect of Scarpa's triangle. If an incision crosses the inguinal crease in this area, excessive scar buildup may be a problem, producing skin irritation when the patient attempts to wear the prosthesis (Fig. 4-17). Vascular surgeons may adequately explore the femoral area by transverse incisions or by incisions parallel to the inguinal crease, thus making the fitting of an above-knee prosthesis easier and more comfortable for the patient.

The popliteal and tibial arteries can be adequately explored through a medial skin incision. If a below-knee amputation is subsequently required, this scar placement will allow the formation of a long posterior skin flap (Fig. 4-18).

The patient who suffers from ischemic limb pain often finds that the flexed position of both the hip and knee is more comfortable. If this hip and knee flexion is allowed to persist, however, fixed contracture of the knee and hip may result (Fig. 4-19). Although flexion contractures of the knee joint of less than 20 degrees can be tolerated in a modern below-knee prosthesis, all too often these knee contractures are in the range of 40 to 60 degrees, making the fitting of a below-knee prosthesis almost an impossibility. In the hip joint, flexion contractures of 20 to 25 degrees in a short stump can be accommodated by increasing the preflexion of the above-knee prosthetic socket, but beyond this point, contracture contributes to significant lumbar lordosis and prevents satisfactory gait. It should be emphasized that a daily effort be made to extend both knee and hip joints fully to prevent fixed contracture.

The geriatric amputee often requires a walker or crutches for ambulation. This requires strong upper limbs. If muscular disuse and deterioration has been allowed to occur in the preamputation phase, rehabilitation to an ambulatory status may be prevented or, at best, greatly prolonged. It

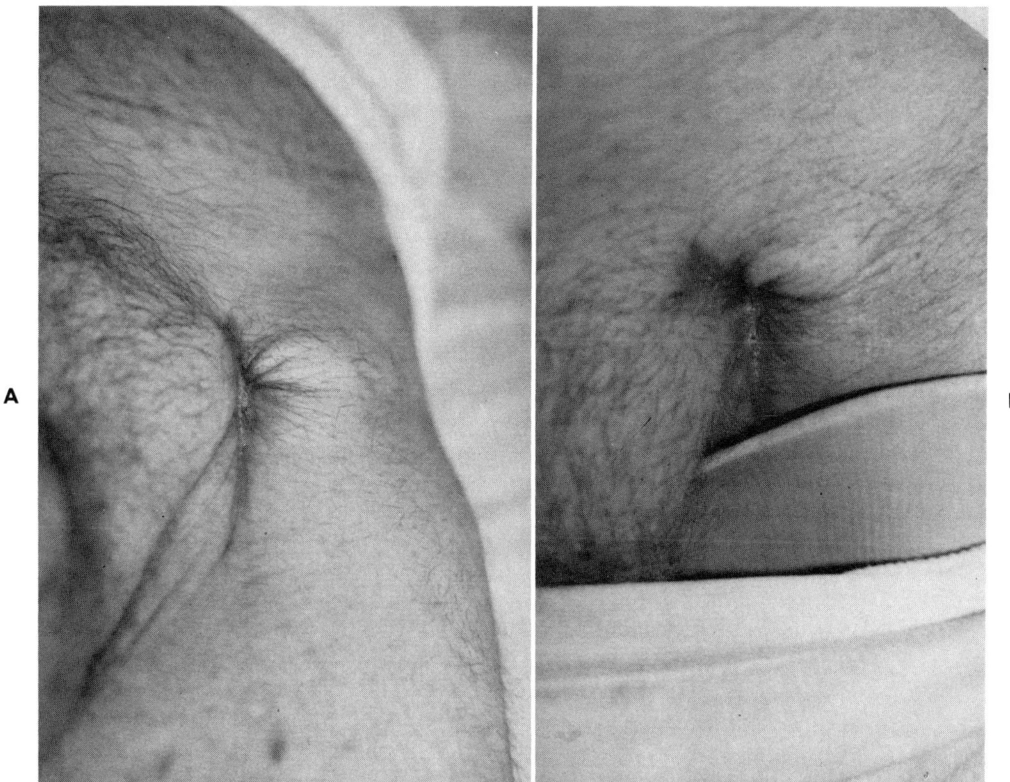

Fig. 4-17. A, Longitudinal scar across inguinal area. **B,** Relationship of socket brim to longitudinal scar.

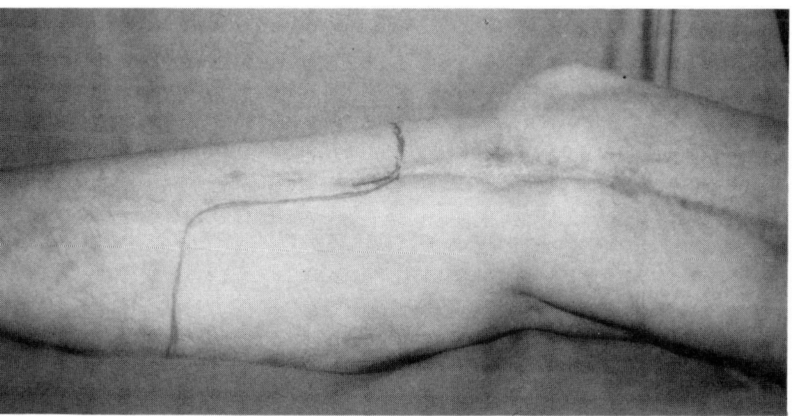

Fig. 4-18. Medial scar allowing satisfactory long posterior skin flap formation for below-knee amputation.

should be emphasized to surgeons treating the patient in the preamputation phase that efforts be made to strengthen or maintain strength in both upper and lower limbs.

The surgeon should be alert to the condition of the opposite leg. Although it may be involved to a lesser degree with vascular insufficiency, the circulation may often be deficient. Ulceration or pressure sores on the opposite "normal" foot can produce major problems for rehabilitation. Healing may be quite slow, especially if ulceration is full thickness. Spenco boots or other soft structures should be used to prevent localized pressure on the vulnerable areas such as the heel, malleoli, or lateral side of the remaining foot.

When it becomes obvious to the vascular or

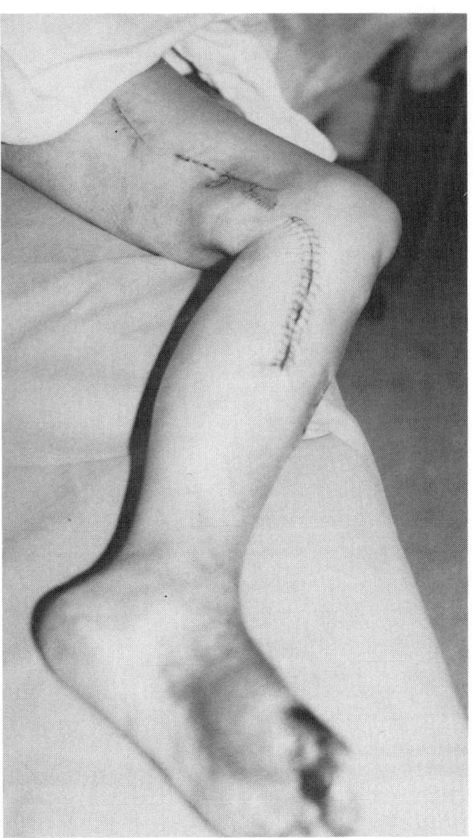

Fig. 4-19. Fixed 80-degree flexion contracture of knee after vascular impairment and ischemic limb pain.

general surgeon that arterial salvage efforts have failed and amputation becomes a necessity, he must be aware that an adequate blood flow at the level of amputation is necessary for proper healing. It is important not only to evaluate circulatory blood flow, but also to correct any cell or volume deficiencies by transfusion. Other blood chemistry abnormalities, for example, low potassium levels, need correction before surgery is performed.[35]

All too often the patient, when informed that the efforts at restoring circulation have been inadequate, gains an impression from the surgeon that a surgical defeat has been encountered and that amputation is an admission of such defeat. This impression should be countered by a constructive attitude, with the careful explanation that in the patient's present condition the gangrenous or painful foot is disabling. Comfortable ambulation is not possible, and essentially, in the present situation the patient is crippled. A properly performed amputation will provide a limb capable of transmitting weight to a prosthesis that allows ambulation. Amputation surgery is but the first step in rehabilitation. It is important to emphasize that removal of the offending dysvascular foot or leg will remove pain, and, with the proper prosthesis, allow ambulation. An optimistic attitude should be engendered in the patient by the surgeon. It is appropriate that the surgeon also undertake the direction of the postoperative care, prosthetic prescription, and subsequent follow-up rehabilitation effort.

The social worker is valuable in reassuring not only the patient, but the family as well, and in reinforcing the attitude of the amputation surgeon. They can, as a team, thus embark on a rehabilitation program that may lead to effective ambulation.

This enthusiasm, of course, is based on the presumption that this is a unilateral amputee, and that every effort will be made to preserve a below-knee level to provide efficient and effective community ambulation. If both legs are removed above the knee in the dysvascular or geriatric patient, rehabilitation is usually limited and will consist, in all probability, of training in transfer techniques for effective wheelchair use.

Operative treatment

Dysvascular or geriatric patients have their general function compromised by limited energy reserve, coordination, and balance. This makes the length of the stump segment that can be preserved most significant. The lowest effective level of primary healing is most important in the rehabilitation of these patients.

Since 1965 the ratio of above-knee to below-knee levels of amputation in the lower limb for vascular disease has been reversed. Prior to 1965, approximately 80% of amputations of the lower limb for vascular disease were above the knee. Since 1965, with increased emphasis on proper rehabilitation and more careful evaluation of the blood-flow status, it is found that approximately 80% of dysvascular limbs are amputated below the knee.[14] Rehabilitation efforts have been more successful since preservation of the knee joint with its proprioceptive feedback, and active balance adjustment is a distinct advantage in using a prosthesis.[33] Recent reports indicate that some selected dysvascular limbs may be suitable for conversion to the Syme amputation.[41]

Many efforts have been made to obtain an accurate method for determining the viability level of a dysvascular lower extremity. In the past such methods as arteriography, the appearance of histamine wheals, the use of xenon 133, and many

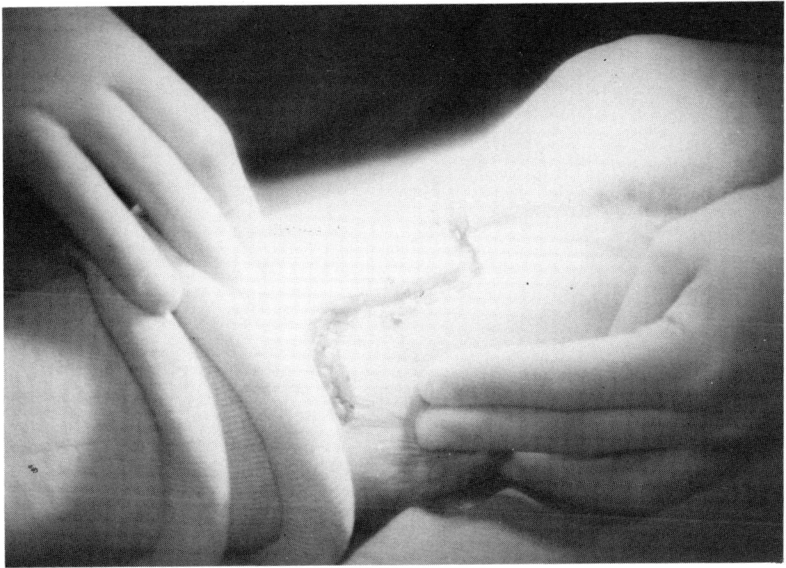

Fig. 4-20. Long posterior skin flap for below-knee amputation secondary to vascular disease.

other techniques have been used in an attempt to evaluate the status of the circulation in order to predict a viable amputation level.[44,45] The recent development of the transcutaneous Doppler ultrasound technique has provided a promising noninvasive method that seems to determine circulatory capacity more accurately.[10] It has been the experience of those working with this technique that a blood flow pressure of 70 mm Hg at the proposed level of amputation will nearly always assure its healing. Wagner[41] at Rancho Los Amigos Hospital reports that of those patients with 70 mm of pressure at the midfoot and heel level, approximately 80% can support a functioning Syme amputation.

Despite the increased sophistication of preoperative testing, however, it is not absolute. Clinical judgment and observation of the tissues at the time of surgery is equally important. In a situation where the circulation is marginal, it is probably wiser to make the attempt to preserve a more functional level of amputation than to commit the patient to an irrevocable higher amputation.

Below-knee incisions in the dysvascular amputee generally require a long posterior flap, since the vascular supply to the posterior skin is superior to that of the anterior skin area. A longer posterior skin flap will survive much better than will anterior and posterior skin flaps of equal length (Fig. 4-20).

All tissues must be handled with extreme gentleness. Any tension in closure of skin or muscle flaps must be avoided. The simplest surgical technique for handling skin, muscle, and fascia is employed. The suggestion has been made in the past that myodesis be performed. Experience has shown, however, that attempts to surgically anchor already compromised muscles to the periphery of the bone lead only to further dysvascularity of the tissue. Sloughing and failure of the amputation stump to heal may ensue. Simple myofascial closure is recommended, suturing the deep fascia from front to back. The skin is approximated without tension.[33]

Postoperative management

Edema is a frequent postoperative complication of the amputation stump. Particularly in the below-knee level it has been found advantageous to apply a rigid plaster dressing after amputation (Fig. 4-21).[9] Rigid plaster dressings provide a number of advantages: (1) prevention of flexion contracture of the knee, (2) reduction of stump edema that can delay wound healing, (3) minimal number of dressing changes, and (4) rest for the stump so that skin healing can proceed without interruption.

The dysvascular amputee generally does not tolerate immediate ambulation with a pylon prosthesis within the first 48 hours. Ambulation starting at about 2 weeks postoperatively, however, has a place in the postamputation phase of the geriatric amputee. The amputation stump is examined approximately 7 to 10 days after the amputation has been performed. If the tissues are viable, and the wound is healing satisfactorily, a

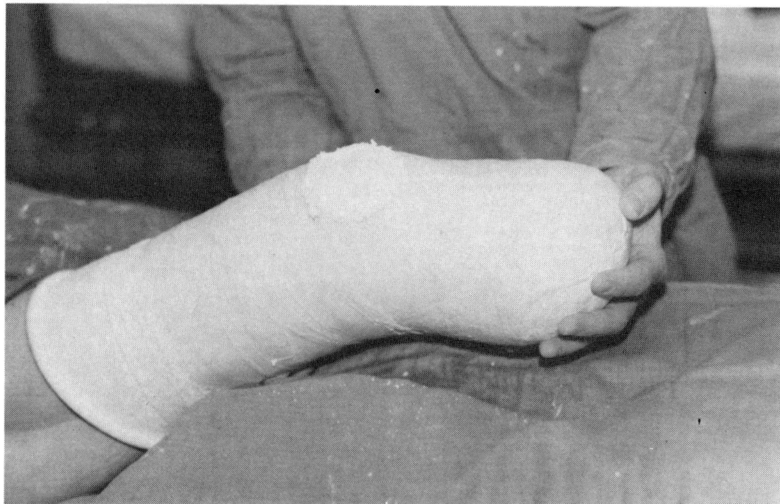

Fig. 4-21. Rigid plaster dressing for below-knee amputation applied over stockinette and cotton sheet wadding.

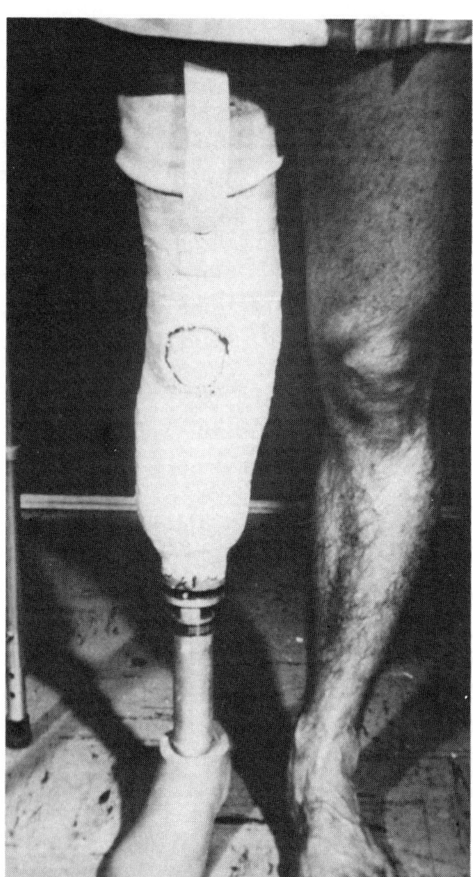

Fig. 4-22. Temporary prosthesis for early postoperative ambulation.

new stump cast with an attached pylon and SACH foot may be applied (Fig. 4-22). The patient may then ambulate with crutches or a walker, taking only as much weight on the pylon as can be comfortably tolerated. Since ambulation maintains muscle tone, stimulates the appetite, and generally improves wound healing, it will help to minimize morbidity.

Although it has been found that with early ambulation, satisfactory stump shrinkage may take place early in the rehabilitation phase, further shrinkage is likely to continue for 3 to 6 months after the amputation. In some instances it might be advantageous to continue with the temporary prosthesis for 3 to 4 months. Most patients, however, treated with a rigid stump dressing will be ready for a definitive prosthesis in approximately 6 to 8 weeks.

If the surgeon does not have sufficient knowledge to prescribe a suitable prosthesis for the lower limb amputee, the patient should be referred to an amputee clinic for further care about 2 to 3 weeks after surgery. It should be emphasized that uninterrupted progress of rehabilitation is important. The earlier active rehabilitation is started, the less disability will result. It is important, therefore, to continue with rehabilitation either through the management of the amputating surgeon or through the facilities of an amputee clinic.

Since many of these amputees have weakened musculature and will show insecurity and lack aggressiveness, it is important to provide them with a prosthesis that provides adequate safety factors. Most above-knee geriatric amputees will not tolerate full suction for suspension and will require a pelvic belt. These belts must be comfortable and well fitted to provide adequate suspension. Many of these patients will have weak hip extensor musculature or may have a flexion contracture at the hip. They will need the knee security afforded by a friction-type safety knee. Some may even require a manually operated positive lock at the knee during the early ambulation phase, so that they have security against knee "buckling." The use of a pickup walker may be preferred to that of crutches, since it provides more stability. This device may also be used in the older patient with the below-knee level if unsteady. Most below-knee amputees, however, can be trained to walk with the use of a cane.

To provide a continued maximum rehabilitation effort, it is important to proceed with ambulation slowly, with careful observation of the residual limb so that skin breakdown may be anticipated and prevented. It is important, particularly in diabetics, who may have anesthetic areas, to carefully observe the skin after each wearing of the prosthesis, to avoid skin ulceration that may take many weeks to heal. Other medical problems in the geriatric patient should be recognized. Loss of hearing may make understanding of directions very poor. Diminished vision may lead to a feeling of insecurity and instability. Poor body balance may lead to stumbling or falling. Deficiency of circulation in the opposite leg may limit walking endurance. If these problems are carefully monitored during the training phase, most can be surmounted, and the patient trained to walk.

Amputees require long-term care. They cannot simply be fitted with a prosthesis, trained, and then discharged. The amputee does require meticulous follow-up care to make sure that socket fit remains satisfactory, to ensure that ambulation is consistent with potential, and that optimum rehabilitation is being maintained. It is important to follow-up on geriatric amputees once the training period has been completed with visits at least every 3 months.

CONCLUSION

If amputation surgery is thought of as constructive surgery, with rehabilitation of the patient to maximum potential as the goal, the necessity of planning the operative approach to achieve this goal can present a major, but rewarding, challenge to the surgeon interested in the welfare of the amputee.

No matter what the type or cause of the amputation, technical skill in the operative procedure, alone, is insufficient; a thorough knowledge of amputee function and careful analytical thought and preparation are required as well.

REFERENCES

1. Ahstrom, J. P.: Pollicization in congenital absence of the thumb. In Ahstrom, J. P., editor: Current practice in orthopaedic surgery, vol. 5, St. Louis, 1973, The C. V. Mosby Co.
2. Aitken, G. T.: Amputation as a treatment for certain lower extremity congenital abnormalities, J. Bone Joint Surg. **41A:**1267-1285, 1959.
3. Aitken, G. T.. Management of severe bilateral upper limb deficiencies, Clin. Orthop. **37:**53-60, 1964.
4. Aitken, G. T.: PFFD, definition, classification and management. In Proximal femoral focal deficiency: a congenital anomaly, Washington, D.C., 1969, National Academy of Sciences.
5. Aitken, G. T.: Surgical amputation in children. In AAOS instructional course lectures, vol. 18, St. Louis, 1973, The C. V. Mosby Co.
6. Aitken, G. T., and Frantz, C. H.: Management of the child amputee. In AAOS instructional course lectures, vol. 17, St. Louis, 1960, The C. V. Mosby Co.
7. Alldredge, R. H., and Thompson, T. C.: The technique of the Syme amputation, J. Bone Joint Surg. **28:**415-426, July, 1946.
8. Amstutz, H. C.: Morphology, natural history, and treatment of PFFD. In Proximal femoral focal deficiency: a congenital anomaly, Washington, D.C., 1969, National Academy of Sciences.
9. Baker, W. H., Barnes, R. W., and Schurr, D. G.: Healing of below-knee amputations: comparisons of soft and plaster dressings, Am. J. Surg. **133:**716-718, 1977.
10. Barnes, R. W., Shanik, G. D., and Slaymaker, E. E.: Index of healing in below-knee amputation: leg blood pressure by Doppler ultrasound, Surgery **79:**13-20, 1976.
11. Brown, F. W.: Construction of a knee joint in congenital total absence of the tibia, J. Bone Joint Surg. **47-A:**695-704, 1965.
12. Brown, F. W.: The Brown operation for total hemimelia tibia, In Aitken, G. T., editor: Selected lower limb anomalies, Washington D.C., 1971, National Academy of Sciences.
13. Brown, P. W., and Kinman, P. B.: Gas gangrene in a metropolitan community, J. Bone Joint Surg. **56-A**(7):1445-1451, Oct., 1974.
14. Burgess, E. M., Romano, R. L., and Zettl, J. H.: The management of lower extremity amputations, Washington, D.C., TR10-6, Aug., 1969, Veterans Administration.
15. Capener, N.: Editorials and annotations. Amputation surgery and prostheses, J. Bone Joint Surg. **45-B:**3-5, Feb., 1963.
16. Cary, J. M.: Traumatic amputation in childhood – the primary management. Inter-Clin. Info. Bull. **XIV**(6):1-10, 1975.
17. Cary, J. M.: Fibular hemimelia with tibial angulation – the identification of a problem, Inter-Clin. Info. Bull. **16**(7-8):1-6, 1977.

18. Cleveland, M., Manning, J. G., and Stewart, W. J.: Care of battle casualties and injuries involving bones and joints. Part V, Amputations, J. Bone Joint Surg. **33-A:**520-521, April, 1951.
19. Dederich, R.: Plastic treatment of the muscles and bone in amputation surgery, J. Bone Joint Surg. **45-B:**60-66, 1963.
20. Entin, M. A.: Reconstruction of congenital abnormalities of the upper extremities, J. Bone Joint Surg. **41-A:**681-701, 1959.
21. Ertl, J.: Über amputationsstümpfe, Chirurg **20:**218-224, May, 1949.
22. Frantz, C. H., and O'Rahilly, R.: Congenital skeletal limb deficiencies, J. Bone Joint Surg. **43-A:**1202-1224, 1961.
23. Gallie, W. E.: The experience of the Canadian Army and Pensions Board with amputations of the lower extremity, Ann. Surg. **113:**925-931, 1941.
24. Haldane, J. B. S.: On being the right size. Reprinted in Newman, J. R.: The world of mathematics, New York, 1956, Simon & Schuster, Inc.
25. Hampton, O. P., Jr.: Wounds of the extremities in military surgery, St. Louis, 1951, The C. V. Mosby Co.
26. Harris, R. I.: Amputations, J. Bone Joint Surg. **26:**626-634, Oct., 1944.
27. Jahnke, E. J., Jr., and Howard, J. M.: Primary repair of major arterial injuries: report of 58 battle casualties, Arch. Surg. **66:**646-649, May, 1953.
28. Kay, H. W.: A proposed international terminology for the classification of congenital limb deficiencies, Inter-Clin. Info. Bull. **13**(7):1-16, April, 1974.
29. Kirk, N. T.: War Department Circular Letter No. 91. Office of the Surgeon General, Washington, D.C., April 26, 1943, U.S. Government Printing Office.
30. Kritter, A. E.: The bilateral upper extremity amputee, Orthop. Clin. North Am. **3:**419-433, 1972.
31. Kruger, L. M.: Fibular hemimelia. In Aitken, G. T., editor: Selected lower limb anomalies, Washington, D.C., 1971, National Academy of Sciences.
32. Mercer, Sir Walter: Reflections on amputation stumps, J. Bone Joint Surg. **45-B:**218-219, Feb., 1963.
33. Moore, W. S., Hall, A. D., and Wylie, E. J.: Below-knee amputation for vascular insufficiency, Arch. Surg. **97:**886-893, Dec., 1968.
34. Nichols, P. J. R., Rogers, E. E., Clark, M. S., and Stamp, W. G.: The acceptance and rejection of prostheses by children with multiple congenital limb deformities, Artif. Limbs **12:**1-13, 1968.
35. Otteman, M. G., and Stahlgren, L. H.: Evaluation of factors which influence mortality and morbidity following major lower extremity amputations for arteriosclerosis. Surg. Gynecol. Obstet. **120:**1217-1220, June, 1965.
36. Panting, A. L., and Williams, P. F.: Proximal femoral focal deficiency, J. Bone Joint Surg. **60-B:**46-52, 1978.
37. Radcliffe, C. W.: Functional considerations in the fitting of above-knee prostheses. Selected articles from Artificial Limbs, Huntington, N.Y., 1970, R. E. Krieger Publishing Co., Inc.
38. Riordan, D. C.: Congenital absence of the radius, J. Bone Joint Surg. **37-A:**1129-1139, 1953.
39. Schmid, H.: Foot skills in children with severe upper limb deficiencies, Am. J. Occ. Therap. **25:**159-163, 1971.
40. Thompson, T. C., and Alldredge, R. H.: Amputations: surgery and plastic repair, J. Bone Joint Surg. **26:**639-644, Oct., 1944.
41. Wagner, F. W.: Orthopaedic rehabilitation of the dysvascular lower limb, Orthop. Clin. North Am. **9**(2):325-349, April, 1978.
42. Westin, C. H., and Gunderson, F. O.: PFFD-a review of treatment experiences. In Proximal femoral focal deficiency—a congenital anomaly, Washington, D.C., 1969, National Academy of Sciences.
43. White, W. F.: Fundamental priorities in pollicization, J. Bone Joint Surg. **52-B:**438-443, 1970.
44. Yao, S. T.: Hemodynamic studies in peripheral arterial disease, Br. J. Surg. **57:**761-766, 1970.
45. Yao, S. T., Hobbs, J. T., and Irvine, W. T.: Ankle systolic pressure measurements in arterial disease affecting the lower extremities, Br. J. Surg. **56:**676-679, 1969.

CHAPTER 5

Prosthetic methods and materials

MICHAEL J. QUIGLEY

In the past 30 years, the field of prosthetics has advanced from a time when all techniques were learned by the apprenticeship method to the present, when most new prosthetists are graduates of university programs. The materials and methods used in 1950 were not unlike those used hundreds of years earlier, with the exception of one or two materials developed in the aircraft industry. Since that time, well-coordinated research programs, coupled with the initiation of educational programs, formed a synergy that resulted in orthotics and prosthetics being recognized as a profession in the 1970s.

The materials and methods used by the prosthetists today are different from those used 30 years ago. In many cases leather has been replaced by polyester resin and thermoplastics, wood has been replaced by polyurethane foams, and steel has been replaced by high-strength aluminum alloys. The new materials and techniques must still conform to the same design criteria as wood, leather, and steel did years ago. Materials used in prosthetics have always needed to be strong, lightweight, biocompatible, and malleable.

The majority of prosthetists are independent small businessmen, with a relatively small amount of capital to invest in fabrication equipment. Although some prefabricated components are available, the shaping and structural strength of each prosthesis is usually custom designed by the prosthetist. New developments in materials and equipment have generally been aimed at the high-volume, mass-production market; therefore water-cooled plastics extruders, blow molders, and carbon fiber structures are often impractical to use because they do not fill the practitioner's need for a custom-designed socket or structure. Similarly, new methods of assessing the efficiency of prostheses, such as force plates, oxygen-consumption measurements, electronic goniometers, and velocity and stance-phase gait analyzers, are impractical to use on a daily basis by the private prosthetist and are also too expensive to use in most hospitals and other institutions. Hopefully, in the near future, small, inexpensive devices will become available that can accurately assess the efficiency of a patient using the prosthesis.

The prosthetist's practice is changing rapidly from the "limb shop" atmosphere to the "private paramedical office" atmosphere for a number of reasons; one is the renewed interest in using central fabrication services. "Central fabrication" means that the patient evaluation, casting, fitting, and delivery of a prosthesis are done in the prosthetist's office and the actual making of a prosthesis is done at a second location, much like the method used for dental prostheses. This separation of the fabrication area from the patient treatment area has the following advantages: (1) the prosthetist's practice can be located in a professional building or other desirable location, which is difficult to do when the fabrication is done in the same facility, since noise, dust, odors, and zoning laws have prevented the prosthetist from acquiring such locations in the past, (2) it is easier to begin new practices because there is no need to hire and manage technicians to fabricate the prostheses, (3) the practitioner's time is used more efficiently because the burden of managing technicians or doing actual fabrication is removed, (4) the time saved by eliminating fabrication work can be used by spending more time with existing patients and by serving more patients, and (5) central fabrication facilities can afford to purchase more sophisticated fabricating machines and learn more techniques so that private practitioners can use newer materials and techniques without having to go through the expense of acquiring new equipment.

Disadvantages of central fabrication include communication problems between the prosthetist and central fabrication laboratory, delays due to shipping time, and difficulty getting special nonstandard devices fabricated. Quality control is more difficult to achieve when central fabrication is used, and often a long learning process is required before the fabrication laboratory can provide prostheses that meet the prosthetist's standards. Central fabrication costs are usually from 25% to 33% of the total cost of prosthetics services. The disadvantages with central fabrication (communication, quality control, nonstandard designs, and costs) are a major reason why the majority of prosthetists in the United States hire their own technicians for fabrication.

Patients are generally seen by the prosthetist a minimum of six times before the fitting is considered to be completed. Although these six visits are discussed in other chapters, it is important to briefly describe each of them here in order to appreciate the different methods that are employed by the prosthetist.

Visit one. The patient is evaluated by a physician or by a clinic team, which mainly consists of a physician, prosthetist, and therapist and often includes a nurse, social worker, and clinic coordinator. At this visit the prescription for the prosthesis is written after input is received from all members of the team. The prosthetist will frequently meet a patient for the first time during the clinic although in many cases the prosthetist may refer the patient to the clinic to receive a prescription.

Visit two. The patient meets with the prosthetist in the prosthetist's office for general orientation, evaluation, and casting.

Visit three. During this visit the patient returns to the prosthetist's office for a test socket fitting. The test socket is evaluated, and all changes are noted for the definitive socket design.

Visit four. The patient is fitted with the prosthesis in an alignment stage. All components of the prosthesis are now in place, the proper length is determined, alignment changes made, and suspension and socket comfort are optimized. Frequently, more than one visit is required to determine the proper alignment.

Visit five. The patient is fitted with the prosthesis, which has now been cosmetically and structurally completed. The patient is given general instruction on how to maintain the prosthesis, and any minor adjustments are made if necessary.

At this point the patient returns to physical therapy, where physical and functional training with the prosthesis are initiated. New patients will have received physical therapy previously to improve their strength, balance, and endurance in preparation for the prosthesis.

Visit six. The patient returns to the physician or the clinic team wearing the prosthesis, and the prosthetist explains the alignment and design of the prosthesis to the team. At this point the physician records the fact that the prescription has been followed and the patient is functioning in the prosthesis. Therapy may be provided before or after this visit.

ORIENTATION

After the initial visit to the clinic, the patient visits the prosthetist's office for orientation, evaluation, measurement, and casting. The first method of patient management employed by the prosthetist is called patient orientation. The prosthetist will meet with the patient privately in his office and explain the design of the prosthesis, what the patient can and cannot expect to do, the amount of time it will take before the patient receives the prosthesis and before the patient should be proficient in the use of the prosthesis, and the different stages (casting, test socket fitting, alignment, etc.) the patient must go through before receiving a prosthesis, as well as discuss other factors with the patient. Frequently, the orientation session will bring out information that was not available to the clinic team when the prescription was prepared. When this occurs the prosthetist contacts the physician to discuss a change in the prescription. Proper orientation relieves the patient of many anxieties and answers a great number of questions that both the prosthetist and patient may have had. The patient's expectations regarding the prosthesis are also discussed, and an attempt is made to reinforce realistic expectations.

The patient's confidence in the prosthetist

should always be improved as a result of this session, since the prosthetist will accurately predict many of the problems the patient will face and suggest solutions (when possible) as these problems occur. In some cases patient orientation may take one visit to the prosthetist's office, and casting and measurement will not take place until the second visit.

EVALUATION

Although the patient is initially evaluated by the clinic team before the prescription is prepared, further evaluation is always required to provide more specific guidelines for prosthesis design. The prosthetist's evaluation includes such items as location of adherent scar tissue and neuromas, range of motion, edema, locations of maximum excursion and power for upper limb amputees, and weight problems (Fig. 5-1).

Measurements are taken of the patient's residual limb and sound limb to be related to the positive mold for proper mold modifications and to establish the proper length of the limb. The measurements of the patient's sound limb related to the length of the residual limb will often determine the components that can be used in the prosthesis and determine the final shape of the prosthesis.

For example, typical measurements of the residual limb for an above-knee prosthesis include

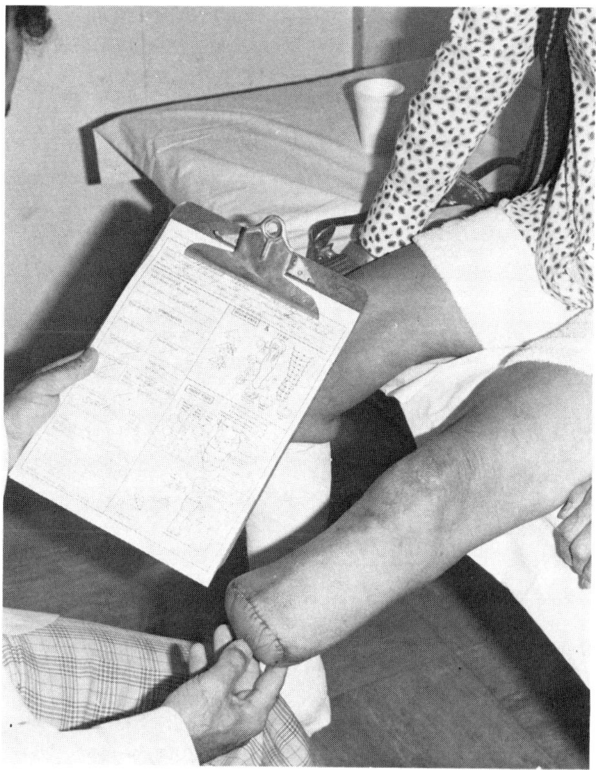

Fig. 5-1. Patient evaluation. Special forms are used by prosthetist during evaluation to indicate patient's measurements, areas of redundant tissue, neuromas, and contractures. Same form is used to indicate all components to be used, socket design, type of suspension, prosthetic sock size, and other information critical to prosthetic treatment.

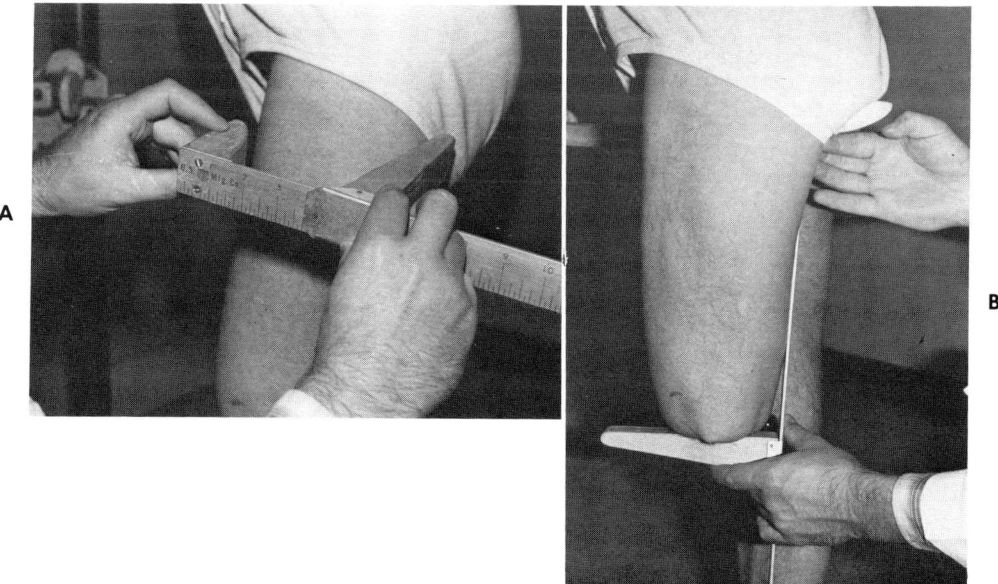

Fig. 5-2. Measurement instrument for above-knee amputations. **A,** Instrument is used to determine anteroposterior dimension of socket, which is taken from adductor longus tendon to ischial tuberosity (not shown here). **B,** Same instrument is used to determine length of amputation from ischial tuberosity.

(1) circumference measurements at the ischial level and distally at 5-cm (2-inch) intervals, (2) the length of the residual limb from the ischial tuberosity to the distal femur and to the end of the amputation (Fig. 5-2), (3) the medial anteroposterior dimension between the adductor longus tendon and the ischial tuberosity, (4) the hip adduction range and hip flexion and extension, and (5) measurements on the sound limb that include circumference measurements at the thigh, calf, ankle, knee diameter, length from the ischial tuberosity to the knee, length from the ischial tuberosity to the floor, and shoe size. The measurements will later be related to both the positive mold taken of the patient and to the final shaping of the prosthesis.

Precise measurements are of the utmost importance. A number of measurement instruments have been developed specifically for the prosthetist, so that measurements can be taken as accurately as possible. One example of such an instrument is the VAPC caliper (Fig. 5-3), a spring-loaded caliper designed specifically to measure the distance from the patellar tendon to the popliteal space for below-knee amputees and to measure the diameter of the femoral condyle. The caliper has a constant tension of about 3 pounds/inch^2 and is calibrated in inches so that any prosthetist would be able to take the same measurements on a given patient.

Patients who are being evaluated for powered upper limb prostheses have myoelectric control sites located with the use of a specially designed electromyograph (EMG) machine (Figs. 5-4 and 5-5). Circumference measurements are taken with a cloth measurement tape and joint range of motion measured with a goniometer.

In summary, accurate measurements of the patient's sound limb and residual limb are required in order to check the dimensions of the mold that has been taken, determine the length of the prosthesis, determine the components that can be used, and provide guidelines for shaping and for the initial alignment of the prosthesis.

CASTING

The purpose of the casting procedure is to provide the prosthetist with an accurate mold of the patient's residual limb. The mold is generally taken of the patient's limb in a specified position and is usually intentionally deformed by the prosthetist to clearly define anatomical landmarks. A number of casting fixtures specifically developed for prosthetics are available (Fig. 5-6). Information on alignment of the prosthesis, such as plumb lines, is also frequently placed on the initial mold. The mold of the patient's residual limb is generally taken in the prosthetist's office during the same visit when the patient receives orientation, evaluation, and measurements.

Plaster of Paris, also called gypsum or calcium sulfate, is the most commonly used material for making impressions of the patient's residual limb. Gauze bandages impregnated with plaster of Paris are available in rolls 2.7 to 4.5 m (3 to 5 yards) long and 5 to 15 cm (2 to 6 inches) wide. Prosthetists use the same type of plaster as physicians do when applying fracture casts. Elastic plaster bandages are also available. These elastic bandages have the advantages of easily adapting to contours and providing a very smooth surface against the skin, but are weaker than the standard type of plaster bandage. These bandages are also available in a variety of setting times that vary from the standard setting time of 8 to 10

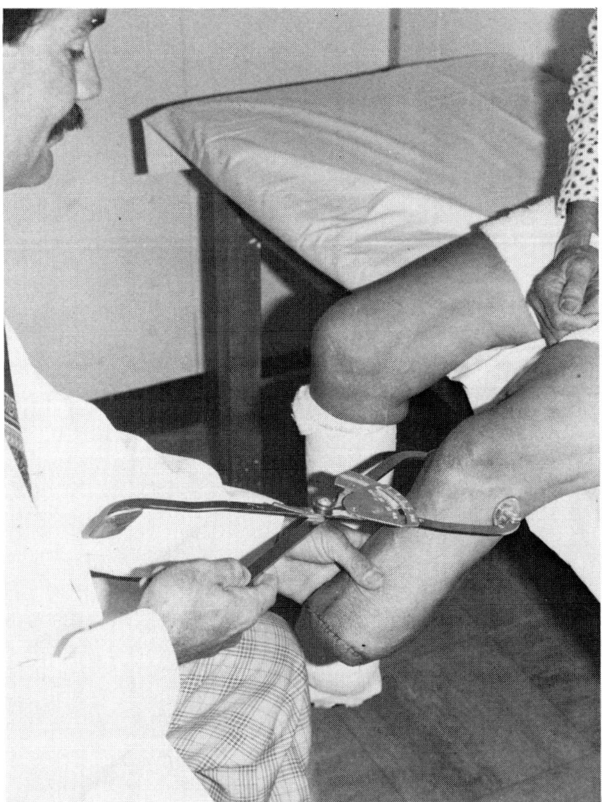

Fig. 5-3. Caliper developed by Veterans Administration to measure width of femoral condyles. Other end of caliper is designed to fit into popliteal space and over patellar tendon to provide anteroposterior dimension. Spring in caliper provides constant compression force on tissue so measurements will be consistent.

minutes to an extra-fast setting time of 3 to 5 minutes. The size and type of plaster bandage to be used depends on the type of mold to be taken, the size of the individual, and the amount of working time that is required before the plaster sets.

Alginate is the second most commonly used material to make impressions of the residual limb. Alginate is a salt of alginic acid, which is extracted from marine kelp and is used elsewhere in the surgical field for absorbable surgical dressings and by dentists for taking tooth impressions. Soluble alginates form a viscous sol that can be changed into a gel by a chemical reaction with compounds such as calcium sulfate, a property that makes it useful for taking impressions. Alginate is used in prosthetics when it is necessary to have a great amount of definition in the im-

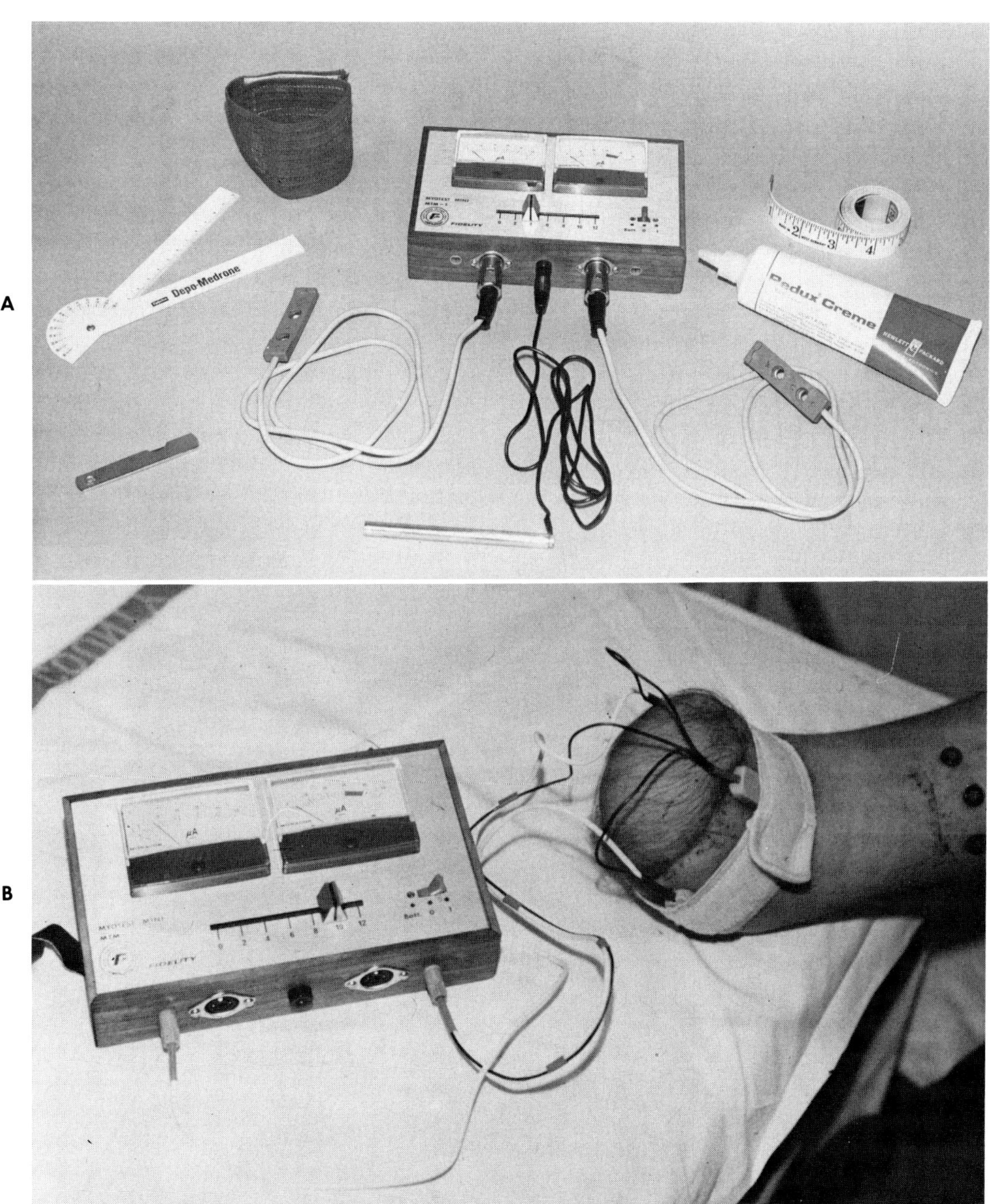

Fig. 5-4. A, Evaluation and measurement tools for myoelectric prosthesis include myotester to evaluate electrical potentials, goniometer, elastic cuff, tape measure, and electrolyte gel. **B,** Myotester (Fidelity Electronics) applied to patient with below-elbow amputation.

pression, such as fingerprints or hair follicles. It is also used to mold body parts with deep undercuts that would make a rigid plaster cast difficult if not impossible to remove without breaking; the gelatin-like set of alginate allows the body part to be pulled out easily. Examples of uses for alginate are casting hands for custom cosmetic gloves, Syme's casts, and casts of facial parts such as ears, noses, and eyes. The disadvantages of alginate are that it is very expensive, it is hard to control the position of the body part while it is being molded, it sets very fast (generally within 1 minute), and the mold shrinks rapidly, which means it should be filled with plaster for the positive mold within a few minutes after the impression has been taken.

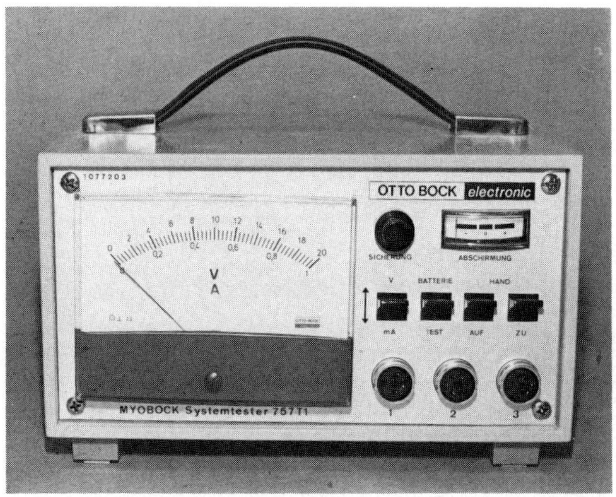

Fig. 5-5. Otto Bock Systemtester, developed to troubleshoot Otto Bock myoelectric prosthesis, comes with set of specialized tools.

A third technique of taking impressions for prosthetic sockets is called the dilatancy or air evacuation technique. This technique employs a receptable that is filled with sand or small plastic beads and is covered with a very loose thin sheet made of rubber or a plastic material (similar to a beanbag chair). A vacuum system is attached to the receptacle, and the body part that is to be molded is placed on the sheet, at the top of the device and pushed into the sand or plastic beads until it is completely enclosed. At this point the air between the sand or plastic beads is evacuated, converting them from a loose fluid-type of mass to a solid structure. The body part is then removed, leaving an impression that is held in place by a continuous vacuum. The impression is filled with plaster, and the vacuum is then released, allowing the sand or plastic beads to settle once again so that the mold can be removed. This technique is used mainly in orthotics for molding

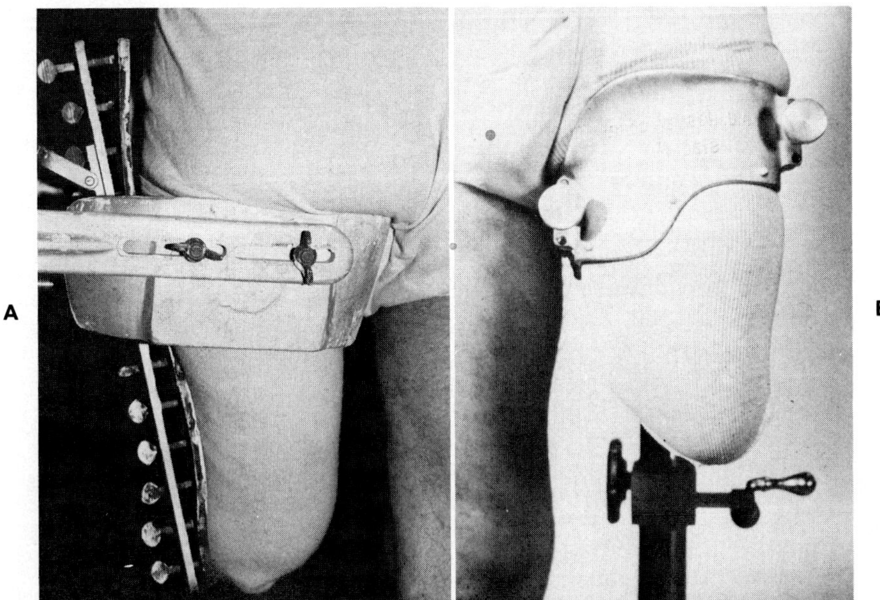

Fig. 5-6. A, Casting instrument developed by Veterans Administration for casting above-knee amputations. Screws on lateral side can be adjusted to mold lateral wall to provide adequate hip adduction and distribute pressures equally on femor. **B,** Casting instrument developed by University of California Biomechanics Laboratory, Berkeley, to cast above-knee amputations. Aluminum-casted quadrilateral brims come in number of right and left sizes.

orthopaedic seats for patients with pressure sores and positioning problems but has been used in prosthetics mainly in Europe.

Any casting procedure provides much more than just a mold of the patient's limb; it also details the possible socket design and provides alignment information. Virtually all molds taken in prosthetics are intentionally deformed by the prosthetist, either by hand or with the use of a special instrument. This deformation of the mold is generally done so that the antomical part, which tends to be more rounded when a circumferential wrap of plastic is placed around it, is flattened in certain dimensions to provide rotational stability and better pressure distribution qualities.

MOLD MODIFICATIONS

After the mold of the patient has been taken it is filled with plaster, and a mandrel, such as a pipe, is placed in the plaster to serve as a handle for the mold. The mold is then modified following certain principles that have been established for each level of amputation. During the mold modification process the prosthetist refers to the measurement form and to the markings made earlier on the patient's limbs, which have been transferred to the plaster. Using these reference marks and other information provided on the measurement form, the prosthetist modifies the positive mold by removing the plaster in areas where increased pressure is needed and adding plaster to the mold in areas where pressure should be relieved.

Pressure applied to the residual limb by the socket will be directly affected by the alignment of the prosthesis, thus the prosthetist must keep biomechanics in mind when modifying the mold. For example, during weight bearing on an above-knee prosthesis the hip abductor muscles pull the femur laterally into the lateral wall of the socket; if the lateral wall is not modified properly, the femur will not be stabilized in this position, and a concentration of pressure will occur at the distal cut end of the femur as it is pulled into the lateral wall. When modifying the mold for an above-knee socket the prosthetist will therefore apply a higher pressure (remove plaster) along the lateral aspect of the femur and leave small relief at the distal end of the femur so that the socket will be designed to stabilize the femur without causing pain or discomfort at the distal end of the femur.

The main purpose of mold modification is to distribute pressure evenly around the socket so that weight-bearing forces and other forces applied through use of the limb may be tolerated without causing discomfort or skin breakdown (Fig. 5-7).

During mold modification trim lines are established around the proximal edge of the socket to either allow complete freedom of motion at the

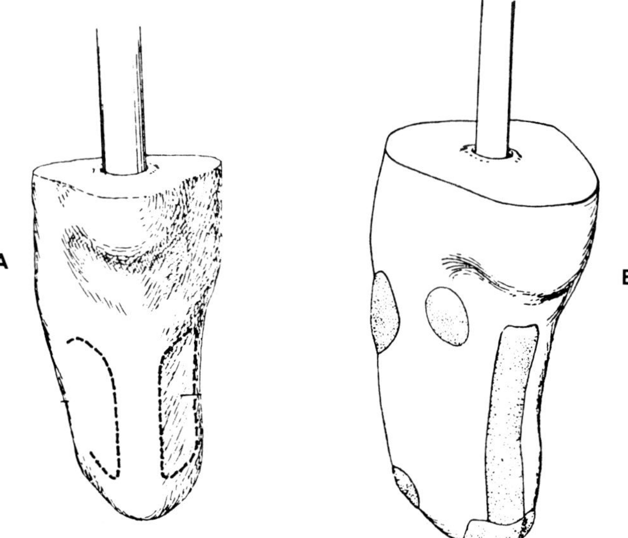

Fig. 5-7. Modification of plaster positive mold for below-knee PTB socket. **A,** Plaster is removed in pressure-tolerant areas, which are usually muscle masses or broad areas of bone, such as medial blade of tibia. **B,** Prominent bones and tendons are relieved by adding plaster. Shown here are reliefs for tibial crest, distal end of tibia, lateral tubercle, fibula head, and distal end of fibula. Hamstring tendons are also relieved. When a plastic socket is formed over this mold, buildups will be recessed.

joint or to allow motion only with a limited range.

Suspension of prostheses can be directly related to mold modification. Suction sockets or sockets held on by tension must be modified to close tolerances. Circumferences of the positive mold are compared to the circumferences recorded on the measurement chart that were taken of the patient. The socket is brought down to these measurements or, in some cases, slightly under these measurements so that an intimate fit occurs and the patient can suspend the prosthesis by contraction of muscles or by forming a perfect seal in the socket that will not allow the introduction of air into the socket so the socket will not be displaced. This type of suspension is commonly used for above-knee amputees and rarely used for below-knee and above-elbow amputees.

Encapsulation of the proximal condyle or bony prominence to provide suspension is also directly related to mold modification procedures. Circumference measurements and mediolateral dimensions from the mold are compared to the measurement chart, and plaster is removed from the mold proximal to the condyle so the socket can clip over the condyle and be suspended from it. Bony prominences that are used for suspension include the malleoli, femoral condyles, iliac crests, styloid processes, and humeral epicondyles. Placement of the undercut areas of the socket are very important; if the mold is modified with the undercut section too high or low, the patient will either have poor suspension or excessive pressure on the bone. The contour of this undercut is also extremely important because it must follow the contour of the bone and have a generous flair to distribute pressure evenly. This type of suspension is used for the PTB below-knee prosthesis with supracondylar suspension, hip disarticulation prostheses suspended over the iliac crest, and for some designs of below-elbow prostheses, particularly the Muenster and Northwestern University design. A similar technique of suspension is used for the Syme amputation, knee disarticulation, wrist disarticulation, and elbow disarticulation prostheses, although in these cases the condyle is encapsulated in the distal end of the socket rather than the proximal end.

Another major consideration in mold modification is to allow for controlled mobility of the nearby anatomical joint. The trim line of the socket must be determined in such a manner that adequate room is left to allow normal range of motion of the joint. For example, in the PTB below-knee prosthesis the patient should be able to sit comfortably or kneel in the prosthesis with the knee joint at approximately 110 degrees of flexion. The patient should also be able to stand in the prosthesis but not be allowed enough extension range to hyperextend the knee. To accommodate the knee during this range of flexion reliefs of plaster are built up at the posterior aspect of the mold to allow for the hamstring tendons during sitting and stair climbing. The mold is trimmed down posteriorly far enough to allow the desired amount of knee flexion. Joint motion is controlled by socket modifications in all prosthetic designs for both the upper and lower limbs.

TEST SOCKETS

The purpose of a test socket fitting is to ensure that the socket fits the patient properly before it is attached to an artificial limb, although many times the test socket is attached to the other components to enable the patient to use the socket functionally while socket fit is being tested. Test sockets are made over the modified positive mold from any number of materials, including plaster bandage, polyester resins, polycarbonate, polypropylene, and wax. One advantage of using a test socket is that the prosthetist is aware that there is no way this particular socket can be used in the final prosthesis and therefore does not hesitate to make changes in the socket to improve the fit.

A separate appointment is made for a test socket fitting. The patient is instructed in the use of prosthetic socks (when applicable), and these are put on the patient's limb before the socket is applied. When weight-bearing test sockets are fitted, the socket is placed on an adjustable stand and raised to the proper level so the patient can bear equal weight on both limbs, or the test socket is attached to the components of the prosthesis. Any number of methods are used to evaluate the socket fit, but, in most cases, holes are made in the socket at strategic areas such as over bony prominences and areas critical to suspension. The tissue is then prodded to check for either excessive pressure or a lack of adequate pressure over that area. A great amount of skill is required to effectively use a test socket. When a test socket is used (Fig. 5-8), areas of excessive or inadequate pressure can be noted by seeing the amount of compression on the prosthetic sock or, when a prosthetic sock is not being used, by blanching of the skin where there is excessive pressure. During the test socket fitting the prosthetist will frequently split the socket to allow for volume adjustments or will heat and deform the socket or trim away portions of the socket. Marks are made in areas that cannot be relieved during the test socket fitting so that when the socket is again filled with plaster the prosthetist can modify the mold in this area to ensure proper fit. Following are the four areas specifically observed during the test socket fitting:

1. Comfort
2. Even distribution of weight-bearing pressure and biomechanical forces
3. Suspension
4. Freedom of motion for the proximal joint

ALIGNMENT AND FITTING

Since each patient has a unique gait pattern and activity level, alignment of the prosthesis must be made on an individual basis. The purpose of aligning a prosthesis is to provide maximum comfort, efficient function, and cosmesis by adjusting the relative position of the components while the patient is using the limb in a number of controlled situations. This stage of prosthesis design is also called a "fitting."

During the alignment stage the prosthesis must be durable and have the ability to function but at the same time must have the ability to be adjusted as many ways as possible. For example, in upper limb prosthetics the suspension and control harnesses are adjustable, the cable hangers are adjustable, attachments for the cable housing are placed on with hose clamps in a temporary manner, special adjustable forearm lift tabs are used and the efficiency of the system is measured by the use of prehension gauges and force scales. In the lower limb, a variety of adjustable components are available, including the Staros-Gardner coupling, the University of California, Berkeley, (UCB) adjustable leg, and endoskeletal pylons that are designed so that they can be readjusted at any time (Fig. 5-9).

Some patients may require more than one visit to optimize the alignment of the prosthesis, since the alignment procedure may take more than 1 hour, and new patients are frequently not able to stand and ambulate for more than 15 minutes at a time. Difficult cases, of course, also require more time. Alignment generally takes place within parallel bars in a private walking room in the prosthetist's office. The following procedures are

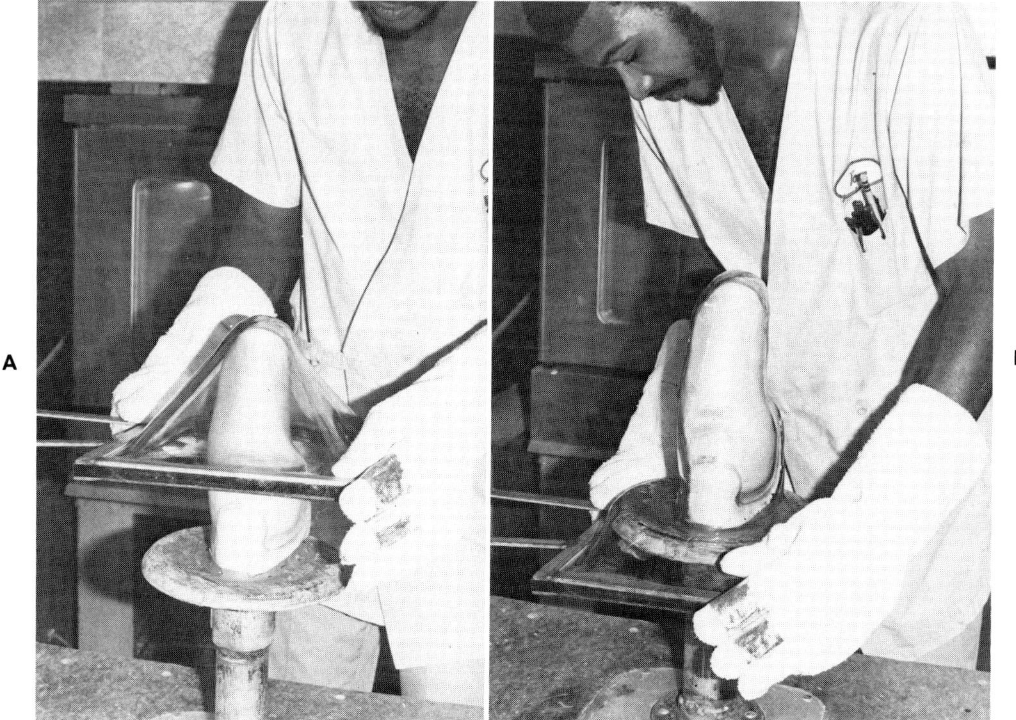

Fig. 5-8. A, Clear polycarbonate test sockets are made by drying material in oven for 1 day to remove all moisture (which causes bubbles) and then placing it in hotter oven until it softens. At this point, material, which has been held in metal frame, is pulled over inverted mold on vacuum-forming table. **B,** Vacuum is then applied, pulling clear plastic onto mold. Prosthetist uses this socket to check for even distribution of pressures before permanent socket is made.

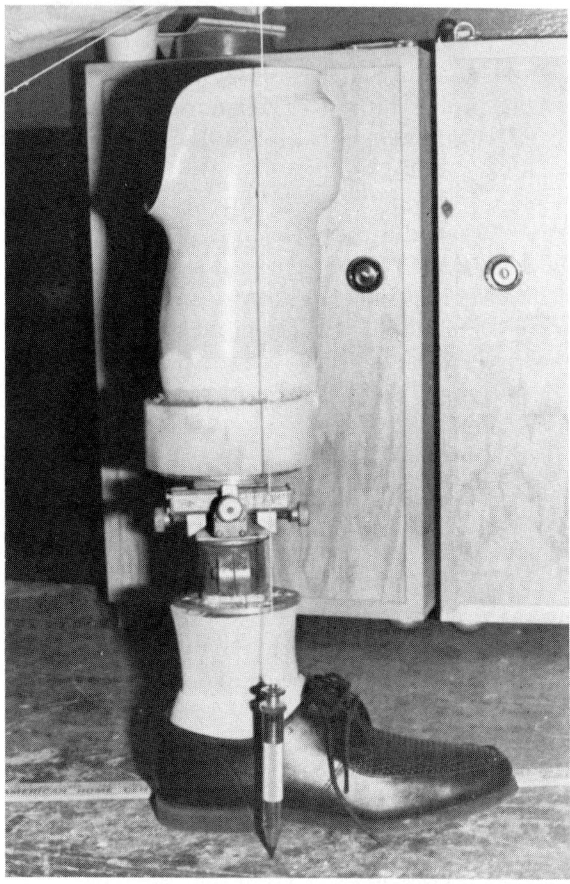

Fig. 5-9. Static alignment of below-knee prosthesis. Plastic socket is bonded to wood or foam, and adjustment device is attached between socket and foot. Static alignment is then established as starting point before patient walks on prosthesis. Alignment is adjusted individually during fitting procedure to allow for comfort, balance, and energy-saving gait. Shown here is UCB alignment device, which allows both angular and sliding adjustments.

generally used during the alignment process for any prosthesis:

1. The function of the prosthesis is explained to the patient. The patient is instructed in how to don the prosthesis properly, including the use of prosthetic socks, if required.
2. Socket fit is checked to ensure that the patient fits into the socket properly.
3. The length of the prosthesis is checked.
4. The suspension is checked.
5. The patient is instructed to try to balance over the prosthesis or to use the prosthesis in a controlled manner.
6. Obviously malaligned components are aligned properly.
7. The patient is requested to walk in the prosthesis or, in the case of an upper limb prosthesis, to flex and open and close a terminal device and operate the prosthesis in a number of different situations. Alignment of components is checked during function and adjusted to provide maximum efficiency, comfort, and cosmesis to the patient.
8. The prosthesis is checked with the patient sitting, and adjustments are made if necessary to increase comfort in this position.

Socket design and alignment complement each other. No matter how sophisticated the components are, how well the prosthesis is finished, or how light it is fabricated, if it is malaligned or has an uncomfortable socket, the patient's function will be drastically reduced.

Fitting and alignment of the prosthesis are not completed until the prosthetist and patient are convinced that the prosthesis is functioning as well as possible. More experienced patients will usually be able to provide feedback concerning the way the prosthesis fits and feels during walking. The prosthetist can then make adjustments in a rapid and accurate fashion, and the fitting procedure takes a minimum of time. New patients, however, cannot always provide accurate feedback, therefore sometimes the patient is referred to physical therapy to use the prosthesis while it is still able to be easily adjusted. The new patient can then practice with the prosthesis, and further adjustments can be made as the patient's endurance and ability to use the prosthesis improve. Generally, 1 week in physical therapy with the prosthesis will afford adequate time for the prosthetist to make decisions concerning the final alignment. The therapist will also be able to provide excellent feedback concerning the patient's use of the prosthesis.

Once fitting and alignment are completed, the alignment device is "transferred out," and lighter foam or wood is used for shaping and strengthening the prosthesis (Fig. 5-10). A final plastic lamination is then applied to the prosthesis. The prosthesis is delivered to the patient in the prosthetist's office after it has been finished. The prosthesis is now structurally sound, shaped to provide maximum cosmesis, and color matched to the patient's skin. The patient is provided the prosthesis and instructed in its care at home. A clinic appointment is frequently made to allow the prescribing physician to see the patient with the prosthesis, and a follow-up appointment is made 1 week later in the prosthetist's office.

FOLLOW-UP MANAGEMENT

Proper patient follow-up is of maximum importance in prosthetics. The new patient in particular requires follow-up at frequent intervals;

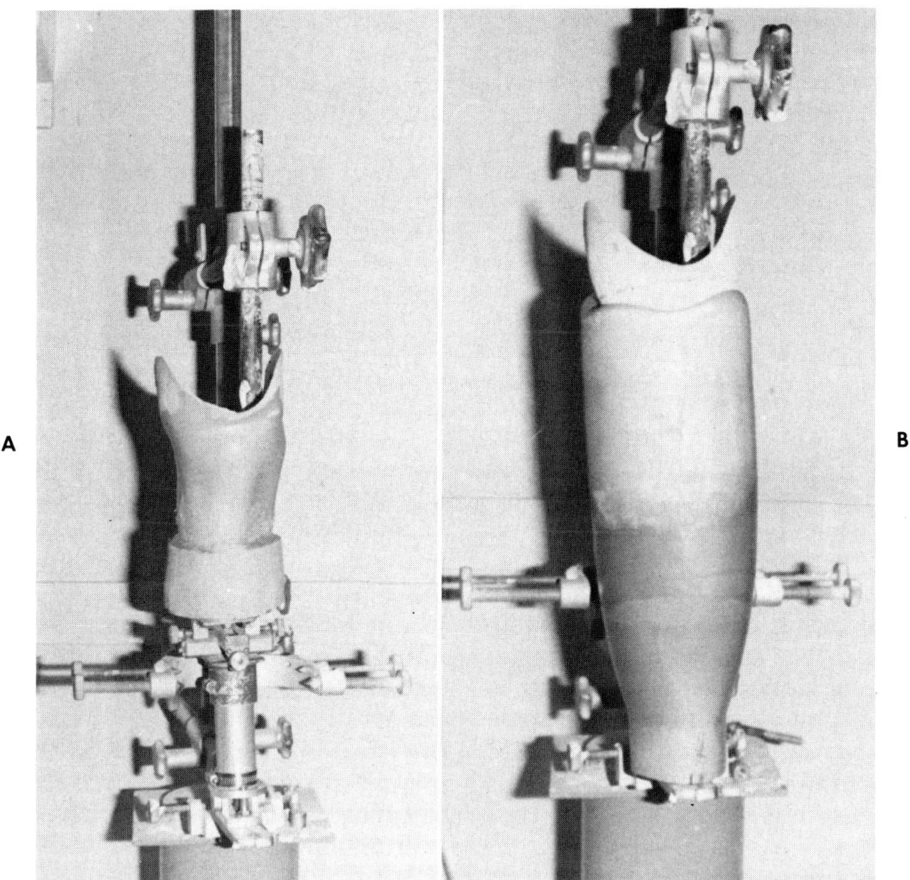

Fig. 5-10. Transfer procedure. **A,** After patient has walked in prosthesis and alignment has been adjusted, mechanical alignment device and pylon are "transferred" out, and foam or wood replaces them to make strong, light cosmetic finish. To prevent alignment (position of socket over foot) from being lost, socket is solidly held in place in this vertical transfer device. Foot is removed, and pylon is bolted to base of transfer device. Adjustable mechanism and pylon are then removed. **B,** Polyurethane foam is used to hold socket in place over foot and to provide strength. Foam will be shaped to match patient's other leg, and plastic lamination will cover it, providing additional cosmesis and strength.

this patient should not only be developing tolerance to pressures of the prosthesis against the skin but also general physical endurance. Patients generally will have many questions after wearing the prosthesis for a week or two. These questions will pertain to such activities as use of the prosthesis while driving a car, during sports activities and dancing, choosing shoes, and wearing the prosthesis to the beach. In addition, a number of small problems can occur during the first couple of weeks of prosthetic wear. These problems will generally be related to pressure areas in the socket, discomfort while sitting, and problems when wearing other shoes. These minor problems are expected by the prosthetist and can be easily corrected during a follow-up visit.

Patients should be seen, at the very minimum, every 4 to 6 months. The prosthesis consists of moving mechanical components and will require cleaning, maintenance, or replacement at some time. Some components, such as hip joints, knee joints, ankle joints, and arm cables, must be cleaned and adjusted on a regular basis because they will directly affect the function of the prosthesis.

Changes in the volume or shape of the patient's residual limb will frequently necessitate socket adjustments, particularly during the first month of wearing a new prosthesis. In some cases the patient can vary the thickness, or ply, of the prosthetic socks to improve the fit of the prosthesis, but in many cases other adjustments are required. Socket adjustments are made only after a careful analysis of the cause of discomfort is completed by the prosthetist. The prosthetist then has two choices; relieving the pressure area by grinding out material from the socket over the area of pressure or by adding material, thereby redistributing the forces over a different area. In some cases minor alignment changes can be made after a prosthesis is completed if the prosthetist believes that the patient's discomfort is related to socket alignment.

New patients will often lose the fit of their initial prosthesis after 1 year. There are a number of reasons for this, with the main reason being the remodeling of the residual limb tissues in response to constant weight-bearing pressures. After 1 year the patient may be wearing two or three thick five-ply prosthetic socks, which results in a bulky-appearing prosthesis that is very hot. The patient's walking habits generally have improved considerably during the first year of prosthetic wear, therefore the prosthetic alignment may not be adequate for the patient's increased activity. For most adults, a replacement prosthesis will last about 3 years.

It is of maximum importance for the prosthetist to keep a good record of all follow-up treatment given to a patient. Follow-up notes will help guide future decisions regarding socket or component modification and prosthetic design.

MATERIALS

A wide variety of natural and man-made materials is used in prosthetics today. Whether the materials are natural or man made, however, they must still conform to the special requirements of the profession: biocompatibility, strength, durability, lightweight, and ease of fabrication. The most common materials used in prosthetics today are wood, plastic, leather, metal, and cloth.

Wood

Wood is often used in lower limb prosthetics to provide shape and interior structural strength. The inherent properties of wood make it a very difficult material to replace. The advantages of wood over many other materials are that it is lightweight, strong, inexpensive, easy to work with, and consistent in texture. Basswood, willow, poplar, and linden wood are most commonly used for prosthetic knees and shins. These woods are lightweight, strong, and free from defects often found in other woods, such as knotholes, warping, and checking. These woods can be shaped easily using standard woodworking tools. When a prosthesis is being finished the shin of the prosthesis is hollowed out until the wood is approximately 0.8 cm (1/4 inch thick), which makes the prosthesis lighter but still has adequate structural strength after it has been covered with a plastic lamination.

Hardwoods are also used in lower limb prosthetics. SACH feet have an interior hardwood keel that provides structural strength to the foot. This keel is bolted to the rest of the prosthesis and provides a strong anterior lever arm for the patient when he stands on the forefoot. Maple and hickory are the most commonly used for keels in SACH feet and to reinforce high stress areas of prosthetic knee units, such as the knee extension stop. Hardwoods are not used in areas where the prosthetist might have to shape or adjust the wood, since the inherent strength of these woods makes them very difficult to work with.

Leather

Leather is another material in common use in prosthetics. Leather is generally used for suspension straps, waist belts, soft inserts on PTB prosthesis, socket linings, and as fairings to provide cosmesis over knee and hip joints. Leather is easy to work with, has a soft natural feel, can stretch in one direction, and is biocompatible. Different variations of cowhide are most commonly used in prosthetics.

Many years ago hides were available from horses, elk, and calves, but today cowhide is modified by the tannery to provide the same feel and working properties as the hides of these other animals; therefore horsehide is actually cowhide that has been treated to provide the thin, soft flexible properties of the original horsehide. The properties of horsehide make it a very attractive material to use when the leather is to contact the skin; therefore it is used to line waist belts, suspension straps, and inserts for PTB sockets. Since horsehide will stretch easily with wear, it must be reinforced with another material such as cowhide or synthetic fabric to prevent stretching.

Other variations of cowhide, such as elk, calf, kip, and rawhide, are used for a variety of purposes in prostheses from such things as dorsiflexion stops in single-axis feet to laces for leather thigh corsets. Plastics such as Naugahyde and thermoplastic foam have replaced leather in some uses but will probably never completely replace this material.

Cloth

Cloth is used for prosthetic socks, waist belts, straps, and harnesses for upper limb prostheses.

Probably the greatest use of cloth is for prosthetic socks, which function in the same manner as athletic socks in that they keep the skin dry, cushion the limb, and take up volume in the socket to improve the fit of the prosthesis. Prosthetic socks are commonly made of wool, cotton, or blends of these natural fibers with nylon, Orlon, acrylics, or other man-made materials.

Wool is the most common material used for prosthetic socks because of its characteristics of elasticity, high absorbency, and ability to hold much moisture without feeling damp. Wool also has a high degree of resistance to acids that are the basis of perspiration and does not wrinkle and stick to the skin, even when it contains a great amount of body moisture. The blend of domestic and foreign wool fleece used in prosthetic socks improves on the basic properties of wool and affords a greater resistance to shrinkage. This material, however, must be washed carefully in a coconut oil–based soap that will dissolve in lukewarm water (38° to 44°C; 100° to 110°F). Wool should be rinsed in lukewarm water as well, since a change in temperature will affect it adversely. Prosthetic socks should also be dried carefully by first removing the excess water, wrapping them in a towel, and then either block drying them away from sunlight or in any other manner that avoids direct heat or cold while the wool is drying. The recent development of machine washable wool will undoubtedly remove the need for hand washing in the near future.

Cotton is also used for prosthetic socks but is in more common use in the form of a cotton stockinette, which is used to protect the limb during casting procedures. Cotton is also blended with wool in prosthetic socks, and some 100% cotton prosthetic socks are available. Cotton is a natural vegetable fiber that is soft, pliable, and absorbant but falls short of wool in all of its properties. Cotton, however, is easier to take care of and more inexpensive than wool, making it more practical for many uses in prosthetics. Cotton stockinette is sometimes used as the final layer in a plastic lamination prosthesis because the cotton fibers will absorb the resin, resulting in an even-colored finish.

Plastics

Nylon is used for prosthetic sheaths, plastic laminations, bushings, suction valves, and nylon stockings to cover prostheses. The major advantages of this man-made fiber are its strength, elasticity, and low coefficient of friction. Nylon prosthetic sheaths are in common use for below-knee amputees. A thin sheath worn directly over the skin drastically reduces shear stresses on the skin from pistoning in the socket and tends to pull moisture away from the skin into the outside prosthetic socks. Nylon stockinette provides inherent strength in nearly all prosthetic laminations. Three to eight layers of nylon are impregnated with polyester or acrylic resins during a lamination to provide both structural strength and a pleasing appearance to the finished prosthesis. Nylon in itself is a thermoplastic material, which means it can be heated and remolded without adversely affecting its physical properties. Nylon is usually laminated with a thermosetting polyester resin that gives the finished prosthesis the properties of thermosetting plastic rather than a thermoplastic.

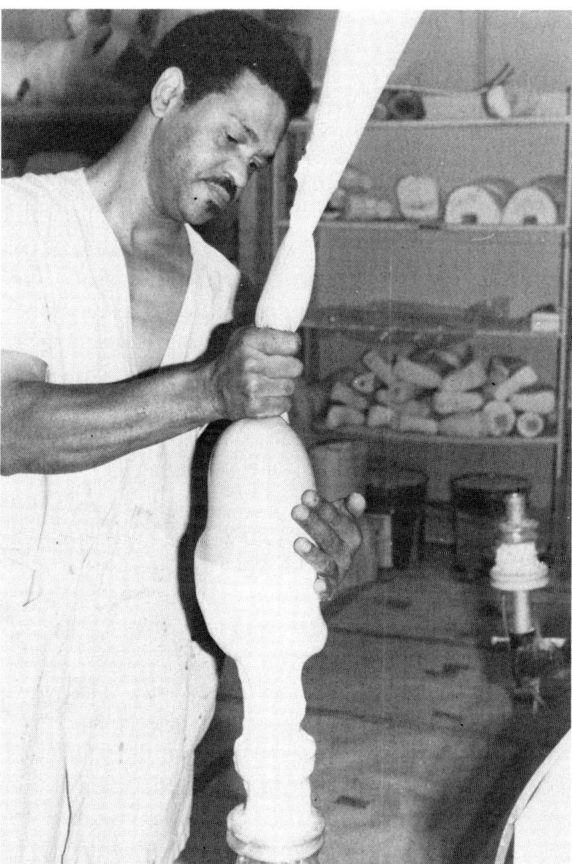

Fig 5-11. Lamination of socket for below-knee prosthesis. Liquid polyester or acrylic resin is mixed with skin-colored pigment, catalyst, and promoter to promote curing. Resin is then poured into polyvinyl alcohol (PVA) sleeve that has been snugly pulled over mold and impregnates layers of Dacron felt and nylon stockinette. Vacuum is applied to pull material into undercuts in mold. After resin sets, solid plastic socket is cut off mold.

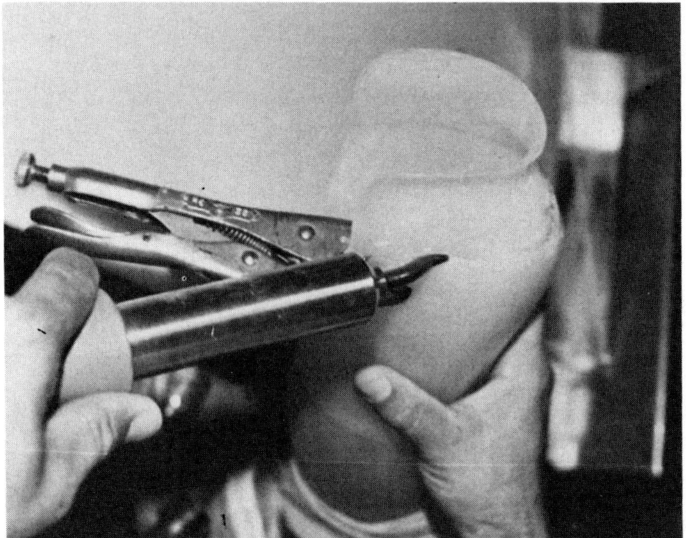

Fig. 5-12. Polypropylene has been recently used for lightweight below-knee prostheses. Here, polypropylene socket is welded to polyprolene shank, using nitrogen and hot air plastic welder. (Courtesy Rancho Los Amigos Hospital.)

Acrylics are thermoplastics that have greater durability and strength than polyester resins. Acrylic fibers are frequently used in the newer synthetic blends of prosthetic socks, since this material is soft, durable, and machine washable. Acrylic resins are finding an increased use for laminations in prosthetics because the high strength allows for a thinner, lighter weight lamination and the thermoplastic properties allow easier adjustments of the prosthesis by reheating the plastic and remolding it. Acrylic resins tend to have a softer feel than polyester resins. Acrylics are more difficult to use during fabrication although they have proven superior qualities. Clear acrylics have been used for years in the sign and building industry for skylights and enclosures for shopping centers; they do not yellow and have the best weather resistance of all plastics.

Polyester resin is a thermosetting plastic that is most commonly used for laminations in prosthetics. Thermosetting plastics cannot be heated and reformed without destroying their physical properties. Polyester resins come in a liquid form that can be pigmented to match the patient's natural skin tone. A benzoyl peroxide catalyst is then added to this resin to initiate the setting process, and a promoting chemical is added to speed up the setting time. The prosthetist will then pour this material into a polyvinyl alcohol (PVA) sleeve that has been pulled snugly over the prosthesis; between the rough-shaped prosthesis and the PVA sleeve are layers of nylon stockinette, Dacron, and fiberglass. A combination of vacuum and the use of the technician's hands mold the resin around the prosthesis to provide a uniformly layered cosmetic plastic lamination. The setting time of the resin is adjusted to allow the technician enough time for the lamination (Fig. 5-11). Once the resin is set, a hard, durable cosmetic finish on the prosthesis results.

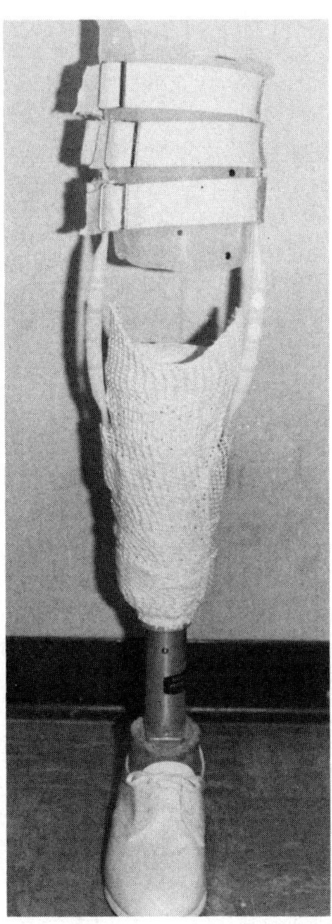

Fig. 5-13. Combination of many new materials, this intermediate prosthesis has thermoplastic Hexcelite socket molded over Orlon-Lycra Spandex prosthetic socket, Plastazote foam padding, ultrahigh-molecular weight polyethylene knee joints, and polypropylene thigh section with polyethylene tongue. Light weight, durability, and ease of adjustments are made possible by these new materials. (Courtesy Rancho Los Amigos Hospital.)

Polyester resins used in prosthetics are mixed with styrene monomer resins to provide flexibility. Styrene is a vinyl compound that has a noxious odor and can exude a potentially dangerous fume; the gases coming from styrene can cause an immediate reaction from the patient if the plastic is not allowed enough time to cure. Therefore

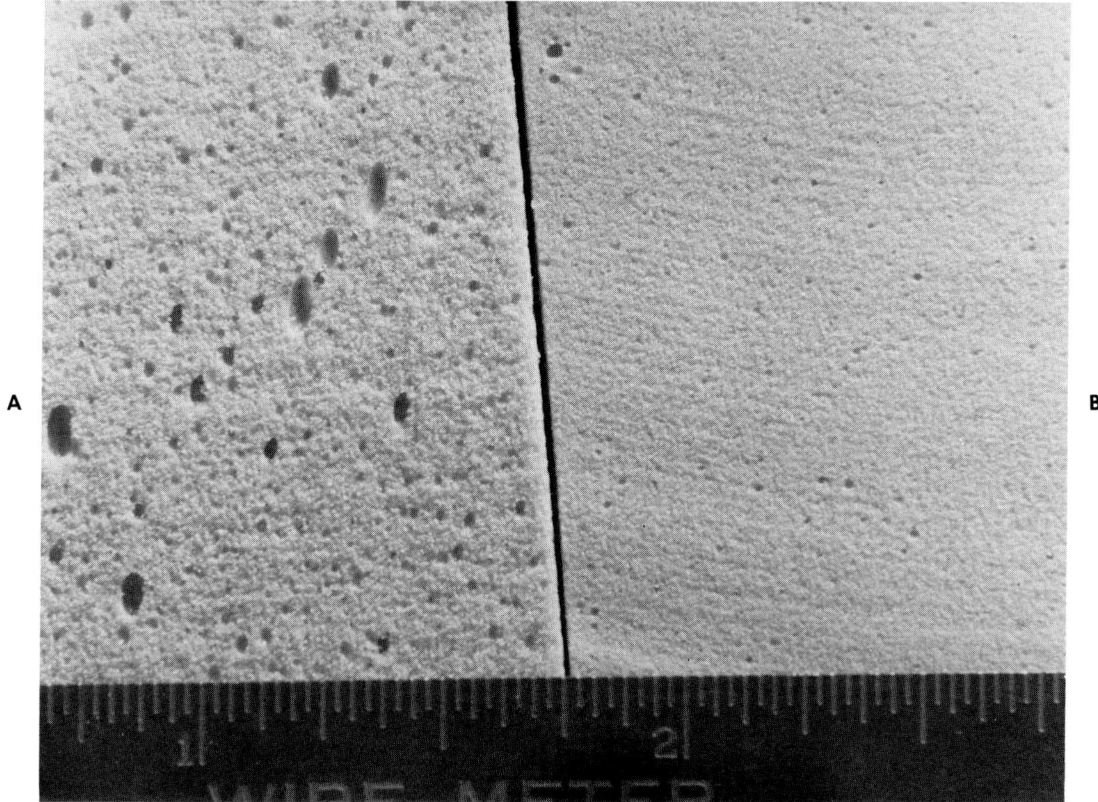

Fig. 5-14. Rigid foam materials are replacing wood in many areas of prosthetics. Same type of foam (usually polyurethane) can be used for different applications by varying setting times and applying heat and/or pressure to foam while it is curing. **A,** Foam was allowed to flow freely while setting, resulting in low-density material that is excellent for filling in voids, but does not have much strength. **B,** Same foam was put under pressure while setting, which prevented expansion and resulted in more uniform material of higher density that can be used to provide structural strength to prosthesis. (Courtesy Hosmer/Dorrance Corp., Inc.)

most prosthetic laminations should be given adequate time to cure before the patient's skin contacts the plastic. Since all polyester resins used in prosthetics contain styrene monomer, these resins should be stored and used in well-ventilated areas. Oven curing is recommended if the resin will not have a few days to cure naturally before a patient fitting is scheduled.

Polypropylene is used for hip joints, pelvic bands, knee joints, and lightweight prostheses. Polypropylene is the single high-volume thermoplastic in the plastic industry for uses varying from fan shrouds in passenger cars to carpets and shipping containers. Polypropylene is an opaque white material that is relatively inexpensive, strong, durable, and easy to mold. The material can be welded using hot air or nitrogen welding guns to bond seams or add reinforcement (Fig. 5-12). Polypropylene sheets 0.3 to 0.9 cm (1/8 to 3/8 inch) thick are usually used in prosthetics and are heated and vacuum formed over the mold of a socket or complete limb.

Polyethylene is an opaque white thermoplastic that looks like polypropylene but feels waxier. The properties of polyethylene vary depending on the density of the material. Low-density polyethylene is very flexible and easy to heat and mold; it is used for triceps cuffs in below-elbow prostheses and for tongues in plastic thigh corsets (Fig. 5-13) and hip disarticulation sockets. High-density polyethylene is more difficult to modify and is usually used to make bushings in joints. Ultrahigh molecular weight (UHMW) polyethylene is used for some knee joints for intermediate prostheses and has other uses in prosthetics because of its good wear characteristics. UHMW polyethylene is used widely in the design of internal hip and knee prostheses.

Polyurethane foams are widely used in prosthetics for cosmetic foam covers and rigid structural sections (Fig. 5-14). Polyurethanes, also called urethanes, are available in three broad groups: flexible foam, rigid foam, and elastomers.

Flexible urethane foams are generally purchased in prefabricated pieces from suppliers as covers for endoskeletal prostheses. The foam is shaped by the prosthetist to measurements and tracings of the patient's limb. Some prosthetists mix these foams themselves and then pour them into a mold of the patient's limb to take advantage of the "skin" that forms around the foam. Using the material in this way is very exacting, time consuming, and can be hazardous, so most prosthetists avoid mixing these foams themselves. Flexible polyurethane foams are used almost exclusively to make SACH feet.

Rigid polyurethane foams compete with wood to provide structural stability to knee units and ankle blocks. Prosthetists routinely use this foam to provide both strength and shape to exoskeletal-type prostheses. A plastic lamination covers the foam to provide additional strength and cosmesis to the prosthesis.

Silicones are used in prosthetics for distal end pads in sockets, to provide a flexible, rubberlike end in air-cushion sockets, and for silicone gel inserts. Silicones can be classified as fluids, elastomers, and resins, all three of which are used in prosthetics. Silicone is synthesized from sand (a combination of silicone and oxygen) and undergoes a number of chemical reactions before liquid or solid silicone results.

The room-temperature vulcanizing (RTV) silicones are used most widely in prosthetics. Silicones have relatively uniform properties over a wide temperature range, repel water, are chemically inert, resist weathering, and have a high degree of slip or lubricity.

Silicone fluid is used for lubrication of moving parts and as a parting agent.

A two-component silicone elastomer is used for foaming end pads in sockets while the patient is wearing the prosthesis to ensure total contact. Silicone alone allows this technique to be done, since no heat or chemical by-product is given off during the cure.

Silicone gel – impregnated gauze is an excellent cushioning and force distribution material in below-knee prosthetic sockets. Although the gel adds weight and bulk to a prosthesis, it has been proven to work well with many problem cases. Silicone gel cushions are frequently used by the disabled to prevent pressure sores from prolonged sitting.

Fiber reinforcements

Basically two types of fiber reinforcements are used in prosthetics today: glass and carbon. The purpose of fiber reinforcements is to strengthen a plastic without adding weight.

Fiberglass is commonly used to reinforce polyester resin laminations where mechanical attachments such as bolts and screws, will fasten. It is also used to stiffen areas of prostheses and to prevent breakage in vulnerable areas. Fiberglass is difficult to finish smoothly and will irritate the patient's skin if it comes in contact, so care must be taken to avoid exposed areas of this material. The added strength fiberglass provides is proportional to the amount used and also depends on the arrangement of the fibers relative to the stresses it must tolerate. A unidirectional arrangement of fibers, as when continuous strand roving is used, allows the best reinforcement loading if the roving is placed directly in line with the stresses. Multidirectional fibers, such as woven mats or fabrics, provide equal strength in all directions, but are less effective when only one stress must be tolerated.

Carbon fibers have not been used in custom fabrication by prosthetists, but are being used by component manufacturers to replace metal. Carbon fibers are generally set in epoxy and can provide a material with a stiffness twice that of steel at one fifth the weight. In addition to this high strength-to-weight ratio, carbon fiber composites have a fatigue resistance twice that of steel, aluminum, and fiberglass. Prefabricated carbon fiber prosthetic components, such as pylon tubes, knee joints, and connectors, could drastically reduce the weight of prostheses while increasing the strength.

CHAPTER 6

The amputee clinic team

ROBERT G. THOMPSON
STEPHEN KRAMER

THE TEAM CONCEPT

The multidiscipline approach to rehabilitation of the amputee, as demonstrated by the amputee clinic team, has yielded superior results during the years of its existence. The evolution of this approach to amputee rehabilitation began during World War II, when the Surgeon General of the Army established a number of amputee centers within Army general hospitals to upgrade the treatment of the combat amputee. When suction suspension for the above-knee amputee was introduced in the United States by the Veterans Administration in 1948, a protocol was established that provided the basis for the amputee clinic team. At that time, the clinic team comprised a physician, prosthetist, and therapist. Gradually, as attention focused on the entire patient and not just on the residual limb, more personnel were added to the clinic team. With improvement in the total care of the amputee, the ablation of a limb no longer can be looked on as the end of treatment, since the rehabilitation program may be initiated at or before the time of surgery.

The clinic team approach has proven to be the most appropriate method of providing prosthetic management. If the team is to render optimum service to the patient, it is essential that each member has an acceptable education and experience in the area of amputee rehabilitation management. Only if all members fully contribute their expertise can the ultimate result be achieved. It is the obligation of the clinic chief to coordinate these efforts during clinical evaluation, prescription, and follow-up. The mechanism employed must assure optimal individual participation of all team members to have the clinic function properly as a unit.

It is the obligation of all team members to make the patient feel at ease and to convey the idea that they are striving to approach prosthetic management in a consistent and knowledgeable manner. The team members should generally refrain from any in-depth discussion of different opinions concerning prescription rationale in the presence of the patient, particularly in the event of difficult problems. It is important that the patient not be alarmed by obvious differences of opinion. Since the physician, prosthetist, and therapist generally provide the most prescription detail, they must maintain control in this area. The patient should be introduced to clinic team members prior to any physical examination or discussion regarding prescription or treatment. Someone should explain to the patient what is going to happen prior to examining the residual limb.

It is imperative that the patient be given realistic rehabilitation goals. Comments that might be construed as indicating an expectation of a level of performance beyond an individual's capabilities are to be carefully avoided. If this is not kept in mind the patient might experience frustration and depression or possibly reject the prosthesis provided.

It is the responsibility of the team to do a thorough examination. A patient who wears a prosthesis, even with no complaints or apparent problems, should not be dismissed without removing the prosthesis for examination. Many prosthesis wearers may not really be aware of problems and may even deny them. Failure to abide by these guidelines can have serious consequences.

The present amputee clinic team consists of the following: a physician knowledgeable in the field of prosthetics and, preferably, amputation surgery; a certified prosthetist; and a physical therapist and an occupational therapist who have been suitably trained at one of the prosthetics education institutions. In addition, a vocational counselor is helpful in providing counseling in the amputee's efforts to obtain gainful employment after rehabilitation. A social worker is of great help in evaluating home and family situations and in easing the transition from disability to function as a member of the family unit. A coordinator to keep notes of clinic meetings and recommendations and schedule future appointments is also needed. Last, but not least, the patient is a crucial member of the team.

THE PATIENT

The patient is the most important member of the team; he is the reason for the clinic's existence and therefore should be the center of attention of the clinic's activities. Some patients thrive on the clinic team approach because they are the object of attention of a number of individuals. Other patients may be overwhelmed by the team, believing themselves to be objects of curiosity, unwanted sympathy, or even derision. Patients should be put at ease in the clinic setting, so that they feel neither threatened nor patronized. All patients should be introduced to the clinic personnel by name rather than by title. If the amputee clinic functions on a serious, professional level, patients will rarely have any complaints as to their care and treatment. If is important that patients remain the center of attention and the clinic personnel do not digress from the immediate problem. Side conversations should be kept to a minimum. The general atmosphere of the clinic should be friendly, and when appropriate, attempts at gentle humor may aid patients in relaxing.

For patients who have already been fitted with a prosthesis and problems have arisen, it is suggested that they be made the center of attention, not just the prostheses. It is probably desirable to restrict the number of people in the clinic team area to those actually required, so that the number of people present is not overwhelming. Some clinics are used for teaching. This is a valuable way to teach the principles of prescription and prosthetic evaluation; however, too many students may detract from the primary reason for the clinic, namely, the care of the amputee. If the problems of the amputee are being explained to the student present, it always wise to refer to the patient and to the limb, rather than simply to refer to the patient's stump as through it were an inanimate object. There should be sufficient time to allow the patient to express himself, both as to needs and problems. The patient should never have the impression of being rushed in and out to finish the clinic on time. It is further emphasized that patients should be considered as individuals. They should be scheduled at staggered intervals so that they are not all present at the opening of the clinic.

It is generally not feasible to examine either an upper or a lower limb amputee who is wearing street clothes, since, in general, it is more distressing to the patient to disrobe in front of the group than it is in a private room with suitable clothing for examining the prosthetic device and remaining limb. The patient's clothing should permit full examination of the involved limb. The lower limb amputee will usually require the use of shorts that are loose fitting over which the suspension apparatus, if present, may be applied. When examining patients with upper limb amputations, it is suggested that women wear a brassiere or halter top so that the harness as well as the prosthesis, can be adequately inspected and evaluated. Decorum, particularly when examining women, should be of the highest quality.

If the clinic team agrees that it is feasible and correct to provide the patient with a prosthesis, this should be done in a very positive manner. It should be emphasized that the prescribed prosthesis will allow functioning in a more desirable manner and thus draw less public curiosity. If all of these criteria are fulfilled, the patient's visit to the amputee clinic should be a pleasant and rewarding experience.

THE PHYSICIAN

The specialized amputee centers that were organized by the Surgeon General during World War II were staffed by orthopaedic surgeons who were extensively trained in amputations and the rehabilitation of the amputee. It was natural for these surgeons to provide medical leadership to amputee clinics as they developed about the country. However, these few trained orthopaedic surgeons were unable to provide coverage for all of the amputee clinic teams that were then beginning operation throughout the United States. Other physicians were called in to staff or consult with the newly developing teams and thus physiatrists, general surgeons, and pediatricians began serving as clinic chiefs.

The physician's role should be that of a coach or manager, responsible for the final decision in case of disagreement. Ideally, the physician should be a surgeon. However, if he is not a surgeon he should certainly have knowledge of amputation surgical techniques and the anatomy beneath the healed skin of the residual limb. The physician should maintain the decorum of the clinic and set the tone of professional attention to the problems of the amputee. At no time should the physician be a dictator, since this generally inhibits full participation by other team members. At all times he should seek consultation of other team members so as to ensure their full participation.

THE PROSTHETIST

The role of the prosthetist has changed for the better during the years of the amputee clinic concept. In some instances, prosthetics was more a business than a profession. The prosthetist in the effective amputee clinic now fulfills a professional role by virtue of having attained a great deal more theoretical, as well as practical, knowledge in prescribing, fabricating, and fitting prostheses. He may frequently be called on to provide initial input for prescription of the prosthesis. The physician is aware that the prosthetist has the greater knowledge of new items in the field of prosthetics and should encourage the introduction of new components or fitting techniques to the clinic team. The prosthetist should require a prescription before providing a patient with a new limb.

Since the prosthetist may be seeing the patient for a longer period than either the physician or therapist, hopefully he will develop a greater rapport with the patient, thus acting as a sounding board for the patient's unspoken or not previously related concerns or hopes for the future.

The prosthetist's role in the amputee clinic is not only to aid in the prescription decision for a particular patient, but to provide expertise in the area of fitting and alignment. The prosthetist should be aware of medical problems that may occur in the residual should be aware of medical problems that may occur in the residual limb and should relay this information to the clinic team. Generally, one prosthetist is sufficient to serve on the amputee clinic team. To avoid favoritism to any one prosthetist in the local area, prosthetist may be asked to staff the amputee clinic on a rotating basis. The truly professional prosthetist may see other prosthetists' patients, make the necessary notes and subsequently contact the patient's prosthetist to relay the clinic team's decision as to the changes suggested.

The modern prosthetist is no longer confined to attendance at amputee clinics and fabrication of prostheses. In many instances he has accompanied the physician into the operating room and sometimes can assist the surgeon in deciding the level of amputation consistent with good prosthetics. The prosthetist usually provides immediate temporary plaster sockets and/or pylons.

It is imperative for prosthetists who participate in the modern clinic atmosphere to be aware of the newest techniques in amputee rehabilitation. They must have a knowledge of biomechanics, as well as newer materials and prosthetic components that may be more efficient in providing function to the amputee.

THE PHYSICAL THERAPIST

The physical therapist has always been a valuable member of the amputee clinic team. Universities have included the therapist in short-term prosthetic courses given to clinic team members, since they are required to know about many of the stump problems with which the physician must deal. The therapist provides pre-prosthetic service in the areas of stump shaping, prevention or elimination of edema, prevention or treatment of joint contractures, and gait training with walkers or crutches. The therapist may also provide a sympathetic ear to the patient's expressed psychological difficulties, particularly relating to his future and ability to use a prosthesis.

Following the prescription procedure, in which the therapist has a part, the prosthesis may be checked by the therapist before the clinic team meets. The therapist will teach the patient how to use it prosthesis in the most efficient manner possible. With this experience, the physical therapist can quickly recognize gait deviations and suggest to the team prosthetist the need for corrective measures. Preferably, the therapist has been educated in these techniques in one of the university programs. In some clinics the physical therapist may share in teaching the upper limb amputee, although in most clinics the upper limb amputee has been directed to the occupational therapist.

THE OCCUPATIONAL THERAPIST

The occupational therapist has assumed a special role in rehabilitating the upper limb amputee, since the use of upper limb prostheses involves many activities of daily living that are the province of the occupational therapist. In some clinics they are not, however, confined to teaching upper limb amputees, but also train lower limb amputees in activities of daily living.

THE NURSE

With the expanding role of nurses in all aspects of care of the disabled patient, some clinics have begun to include a nurse in the amputee clinic setting. It is quite true that the nurse's primary role has been caring for the amputee in the hospital and thus has a very important role in the immediate postoperative phase. A nurse who is well versed in rehabilitation of the amputee is quick to recognize possible complications, such as pressure sores, contractures of knee or hip joints, persistent edema or stasis, and generalized weakness that may inhibit the patient's ambulation using a walker or crutches. The nurse may be the first to recognize a psychological problem resulting from the trauma of the amputation surgery.

In the amputee clinic setting the nurse can interview and observe the patient and is afforded an opportunity to assess ability in activities of daily living. Before each patient is called into the clinic area, the rehabilitation nurse might relate information that the patient hesitates to mention to the team. Under optimal conditions the nurse should visit the patient preoperatively and postoperatively. During these visits the concept of the amputee clinic should be introduced, and its operation explained. Thus the nurse's personal acquaintance may provide some degree of insight into each patient's problems prior to definitive evaluation.

THE VOCATIONAL COUNSELOR

Many clinics, particularly those servicing patients injured at work or young adults who may need to make an adjustment in their job situation, will benefit from the services of a vocational rehabilitation counselor. These individuals will be able to assess the work ability of the amputee and suggest necessary job adjustments based on their knowledge of various job requirements. They also have knowledge of the many training or retraining courses available to these individuals. Many states have active rehabilitation counseling programs that can furnish consultation either while the patient is physically in the clinic or later by referral to their offices.

THE SOCIAL WORKER

Social workers have become an important part of medical practice generally, but are very important in situations involving amputees. They are trained to observe patient behavior and quickly recognize areas that may provoke anxiety, such as loss of body image, fear or job loss or work ability, fear of family rejection, and fear of inability to pay for the cost of their treatment, including prostheses. Social workers have special knowledge of agencies that can help support the patient in recovery and provide financial aid for obtaining a prosthesis. Social workers are a valuable liaison between the clinic and the patient's family and may relay to the clinic team family fears that may undermine a patient's progress in rehabilitation.

THE COORDINATOR OF AMPUTEE CLINIC ACTIVITIES

Most amputee clinics have a member who coordinates the activities of the clinic, arranges appointments for the patient, contacts the prosthetic facilities for future or present appointments, provides the necessary records for each clinic visit, and schedules appointments for therapy. In the Veterans Administration, this role has been performed by the prosthetics representative, a full-time employee of the Veterans Administration, with primary responsibilities in the area of prosthetics and orthotics. The coordinator supervises activities in the amputee clinics and provides the necessary liaison between the patient and team members.

In conclusion, the amputee clinic has proven to be the most appropriate mechanism for providing amputees with the short-term and long-term management necessary for optimal rehabilitation.

PART TWO

The upper limb

CHAPTER 7

Kinesiology and functional characteristics of the upper limb

SHAHAN K. SARRAFIAN

The functional capacity of the upper limb is determined by the shoulder complex, elbow, wrist, and hand, developing multiple integrated spheres of action. Given the normal proportion of limb segments, this capacity is limited in relationship to the surrounding space. In the standing position the upper limb field of motion reaches the midthigh region. Any more distal point on the lower extremity or on the ground is reached through mobility provided by the hip, knee, ankle, and trunk (Fig. 7-1). Furthermore, a distant point in space comes within the reach of the upper limb action through a functional integration with gait.

A maximum arcuate field or envelope of action termed "E_1" (Fig. 7-2) is traced by the most distal point of the upper extremity through the motion of the shoulder complex, all other joints being held in extension. Within this envelope, the elbow, wrist, and hand develop their own fields of motion, E_2, E_3, and E_4. These contained capabilities enrich the functional performances of the upper extremity.

SHOULDER COMPLEX

Motion in the frontal or coronal plane

When the arm and forearm are held in the anatomic position, the antecubital surface facing anteriorly, the upper limb sweeps a circular surface in the frontal plane. The very distal point of the extremity traces an envelope of action E_1 (Fig. 7-3).

In position 1 the shoulder is in neutral rotation, and the extremity can be elevated in the outer half of the circle to positions 2 and 3. The elbow does not contribute to the functional exploration in this segment of the arc of motion. If the wrist is initially held in neutral rotation, the hand sweeps the space E_3, and the digits explore the interior of this space through E_4. Beyond position 3 the shoulder externally rotates, and complete elevation is achieved at position 4. In this second arc of motion the elbow explores the segment of the space through its action envelope E_2. The sweeping of the inner half of the coronal circle is now possible from position 4 to 5 through internal rotation of the shoulder. The elbow action dissipates. From position 5 to 6 the shoulder externally rotates, and elbow functional capability in this plane reappears, whereas with further external rotation from position 6 to 1, the elbow action dissipates again.

When the upper limb is maintained in neutral rotation at the shoulder, the motion is quite restricted (Fig. 7-4), and no elbow action is possible in this plane. Maintaining the extremity in complete external rotation permits the exploration of the outer half of the frontal circle with ease whereas any functional development in the inner half is very restricted. The elbow envelope of action is clearly visible now in all positions (Fig. 7-2).

Placement of the limb in complete internal rotation restricts significantly the field of motion

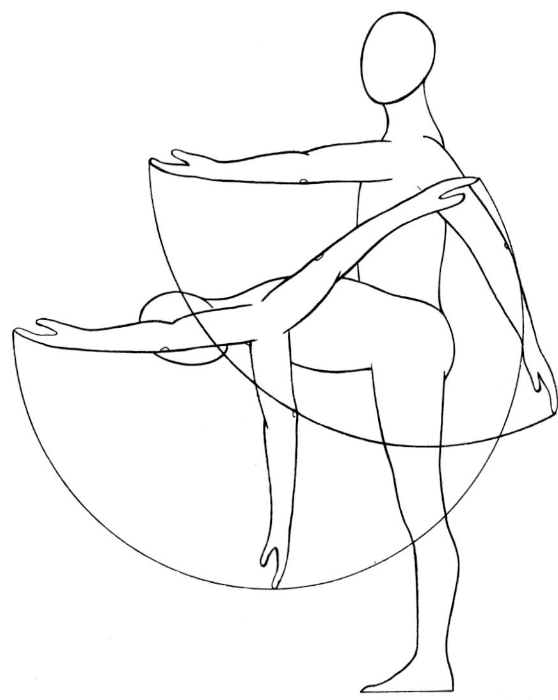

Fig. 7-1. Field of motion of upper limb is circle, and length of extremity is radius. Any further point in space or distal to midthigh is reached through associated hip, knee, ankle, and trunk motion.

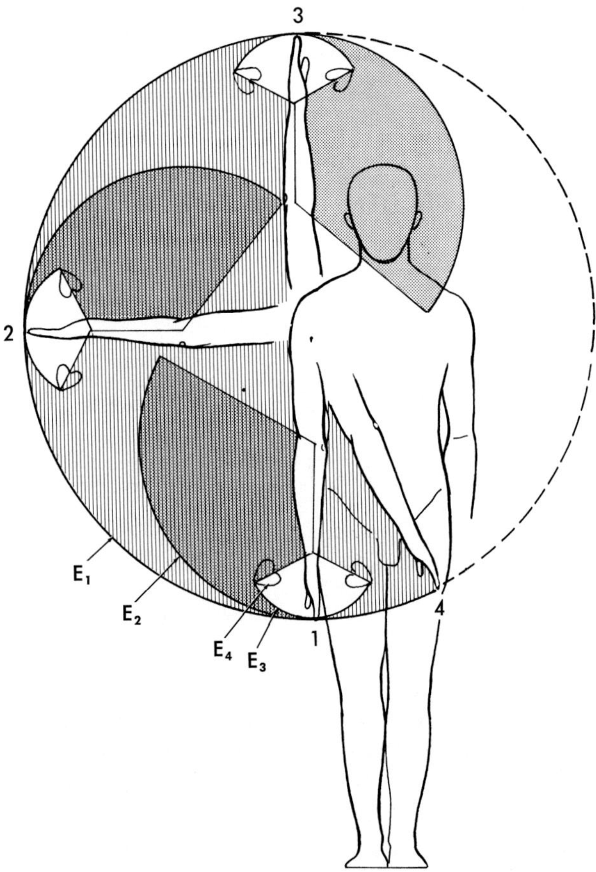

Fig. 7-2. Elevation of externally rotated upper limb in frontal plane. Complete exploration of outer half of circle is possible through envelope of action E_1. Elbow allows sweeping of space E_2. Wrist develops motion field E_3. Spiral envelope of motion E_4 is determined by finger motion.

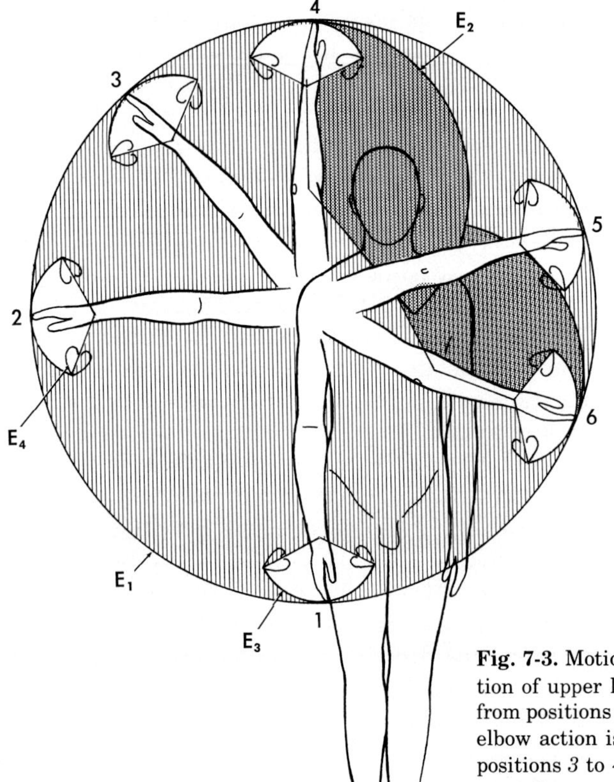

Fig. 7-3. Motion in frontal plane, starting with neutral position of upper limb, position *1*. It is possible to explore space from positions *1* to *2* without associated external rotation. No elbow action is possible then. Limb is further elevated from positions *3* to *4* through association of external rotation. Descent from positions *4* to *5* involves internal rotation. From positions *5* to *6* and *1*, extremity derotates to reach neutral position.

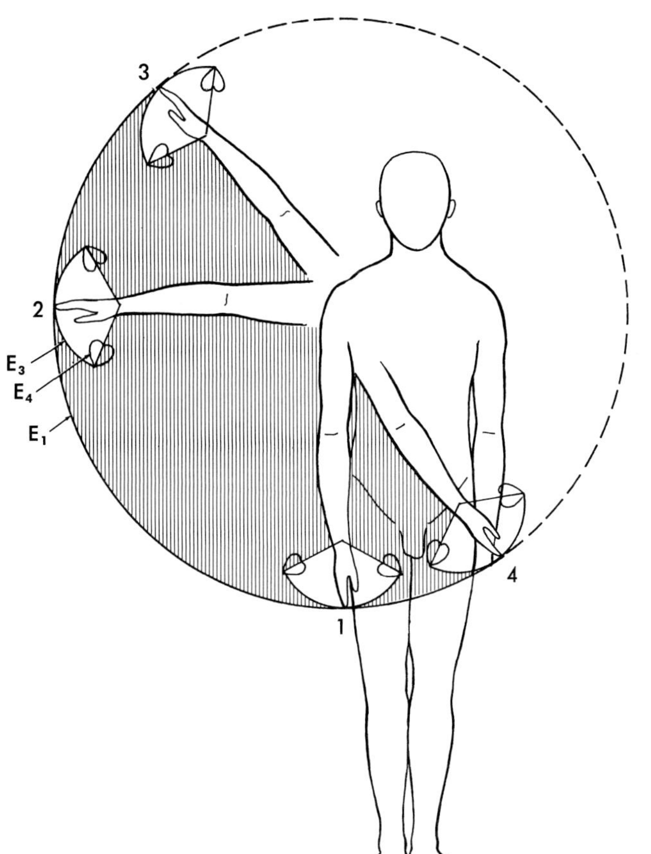

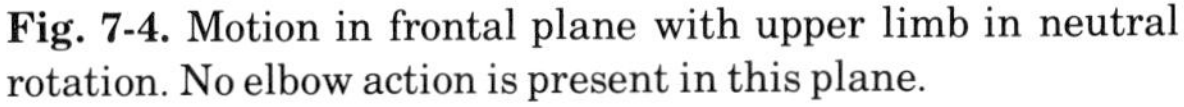
Fig. 7-4. Motion in frontal plane with upper limb in neutral rotation. No elbow action is present in this plane.

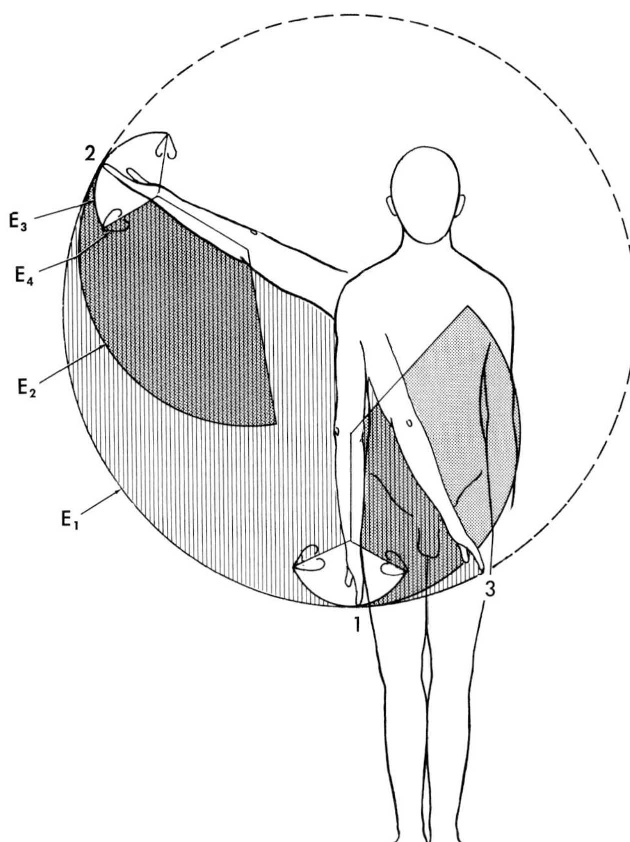

Fig. 7-5. Motion in frontal plane with upper limb in complete internal rotation. Field of motion E_1 is limited, but elbow motion is possible exploring space E_2. Wrist and digits are continuously functional.

(Fig. 7-5). Elbow action is possible from position 1 to 2. The coronal plane is also explored posteriorly in the inner half space (Fig. 7-6). With a position of internal rotation at the shoulder the limb traces a small arc of displacement just enough for the elbow, wrist, and hand to sweep the surface corresponding to the gluteal area and up to the opposite scapular region. From position 3 the elbow envelope of action scans the posterior aspect of the head, neck, and shoulder.

During the elevation of the upper extremity in the frontal plane, the motion is determined by the scapulohumeral joint and the scapulothoracic upward rotation. The acromioclavicular and sternoclavicular joints participate also in a synchronized manner (Fig. 7-7). External rotation accompanies the elevation for the performance of a smooth motion. Beyond 90 degrees of elevation this external rotation is necessary to free the greater tuberosity from the acromial process, and more humeral articular surface is offered to the opposing glenoid (Fig. 7-8).

From 0 to 30 degrees of elevation (Fig. 7-7) the motion occurs at the scapulohumeral joint, and the scapular motion is variable. This is the "setting phase" of the scapular motion. In the remaining arc of motion of 150 degrees the scapulohumeral (SH) joint motion and the scapulothoracic (ST) motion of upward rotation participate with the ratio of $\frac{SH}{ST} = \frac{2}{1}$ as measured in the frontal plane. The total contribution of the scapulohumeral joint is 130 degrees. The clavicle does not remain still. In the initial 90 degrees of motion the clavicle is elevated at the sternoclavicular joint for about 40 degrees, and in the second half of the arc of motion the clavicle rotates on its long axis for another 40 to 50 degrees.[8] A combined acromioclavicular motion of 20 degrees

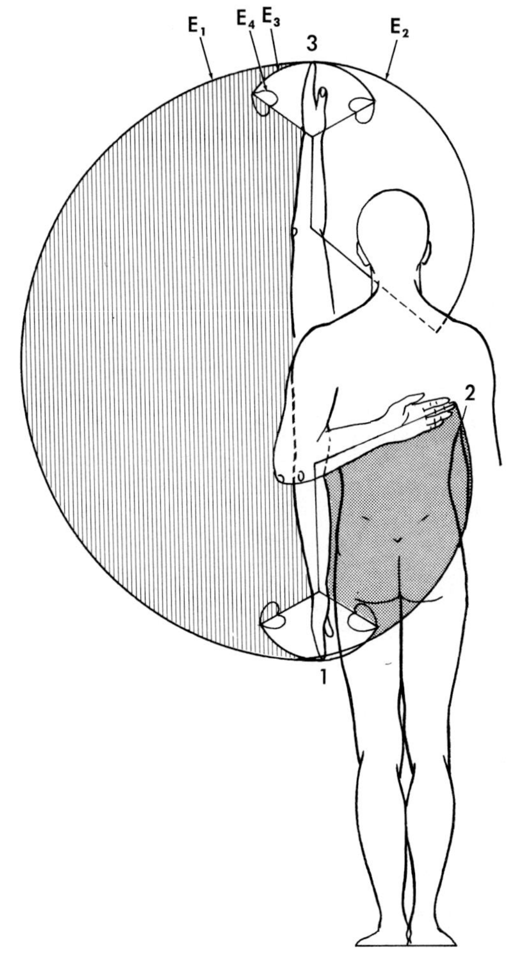

Fig. 7-6. Motion in frontal plane posterior to body. Gluteal area and mid and lower back are within reach of internally rotated upper limb, position *1*, combined to elbow field of motion, position *2*. Posterior aspect of neck and shoulders is reached by external rotation, position *3*, combined to elbow field of motion E_2.

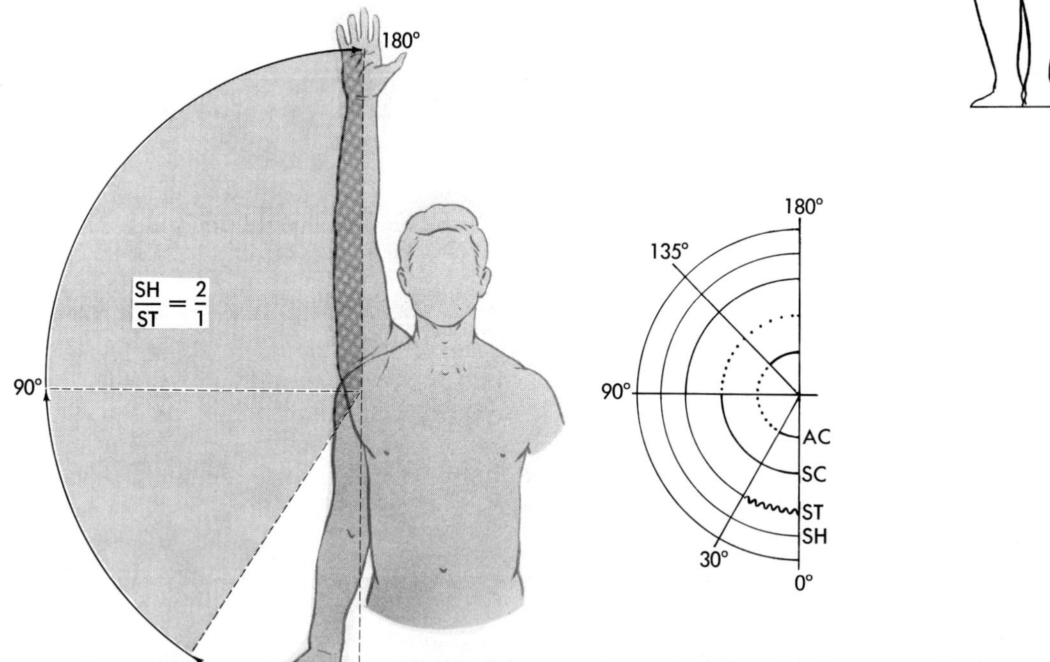

Fig. 7-7. Elevation of upper limb from 0 to 180 degrees. From 0 to 30 degrees, motion is mostly scapulohumeral. Scapulothoracic motion is variable. From 30 to 180 degrees, there is relationship between scapulohumeral and scapulothoracic motion with ratio $\frac{\text{SH}}{\text{ST}} = \frac{2}{1} = \frac{100 \text{ degrees}}{50 \text{ degrees}}$. Sternoclavicular motion in form of clavicular elevation of 40 degrees occurs during initial 90 degrees. From there on clavicular rotation on long axis of 40 to 50 degrees occurs. Acromioclavicular motion occurs from 0 to 30 degrees and then from 135 to 180 degrees with range of motion of 20 degrees.

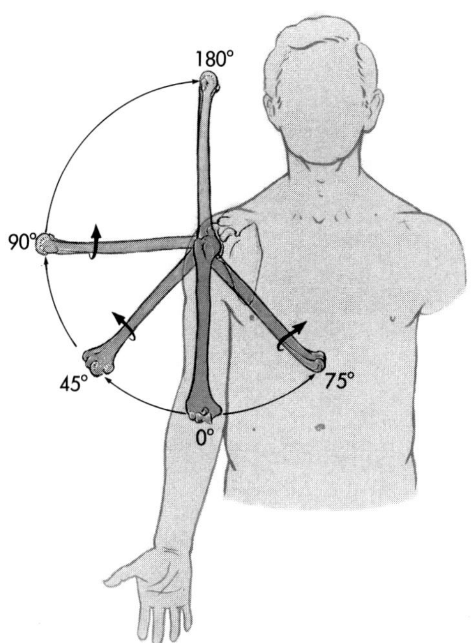

Fig. 7-8. Natural elevation of upper limb in frontal plane involves 90 degrees of external rotation. Elevation in lower and inner segment of circle involves internal rotation.

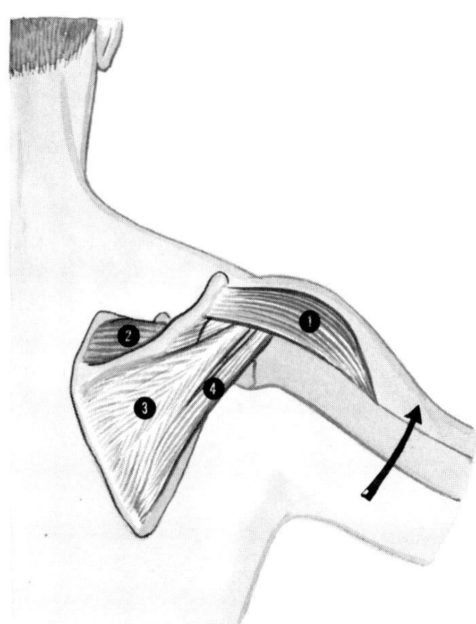

Fig. 7-9. Elevators at scapulohumeral joint in frontal plane: *1*, middle deltoid; *2*, supraspinatus; *3*, infraspinatus; *4*, teres minor; and subscapularis (not shown), anteriorly.

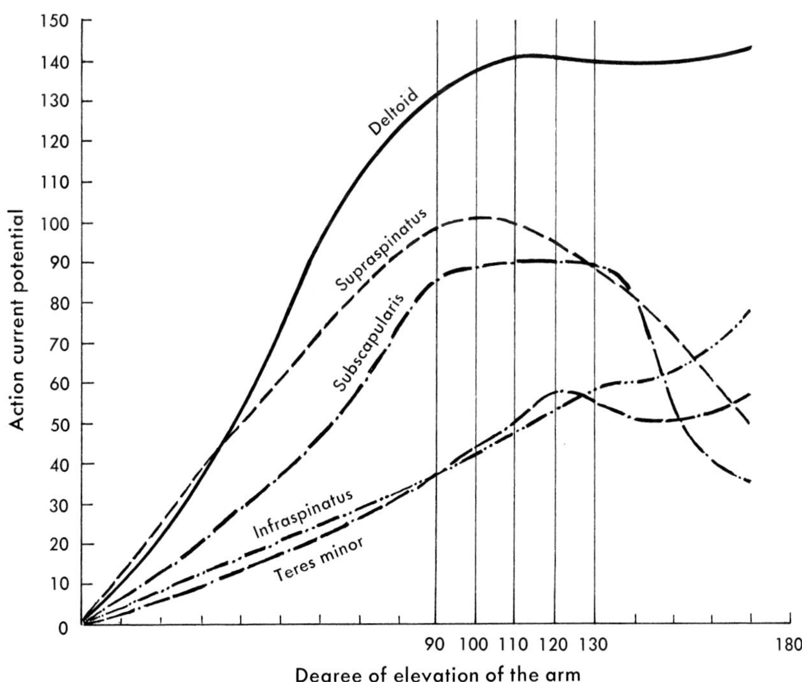

Fig. 7-10. Electromyographic activity of elevators at scapulohumeral joint in frontal plane. All five muscles are active from 0 to 90 degrees. Beyond 110 degrees deltoid holds maximum level of activity. Supraspinatus decreases in activity after 100 degrees. Infraspinatus and teres minor maintain high levels of activity during second half of elevation to ensure necessary external rotation of shoulder. (From Inman, V. T., Saunders, M., and Abbott, L. C.: J. Bone Joint Surg. **26**:1-30, Jan., 1944.)

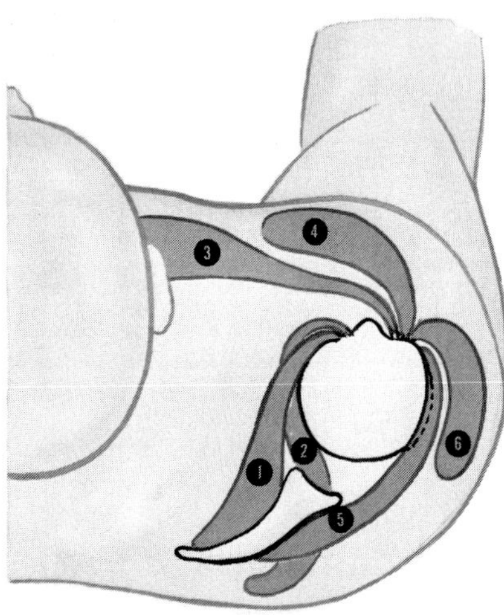

Fig. 7-11. Rotators at scapulohumeral joint. Internal rotators: *1*, subscapularis; *2*, latissimus dorsi and teres major; *3*, pectoralis major; *4*, anterior deltoid. External rotators: *5*, infraspinatus and teres minor; *6*, posterior deltoid.

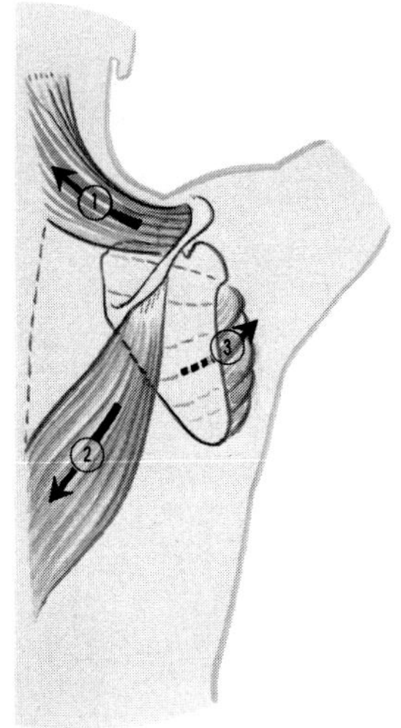

Fig. 7-12. Upward rotation of scapula: *1*, upper trapezius; *2*, lower trapezius; *3*, serratus anterior.

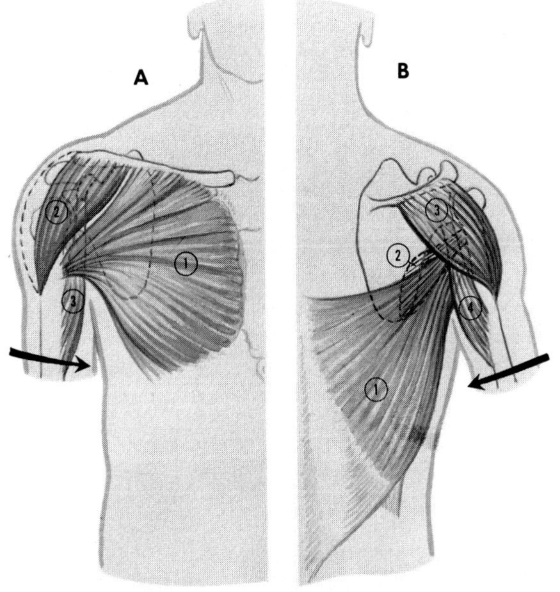

Fig. 7-13. Adductors at scapulohumeral joint. A, Anterior adductors: *1*, pectoralis major; *2*, anterior deltoid; *3*, coracobrachialis. B, Posterior adductors: *1*, latissimus dorsi; *2*, teres major; *3*, posterior deltoid; *4*, long head triceps.

occurs during the initial and terminal phases of the elevation.

The motor units responsible for the scapulohumeral elevation are the middle segment of the deltoid muscle and the components of the rotator cuff: the supraspinatus, infraspinatus, teres minor, and subscapularis muscles (Fig. 7-9).

The deltoid acts as the upper vector component of a force couple, whereas the rotator cuff stabilizes the humeral head and acts as the lower vector force of the couple. The electromyographic study of these muscles (Fig. 7-10)[8] indicates that the deltoid action potential increases steadily with elevation, reaches a maximum at 110 degrees, and maintains a plateau level of activity with a final peak at full elevation. The supraspinatus also reaches a peak at 110 degrees, and beyond this point its activity diminishes tracing a sine wave. The subscapularis reaches the peak activity at 100 degrees, maintains a plateau level up to 130 degrees, and diminishes rapidly in action. The teres minor reaches the maximum at 120 degrees and from there maintains the high level of activity, whereas the infraspinatus increases steadily in activity from the initial position to that of full elevation. The action of these two last muscles is necessary to continue the external rotation of the humerus during the last stage of the elevation. The posterior segment of the deltoid also participates as an external rotator (Fig. 7-11).

The motor units acting during the upward rotation of the scapula are the upper and lower segments of the trapezius and the lower digitations of the serratus anterior. They act on the scapula as a force couple (Fig. 7-12).

When the upper limb moves in the lower and inner quadrant of the envelope of action E_1, it is adducted and internally rotated. The internal rotation is brought about by the subscapularis, pectoralis major, and anterior segments of the deltoid (Fig. 7-11). Adduction is determined by the latter two muscles, supplemented by the ac-

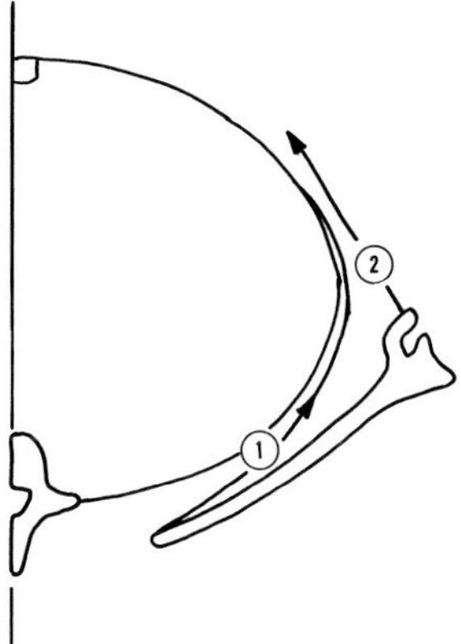

Fig. 7-14. Abductors or protractors of scapula: *1,* serratus anterior; *2,* pectoralis minor.

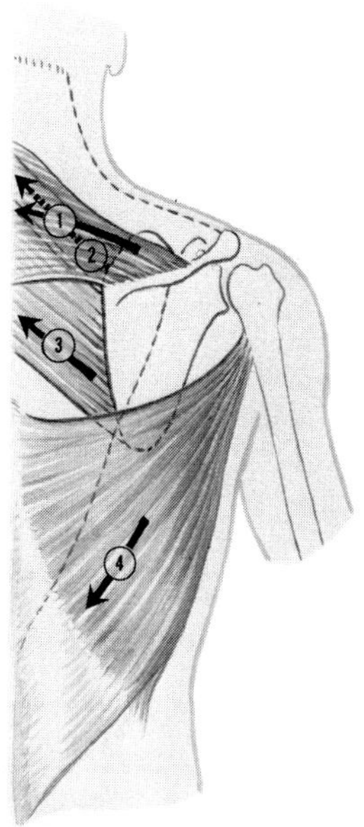

Fig. 7-15. Adductors or retractors of scapula: *1,* middle trapezius; *2* and *3,* rhomboidei minor and major; *4,* latissimus dorsi.

tion of the coracobrachialis (Fig. 7-13). During the anterior adduction–internal rotation, the scapula is abducted. This motion is controlled by the serratus anterior and the pectoralis minor (Fig. 7-14). When the upper limb moves in a similar lower and inner quadrant, but posterior to the body, the limb is once more adducted and internally rotated. The posterior adduction is brought about by the latissimus dorsi, teres major, long head of the triceps, and posterior segment of the deltoid (Fig. 7-13). The latissimus dorsi and teres major determine also the associated internal rotation (Fig. 7-11). During this same motion, the scapula is adducted by the middle segment of the trapezius and the combined action of the rhomboidei and latissimus dorsi (Fig. 7-15). When the upper limb is in a maximum position of elevation and is brought down in the frontal plane in the outer half circle, the scapula makes a downward rotation. This is determined by the combined action of the latissimus dorsi, lower segment of the pectoralis major, the pectoralis minor acting as the lower component for a force couple, and the levator scapulae, with the rhomboidei acting as the upper component of the rotational couple (Fig. 7-16). Downward stabilization of the limb in the frontal plane is also of important functional significance, such as in crutch walking or parallel bar exercising. This function is determined by the depressors of the shoulder complex: latissimus dorsi, lower segment of trapezius, lower segment of pectoralis major, pectoralis minor, and subclavius (Fig. 7-17).

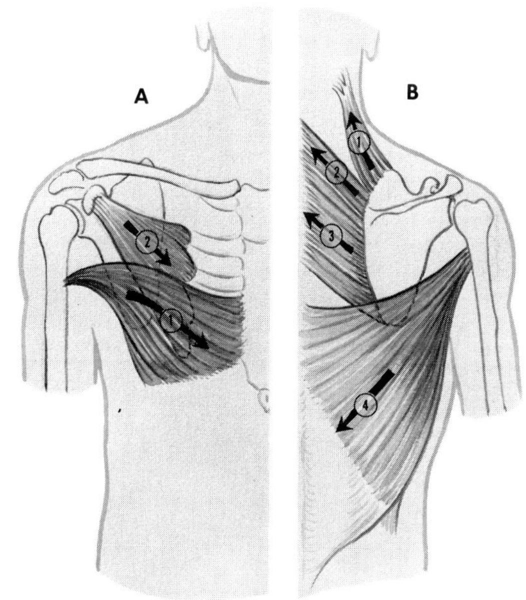

Fig. 7-16. Downward rotation of scapula. **A,** Anterior: *1,* lower segment pectoralis major; *2,* pectoralis minor. **B,** Posterior: *1,* levator scapula; *2* and *3,* rhomboidei minor and major; *4,* latissimus dorsi.

The upward stabilization in the frontal plane is also necessary for functional purposes, as in carrying heavy loads on the shoulders. This is controlled by the elevators of the scapula: levator scapulae, upper segment of trapezius, and rhomboidei (Fig. 7-18).

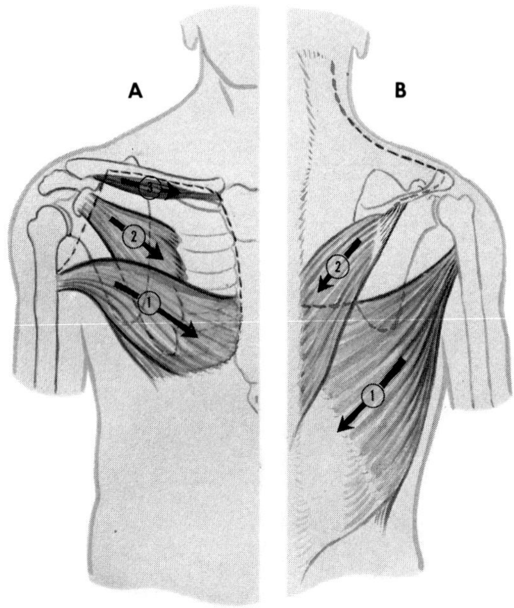

Fig. 7-17. Depressors of scapula. A, Anterior: *1,* lower segment pectoralis major; *2,* pectoralis minor; *3,* subclavius. B, Posterior: *1,* latissimus dorsi; *2,* lower segment trapezius.

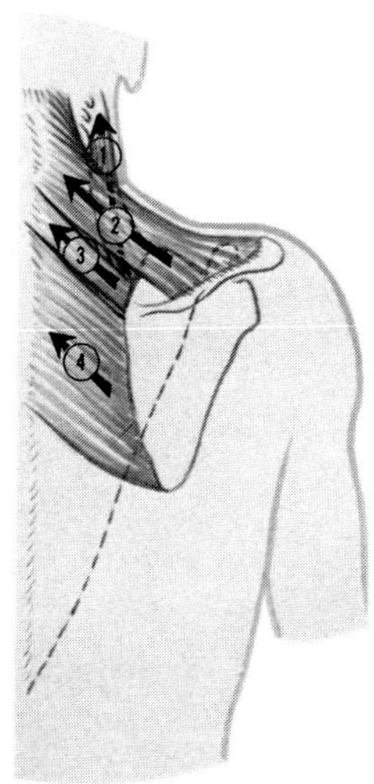

Fig. 7-18. Elevators of scapula: *1,* levator scapulae; *2,* upper segment of trapezius; *3* and *4,* rhomboidei minor and major.

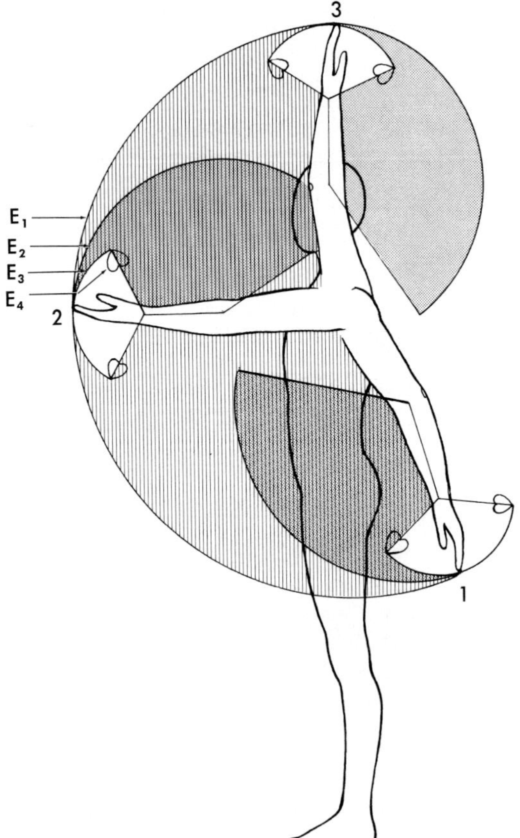

Fig. 7-19. Elevation in sagittal plane. Exploration of space from positions *1* to *3* is possible in neutral rotational position of shoulder. Elbow action E_2 is present in plane. In position *3* posterior segment of space is reached through elbow action.

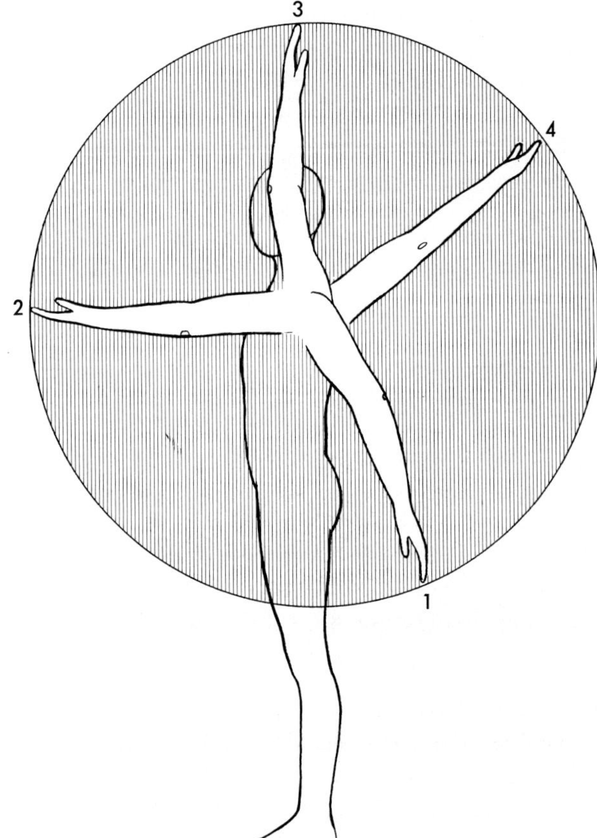

Fig. 7-20. Motion in sagittal plane. Posterior arc of motion from positions *3* to *4* is possible through internal rotation. From positions *4* to *1* extremity derotates to reach neutral position.

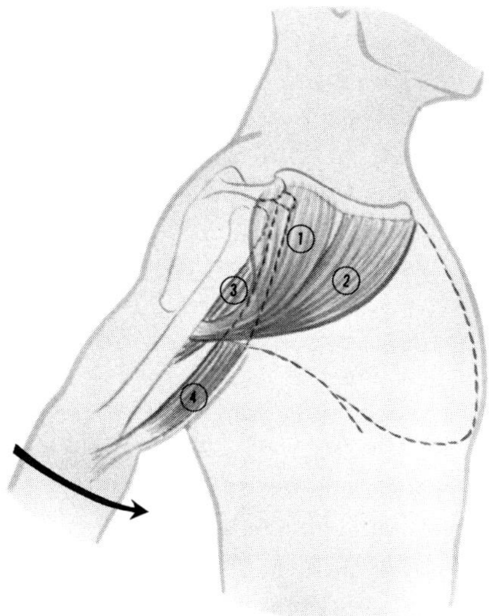

Fig. 7-21. Flexors at scapulohumeral joint: *1,* anterior segment of deltoid; *2,* clavicular segment of pectoralis major; *3,* coracobrachialis; *4,* biceps. Arrow indicates flexion.

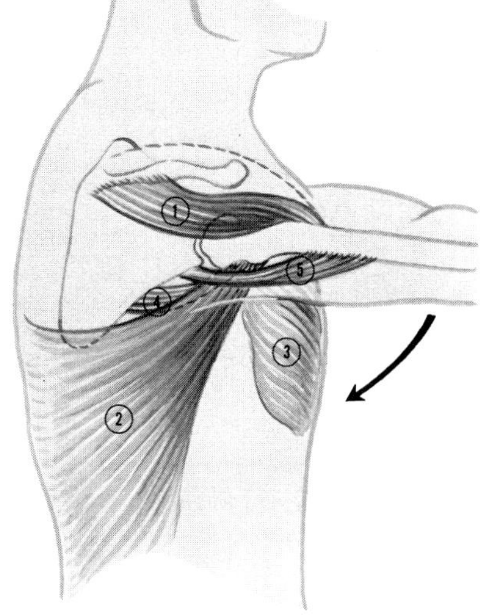

Fig. 7-22. Extensors at scapulohumeral joint: *1,* posterior deltoid; *2,* latissimus dorsi; *3,* pectoralis major; *4,* teres major; *5,* long head triceps.

Motion in the sagittal plane

From a neutral rotational position the upper limb moves in the sagittal plane sweeping the surface from position 1 to 3 (Fig. 7-19). The elbow, wrist, and hand are capable of functioning in this plane through their envelopes of action, E_2, E_3, and E_4.

In position 3 the elbow action extends farther posteriorly, the hand reaching the posterior aspect of the shoulder. Further movement in the posterior half of the field is possible through the internal rotation of the shoulder followed by gradual external rotation to bring the limb to its neutral initial position (Fig. 7-20). The elevation of the upper limb or flexion from position 1 to 3 is determined by the anterior segment of the deltoid, biceps, coracobrachialis and clavicular head of the pectoralis major (Fig. 7-21). The rotator cuff is also active in stabilizing the humeral head. The scapulothoracic mechanism participates in the motion through upward scapular rotation in the ratio of $\frac{SH}{ST} = \frac{2}{1}$.[8] From the elevated position 3 the upper limb is brought down by the posterior segment of the deltoid, long head of the triceps, latissimus dorsi, and pectoralis major (Fig. 7-22). Beyond neutral the motion continues as extension, and all motors continue their action except the pectoralis major. The range of extension is 60 degrees (Fig. 7-23).[1] Contributors to this motion are gravity and downward rotators of the scapula.

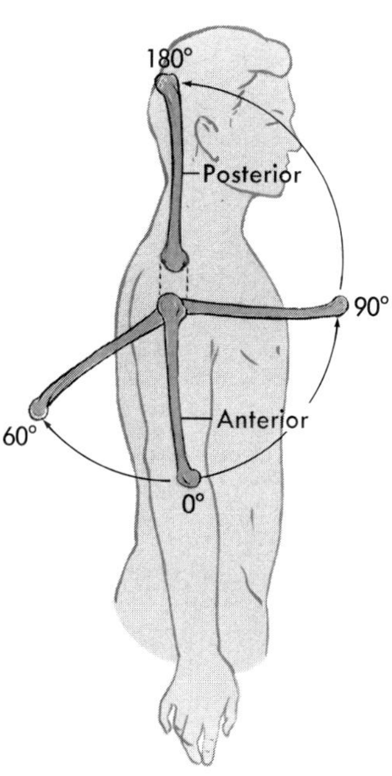

Fig. 7-23. Flexion at scapulohumeral joint is 180 degrees, and no combined rotation is necessary. Extension is 60 degrees.

Motion in the horizontal plane

When the upper extremity is elevated to 90 degrees in the frontal plane, the distal point of the limb scans the horizontal plane, tracing an arc of 165° degrees (Fig. 7-24).[1] The flexors and extensors of the scapulohumeral joint control the motion.

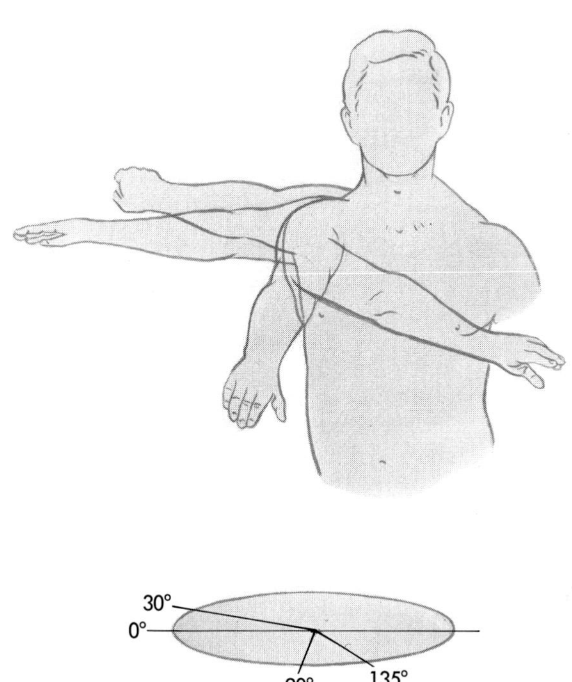

Fig. 7-24. Motion in horizontal plane: flexion of 135 degrees and extension of 30 degrees.

Rotary capability of the shoulder complex

When the upper extremity is held in the neutral rotational position at the shoulder and the elbow is flexed at 90 degrees, the distal point traces an arc of internal rotation of 80 degrees and an arc of external rotation of 60 degrees. With the shoulder elevated 90 degrees in the frontal plane, this rotary capability changes to 90 degrees of external rotation and 70 degrees of internal rotation (Fig. 7-25).[1]

ELBOW

The elbow joint determines an arc of motion, E_2, of 150 degrees. The orientation of the plane of action is closely influenced by the rotational position of the shoulder joint. When the arm is elevated in the frontal plane, for example, the envelope of action E_2 of the elbow is located in this plane if the shoulder is in external or internal rotation.

The main flexors of the elbow are the brachialis and the biceps. The brachioradialis and pronator teres are the accessory flexors (Fig. 7-26). There is an intricate interplay and a wide range of participation in the elbow flexors.[13] The brachialis is the baseline flexor, being active at any rotational position of the forearm and any speed and with or

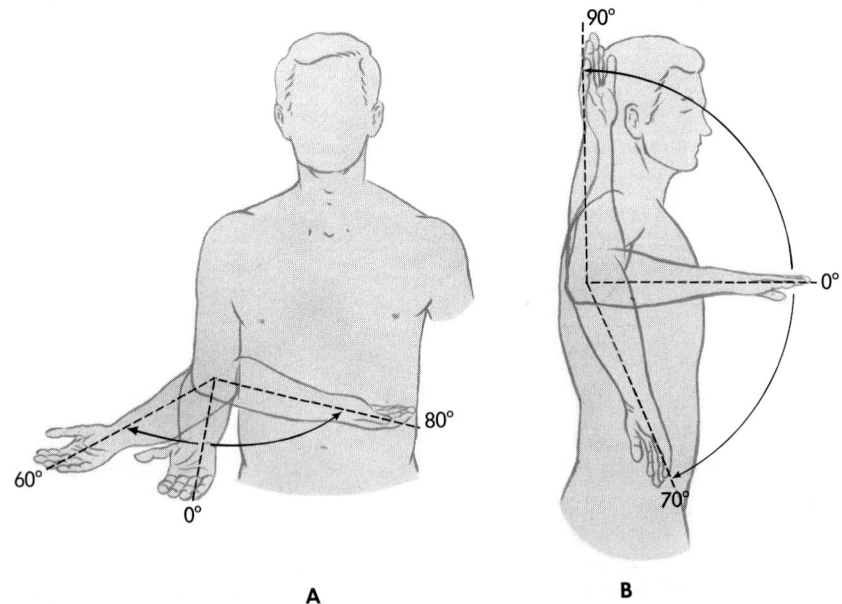

Fig. 7-25. Rotation at scapulohumeral joint. **A,** Rotation with arm in neutral elevation: external rotation 60 degrees and internal rotation 80 degrees. **B,** Rotation with arm elevated 90 degrees: external rotation 90 degrees and internal rotation 70 degrees.

without load applied to the flexing forearm (Fig. 7-27). It is also active in flexed elbow posture or during extension of the forearm, acting then as an antigravity muscle. The biceps is a flexor of the supine forearm, and its activity is evident as soon as slight resistance is applied. Deactivation occurs when the forearm is pronated, unless significant resistance is applied to the pronated flexing forearm.[14]

The biceps is minimally active as antigravity muscle or in maintaining a static flexed position. The brachioradialis is active when the forearm is flexing rapidly at any rotational position. It is also a reserve flexor during flexion against resistance, especially in neutral rotation of the forearm. The pronator teres does not participate as a flexor unless resistance is encountered during flexion.

The extensor of the elbow is the triceps assisted by the anconeus (Fig. 7-28). The baseline worker during extension is the medial head of the triceps. Without load being applied, the long head is not active, whereas the lateral head is minimally active. These last two reserve extensors come into play when resistance is applied to the motion of extension (Fig. 7-29).[19]

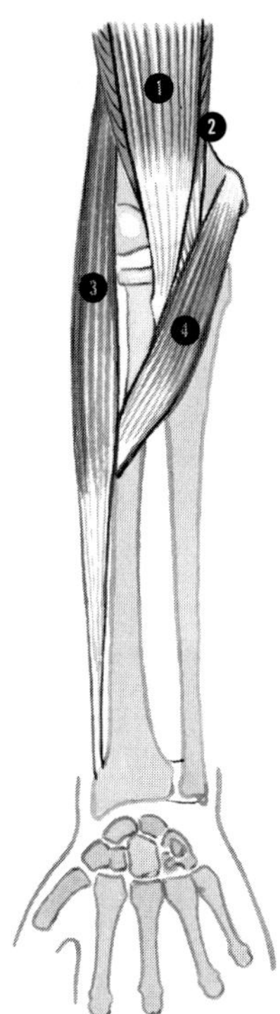

Fig. 7-26. Elbow flexors: *1,* biceps, reserve flexor; *2,* brachialis, main flexor; *3,* brachioradialis, accessory flexor; *4,* pronator teres, accessory flexor.

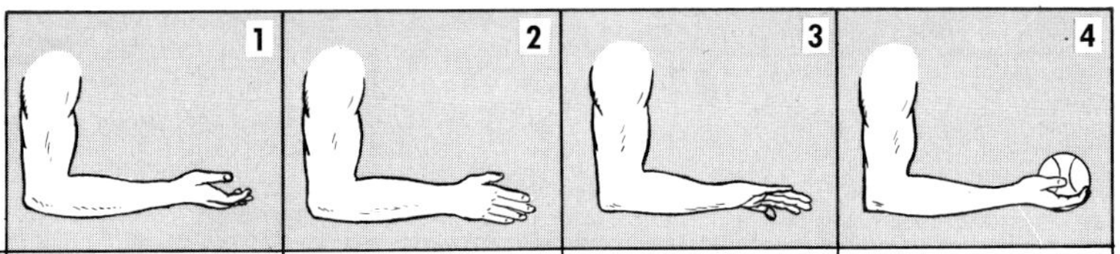

	1	2	3	4
BRACHIALIS	+ +	+ +	+ +	+ + +
BICEPS	+	+	− to ±	+ + +
BRACHIORADIALIS	+	+ +	+	+ +
PRONATOR TERES	−	−	−	+ +

Fig. 7-27. Elbow flexion; *1,* flexion in supination without resistance; *2,* flexion in neutral without resistance; *3,* flexion in pronation without resistance; *4,* flexion in supination with resistance. Brachialis is baseline flexor. Biceps is reserve flexor. It is flexor of supine forearm especially when resistance is encountered. Its action is minimum in pronation. Brachioradialis is more active in neutral and against resistance. Pronator teres is active only against resistance. +++, Maximum activity; ++, mild activity; +, minimal activity; −, no activity.

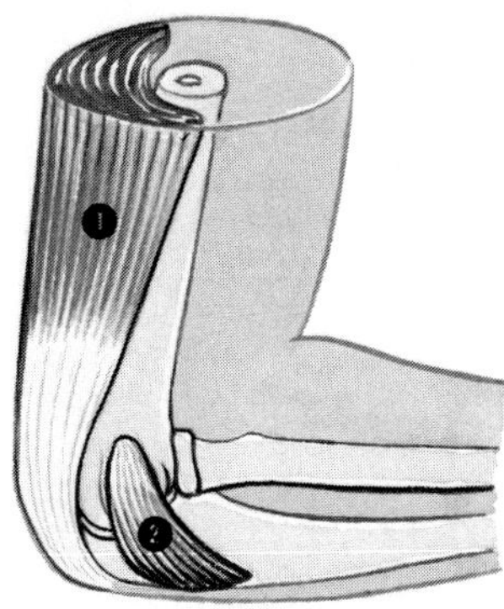

Fig. 7-28. Elbow extensors: *1,* triceps; *2,* anconeus.

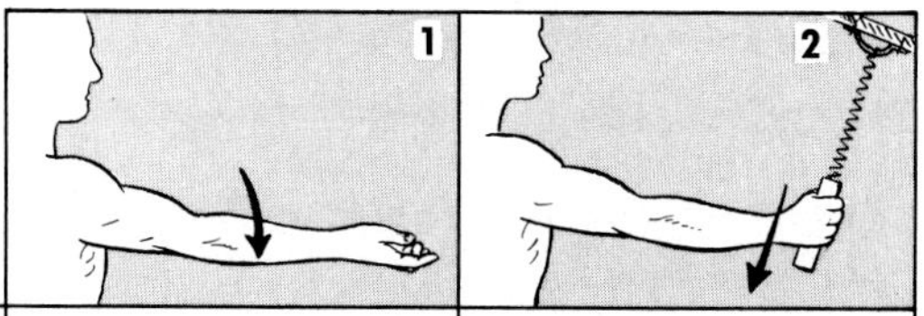

	1	2
TRICEPS MEDIAL HEAD	+ +	+ +
LATERAL HEAD	+	+ +
LONG HEAD	—	+ |

Fig. 7-29. Elbow extension: *1,* without resistance, medial head of triceps is main extensor assisted by lateral head; *2,* against resistance, all three heads of triceps are active. +++, Maximum activity; ++, mild activity; +, minimal activity; − no activity.

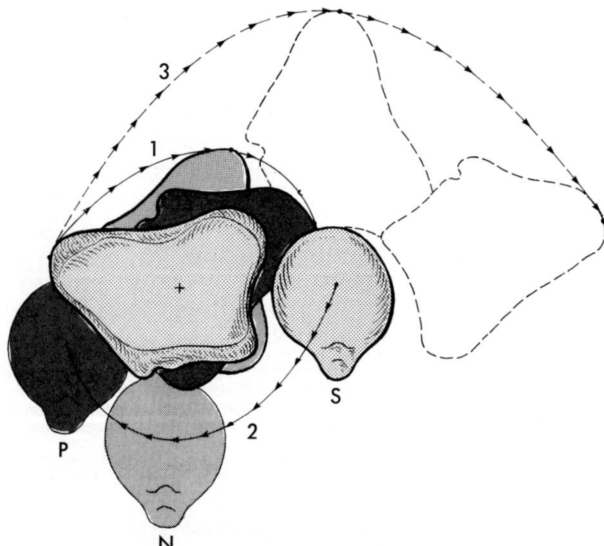

Fig. 7-30. Rotation at distal radioulnar joint. In habitual rotation axis passes through middle of distal radius, +. From supination to pronation radial styloid traces curve *1,* and head of ulna traces curve *2.* From supination, *S,* to neutral, *N,* head of ulna is extended and laterally displaced. From neutral, *N,* to pronation, *P,* it is flexed and further laterally displaced. When axis of motion passes through center of ulnar head, latter stays still during rotation, whereas radial styloid traces very large curve *3.* Location of axis of rotation is determined by peripheral point of fixation.[2]

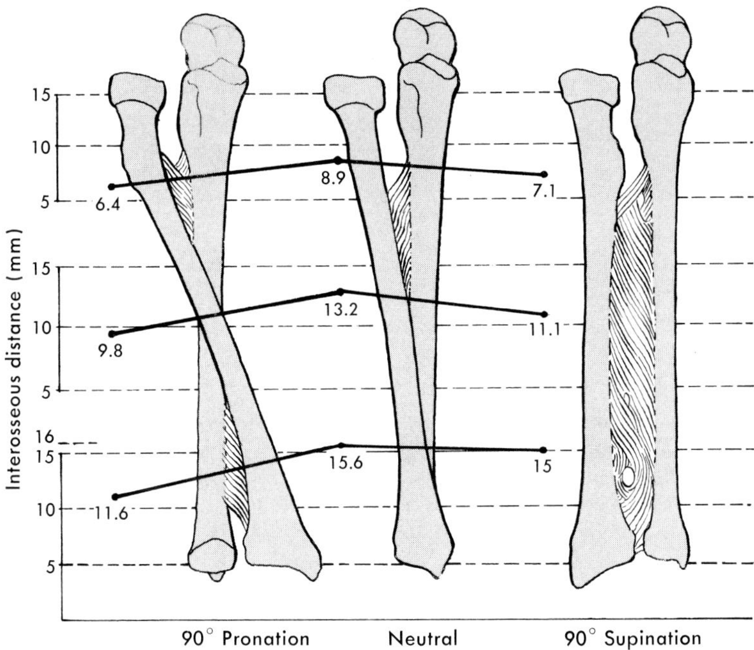

Fig. 7-31. Interosseous distance in pronation, neutral, and supination. Distance is maximum in neutral and minimum in pronation. (Modified from Christensen, J. B., Adams, J. P., Cho, K. O., and Miller, A.: Anat. Rec. **160**:261-271, 1968.)

FOREARM ROTATION

The average range of pronation-supination of the forearm with the elbow flexed at 90 degrees is 173 degrees measured at the level of the hand. The corresponding rotation measured at the wrist is 156 degrees.[4] The difference of 17 degrees indicates the participation of the radiocarpal and midcarpal joints. When the distal radius and the head of the ulna are aligned in the vertical plane delineating the neutral position at the level of the wrist, the hand is in a position of minimal supination of 11 degrees. The average range of pronation is 62 degrees, ranging from 49 degrees to 84 degrees. The average range of supination is 104 degrees, ranging from 86 degrees to 122 degrees.[4]

The axis of pronation-supination is variable in location. It extends from the center of the radial head to the distal end of the radius and ulna, passing "anywhere between the radial and ulnar styloid processes."[2] In the average habitual motion, the axis passes through the distal radius in line with the third metacarpal or the long finger. During this rotary motion the distal radius and the head of the ulna trace arcs of motion quite comparable in size (Fig. 7-30). Starting from the position of supination, the head of the ulna is extended and laterally displaced in the neutral position. In pronation the ulnar head is flexed and

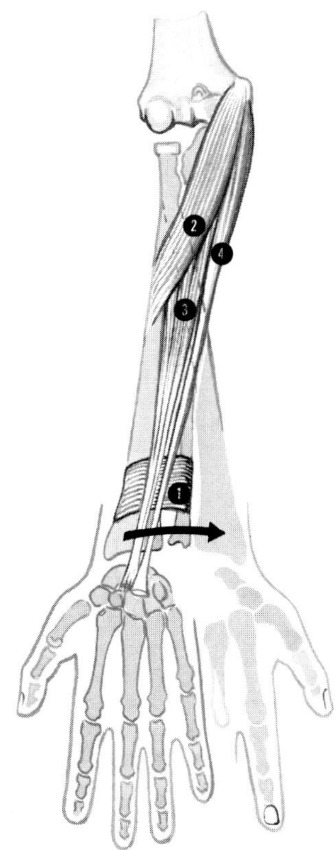

Fig. 7-32. Pronators of forearm: *1,* pronator quadratus: main pronator; *2,* pronator teres: reserve pronator; *3,* flexor carpi radialis: accessory pronator; *4,* palmaris longus: accessory pronator.

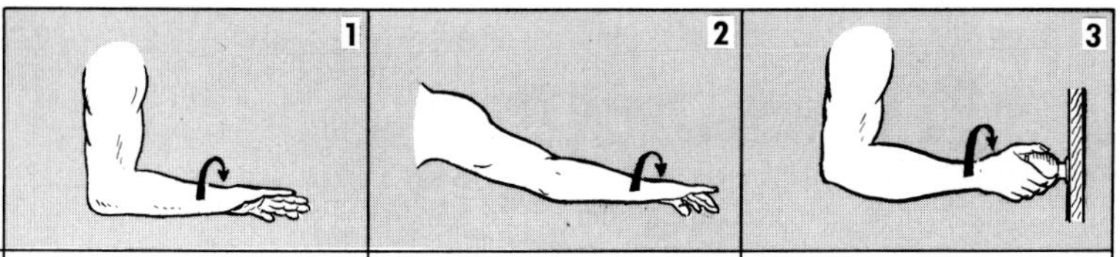

	1	2	3
PRONATOR TERES	+	+	+ + +
PRONATOR QUADRATUS	+ +	+ +	+ + +

Fig. 7-33. Pronation of forearm: *1,* with elbow flexed without resistance; *2,* with elbow extended without resistance; *3,* against resistance. Pronator quadratus is main pronator active at any position of elbow. Pronator teres increases in activity only against resistance or when speed is required. +++, Maximum activity; ++, mild activity; +, minimal activity.

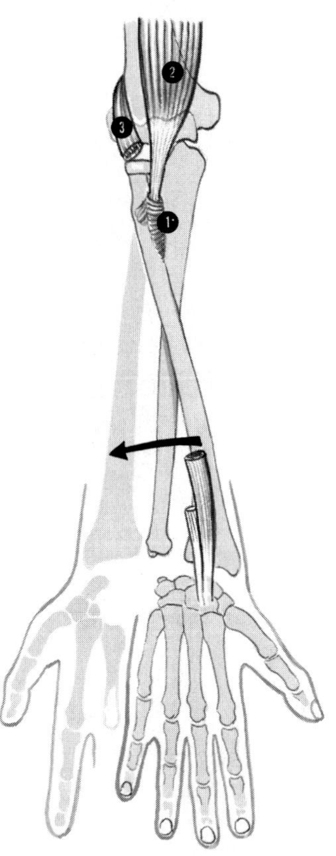

Fig. 7-34. Supinators of forearm: *1,* supinator: main supinator; *2,* biceps: reserve supinator; *3,* extensor carpi radialis longus and brevis: questionable accessory supinators. Arrow indicates supination.

further displaced laterally. When the hand rests on its ulnar border on a surface and rotation is initiated, the motion occurs around the axis passing through the head of the ulna and the little finger. The head of the ulna remains still. The hand then makes a circumferential transposition. The styloid process of the radius traces a large arc of motion (Fig. 7-30). When rotational motion occurs along an axis passing through the middle finger and near the radial styloid process, the head of the ulna traces a much larger arc of motion than the radius. One can easily appreciate the shift of the rotational axis by supinating and pronating the forearm, the elbow being held at 90 degrees flexion, with the tip of an extended finger applied against the wall or the border of a table. In other words, the peripheral point of fixation, through the finger or through the tool held in the hand, determines the location of the axis or pronation-supination. When the rotation occurs along the oblique axis, passing through the head of the ulna, the radial styloid traces an arc corresponding to the base of a cone. In full pronation the styloid process appears then to be less distal relative to the head of the ulna.[6]

The interosseous membrane uniting the radius and ulna relaxes or tenses during pronation-supination. The interosseous distance measured in the distal, middle, and proximal thirds of the forearm is the largest in neutral position and the smallest in full pronation (Fig. 7-31).[3] The tension in the membrane is thus minimal in full pronation. During a fall on the outstretched pronated hand, the interosseous membrane is not the main element of pressure transmission to the elbow through the ulna. When load is applied to the forearm from a distoproximal direction, the radius transmits directly to the humerus 57% of the load and to the ulna 43%.[7]

The forearm is pronated by the pronator quad-

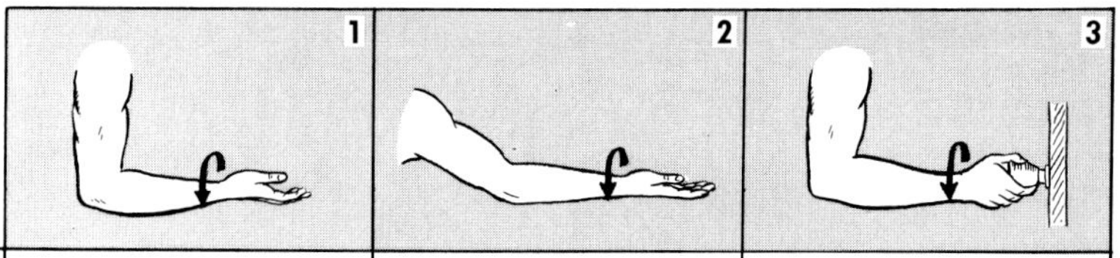

	1	2	3
SUPINATOR	+ +	+ +	+ + +
BICEPS	+	±	+ + +

Fig. 7-35. Supination of forearm: *1,* with elbow flexed without resistance; *2,* with elbow extended without resistance; *3,* against resistance. +++, Maximum activity; ++, mild activity; +, minimal activity; –, no activity. Supinator is main supinator. Biceps is reserve supinator functioning best with elbow flexed at 90 degrees or when speed and/or power is required.

ratus and pronator teres (Fig. 7-32). The main pronator is the pronator quadratus, the action of the muscle being independent from the position of the elbow. The pronator teres is a reserve pronator reinforcing the power when speed is required or resistance is applied to the motion (Fig. 7-33).[14] The participation of the accessory pronators, flexor carpi radialis and palmaris longus, is controversial. The forearm is supinated by the supinator (Fig. 7-34). The biceps is the reserve supinator, reinforcing the action when fast supination is required or resistance is encountered (Fig. 7-35). The extensor carpi radialis longus and brevis are to be mentioned as accessory supinators.

WRIST

The wrist acts as a universal joint. It develops a spheroid type of motion envelope E_3 (Fig. 7-36), which permits the hand to move without digital motion. The wrist flexes, extends, deviates laterally, and participates minimally in pronation-supination. The wrist traces an arc of 121 degrees of flexion-extention with a minimum of 84 degrees and a maximum of 169 degrees. The average arc of extension is 55 degrees, ranging from 31 degrees to 79 degrees, and the average arc of flexion is 66 degrees, ranging from 38 degrees to 102 degrees, as measured on fifty-five normal adult wrists.[18] The radiocarpal and midcarpal joints participate in this motion, and both flexion and extension are initiated in the midcarpal joint (Fig. 7-37). Starting from the neutral position, when the wrist flexes, the average range of flexion is 40 degrees at the midcarpal joint and 26 degrees at the radiocarpal joint. The midcarpal joint contributes 60% of the arc of flexion, and the radiocarpal joint contributes 40%. During extension the average range of extension is 19 degrees at the midcarpal joint and 37 degrees at the radiocarpal joint. The midcarpal joint contributes 33.5% of the arc of extension, and the radiocarpal joint contributes 66.5% (Fig. 7-38).[17] The scaphoid belongs anatomically to both rows, and yet functionally it is part of the distal row in extension and of the proximal

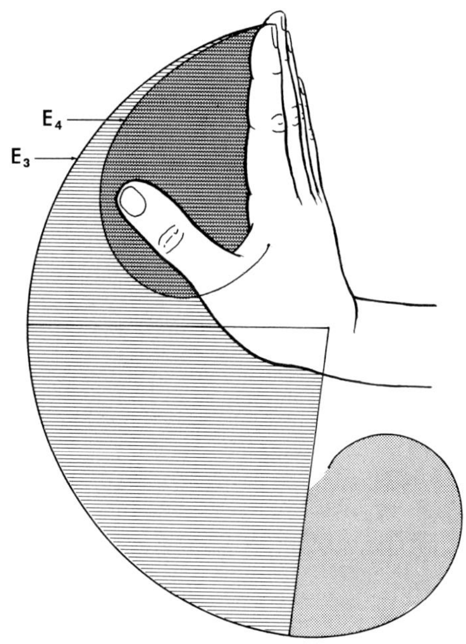

Fig. 7-36. Field of motion of wrist and hand: E_3, action envelope of wrist; E_4, action envelope of finger tracing equiangular spiral.[11] Field of motion of finger is within E_3 when wrist is extended or projects proximally when wrist is flexed.

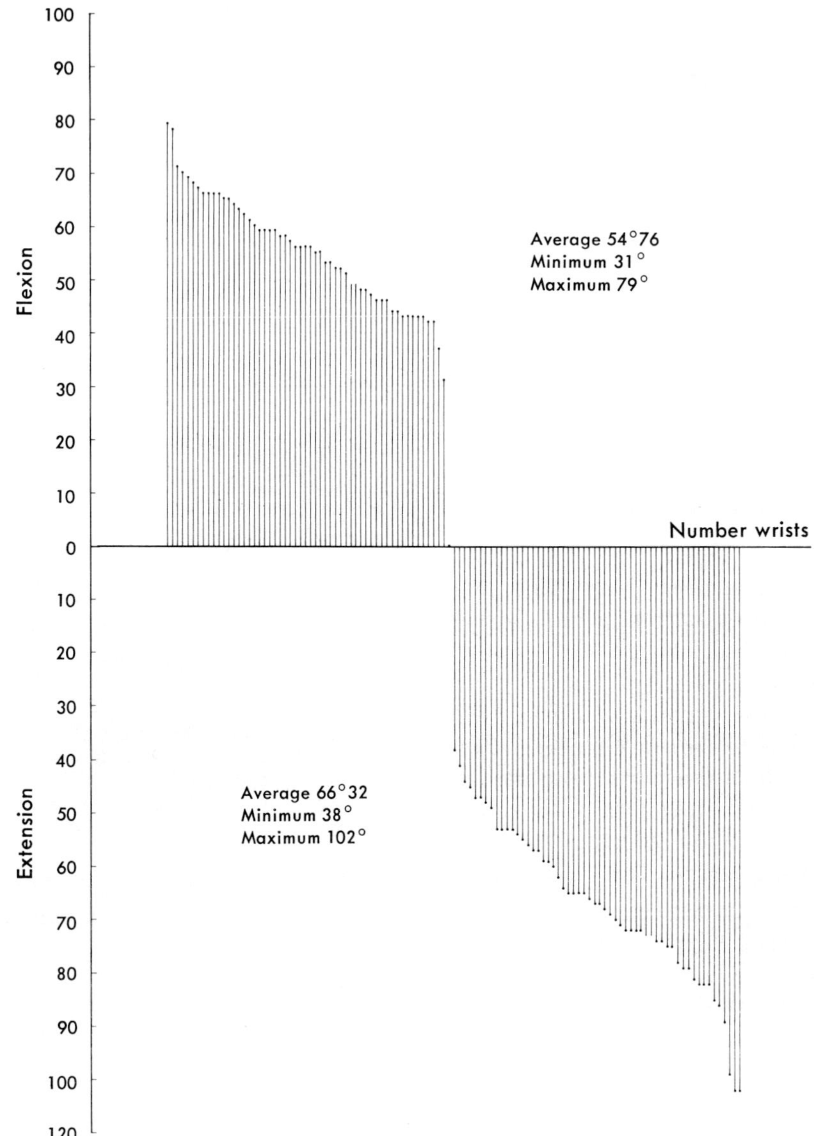

Fig. 7-37. Radiocapitate motion in extension and flexion of wrist. (From Sarrafian, S. K., and Melamed, J. L.: Unpublished data, 1975.)

row in flexion.[17] This behavior of the scaphoid correlates well with the concept of the carpus becoming a rigid "close-pack" mass in extension and "loose-pack" mass in flexion.[14] The rigidity of the carpal mass in extension favors the fracture of the scaphoid or the distal end of the radius on impact. The combination of wrist extension and pronation-supination permits the hand to explore the outer half of a circle (Fig. 7-39). The flexed wrist when rotated permits the hand to explore the inner half of the circle (Fig. 7-40). This latter motion is concerned more with functional activities related to our body. Functionally the hand is used more frequently with the wrist extended and radially deviated or with flexion combined to ulnar deviation.

The wrist is flexed by the flexor carpi radialis, flexor carpiulnaris, and palmaris longus. The long digital flexors are the accessory flexors of the wrist. The wrist extenders are the extensor carpi radialis longus, brevis, and the extensor carpiulnaris. The digital extensors are the accessory extensors of the wrist. The motion of lateral deviation of the wrist averages 40 degrees, with 30 degrees in the ulnar direction and 15 degrees on the radial side. The proximal and distal rows of the carpus participate and move in the opposite direction. During ulnar deviation the distal row

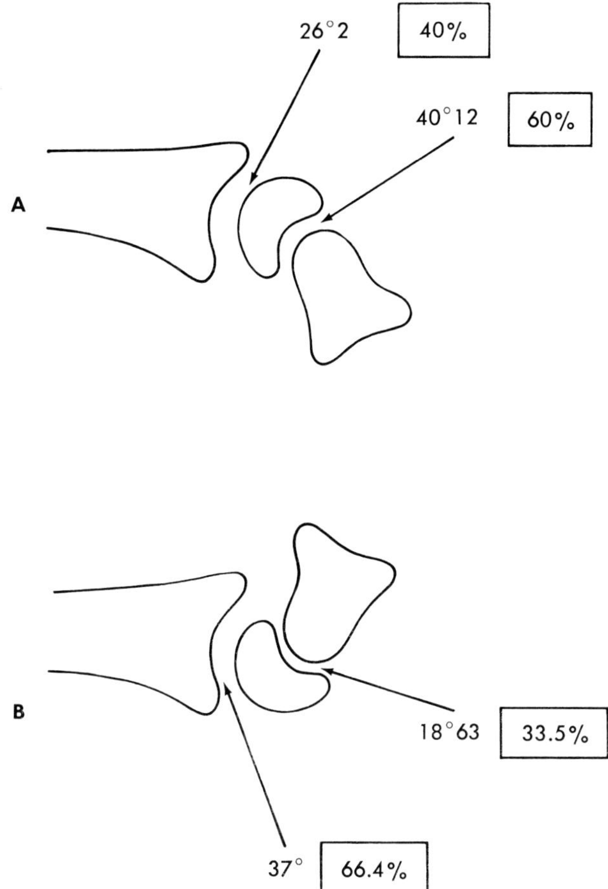

Fig. 7-38. Contribution of radiocarpal and midcarpal joints to flexion-extension. A, Flexion: 60% is midcarpal, and 40% is radiocarpal. B, Extension: 33.5% is midcarpal, and 66.4% is radiocarpal. (From Sarrafian, S. K., Melamed, J. L., and Goshgarian, G. M.: Clin. Orthop. 126:153-159, July-Aug., 1977.)

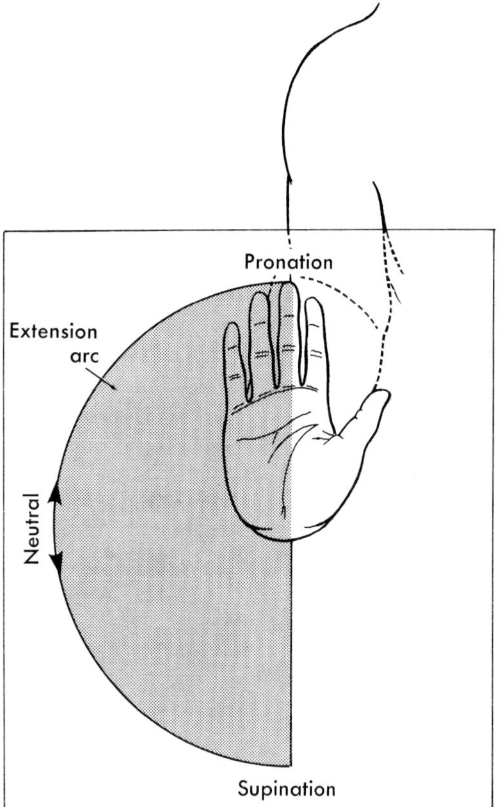

Fig. 7-39. Extended wrist, when rotated, explores outer half of circle, which is base of spheroid E_3.

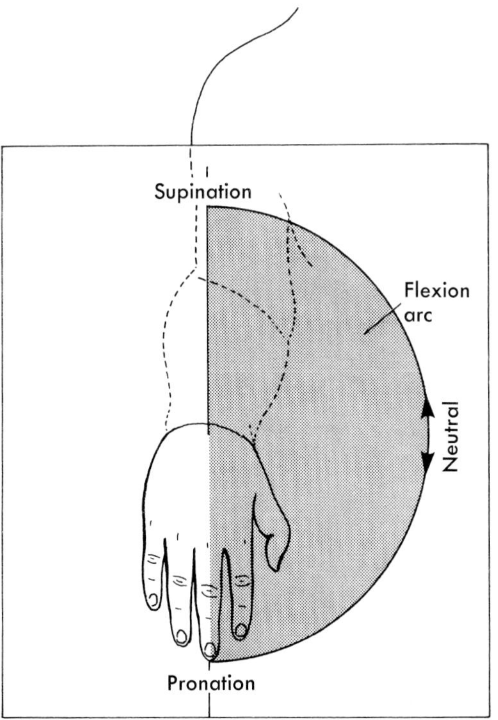

Fig. 7-40. Flexed wrist, when rotated, explores inner half of circle, which is base of spheroid E_3.

rotates with the metacarpals ulnaward, and the proximal row, including the scaphoid turns radialward. The reverse motion occurs during radial deviation. The range of ulnar deviation is greater when the hand is supinated. During radial deviation the scaphoid rotates posteroanteriorly, the proximal pole turning dorsally and the distal pole with its tuberosity anteriorly. The lunate follows the scaphoid and flexes. In ulnar deviation, the scaphoid derotates and exposes its full profile (Fig. 7-41).

Pronation occurs when the hand extends in a radial direction starting from a neutral rotation position. Supination accompanies the motion of flexion with ulnar deviation. This combination of motion becomes quite evident during manipulative functions of the hand and wrist when involved in a power-type performance (hammering, casting a fishing line, swinging a club, etc.).

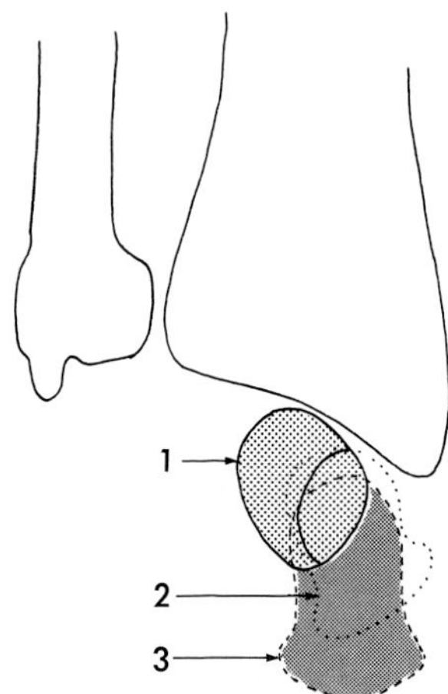

Fig. 7-41. Position of scaphoid: *1,* in radial deviation, tuberosity points anteriorly; *2,* in neutral; *3,* in ulnar deviation derotation occurs, and scaphoid exposes its full profile.

The center of rotation during radioulnar deviation is located in the head of the capitate.[20] The radial deviators of the wrist are the abductor pollicis, extensor pollicis brevis, extensor carpi radialis longus and brevis, long extensors of the index, and the flexor carpi radialis. The ulnar deviators are the extensor carpi ulnaris, flexor carpi ulnaris, and long extensors of the middle, ring, and little fingers.

The wrist is a key joint with regards to the functional activities of the hand. Grip power is maximal when the wrist is extended to 35 degrees and minimal with the wrist maximally flexed. The degree of participation of the digital motors determines, on the other hand, the recruitment of the wrist motors. When the wrist is in extension and the fingers make a soft fist, the following

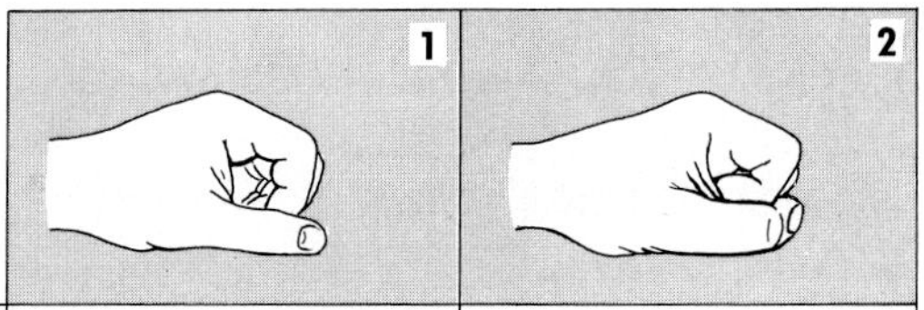

	1	2
EXTENSOR CARPI RADIALIS BREVIS	+ + +	+ + +
EXTENSOR CARPI ULNARIS	+ +	+ + +
EXTENSOR CARPI RADIALIS LONGUS	+	+ + +

Fig. 7-42. Wrist extension: *1,* with soft fist; *2,* with tight fist. +++, Maximum activity; ++, mild activity; +, minimal activity.

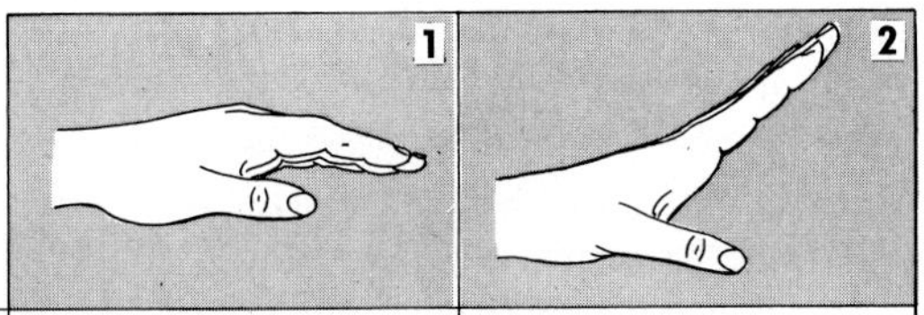

	1	2
EXTENSOR CARPI ULNARIS	+ + +	+ + +
FLEXOR CARPI ULNARIS	+ + +	+ + +
EXTENSOR CARPI RADIALIS BREVIS		+ +
PALMARIS LONGUS		+ +
EXTENSOR CARPI RADIALIS LONGUS		+
FLEXOR CARPI RADIALIS		+

Fig. 7-43. Wrist extension: *1,* with gentle opening of fingers; *2,* with forceful opening of fingers. + + +, Maximum activity; ++, mild activity; +, minimal activity.

wrist motors are active in a descending order: extensor carpi radialis brevis, extensor carpi ulnaris, and extensor carpi radialis longus. With a tight fist, all three extensors are maximally active (Fig. 7-42).[16]

When the fingers are gently extended and the wrist is held in extension, the extensor carpi ulnaris and flexor carpi ulnaris are active. The forceful opening of the fingers brings into action, in a descending order, the following additional wrist motors: extensor carpi radialis brevis, palmaris longus, extensor carpi radialis longus, and flexor carpi radialis (Fig. 7-43).[16]

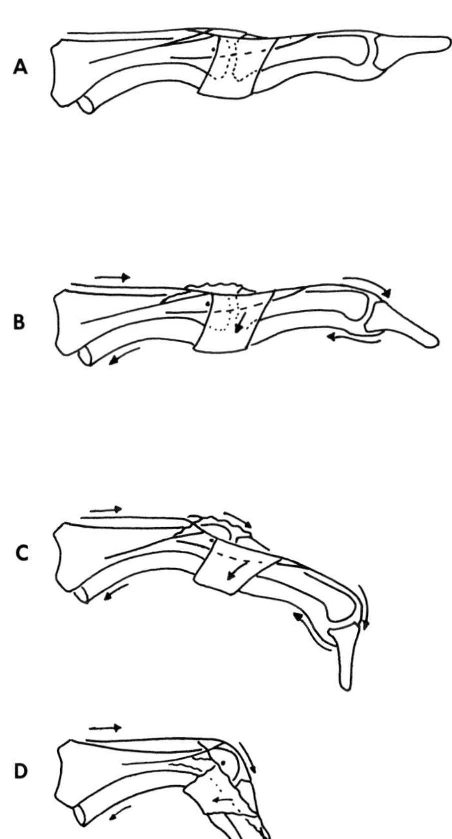

Fig. 7-44. Landsmeer's[10] concept of coordination of interphalangeal joint flexion. **A,** Finger in extension. **B,** Active flexion at distal interphalangeal joint increases tension in terminal extensor tendon and oblique retinacular ligament. Extensor trifurcation advances distally, extensor middle slip relaxes, and middle joint flexes automatically to same degree. **C** and **D,** As flexion continues middle slip increases in tension. Trifurcation advances further distally, thus relaxing lateral tendons and terminal tendon, including oblique retinacular ligament. Distal joint then flexes without encountering extensor resistance.

HAND

Fingers

The hand located at the end of a multisegmented system functions within the action envelope E_3 of the wrist. The flexing finger traces an action envelope, E_4, which is an equiangular spiral (Fig. 7-36).[11]

When the wrist is extended the field of motion of the fingers is within the wrist envelope E_3. With wrist flexion the action envelope E_4 of the fingers extends beyond the field of motion of the wrist (Fig. 7-36).

If the fingers are to be used for the purpose of prehension, the interphalangeal and metacarpophalangeal joints are to flex in a coordinated fashion to permit the wrapping of the digital palmar surface over the surface of the object. Separately the distal joint is flexed by the flexor profundus, the middle joint by the flexor superficialis and the metacarpophalangeal joint by the intrinsic muscles. The coordination of flexion at the interphalangeal joints and the metacarpophalangeal joint is brought about by the instantaneous participation of the extrinsic-intrinsic motors commanded by the motor cortex.

Furthermore, a fine mechanism of coordination is present locally in the fingers at the level of the interphalangeal joints as presented by Landsmeer.[10] As soon as flexion is initiated at the level of the distal joint (Fig. 7-44) by the flexor profundus, the terminal extensor tendon is displaced distally, and through the lateral tendons the extensor trifurcation is carried distally, thus relaxing the middle slip. Simultaneously, the oblique retinacular ligament attached to the terminal tendon increases also in tension and, passing volar to the axis of motion at the proximal interphalangeal joint, flexes automatically the middle phalanx. This is a passive mechanism of interphalangeal joint coordination. When the finger reaches a position of flexion close to 70 degrees at the proximal interphalangeal joint, the previously relaxed middle slip goes under tension, and the extensor trifurcation is displaced further distally. This displacement relaxes the lateral slips, lateral tendons, and terminal tendon. This unloading of the extensor tendon at the distal joint allows completion of the flexion at this joint without encountering undue resistance. Any break in this system of activation and coordination interferes immediately with the function of prehension.

The absence of intrinsic muscle action not only breaks the contour of the longitudinal arch of the finger, but also creates an abnormal pattern of function. The three joints flex successively from a distoproximal direction rather than simultaneously, and this pattern of flexion prevents the palmar skin from making the necessary surface contact with the object.

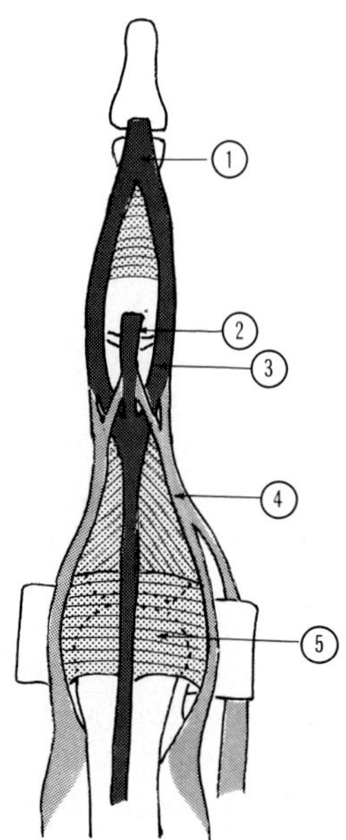

Fig. 7-45. Extensor system: *1,* terminal tendon; *2,* middle slip; *3,* lateral slip; *4,* intrinsic tendon; *5,* quadrilateral lamina.

The opening of the fingers is an essential prerequisite for the act of prehension. The extension of the metacarpophalangeal joint is controlled by the long extensor. The mechanism is dual. An indirect action of extension is exerted by the long extensor on the proximal phalanx through the volar attachment of the transverse or quadrilateral lamina. A direct action is present through a tendinous attachment of the long extensor to the dorsum of the proximal phalanx. This band is present in only 38.5% of dissected hands.[9]

The proximal interphalangeal joint is extended by the long extensor middle slip and spiral fibers arising from the intrinsic tendons. The distal joint is extended by the terminal tendon, which is essentially formed by the long extensor lateral slip, receiving also contribution from the corresponding intrinsic tendons. The oblique retinacular ligaments participate in the constitution of this tendon (Fig. 7-45).

When the middle joint extends actively, the oblique retinacular goes under tension and automatically extends the distal joint.[10] This is another mechanism of coordination on the extensor side of the finger. The flexing finger increases gradually in skeletal length due to the noncircular contour of the metacarpal head. This creates undue tension in the extensor system, but immediate adjustment occurs by the distal shift of the entire extensor mechanism and the volar displacement of the lateral slips at the level of the middle joint.

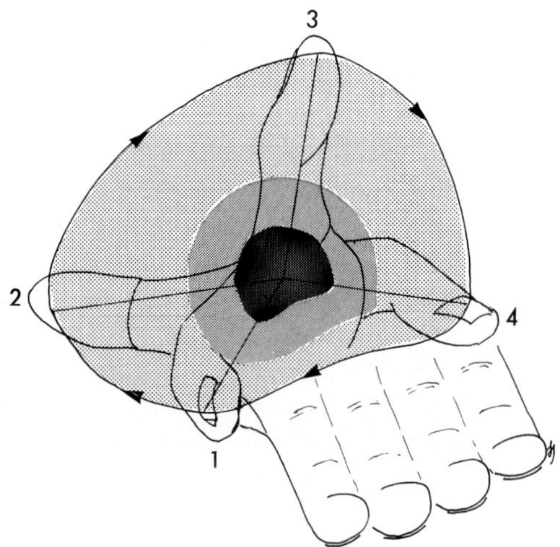

Fig. 7-46. Conoid field of motion of thumb. All functional activities occur within this field of motion. Basic motions are as follows: *1* to *2,* extension and abduction in palmar plane; *2* to *3,* abduction in plane perpendicular to palm with pronation; *3* to *4,* flexion, adduction, and further pronation; *4* to *1,* extension palmar abduction with supination; *1* to *4,* flexion, adduction, and pronation.

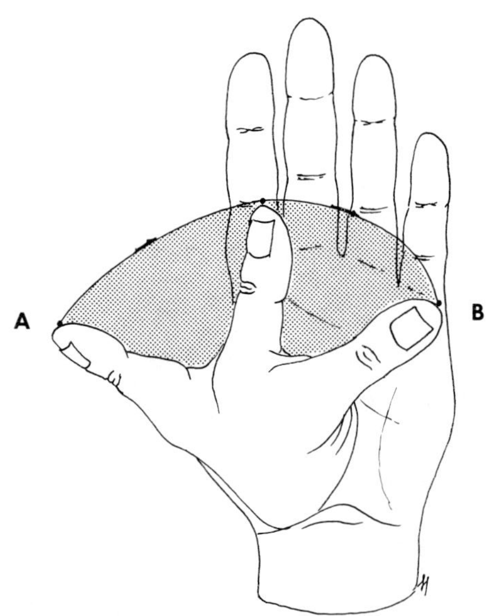

Fig. 7-47. Thumb traces equiangular spiral[12] when sweeping palmar surface from *A* to *B.*

In maximum flexion, the lateral slips are at the level of the axis of motion of the joint. The side motion and rotation of the fingers are determined by the intrinsic muscles. The dorsal interossei abduct or spread the fingers, whereas the volar interossei adduct the fingers relative to a functional axis passing through the third metacarpal. There is more abduction to the finger in extension and less in flexion.

A final passive mechanism of flexion-extension of the finger is present through a tenodesis effect: wrist extension flexes, and wrist flexion extends the fingers.

Thumb

The thumb sweeps a conoid surface[12] through circumduction. This curved surface is flattened on the palmar aspect (Fig. 7-46). All functional activities of the thumb occur within this envelope. Through flexion-adduction the thumb traces the segment of the base of the cone along the palmar surface. The curve traced during this motion is an equiangular spiral[12] (Fig. 7-47). Through extension-abduction the ray returns to its initial position.

A fundamental function of the thumb is opposition with the fingers. This occurs as the pad of the thumb is set against the pulp of a corresponding finger. To bring about this opposition, the thumb is abducted in a plane perpendicular to the palm, flexed and rotated (pronated) on its long axis (Fig. 7-48). The thumb and the pulp of the finger make contact along the equiangular spiral curve of the finger.

There are two phases to the opposition. In phase one, the thumb is positioned against the pulp of a corresponding finger. This is determined by the abductor pollicis brevis, opponens, and superficial head of the short flexor. Phase one is a function of the median nerve. Phase two of the opposition is the clamping of the thumb pad against the opposed finger. This phase provides the power to the opposition. It is controlled by the adductor and deep head of the short flexor. It is a function of the ulnar nerve (Fig. 7-48).

Functional activities

The functional activities of the hand are extensive but can be grouped into nonprehensile and prehensile activities. The former includes touching, feeling, pressing down with the fingers, tapping, vibrating the cord of a musical instrument, lifting or pushing with the hand, stirring, etc. Prehensile activities are grouped into precision and power grips.[15] The precision grip involves the participation of the radial side of the hand with the thumb, index, and middle finger forming a three-jaw chuck. When the pulp of these digits comes into contact, the grip is of the palmar type, whereas contact with the tip of the same digits, for very precise work, creates a tip-type of grip. A lateral, or key, grip involves contact of the pulp of the thumb with the lateral aspect of the corresponding finger in its distal segment.

The power grip involves more the ulnar aspect of the hand with involvement of the little and ring fingers. The radial three digits participate also actively either in pure power pattern form or by adding an element of precision to the power grip. A typical power grip is the cylindrical grip. All fingers are flexed maximally, for example, around the handle of a tool, and the counterpres-

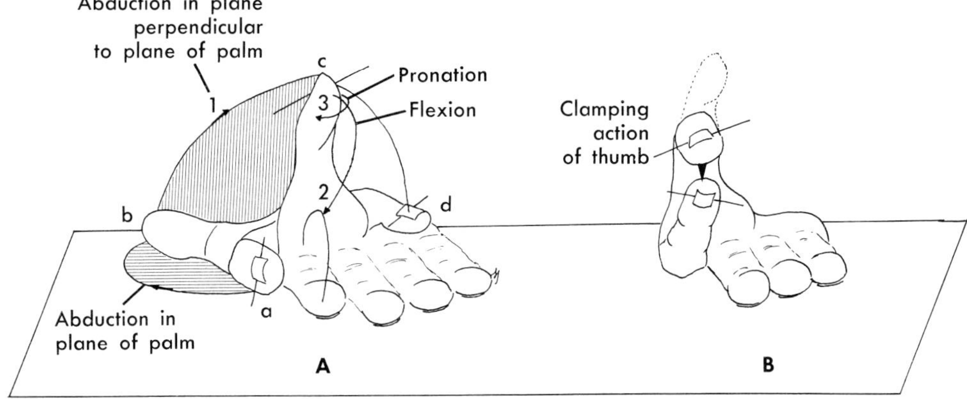

Fig. 7-48. Opposition of thumb. **A,** Stage I is positioning of thumb against corresponding finger. This motion involves curve *1*, abduction in plane perpendicular to palm; curve *2*, flexion; curve *3*, pronation. **B,** Stage II involves clamping of opposed digits. This provides power to opposition.

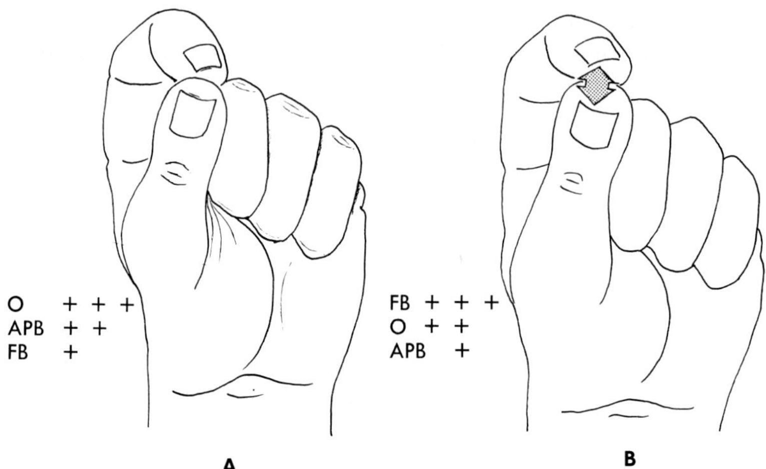

Fig. 7-49. Electromyographic activity during opposition. **A,** Soft opposition. **B,** Hard opposition. *O,* Opponens; *APB,* abductor pollicis brevis; *FB,* flexor pollicis brevis. +++, Maximum activity; ++, mild activity; +, minimum activity.

sure to the flexing fingers is provided by the thenar eminence. More power is provided to this grip when the thumb wraps around the flexed fingers. If an element of precision is necessary, the thumb will adopt a longitudinal position of adduction, allowing for small adjustments of posture. In general, the pattern of the grip during prehension is determined by the intention and not necessarily by the shape of the object.[15] A scalpel is held in a precision grip for exact work or in a power grip for bold cuts.

The hook power grip involves flexion of both interphalangeal joints and minimal participation of the metacarpophalangeal joint. This pattern is used in carrying a suitcase.

The spherical grip is an interesting grip. If the object held by the digits is large, the grip is of the power type with minimal flexion of the fingers, which are abducted and rotated, and the thumb participates at the opposite pole, stabilizing the object and providing the necessary counterpressure. With a smaller spherical object the fingers are adducted, and the thumb is in opposition, and the pattern of the prehension is of the precision type.

Despite the multitude of functional activities of the hand, any prehensile act when arrested instantaneously might fit in one of these patterns in a pure or combined form. In the cylindrical grip the motors responsible are the flexor profundi and the intrinsic muscles except for the second dorsal interosseous and the three radial lumbricales. The flexor superficialis is a reserve flexor and participates when more power is necessary. The index finger is the exception where the flexor superficialis pattern predominates.[13] The thumb brings its contribution with the thenar muscles and the long motors, except for the abductor pollicis longus.

In the hook type of prehension, the radial intrinsics are silent. The long flexors, fourth dorsal interosseous, lumbricales, and the abductor digiti quinti, are active.[13]

During soft opposition of the thumb with the index finger—palmar prehension—the opponens, abductor pollicis brevis, and short flexor are active in a decreasing order (Fig. 7-49).[5] When pressure is exerted the short flexor becomes the more active, followed by the opponens and abductor pollicis brevis. In the lateral grip the flexor pollicis brevis and the opponens are very active. The activity of the abductor pollicis brevis is negligible.[5]

REFERENCES

1. American Academy of Orthopaedic Surgeons: Joint motion—method of measuring and recording, Chicago, 1969.
2. Capener, N.: The hand in surgery, J. Bone Joint Surg. **38B**(1):128-151, Feb., 1956.
3. Christensen, J. B., Adams, J. P., Cho, K. O., and Miller, L.: A study of the interosseous distance between the radius and ulna during rotation of the forearm, Anat. Rec. **160:**261-271, 1968.
4. Darcus, H. D., and Salter, N.: The amplitude of pronation and supination with the elbow flexed to a right angle, J. Anat. **87:**169-184, 1953.
5. Forrest, W. J., and Basmajian, J. V.: Functions of human thenar and hypothenar muscles: and electromyographic study of 25 hands, J. Bone Joint Surg. **47A**(8):1585-1594, 1965.

6. Gemmill, J. F.: On the movement of the lower end of the radius in pronation and supination and on the interosseous membrane, J. Anat. Physiol. **35:**101-109, 1901.
7. Halls, A. A., and Travill, A.: Transmission of pressures across the elbow joint, Anat. Rec. **150:**243-247, 1964.
8. Inman, V. T., Saunders, M., and Abbott, L. C.: Oberservations on the function of the shoulder joint, J. Bone Joint Surg. **26:**1-30, Jan., 1944.
9. Kaplan, E. B.: Functional and surgical anatomy of the hand, ed. 2, Philadelphia, 1965, J. B. Lippincott Co.
10. Landsmeer, J. M. F.: The anatomy of the dorsal aponeurosis of the human finger and its functional significance, Anat. Rec. **104:**31-44, 1949.
11. Littler, J. W.: On the adaptability of man's hand, Hand **5**(3):187-191, 1973.
12. Littler, J. W.: Hand structure and function, Symp. Reconstr. Hand Surg. **9:**3-12, 1974.
13. Long, C., Conrad, P. W., Hall, E. A., and Furler, S. L.: Intrinsic-extrinsic muscle control of the hand in power grip and precision handling: an electromyographic study, J. Bone Joint Surg. **52A**(5):852-867, July, 1970.
14. MacConaill, M. A., and Basmajian, J. V.: Muscles and movements—a basis for human kinesiology, Baltimore, 1969, The Williams & Wilkins Co.
15. Napier, J. R.: The prehensile movements of the human hand, J. Bone Joint Surg. **38B**(4):902-913, Nov., 1956.
16. Radonjic, D., and Long, C.: Kinesiology of the wrist. Am. J. Phys. Med. **50**(2):57-71, 1971.
17. Sarrafian, S. K., Melamed, J. L., and Goshgarian, G. M.: Study of wrist motion in flexion and extension, Clin. Orthop. **126:**153-159, July-Aug., 1977.
18. Sarrafian, S. K., and Melamed, J. L.: Unpublished data, 1975.
19. Travill, A. A.: Electromyographic study of the extensor apparatus of the forearm, Anat. Rec. **144:**373-376, 1962.

CHAPTER 8

Principles of amputation surgery in the upper limb

ERNEST M. BURGESS

Function of the upper limb is, in essence, function of the hand. Elements of the arm proximal to the wrist act to place the hand in an attitude and position appropriate to the desired motor and sensory objective. It has been said that humans live through their eyes and hands. Artists, anthropologists, anatomists, authors, all of us, look with reverence and respect at that remarkable instrument of work and expression, the hand. Little wonder that major amputation through the upper limb is so overwhelming a challenge for functional restoration.

A great deal of upper limb use is bimanual, yet loss of one hand and arm does not preclude free movement within the environment and the performance of a large degree of necessary and discretionary function with the remaining normal arm and hand. This is in contrast to unilateral lower limb loss, in which the individual must have prosthetic substitution to move about effectively or alternatively uses the upper limbs through assistive devices to walk. These two reasons, the complexity of upper limb prosthetic substitution and the ability of the patient to function quite effectively with the remaining normal arm, combine to decrease motivation for prosthetic fitting and training of amputees with unilateral amputations. This circumstance is particularly true for higher levels of amputation with increasing prosthetic design and training demands. It is usually much easier for the amputee to enlarge the functional capability of the remaining arm and hand than to learn to use what appears to be a cumbersome, heavy , unsightly, and functionally inadequate limb substitute. Many amputees with unilateral upper limb amputations, especially in older persons whose amputation is at the above-elbow level, find it more satisfactory to forgo compromised bimanual function rather than go down the hard, long road of modest functional use. This situation is reversed completely with bilateral amputations. The disability is so severe and life so stark that most people with bilateral amputations will be motivated to maximum effort. The alternative, which is severe dependency on others for very personal activities of daily living, usually drives these individuals to meet the challenge with great cooperation, patience, and effort.

Engineers and prosthetists are fascinated by the opportunity to duplicate hand function, but as yet have been unsuccessful. Since the end of World War II, this effort has proceeded at a rapid pace throughout the world. National pride and prestige have, in some instances, become involved. Prostheses powered by external sources of energy have been widely publicized and identified with national, regional, and institutional names.

The thalidomide experience, which produced a considerable number of infants born with both upper limbs missing, further accelerated the demand for innovative prosthetic design. Unfortunately, many avenues of investigation, often expensive, terminated in blind alleys of frustration and disappointment. We have now entered a stage of solid progress involving a high level of national and international cooperation. The surgeon called on to perform an upper limb amputation is required to have a working knowledge of currently available prostheses. This is one of the basic principles of amputation surgery.

It has been pointed out that upper limb function centers primarily around the hand. The principles of hand surgery, then, apply to amputations throughout the upper limb. Since the amputation site now becomes that primary portion of the limb through which the prosthesis will contact the environment and perform useful function, the surgeon, as in hand surgery, ablates no portion of the limb that has potential capacity for use. There are certainly no sites of elective amputation in the upper limb; with very few exceptions maximum conservation of bone length and soft tissues is practiced.

Amputations through the fingers and metacarpals usually require no prosthetic replacement. Surgical principles as they apply to both congenital and acquired amputations are thoroughly described in texts and articles on hand surgery. The remarkable accomplishments in the field of traumatic and reconstructive hand surgery are well known. The many details of surgical hand reconstruction are not covered in this book. Principles of upper limb amputations now described apply to levels above the finger and thumb rays.

The general principles of amputation surgery have been outlined earlier and hold for both upper and lower limbs. Variations and modifications useful in upper limb amputation will now be described.

TRANSCARPAL AMPUTATION

Amputations distal to the metacarpophalangeal joints are included in Chapter 10. When it is necessary to amputate through or proximal to the carpometacarpal joints and when no functional rays remain, the surgeon is confronted with a decision of level selection. If wrist function is uninvolved, the amputee is left with a strong, sensorimotor end-organ, permitting hook and carrying capacity by active wrist flexion or extension. The terminal limb can also stabilize independently and act in a supportive manner with the opposite hand for many functions not requiring pinch and grasp. The residual sensory function is of great importance. Transcarpal amputation can be fitted with an attractive, nonfunctioning glove-style prosthesis. In general, the amputee chooses to wear such a device only for cosmetic purposes. Although functional partial hand prostheses will be discussed later, they are generally a poor trade-off for the loss of natural residual limb sensation inherent in wearing a prosthesis. Certain specialized tasks, however, can be efficiently carried out when the patient wears a partial hand substitute. Such prostheses may be designed for use in both vocational and recreational activities.

On occasions, the amputee will request revision to wrist disarticulation to wear a more conventional prosthesis. This circumstance occurs infrequently. Before even considering such a revision in the presence of a functional transcarpal amputation, the surgeon should thoroughly acquaint the amputee with all relevant facts and should also have the patient talk to and see other amputees wearing a prosthesis fitted to the anticipated level of revision.

WRIST DISARTICULATION

Wrist disarticulation is an excellent amputation when adequate soft tissues are present for wound closure and healing. If normal distal radioulnar joint function remains and prosthetic socket fit is correct, the amputee will translate at least 50% of normal forearm rotation to the terminal device. Certain forearm tendons, which are sectioned at the amputation level, can be stabilized distally. Specific stabilizing techniques are detailed in Chapter 11. Distal radial and ulnar styloid processes should be rounded moderately to avoid unusual prominences, but specific care must be taken to avoid damage to the distal radioulnar joint. When possible, a volar skin and soft tissue pad is retained for distal coverage, with the skin scar dorsal. When using total-contact design prostheses, placement of the skin suture line is less relevant, provided that the scar is nonadherent and nontender.

FOREARM AMPUTATION

Amputations through the forearm are carried out at the lowest effective level consistent with adequate soft tissue coverage. Bone ends are carefully rounded to remove sharp edges. Distal muscle stabilization is most important. By this means, forearm muscle function is retained. This is especially true when a myoelectric prosthesis is to be used, and the electrical muscle signal will initiate terminal device control. Forearm bones are sectioned distally at the same level unless anomaly, trauma, infection, or other pathological conditions dictate otherwise. Management of other tissues, including nerves, has been described in Chapter 2. Surgical treatment of the cutaneous sensory nerves, particularly the superficial branch of the radial nerve, requires careful technique. Painful subsutaneous neuromata are not uncommon in the forearm.

The very short below-elbow amputation can be functionally lengthened by dividing the radial insertion of the biceps tendon and allowing it to retract, thus increasing the depth of the antecubital area. This increased depth allows better suspension of the prosthesis. The brachialis muscle is of adequate strength to provide forearm flexion.

ELBOW DISARTICULATION

Elbow disarticulation is preferred to a higher above-elbow amputation. Muscle stabilization is routinely performed, and moderate contouring of the humeral condyles is carried out, just sufficient to remove sites of pressure intolerance against the socket, yet retain sufficient enlargement and contour to provide stability within the prosthesis, a major advantage of both wrist and elbow disarticulation.

ABOVE-ELBOW AMPUTATION

Above-elbow diaphyseal amputation through the humerus is carried out at the lowest effective level surgically feasible. Bone ends are moderately rounded, and muscle stabilization is accomplished whenever possible. The short above-elbow amputation is preferred to shoulder disarticulation even though little useful shoulder joint function is retained. The added surface and shoulder contour provided by the retained head of the humerus simplifies prosthetic fitting both functionally and from the cosmetic standpoint.

SHOULDER DISARTICULATION AND FOREQUARTER AMPUTATION

Shoulder disarticulation and forequarter amputation present no unusual problems. The general principles that have been outlined apply here. Specific techniques will be described under appropriate sections in Chapter 13.

BIBLIOGRAPHY

Burgess, E. M.: Major amputations. In Nora, P. F., editor: Operative surgery—principles and techniques, Chapter 49, 1972, Lea & Felieger.

Burkhalter, W. E., Mayfield, G., and Carmona, L. S.: The upper extremity amputee—early and immediate postsurgical prosthetic fitting, J. Bone Joint Surg. **58A**:46-51, Jan., 1976.

Dederich, R.: Amputationen der unteren extremitat, operationstechnik und prothetiscke sofortversorgung, Stuttgart, 1970, George Thieme Verlag.

Edmonson, A. S., and Crenshaw, A. H., editors: Campbell's operative orthopaedics, ed. 6, St. Louis, 1980, The C. V. Mosby Co.

Loughlin, E., Stanford, J., and Phelps, M.: Immediate postsurgical prosthetic fitting of a bilateral below-elbow amputee—a report, Artif. Limbs **12**:17-19, Spring, 1968.

Sarmiento, A., McCollough, N., Williams, E., and Sinclair, W.: Immediate postoperative prosthetic fitting in the management of upper extremity amputees, Artif. Limbs **12**:14-19, Spring, 1968.

Slocum, D. B.: An atlas of amputations, St. Louis, 1949, The C. V. Mosby Co.

CHAPTER 9

Upper limb prosthetic systems

Section I

Socket designs

NORMAN BERGER

The socket is the portion of the prosthesis that covers the residual limb or stump. Distal to the socket, a prosthetic extension replaces the void between the end of the stump and the wrist unit, in the case of the below-elbow prosthesis, or between the end of the stump and the elbow unit, in the case of the above-elbow prosthesis. When the amputation is through a joint (that is, disarticulation at the shoulder, elbow, or wrist), the socket covers the remaining segment, but no prosthetic extension is needed to replace segment length, since none is lost.

Assuming an unimpaired joint immediately proximal to the site of amputation, the stump will retain motions normally associated with the remaining anatomy. The forearm stump will flex and extend at the elbow joint and rotate at the proximal radioulnar joint. The humeral stump will flex and extend, abduct and adduct, and rotate at the glenohumeral joint. The socket that covers the residual segment must transmit these remaining stump motions to the prosthesis to the maximum possible extent. The socket is thus a major determinant of functional effectiveness and an indispensable link in the series of events summarized by the phrase "prosthesis control," which refers both to positioning the prosthesis in space and to operation of the components of the prosthesis. As a corollary to transmission of stump motion, the socket should not impede use of any residual function. Furthermore, the socket must have a sufficiently stable purchase on the stump to avoid inadvertent motion of the prosthesis and to preclude painful concentrations of pressure as the stump resists torques and bending moments produced by normal operation of the prosthesis.

It is clear, then, that socket design must provide for motion, stability, and comfort if prosthetic function is to be optimal. Two points should be emphasized as significant aids in achieving these somewhat contradictory goals:

1. Basic biomechanical principles of socket design must be kept in mind. These include the principle of total contact (often referred to in upper limb prosthetics as "double-wall sockets") to avoid edema and distribute pressure as widely as possible; recognition of differential tolerance to pressure and differential compressibility of tissues; provision of adequate reliefs for bony prominences, tender spots, and areas of high pressure concentrations; and provision of buildups for soft, compressible, and tolerant areas. These fundamentals have been most clearly delineated in relation to sockets for lower limb prostheses,[2] but are equally relevant to the upper limb.

2. The prosthetist should use trial or check socket procedures to verify the adequacy of socket fit before finalizing and fabricating the prosthesis. Commonly, a check socket is made of a malleable, easily modified material such as beeswax; a careful and detailed evaluation is performed; changes in shape, contour, and extent are introduced as needed; and a final, permanent socket is fabricated only when these goals have been adequately realized.

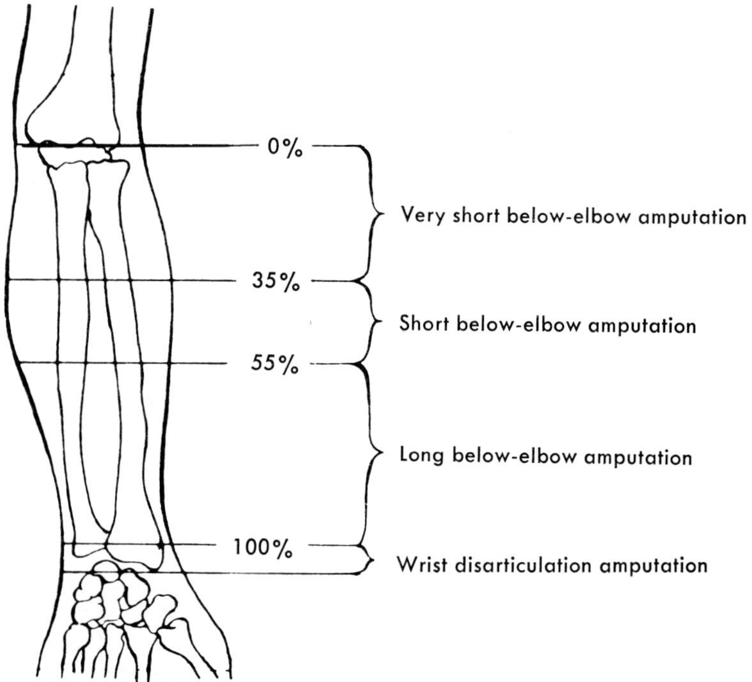

Fig. 9-1. Below-elbow classification system. (Modified from Upper-limb prosthetics, New York, 1971, New York University, Post-Graduate Medical School, Prosthetics and Orthotics.)

BELOW-ELBOW AMPUTEE CLASSIFICATIONS AND SOCKET DESIGNS

The amputee classification system promulgated by the university teaching centers in the United States[9,10] defines four fundamental types of below-elbow stumps (Fig. 9-1). For unilateral amputations, the percentage figures derive from (1) measurement of the residual limb and intact forearm on ths sound side and (2) application of a simple formula: stump length times 100, divided by sound forearm length. Obviously, the four types differ from each other in the percentage of remaining length but, more important, each type presents a different prosthetic problem and therefore requires a different socket design.

Wrist disarticulation

The forearm stump in wrist disarticulation can be expected to retain excellent range of motion and strength in elbow flexion-extension and in pronation-supination. Therefore a primary consideration in socket design is the provision of a stable stump-socket relationship that at the same time allows use of these residual motions. To encourage efficient transmission of stump rotation to the socket, the prosthetist flattens the medial and lateral sides of the malleable check socket near the distal end,[6] thus producing an elliptical cross section (Fig. 9-2). Despite this contouring, pronation-supination will still be restricted if the proximal socket border extends too far over the

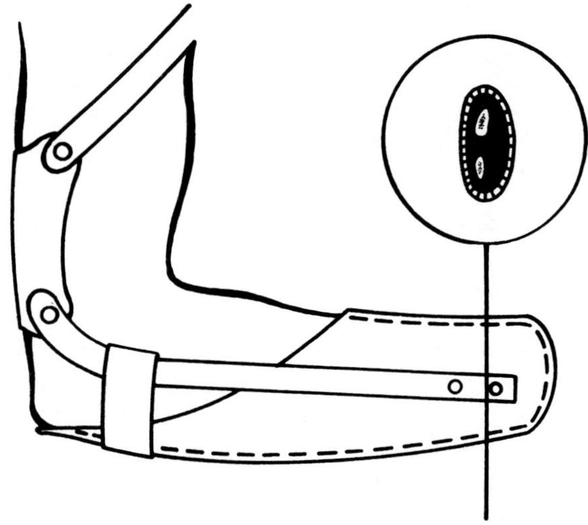

Fig. 9-2. Schematic of wrist disarticulation socket. Inset gives cross-sectional anatomy 2.5 cm (1 inch) from stump end. (Modified from Taylor, C. L.: The biomechanics of the normal and of the amputated upper extremity, Chapter 7. In Klopsteg, P. E., and Wilson, P. D., editors: Human limbs and their substitutes, New York, 1954, McGraw-Hill Book Co., Inc.)

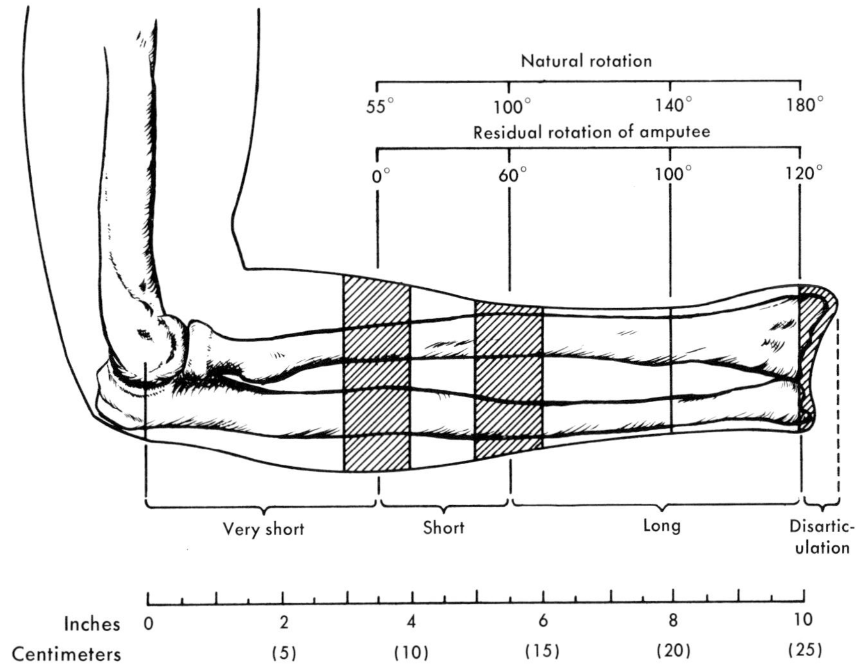

Fig. 9-3. Residual rotation in amputation stump and intact forearm. (Modified from Taylor, C. L.: The biomechanics of the normal and of the amputated upper extremity, Chapter 7. In Klopsteg, P. E., and Wilson, P. D., editors: Human limbs and their substitutes, New York, 1954, McGraw-Hill Book Co., Inc.)

radius toward the elbow crease. Note in Fig. 9-2 that the socket covers approximately 50% (or slightly more) of the radial surface. This trim line also ensures that there will be no restriction of elbow flexion. Do not, however, sacrifice socket stability by excessive trimming of this proximal border.

Also in Fig. 9-2, the proximal socket border extends over the ulna up to the olecranon. This proximal extension, which is characteristic of virtually all below-elbow sockets, aids in resisting bending moments, as in lifting, when a downward force is applied at the terminal device. Care must be taken, however, to avoid contact of this aspect of the socket with the humeral epicondyles at the extremes of pronation and supination.

Finally, some wrist disarticulation patients may exhibit prominent radial and ulnar styloids, in which case the socket will need local reliefs over these bony protuberances. In addition, the width of the styloids may make entry of the stump into the socket difficult, in which case channels or cutouts may be required.

Long below-elbow stump

Since the range of residual pronation-supination is proportional to remaining length (Fig. 9-3), the long below-elbow stump can be expected to retain sufficient rotation to be of functional value in prosthesis use. In fact, this is the primary reason that the boundary for this amputee type is established at 55% of forearm length.

The goals of socket design are essentially the same as for the wrist disarticulation, and, with the exception of features relating to the width and prominence of the styloids, the socket has the same characteristics: medial and lateral flattening to produce an elliptical cross section near the distal end, a relatively low trim line over the radius, and a relatively high trim line over the ulna. The precise degree to which a particular socket will exhibit these characteristics depends on whether the stump length is toward the shorter or longer end of the 55% to 100% range, softness or firmness of stump tissue, strength and range of residual motion, and cross-sectional shape of the stump. These variables place heavy demands on the experience, skill, and art of the prosthetist in achieving a compromise between the requirements of motion and stability. As mentioned earlier, the malleable check socket is the most efficient tool available to help the prosthetist finalize the socket design.

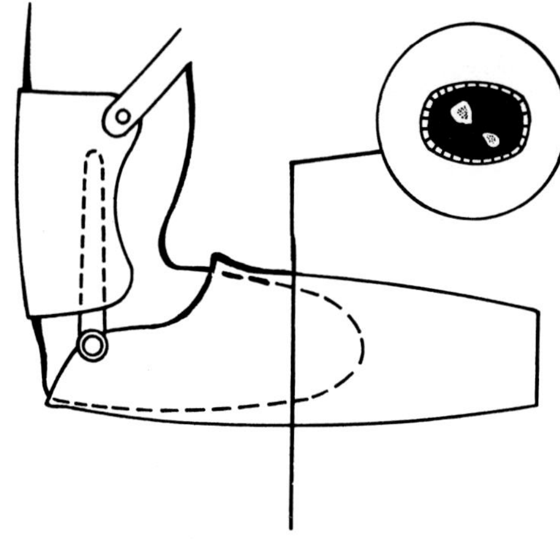

Fig. 9-4. Schematic of socket for short below-elbow amputee. Inset gives cross-sectional anatomy 2.5 cm (1 inch) from stump end. (Modified from Taylor, C. L.: The biomechanics of the normal and of the amputated upper extremity, Chapter 7. In Klopsteg, P. E., and Wilson, P. D., editors: Human limbs and their substitutes, New York, 1954, McGraw-Hill Book Co., Inc.)

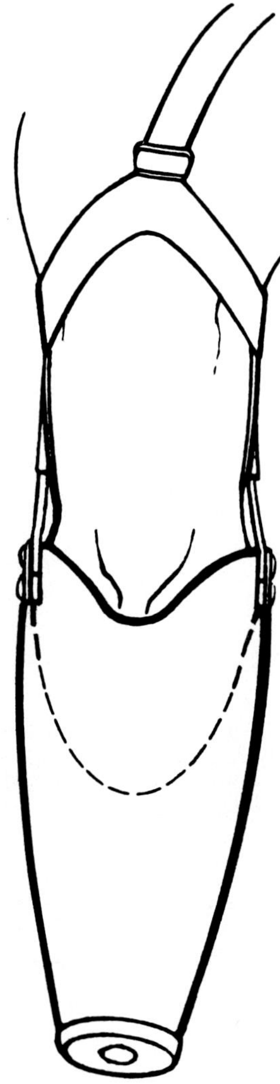

Fig. 9-5. V-shaped anterior trim of short below-elbow socket. (From Bechtol, C. O.: Anatomical and physiological considerations in the clinical application of upper-extremity prosthetics, Chapter 8. In Orthopedic appliances atlas, vol. 2, Artificial Limbs, Ann Arbor, Mich., 1960, J. W. Edwards.)

Short below-elbow stump

With 35% to 55% of forearm length remaining, the short below-elbow stump will retain only a negligible amount of rotation (Fig. 9-3) and will more nearly approach a circular cross section (Fig. 9-4). Under these circumstances, mediolateral flattening of the socket is dispensed with, pronation-supination is sacrificed, and comfortable and strong flexion becomes the primary goal. This implies a higher proximal socket border over the radius, with the trim line as close as possible to the biceps tendon as is consistent with full range of elbow flexion (135 degrees). If necessary, it is preferable to sacrifice a small amount of this range rather than minimize stump-socket contact. For such problems, a V-shaped notch over the biceps tendon is a useful technique,[1] as illustrated in Fig. 9-5.

Very short below-elbow stump

This shortest of below-elbow stumps presents the most difficulty in achieving the basic goals of motion, stability, and comfort. Not only is pronation-supination lost, but elbow flexion is inevitably interfered with by the need to cover as much as possible of the stump for socket stability and distribution of force over a wide area. Solutions to this formidable problem relate to the provision of special socket designs and mechanical hinges.

The split socket. The greater the range of flexion, the more impingement of the proximal socket brim on the biceps tendon and the elbow crease, with consequent discomfort and displacement of the socket. Would it not be desirable to provide a socket that encases the stump, a separate forearm to which the wrist unit and terminal device are attached, and a mechanical coupling between the two, which amplifies or steps up the range of motion of the forearm in relation to the stump (Fig. 9-6). For example, a step-up ratio of 2:1 means that the forearm and terminal device will be driven through a flexion range of 130 degrees by only 65 degrees of stump motion, thus considerably alleviating the impingement problem. The disadvantage of this split-socket arrangement, however, is that approximately twice the force is re-

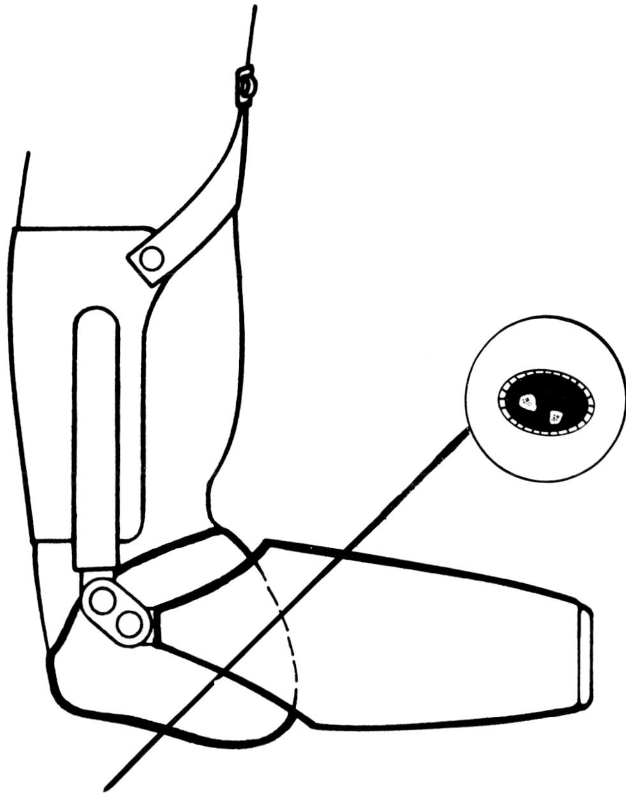

Fig. 9-6. Schematic of split socket. Inset gives cross-sectional anatomy 2.5 cm (1 inch) from stump end. (Modified from Taylor, C. L.: The biomechanics of the normal and of the amputated upper extremity, Chapter 7. In Klopsteg, P. E., and Wilson, P. D., editors: Human limbs and their substitutes, New York, 1954, McGraw-Hill Book Co., Inc.)

quired from the stump than would be needed with no step-up to power the same amount of flexion. Although flexion range is amplified, flexion force is decreased in the same ratio.

If the stump is so weak or so limited in range of motion that it cannot drive the forearm through a functional flexion range, the split socket may be used with an alternate mechanical coupling that provides an elbow lock. In this case, flexion of the forearm is produced by the harness and cable control system, whereas the short, weak, limited stump functions only to trip the locking mechanism. Several designs of step-up and locking hinges are commercially available, and further information may be found in Section III of this chapter.

Whatever the hinge mechanism, the socket (Fig. 9-6) should be somewhat flattened anteroposteriorly, encompass the olecranon and epicondyles, and include a V-shaped relief for the biceps tendon. The flattening and firm fit in the area of the elbow will provide effective stump-socket stability, while any resulting restriction in motion about the elbow is compensated for by the specially designed hinges previously mentioned.

The Muenster socket. To overcome problems inherent in the step-up prosthesis, particularly the decrease in lifting power available to the amputee, Drs. Hepp and Kuhn of Muenster, Germany, devised in the 1950s a socket that provided a more intimate encapsulation of the very short below-elbow stump.[4] This Muenster socket (Fig. 9-7) was successfully evaluated by New York University[8] and continues to be used for the unilateral amputee as a preferred alternative to the split socket.[3]

The socket is characterized by an anterior trim line that extends to the level of the antecubital fold with a channel provided for the biceps tendon, and a posterior trim line, which hooks over the olecranon. These high socket borders and the overall intimate fit produce excellent stump-socket stability and considerable lifting force, but also restrict flexion range of motion to approximately 70 degrees (from an initial flexion position of 35 degrees to 105 degrees).[8] Donning the socket

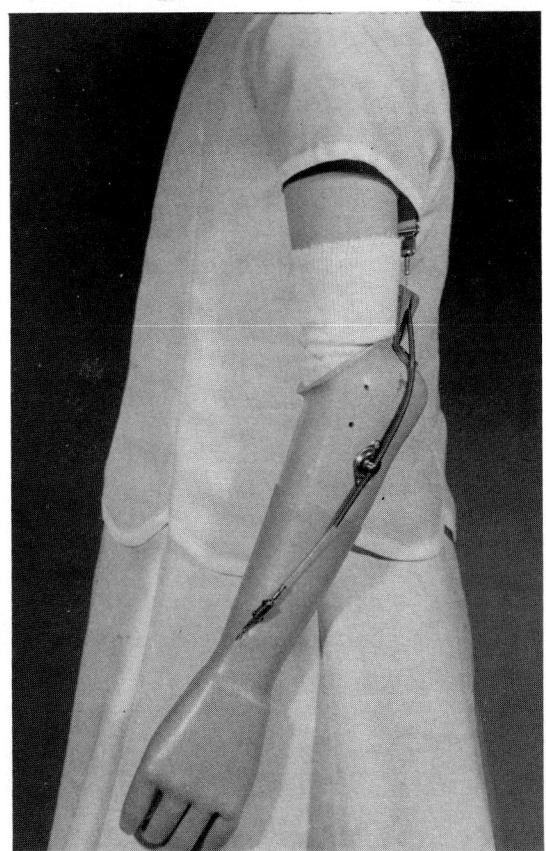

Fig. 9-7. The Muenster socket. (From Upper-limb prosthetics, New York, 1971, New York University, Post-Graduate Medical School, Prosthetics and Orthotics.)

may require pulling the stump in with a stump sock because of the high trim lines and the 35-degree angle between the humeral and forearm sections. These factors are of little concern to most unilateral patients; however, for the bilateral amputee, the restricted flexion range and the donning problem must be carefully considered before a prescription decision is reached.

A comfortable and functional fit of the Muenster socket requires special skills on the part of the prosthetist, particularly in forming the plaster wrap of the stump. As the plaster hardens, a molding grip is applied (Figs. 9-8 and 9-9) to ensure that the socket will exert moderate pressure on the cubital fold on either side of the biceps tendon, moderate downward pressure on the anterior surface of the stump, although avoiding the anterodistal end, and gentle pressure on the posterior surface of the humerus just above the level of the condyles.

ABOVE-ELBOW AMPUTEE CLASSIFICATIONS AND SOCKET DESIGNS

Based on the same procedures of measurement and computation of the percentage of sound side length remaining, the amputee classification system defines six types of above-elbow and shoulder stumps (Fig. 9-10). The three longest types, ranging from 30% to 100% of length remaining, retain a bony lever arm and musculature sufficient to move a socket through a considerable range of shoulder flexion-extension and abduction-adduction. The harness and control cable system (Section II) is designed to use these motions for opera-

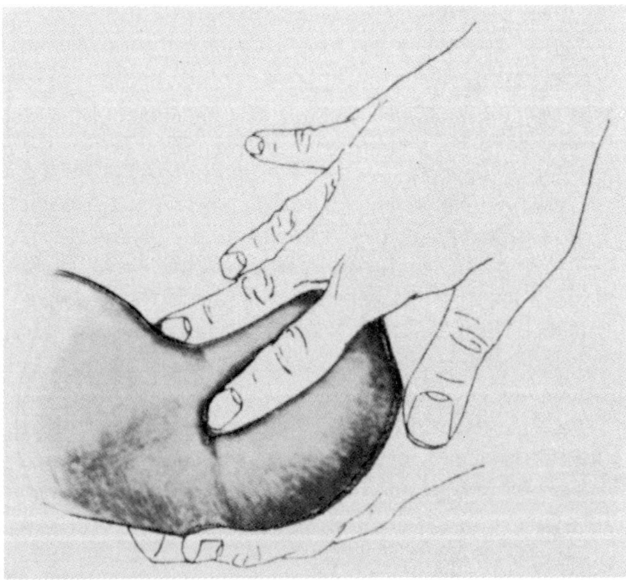

Fig. 9-8. Anterior molding grip. (From Upper-limb prosthetics, New York, 1971, New York University, Post-Graduate Medical School, Prosthetics and Orthotics.)

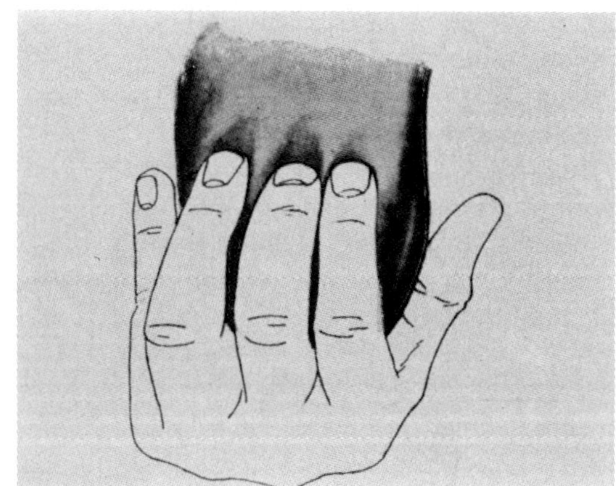

Fig. 9-9. Posterior molding grip. (From Upper-limb prosthetics, New York, 1971, New York University, Post-Graduate Medical School, Prosthetics and Orthotics.)

tion of the terminal device, elbow flexion and extension, and elbow locking and unlocking. Secondarily, these motions also position the entire prosthesis in space.

It will be noted that rotation of the humerus about its long axis has not been mentioned. This motion, although taking place in the glenohumeral joint and therefore anatomically intact, is usually not useful for either control of prosthetic components or positioning the entire prosthesis. Reasons for this are (1) the harness straps and cables that suspend and control the prosthesis tend to restrict rotation of the socket and (2) by its nature, the humeral stump has fewer bony prominences, a thicker layer of soft tissue that tends to move easily around the humerus, and a rounder cross-sectional shape as compared to forearm stumps. Therefore, although rotational stability is important, less strenuous efforts are made to capture this motion as an active mover of the prosthesis than are made to capture pronation-supination in the below-elbow case.

The exception to these statements is the elbow disarticulation in which the flaring condyles of the humerus provide an excellent opportunity for improved socket purchase and virtually normal control of rotation. It has even been suggested by Drs. Marquardt and Neff[5] of Heidelberg, Germany, that this function of the condyles may be provided surgically for the standard above-elbow type by means of an angulation osteotomy, which creates a bone hook at the end of the humerus for improved socket purchase, efficient motion transmission, and elimination of pseudoarthrosis.

Sockets for elbow disarticulation, standard, and short above-elbow stumps

To allow full use of remaining stump motions for control of the entire prosthesis and its components, a close and extensive socket fit is required. Although overall intimacy of fit is essential, particular attention should be paid to the anterodistal segment, since this socket area is largely responsible for picking up and transmitting stump motion in a flexion direction, which is the single most important control motion. Care must be taken, however, to avoid pressure at the sensitive cut end of the humerus.

Since the major portions of muscle bulk lie anterior and posterior to the humeral shaft, sockets tend to be oval in a cross section, that is, wider anteroposteriorly than mediolaterally (Fig. 9-11). Typically, the medial wall is flattened in the sagittal plane, which permits shoulder adduction,

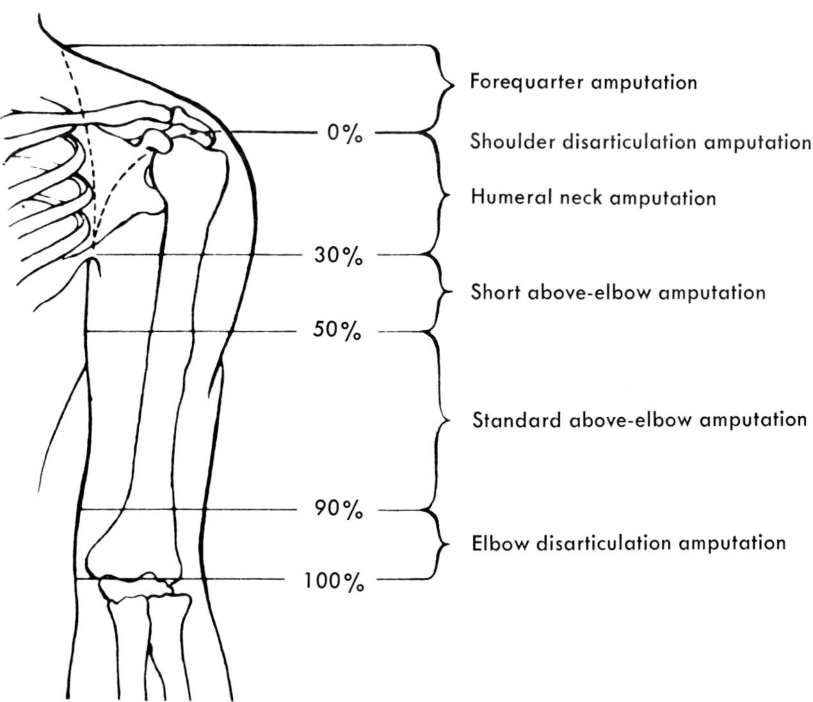

Fig. 9-10. Above-elbow classification system. (Modified from Upper-limb prosthetics, New York, 1971, New York University, Post-Graduate Medical School, Prosthetics and Orthotics.)

helps rotational stability, and widens the anteroposterior stump diameter by some displacement of tissue. This medial flattening must not be overdone for fear of placing undue pressure on major blood vessels and nerves in the upper humeral area. Nor should the anteroposterior width be overdone. Maintenance of a snug anteroposterior fit will enable some patients to "grip" the socket by deliberate bulging of remaining musculature, particularly the biceps, with consequent improvement of stump-socket stability.

To obtain maximum purchase, the proximal socket border on the lateral side should reach the level of the acromion, except in the case of a short above-elbow amputation. In this situation it is necessary to extend the socket border approx-

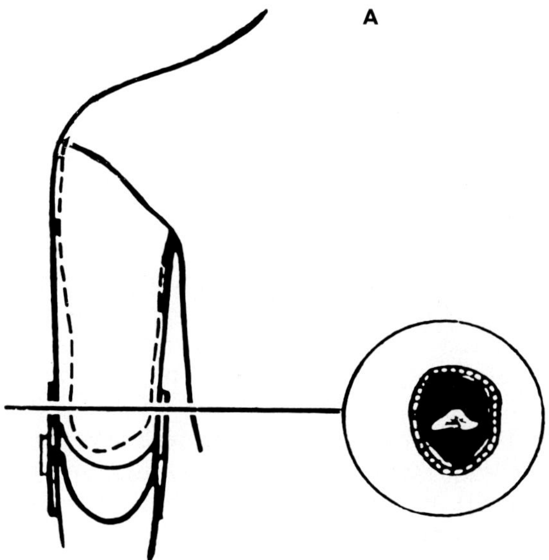

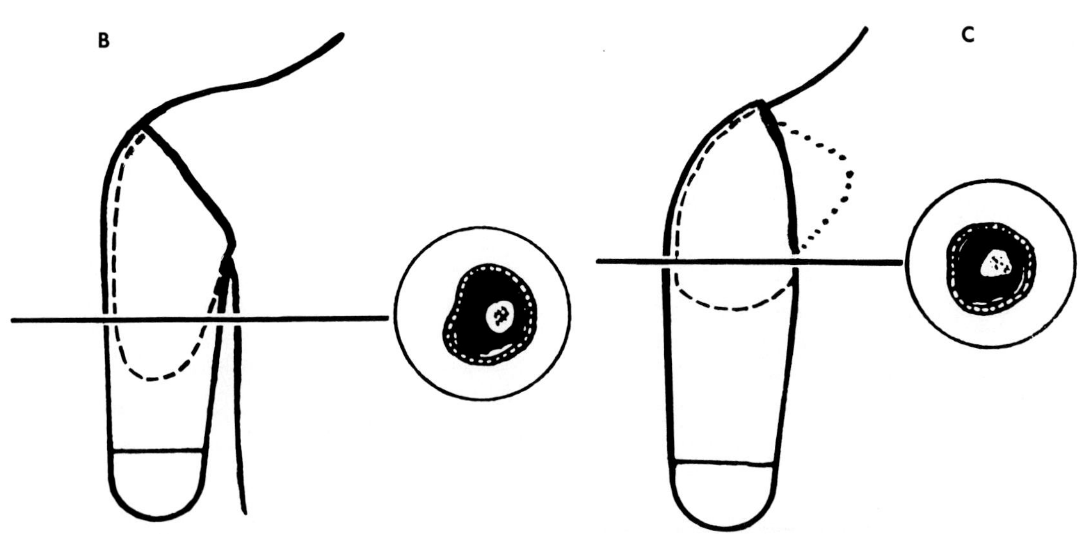

Fig. 9-11. Schematics of above-elbow sockets. Inset gives cross-sectional anatomy at indicated level. Dashed lines show stump contour and inner wall of socket. (Modified from Taylor, C. L.: Artif. Limbs 2(3):4-25, Sept., 1955.)

imately 5 cm (2 inches) beyond the acromion. Between the highest lateral point and the axilla, the anterior and posterior socket margins display a variable contour depending primarily on stump length and tissue consistency. The shorter, softer stumps will require anterior and posterior socket projections or wings for maximum support (Fig. 9-11, *C*, dotted line). Such wings should not extend past the deltopectoral line anteriorly, nor more than 5 cm (2 inches) medial to the axilla posteriorly. These margins, however, are considerably reduced for the longer, firmer stumps.

Sockets for shoulder amputations: humeral neck, disarticulation, and forequarter types

The extensive anatomical loss in shoulder amputations leaves virtually no motions that are useful for actively positioning the entire prosthesis. Motions that do remain (essentially scapular abduction-adduction and shoulder elevation) must be used for control of the terminal device and elbow unit, a difficult task because of the limited displacement or excursion of these motions as compared to the displacements required for operation of prosthetic components. For example, scapular abduction (shoulder shrug) produces an average anatomical displacement of 5.6 cm (2.24 inches) in the adult,[7] whereas a total control cable displacement of 9.7 cm (3.87 inches) is required to fully flex the prosthetic elbow *and* to fully open a voluntary opening hook, such as the Dorrance 5XA. It is therefore imperative that the socket capture and transmit efficiently the remaining anatomical motions. At the same time, the socket must provide stability for itself and the prosthesis by achieving a firm seat on the remaining segments of the shoulder girdle.

Fortunately, these two requirements are not contradictory, since the extensive fit needed for stability will not impede scapular motions. Rather, a socket that covers the scapula snugly will be better able to transmit its motion. Posteriorly, therefore, the shoulder socket should extend to the medial border of the scapula, whereas anteriorly it remains lateral to the nipple with care taken to ensure that this socket margin does not interfere with scapular abduction. Inferiorly, the socket conforms to the thoracic wall and extends 7.5 to 10 cm (3 to 4 inches) below the axilla to help stabilize against rotation around the point of the shoulder. For the same reason, as well as for resistance against axial loads, the superior-medial socket border extends as close to the neck as possible without impingement as the patient moves.

For true shoulder disarticulation (Fig. 9-12, *B*), the socket must be carefully relieved over the coracoid and acromion processes. These bony prominences of the scapula, as well as the lateral end of the clavicle, are potential sources of discomfort and hence require special attention during fitting. An advantage of the humeral neck amputation (Fig. 9-12, *A*) is the rounding out of the shoulder, which minimizes this fitting problem and also provides additional socket stability.

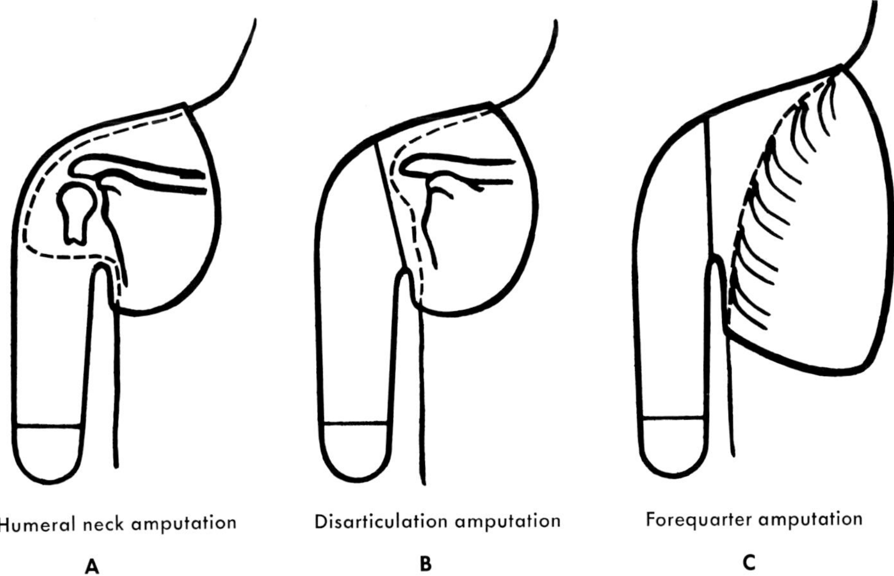

Fig. 9-12. Schematics of shoulder sockets. Solid lines show residual bony structure; dashed lines show body contour and inner wall of socket. (Modified from Taylor, C. L.: Artif. Limbs 2(3):4-25, Sept., 1955.)

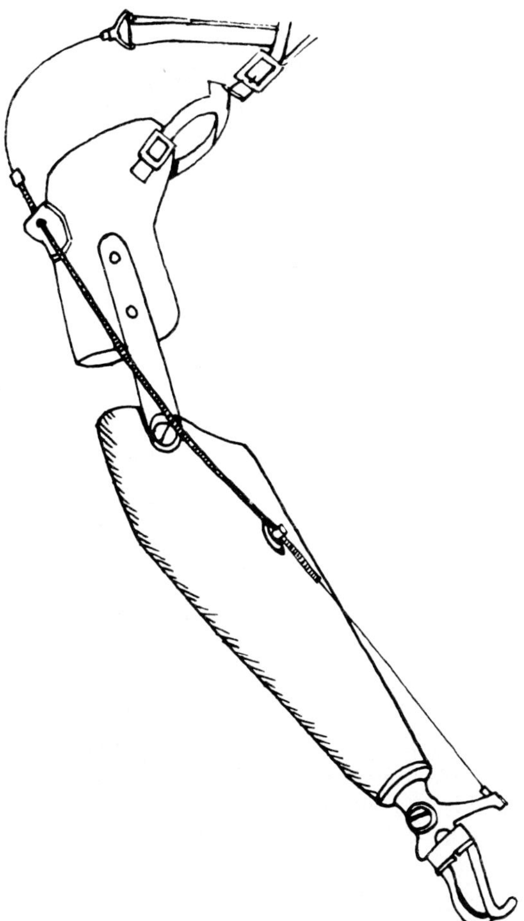

Fig. 9-13. Below-elbow prosthetic control system. (From Below and above elbow harness and control system, Evanston, Ill., 1966, Northwestern University Prosthetic-Orthotic Center.)

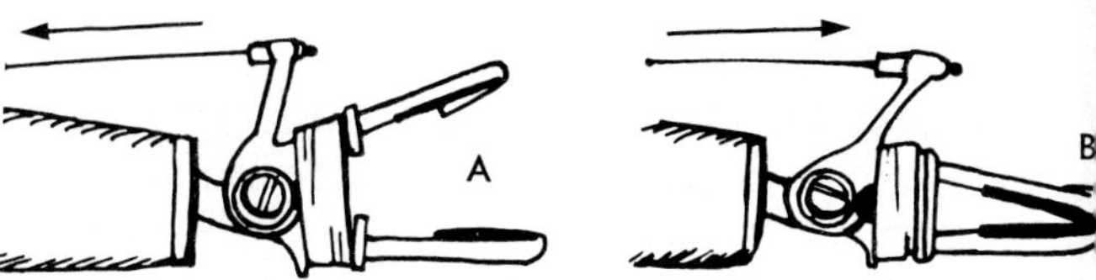

Fig. 9-14. Prehension device with cable tensed (A) and with cable relaxed (B). (From Below and above elbow harness and control system, Evanston, Ill., 1966, Northwestern University Prosthetic-Orthotic Center.)

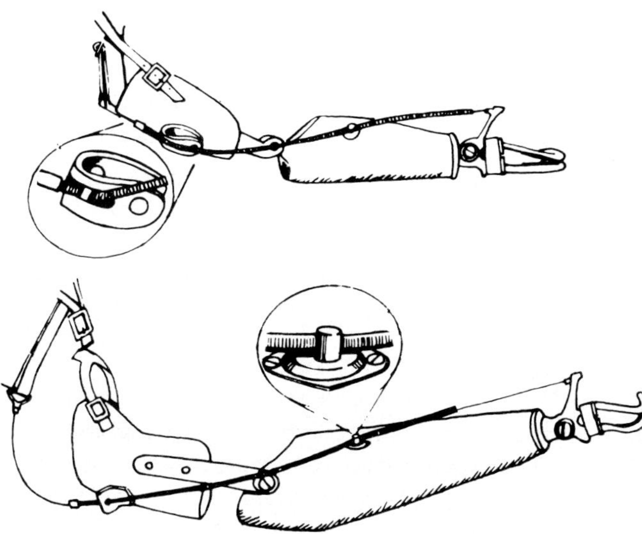

Fig. 9-15. Control cable housing. (From Below and above elbow harness and control system, Evanston, Ill., 1966, Northwestern University Prosthetic-Orthotic Center.)

It should be pointed out that Fig. 9-12 illustrates socket trim lines and remaining anatomy, but does not depict the various mechanical joints that are often used to provide motion between the humeral and socket segments of the prosthesis. Further information about these mechanical shoulder joints (in which the motions are passively, not actively, controlled) will be found in Section III of this chapter.

Finally, the forequarter amputation (Fig. 9-12, *C*) must be separated from the other two shoulder types, since the problems are unique. In the absence of a shoulder on which to obtain purchase, the socket will have to cover considerably larger portions of the thorax, both anteriorly and posteriorly, and may extend behind the neck and over the sound shoulder to afford stability. Furthermore, the loss of shoulder girdle motions leaves little that can be used for prosthesis control. In these circumstances, the provision of a functional, body-powered prosthesis is not feasible, and the usual recourse is to a socket (and perhaps prosthesis) whose major purpose is the restoration of symmetry. Design goals thus relate to lightness and cosmesis rather than to stability, motion transmission, component control, and function. There is no question that successful, functional, prosthetic restoration for the forequarter and other high-level amputations awaits the further development of external power and highly sophisticated control methods.

Section II

Harnessing and controls

CHARLES M. FRYER

In most upper limb prosthetic applications, the functions of control and suspension are closely interrelated. The prosthesis is suspended on the residual limb by the intimacy of the socket fit and by a system of Dacron straps collectively referred to as a "harness." In a well-designed harness the

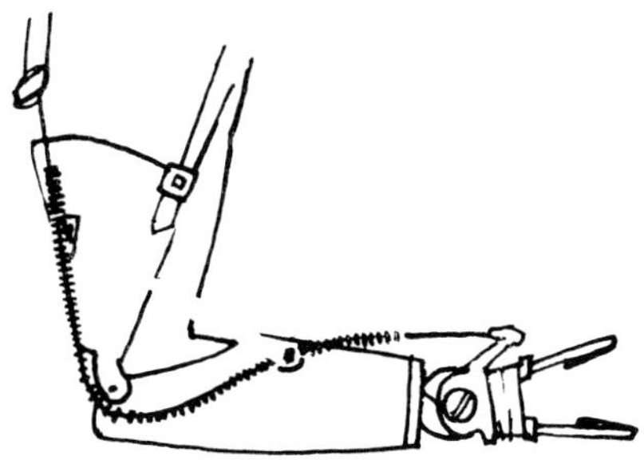

Fig. 9-16. Length of control cable remains constant. (From Below and above elbow harness and control system, Evanston, Ill., 1966, Northwestern University Prosthetic-Orthotic Center.)

same straps are strategically positioned in relation to the shoulder girdle and/or thorax, enabling the amputee to control the prosthetic components with a minimum of exertion and body motion. To understand the two main functions of a prosthetic harness it is first necessary to examine the mechanical operating principles of prosthetic control systems.

MECHANICS OF THE BELOW-ELBOW CONTROL SYSTEM

The below-elbow prosthetic control system is a one-cable or "single-control" system. A stainless steel control cable is firmly attached at its proximal end to one of the Dacron straps of the harness (Fig. 9-13). Distally, the cable terminates at some type of prehension device (Fig. 9-14).

Prehension devices, usually referred to simply as "terminal devices," may be either prosthetic hands with one or more movable fingers or two-fingered devices with a hook-type configuration. With this type of terminal device the amputee uses shoulder motion on the amputated side to apply tension to the control cable (Fig. 9-14). The cable tension is transmitted to the operating lever or "thumb" of the terminal device, causing one finger of the hook to move away from the other stationary finger (Fig. 9-14, *A*). When cable tension is relaxed, the movable finger closes on the stationary finger (Fig. 9-14, *B*). The force of prehension is, in this particular case, determined by the number of rubber bands located at the bases of the hook fingers. As a general rule each rubber band produces approximately 0.45 kg (1 pound) of prehensile force between the hook fingers.

For most of its length the control cable is encased in a flexible stainless steel housing (Fig. 9-15). At its upper end, the housing through which the control cable passes is attached to the triceps pad (Fig. 9-15) of the prosthesis by a fixture called a "crossbar assembly" (Fig. 9-15). A baseplate and retainer serve to anchor the distal end of the cable housing at approximately the midforearm level of the prosthesis (Fig. 9-15).

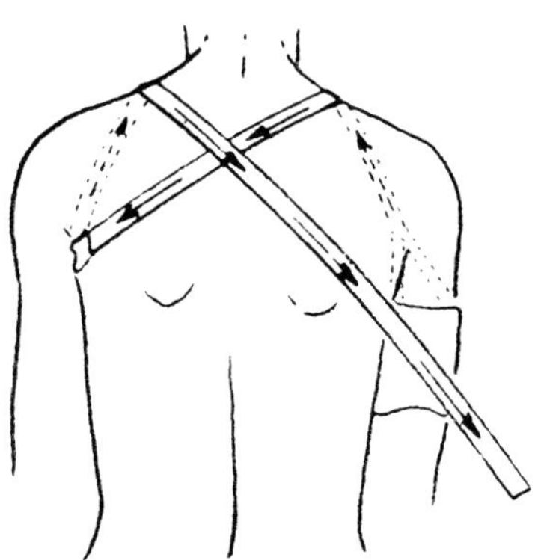

Fig. 9-17. Figure-of-eight configuration of standard below-elbow harness. (From Santschi, W. R., editor: Manual of upper extremity prosthetics, ed. 2, Los Angeles, 1958, University of California Department of Engineering.)

The cable housing is an integral part of the below-elbow single-control system. In effect, the housing maintains a constant length of the control cable regardless of the angular attitude of the anatomical elbow joint. The amount of body motion used to operate the terminal device remains essentially the same with the elbow flexed to 135 degrees or with the elbow completely extended (Fig. 9-16).

STANDARD BELOW-ELBOW HARNESS

The standard harness for the unilateral adult below-elbow amputee is composed of 2.5-cm (1-inch) wide Dacron webbing. The webbing is arranged to form a horizontally oriented figure of eight (Fig. 9-17).

The axilla loop serves as the primary anchor from which two other straps originate. As indicated by its name, the axilla loop encircles the shoulder girdle on the nonamputated side (Fig. 9-18).

The second component of the below-elbow harness is the anterior support strap or, as it is sometimes called, "the inverted Y suspensor." The anterior support strap originates at the axilla loop, passes over the shoulder on the amputated side and is attached to the anteroproximal margins of the triceps pad of the prosthesis. The primary function of the anterior support strap is to resist displacement of the socket on the residual limb when the prosthesis is subjected to heavy loading (Fig. 9-19).

The control attachment strap originates at the axilla loop and terminates at the proximal end of the prosthetic control cable (Fig. 9-20). Anchored

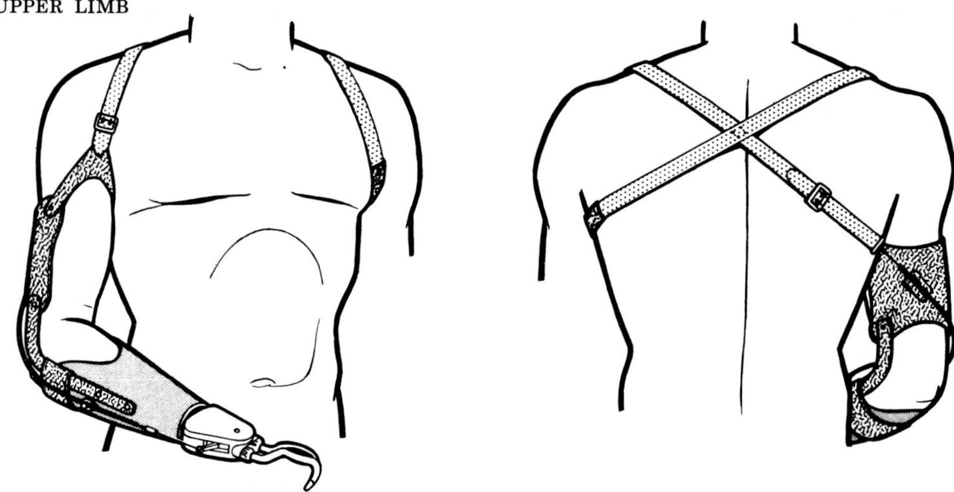

Fig. 9-18. Axilla loop. (From Pursley, R. J.: Harness patterns for upper-extremity prostheses, Chapter 4. In American Academy of Orthopaedic Surgeons: Orthopaedic appliances atlas, vol. 2, Artificial limbs, Ann Arbor, Mich., 1960, J. W. Edwards.)

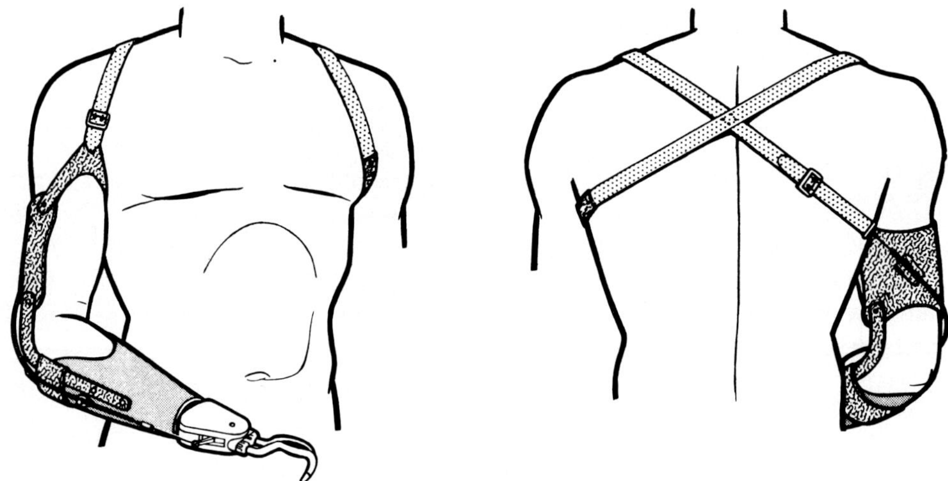

Fig. 9-19. Anterior support strap. (From Pursley, R. J.: Harness patterns for upper-extremity prostheses, Chapter 4. In American Academy of Orthopaedic Surgeons: Orthopaedic appliances atlas, vol. 2, Artificial limbs, Ann Arbor, Mich., 1960, J. W. Edwards.)

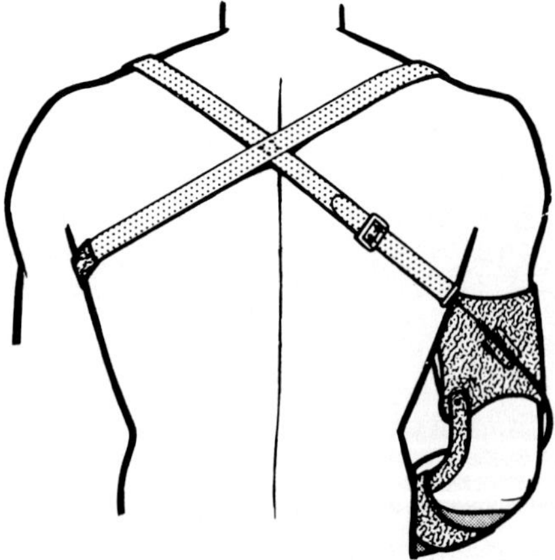

Fig. 9-20. Control attachment. (From Pursley, R. J.: Harness patterns for upper-extremity prostheses, Chapter 4. In American Academy of Orthopaedic Surgeons: Orthopaedic appliances atlas, vol. 2, Artificial limbs, Ann Arbor, Mich., 1960, J.W. Edwards.)

by the axilla loop, the control attachment strap acts, in effect, as an extension of the control cable. Located between the spine and inferior angle of the scapula, the control attachment strap permits the use of scapular abduction and shoulder flexion on the amputated side for operation of the terminal device.

The posterior junction of the axilla loop with the anterior support and control attachment straps—the crosspoint of the harness—may be either sewn together (Fig. 9-21) or connected by a stainless steel ring (Fig. 9-22). In the latter case, the harness is referred to as a "below-elbow, ring-type harness." (Because they are less restrictive, ring-type harnesses enjoy a high degree of acceptability by most below-elbow amputees.)

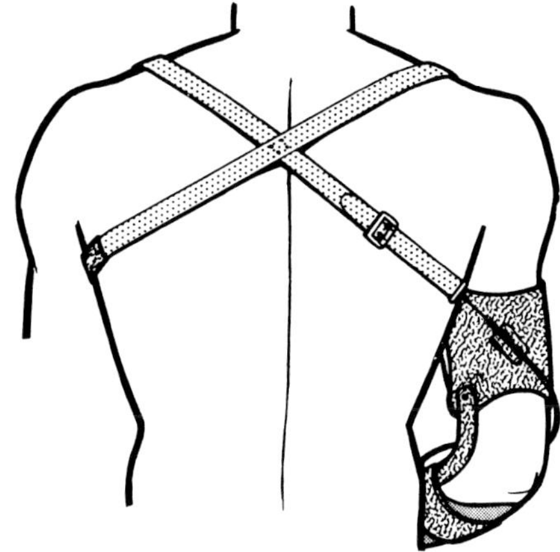

Fig. 9-21. Cross point of harness sewn together. (From Pursley, R. J.: Harness patterns for upper-extremity prostheses, Chapter 4. In American Academy of Orthopaedic Surgeons: Orthopaedic appliances atlas, vol. 2, Artificial limbs, Ann Arbor, Mich., 1960, J. W. Edwards.)

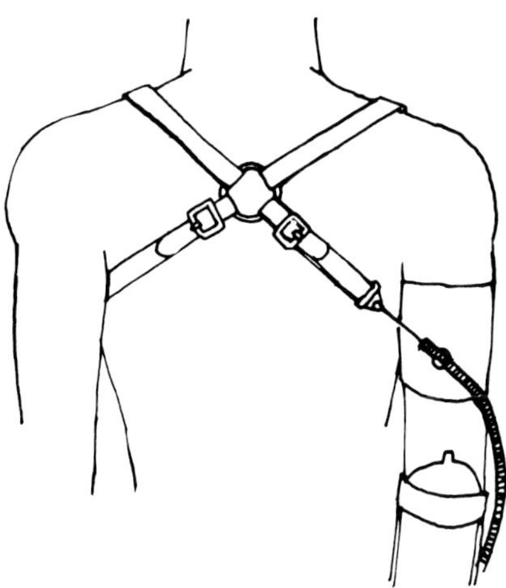

Fig. 9-22. Cross point of harness connected by stainless steel ring. (From Below and above elbow harness and control system, Evanston, Ill., 1966, Northwestern University Prosthetic-Orthotic Center.)

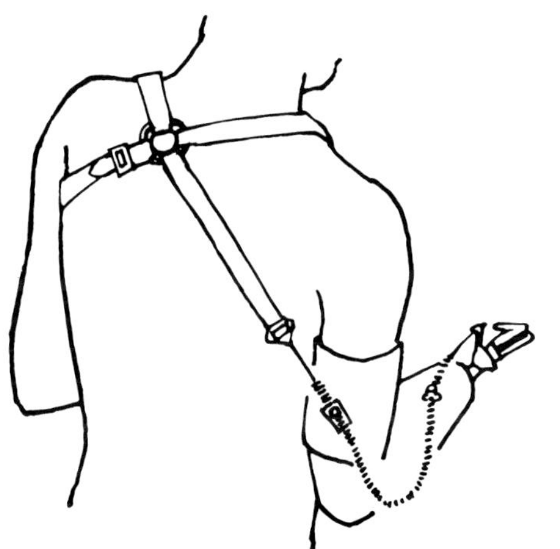

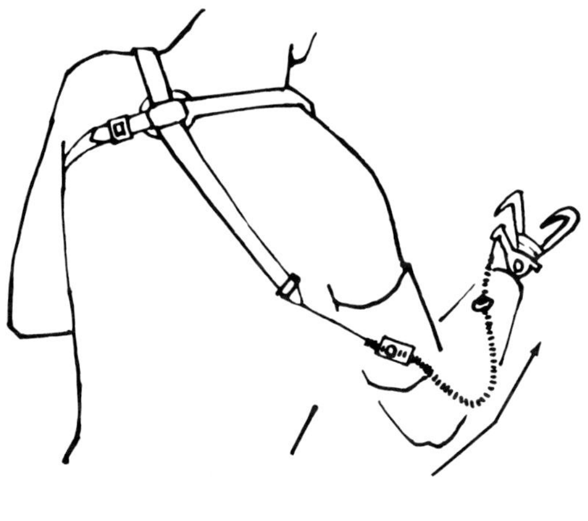

Fig. 9-23. Glenohumeral joint flexion for operating terminal device. (From Below and above elbow harness and control system, Evanston, Ill., 1966, Northwestern University Prosthetic-Orthotic Center.)

Whether the harness straps are sewn together or attached to the axilla loop by a steel ring, mechanical efficiency will be enhanced if the cross point is located below the spinous process of C-7 and slightly toward the nonamputated side.

The primary body control motion for operating the terminal device of a below-elbow prosthesis is flexion of the glenohumeral joint (Figs. 9-23). Glenohumeral flexion is excellent for the generation of force and provides more than enough cable travel for full terminal device operation. When terminal device operation close to the midline of the body is required, as when buttoning a shirt, the standard below-elbow harness permits the amputee to use biscapular abduction for terminal device operation (Fig. 9-24).

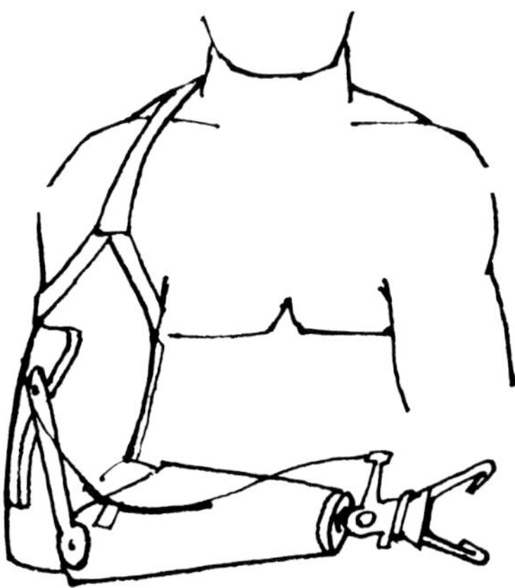

Fig. 9-24. Biscapular abduction for terminal device operation. (From Below and above elbow harness and control system, Evanston, Ill., 1966, Northwestern University Prosthetic-Orthotic Center.)

HEAVY-DUTY BELOW-ELBOW HARNESS

A major disadvantage of the standard figure-of-eight harness for below-elbow amputees relates to the axilla loop. The axillary portion of the loop should always be padded and worn on top of an undergarment. Even so, whenever significant tension is applied to the anterior support and control attachment straps, the tension drives the loop vertically upward into the axilla on the nonamputated side. Over a period of time, excessive pressure in the axillary area may cause skin irritation and, in extreme cases, produce neurotrophic changes from brachial plexus pressure. When it is anticipated that the below-elbow amputee will engage in very strenuous work activities, particularly the repeated lifting of heavy objects, it is

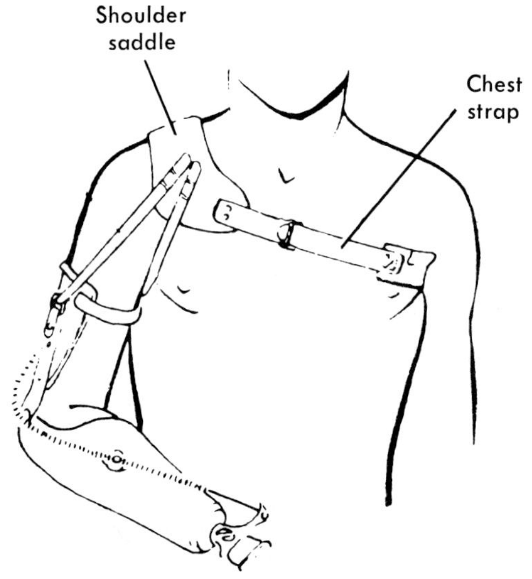

Fig. 9-25. Shoulder-saddle harness. (From Santschi, W. R., editor: Manual of upper extremity prosthetics, ed. 2, Los Angeles, 1958, University of California Department of Engineering.)

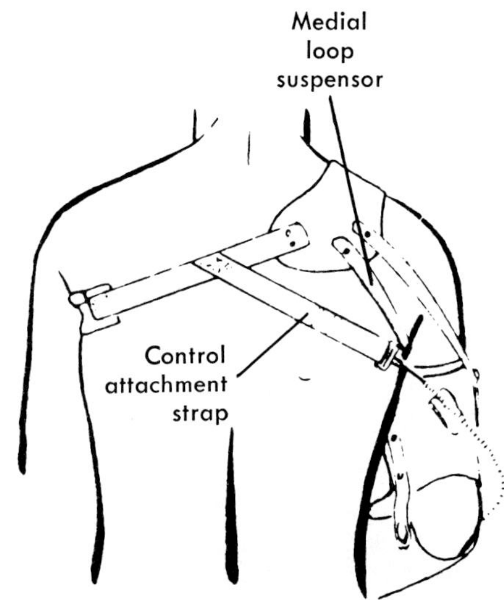

Fig. 9-26. Location of control attachment strap on shoulder-saddle harness. (From Santschi, W. R., editor: Manual of upper extremity prosthetics, ed. 2, Los Angeles, 1958, University of California Department of Engineering.)

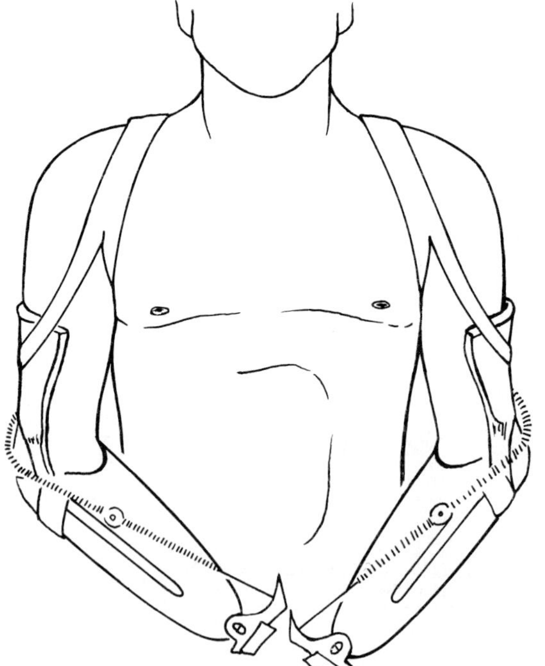

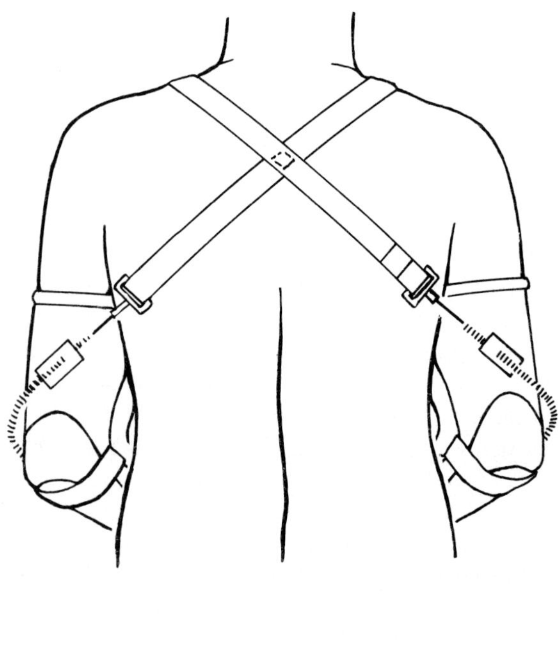

Fig. 9-27. Bilateral below-elbow harness. Note location of control attachment strap in back view. (From Santschi, W. R., editor: Manual of upper extremity prosthetics, ed. 2, Los Angeles, 1958, University of California Department of Engineering.)

recommended that a nonstandard below-elbow harness system be considered.

The nonstandard below-elbow harness is generally referred to as a "heavy-duty" or "shoulder-saddle" harness. With the heavy-duty harness, tension loading on the prosthesis is distributed over the shoulder on the amputated side, rather than being transmitted to the axilla on the non-amputated side. This redistribution of loading is accomplished by fitting a fairly wide, leather shoulder saddle on the amputated side. Two support straps are extended from the posterior portion of the shoulder saddle through D rings located on the medial and lateral surfaces of the triceps pad and terminate on the anterior surface of the saddle. The shoulder saddle is anchored in place by the use of a chest strap. Since the control attachment strap is located in essentially the same place as in the standard harness, midscapular level, the amputee uses glenohumeral flexion and/or scapular abduction for terminal device operation (Figs. 9-25 and 9-26).

BILATERAL BELOW-ELBOW HARNESS

The harness pattern for the bilateral below-elbow amputee differs only slightly from the previously described standard below-elbow harness. Viewed from the rear, the control attachment strap for operation of the right terminal device extends obliquely upward across the back and terminates as the anterior support strap for the left prosthesis (Fig. 9-27). Likewise the control attachment strap for operation of the left terminal device becomes the anterior support strap for the left prosthesis. As in the case of the standard unilateral harness, the posterior cross point may be sewn together or connected by a stainless steel ring. The bilateral below-elbow amputee uses the same body control motions, glenohumeral flexion and/or biscapular abduction, for terminal device operation as does the unilateral below-elbow amputee.

BELOW-ELBOW HARNESS MODIFICATIONS

Step-up hinges used with a split socket may be used in a short below-elbow amputee to provide increased (double) excursion of the forearm and terminal device, but require the amputee to use approximately twice as much force to flex the prosthetic forearm. Since split sockets are used only at very short below-elbow levels of amputation, the extra force requirement may cause considerable discomfort on the volar or radial surfaces of the remaining portion of the amputee's forearm. In such instances, a relatively simple control system modification may be used to minimize discomfort and facilitate elbow flexion.

The modification consists of splitting the cable housing into proximal and distal segments simi-

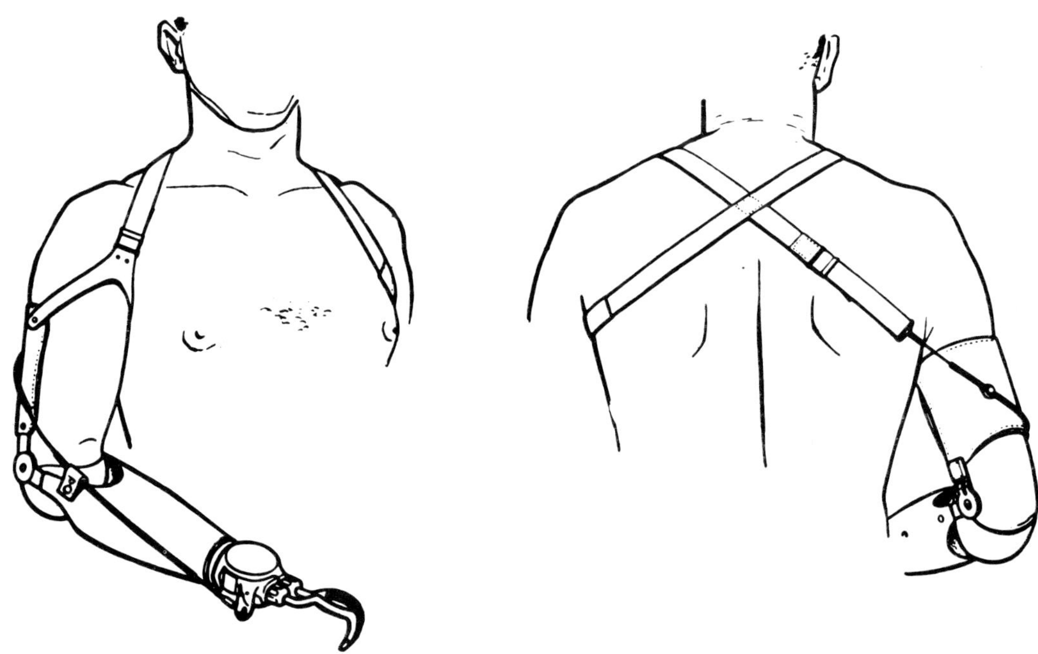

Fig. 9-28. Modification of cable housing in below-elbow harness. (From Bechtol, C. O.: Anatomical and physiological considerations in the clinical application of upper-extremity prosthetics, Chapter 8. In American Academy of Orthopaedic Surgeons: Orthopaedic appliances atlas, vol. 2, Artificial limbs, Ann Arbor, Mich., 1960, J. W. Edwards.)

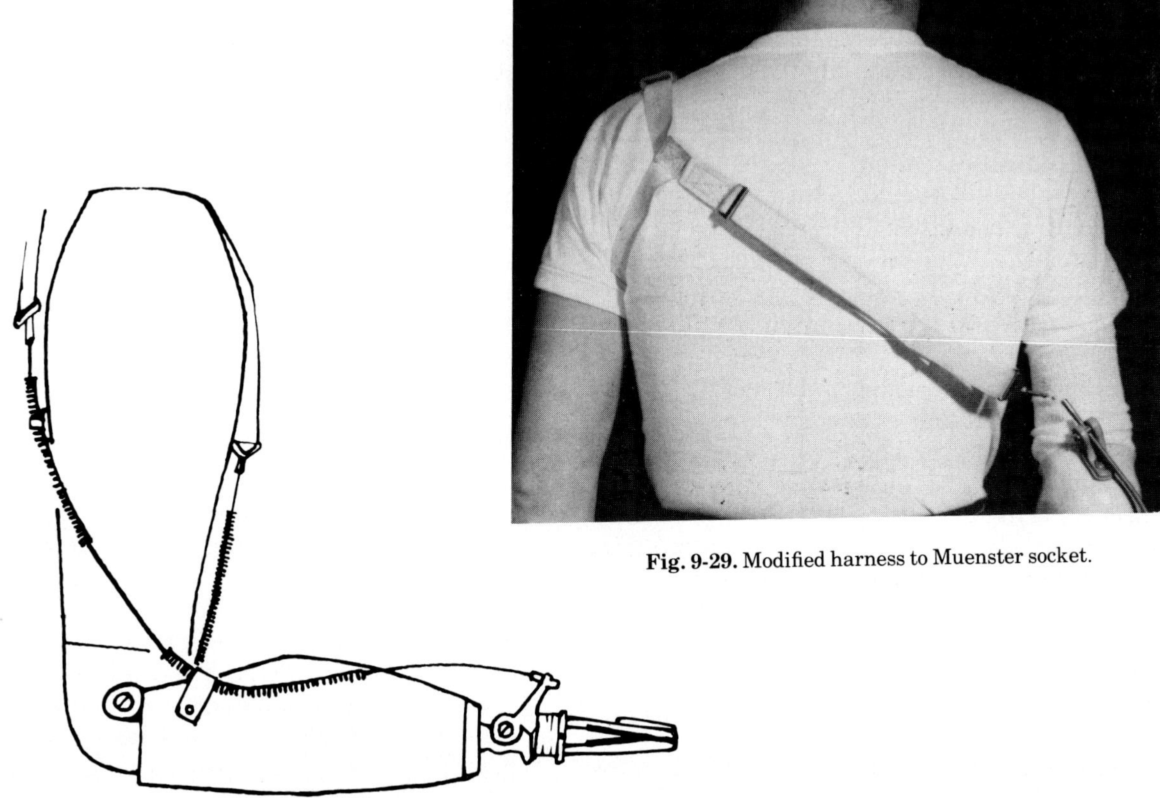

Fig. 9-29. Modified harness to Muenster socket.

Fig. 9-30. Above-elbow control system. Note use of two cables. (From Below and above elbow harness and control system, Evanston, Ill., 1966, Northwestern University Prosthetic-Orthotic Center.)

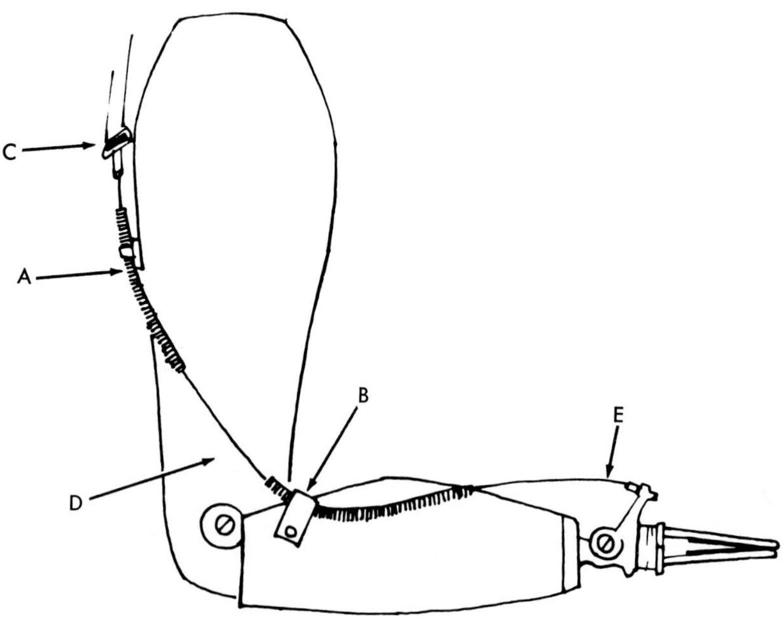

Fig. 9-31. Split housing for cable in elbow flexion/terminal device. (From Below and above elbow harness and control system, Evanston, Ill., 1966, Northwestern University Prosthetic-Orthotic Center.)

lar to those used for the above-elbow prosthesis. The proximal piece of housing is attached to the triceps pad and the distal piece to the prosthetic forearm. The control cable is now exposed as it passes anterior to the elbow joint. Tension applied to the control cable by glenohumeral flexion on the amputated side assists in elbow flexion (Fig. 9-28).

In selected instances the unilateral below-elbow amputee can be fit with a socket (Muenster), which obviates the need for the suspensory function of a harness. Such self-suspending prostheses are held on the residual limb by the intimacy of the socket fit proximal to the olecranon and humeral epicondyles and in the antecubital fossa. Since these fittings eliminate the need for a triceps pad and anterior support strap, the harness consists of a simple axilla loop around the shoulder on the nonamputated side. Extending obliquely downward across the amputee's back, the control attachment strap runs from the axilla loop to the terminal device control cable. As in the case of the standard harness, shoulder flexion and/or scapular abduction on the amputated side are the control motions for terminal device operation (Fig. 9-29). The disadvantage of this type of harnessing is that long-sleeved clothing is difficult to wear.

MECHANICS OF THE ABOVE-ELBOW CONTROL SYSTEM

Above-elbow prostheses are usually operated by two distinctly separate control cables (Fig. 9-30). One cable serves both to flex the prosthetic elbow joint and to operate the terminal device. A second cable permits the amputee to lock and unlock the prosthetic elbow.

Elbow flexion/terminal device control cable

The housing through which the elbow flexion/terminal device cable passes is split into two separate parts (Fig. 9-31). The proximal portion of the split housing is attached to the posterior surface of the humeral section of the prosthesis. The distal portion of the split housing is fixed to the prosthetic forearm by a device called an "elbow flexion attachment."

The elbow flexion/terminal device control cable originates at the control attachment strap of the harness (Fig. 9-31, *C*). Passing through the proximal portion of the split housing, the control cable continues exposed anterior to the mechanical elbow axis (Fig. 9-31, *D*). The elbow flexion/terminal device control cable continues through the distal portion of the split housing and terminates with its attachment at the terminal device (Fig. 9-31, *E*). Since the housing is in two separate pieces and the control cable passes in front of the elbow axis, tension applied to the cable causes the prosthetic elbow to flex. The extension is limited to the gap between the two cable housings.

The ease with which the amputee can operate the elbow unit and terminal device depends, to a considerable extent, on the location of the elbow flexion attachment. Greater force and less cable excursion are required where the elbow flexion attachment is closest to the elbow axis. Converse-

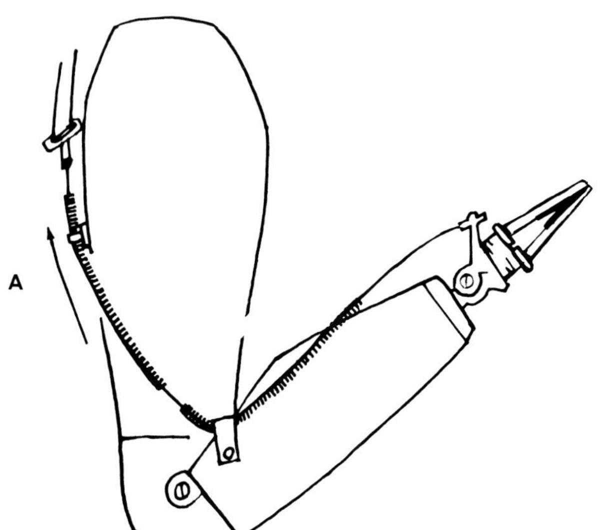

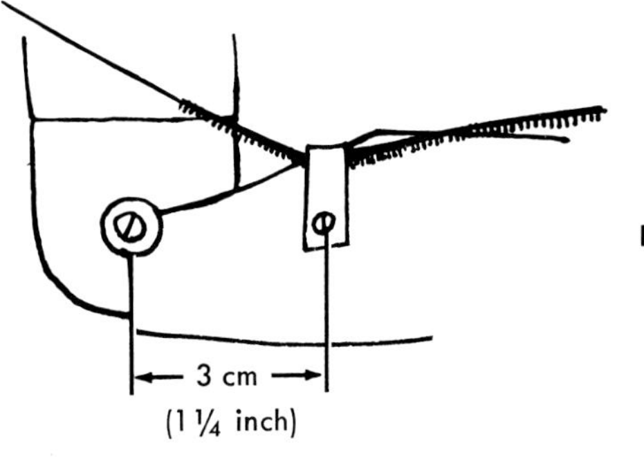

Fig. 9-32. A, Prosthetic elbow flexed because of split cable housing. **B,** Location of elbow flexion attachment should be determined on individual basis. (From Below and above elbow harness and control system, Evanston, Ill., 1966, Northwestern University Prosthetic-Orthotic Center.)

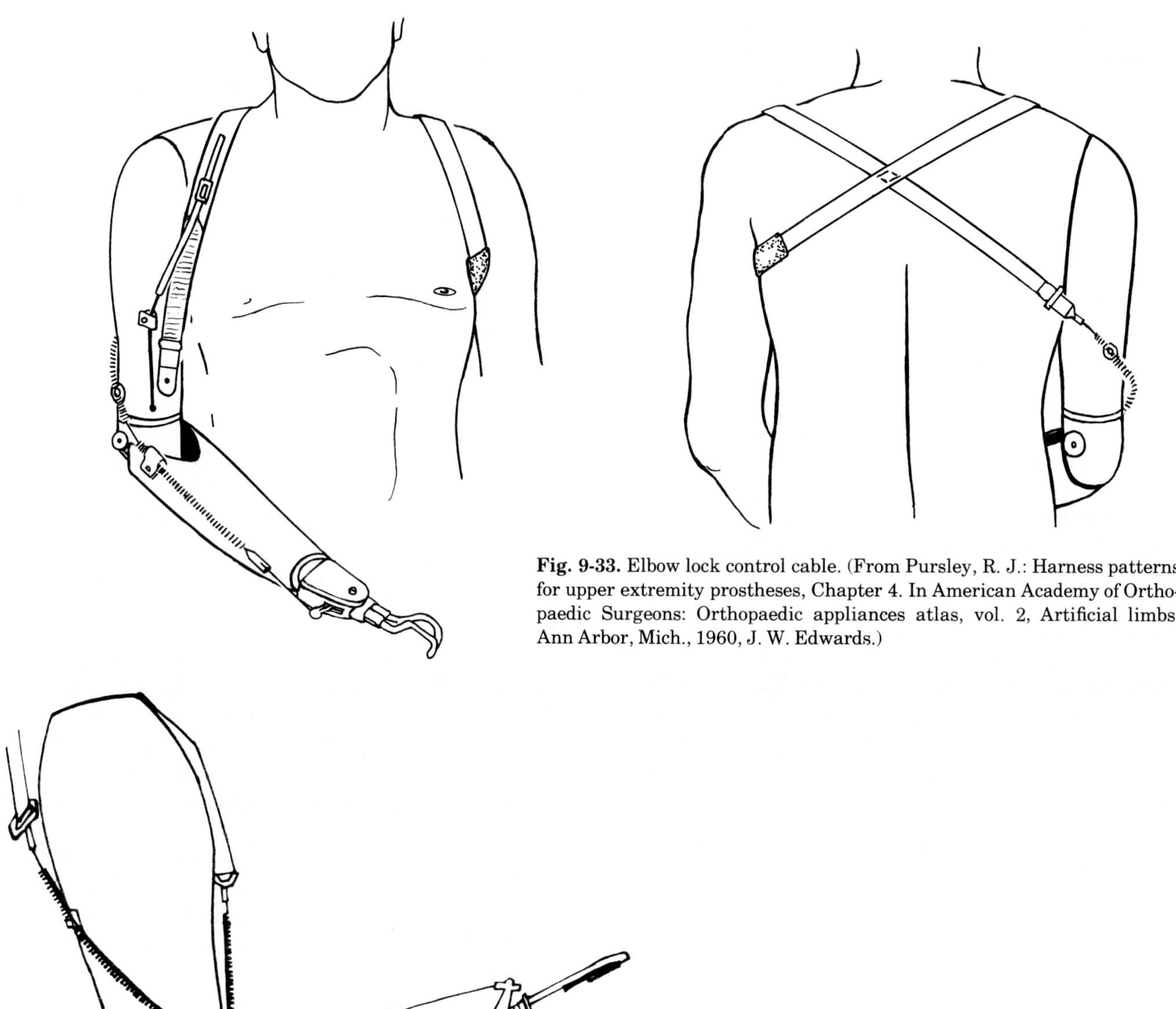

Fig. 9-33. Elbow lock control cable. (From Pursley, R. J.: Harness patterns for upper extremity prostheses, Chapter 4. In American Academy of Orthopaedic Surgeons: Orthopaedic appliances atlas, vol. 2, Artificial limbs, Ann Arbor, Mich., 1960, J. W. Edwards.)

Fig. 9-34. Reapplication of tension on elbow flexion/terminal device control cable permits operation of terminal device. (From Below and above elbow harness and control system, Evanston, Ill., 1966, Northwestern University Prosthetic-Orthotic Center.)

ly, a more distal placement of the attachment requires less force but greater cable excursion.

Generally, the longer the residual limb, the closer the elbow flexion attachment may be placed to the elbow axis. Higher above-elbow levels of amputation require a more distal placement of the attachment.

Although the initial placement of the elbow flexion attachment 3.1 cm (1¼ inches) distal to the elbow axis is usually satisfactory, in most instances, its precise location should be determined on an individual basis (Fig. 9-32).

Elbow lock control cable

The proximal end of the elbow lock control cable originates at the anterior suspension strap (Fig. 9-33). Passing down the anteromedial surface of the humeral section of the prosthesis, the distal end of the cable engages the elbow locking mechanism. The elbow lock works on an alternator principle: pull and release to lock, pull and release to unlock. An excursion of 1.3 cm (½ inch) and a force of approximately 0.9 kg (2 pounds) are necessary to cycle the elbow unit.

In summary, the operating sequence of the two-cable system used with most above-elbow prostheses is as follows: (1) tension applied to the elbow flexion/terminal device control cable causes the elbow to flex; (2) when the desired angle of elbow flexion is achieved, the rapid sequential application and release of tension on the elbow lock control cable locks the elbow; and (3) with the elbow locked, the reapplication of tension on the elbow flexion/terminal device control cable permits operation of the terminal device (Fig. 9-34).

STANDARD ABOVE-ELBOW HARNESS

Full operation of the terminal device of a below-elbow prosthesis requires only 5 cm (2 inches) of cable excursion. More than twice that amount of excursion is required for full elbow and terminal device operation of an above-elbow prosthesis. Consequently, much greater attention must be paid to the details of fitting the above-elbow harness. Precision in the location of the harness and control system components is essential for achieving satisfactory comfort and function.

Like the standard below-elbow harness, the above-elbow harness consists of a system of interconnected Dacron and elastic straps laid up in a figure of eight (Fig. 9-33). The common elements of the standard above-elbow harness are the axilla loop, anterior support strap, lateral support strap, control attachment strap, and elbow lock control strap.

The axilla loop acts as the fixed anchor from which other harness components originate. Some of the straps originating at the axilla loop serve to suspend the prosthesis on the residual limb, others provide the amputee with volitional control of the prosthetic components.

The anterior support strap, sometimes referred to as the elastic suspensor, originates at the axilla loop (Fig. 9-33, *A*). Passing over the shoulder on the amputated side, the strap continues down the anteromedial surface of the humeral section of the prosthesis. The anterior support strap terminates with its attachment on the anterior surface of the prosthetic socket slightly proximal to the mechanical elbow joint (Fig. 9-33, *B*). Viewed from the front, it should be noted that the distal two thirds of the anterior support strap consist of elastic rather than Dacron webbing (Fig. 9-33, *C*).

The anterior support strap serves several functions in the above-elbow harness systems. Anchored to the axilla loop posteriorly and to the humeral section anteriorly, this strap helps to suspend the prosthesis against axial loading. However, since the anterodistal two thirds of the strap consist of elastic webbing, suspensory function is obviously limited.

A second function of the anterior support strap is to help prevent rotation of the prosthetic socket on the residual limb during prosthetic usage. The above-elbow amputee uses glenohumeral flexion on the amputated side to flex the prosthetic elbow and/or operate the terminal device. Since the proximal control cable housing is attached on the posterolateral surface of the humeral section of the prosthesis, glenohumeral flexion tends to

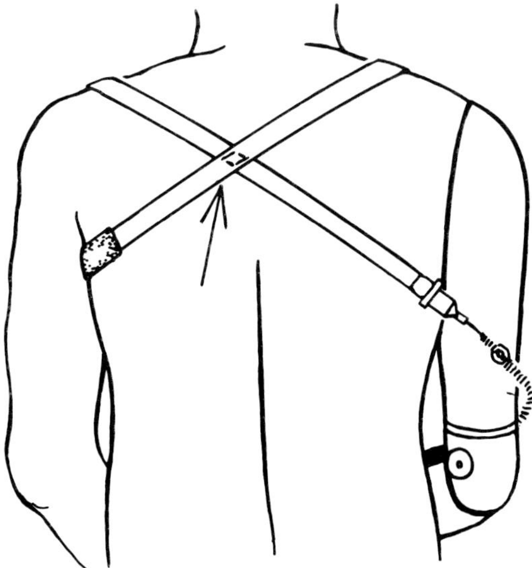

Fig. 9-35. Posterior intersection of harness straps (arrow) should be positioned toward nonamputated side of body. (From Pursley, R. J.: Harness patterns for upper extremity prostheses, Chapter 4. In American Academy of Orthopaedic Surgeons: Orthopaedic appliances atlas, vol. 2, Artificial limbs, Ann Arbor, Mich., 1960, J. W. Edwards.)

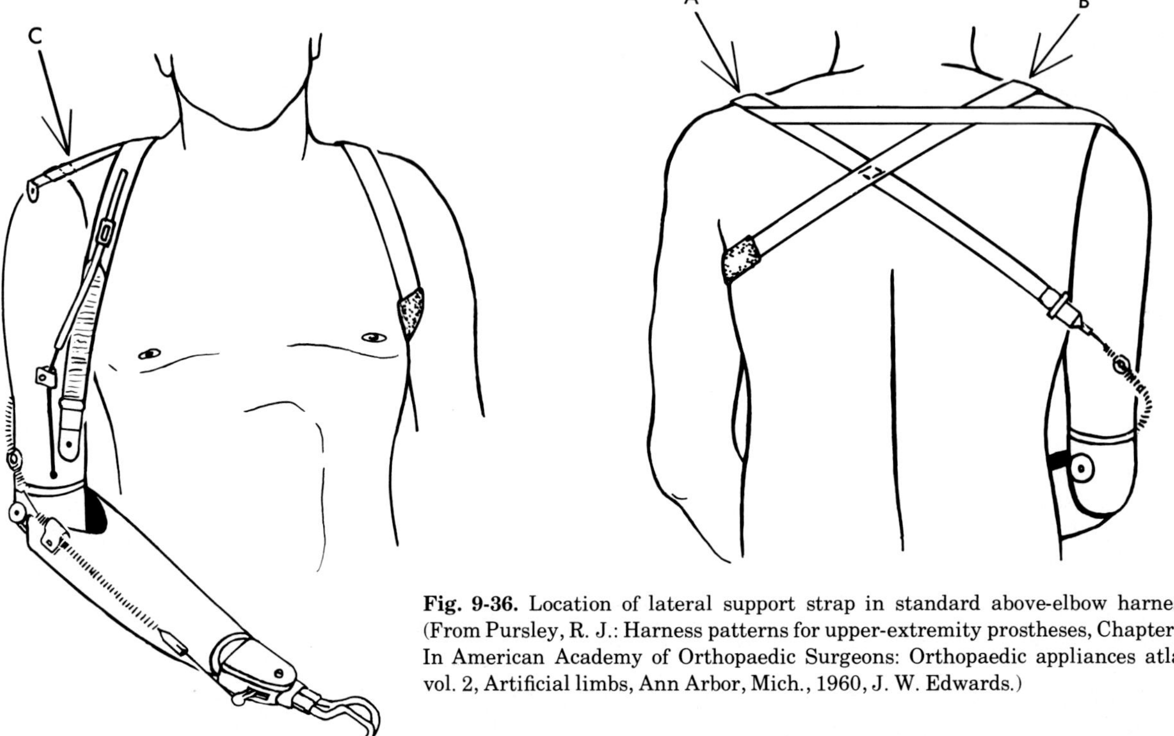

Fig. 9-36. Location of lateral support strap in standard above-elbow harness. (From Pursley, R. J.: Harness patterns for upper-extremity prostheses, Chapter 4. In American Academy of Orthopaedic Surgeons: Orthopaedic appliances atlas, vol. 2, Artificial limbs, Ann Arbor, Mich., 1960, J. W. Edwards.)

cause the socket to externally rotate on the residual limb. The anterior support strap running downward mediolaterally resists external rotation of the socket.

As a key element of the entire harness, the axilla loop should encircle and fit the shoulder on the nonamputated side as securely as possible. A small, snug axilla loop, one that does not compromise amputee comfort to an excessive degree, provides the most positive prosthetic suspension and control. To maintain a fairly snug axilla loop, the posterior intersection of the harness straps should be positioned toward the nonamputated side of the body (Fig. 9-35).

The lateral support strap is the primary suspensory element of the harness. Originating posteriorly from the upper portion of the axilla loop, the strap is directed horizontally and stitched to the anterior support strap at their intersection (Fig. 9-36, *A* and *B*). The lateral end of the strap passes just anterior to the acromion and is attached close to the proximal trim line of the prosthetic socket (Fig. 9-36, *C*). In addition to its suspensory function, the strap helps to prevent external rotation of the socket on the limb when tension is applied to the elbow flexion/terminal device control cable.

The control attachment strap originates at the posterior intersection of the axilla loop. Running obliquely downward across the amputee's back, the control attachment strap terminates with its direct attachment to the elbow flexion/terminal device control cable (Fig. 9-37).

With the control attachment strap firmly fixed at its proximal end by the axilla loop, it is easy to visualize how shoulder flexion on the amputated side creates both the cable tension and cable excursion required for elbow flexion and terminal device operation.

The proper location of the control attachment strap as it passes from the axilla loop to the elbow flexion/terminal device control cable is important. If the control attachment strap lies too high on the amputee's back, shoulder flexion will not produce sufficient cable excursion for full operation of the mechanical elbow and terminal device. Too low a strap position requires the amputee to use unnecessarily forceful shoulder flexion for full operation. With the control attachment strap located at approximately midscapular level, midway between the spine and inferior angle, the amputee will usually be able to achieve full operation of the components through the application of a moderate amount of force.

A cross back strap is sometimes used as an adjunct to the standard above-elbow harness (Fig. 9-38). Originating at the axilla loop close to the posterior axillary fold, the cross back strap passes horizontally across the amputee's back and terminates at the distal end of the control attachment

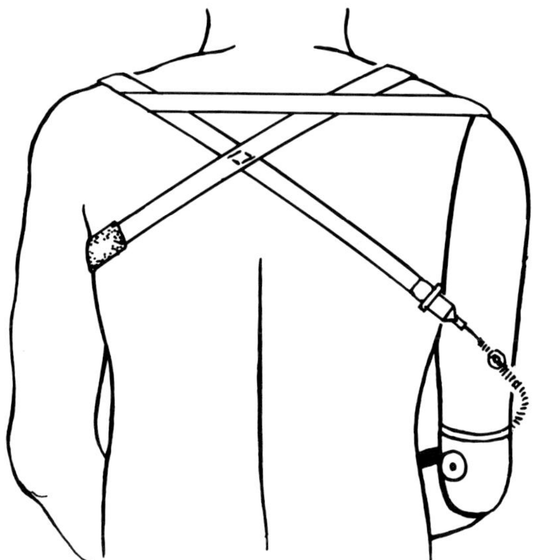

Fig. 9-37. Location of control attachment strap in standard above-elbow harness. (From Pursley, R. J.: Harness patterns for upper-extremity prostheses, Chapter 4. In American Academy of Orthopaedic Surgeons: Orthopaedic appliances atlas, vol. 2, Artificial limbs, Ann Arbor, Mich., 1960, J. W. Edwards.)

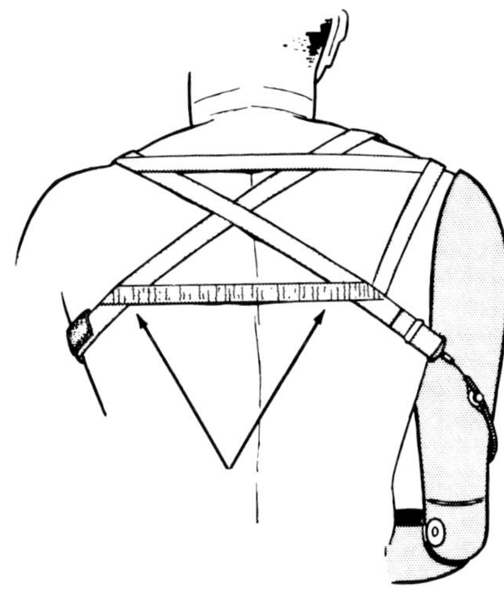

Fig. 9-38. Cross back strap (arrows) used as adjunct to standard above-elbow harness. (From Pursley, R. J.: Harness patterns for upper-extremity prostheses, Chapter 4. In American Academy of Orthopaedic Surgeons: Orthopaedic appliances atlas, vol. 2, Artificial limbs, Ann Arbor, Mich., 1960, J. W. Edwards.)

strap. Indications for the use of this strap relate primarily to amputee comfort and ease of prosthetic operation.

At midhumeral and higher levels of above-elbow amputation it becomes increasingly important that the harness be fitted as intimately as possible. Since a snug harness fit requires a relatively small axilla loop, the loop may tend to cause axillary discomfort on the nonamputated side. This discomfort is due, primarily, to vertical compression of the pectoral, teres major, and latissimus dorsi tendons by the axilla loop during strenuous prosthetic usage. The use of a cross back strap in such instances helps to reduce the magnitude of the vertically directed force created by a snug axilla loop.

Another indication for the addition of a cross back strap is when the posterior intersection of the harness rides too high on the amputee's back. With the posterior intersection of the harness on, or superior to, the spinous process of C-7, the amputee is uncomfortable, and the work efficiency of the entire harness and control system is diminished. The cross back strap helps to maintain the posterior intersection of the harness below the spine of C-7.

As noted earlier in this chapter, the standard above-elbow prosthetic control system requires approximately 11.3 cm (4½ inches) of cable excursion for full elbow and terminal device operation. Whether or not the amputee is able to generate this much cable excursion depends to a great extent on the path of the control attachment strap as it crosses the amputee's back. Ideally, the path of the control attachment strap should run between the spine and inferior angle of the scapula. Cable excursion, normally produced by glenohumeral flexion on the amputated side, diminishes as the path of the control attachment strap moves closer to the shoulder joint. The addition of a cross back strap helps to keep the path of the control attachment strap positioned lower on the back.

Cross back straps may be made of either elastic or Dacron webbing. The nonelastic strap provides the amputee with more positive control of the prosthetic components and overall tautness of the harness. An elastic strap provides less positive control but greater degrees of comfort and mobility of the shoulder girdle.

The elbow lock control strap originates at the upper, nonelastic portion of the anterior support strap and is attached at its distal end to the elbow lock control cable (Fig. 9-39).

To either lock or unlock the prosthetic elbow the amputee must first apply tension and then, in rapid sequence, relax tension on the elbow lock control cable. Although the cable excursion requirement for prosthetic elbow operation is small, approximately 1.3 cm (½ inch), the body motion is somewhat complex. The amputee applies tension to the elbow lock control strap and cable by slight extension and abduction of the glenohumeral joint combined with equally slight shoulder depression on the amputated side. This motion, in addition to exerting tension on the elbow lock control strap and cable, also stretches the elastic portion of the anterior support strap. With the rapid return of the prosthesis to the starting position, the elastic tension of the anterior support strap serves to complete the lock/unlock cycle.

The ring-type harness does not enjoy the same degree of acceptability in above-elbow harnessing as it does at the below-elbow level. At midhumeral and higher levels of amputation it becomes increasingly important that the harness fit be as snug as possible. Ring-type harnesses do not permit the same degree of tautness in the straps of the system as do stitched harnesses. Consequently, at the higher above-elbow levels the ring-type harness is found wanting in that it does not provide a very high degree of positive control of the prosthetic components, unless after adjustment the straps are sewn in place.

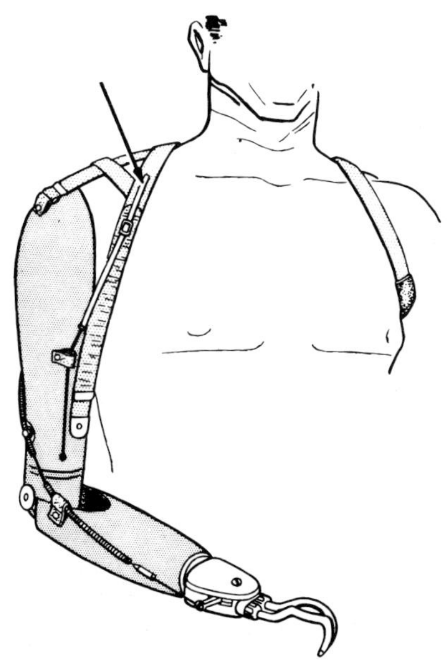

Fig. 9-39. Elbow lock control strap (arrow) on above-elbow harness. (From Pursley, R. J.: Harness patterns for upper-extremity prostheses, Chapter 4. In American Academy of Orthopaedic Surgeons: Orthopaedic appliances atlas, vol. 2, Artificial limbs, Ann Arbor, Mich., 1960, J. W. Edwards.)

The standard figure-of-eight harness is suitable for and acceptable to the great majority of unilateral above-elbow amputees. However, the unilateral above-elbow amputee who, on a regular basis, engages in unusually strenuous physical activity may find the standard harness uncomfortable. During periods of heavy work, the relatively narrow straps of a standard above-elbow harness tend to subject the soft tissues over which they pass to inordinately high unit pressures. Particularly vulnerable are the skin, tendons, and neurovascular structures of the axilla on the nonamputated side. The problem is further compounded at the above elbow level because maximal control of the components of the prosthesis requires the use of a small, snug axilla loop.

Alleviation of axillary discomfort for the above-elbow amputee who engages in unusually heavy work is best achieved through the use of a shoul-

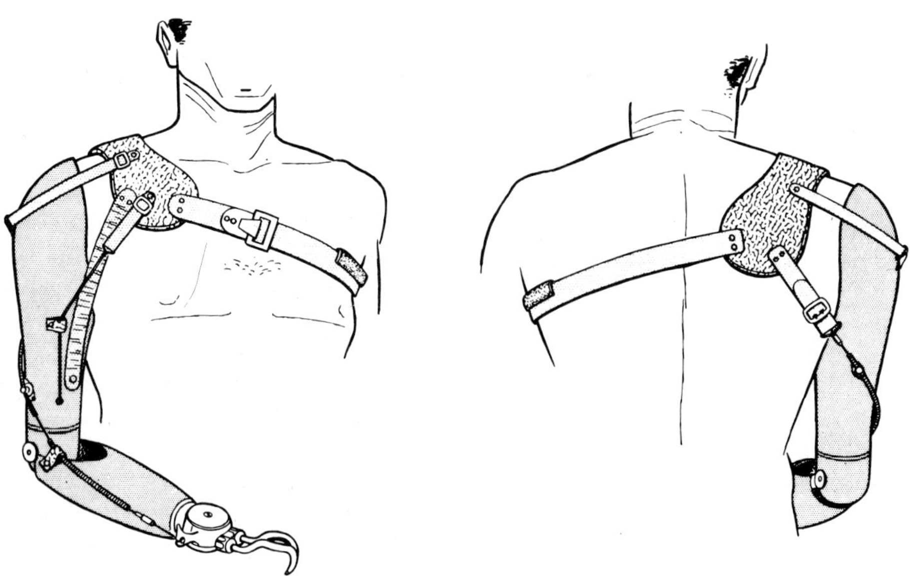

Fig. 9-40. Above-elbow shoulder-saddle harness. (From Pursley, R. J.: Harness patterns for upper-extremity prostheses, Chapter 4. In American Academy of Orthopaedic Surgeons: Orthopaedic appliances atlas, vol. 2, Artificial limbs, Ann Arbor, Mich., 1960, J. W. Edwards.)

der-saddle harness. The above-elbow shoulder harness distributes tension loading on the prosthesis to the shoulder on the amputated side. Since the control attachment and elbow lock control straps run along the same paths as they do in the standard harness, the body control motions for prosthetic operation remain essentially unchanged (Fig. 9-40).

The harness for the bilateral above-elbow amputee consists essentially of two figure-of-eight harnesses without axilla loops (Fig. 9-41). The control attachment strap for the right prosthesis is continued over the amputee's left shoulder and becomes the anterior support strap for the left prosthesis. Likewise, the left control attachment strap becomes the right anterior support strap. At their intersection in the midline of the amputee's back the two straps are sewn together. As in the unilateral harness system, the elbow lock control straps of the bilateral harness originate on the nonelastic portion of the anterior support strap. The lateral support straps consist of a continuous piece of Dacron webbing attached close to the proximal trim lines of both sockets and pass slightly anterior to the acromion processes. Posteriorly, the lateral support straps are stitched to the anterior support straps. Whereas a cross back strap is considered optional in the standard unilateral above-elbow harness, it is an essential component in the bilateral harness. As seen in Fig. 9-41, the cross back strap runs horizontally between the two control attachment straps. Two over-the-shoulder straps complete the bilateral figure-of-eight harness for the bilateral above-elbow amputee.

At their posterior origins the over-the-shoulder straps are sewn to the control attachment straps. Prior to passing over the amputee's shoulder, the straps are also stitched to the lateral support straps. The over-the-shoulder straps terminate anteriorly by attachment to the nonelastic portions of the anterior support straps (Fig. 9-42).

The bilateral above-elbow harness permits the amputee to use glenohumeral flexion and/or scapular abduction for elbow flexion and terminal device operation. Elbow lock control is effected by slight glenohumeral extension and abduction combined with shoulder depression. Two major problems confront the bilateral amputee with the harness just described. First, there is some difficulty in operating both prostheses simultaneously. Tension applied to both elbow flexion/terminal device cables permits opening (or closing) of both terminal devices, but both terminal devices cannot be operated to effect simultaneous opening and closing on opposite sides without relaxing tension on one of the cables. Consequently, the possibility of active bimanual manipulation of

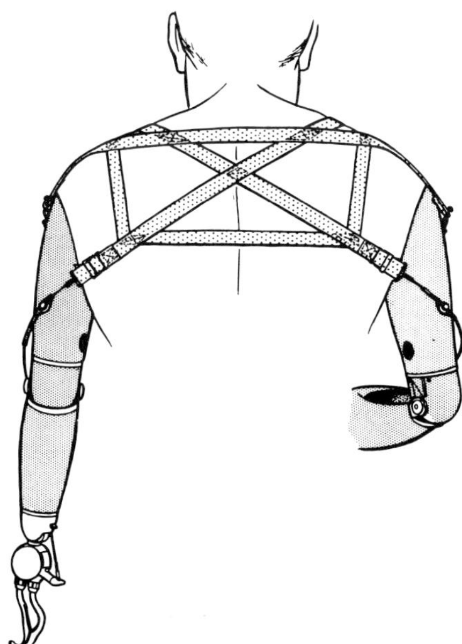

Fig. 9-41. Harness for bilateral above-elbow amputee (posterior view). (From Pursley, R. J.: Harness patterns for upper-extremity prostheses, Chapter 4. In American Academy of Orthopaedic Surgeons: Orthopaedic appliances atlas, vol. 2, Artificial limbs, Ann Arbor, Mich., 1960, J. W. Edwards.)

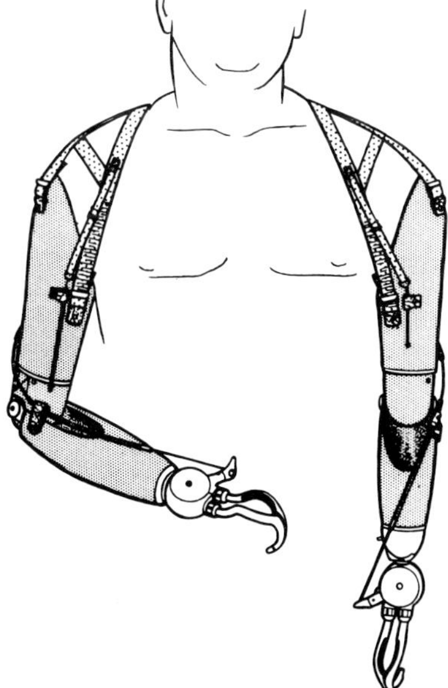

Fig. 9-42. Harness for bilateral above-elbow amputee (anterior view). (From Pursley, R. J.: Harness patterns for upper-extremity prostheses, Chapter 4. In American Academy of Orthopaedic Surgeons: Orthopaedic appliances atlas, vol. 2, Artificial limbs, Ann Arbor, Mich., 1960, J. W. Edwards.)

objects is minimal. A second major deficiency of this harness system is that it does not permit the amputee to lift any significant amount of weight in the terminal device of either prosthesis.

SHOULDER DISARTICULATION HARNESS

At the shoulder disarticulation level of amputation the absence of glenohumeral flexion as a control source requires the use of other body motions for prosthetic operation. Biscapular abduction is, at least for most adult male amputees, a satisfactory body motion for generating sufficient cable tension to flex the elbow and operate the terminal device of the prosthesis.

The force generated by active biscapular abduction is best harnessed through use of a chest strap (Fig. 9-43). Composed of 3.8-cm (1½-inch) wide nonelastic webbing, the chest strap originates by a buckle on the anterior surface of the shoulder cap of the socket. Running horizontally across the amputee's thorax, the strap passes immediately inferior to the axilla on the nonamputated side. The chest strap terminates posteriorly with its attachment to the proximal end of the elbow flexion/terminal device control cable.

Vertical suspension of the chest strap and prosthetic socket is augmented by the use of an elastic suspensor strap. The anterior suspensor originates posteriorly on the chest strap (Fig. 9-44). Passing over the shoulder on the amputated side along a diagonal path, the suspensor terminates with its attachment to the proximal surface of the shoulder cap. In addition to assisting with vertical support, the anterior suspensor helps prevent external rotation of the socket on the shoulder during use of the prosthesis.

Biscapular abduction is usually more than adequate to produce sufficient cable tension for fully operating the elbow and terminal device of a shoulder disarticulation prosthesis. Abduction of the scapulae is, however, a poor body motion for generating adequate cable excursion. Very few shoulder disarticulation amputees are capable, through biscapular abduction, of creating enough cable excursion to permit complete elbow and terminal device operation.

Since biscapular abduction is a good source for generating cable tension but a poor source of cable excursion, shoulder disarticulation harnesses frequently require the addition of an excursion amplifier (Fig. 9-45). A simple excursion ampli-

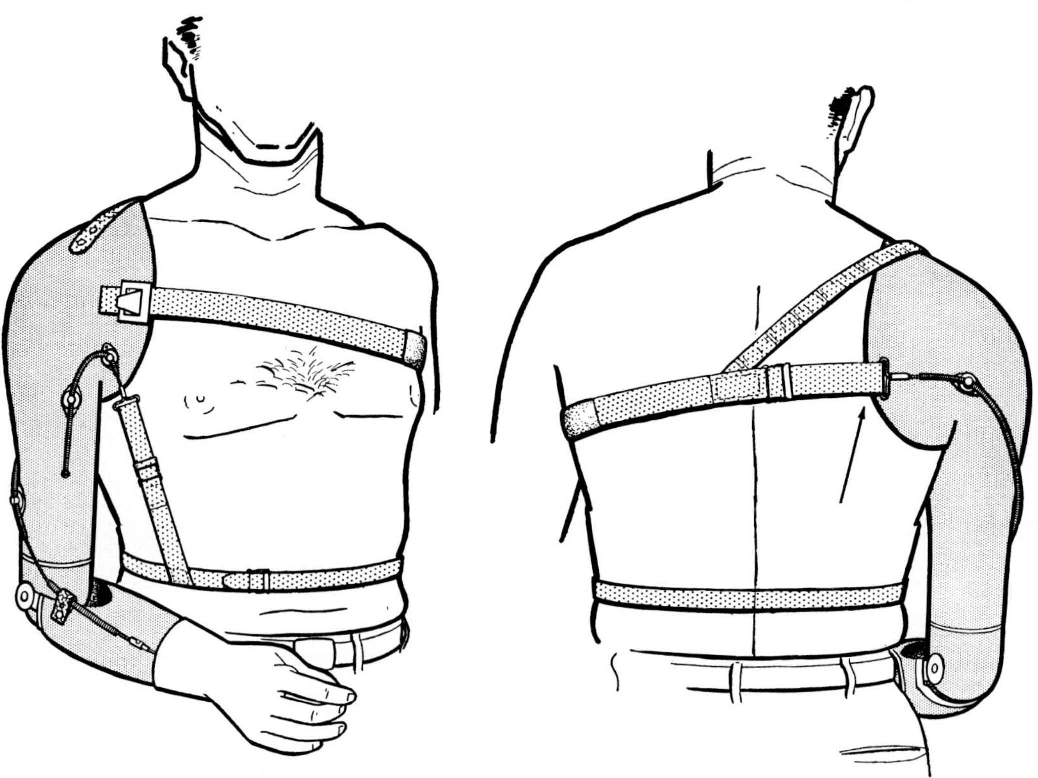

Fig. 9-43. Chest strap (arrow) on shoulder disarticulation harness. (From Pursley, R. J.: Orthop. Prosthet. Appl. J., March, 1955, p. 15.)

fier consists of a small pulley attached near the posterior end of the chest strap of the harness. The proximal end of the elbow flexion/terminal device cable passes through the pulley and is attached to the posterior surface of the prosthetic shoulder cap. With this type of amplifier each 2.5 cm (inch) of cable excursion generated by biscapular abduction causes the elbow flexion/terminal device control cable to move through an excursion of 5 cm (2 inches). Consequently 5.6 cm (2¼ inches) of chest expansion produces the 11.3 cm (4½ inches) of cable excursion required for full elbow and terminal device operation.

It should be noted that although the incorporation of a pulley in the harness system doubles the cable excursion, it also doubles the input force required for elbow flexion and/or terminal device operation. Since biscapular abduction is a good source of force generation, this increased force requirement does not generally pose a major problem for most adult shoulder disarticulation amputees. Nevertheless, an effort should be made to maximize the mechanical efficiency of the cable system by reducing friction to its lowest possible level.

Depending on factors such as body build, availability of adequate range of scapulothoracic motion, and the neuromuscular coordination of the amputee, locking and unlocking of the elbow unit of a shoulder disarticulation prosthesis can be effected in one of several different ways. The preferred method involves the incorporation of the elbow lock control strap as an anterior extension of the chest strap.

In this method the anterior attachment of the chest strap is bifurcated (Fig. 9-46). The upper leg of the split strap consists of nonelastic webbing. The lower leg is nonelastic at its extremities – its origin on the chest strap and attachment on the socket – but has a segment of elastic webbing at its center. A nonelastic elbow lock control strap originates at the chest strap, passes laterally between the two legs of the split strap and attaches directly to the proximal end of the elbow lock control cable. With this harness arrangement, cable tension for locking and unlocking the elbow is created by scapular adduction on the amputated side.

Incorporation of the elbow lock control strap with the chest strap makes it easier to don the prosthesis but requires a fairly high level of neuromuscular coordination for successful operation.

An alternative arrangement for elbow lock con-

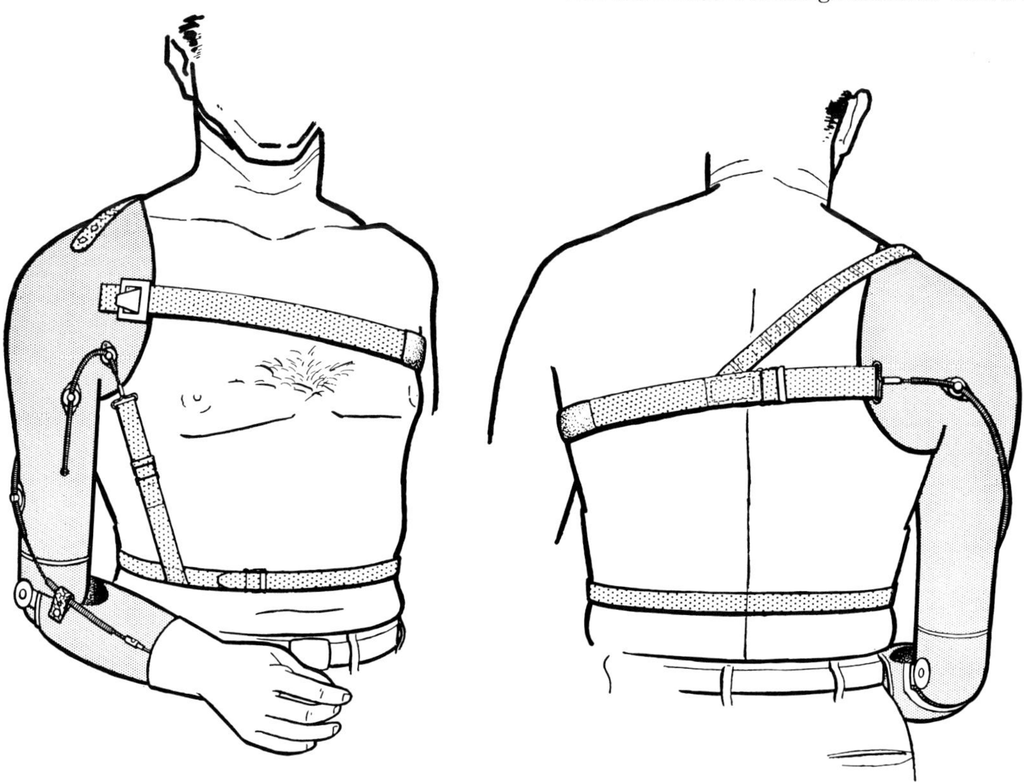

Fig. 9-44. Elastic suspensor strap on shoulder disarticulation strap. (From Pursley, R. J.: Orthop. Prosthet. Appl. J., March, 1955, p. 15.)

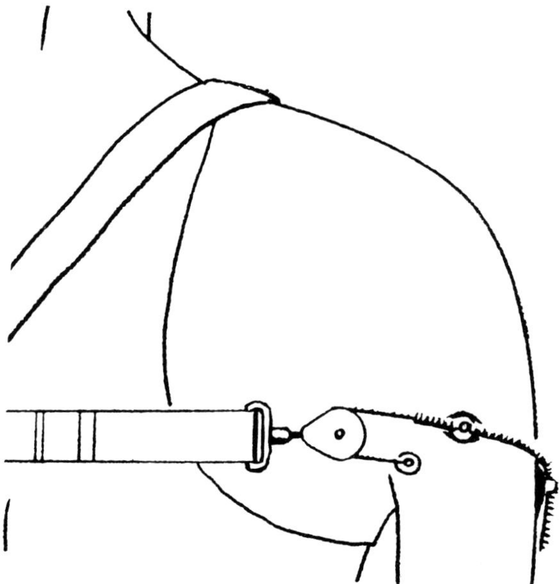

Fig. 9-45. Excursion amplifier on shoulder disarticulation strap. (From Santschi, W. R., editor: Manual of upper extremity prosthetics, ed. 2, Los Angeles, 1958, University of California Department of Engineering.)

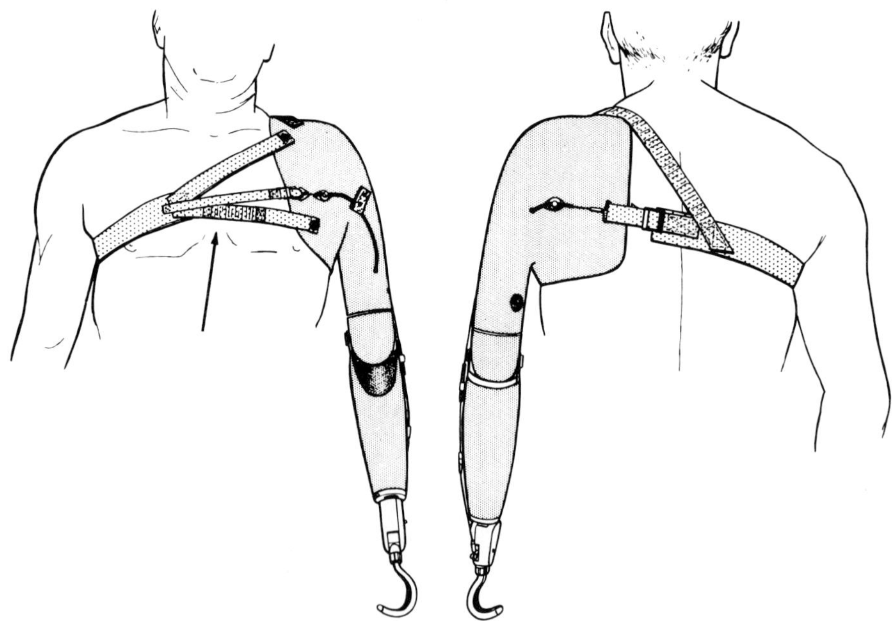

Fig. 9-46. Elbow lock control strap (arrow) incorporated as anterior extension of chest strap on shoulder disarticulation prosthesis. (From Pursley, R. J.: Harness patterns for upper-extremity prostheses, Chapter 4. In American Academy of Orthopaedic Surgeons: Orthopaedic appliances atlas, vol. 2, Artificial limbs, Ann Arbor, Mich., 1960, J. W. Edwards.)

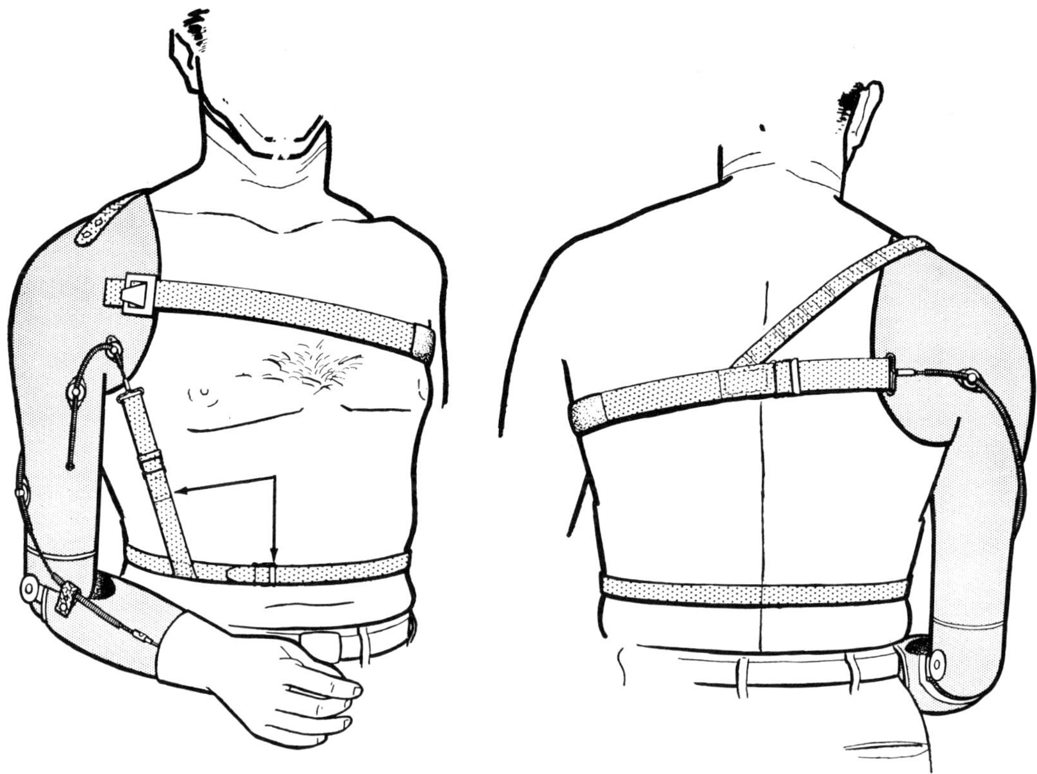

Fig. 9-47. Waist belt on shoulder disarticulation prosthesis as alternative elbow lock control. (From Pursley, R. J.: Orthop. Prosthet. Appl. J., March, 1955, p. 15.)

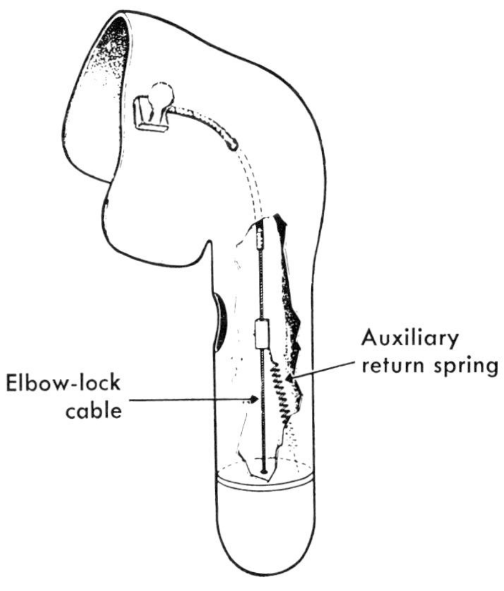

Fig. 9-48. Nudge control is alternative elbow lock control on shoulder disarticulation prosthesis. (From Santschi, W. R., editor: Manual of upper extremity prosthetics, ed. 2, Los Angeles, 1958, University of California Department of Engineering.)

trol requires the use of a waist belt (Fig. 9-47). The waist belt serves to anchor the distal end of the elbow lock control strap. From its anchor on the waist strap the control strap runs obliquely upward where it is attached to the proximal end of the elbow lock control cable. With the waist belt system, the primary body control motion for cycling the elbow unit is shoulder elevation on the amputated side.

A third option for achieving elbow lock control requires the use of a nudge control mounted on the anteroproximal surface of the prosthetic shoulder cap (Fig. 9-48). The nudge control for locking and unlocking the elbow is operated by force exerted by the amputee's chin. Nudge control is usually reserved for severely disabled persons such as bilateral shoulder disarticulation amputees. Realistically, the functional expectations for persons with acquired bilateral shoulder disarticulation amputations are extremely limited. With the help of adaptive equipment, environmental modifications, modifications of clothing, and a unilateral prosthetic replacement, it may be possible to achieve a reasonable degree of partial independence in the basic functions of personal hygiene, dressing, and eating.

There is no such thing as a "standard" harness for bilateral shoulder disarticulation amputees. Although most authorities agree that fittings should be unilateral rather than bilateral, the specifics of the harness and control system are left to the experience and ingenuity of the prosthetist, therapist, physician, patient, and members of the patient's family.

The unilateral prosthesis should permit active operation and passive prepositioning of a lightweight terminal device, active or passive flexion of the wrist unit, active flexion and locking of the elbow unit, passive external and internal rotation of the humeral section, and passive prepositioning of the shoulder joint in flexion and abduction.

Absence of the humeral heads narrows the girth of the shoulder girdle and reduces the effectiveness of biscapular abduction as a work source. A small well-padded plastic cap covering the apex of the acromion on the side opposite the prosthesis enhances the available range of biscapular motion, thereby preserving this important control source (Fig. 9-49).

Biscapular abduction and the use of an excursion amplifier should permit adequate cable excursion for producing a reasonable degree of elbow flexion and terminal device operation. Shoulder elevation on the amputated side may be used for elbow lock control.

Harnessing patterns for the forequarter amputation do not differ significantly from those used in the shoulder disarticulation, except that the efficiency of operation is less.

Section III

Upper limb prosthetic components

CHARLES M. FRYER

Prosthetic components that are most frequently prescribed in the management of persons with upper limb amputations are (1) terminal devices (hand substitutes), (2) wrist units, (3) elbow units, and (4) shoulder units. Although an attempt is made to discuss the general functional characteristics of each group of components, the specifics of mechanical design will not be detailed in this section.

TERMINAL DEVICES

Commercially available terminal devices fall into two general categories: hooks and hands. From the standpoint of function, hook devices are more versatile, durable, and lighter in weight than hand devices. Hand devices are obviously more aesthetically acceptable. All terminal devices manufactured in the United States, both hooks and hands, have a standard stud (1.3 to 50 cm; 1/2 to 20 inches) for attachment to the prosthetic forearm and are therefore interchangeable.

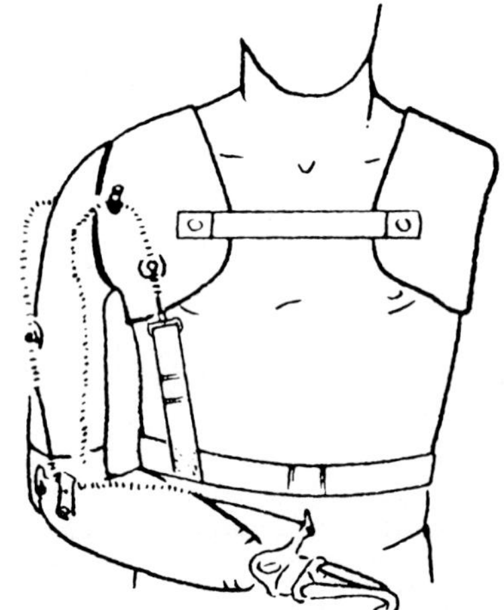

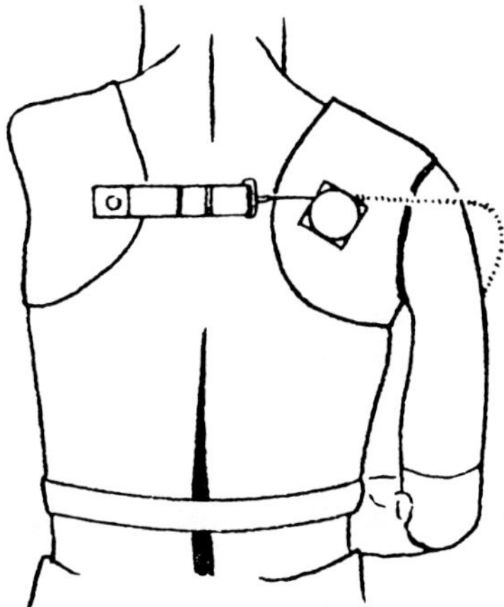

Fig. 9-49. Small, well-padded plastic cap covers apex of acromion on side opposite prosthesis. (From Santschi, W. R., editor: Manual of upper extremity prosthetics, ed. 2, Los Angeles, 1958, University of California Department of Engineering.)

Hooks

Hook devices are available in either "voluntary opening" or "voluntary closing" models. Because of their mechanical simplicity, ease of operation, functional versatility, and availability in a wide range of sizes, voluntary opening hooks are prescribed more frequently than any other terminal device.

Voluntary opening hooks come in right-hand and left-hand models (Fig. 9-50). Handedness is determined by the position of the operating lever or "thumb" of the hook; the thumb being located on the radial side of the hook.

Hosmer/Dorrance hooks. The Hosmer/Dorrance name is associated with a wide range of functional, voluntary opening hooks. Most adult male amputees can be satisfactorily fit with series 5 hooks. The major similarities among all hooks in the 5 series are that all are voluntary opening and between 12.5 to 15 cm (4⅞ and 5 inches) long (Fig. 9-51).

As a general rule, and particularly in the case of the above-elbow amputee, the more proximal the level of amputation, the more desirable it becomes to prescribe a lightweight terminal device. Hooks, 5, 5X, 5P, SS-555, and SSS-555 weigh approximately twice as much as do hooks 5XA and 555.

Hooks 5, 5X, 5XA, and 5P have canted finger configurations; hooks 555, SS-555, and SSS-555 have lyre-shaped fingers. Canted fingers permit

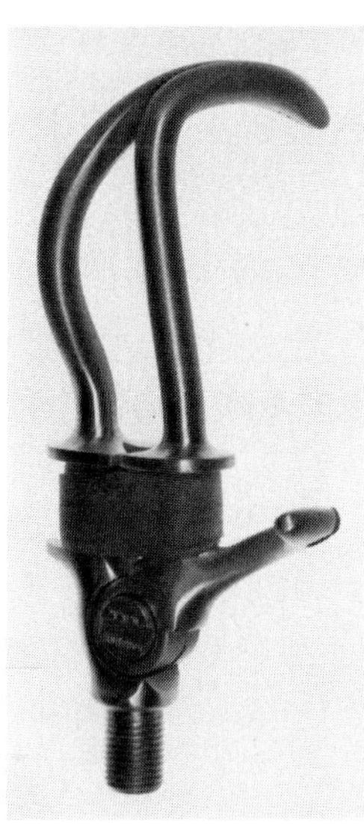

Fig. 9-50. Left, voluntary opening hook-type terminal device. (Courtesy Hosmer/Dorrance Corp., Campbell, Calif.)

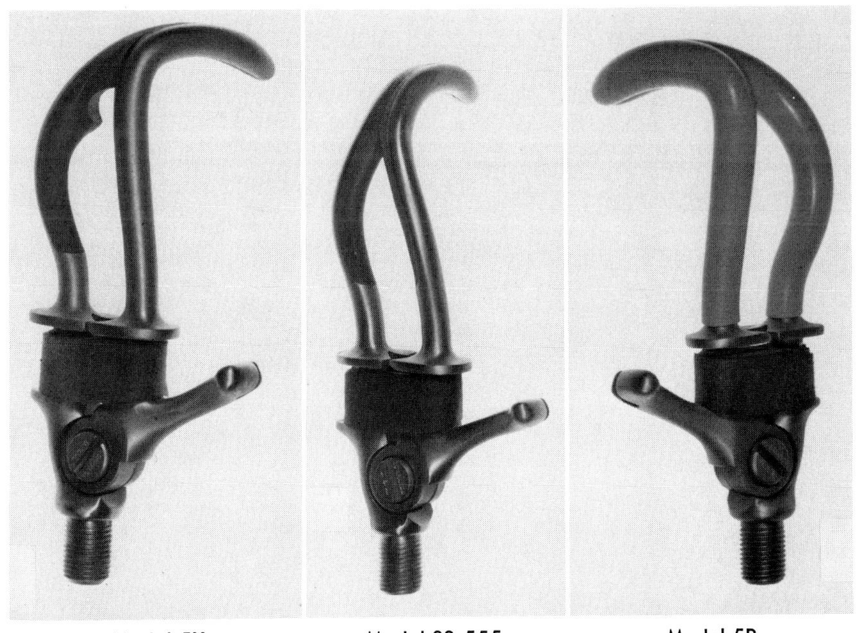

Model 5X

Model SS-555

Model 5P

Continued.

Fig. 9-51. Hosmer/Dorrance voluntary opening hooks for adult male amputees. (Courtesy Hosmer/Dorrance Corp., Campbell, Calif.)

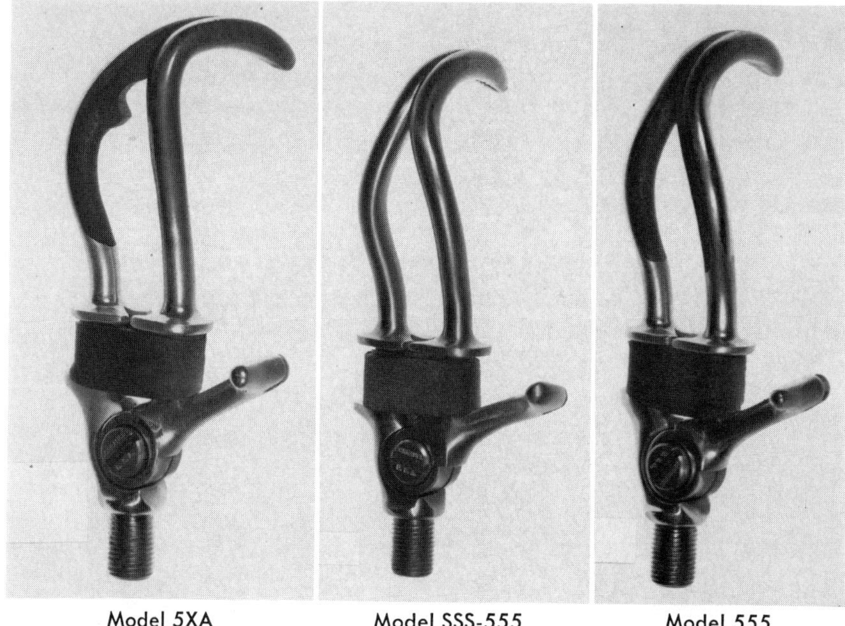

Fig. 9-51, cont'd. Hosmer/Dorrance voluntary opening hooks for adult male amputees. (Courtesy Hosmer/Dorrance Corp., Campbell, Calif.)

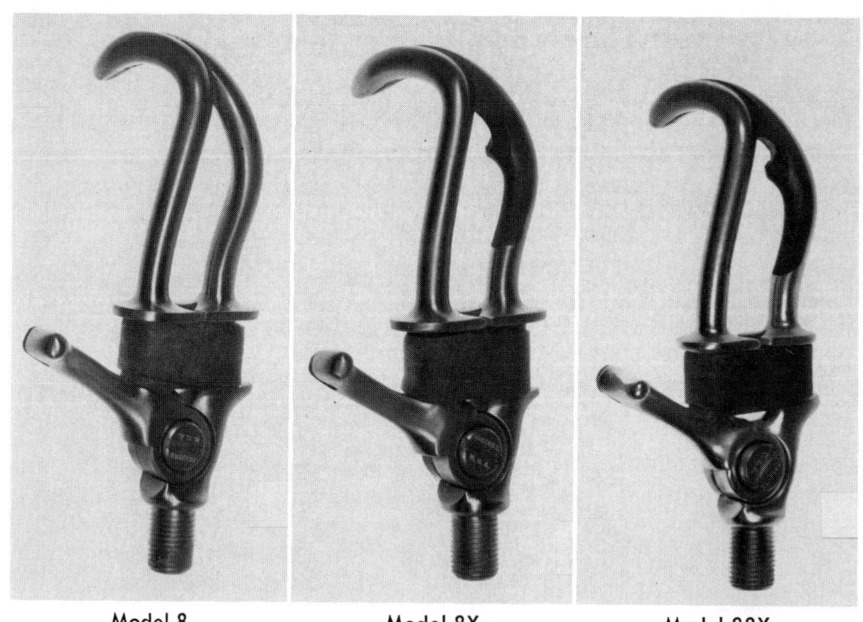

Fig. 9-52. Hosmer/Dorrance hooks for female and teenage amputees. (Courtesy Hosmer/Dorrance Corp., Campbell, Calif.)

better visualization of the work field as the amputee attempts to manipulate small objects. Lyre-shaped fingers make it somewhat easier to grasp or hold rounded objects.

The fingers of hooks 5 and SSS-555 are unlined and have serrated holding surfaces. All other hooks in series 5 are lined with neoprene or covered with plastisol. Finger linings and coverings provide increased traction for holding objects and minimize damage when manipulating delicate

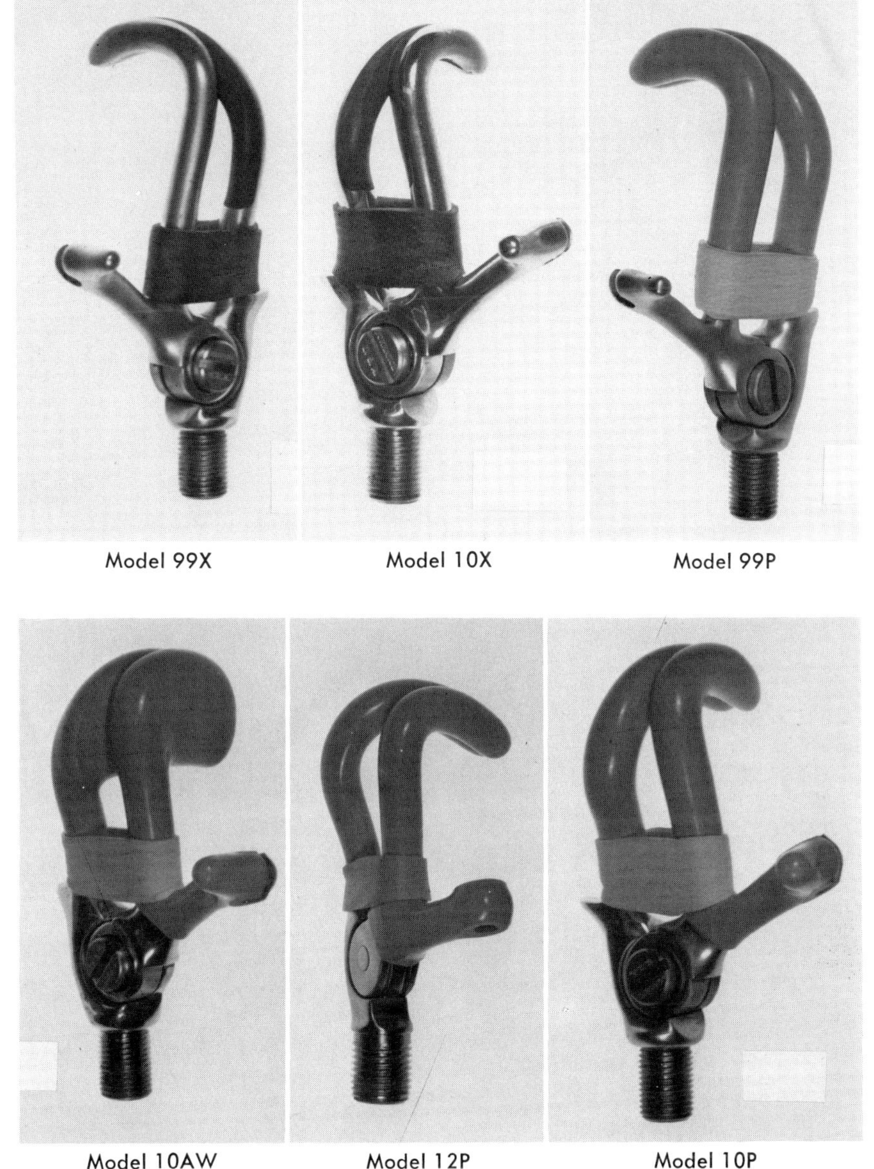

Fig. 9-53. Hosmer/Dorrance hooks for children and infants. (Courtesy Hosmer/Dorrance Corp., Campbell, Calif.)

structures and surfaces. A disadvantage of lined or covered fingers is that, once worn-out through usage, the hook must be returned to the manufacturer for replacement of the neoprene or plastisol.

Most female and small teenage amputees can be fit with series 8 hooks: 8, 8X, and 88X (Fig. 9-52). Hooks 99X, 99P, 10X, 10AW, 10P, and 12P are indicated for children and infants (Fig. 9-53).

Hook models 3, 6, 6LO, 7, and 7LO are heavy-duty terminal devices prescribed almost exclusively for adult male amputees (Fig. 9-54). These models have special features that facilitate the holding, grasping, and carrying of buckets, chisels, knives, and carpentry tools. An especially attractive feature for heavy-duty users is the large, circular opening between the hook fingers that facilitates the manipulation of long-handled implements such as shovels, rakes, and brooms.

Trautman Locktite hook. This voluntary-opening, heavy-duty hook is prescribed mostly for adult male amputees (Fig. 9-55). Like Hosmer/Dorrance's 3, 6, 6LO, 7, and 7LO hooks, the Trautman Locktite hook also has a large circular opening between the fingers that facilitates hold-

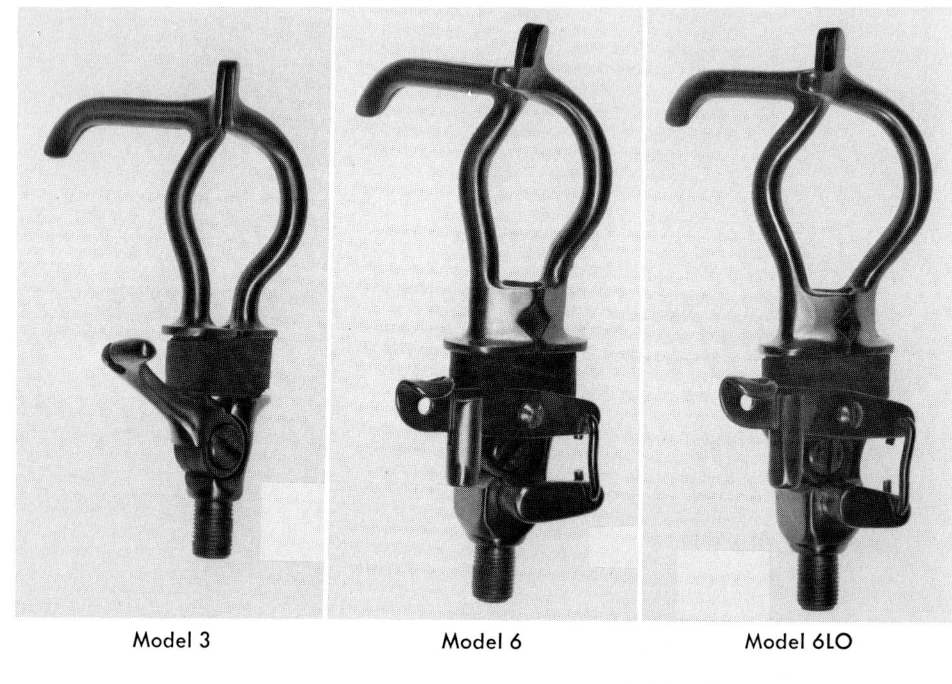

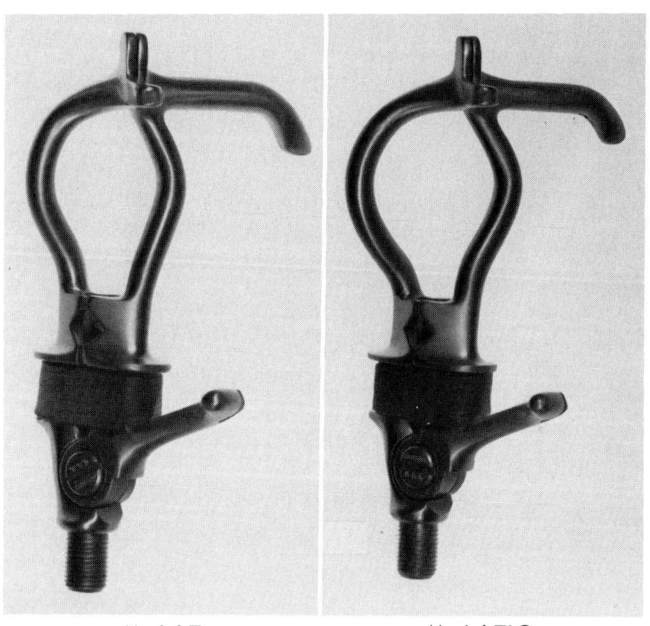

Fig. 9-54. Hosmer/Dorrance hooks for adult male amputees. (Courtesy Hosmer/Dorrance Corp., Campbell, Calif.)

ing long-handled tools. This stainless steel hook has a cam and lever mechanism that locks the hook when the fingers are in the nearly closed position. Once grasped, an object can be released only by reapplying force on the operating lever of the device.

Sierra two-load hook. Available in the adult size only and with lyre-shaped fingers, this voluntary opening terminal device permits the amputee to preselect a prehension force of either 1.6 or 3.2 kg ($3^1/_2$ or 7 pounds) (Fig. 9-56). A small switch at the base of the thumb permits the amputee to engage either one spring (1.6 kg; $3^1/_2$ pounds) or two springs (3.2 kg; 7 pounds) encased in an aluminum housing. The two-load hook is not considered to be a heavy-duty terminal de-

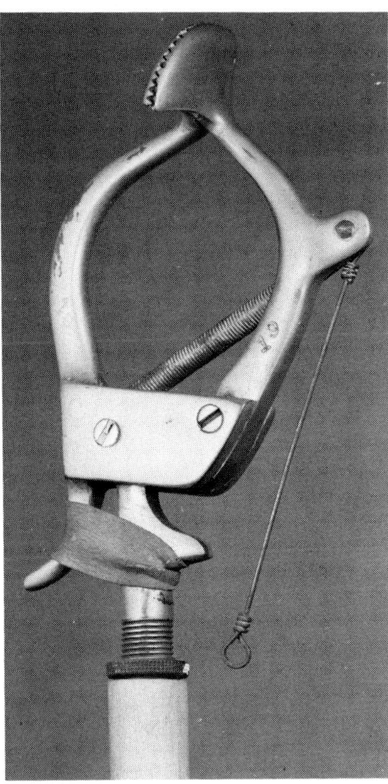

Fig. 9-55. Trautman Locktite hook for adult male amputees.

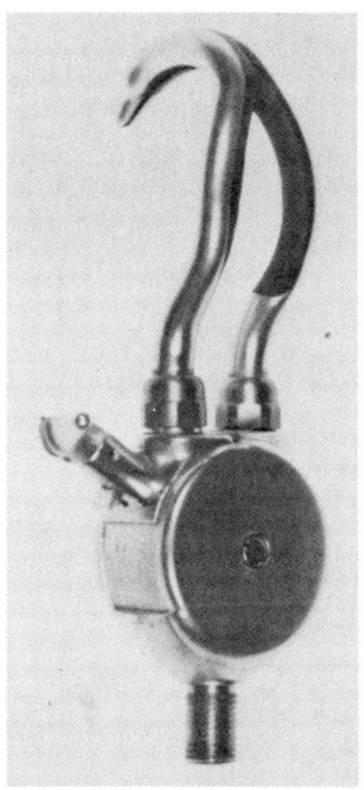

Fig. 9-56. Sierra two-load hook.

vice. Like all previously discussed terminal devices, the thumb is on the radial side of the hook.

APRL hook. The APRL (Army Prosthetic Research Laboratory) hook (Fig. 9-57) differs from all previously discussed hooks in several major respects:

1. The APRL hook is a voluntary closing rather than a voluntary opening mechanism.
2. The fingers can be locked at any position throughout the range of finger motion. (The reader may recall that the Trautman Locktite hook and Hosmer/Dorrance's models 6 and 6LO are locked with the fingers in the closed positions only.)
3. A selector switch on the hook housing permits the amputee to choose either:
   a. A large (7.5 cm; 3 inch) finger-opening position while retaining the locking mechanism.
   b. A small (3.4 cm; 1$^{3}/_{8}$ inch) finger-opening position while retaining the locking mechanism.
   c. A small (3.4 cm; 1$^{3}/_{8}$ inch) finger-opening position with the locking mechanism eliminated.
4. The operating lever, or thumb, is located on the ulnar rather than the radial surface of the device.

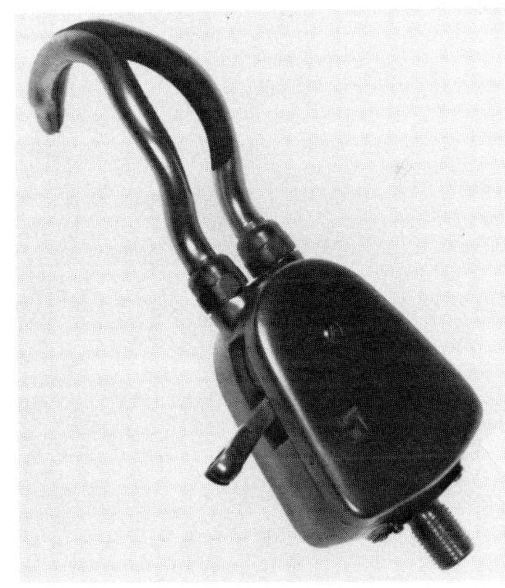

Fig. 9-57. Army Prosthetics Research Laboratory hook.

5. The APRL hook is the longest (32 cm; 6$^{1}/_{2}$ inches) of the commercially available terminal devices.

The APRL hook is available only with lyre-shaped, neoprene-lined fingers and only in the adult size. As in the case of most of the previously discussed terminal devices, the APRL hook has a stationary finger and a movable finger. The movable finger of the APRL hook is maintained in the fully opened position by a spring. Tension on the control cable causes the movable finger to oppose the stationary finger. When cable tension is relaxed, the movable finger is locked in its new position. Reapplication of tension on the control cable unlocks the movable finger, and the spring returns it to the fully opened position. Because of its fragility, mechanical complexity, length, and cost, the APRL hook is seldom prescribed for amputees other than those previous wearers of an APRL hook.

Hands

Hand terminal devices are available in both voluntary opening and voluntary closing models. Like hooks, the most frequently used hand devices are those with voluntary opening mechanisms. Regardless of the operating mode, whether voluntary opening or voluntary closing, all commercially available hands share the following characteristics:

1. All hands and hooks have 1.3- to 50-cm (1/2- to 20-inch) studs for attachment to the prosthetic forearm. Consequently, all commercially available terminal devices are interchangeable.
2. The basic pattern of finger motion for grasping and holding objects is that of palmar prehension. For carrying objects such as suitcases, all hands provide, to a greater or lesser extent, some hook prehension capability.
3. Correct hand size is selected by the circumferential measurement around the metacarpophalangeal joints of the nonamputated hand.
4. All prosthetic hands discussed in this chapter can be covered with a cosmetic glove.

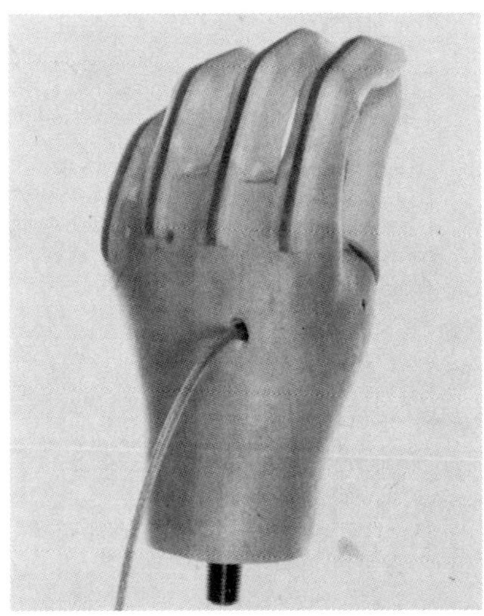

Fig. 9-58. Becker Plylite hand.

Becker Plylite hand. The Becker Plylite hand (Fig. 9-58) is a simple, lightweight, voluntary opening hand that is available in sizes 6 to 10 in 1.3-cm (1/2-inch) increments (e.g., 6, 6 1/2, 7, 7 1/2, 8). The only moving component is the thumb. The larger models permit sufficient thumb movement to grasp objects of up to 7.5 cm (3 inches) in thickness. An optional locking mechanism is available, which locks the thumb in the closed position.

Becker Lock-Grip and Imperial hands. The Becker Lock-Grip and Imperial hands (Fig. 9-59) are voluntary opening hands with control cable tension that causes all five fingers to open. The

A

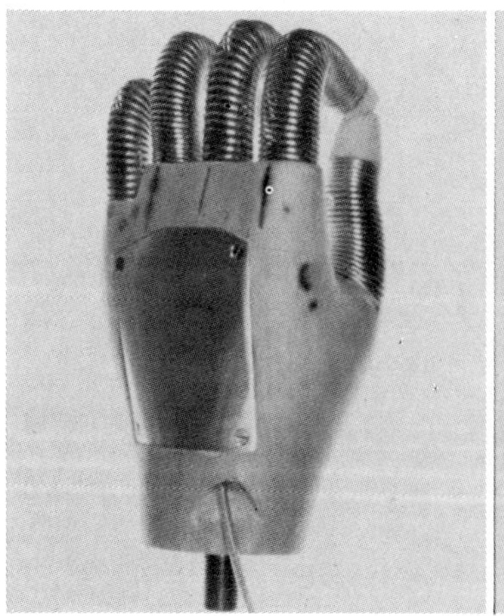

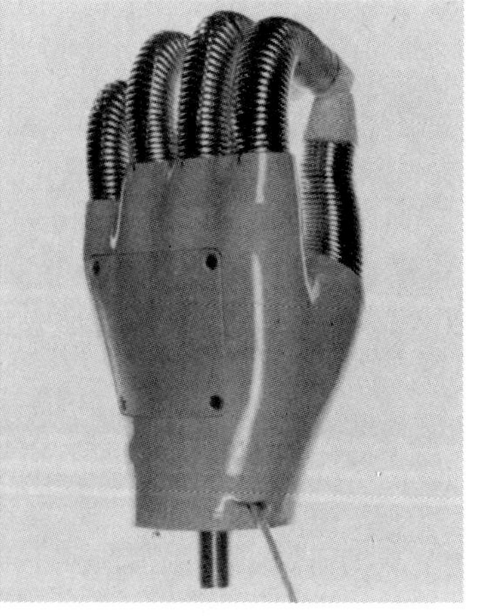

B

Fig. 9-59. A, Becker Lock-Grip hand. **B,** Imperial hand.

Lock-Grip model contains a mechanism that locks the fingers in the closed position. Finger opening from the fully closed position can be effected only by control cable tension. Lock-Grip hands are available in 1.3-cm (1/2-inch) increments from size 6 1/2 to size 10. The Imperial model, available in size 8 only, permits easy adjustment of finger prehension force with the use of a screwdriver.

Robin-Aids mechanical hand. The Robin-Aids mechanical hand (Fig. 9-60) is a voluntary opening hand with control cable tension that causes digits two, three, four, and five to move away from a stationary thumb. The thumb can be manually prepositioned for normal or large opening prehension. The force of prehension is generated by springs and may easily be increased or decreased by the prosthetist. This is the only commercially available hand with an adjustable length feature that permits its use with very long below-elbow and wrist disarticulation amputation levels.

Robin-Aids soft mechanical hand. The Robin-Aids soft mechanical hand (Fig. 9-61) is a voluntary opening hand. Tension on the central cable causes the thumb and first two fingers to open. The endoskeletal frame is encased in plastisol and covered with a urethane foam of low density that provides "softness." Both of the Robin-Aids hands are available in sizes 7, 7 1/2, 8, 8 1/2, and 9.

Sierra mechanical hands. Sierra mechanical hands are available in two models: the APRL vol-

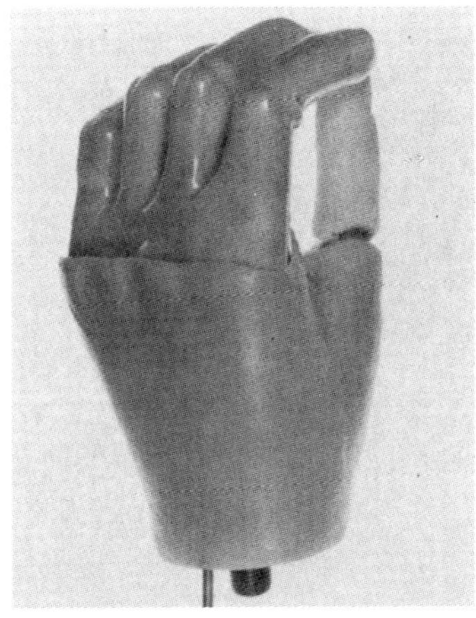

Fig. 9-60. Robin-Aids mechanical hand.

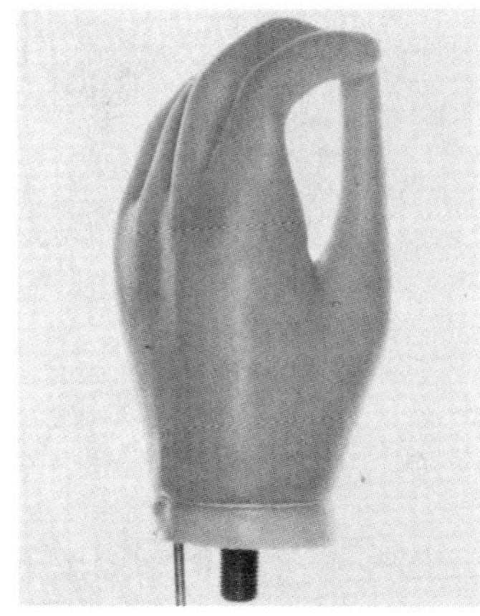

Fig. 9-61. Robin-Aids soft mechanical hand.

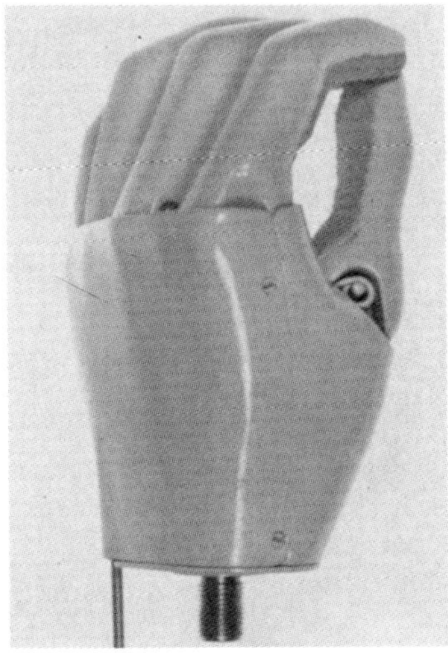

Fig. 9-62. Sierra mechanical hand, APRL voluntary closing model.

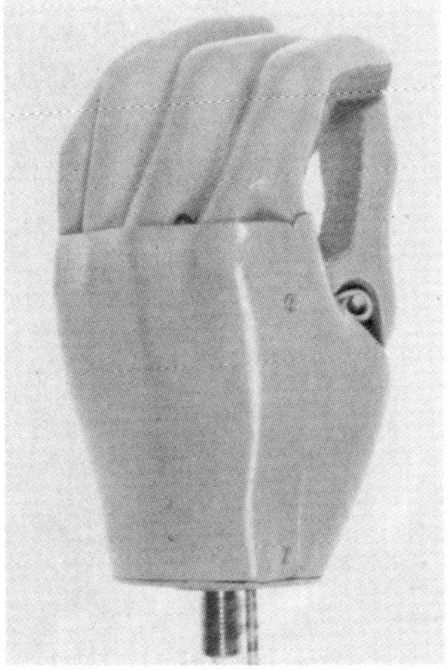

Fig. 9-63. Sierra voluntary opening hand.

untary closing hand (Fig. 9-62) and the Sierra voluntary opening hand.

APRL voluntary closing hand. With the APRL hand in the fully opened position, tension on the control cable causes the first two fingers to begin to move toward a stationary thumb. When control cable tension is relaxed, the fingers automatically lock in position. Thus the amputee can grasp various-sized objects and hold them without having to maintain tension on the control cable. The reapplication of tension to the cable causes the fingers to unlock, permitting release of the objects. The stationary thumb may be manually prepositioned to provide normal or large opening prehension. The voluntary closing APRL hook is available in size 8 only.

Sierra voluntary opening hand. The Sierra voluntary opening hand (Fig. 9-63), like the APRL hand, has a two-position stationary thumb. From the fully closed position, control cable tension causes the first two fingers to move away from the thumb. As tension on the control cable is relaxed, springs cause the fingers to move close toward the thumb. A "Bac Loc" feature operates in all finger positions and permits the amputee to hold heavy objects securely. Finger opening and release of the Bac Loc mechanism are operated simultaneously through a single control cable. The Sierra voluntary opening hand is available in size 8 only.

Hosmer/Dorrance functional hands. Hosmer/Dorrance functional voluntary opening hands (Fig. 9-64) permit the prosthetist to adjust finger prehension by the installation of different tension springs. The hands are available in four sizes: 8, 7, 6½, and 5½.

Otto Bock system hands. Otto Bock system hands (Fig. 9-65) consist of four basic elements: (1) standard chassis and wrist plate (Fig. 9-65, *A*), (2) operating mechanism (Fig. 9-65, *B*), (3) inner hand (Fig. 9-65, *C*), and (4) cosmetic glove (Fig. 9-65, *D*). The standard chassis and wrist plate consist of a lightweight, endoskeletal frame capable of accommodating various types of operating mechanisms. The standard chassis is available in size 6¾ for children, 7¼ for women, and 7¾ for men. Following are operating mechanisms that can be accommodated in the standard chassis:

1. Cable-operated, voluntary opening mechanism
2. Cable-operated, voluntary closing mechanism
3. Mechanism for electrically powered hand operation
4. Mechanism for pneumatically powered hand operation
5. Passively operable hand with a spring-activated thumb and fingers

The inner hand consists of flexible plastic, which covers and protects the operating mechanism. A cosmetic glove covers the inner hand.

Nonfunctional cosmetic hand. Nonfunctional cosmetic hands (Fig. 9-66) usually consist of a malleable wire frame embedded in a flexible, foamed plastic, which is covered by a cosmetic skin of polyvinylchloride (PVC). The inner wire

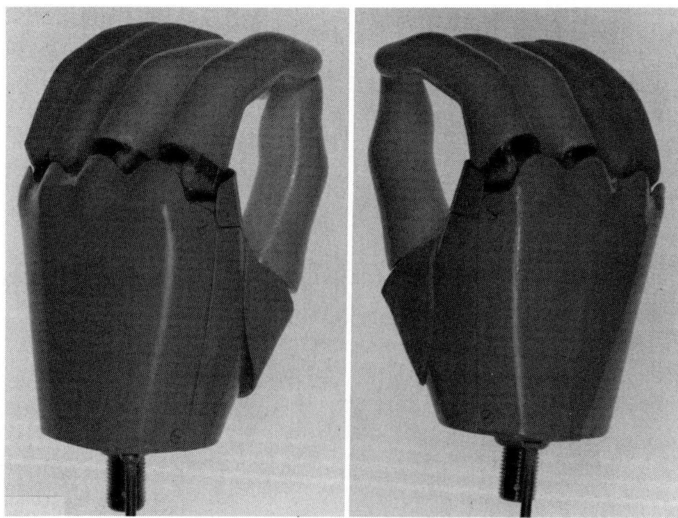

Fig. 9-64. Hosmer/Dorrance functional hands. (Courtesy Hosmer/Dorrance Corp., Campbell, Calif.)

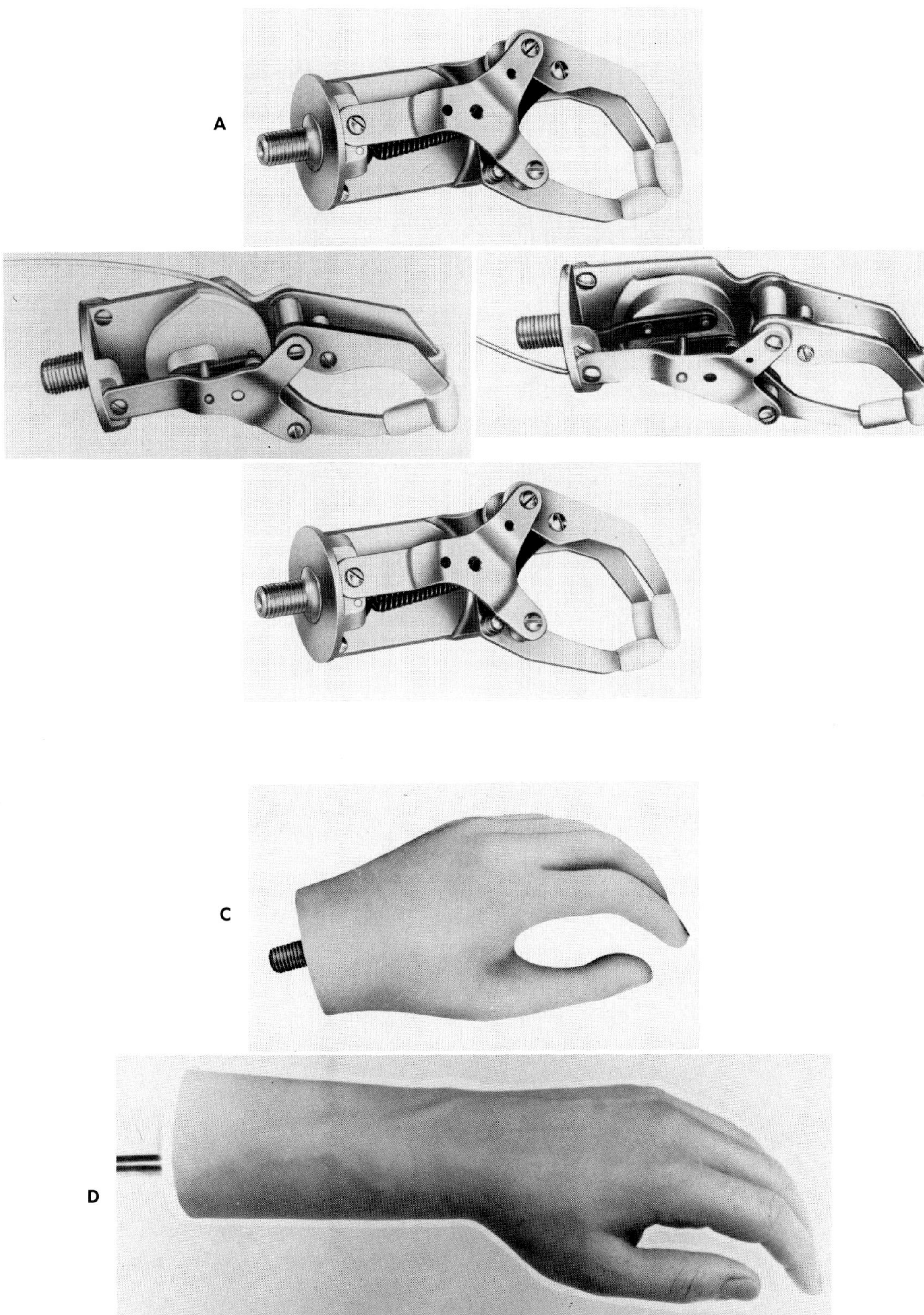

Fig. 9-65. Otto Bock system hands. **A,** Standard chassis and wrist plate. **B,** Operating mechanism. **C,** Inner hand. **D,** Cosmetic glove. (Courtesy Otto Bock Orthopedic Industry, Inc., Minneapolis, Minn.)

frame permits passive finger positioning of the finished hand. A reasonably high degree of accuracy in matching the anatomical detail of the remaining hand is possible with alginate or Silastic casting techniques.

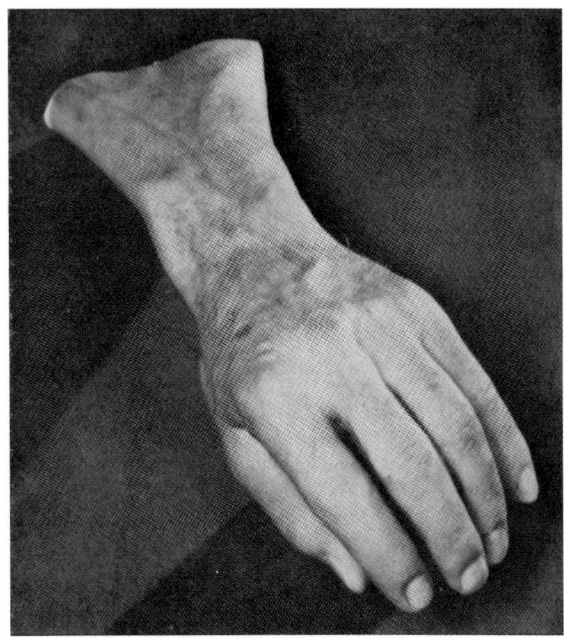

Fig. 9-66. Nonfunctional cosmetic hand. (Courtesy Hosmer/Dorrance Corp., Campbell, Calif.)

WRIST UNITS

Prosthetic wrist units are designed to serve two basic functions: to attach a terminal device to the forearm of the prosthesis and to permit the amputee to preposition the terminal device prior to operation. The need for the first function is obvious. To the uninitiated, the importance of the second function of wrist units may be less clear.

The above-elbow amputee has lost all ability to supinate and pronate the prosthetic forearm. The below-elbow amputee with a short residual forearm (50% or less than the length of the nonamputated forearm) no longer retains active, transmissable supination and pronation. Even at the very long below-elbow levels of amputation, the motions of supination and pronation are severely restricted. Consequently, the upper limb amputee must be provided with a device that permits some form of substitution for active forearm rotation.

Friction wrist units

Commercially available wrist units (Fig. 9-67) permit the amputee to substitute for supination and pronation by manually rotating the terminal device with the remaining normal hand. Bilateral amputees usually preposition the terminal devices for use by striking one device against the other, thereby rotating it to the desired position of function.

Friction wrist units are available in aluminum or stainless steel in the adult size (5-cm; 2-inch diameter) and medium size (4.4-cm; 1¾-inch diameter).

Oval-shaped friction wrist units are available in adult and medium sizes (Fig. 9-68). The oval configuration provides better cosmesis in cases of long below-elbow levels of amputation. Also,

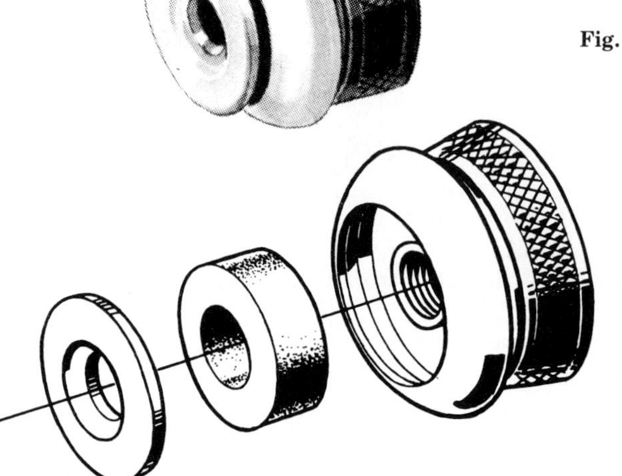

Fig. 9-67. Friction wrist units. (Courtesy Hosmer/Dorrance Corp., Campbell, Calif.)

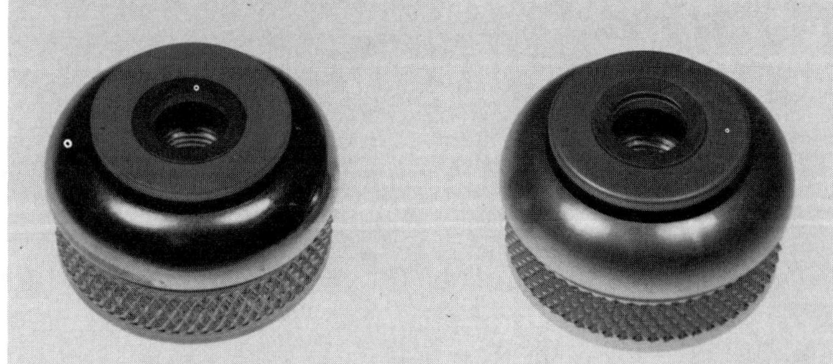

since most prosthetic hands have an oval base, the oval-shaped wrist unit provides for a smoother transition from the prosthetic hand to the prosthetic forearm. This wrist unit does not provide constant friction.

Friction wrist units designed specifically for wrist disarticulation levels of amputation are made as thin as possible to conserve the length of the prosthetic forearm (Fig. 9-69). These wrists do not provide constant friction and function in the same manner as previously described units. The units are available in two sizes: adult (5-cm; 2-inch diameter) and medium (3.4-cm; 1$^3/_8$-inch diameter).

The foregoing wrist units do not provide constant friction. As the terminal device stud is screwed into the wrist unit, a rubber washer is compressed, creating friction. As the terminal device is unscrewed, friction is reduced. It is highly desirable that wrist units provide constant fric-

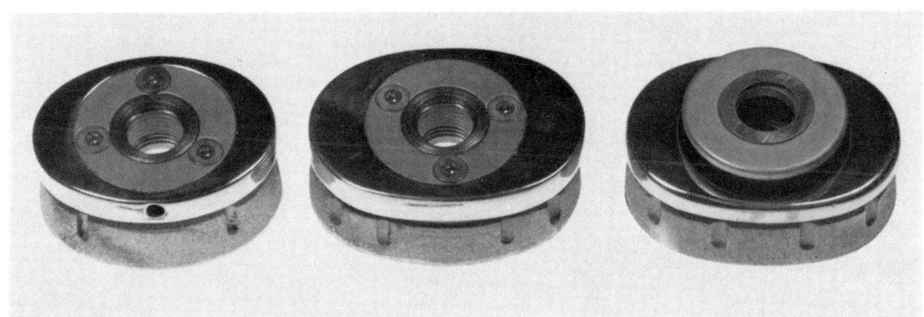

Fig. 9-68. Oval-shaped friction wrist units. (Courtesy Hosmer/Dorrance Corp., Campbell, Calif.)

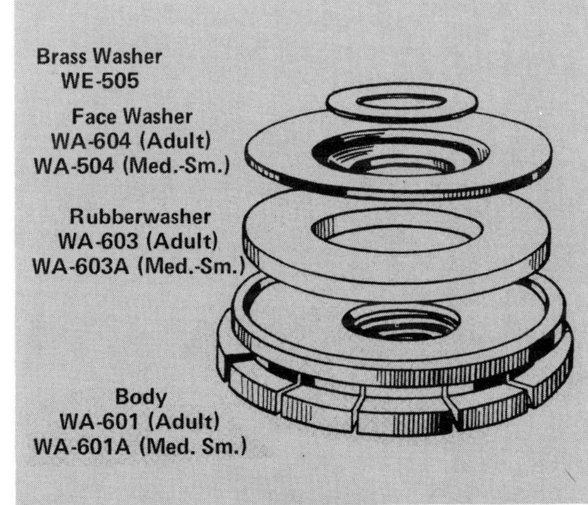

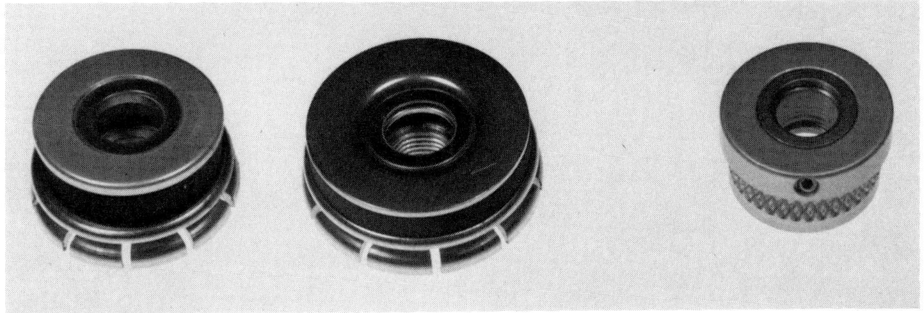

Fig. 9-69. Friction wrist unit designed for wrist disarticulation. (Courtesy Hosmer/Dorrance Corp., Campbell, Calif.)

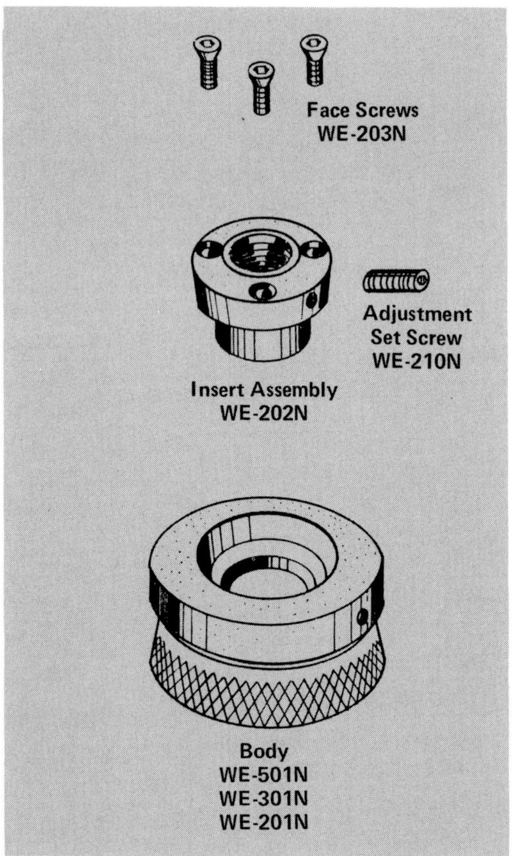

Fig. 9-70. Constant friction wrist unit. (Courtesy Hosmer/Dorrance Corp., Campbell, Calif.)

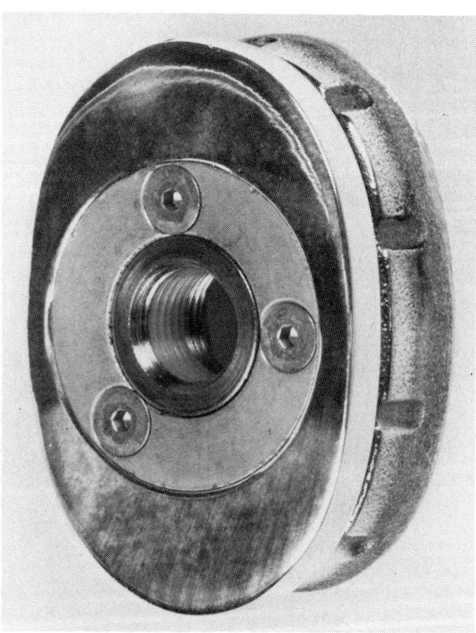

Fig. 9-71. Round and oval configurations of constant friction wrist units.

tion. Modern units permit the amputee to rotate the terminal device through 360 degrees of motion without a change in the effective friction.

Constant friction wrist units

Constant friction wrist units are designed to provide constant friction throughout the range of rotation of the terminal device. Most units of this type employ a nylon-threaded insert with steel lead threads (Fig. 9-70). Turning a small set screw in the body of the wrist causes the nylon thread to be deformed against the stud of the terminal device, creating constant friction. Damage to the insert threads may be repaired by simply removing and replacing the entire insert.

Constant friction wrist units are available in both the round and oval configurations (Fig. 9-71). In the round configuration, four sizes are available: infant (3.1 cm; 1¼ inch), child (3.8 cm; 1½ inch), medium (4.4 cm; 1¾ inch), and adult (5 cm; 2 inches). In the oval configuration two sizes are available: adult and medium.

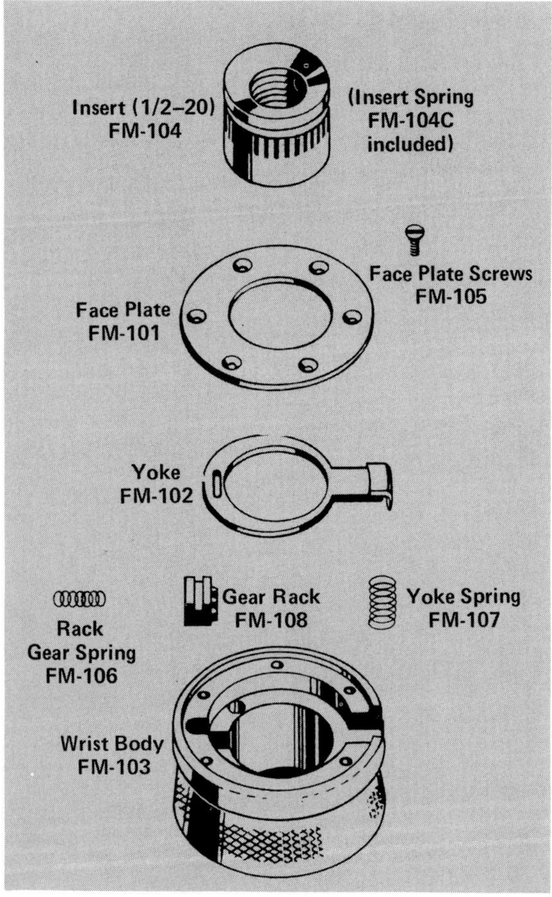

Fig. 9-72. Quick-change wrist units. (Courtesy Hosmer/Dorrance Corp., Campbell, Calif.)

Quick-change wrist units

Quick-change wrist units are designed to facilitate rapid interchange of different terminal devices, usually a hook and a hand (Fig. 9-72). All commercially available quick-change units permit the amputee to do the following:

1. Remove the terminal device from the wrist unit.
2. Replace the terminal device with a different terminal device.
3. Manually position the terminal device in supination or pronation.
4. Lock the terminal device in the desired altitude of supination or pronation.

Most quick-change units employ an adapter, which is screwed tightly on the studs of the two (or more) terminal devices to be interchanged. In Fig. 9-72, light downward pressure on the activating lever by the amputee unlocks the terminal device but does not cause its ejection. With the terminal device unlocked, the amputee manually rotates the hook or hand to the desired altitude of pronation or supination. Next, the application of a proximally directed axial force, with the sound hand, causes the terminal device to be locked in the new position. Heavy downward pressure on the activating lever causes ejection of the adapter and attached terminal device.

Quick-change units are available from the Hosmer/Dorrance Corporation in the adult size and round configuration only (Fig. 9-73).

Modern wrist flexion units permit terminal device operation in any of three positions: neutral, 30 degrees of volar flexion, or 50 degrees of volar flexion (Fig. 9-74). An activating lever, which the amputee depresses with the sound hand, unlocks the terminal device. Gravity, or tension on the terminal device control cable, causes the wrist unit to flex. The wrist automatically locks in neutral, 30 degrees of flexion, or 50 degrees of flexion. These units also provide constant friction for manual positioning of the terminal device in supination or pronation.

Because of the flattened, oval-shaped base of prosthetic hands, wrist flexion units are recommended for use with hook terminal devices only. In addition, the activating lever is more difficult to manipulate because of the cosmetic glove used with prosthetic hands. Wrist flexion units incorporating a constant friction mechanism for supination and pronation are available in adult (5 cm; 2 inches), medium (4.4 cm; 1¾ inch), and child (3.8 cm; 1½ inch) sizes.

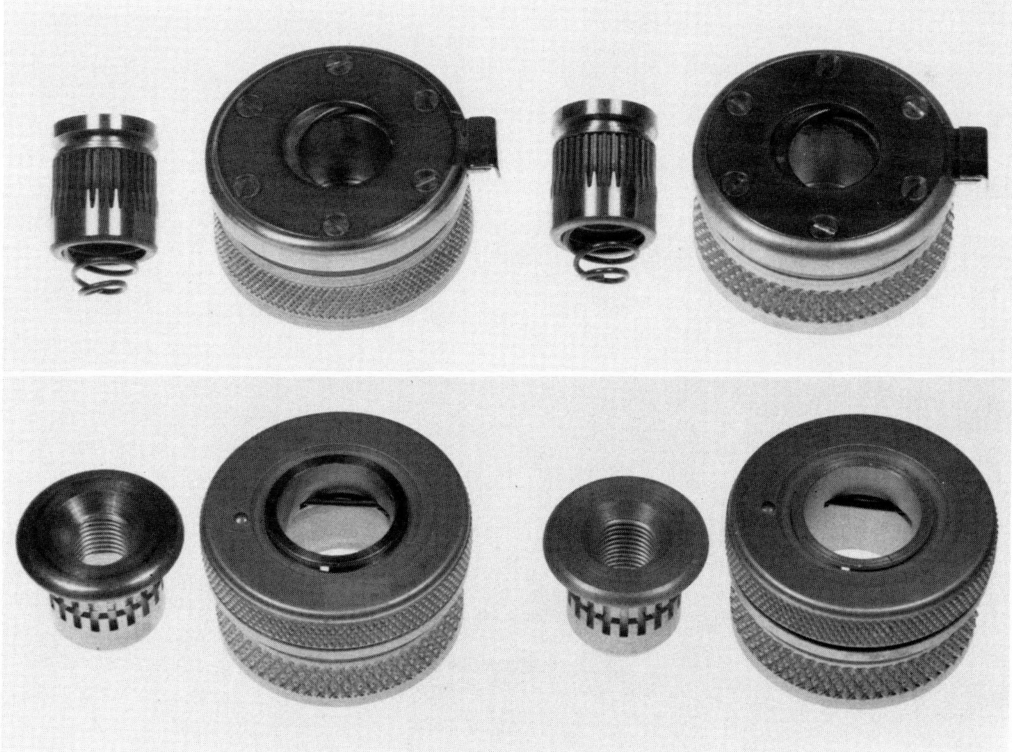

Fig. 9-73. Quick-change wrist units. (Courtesy Hosmer/Dorrance Corp., Campbell, Calif.)

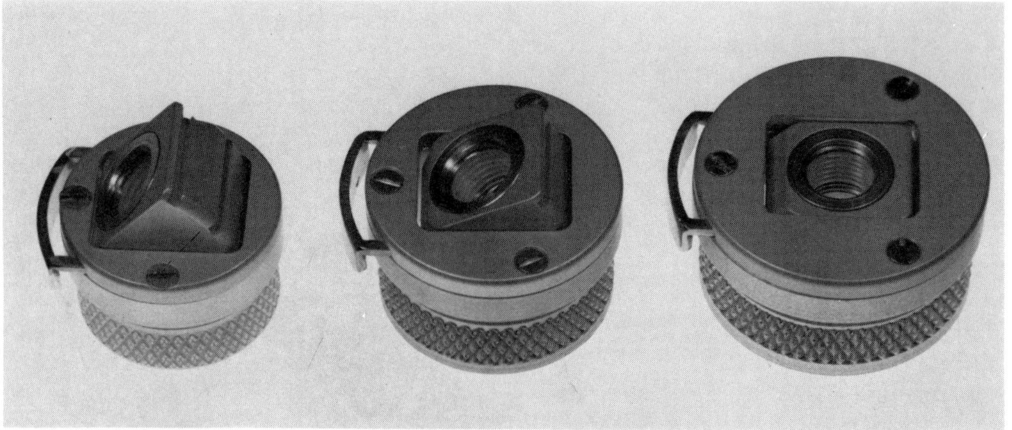

Fig. 9-74. Wrist flexion units. (Courtesy Hosmer/Dorrance Corp., Campbell, Calif.)

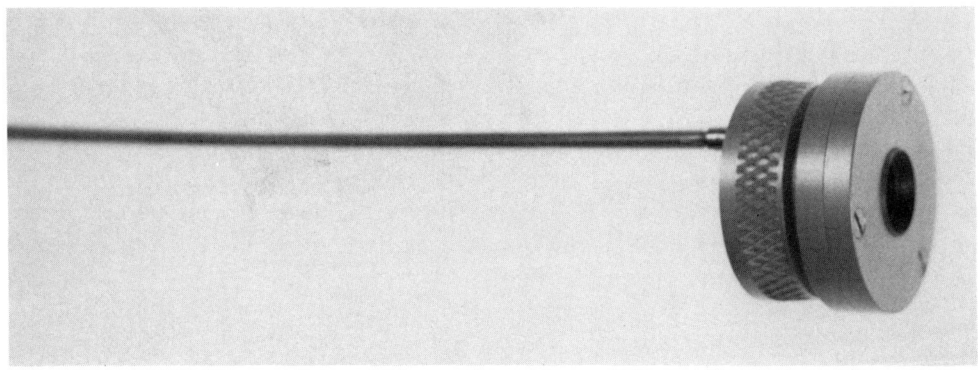

Fig. 9-75. Rotational wrist unit. (Courtesy Hosmer/Dorrance Corp., Campbell, Calif.)

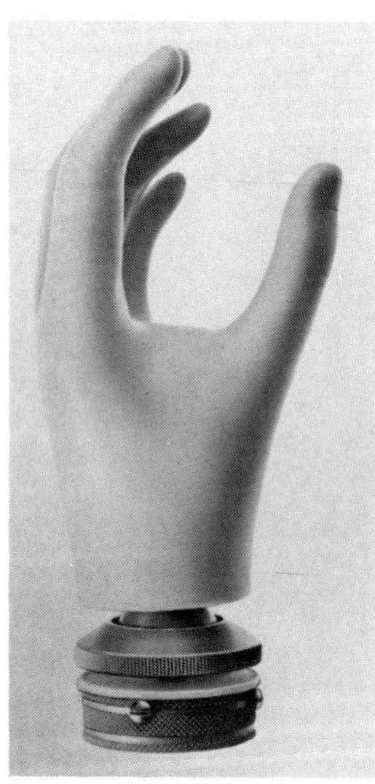

Fig. 9-76. Ball and socket wrist unit. (Courtesy Otto Bock Orthopedic Industry, Inc., Minneapolis, Minn.)

Rotational wrists

Previously discussed friction wrist units may present difficulties for those amputees who engage in work or avocational activities that exert high rotational loads on the terminal device. Friction and constant friction wrist units tend to permit unwanted rotation when subjected to very high torsional loading.

Rotational wrist units are cable controlled, positive-locking mechanisms (Fig. 9-75). In the unlocked mode, these units permit manual prepositioning of the terminal device in almost any attitude of supination or pronation through a 360-degree range. Once locked in position, these units provide much greater resistance to rotation than do friction units.

The bilateral amputee may find that rotational wrist units facilitate prepositioning of the terminal devices. With the wrist unit unlocked and the terminal devices fully supinated or pronated, ten-

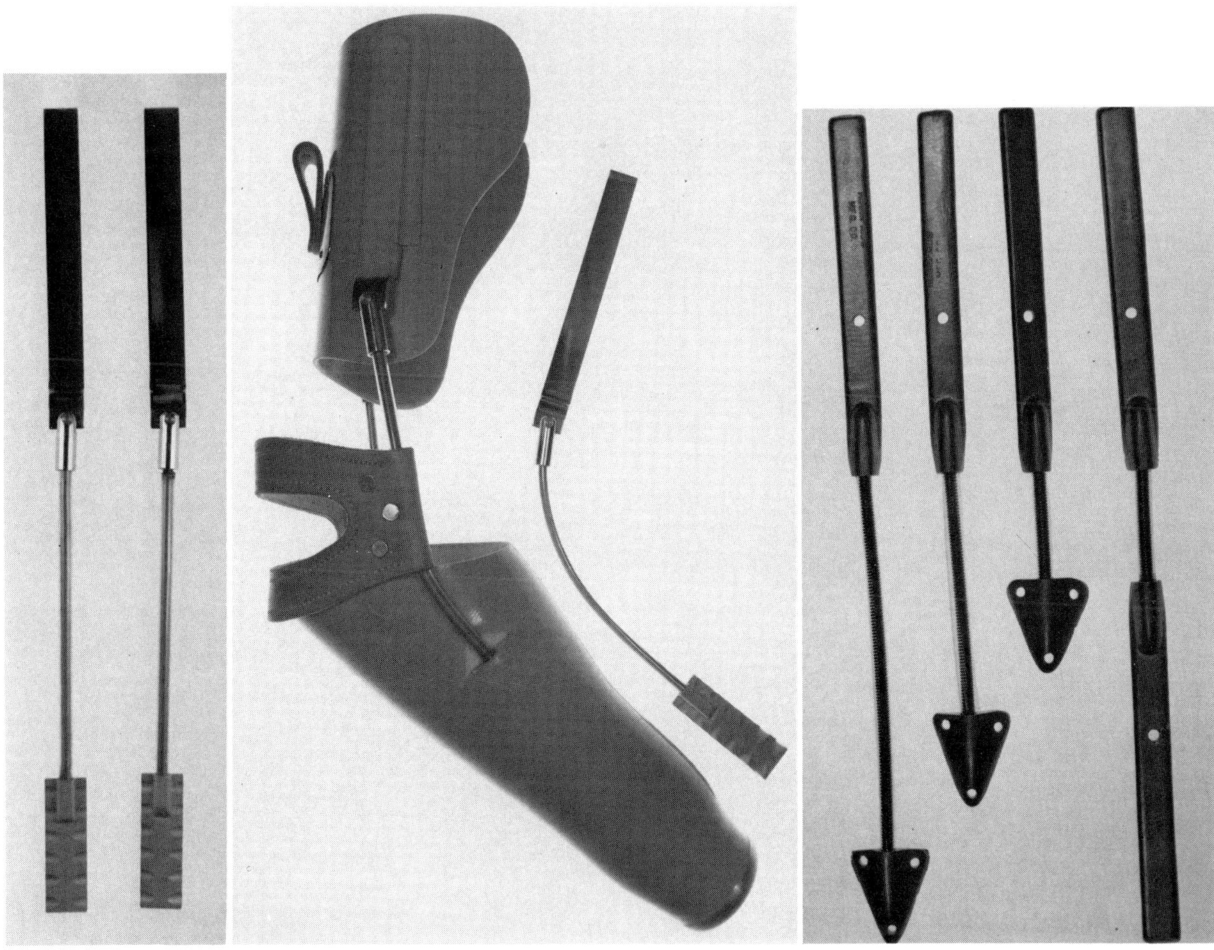

Fig. 9-77. Flexible hinges used in elbow units for below-elbow amputee. (Courtesy Hosmer/Dorrance Corp., Campbell, Calif.)

sion on the terminal device control cable causes the terminal device to rotate back to the "neutral" position.

Ball and socket wrist

A ball and socket wrist unit is available for use with terminal devices equipped with metric threads (12 × 1.5 mm) (Fig. 9-76). The unit permits universal prepositioning of the terminal device with constant friction. The magnitude of the friction loading can be easily adjusted by the amputee.

ELBOW UNITS

Elbow units for the below-elbow amputee

With amputation through the distal third of the forearm, the amputee retains a limited amount of active supination and pronation. Flexible hinges facilitate the transmissions of this residual forearm rotation to the terminal device, thereby minimizing the requirement for manual prepositioning by the amputee.

Flexible hinges. Flexible hinges of metal or leather are commercially available. Dacron webbing may also be used. Attached proximally to the triceps pad and distally to the prosthetic forearm, these hinges permit the transmission of approximately 50% of the residual forearm rotation to the terminal device (Fig. 9-77).

Rigid hinges. For all practical purposes, amputations at or above the midforearm level obviate the possibility of transmitting active supination or pronation to the terminal device. At these levels of amputation the amputee must resort to manual prepositioning of the terminal device.

Single-axis hinges. Single-axis hinges are designed to provide axial (rotational) stability between the prosthetic socket and residual forearm

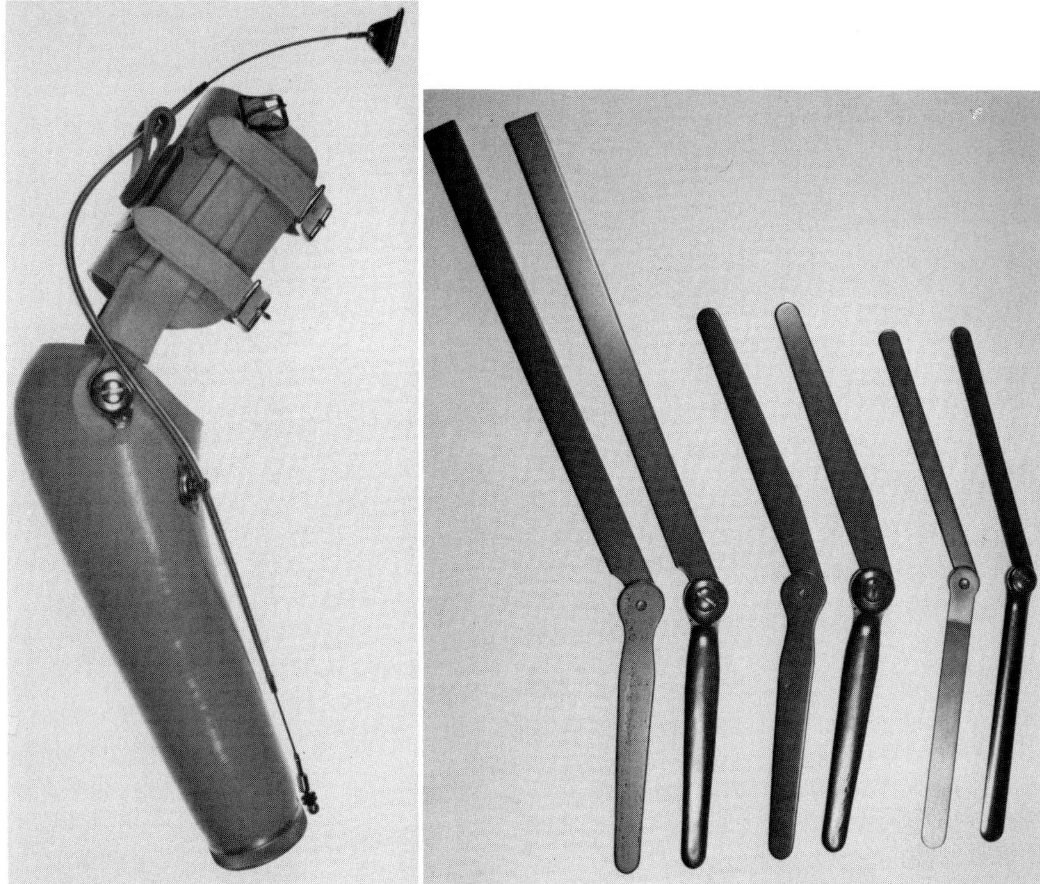

Fig. 9-78. Rigid, single-axis hinges provide axial stability between prosthetic socket and residual forearm. (Courtesy Hosmer/Dorrance Corp., Campbell, Calif.)

during active prosthetic use (Fig. 9-78). Correctly aligned single-axis hinges should not restrict the normal flexion-extension range of motion of the anatomical elbow joint. Single-axis hinges are available in both adult and child sizes.

Polycentric hinges. Short below-elbow levels of amputation require that the anteroproximal trim line of the prosthetic socket be close to the elbow joint. With a high anterior socket wall, complete elbow flexion tends to be restricted by the bunching of soft tissues in the antecubital region. Polycentric hinges (Fig. 9-79) help to increase elbow flexion by reducing the tendency for bunching of the soft tissues. Polycentric hinges are available in adult, medium, and child sizes.

Step-up hinges. Amputations immediately distal to the elbow joint require a prosthetic socket with extremely high trim lines. Consequently, flexion of the anatomical elbow joint is often restricted to 90 degrees or less. In those situations in which a full range of elbow flexion is essential, step-up hinges may be employed (Fig. 9-80).

The use of step-up hinges requires that the prosthetic forearm and socket be separated. Consequently, protheses employing step-up hinges are frequently referred to as split sockets prostheses. Step-up hinges amplify the excursion of anatomical elbow joint motion by a ratio of approximately 2:1. Sixty degrees of flexion of the anatomical elbow joint causes the prosthetic forearm (and terminal device) to move through a range of approximately 120 degrees of motion. The increased range of motion requires that the amputee exert twice as much force to flex the step-up hinge. Step-up hinges are available in adult, medium, and child sizes.

Stump-activated locking hinge. Amputees with very high below-elbow levels of amputation are often unable to operate a conventional below-elbow prosthesis for the following reasons:

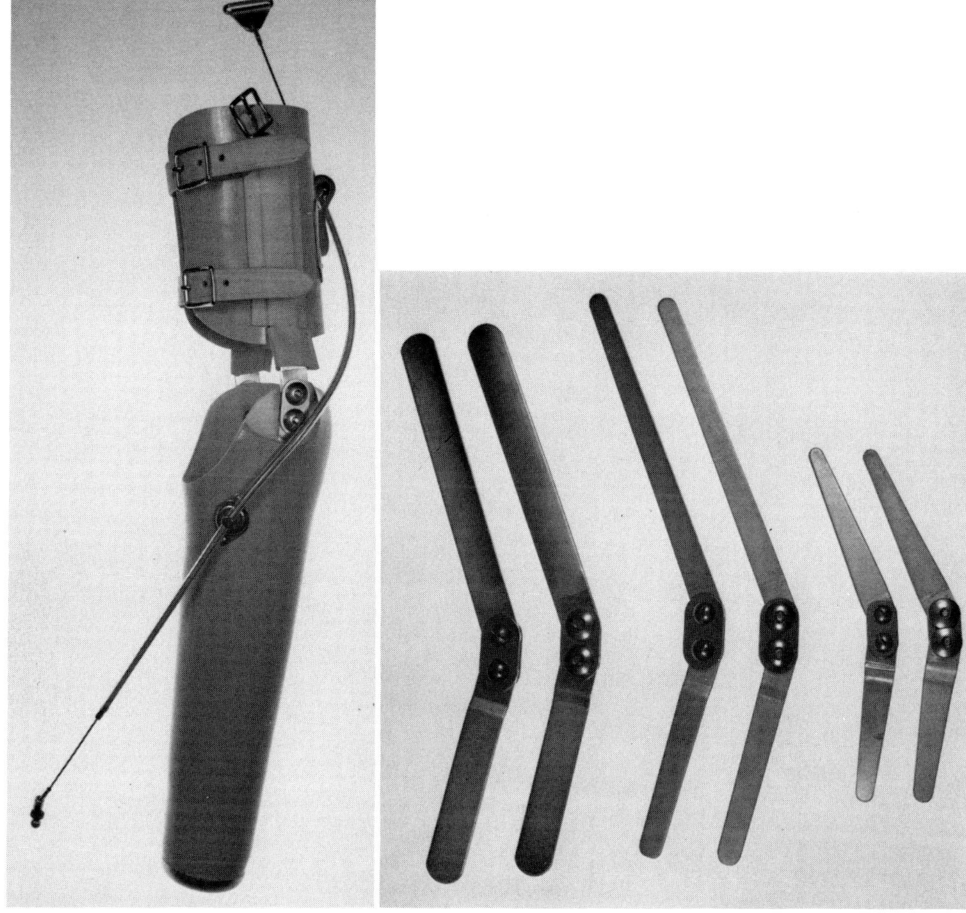

Fig. 9-79. Rigid, polycentric hinges help increase elbow flexion. (Courtesy Hosmer/Dorrance Corp., Campbell, Calif.)

1. Inadequate strength of the elbow flexors
2. Inadequate range of elbow flexion
3. Inability to tolerate the high unit pressure on the volar surface of the forearm when step-up hinges are used

With stump-activated locking hinges, the below-elbow prosthesis is controlled in much the same manner as an above-elbow prosthesis. As in the case of step-up hinges, a split-socket prosthesis is used (Fig. 9-81). Shoulder flexion on the amputated side flexes the mechanical elbow joint. The residual limb is used only for locking and unlocking the mechanical joint. Stump-activated locking hinges are available in two sizes, adult and small.

Elbow units for elbow, above-elbow, and below-shoulder disarticulation amputees

Loss of function of the anatomical elbow joint requires a mechanical substitute that permits controlled flexion and extension through a range of approximately 135 degrees. In addition, the unit must permit the amputee to lock and unlock the elbow at numerous points throughout the 135-degree range of motion.

Outside-locking hinges. Elbow disarticulation and transcondylar levels of amputation usually require the use of a specially designed elbow unit. The length of the residual humerus precludes, for both aesthetic and functional reasons, the use of standard prosthetic elbow units.

Outside-locking hinges are available in standard and heavy-duty models (Fig. 9-82). The standard units provide seven different locking positions throughout the range of flexion and come in adult, medium, and child sizes. The heavy-duty model provides five locking positions and comes in the adult size only.

Inside-locking elbow units. Amputations through the humerus approximately 5 cm (2 inch-

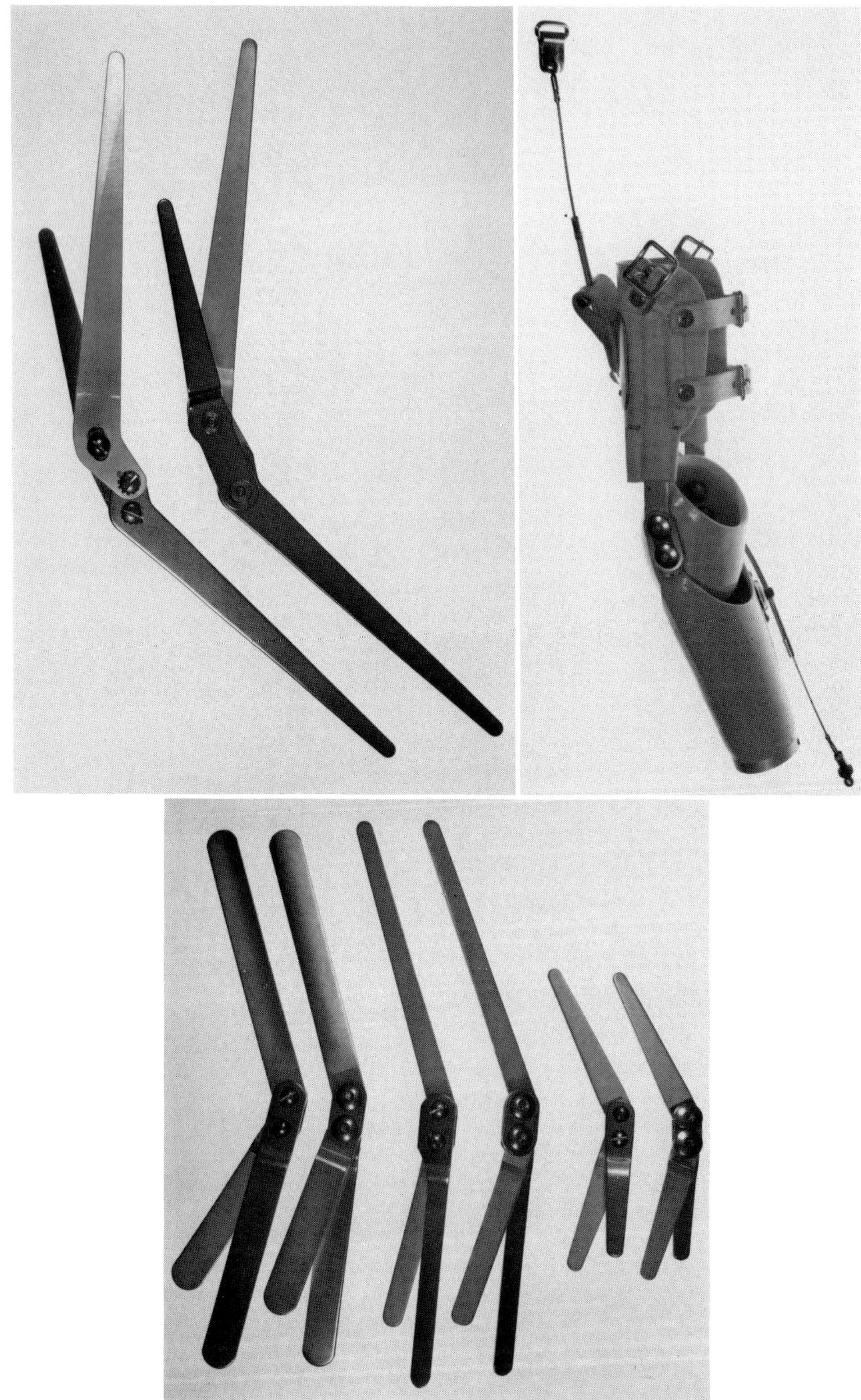

Fig. 9-80. Rigid, step-up hinges for full range of elbow flexion. (Courtesy Hosmer/Dorrance Corp., Campbell, Calif.)

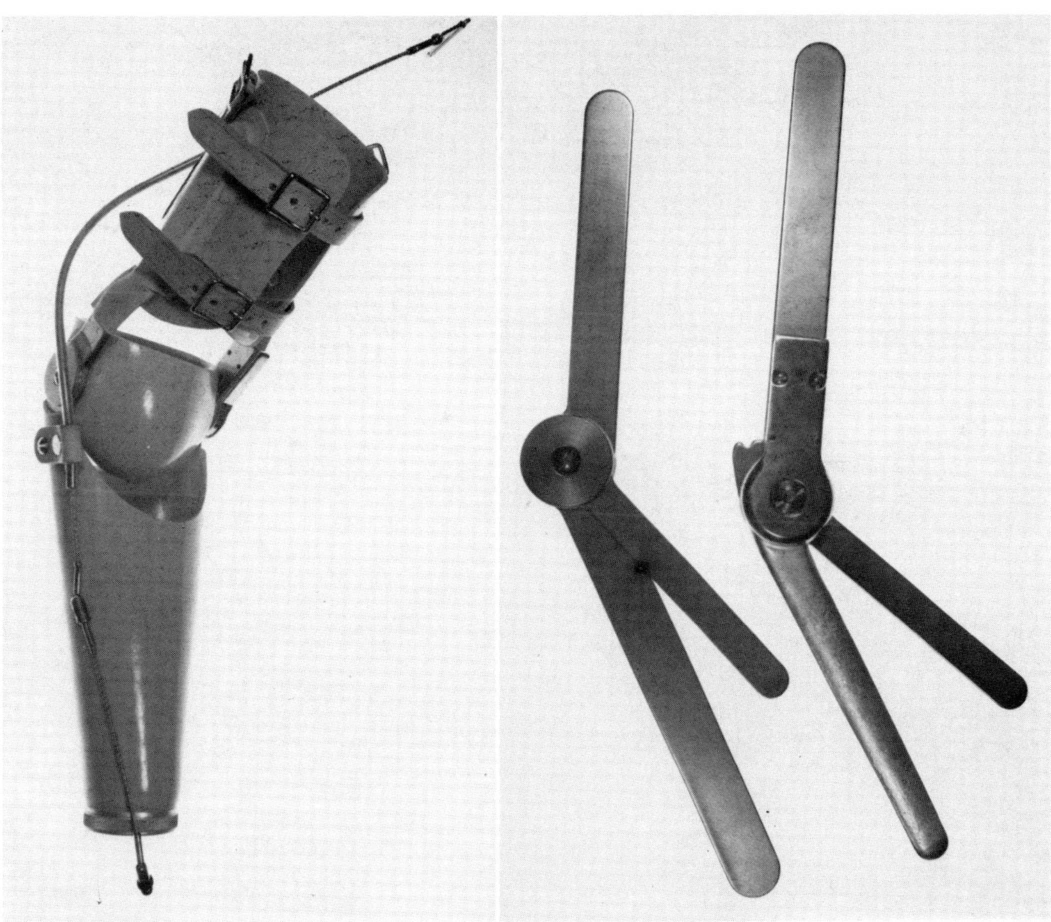

Fig. 9-81. Rigid, stump-activated locking hinge. (Courtesy Hosmer/Dorrance Corp., Campbell, Calif.)

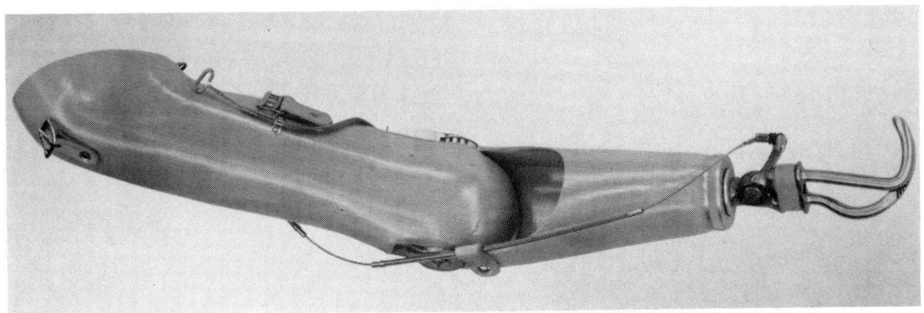

Fig. 9-82. Outside-locking hinges used in elbow unit designed for elbow disarticulation and transcondylar levels of amputation. (Courtesy Hosmer/Dorrance Corp., Campbell, Calif.)

es) proximal to the elbow joint provide adequate space to accommodate inside-locking elbow mechanisms. Inside-locking units permit the amputee to lock the elbow in any of eleven positions of flexion (Fig. 9-83). In addition, inside-locking units incorporate a friction-held turntable. The turntable permits manual prepositioning of the prosthetic forearm as a substitute for external and internal rotation of the humerus.

SHOULDER UNITS

Functional use of a body-powered prosthesis by the unilateral shoulder disarticulation amputee is, at best, extremely limited. Passively operated,

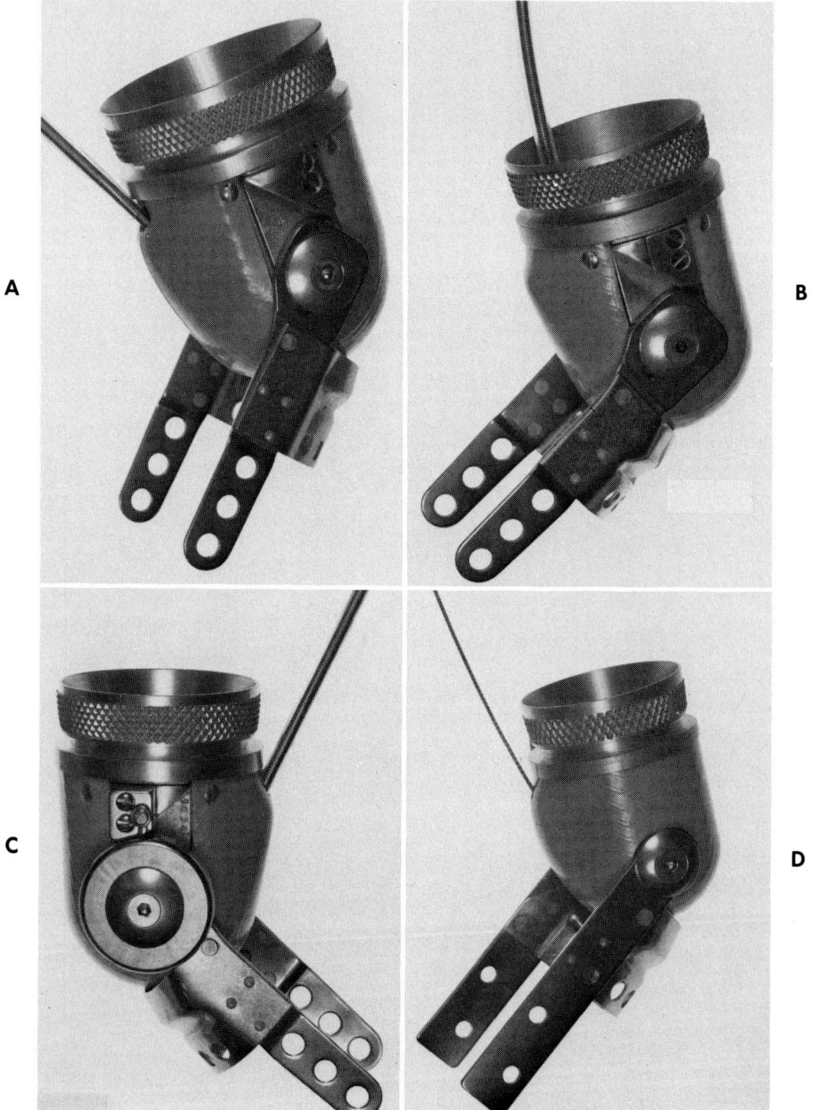

Fig. 9-83. Inside-locking elbow units permit amputee to lock elbow in eleven positions of flexion. **A,** Inside-locking units are available in adult, medium, and child sizes. **B,** Unit with internal exit for elbow-lock control cable. **C,** Externally attached, spring-loaded, forearm lift assist. (On elbows made by Pope Brace Co., spring assist is mounted internally.) Forearm lift assist reduces amount of cable excursion and force required to flex prosthetic elbow. **D,** Noncable-controlled, friction-held elbow unit for very young child. (Courtesy Hosmer/Dorrance Corp., Campbell, Calif.)

friction-loaded shoulder units do, however, provide some assistance with dressing, eating, writing, and other activities of daily living (Fig. 9-84).

Manually positionable shoulder units with adjustable friction loading are available in single axis, double-axis (Fig. 9-85, *A*), triple-axis (Fig. 9-85, *B*), and ball and socket configurations. Single-axis units permit passive abduction. Double-axis units allow for positioning in flexion and abduction. Triple-axis and ball and socket configurations permit universal passive motion. Shoulder units are available in large, medium, and small sizes.

MODULAR UPPER LIMB PROSTHESES

Two modular upper limb prosthetic systems are currently available in the United States. They are composed of tubular humeral and forearm elements, and the components allow for encasement in cosmetic foam covers. After final shaping and

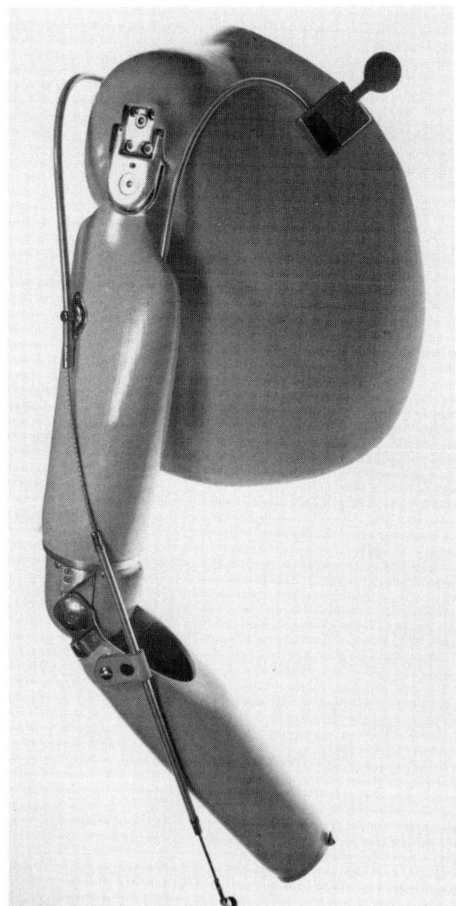

Fig. 9-84. Passively operated, friction-loaded shoulder unit. (Courtesy Hosmer/Dorrance Corp., Campbell, Calif.)

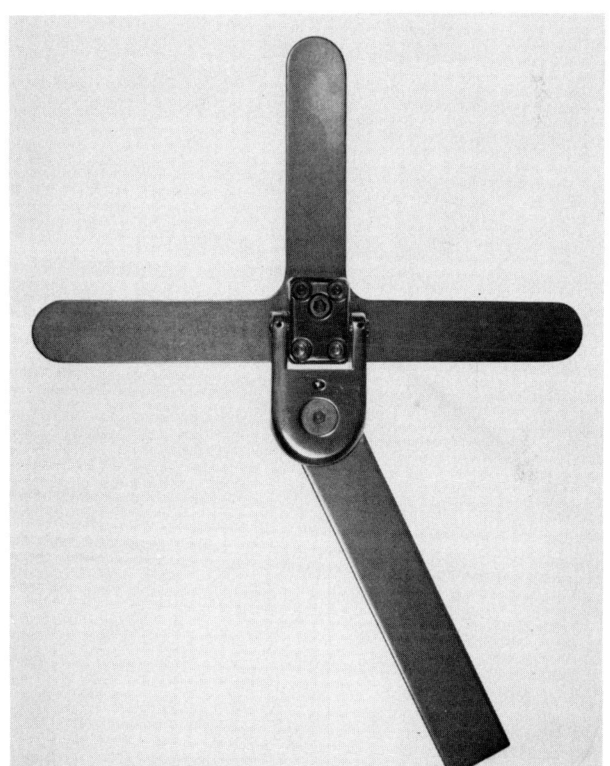

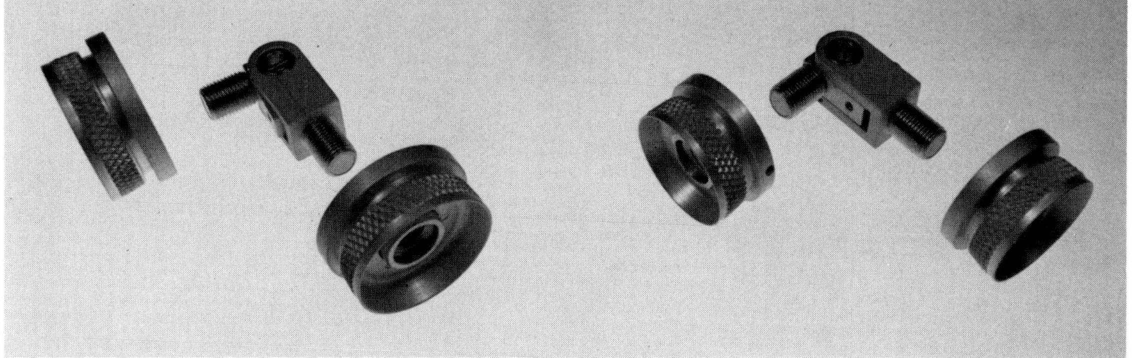

Fig. 9-85. Configurations available in manually positionable shoulder units. **A,** Double axis. **B** and **C,** Triple axis. (Courtesy Hosmer/Dorrance Corp., Campbell, Calif.)

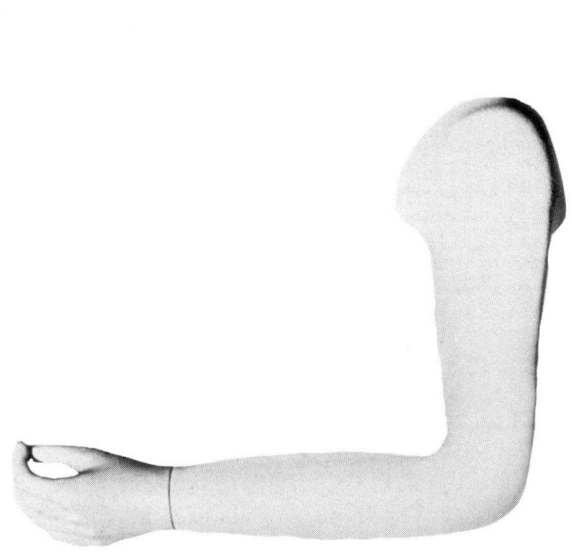

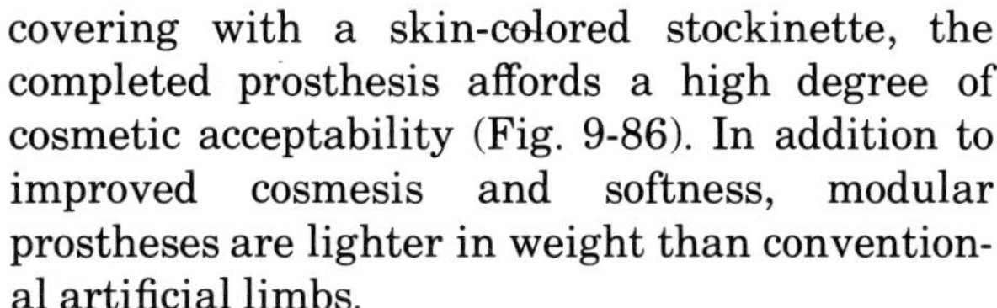

Fig. 9-86. Modular upper limb prosthesis covered with skin-colored stockinette. (Courtesy Otto Bock Orthopedic Industry, Inc., Minneapolis, Minn.)

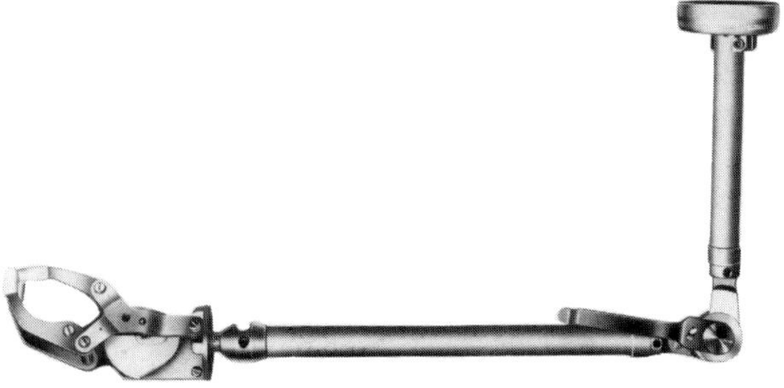

Fig. 9-87. Otto Bock Pylon Arm system. (Courtesy Otto Bock Orthopedic Industry, Inc., Minneapolis, Minn.)

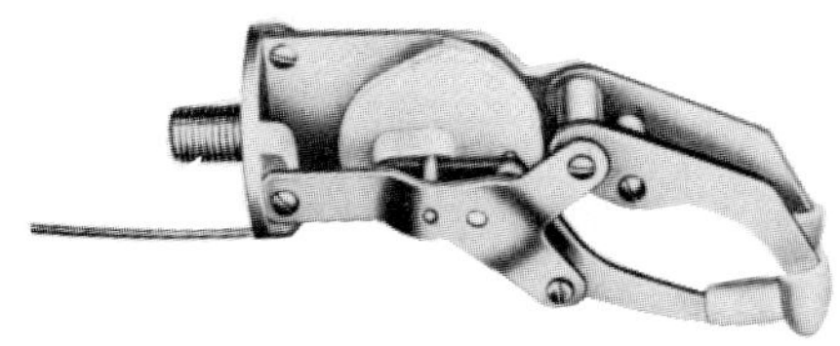

Fig. 9-88. Hand for Otto Bock Pylon Arm system.

covering with a skin-colored stockinette, the completed prosthesis affords a high degree of cosmetic acceptability (Fig. 9-86). In addition to improved cosmesis and softness, modular prostheses are lighter in weight than conventional artificial limbs.

The Otto Bock Pylon Arm system for above-elbow and shoulder disarticulation amputees permits passive or cable-operated elbow flexion, with manual locking (Fig. 9-87). Passive prepositioning of the humeral segment in internal or external rotation and the forearm in supination or pronation is achieved by the use of rotation adaptors.

The system hands (Fig. 9-88) provide a wide variety of terminal device options: cable-controlled, voluntary opening or closing units, and a passive hand unit with a spring-activated thumb and fingers. For the shoulder disarticulation level, the Otto Bock system offers two friction-loaded, passively positionable shoulder units: a ball and socket joint and a flexion-extension, abduction-adduction hinge (Fig. 9-89).

The endoskeletal system of the Hosmer/Dorrance Corporation includes components for below-elbow, above-elbow, and shoulder disarticulation levels of amputation (Fig. 9-90). All terminal devices with the standard 1.3- to 50-cm (½- to 20-inch) thread can be used with the Hosmer/Dorrance system. Socket attachment turntables permit passive rotation of the humeral and forearm segments. A separate wrist unit allows for manual prepositioning of the terminal device in flexion.

Three elbow units are available for either cable-controlled or manual operation: a constant friction elbow, an elbow with a manual lock, and an elbow joint with a cable-controlled locking mechanism. For the shoulder disarticulation level, a manually positionable flexion-extension, abduction-adduction hinge is available.

Section IV

External power in upper limb prosthetics

DUDLEY S. CHILDRESS

The concept of powered upper limb prostheses began in the early part of the twentieth century. Published in 1919, the classical *Ersatzgleider und Arbeitshilfen* contains drawings of a hand powered by compressed gas and a hand driven by electric current. The lack of portable energy sources suitable to power these devices was partly responsible for the failure of these powered hands to be used to any extent at that time. Subsequently, little was done with respect to powered upper limb systems until after World War II.

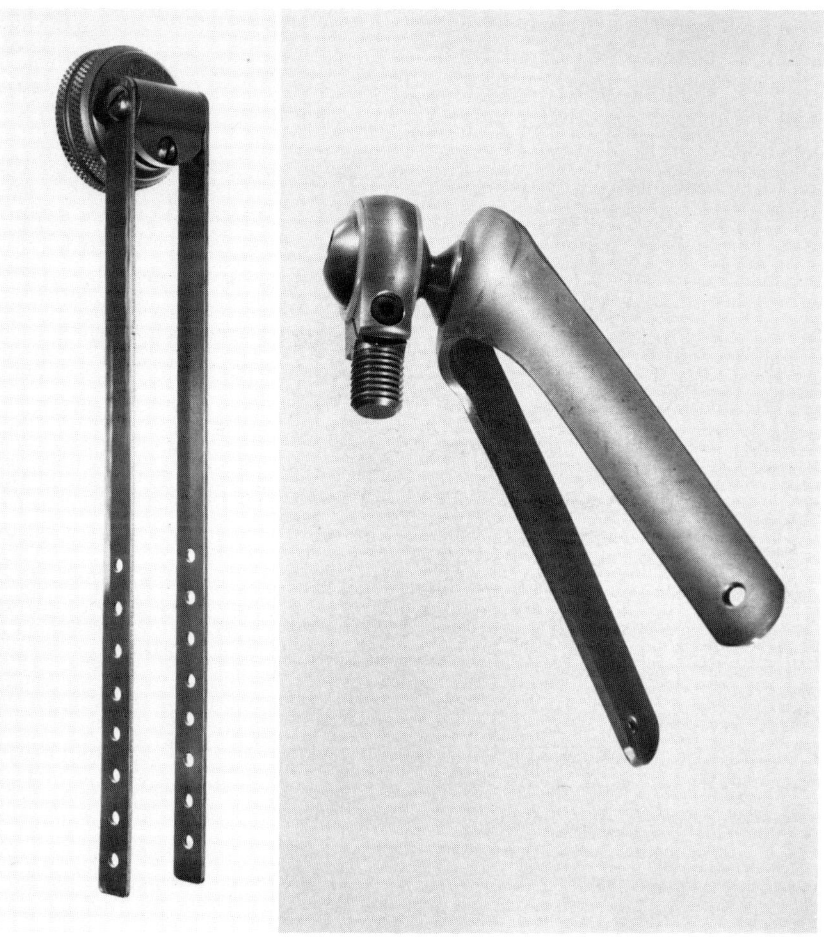

Fig. 9-89. Passive shoulder units for Otto Bock system. (Courtesy Otto Bock Orthopedic Industry, Inc., Minneapolis, Minn.)

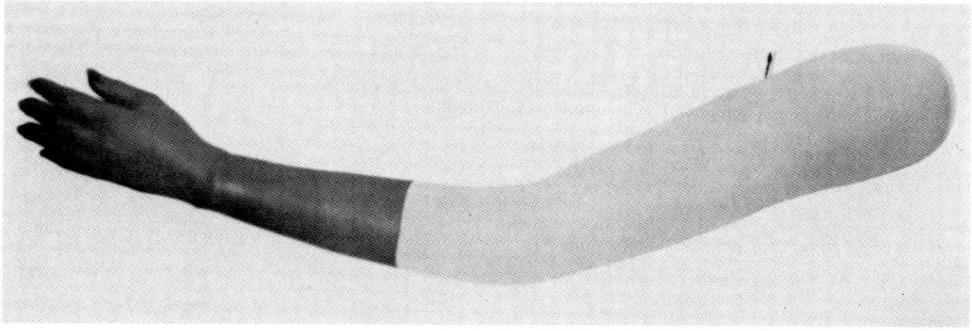

Fig. 9-90. Cosmetic endoskeletal arm system with passive elbow lock.

Wilson[13] and Childress[4] have summarized the development of powered limbs during the postwar era. Unfortunately, developments in this field have been more promising than practical. Apologists for the field believe the slow progress results (among a host of other practical problems) from the great difficulty associated with building adequate replacements for the human hand and arm from technological components.

Two events seem to stand as landmarks in the development of powered upper limb prostheses: (1) congenital amputations resulting from prescription of the drug thalidomide for expectant mothers and (2) public announcements (about 1959) by scientists in the Soviet Union of the development of a myoelectrically controlled, electric hand prosthesis for below-elbow amputees. The problem created by the use of thalidomide galvanized governmental support for research and development of powered upper limb prostheses, particularly in several European countries. The Soviet Union announcements and their demonstrations of an electric hand (myoelectrically controlled) captured the imagination of scientists and engineers around the world and ignited a new interest in powered upper limb research.

Throughout history, humans have been fascinated with the hand and with the possibility of constructing artificial replacements. The idea of using the limbs' own muscle signals to control these hands seemingly made the concept even more interesting.

The idea of using the residual neuromuscular system to control prostheses or to control a grasping action is not new. The Krukenberg procedure, in which the radius and ulna are surgically fashioned into two large fingers for gripping, and the tunnel kineplasty, in which a direct mechanical attachment to a muscle is surgically constructed, use this concept. Myoelectric control follows the pattern set by these precursors by also making use of the residual neuromuscular system for control.

Myoelectric control is emphasized because this control concept appears to have been the stimulus for the development of many of the electrically powered hands now commercially available. These hands may, of course, be controlled in many other ways, and so this stimulus has had a general impact on the upper limb field.

Myoelectric control originated in Germany, and the work was published in 1948,[7] the same year in which Bell Laboratories (United States) announced the development of the transistor. This latter development was to make myoelectric control clinically practical and to have significant impact on powered prostheses through the development of other practical electronic controllers. Scientists in the United Kingdom rediscovered myoelectric control in the 1950s, but they did not carry through to practical applications until after the Soviet Union system was announced. Bottomley[2] and associates later developed the first practical myoelectric prosthesis that was proportionally controlled. The late 1960s saw commercial development of electric hand prostheses, primarily in association with myoelectric control systems. Except for a few locations, however, these devices have not been prescribed in routine amputee clinics of North America until recent years.

Electric hands, myoelectrically controlled, have not had much impact on prostheses for children, although some congenital below-elbow amputees are now successfully using these systems.[11] The congenital amputee with high-level amputation sites has not been helped much by this control method. Electric elbows (largely switch-controlled) developed in Canada have had some impact on this problem, but no multifunctional powered limbs are commercially available in North America that adequately solve the problems of the high-level arm amputee (adult or child).

Generally, the control of multiple-powered joints is difficult for amputees. Schmidl[8] has had some success applying myoelectric control of three powered functions, but this technique is not widely applied. Other attempts, some very sophisticated, are still experimental or in prototype stages of development (e.g., Herberts).[6] The work of Simpson[10] in the United Kingdom has been fruitful using unbeatable position servomechanisms and kinematic coupling[3] of some joints in the design of multifunctional limbs, based on a principle called "extended physiological proprioception." His gas-powered prostheses, however, have not been available in North America and have not been applied to adult amputees. Nevertheless, this pioneering work and other work of European and Canadian centers, originally directed toward thalidomide-induced problems, will undoubtedly have a significant impact on the future direction of powered-limb development.

POWERED PROSTHETIC COMPONENTS

Hands

From a kinematic viewpoint, all available powered hands are essentially the same as nonpowered hands. All use palmar prehension, and most are basically constructed around a metal (aluminum) frame, covered by a soft liner of PVC, which is in turn covered by a PVC cosmetic glove. The thumb opposes the index and middle fingers of the hand in an active manner, whereas the ring and little finger are usually passive. Finger velocities of the electric hands generally approximate 1 radian/sec (approximately 60 degrees/sec) with the pinch force in adult hands between 90 and 130 newtons (approximately 9 to 13.5 kg; 20 to 30 pounds). Child-size hands usually have proportionally less pinch force.

It is important for the person experienced with body-powered hands to realize the enormous difference between mechanical hands and powered hands. Body-powered hands, particularly the voluntary opening variety, have traditionally not been very functional because they require considerable effort to achieve nominal opening and pinch force. They have largely complemented the prosthetic hook as a cosmetic replacement. Powered hands, however, generally open widely, have high pinch forces, and require minimal effort to operate. Consequently, the powered hand usually can be much more functional for an amputee than the body-powered hand (mechanical hand).

Major contributors to the powered hand market in North America are Otto Bock Orthopedic Industries, Inc. (Germany and the United States), Fidelity Electronics (VANU and Viennatone hands, the United States and Austria), Variety Village Electro Limb Production Centre (child size, Canada), and Systemtechnik (child size, Sweden). Otto Bock Orthopedic Industries, Inc., has been a major designer of powered hands (electric and pneumatic) and was originally involved with the first models of the Viennatone hand. This company has developed a hand system, which incorporates design similarity into body-powered, gas-powered, and electric-powered devices. They have three sizes of electric hands: (1) adult male, (2) adult female, and (3) child. Female and male hands are mechanically identical, except the female hand is shorter, and the inner liner has a smaller circumference.

Adult models of the Otto Bock electric hand have a unique automatic gearshift mechanism. The gearshift is force activated so that when the fingers are moving in space (not gripping), the hand is in high gear. When the fingers close on an object and the gripping force exceeds about 9 newtons (approximately 0.9 kg; 2 pounds), the system shifts to low gear to more easily generate a strong pinch force. The shifting of gear ratios is an economical approach for single-motor hand designs in which a trade-off is usually necessary between speed and pinch force (higher speed, less pinch force). With the gearshift, a designer can more easily achieve the desirable speed, as well as the desired pinch force, while retaining a reasonably small drive motor. This is particularly true in prosthetic hand design when the fingers usually operate with velocity at low force (torque) or with low velocity (pinching) at high force (torque). The child-size Otto Bock hand does not use the automatic gearshift design. It, as well as the other electric hands, are basically driven by permanent magnet motors driving spur gears.

Powered hand designs all incorporate a back-locking mechanism, which keeps the hand from opening due to outside forces at the finger tips, after an object has been grasped. This vise-type action permits the hand to grip objects after initial closure without the continuous application of power. This is extremely important in electrically powered hands in which the motor is stalled during grip; drawing a high stall current, but generating no output power. Adults may be informed not to draw stall currents for long periods so as not to quickly deplete the battery. Similar hand systems for children may need current cutoff systems that automatically turn the drive current off after stall conditions are reached. The back-locking feature is one of the few characteristics of an artifical hand that is superior to the normal physiological hand. It permits an object to be held and carried for long periods without expenditure of effort.

The skeletal structures of the Veterans Administration and Otto Bock electric hands are shown in Fig. 9-91. The Veterans Administration hand is a modification of the Viennatone Hand. The changes include break-away fingers that release under extreme loads (about 22.5 kg; 50 pounds of force), as well as different drive motor, gears, and back lock.

Fig. 9-92 shows several electric hands as they appear with their inner liners. A glove, which matches the user's skin tone, is worn over the liner. This glove must be carefully looked after for it to remain serviceable over a reasonable period of time (e.g., 6 months) when used by an active wearer. Stains should be removed immediately to prevent migrations into the plastic material. Also, a cleanser and protective agent (e.g., silicone cream) should be used on the glove each evening. If heavy work (shoveling, raking, etc.) is performed, the wearer should don a protective mitten over the hand. An oven mitten, with the thumbpiece properly positioned, may be used as a convenient and effective protective cover.

The child-size hands available from Variety Village Electro Limb Production Centre, Systemtechnik, and Otto Bock Orthopedic Industries, Inc., make it possible to make a reasonable size transition during growth. The Electro Limb and Systemtechnik hands can be used with very young children (3 to 6 years old). This can be fol-

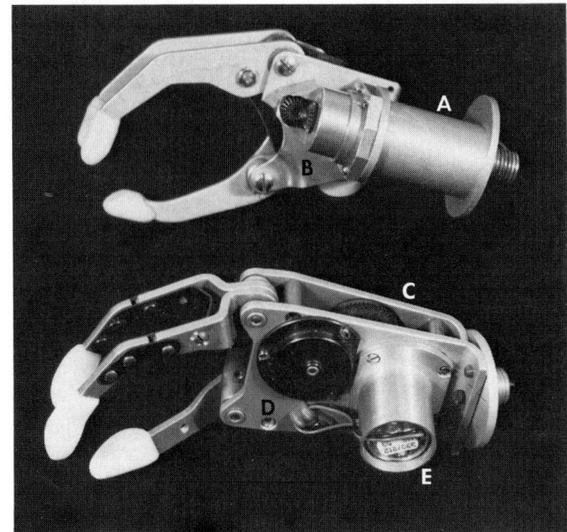

Fig. 9-91. Skeletal structures of Otto Bock and Veterans Administration (VA) hands. *A*, Permanent magnet motor within housing. *B*, Automatic force-actuated gearshift. *C*, Spur gear train. *D*, Back lock. *E*, Permanent magnet motor and housing.

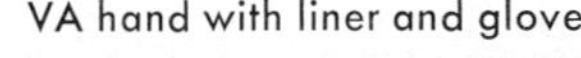

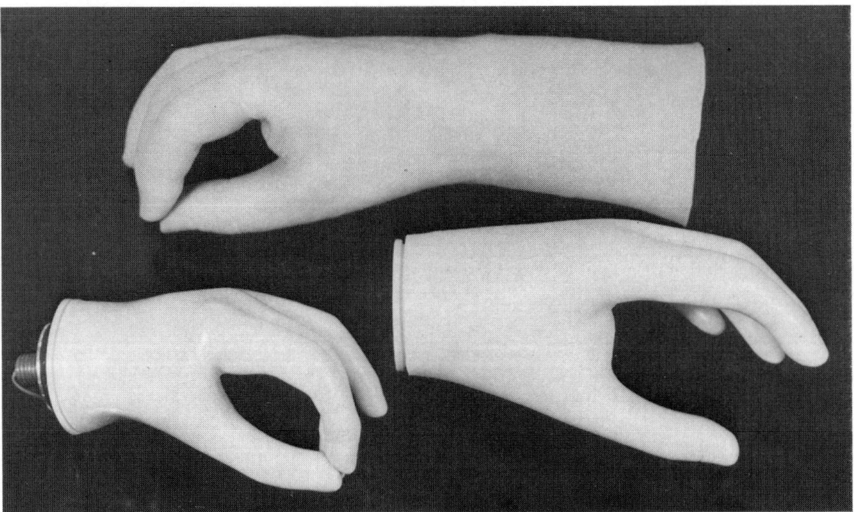

Fig. 9-92. Electric hands, liners, and cosmetic glove.

lowed by the Otto Bock child-size hand, then the Otto Bock female hand, and finally the adult male hands. A system whereby these hands may be passed down to other children appears to have merit because of the significant expense associated with purchasing new powered hands.

Electric hands generally have acceptable maintenance records. The fingers, finger pivots, and finger gears generally wear first. The fingerpieces are sometimes abused by amputees who use them for prying. The other vulnerable part is the electric drive motor. A motor should serve for several years, and an electric hand should serve for 3 to 5 years, if it is not abused. Appropriate repairs can result in a significantly longer lifetime. Projected life is, of course, based on usage. An amputee who must use the prosthesis for all grasping activities will wear component parts more rapidly than a unilateral amputee who uses the hand only for assistance.

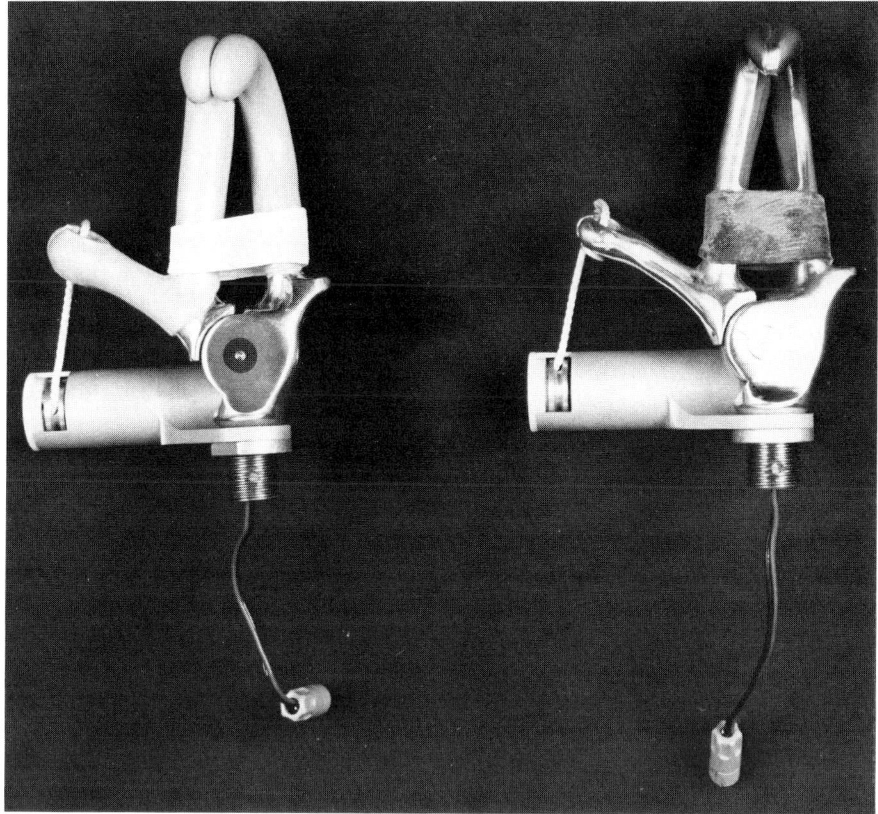

Fig. 9-93. Michigan electric hooks showing electric motor housing, pulley, and pull cord.

Powered hooks

The use of external power for hook terminal devices has not been as popular as for hand prostheses. Various powered hooks have been designed, but few are available for general use. Perhaps this is because hooks are not used as avidly in Western European countries as in North America. The European sources of powered terminal devices therefore have favored powered hand development.

The Michigan hook (Fig. 9-93), a simple powered hook for children, is available from commercial sources and has been used with some success. As with many powered components, it is used, not so much on the basis of its own merits, but because it is available.

The Michigan hook was designed originally as a terminal device for a redesigned version of the Michigan Feeding Arm, developed by the Area Amputee Center in Grand Rapids, Michigan. It was designed for simplicity of construction and simplicity of control, not efficiency. Closing one electrical switch opens the hook fingers against a rubber band, and releasing the switch permits the fingers to close through recovery of the stored energy. The hook is constructed around a standard (child size) hook prosthesis with attached motor. Spur-gear assembly, pulley, drive housing, pull cord, motor damping circuit, switch, and battery. No back lock is required because the spring action of the rubber band holds the fingers closed.

Several powered hooks are now under development or in prototype evaluation. Such terminal devices should be in the prothetics armamentarium. They will be particularly useful if they can be quickly interchanged with hand components, so the appropriate device could be chosen that best serves the user's needs. Powered hands are excellent for gripping medium to large objects. Their soft linings mold over the surfaces to permit firm gripping action. They also have a pleasing appearance. In contrast, the hook, which permits much greater visibility when handling objects, is capable of picking up small items, but is not as effective with large objects. Unfortunately, the form of the hook that follows its function is not aesthetically pleasing in the eyes of many.

Otto Bock has available a pincer (specially shaped tweezers) that facilitates handling small objects with an electric hand (Fig. 9-94). Regular tweezers may also be used, but they will fall from the hand if the fingers open too widely. The special pincers have a finlike structure on their dorsal side, which wedges between the index and middle fingers of the hand.

The powered hook and powered hand, as with their nonpowered counterparts, are not comparable devices. Each has functional advantages and disadvantages that relate to the type of task being performed, and each imparts its own peculiar subjective response to the user and to others.

Wrist rotators

In powered prostheses, supination and pronation (roll) of the artificial hand/hook is usually achieved through use of a wrist rotator device. This device rotates the terminal device with respect to the wrist and is normally located in the vicinity of the anatomical wrist.

Otto Bock markets the only commercially available wrist rotator (Fig. 9-95). This rotator is intended to be used for "prepositioning" activites. That is, it positions the hand or other terminal device for optimal usage. It does not generate enough torque for such activities as turning doorknobs or loosening jar caps.

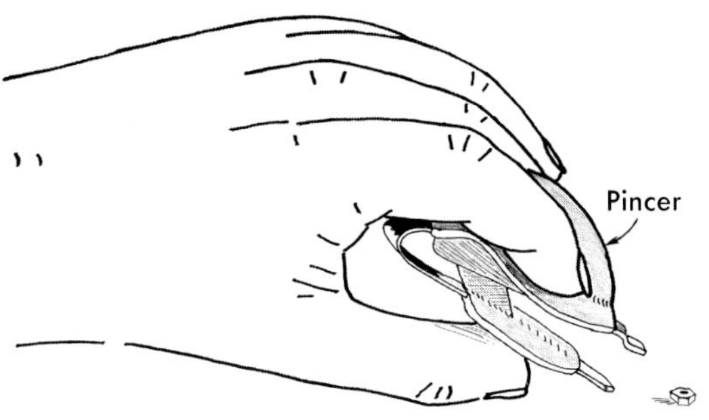

Fig. 9-94. Prosthetic hand using Otto Bock pincer for gripping small objects. Note dorsal wing for wedging between fingers.

Wrist rotators add weight distally to a prosthesis and add to system complexity. Consequently, it is often appropriate to seek alternate solutions for wrist rotation. Wrist disarticulation amputees are often best fitted with styloid suspension that permits natural supination-pronation to occur. Long below-elbow amputees can sometimes use a split socket (supracondylar suspension) to directly rotate the hand. Below-elbow amputees with moderate length limbs who have but little residual forearm rotation may be fitted with a split socket, and this residual motion can be used to activate electrical switches that control the wrist rotator. Short below-elbow amputees require an alternate control for wrist rotation, and this can sometimes be achieved myoelectrically. Medium and short below-elbow amputees may consider using compensatory motions to pronate the hand. For example, humeral abduction will effectively bring about a pronated position of the hand. Of course, passive rotation is also very practical. Although potentially avoidable, compensatory actions by the amputee can decrease prosthesis cost, complexity (improving reliability), and weight without much change in functional performance and therefore should be viewed as a practical alternative when powered prostheses are fitted.

Powered wrist rotators have always been considered important powered components. Nevertheless, in practice their effective control is a problem, and their usefulness may be questioned when they are used with unilateral arm amputees.

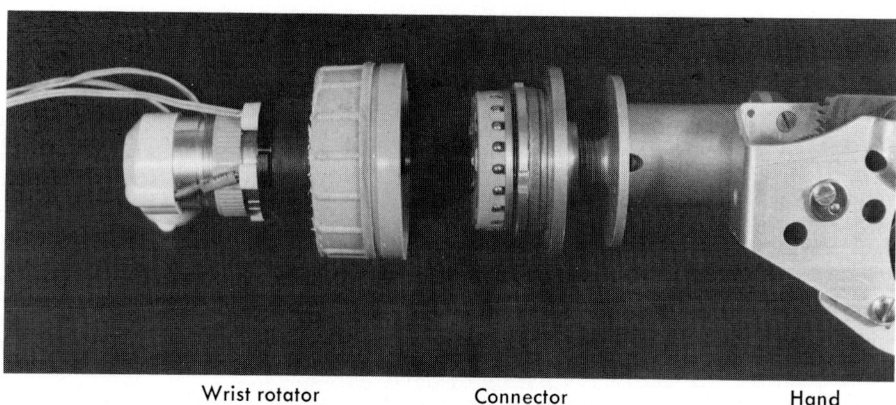

Fig. 9-95. Otto Bock electric wrist rotator shown with wrist connector and electric hand.

Electric powered elbows

Although numerous electric powered elbows have been designed and evaluated during recent years, only a few are readily available to prosthetics practitioners (Fig. 9-96). The Veterans Administration electric elbow (adult size) may be purchased through Fidelity Electronics, and a Canadian-designed, child-size, electric elbow is available from Electro Limb in Toronto.

The electric elbows currently available have typical angular velocities (lightly loaded) of 1 to 2 radians/sec and stall torques in the vicinity of 3 to 9 newton-meters.

Bilateral amputees (high-level) are compelled to use powered elbows for lifting, but unilateral amputees use the elbow primarily for positioning the forearm. A back-locking mechanism is important on the elbow so the forearm may be used passively to hold objects (e.g., a coat over the arm) or to press against objects (e.g., paper on a desk). Nevertheless, amputees prefer the elbow to be free swinging when they walk. As a result, most powered elbows have been designed to be free swinging when the elbow is fully extended.

Although powered hands and wrists can operate effectively at reasonably low power levels (e.g., 3 to 6 watts input to motor), elbows require significantly greater power during active lifting (e.g., 20 to 25 watts input to the motor). The weight of the forearm can be balanced by springs, but if work is done in lifting, it must be supplied by the elbow.

Good users of body-powered elbows generally find powered elbows to be slow and noisy. Nevertheless, amputees who require powered elbows usually find them useful, even though much remains to be done with improvement of the designs.

Existing electric elbows use permanent magnet motors for their driving torque. The Electro Limb elbow and a newly developed elbow at New York University (Hosmer/Dorrance Corp. has manufactured prototypes) use spur-gear drive trains. The Veterans Administration elbow and an elbow developed by Liberty Mutual Insurance Company (Boston arm) use the harmonic drive as a gear reducer. This mechanism is lightweight and physically amenable to a powered elbow.

High-speed permanent magnet motors require considerable gearing down for use in powered prosthetic joints. An alternative approach is to use low-speed torque motors. This obviates the need for multiple gear stages, and noise can therefore be greatly diminished. These motors are designed to operate at or near stall conditions. Their main drawback has been high cost. Several powered elbows (Utah arm and Johns Hopkins arm) now under development and evaluation use this approach, and it appears to be the direction future electric elbow design will take. Quiet, but rapid, response at appropriate torque levels may be achieved with this approach.

Shoulder joints and humeral rotators

No powered shoulders or powered humeral rotators are available to clinicians, although humeral rotators have been used experimentally and gas-powered shoulder joints have been used in prosthetic arm systems.[10] The glenohumeral joint is important in arm movement, and if shoulder disarticulation amputees are ever to be fitted well with powered limbs, powered gleno-

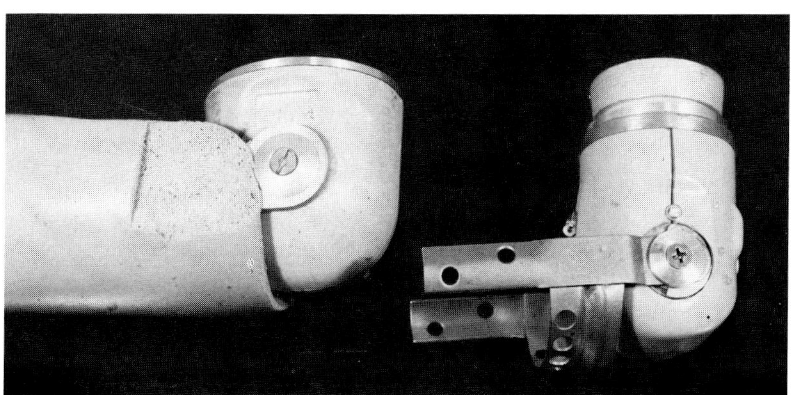

VAPC electric elbow　　　Electro-Limb electric elbow

Fig. 9-96. Commercially available electric elbows.

humeral joints will be necessary. The joint requires a high torque and has not been amenable to electric actuators. Also, amputees with high-level amputations are relatively few in number and therefore the stimulus for commercial development has been low.

Powered sources and actuators

Compressed gas and electric batteries are the main energy sources for powered prosthetic limbs. Compressed gas has been widely used in the United Kingdom and in Western Europe, but little used in North America. This is partially because a distribution and maintenance system for gas cylinders was never developed in America.

Compressed gas systems are advantageous in prosthetic systems because the actuators are lightweight in relation to their power output. They also do not require locking mechanisms because the actuators can generate constant forces or torques without energy expenditure. Gas systems also are mechanically compliant when compared with many electrical systems, and this makes them more like normal physiological systems. The actuators have excellent dynamic response, and they are quiet. (Early systems had an exhaust "hiss," but this was eliminated by laminar exhaust flow through multiple openings.) The main technical disadvantage of gas systems has been low-energy density and low energy-to-weight ratios for the storage containers.

Electric storage in secondary cells (rechargeable batteries) is used most widely in powered prosthetic systems. Nickel-cadmium (Ni-Cd) batteries are most commonly used. These batteries may be replaced in coming years by the nickel-zinc battery or some other battery of greater energy density. Nevertheless, the Ni-Cd unit has proven to be acceptable for a variety of prosthetic applications. They have a lifetime of over 1000 recharge cycles, and the typical Ni-Cd used in prosthetic applications is rated at between 100 and 400 milliampere/hour (mA/hour). A 100 mA/hour battery should sustain its voltage for approximately 1 hour at a current of 100 mA. At higher currents, the capacity is diminished, but the intermittent currents typically required by prostheses may be handled well.

Some Ni-Cd batteries need to be charged at a capacity over 10 rate (C/10), where C is the capacity in mA/hour. For example, a 100 mA/hour battery would be charged at 10 mA. A typical charging time is therefore about 10 to 12 hours. Some modern designs may be charged at the C/1 rate. A 100 mA/hour battery would then be charged at 100 mA over a period slightly longer than 1 hour. When the fast charging is complete, the charger automatically drops to a trickle charging rate. These fast-charge batteries are convenient for amputees because they assure a complete charge may be delivered during overnight charging.

The wide use of rechargeable batteries in portable appliances assures their continued technical development and moderate price. Consequently, it appears that electric energy will continue to be the power source of choice for powered prostheses of the future. Another advantage of electric power is that electronic control circuits may also be operated from this energy source.

A rule of thumb concerning battery drain is to

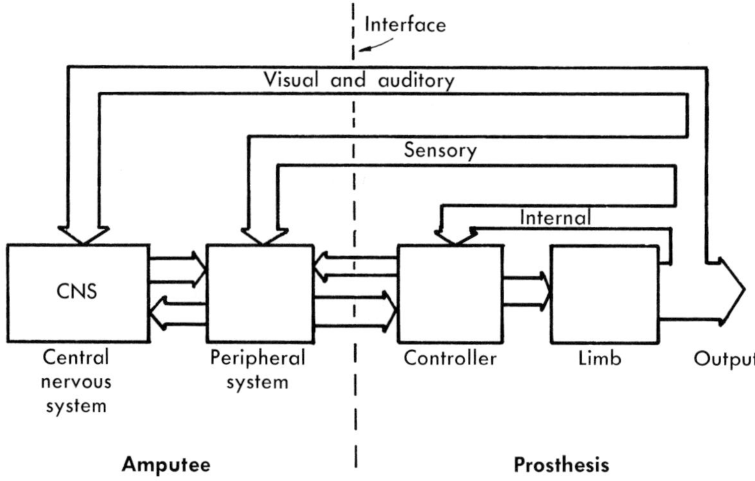

Fig. 9-97. Information flow pathways in amputee-prosthesis system. Most powered systems available commercially have only visual and auditory feedback. They commonly use switch closures or myoelectric signals for inputs to controller.

maintain the quiescent (standby) energy consumed in a day's operation below 10% of the stored energy (preferably below 5%). In this way, 90% or more of the stored energy is available for use by actuators of the powered limb. Otto Bock Orthopedic Industries, Inc., has chosen to use a modular battery arrangement so the amputee can carry a spare battery replacement. This idea also facilitates repair in case of battery failure and appears to have merit.

Most electrical systems for prostheses are now based on 6 or 12 volts (V). There is a tendency toward 6 V for below-elbow prosthetic systems because the hand operates at low power and because there is frequently little space available for the battery. Other than potentially smaller size, advantages that can accrue with 6 V are (1) greater battery reliability because of fewer cells (1.25 V/cell) and (2) a greater energy-to-weight ratio because the ratio of active battery chemicals to container materials can be increased.

Electric storage can also be used to operate hydraulic pumps, and the use of hydraulic actuators makes technical sense for prosthetic arm design. Nevertheless, hydraulic systems for arms are difficult to construct because commercial hydraulic components are generally to large and heavy for artificial arms. Problems with component availability have therefore held back advances in this direction.

CONTROL

Even if it were possible to build excellent mechanical or electromechanical replacements for the hand and arm, with all the complex motions of the normal hand, there would remain the monumental problem of controlling such an arm. Compounding this control problem is the need for the control to be subconscious in nature, with the limb serving the user, not the user serving the limb.

Harris[5] has said, "In almost all activities, as long as you have to think about what you're doing, you're not doing it very well." This is particularly true in an amputee's use of a prosthesis. Control methods are, in fact, as important in prosthetic limb design as the arm components themselves, perhaps more so. Wiener[12] has suggested that lack of good control in a prosthesis may be due to the absence of sensory feedback. If this is so, it remains a grievous fault because appropriate kinds of sensory feedback in powered arm prostheses are still missing.

Fig. 9-97 shows the flow of information in a man-prosthesis system. Most powered prostheses in clinical use have only visual and auditory feedback pathways. The input control signals are most frequently small movement of on-off electric switches or myoelectric potentials.

The man-prosthesis combination is a special type of man-machine system in which the machine is effectively a replacement part of the man. Whereas the control of most man-machine systems is through the hands or feet, the control of prosthetic devices must usually come from some other source, and this makes the man-prosthesis system unique.

Switch control

Control of powered prosthetic actuators by switches (on-off control) is the simplest and least expensive electrical control method available. Switch control is a form of velocity control because the switch usually controls the off or the on velocity state. Visual feedback is used to monitor position and derive information concerning when to operate the switch or switches. This operation is through some type of body motion.

Two switches are generally used to operate an electric motor actuator. They can be arranged as shown in Fig. 9-98. This circuit also provides dynamic braking of the motor when the power is off.

Because it is sometimes more convenient to harness motion in a single direction, a three-state switch arrangement is frequently used to control an actuator. A small excursion produces motor rotation in one direction, and a larger excursion (same direction) produces the oppostie motor action. The VAPC pull switch may be purchased for this type of control (Fig. 9-99). This switch may be harnessed in many ways. Fig. 99-100 shows examples of switch control by shoulder elevation, chest expansion, and biscapular abduction. The resourceful prosthetist can develop other schemes as needed for switch control.

Switch controls are also available from Variety Village Electro Limb Production Centre (for pow-

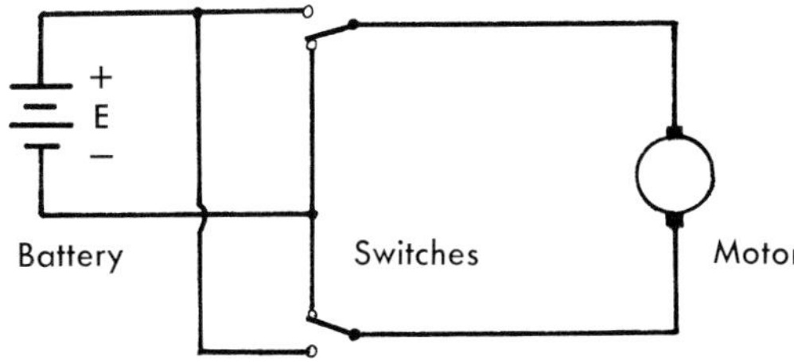

Fig. 9-98. Simple electrical circuit for two-switch control of electric motor.

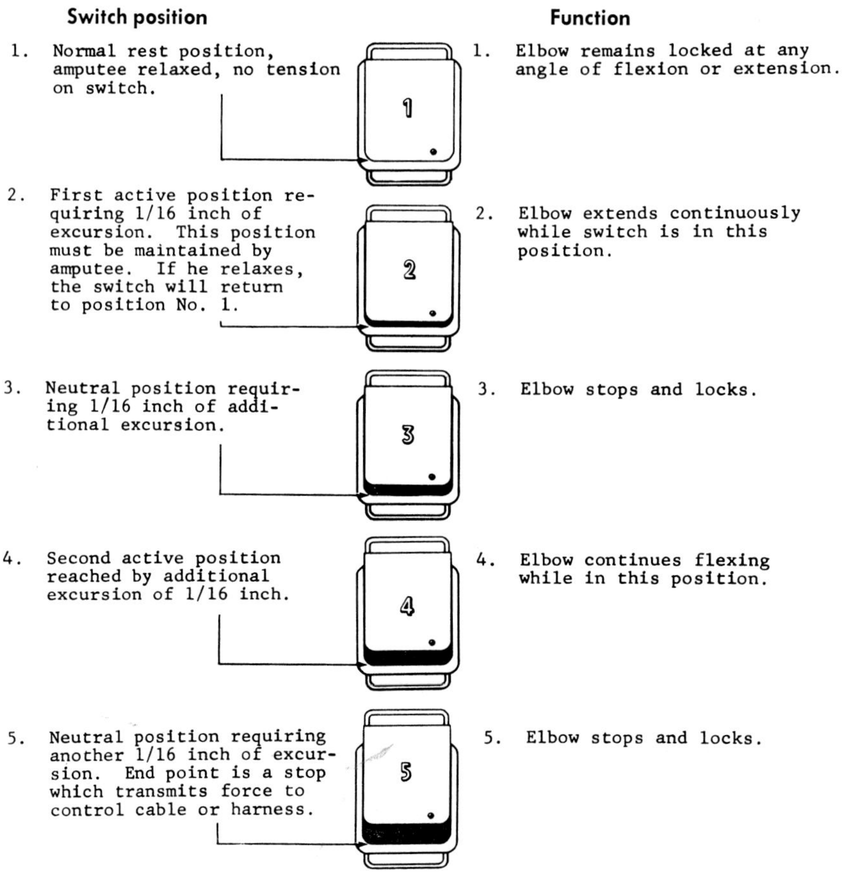

Switch position		Function
1. Normal rest position, amputee relaxed, no tension on switch.	1	1. Elbow remains locked at any angle of flexion or extension.
2. First active position requiring 1/16 inch of excursion. This position must be maintained by amputee. If he relaxes, the switch will return to position No. 1.	2	2. Elbow extends continuously while switch is in this position.
3. Neutral position requiring 1/16 inch of additional excursion.	3	3. Elbow stops and locks.
4. Second active position reached by additional excursion of 1/16 inch.	4	4. Elbow continues flexing while in this position.
5. Neutral position requiring another 1/16 inch of excursion. End point is a stop which transmits force to control cable or harness.	5	5. Elbow stops and locks.

Fig. 9-99. VAPC electric switch showing various control states possible from single-site input.

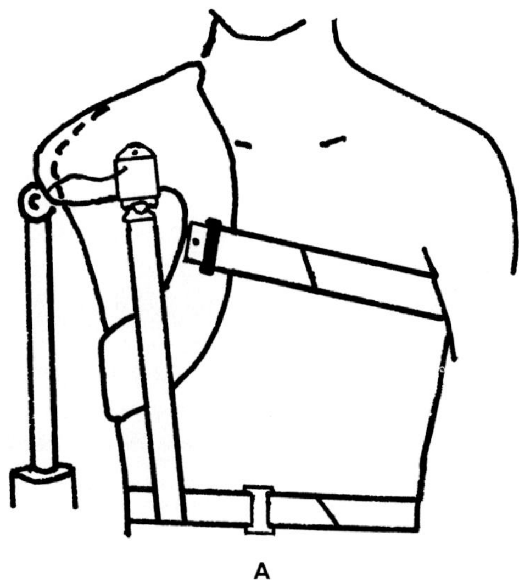

Fig. 9-100. Three possible switch-control configurations for powered prosthetic joints. **A,** Shoulder-elevation control for shoulder disarticulation amputee (anterior view).

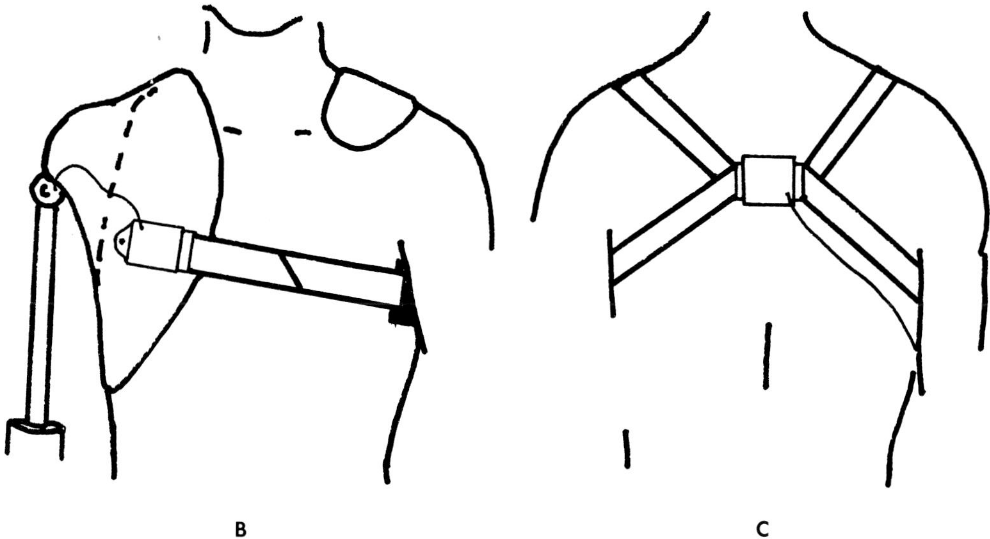

Fig. 9-100, cont'd. B, Chest-expansion control for interscapulothoracic amputee (anterior view). **C,** Biscapular control with "butterfly" harness for below-elbow or above-elbow amputee (posterior view).

ered elbows and powered hands) and from Otto Bock Orthopedic Industries, Inc. (for wrist rotators). They can be fabricated easily for special requirements. Despite their simplicity and low cost, electric switches are only marginally adequate for prosthesis control. They can work well when controlling a single actuator, but their efficacy diminishes when applied to multifunctional powered limbs (two or more powered actuators).

Myoelectric control (below-elbow amputee)

To develop subconscious control, one approach is to use the residual neuromuscular system remaining after amputation. Myoelectric control can do this fairly effectively, at least for below-elbow amputees. Amputees report subconscious control after wearing the prosthesis a few months. By using the finger or wrist flexor muscles to generate a control signal for closing the artificial hand and finger or wrist extensor muscles for the signal to open the hand, it may be controlled in a seminatural way.

Amputees with acquired amputations can often use their phantom limb sensation to help bring about correct muscle contractions to control the hand. Therapists can use this phantom sensation in training the amputee with an acquired amputation but the amputee with a congenital amputation must learn through trial and error procedures.

The electric powered hand prosthesis for

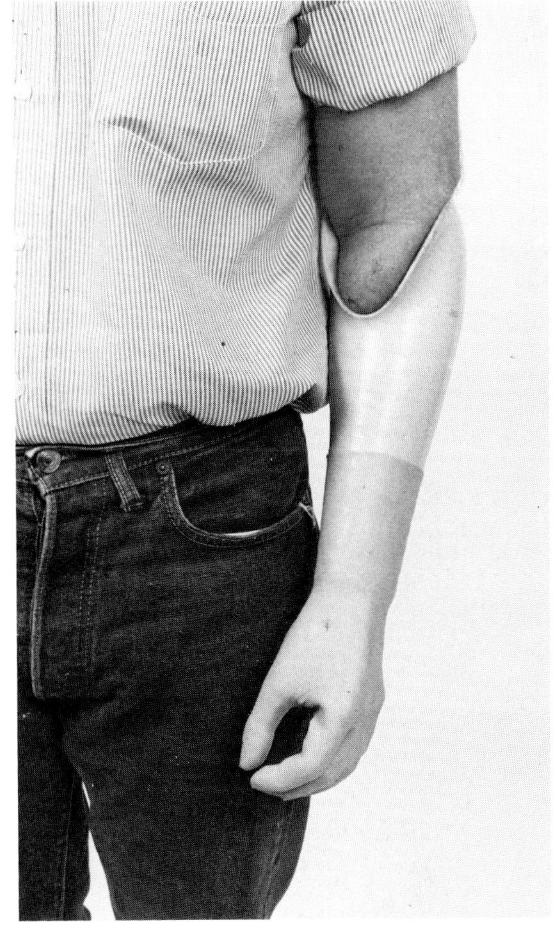

Fig. 9-101. Below-elbow amputee wearing myoelectric below-elbow prosthesis (self-contained and self-suspended).

the below-elbow amputee has been the most widely used in clinical practice. When this unit is properly fitted as a self-suspended and self-contained unit, it is a well-appointed prosthesis (Fig. 9-101).

The below-elbow myoelectric system is particularly well suited for amputees who do light work (e.g., salespersons, students, and persons in business or in professions). It is usually not recommended for someone doing heavy work (e.g., farming, construction), although it might be used as a second prosthesis. It should not be immersed in water and may not be useful for activities such as dishwashing. This powered system requires more care than most body-powered, hook prostheses. The batteries must be charged regularly and care given to the cosmetic glove. An amputee who is attentive to care of the prosthesis can maximize its performance.

Myoelectric control systems take many forms and vary greatly in technical detail, but the most common approach is illustrated in Fig. 9-102. Scott[9] has given a good introductory explanation of the myoelectric control approach.

Good results with powered prostheses, particularly myoelectric prostheses, seem to come about more as the result of good prosthetic fitting and training techniques than from technical considerations. It is recommended that a prosthetist secure special training before fitting powered prostheses and that skills in this area be maintained through the experience of regular involvement with fittings of this nature. Aperiodic involvement is not sufficient. Therefore, because the number of powered protheses fitted is relatively small, it seems appropriate for a few individuals to become highly skilled in fitting these systems, because the prosthetist holds the key to successful clinical results.

Check sockets are required both to obtain an intimate fit and to check electrode positions. The socket must be well fitted, like the PTB socket for the below-knee amputee. (Clear check sockets are particularly useful.) It is important to have the amputee operate the prosthesis from the check socket with the arm in various positions and under load conditions. The below-elbow amputees should be able to operate the system at any angle of elbow flexion (with or without elbow loading) and in any arm position. Electrode contact must be maintained at all positions and under all loads. Electrode position and amplifier gain must be adjusted so that muscle activity other than from the control muscles does not activate the prosthetic hand.

The socket should be comfortable and permit the amputee to use it for lifting heavy objects (e.g., suitcases). Suspension forces can be tolerated over the anterior surface of the forearm and over the triceps tendon. Suspension from the bony prominences such as the medial and lateral epicondyles of the humerus should be avoided. Preflexion of the elbow (20 to 30 degrees) can improve weight-lifting properties at the socket-arm interface.

Billock[1] has developed a supracondylar socket specifically for below-elbow amputees using myoelectric prostheses. Otto Bock Orthopedic Industries, Inc., has also developed appropriate fitting techniques for use with myoelectric systems. The importance of the interface between people and their prostheses cannot be overemphasized. New techniques such as atmospheric pressure suspension need more investigation.

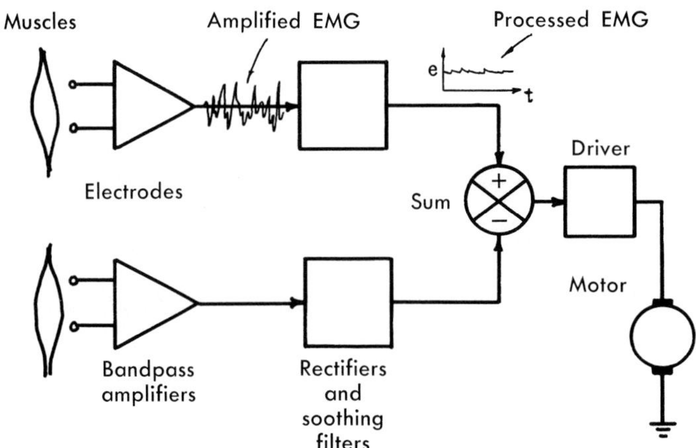

Fig. 9-102. General concept of myoelectric control of single electric actuator from two muscle sites.

Amputees with long to medium residual forearms generally have no trouble operating myoelectric prostheses. Amputees with short to very short forearms may not have enough residual muscle mass remaining to control the prosthesis, and their arms may not be long enough to efficiently support the weight of the prosthesis (approximately 0.9 kg; 2 pounds). Also, with a short limb it sometimes is difficult to place the electrodes and still have room for socket relief areas around bony prominences.

Adequate muscle mass can be tested by palpation and myoelectric signal testers. The myoelectric system itself can also be used as an evaluation system of myoelectric activity.

Myoelectric control (above-elbow amputee)

Two approaches to myoelectric control for the above-elbow amputee are now used. Both require the presence of a myoelectric signal from the biceps brachii and triceps brachii. Both are hybrid-powered prostheses because they use body power and external power (electricity) in the same prosthesis.

In the first case, the myoelectric signal from the biceps is used to control flexion of a powered elbow, and the triceps signal controls elbow extension. A conventional harness and cable are used to control a body-powered terminal device. This technique is used with the Boston arm and with a limb being developed at the University of Utah. It is an approach with merit, permitting simultaneous control of two functions in a somewhat subconscious way.

The second approach is the converse of the first. A body-powered elbow and harness are used in conjunction with an electrically powered hand, which is controlled by myoelectric signals from the biceps and triceps. (The biceps signal closes the hand, and the triceps signal opens it.) This approach seems incorrect at first thought; however, several advantages make it a practical approach: (1) the same commercial systems available for below-elbow amputees may be used for

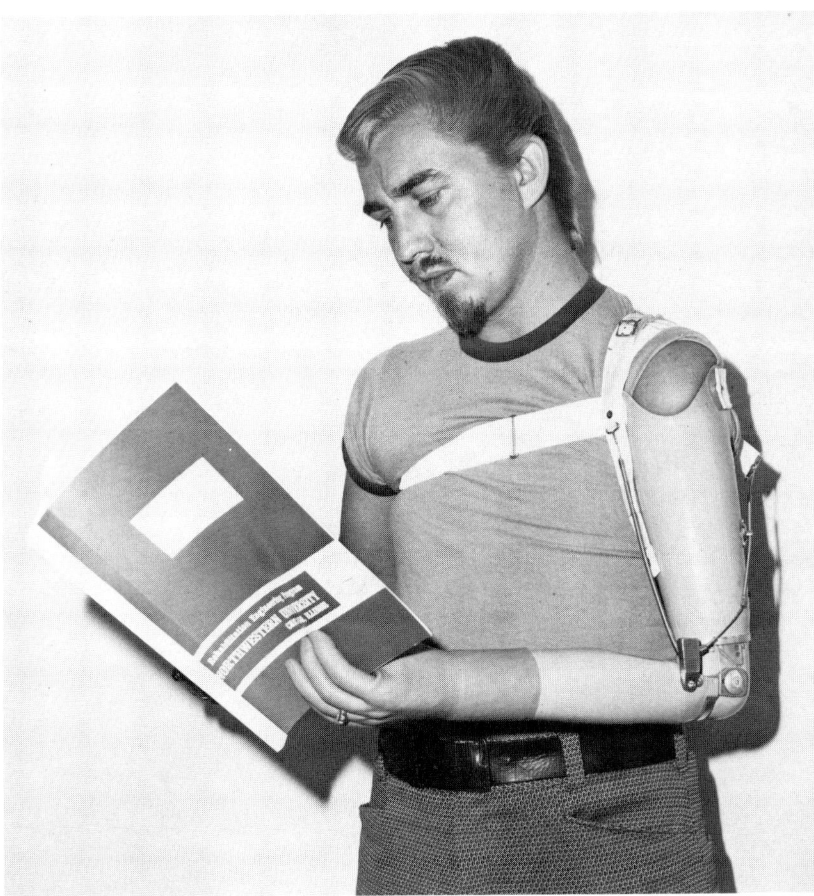

Fig. 9-103. Above-elbow amputee wearing hybrid prosthesis. Elbow is body powered through cable and harness, whereas electric hand is controlled by myoelectric signals from biceps and triceps.

above-elbow amputees, (2) the body-powered elbow is quiet and fast, (3) the arm is cosmetically pleasing, and (4) the control is surprisingly somewhat natural. This approach has been used extensively in several European countries over the past 10 years with good success and similar results have been obtained with limited fittings in North America. Fig. 9-103 shows this approach in conjunction with a thoracic suspension harness.

HIGHER LEVEL AMPUTATIONS

Although powered prostheses should have their greatest value for people with shoulder disarticulation or intrascapulothoracic amputations, this promise has not yet been fulfilled. One reason is that a firm theoretical base for prosthetics design has not yet developed. Consequently, design remains on an empirical basis. Nevertheless, several theories are now extant, and there is continued hope that the promise of external power for the high-level upper limb amputee will ultimately be a reality.

One of the problems limiting development of powered limbs for the high-level amputee is cost. Indeed, high costs are a factor inhibiting clinical use of external power at all amputation levels. Multifunctional powered prostheses are particularly costly and require an effective service and maintenance organization for their support. However, if powered limbs can be designed that are obviously superior to existing prostheses, then the problem of cost will subside.

SUMMARY

Powered artificial limbs are now having an impact in the field of prosthetics at the clinical level. These prostheses are not a panacea. They remain primitive but are still useful when applied in the right way, under proper circumstances. They should complement body-powered prostheses, offering another option for better service of the upper limb amputee.

REFERENCES

Socket designs

1. Bechtol, C. O.: Anatomical and physiological considerations in the clinical application of upper-extremity prosthetics, Chapter 8. In Orthopedic appliances atlas, vol. 2, Artificial limbs, Ann Arbor, Mich., 1960, J. W. Edwards.
2. Biomechanics of below-knee prostheses, Chapter 8. In Lower-limb prosthetics, New York, 1975 revision, New York University, Post-Graduate Medical School, Prosthetics and Orthotics.
3. Epps, C. H. Jr., and Hile, J. H.: Experience with the Muenster-type below-elbow prosthesis: a preliminary report, Artif. Limbs **12**(1):20-24, Spring, 1968.
4. Hepp, O., and Kuhn, G. G.: Upper extremity prostheses. In Prosthetics International, Copenhagen, 1960, Committee on Prostheses, Braces and Technical Aids, International Society for the Welfare of Cripples.
5. Marquardt, E., and Neff, G.: The angulation osteotomy of above-elbow stumps, Clin. Orthop. **104**:232-238, Oct., 1974.
6. Staros, A., and Pirrello, T.: The construction and fitting of Upper-extremity prostheses, Chapter 3. In Orthopedic appliances atlas, vol. 2, Artificial limbs, Ann Arbor, Mich., 1960, J. W. Edwards.
7. Taylor, C. L.: The biomechanics of the normal and of the amputated upper extremity, Chapter 7. In Klopsteg, P. E., and Wilson, P. D., editors: Human limbs and their substitutes, New York, 1954, McGraw-Hill Book Co., Inc.
8. The "Muenster-type" fabrication technique for below-elbow prostheses, New York, June; 1964, New York University, College of Engineering, Research Division, Adult Prosthetic Studies.
9. Upper-extremity prosthetics, Evanston, Ill., Northwestern University Medical School, Prosthetic-Orthotic Education.
10. Upper-limb prosthetics, New York, 1971 revision, New York University, Post-Graduate Medical School, Prosthetics and Orthotics.

External power in upper limb prosthetics

1. Billock, J. N.: The Northwestern University supracondylar suspension technique for below-elbow amputations, Orthot. Prosthet., pp. 16-23, Dec., 1972.
2. Bottomley, A., Kinnier Wilson, A. B., and Nightingale, A.: Muscle substitutes and myo-electric control, J. Br. IRE **26:** 439, 1963.
3. Carlson, L. E., and Radcliffe, C. W.: A multi-mode approach to coordinated prosthesis control, Adv. Ext. Control Human Extremities, 1973, pp. 185-196. (Proceedings of the Fourth International Symposium, Dubrovnik, Yugoslavia, 1972.)
4. Childress, D. S.: Powered limb prostheses: their clinical significance, IEEE Trans. Biomed. **20**(3):200-207, 1973.
5. Harris, S. J.: Chicago Sun-Times, March, 1978.
6. Herberts, P., Almström, C., Kadefors, R., and Lawrence, P.: Hand prosthesis control via myoelectric patterns, Acta. Orthop. Scand. **44**:389-409, 1973.
7. Reiter, R.: Eine neue electrokunsthand, Grenzgebiete der Medizin **4**:133, 1948.
8. Schmidl, H.: The INAIL experience fitting upper-limb dysmelia patients with myoelectric control, Bull. Prosthet. Res. **10**(27):17-42, Spring, 1977.
9. Scott, R. N.: Myo-electro control, Science J., March, 1966.
10. Simpson, D. C.: The choice of control system for the multimovement prosthesis: proprioception (e.p.p.). In Herberts, P. et al., editors: The control of upper-extremity prostheses and orthoses, Springfield, Ill., 1974, Charles C Thomas, Publisher.
11. Sörbye, R.: Myoelectric controlled hand prostheses in children, Int. J. Rehab. Res. **1**:15-25, 1977.
12. Wiener, N.: Cybernetics (Introduction), MIT Press, 1948.
13. Wilson, A. B., Jr.: Externally powered upper-limb prostheses, Newsletter, Prosthet. Orthot, Clin. **2**(1):1-4, 1978.

CHAPTER 10

Partial hand amputation

SIDNEY J. BLAIR
STEPHEN KRAMER

HAND FUNCTION

Since it is the objective of hand amputation surgery to preserve and restore function, it is important for the surgeon who undertakes this task to understand hand function. Hand function includes four separate but interrelated ideas: (1) individual digit function, (2) the effect of the loss of each amputated segment on the hand, (3) the functional requirements an individual places on the hands, regarding appearance and occupation, and (4) the integrated use of the hand elements.

Functions and movements of the hand can be divided into two main headings: nonprehensile functions and prehensile functions.[15] In nonprehensile functions, the hand is used to push, lift, hold, hook, and scoop objects. Other nonprehensile movements include percussive motions of the fingers as in piano playing and typing.

Prehensile movements and activities are those in which an object is seized and held partly or wholly within the compass of the hand.[15] All of the prehensile activities of the hand can be described in terms of the precision grip, power grip, or a combination of both.

In the precision grip, the object is held between the flexor aspect of the fingers and opposing thumb. Frequently this is accomplished with motion occurring only in the metacarpophalangeal joints. Precision grip can be divided into three types of pinch.

Pulp-to-pulp pinch can be either single or multiple and is the most common type used in daily activity. In single pulp-to-pulp pinch the pad of the thumb opposes the pad of a single finger, as when picking up a piece of paper. In multiple pinch, the pad of the thumb opposes the pad of two or more fingers as when picking up small objects. Another variation of the multiple pinch is the three-chuck action pinch in which the thumb holds the object against the side of the middle finger and the pad of the index finger.

In *key, or lateral, pinch* the pad of the thumb holds the object against the index finger. The most common example is holding a key or a coffee cup. The third type is *tip-to-tip,* or *fingernail, pinch,* which is used mainly to grasp small objects.

In power grip, a clamping force is produced in which the flexed fingers act against counterpressure from the palm or thenar eminence, and distal segment of the thumb. Objects that are small in diameter can be grasped very tightly, since wrapping the thumb around the flexed fingers will increase the power of the grip.

Besides the grips described, the fingers can be used in free movements such as flicking, brushing, buttoning and unbuttoning, typing, and playing various musical instruments. These activities depend on the interaction of movements and stability at the metacarpophalangeal and interphalangeal joints. When immobilization of any joint is necessary, the position of immobilization is important. For example, a hook grip is the only grip possible when the metacarpophalangeal joints are stiff and the interphalangeal joints are mobile. In contrast, the hand with mobile metacarpophalangeal joints and stiff interphalangeal joints has more combinations of function possible.

The key to muscle action is sensory feedback. Various motor actions are guided by the intrinsic sensation of position, tension, motion, and touch. In addition, the hand is also a vital source of information as to the character and quality of objects. The term "tactile gnosis" has been coined by Moberg[13] to describe the quality of sensation that makes a precision sensory grip possible without the help of sight. When this function is impaired, actions cannot be performed as rapidly or skillfully.

THE THUMB

Since the thumb forms one of the two essential poles both for power and precision grip, it becomes the most important single digit of the hand. The loss of the thumb constitutes a 40% functional loss of the hand.

Four major requirements of a functioning thumb are sensibility, length, opposability, and stability.[18] The goal in sensibility is to obtain fine two-point discrimination and stereognosis. All flap procedures should be designed to achieve that end. Unfortunately, at times, one has to settle for protective sensibility. With the thumb adducted, the ideal length should reach the middle portion of the proximal phalanx of the index finger. Less length decreases opposability proportionally. Stability of the joints by ligaments and muscle control is important when the thumb is in action. For this reason careful attention to ligament reconstruction and muscle reattachment is necessary. The thumb must be capable of being placed in a position to meet the remaining fingers of the hand. This depends on a supple web space, in addition to a supple and stable first carpometacarpal joint.[18]

In reconstruction of the thumb the length of the remaining stump determines the type of treatment to be given. Amputations distal to the midportion of the proximal phalanx are somewhat similar to finger amputations. However, since length is so important, bone should not be sacrificed for skin coverage. Therefore local skin mobilization, transpositions, and distant flaps are done much more frequently on the thumb. Amputations at the proximal portion of the proximal phalanx can be functionally lengthened by deepening the web space. The critical functional length of thumb amputations, however, is at the metacarpophalangeal joint. Various procedures are available to restore length and thumb function to these most serious amputations.

Amputation through the distal phalange

Loss of the tip of the thumb, which cannot be closed primarily without shortening the bone, will require a split-thickness graft. When more than the tip is lost, various types of flaps are necessary to provide sensation and coverage of the tip. These can be provided by the lateral V-Y flap[8] or the volar V-Y flap,[1] which will be described in the discussion on fingertip amputations.

If additional coverage beyond the capability of the V-Y flaps is needed, more sophisticated techniques are employed. Many surgeons refer patients needing these procedures to specialists rather than attempt the surgery themselves. Three techniques are outlined: advancement pedicle flap, cross-finger flap, and neurovascular island transfer. Each of these can also be used for secondary resurfacing of scarred, tender tips.

Advancement pedicle flap for thumb injuries.[16] Under tourniquet control, midaxial incisions are made on the radial and ulnar aspects of the thumb. The volar skin with its subcutaneous tissue and both neurovascular bundles is elevated without disturbing the underlying tendon or its sheath. Flexion of the interphalangeal joint will usually allow the flap to be mobilized up to 2 cm if it is elevated to the proximal crease of the thumb. Both the interphalangeal and metacarpophalangeal joints are immobilized in 30 or 40 degrees of flexion for 3 weeks. Several months are required for motion to be regained.

Posner and Smith[16] indicated that the advancement pedicle flap could be used on the finger, but that the dorsal skin of the finger depends more on volar venous drainage than the thumb. If this technique is to be used in the finger, the flaps should not be raised proximal to the proximal interphalangeal joint.

Cross-finger flap. The cross-finger flap[3] differs from the advancement pedicle flap in that it is taken from another finger, usually the long finger. In this technique, the pattern of the defect is fashioned from gauze or paper, and the proposed flap is placed over the thumb and against the long finger. This will help to determine where the flaps should be placed and the pattern can be outlined with a skin marker. The flap is dissected in the areolar plane, over the extensor tendon, preserving the veins. A split-thickness graft is used to close the donor site.

Neurovascular island transfer. The neuro-

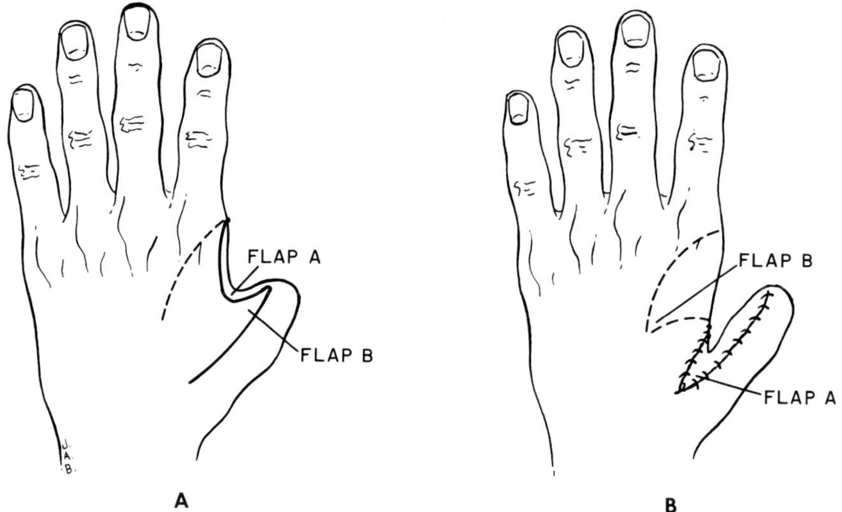

Fig. 10-1. Deepening of web space by means of Z-plasty. Flaps are outlined in **A** and then transposed in **B**.

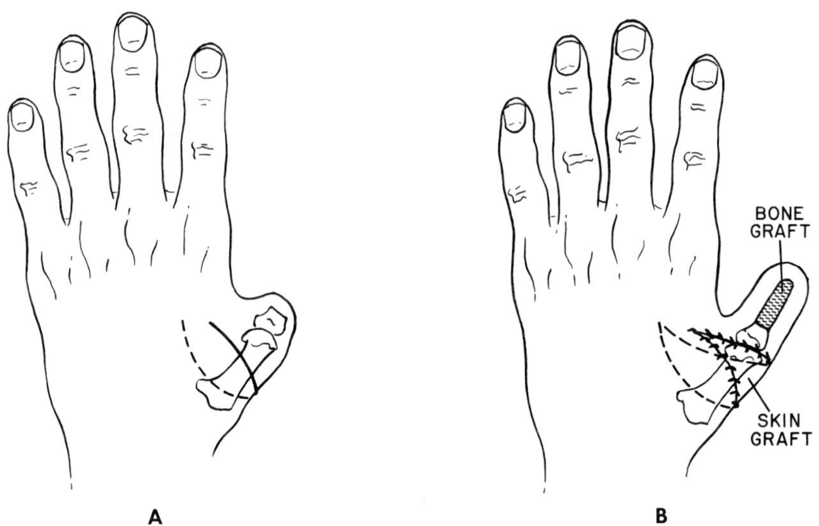

Fig. 10-2. Gillies-Millard procedure allows lengthening of residual thumb by means of bone graft and raised flap. **A**, Level of incision for flap. **B**, Completed flaw with inserted graft and skin graft to defect.

vascular island transfer[9] is a reconstructive technique in which a composite graft of neurovascular pedicle is dissected from the ulnar side of the long or ring finger and transferred across the palm to the volar aspect of the thumb. This technique is infrequently done at present.

Amputation between the midproximal phalange and middistal phalange

As the level of amputation opposes the metacarpophalangeal joint of the index finger, a deepening of the web space by Z-plasty (Fig. 10-1) is recommended.[18] Essentially the two flaps are created in the dorsal and volar aspects of the hand. The apex of flap A is at the index finger, and the other is on the thumb. The midpoint of the thenar crease is the site of the beginning incision, which follows the course to the index finger. By following the height of the skin fold of the web space, the incision is carried to the dorsal ulnar aspect of the thumb. This is the apex of the dorsal flap. The flaps are mobilized, and the dorsal flap wraps around the base of the index finger, while the volar flap wraps around the base of the thumb. The scar in the web space will be in an anteroposterior direction. Sometimes it will be necessary to release the fascia in the first web space and the adductor pollicis, so that the indention may be brought more proximal.

Amputation at the metacarpophalangeal joint

When the level of amputation is at the metacarpophalangeal joint, it is necessary to increase the length of the thumb and to provide adequate skin coverage (Fig. 10-2). Three methods are available to achieve this.

Gillies and Millard[6] describe a procedure in which a horseshoe flap of skin and subcutaneous tissue is made on the dorsum of the first metacarpal. A bone graft is inserted into the amputation stump, and the flap is positioned to cover the graft. The indication for this procedure is the presence of good adjacent tissues.

Matev[10] describes a technique for lengthening the thumb when the skin of the metacarpal is poor. In this procedure flaps are raised and rotated, and the donor areas are covered with split-thickness skin grafts. In addition, Matev[10] has also described a technique of lengthening the metacarpal by osteotomy of the shaft and distraction by means of crossed Kirschner wires. The lengthening is carried out for 1 month. A good mobile skin cover in a young person is a necessary requisite for any lengthening procedure. A lengthening procedure by means of a tube flap and bone graft can be performed. Recently, McGregor[11] described a groin flap that could be made into a tube and a bone graft inserted. Disadvantages of these procedures are the instability of the skin over the bone and absorption of the graft.

FINGERS

Fingertip amputation

Fingertip amputations are defined as those amputations of the terminal phalanx distal to the insertions of the flexor and extensor tendons. These constitute the most common partial hand amputation.

For transverse lacerations in which there are no flaps, the treatment depends on the age of the patient. The bone in children can be trimmed to 1 mm below the skin and allowed to epithelize. It will heal rapidly with few problems.

In adults with larger transverse defects, sensation takes precedence over length. Generally, bone should not be retained to be covered by various plastic procedures, but should be trimmed slightly below the soft tissue level and then covered with a thin split-thickness graft taken from the inner side of the forearm. (Some surgeons take these grafts from the side of the same finger.) This technique can be done in about 90% of the adult fingertip injuries. The skin will contract to a narrow area and bring normal innervated non-hypersensitive skin over the tip.[12]

Traumatic amputation through the proximal or middle phalanges

When resurfacing is needed over exposed tendon, joint, or bone, skin with subcutaneous tissue and blood supply through the base of the flap is used. The dissection plane is through the areolar tissue overlying the tendons with the veins included in the flap. The skin flaps have the same thickness throughout as compared to flaps in other parts, which are thinner at the tips and thicker at the base. The type of flap used is dictated by the direction of the amputation and the digit involved.

With perpendicular or transverse transections, triangular flaps from the side can be used.[8] Using digital block anesthesia, and using a red rubber catheter as a tourniquet, two triangular flaps measuring 3 to 4 mm in height are developed. They are centered in the midlateral line on each side of the finger with the apices directed proximally. The incision through the skin and pulp should be deep enough to free the flap for mobilization. Not more than 50% of the thickness of the proximal part of the pulp need be severed. The base of the flaps are sutured with 5-0 nylon and the dorsal margins are sutured to the nail. The remaining fishmouth gaps can be closed with interrupted nylon sutures.

The second technique, which is preferred, is the triangle flap from the volar surface described by Atasoy and Kleinert.[1] The flap's base, which is the amputation skin edge, should be the same width as the amputated edge of the nail matrix. The apex of the triangle can extend to the distal flexion crease. The flap is developed by cutting through the skin and separating the subcutaneous tissue from the periosteum and flexor tendon sheath. The stump is debrided, and the bone ends are smoothed. The flap is advanced and sutured to the nail bed with 6-0 nylon.

Volar oblique amputation requires more extensive resurfacing. When these occur on the index finger they are best managed with a volar advancement flap. The incisions are made in the midlateral line, and the soft tissues with the neurovascular bundle intact are elevated with

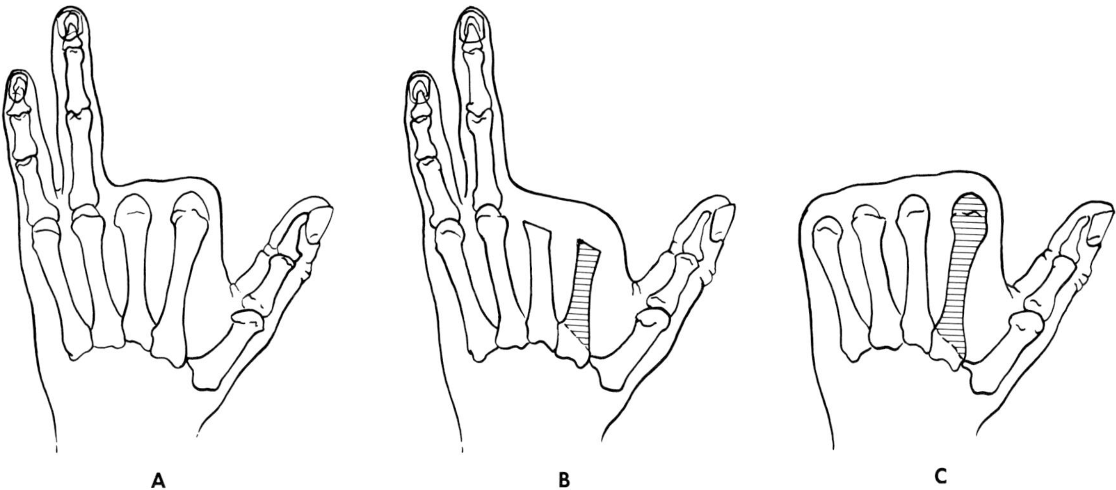

Fig. 10-3. A, Problem 1. **B,** Problem 2. **C,** Problem 3. (See text.)

the neurovascular bundle. A 5-mm back cut can be made to allow advancement. Sometimes a complete transverse cut will have to be made to obtain further advancement. It may be necessary to flex the distal interphalangeal joint to advance the flap, 1.5 to 2 cm. A split-thickness graft can be placed over the base of the finger.

Oblique defects of the long, ring, and little fingers can be covered with cross-finger flaps. This type of flap provides good coverage that will allow return of some protective sensibility. This flap is usually taken from the dorsal aspect of the middle phalanx. The flaps should be elevated from midlateral line to midlateral line with the bases on the side adjacent to the injured digit. The flap should be elevated in the areolar tissue plane overlying the extensor tendons. The donor pedicle site is covered with a split-thickness skin graft. The pedicle is left in place for 3 weeks.

Traumatic multiple digit amputation

When treating a hand with multiple digit amputations, all efforts are directed to salvaging the basic functional unit of the hand.[4] This has been defined as a hand that has a stable wrist, a radial digit with good sensation, and mobility in at least one or two fingers on the ulnar aspect of the hand. In addition, the radial and ulnar digits should be separated by a cleft deep enough to allow useful prehensile movements. The general objectives in attempting to salvage and restore the basic hand include the following:

1. Preservation of length of the surviving fingers
2. Salvage of remnants of the fingers and their remaining portions
3. Restoration of normal sensation
4. Provision of adequate skin coverage and an adequate cleft between the remaining fingers
5. Restoration of sufficient number of movable parts to execute power and precision grips
6. Ability to approximate the polar elements

Multiple traumatic amputations can leave a wide variety of residual hand deformities. The reconstruction requires ingenuity and resourcefulness. Following is a list of more common residual hands and a proposed solution, all of which are better than any prosthesis.

Problem 1: Amputated index and middle finger with a normal thumb and little and ring fingers (Fig. 10-3, *A*).[18]

SOLUTION: There is no cleft problem. Stability for grasp is fair.

Problem 2: Amputated central digits at level of metacarpal shafts with a normal thumb and ulnar digits (Fig. 10-3, *B*).

SOLUTION: The projecting second metacarpal is excised by a zigzag incision that does not cause a web-space contracture.

Problem 3: Amputation of all the digits at the level of the metacarpophalangeal joint with the thumb intact (Fig. 10-3, *C*).

SOLUTION: Deepen the cleft in the web space at the first and second metacarpals.

Problem 4: Intact thumb with a second metacarpal midshaft amputation, and the third, fourth, and fifth metacarpal heads intact (Fig. 10-4, *A*).

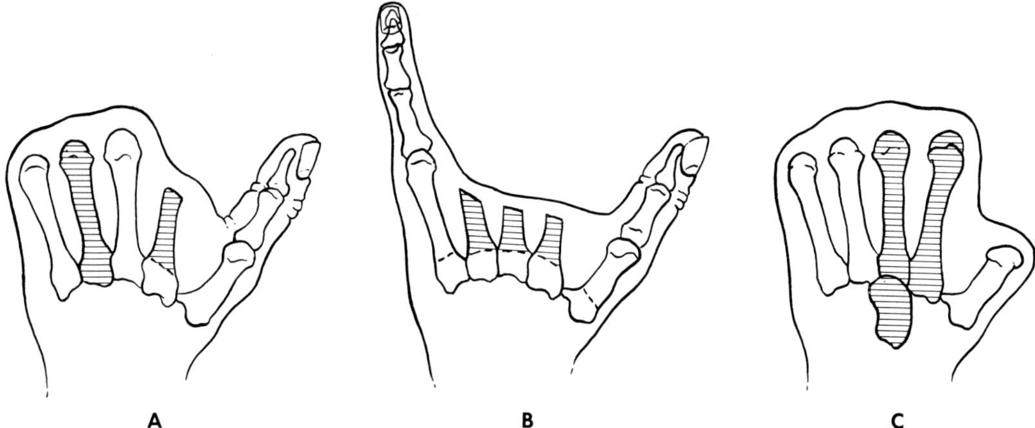

Fig. 10-4. A. Problem 4. **B**, Problem 5. **C**, Problem 6. Scheduled portions are to be resected. (See text.)

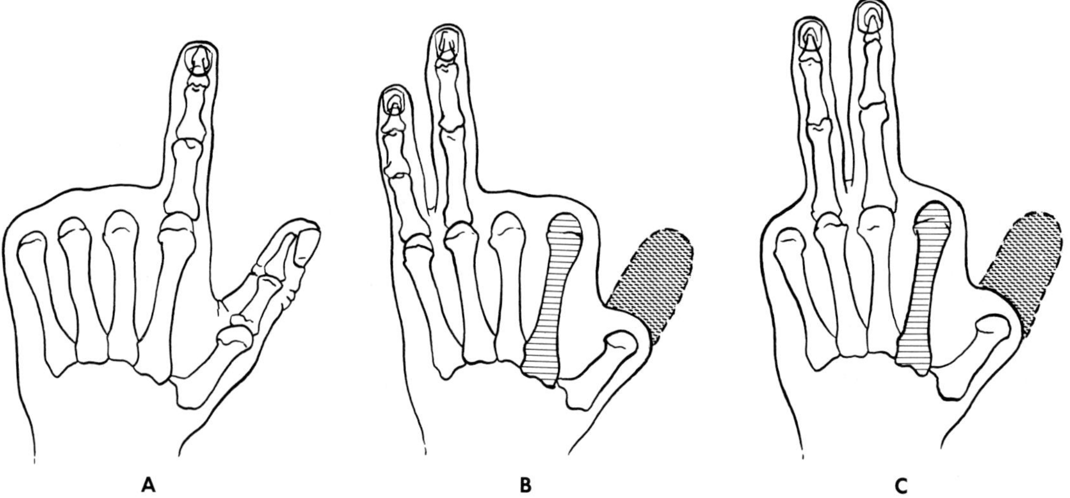

Fig. 10-5. A, Problem 7. **B,** Problem 8. **C,** Problem 9. Cross-hatched areas represent elongation of thumb by various procedures. (See text.)

SOLUTION: Clear the web space, resect the metacarpal heads, and perform a pollicization of the fourth and fifth metacarpals. It may be necessary to resect the fourth metacarpal and phalangize the fifth metacarpal.

Problem 5: Thumb and little fingers intact; all others have been amputated at the shaft or bases (Fig. 10-4, *B*).

SOLUTION: Clear the web space, perform an osteotomy on the thumb and little finger, and provide for motor power.

Problem 6: All fingers and thumbs are amputated; joints form mitten hands (Fig. 10-4, *C*).

SOLUTION: Create a two-digit hand by resecting the second and third metacarpals and capitate bone. Motor power must be furnished. A second solution is to create a three-digit hand by resecting the second and fourth metacarpals.

Problem 7: Intact thumb and index finger with amputated middle, ring, and little fingers (Fig. 10-5, *A*).

SOLUTION: If the level is at or distal to the metacarpophalangeal joint, preserve all length. The distal ends of the metacarpal shafts should be padded well.

Problem 8: Intact ring and little fingers with amputated thumb, index, and middle fingers at the metacarpophalangeal joint (Fig. 10-5, *B*).

SOLUTION: Create a cleft between the thumb and metacarpals. Create mobility and disarticulate the second metacarpal bone with a modified z-plasty. Lengthen the thumb using various elongation procedures.

Problem 9: Middle and ring fingers remain, but the thumb, index, and little fingers are amputated (Fig. 10-5, *C*).

SOLUTION: Provide grasping surface by removing the second metacarpal and performing a Z-plasty between the stumps and remaining fingers. This can be accomplished through à posterior shift of the third and fourth metacarpals at their carpometacarpal articulations and arthrodesis.

Elective amputation of a finger

The goal in elective amputation of a finger is a smooth, pain-free, nontender, mobile stump covered with mobile skin. Incisions should be planned so that the scar will not cross flexure lines at the right angles. Volar flaps should be tongue shaped rather than semicircular and approximately twice the length of the dorsal flap. The dorsal flap may be cut with the finger in flexion and the palmar flap in extension.

The bone should be cut cleanly without leaving spikes or splintering. It should be divided 3 or 4 mm proximal to the soft tissues, allowing approximation of the flaps without tension. In children, disarticulation is recommended. The protuberance of the condyles, both anteriorly and laterally, must be removed in order to prevent a bulky stump. Usually articular cartilage is removed to allow fixation of the soft tissues to the stump ends. However, Harris[7] has indicated that removal of cartilage was not necessary and not advisable.

The nerves should be gently exposed by spreading the tissues with an instrument and then transecting them with a sharp knife about 0.5 cm from the tip. No traction should be applied to the nerve, and no ligature should be used.

Tendons are severed by simple transverse section, and retraction will occur. Because fixation of a tendon to the stump can cause considerable interference with function, the tendons must be sutured to each other or to the end of the stump. Since there are attachments of the intrinsic muscle to the proximal phalanges, these phalanges will move satisfactorily. The tourniquet is released prior to closure, and the remainder of the bleeding is controlled. Final closure is by means of carefully placed 5-0 or 6-0 nylon sutures. All patients are treated with volar splints postoperatively to minimize plain and edema. Circular dressings are not placed about the stumps.

Complications of amputations

Complications of amputations[17] include the unhealed, painful, or tender stump, reduction in the function of the hand, or an unsightly stump. Frequently a discharging sinus will be present at the end of the stump. This is either due to a foreign body or to a free avascular piece of bone acting as a sequestrum. Removal of separated fragments and foreign bodies will usually allow healing. With persistent ulceration of the stump, reamputation is best for the single amputation of the middle, ring, and little fingers. When the thumb or index fingers are involved or with multiple amputations, coverage by local flaps or finger flaps should be considered.

Painful stumps are usually due to neuroma formation or a reflex sympathetic dystrophy. Pain in amputation stumps may be due to defects in healing or failure to provide adequate soft tissue coverage for nerves. Other causes of painful stumps include retention of nail bed remnants, inclusion cysts, retained foreign bodies, and cartilage under the terminal scar. A well-padded stump devoid of scars is the goal.

Some amputations cause functional impairment. When an index finger is shortened beyond the point the thumb can oppose, it will stick out and be exposed to injury. A rigid extended index or middle finger that cannot oppose the thumb will interfere with function. This also occurs in fingers that are overflexed and overangulated.

Perception of a stump as unsightly is influenced by occupation, age, and social status. For women who have had their index finger or little finger amputated through the metacarpophalangeal joint, the appearance of the stump may be improved by excising the remaining metacarpal. The gap left by total loss of the ring finger may be improved by removing the fourth metacarpal. A shift of the second metacarpal to improve the appearance of an amputated middle finger is occasionally indicated.

TRANSMETACARPAL AND RAY AMPUTATION

The technique of index metacarpal amputation is as follows: an asymmetrical dorsal racket-shaped incision is made. This incision, which parallels the ulnar border of the index metacarpal, swings about the metacarpal head, follows the proximal crease of the fingers, and then continues dorsally to meet the dorsal incision. The subcutaneous tissue is preserved with the flaps. The extensor tendons are sectioned in the proximal portion of the wound. The interossei are separated from the shaft of the metacarpal. The nerves are sectioned 2 cm distal to the incision and transferred beneath the interosseous muscle. Mobilization of the digital nerves proximal to the incision should be avoided. The periosteum of the metacarpal is incised and osteotomy is performed at the junction of the proximal and middle third. The bevel of the osteotomy is dorsal and radial (Fig. 10-6). The flexor tendons are dissected

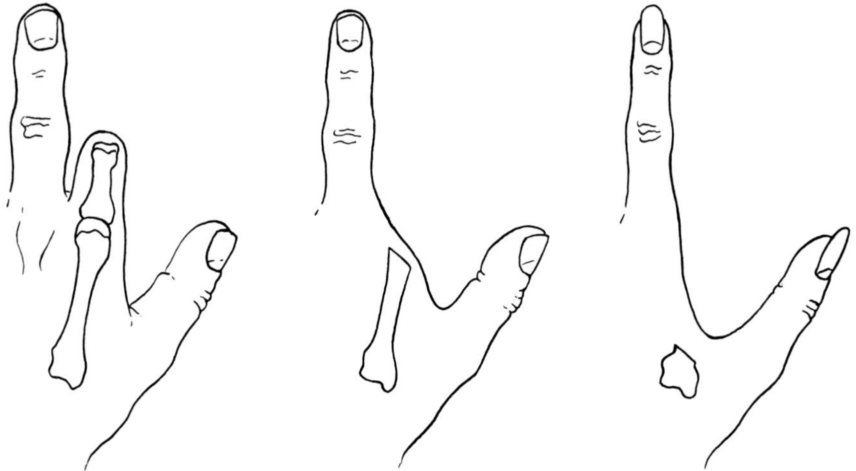

Fig. 10-6. Preamputation is contrasted with two levels of amputation. If second metacarpal is too long, web space is compromised. Proper level is shown on right.

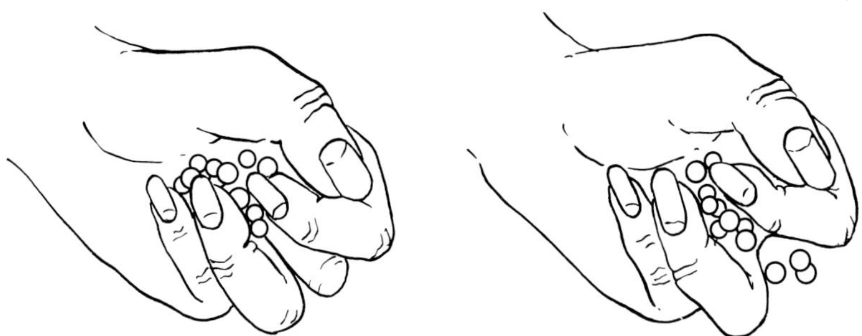

Fig. 10-7. Loss of long finger allows small objects to fall out of hand.

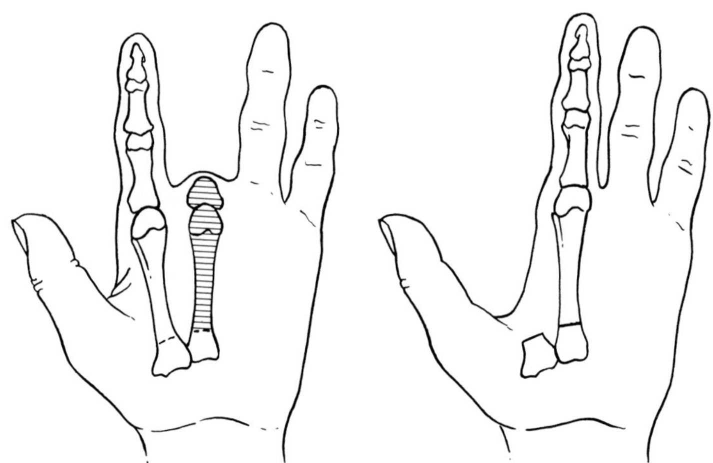

Fig. 10-8. Procedure combines ablation of third metacarpal with transposition of index ray.

from the flap by transecting the transverse metacarpal ligament. The tendon of the dorsal interosseous is sutured to the tissue at the base of the long finger but not into the second dorsal interosseous muscle. After hemostasis has been obtained, the wound is closed with 5-0 nylon. A drain may be used proximally and removed in 24 hours.

The long, or middle, finger

The long, or middle, finger is the most powerful finger and because of this it is considered to be functionally 20% of the hand. Besides reinforcing the index finger in key pinch, it provides strength and stability for the power grip. As with the other fingers, the more proximal the amputation, the more severe the impairment. When the amputation occurs at the proximal portion of the proximal phalanx or at the metacarpophalangeal joint, small objects will fall out of the hand when the fingers are brought together (Fig. 10-7).

Strength is lost in key pinch because of the lack of support, which allows the index finger to bend ulnarward. Since the second metacarpal forms part of the rigid skeleton and will not move to collapse the space, ablation of the third metacarpal will not solve the problem. Therefore when the long finger is damaged to the extent that amputation must occur at a site proximal to the distal quarter of the proximal phalanx, the function of the finger, and also the entire hand, is disturbed.

Therefore Carroll[2] has recommended a procedure of transposing the index finger onto the base of the third metacarpal (Fig. 10-8). Essentially the third metacarpal is revised, and through the same incision the second metacarpal is exposed and transposed to the base of the third metacarpal. The incision used for elective amputation of the third metacarpal when no transposition occurs begins at the base. It then continues distally on the dorsum to the head and swings to the side of the finger at the web space, where it crosses the volar aspect of the finger at the level of the proximal flexor crease, and then goes through the opposite web space to join the dorsal incision.

The extensor tendon is transected at the proximal margin of the wound. The periosteum is incised, and the third metacarpal is osteotomized at the base, avoiding the insertion of the extensor carpi radialis brevis. The shaft is then dissected distally. The transverse metacarpal ligaments are transected, and the neurovascular bundles are identified. The arteries are ligated and the nerves are left long so that they can be brought dorsally into interosseous space. The flexor tendons are transected and allowed to retract. The periosteal sleeve is sutured and the wound is closed with interrupted 5-0 nylon sutures.

The ring finger

The ring finger also fills in the span and with the little finger provides the arch with mobility. The finger functionally represents 10% of the hand. Proximal amputation of the proximal interphalangeal joint may be an indication for subperi-

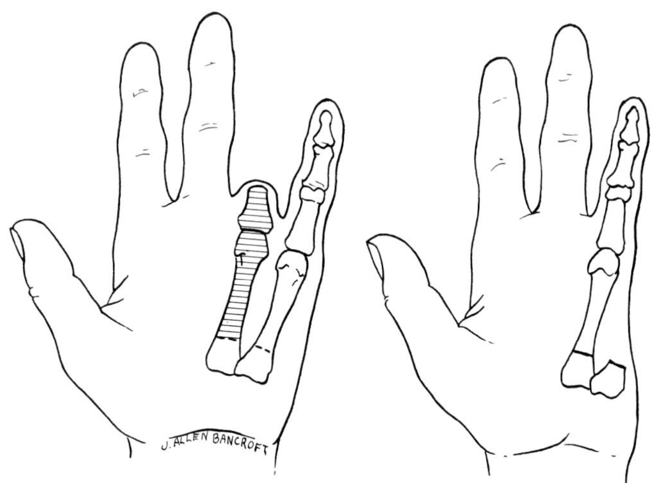

Fig. 10-9. Two approaches to partial amputation of fourth ray. Metacarpal may be amputated as primary procedure (left) or combined with transposition of fifth ray.

osteal resection of the ray down to the metacarpal base.

Injury to this finger is common because when a ring gets caught the entire weight of the body is transmitted through the ring to the digit, resulting in avulsion of the tissues. There are various degrees of injury. Those categorized as class I are crush injuries with minimal trauma to the neurovascular structures. Class II injuries are those with extensive lacerations, but with the neurovascular bundles intact. Crushing avulsions with laceration of the neurovascular bundles make up class III injuries. Class IV injuries are similar to class III but with bone and joint destruction. Classes I and II have a good prognosis, whereas the other two will require immediate intrapalmar amputation.[2]

Some believe that the fourth metacarpal is necessary to preserve the broad palm for power grip. However, Carroll[2] believes that it is not necessary to preserve the metacarpal in ring injuries in which extensive damage has been done to that finger. He also believes that the procedure of transferring a normal fifth finger to replace the ring finger for cosmetic purposes is unnecessary and hazardous and recommends intrapalmar amputation of the fourth ray (Fig. 10-9).

The little finger

Because of the ulnar position, the little finger lends breadth and stability to the grasp. It also provides the palm with mobility. A good share of the stability of the palm in grasp is afforded by the fifth metacarpal, and it is the key of the medial locking in the power grip. The little finger is considered to be by some an unimportant finger; however, Flatt[5] and many other surgeons consider this to be a very important finger, and its preservation is of great importance. Again, length is important, and maintaining as much length as possible beyond the proximal interphalangeal joint is indicated. When amputation occurs proximal to the proximal interphalangeal joint, some patients find the stump useful, but for many it is useless and unsightly and may catch in a pocket.

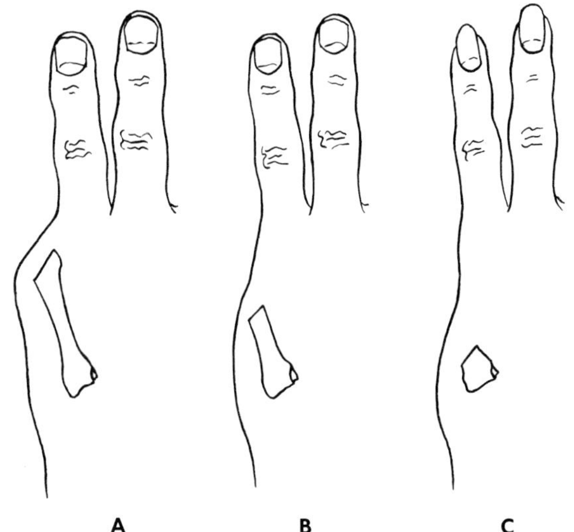

Fig. 10-10. Levels of amputation of fifth ray. Long residual segment (**A**) provides maximum width of hand and power grip. Cosmesis is improved with more proximal osteotomy and beveling (**B**). If prominence from residual metacarpal is undesirable, osteotomy may be at base (**C**).

When it becomes necessary to reamputate at a more proximal level, the sex and occupation of the patient must be considered. In laborers, reamputation should be carried out by disarticulation at the metacarpophalangeal joint so that the maximum width of the hand is maintained for power grip. A bony prominence will remain over the metacarpal head, which may be corrected by beveling the lateral posterior aspect of the metacarpal head. It has been found that in disarticulations removal of the cartilage is not necessary and tends to give a less painful amputation stump. The profundus tendon at resting length can be sutured to the metacarpal head to provide increased mobility.

Amputations through the midportion of the metacarpal are carried out when cosmesis is more important than power grip (Fig. 10-10, *A*). In this case amputation is done through a dorsal incision on the radial aspect of the fifth metacarpal and loops around the stump. The amputation should be carried out at the proximal half of the metacarpal and the bone beveled to give a smooth surface (Fig. 10-10, *B*). If this cannot be accomplished, amputation can be carried out near the base of the metacarpal (Fig. 10-10, *C*).

The technique for fifth-ray resection of the metacarpal is begun with a dorsal racket incision. The incision begins at the proximal portion of the fifth metacarpal on the radial side. It then proceeds distally and rings the base of the little finger at the proximal crease. Dissection of the dorsal branches of the ulnar nerve is performed to avoid an area of anesthesia over the residual peripheral ulnar side of the hand.

The periosteum of the fifth metacarpal is incised and elevated from the metacarpal. An oblique osteotomy is performed. The extensor digiti minimi tendon is cut near the proximal edge of the wound. The small slip from the ring extensor to the little finger is carefully transected, as well as insertion of the abductor digiti minimi. The digital vessels are ligated and the digital nerves are placed deep in the interosseous space to avoid neuromas on the ulnar and palmar side of the hand. The flexor tendons are then pulled distally and transected. The abductor digiti minimi tendon is sutured to the lateral band on the ulnar side of the ring finger. The flaps that have been fashioned are then sutured so that the suture line is on the dorsal aspect of the ulnar side of the hand.

PARTIAL HAND PROSTHESES

Partial hand prostheses are seldom necessary. Almost any residual limb that provides sensation and opposition is better than hand prostheses. However, there are a few very specific indications for partial hand prostheses: cosmesis, protection of sensitive skin, and functional considerations.

The patient who has sustained a partial hand amputation may be extremely self-conscious of the loss. Attention to cosmesis may relieve these feelings of self-doubt and be a worthwhile addition to total patient care. Normal prosthetic management consists of a cosmetic glove, generally with residual digit fillers, wires, and a hidden zipper (Fig. 10-11). If the system is designed to terminate just proximal to the styloids, a bracelet or wide watchband eliminates the immediate transition zone between the glove and the patient. Often the patient feels somewhat more comfortable with the snug, intimate fit of the glove, much as do patients with other levels of amputation when wrapped in a compression bandage.

The patient who has more residual function should not be fitted with an entire glove, but only cosmetic digits. Although this prosthesis is restrictive to some degree, since the sense of touch is compromised, improved cosmesis made the patient shown in Fig. 10-12 feel more secure in cer-

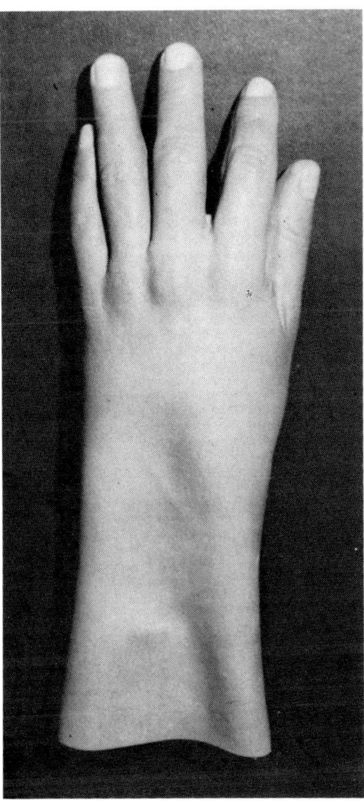

Fig. 10-11. Prosthetic management or partial hand amputation often consists of cosmetic glove, generally with residual digit fillers, wires, and hidden zipper. If system is designed to terminate just proximal to styloids, bracelet or wide watch band eliminates immediate transition of glove.

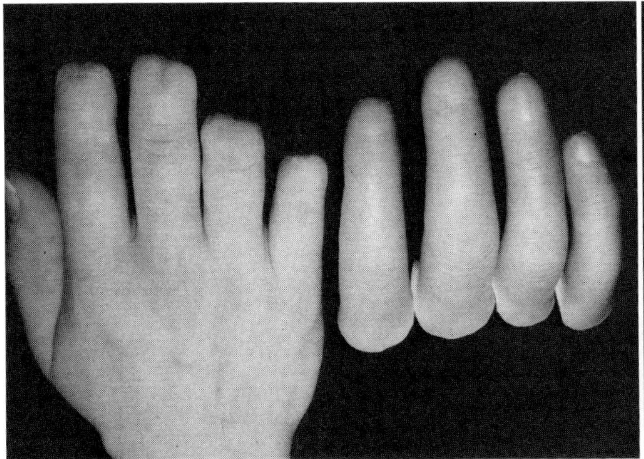

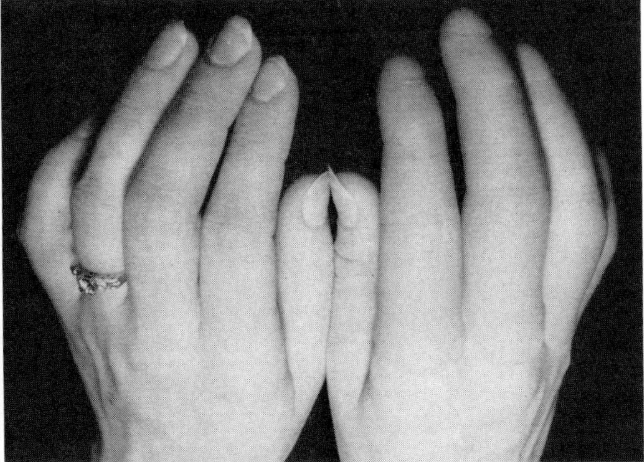

Fig. 10-12. Although restrictive to some degree, especially since sense of touch is compromised, cosmetic partial replacements designed with firm fillers and wired to permit passive positioning of digits may maintain some functional characteristics.

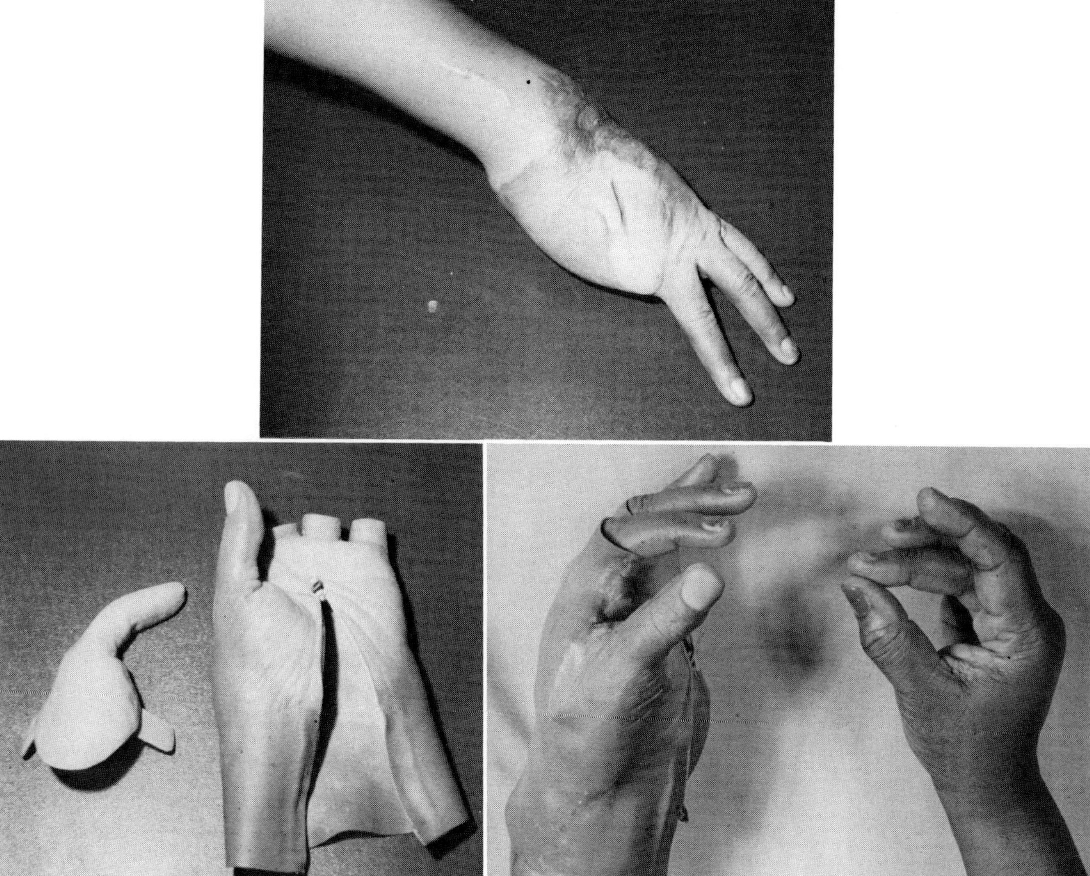

Fig. 10-13. Cosmetic partial hand replacements for missing thumb can be constructed similar to those for absent fingers.

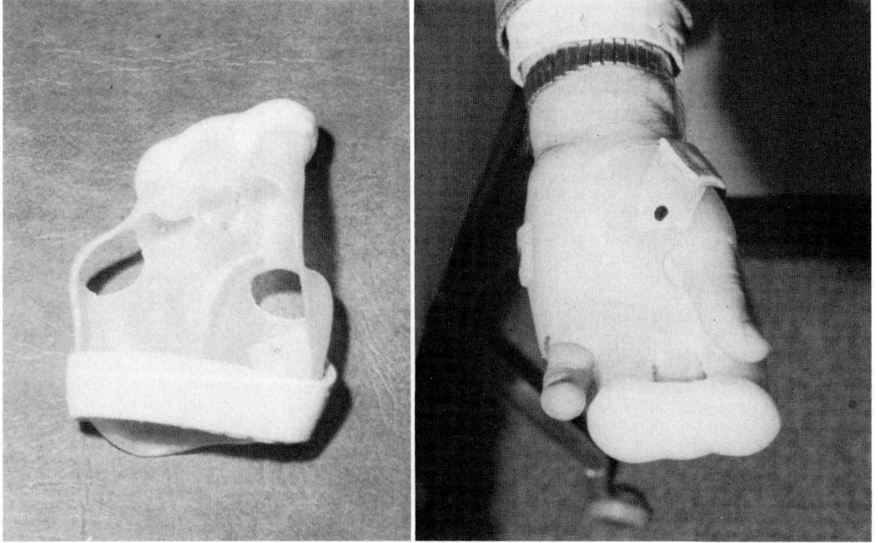

Fig. 10-14. This device provides foam and rigid plastic protection for ends of residual digits, which are extremely sensitive. With this device wearer, who is a manual laborer, can lift and push heavy objects without pain.

tain social situations. Cosmetic partial replacements are designed with firm fillers and wired to permit passive positioning of the digits, thus maintaining some of the functional characteristics of the hand. When the missing digit is the thumb, a similar device can be constructed (Fig. 10-13). Because of the importance of the thumb in prehension, cosmetic thumbs are less functional than cosmetic devices for fingers.

The sensitive skin of a partial hand amputation or the point tenderness of a painful neuroma may need to be protected by a prosthetic device. This is usually a short-term application until further surgery corrects the problem or additional skin healing has occurred. In an occasional patient may be a long-term need (Fig. 10-14).

The third application of prosthetics to partial hand amputation is to provide increased function. Functional prostheses may be considered in three classes. The prosthesis may be used purely as a post to provide opposition. It may have specialized features to aid in certain occupations, or it may be the conventional type of hook and harness arrangement.

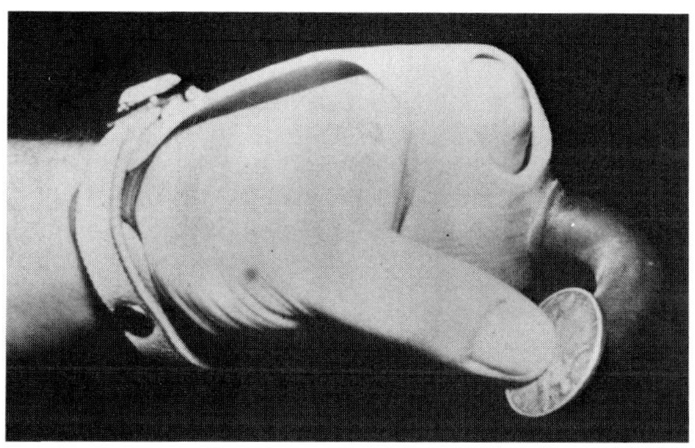

Fig. 10-15. Device designed to provide opposition for mobile thumb and no other phalanges.

In the patient who has a mobile, sensate thumb but no other phalanges, the need for opposition is most acute. Fig. 10-15 depicts one of the various designs employed to provide prehension in a precision manner for the partial hand amputee. A device such as this can be donned and doffed with little nuisance and is well accepted. Variations of this theme abound.

It is important that the prosthetic device for a partial hand amputee not serve so many functions that it does none of them well. Occasionally a custom-designed system that serves only one basic function will be very well received and add to the abilities of the wearer. In such cases the prosthetic device will be used on those occasions when the specific need arises. This nonstandard device is limited only by the ingenuity and design capabilities of the prosthetist. Fig. 10-16 is an example of two nonstandard custom devices designed for an individual with severe hand loss, who earned his living doing heavy labor. These systems make full use of the sensation available and combine it with stability and provide for power grip.

If the partial hand amputation is so extensive that an insufficient residual limb makes opposition possible, a hook with harnessing and a cable is the most functional device. This approach is often the one of choice when confronted with a patient with bilateral partial hand amputations. The cable control system and figure-of-nine harness are incorporated with the appropriate terminal device for the patient's needs (Fig. 10-17).

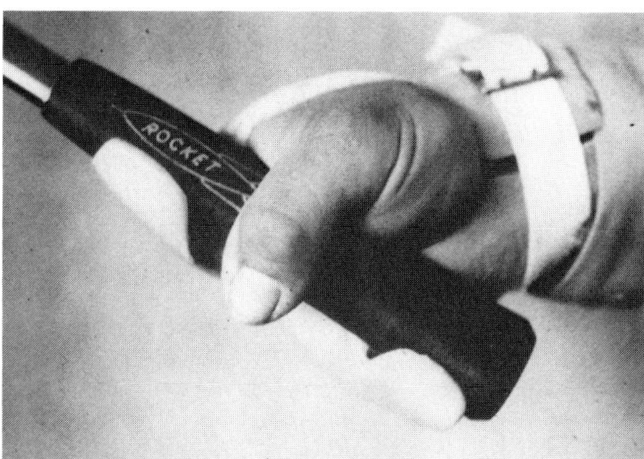

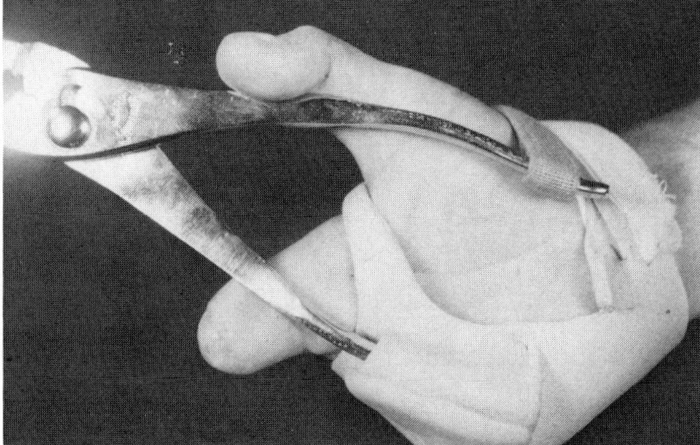

Fig. 10-16. Depending on patient's vocation or avocation, nonstandard approach may be indicated.

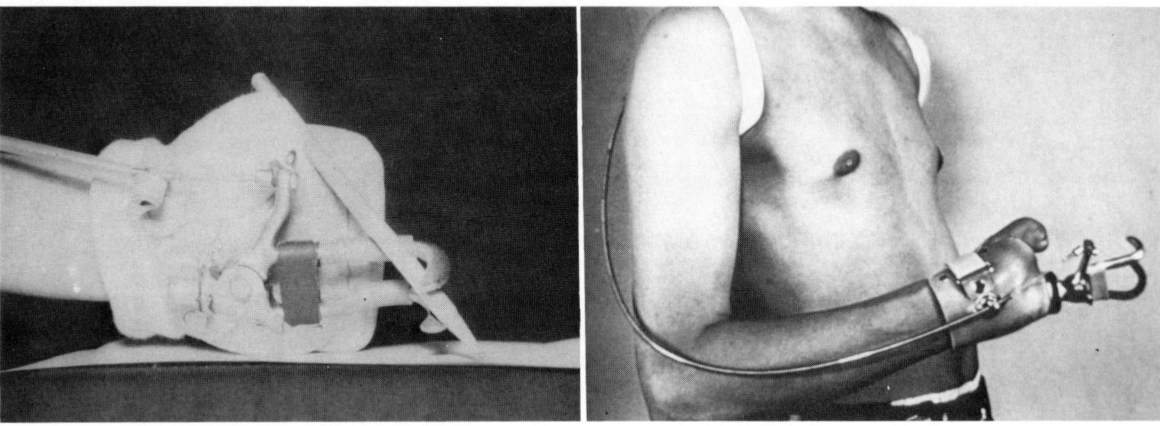

Fig. 10-17. Cable control system and figure-of-nine harness incorporated with appropriate terminal device for patient's needs.

Although research and development continues, no powered hook terminal device is presently available. This component would allow a handy hook-type fixation, while eliminating the necessity of a harness and cable control system.

The advent of myoelectric upper limb prosthetics has not as yet been of benefit to the partial hand amputee. The vast percentage of mechanical hands available are not suitable for the partial hand amputee because achieving length equal to the sound side presents a problem. Also, the inability to eliminate mechanical fingers to accommodate for remaining digits renders these standard hands useless for prosthetic management.

When challenged to fill both cosmetic as well as functional needs for the partial hand amputee, the one acceptable system available is the Robin-Aids hand, which consists of mechanical fingers with interchangeable components. Patients with the thumb intact, small, small and ring, or no fingers remaining can be managed successfully. The thumb is an independent two-position variety that allows larger grasp for items such as a glass or bottle after passive prepositioning.

Fingers are individually adjustable at the metacarpophalangeal and proximal interphalangeal joints and maintain prepositioning through the use of constant friction. This possibility enhances the system's ability to deal with objects of varying size.

Like most standard mechanical hands, the Robin-Aids hand is of the voluntary opening variety. Prehension force is adjustable by means of varying spring tension. Leather gloves are interchangeable with cosmetic zipper gloves for work or dress. The overall length is adjustable to accomodate precise length for individual amputees.

Training for the patient with a prosthetic system is usually quite simple. Patients who have been fitted with cosmetic restoration usually require little, if any therapy. Some degree of follow-up may be indicated to ensure patient understanding and acceptance.

The vast majority of functional partial hand systems employ no complicated or elaborate cable control or harness components. If the device is correctly designed, it is easy to don and doff and require little training. However, it is important that these patients be seen and treated in therapy to assure acceptance and gain optimal use of the prosthesis. After a short period of training occasional visits are usually sufficient.

In summary, the clinic team is rarely called on to provide a prosthesis for partial hand amputation patients. When required they are generally nonstandard, highly personal devices. The patient should be carefully questioned about expectations and needs. The simplest device consistent with these needs will provide the most acceptance, function, and patient satisfaction.

REFERENCES

1. Atasoy, E., Iokimidis, E., Kasdan, M., Kutz, J. E., and Kleinert, H. E.: Reconstruction of the amputated finger tip with a triangular volar flap. J. Bone Joint Surg. **52A:** 921, 1970.
2. Carroll, R. E.: Transposition of the index finger to replace the middle finger. In DePalma, A. F., editor: Clinical orthopaedics, vol. 15, Philadelphia, 1959, J. B. Lippincott Co.
3. Chase, R. A.: Atlas of hand surgery, Philadelphia, 1973, W. B. Saunders Co.

4. Entin, M. A.: Salvaging the basic hand, Surg. Clin. North Am. **38:**1063-1081, 1968.
5. Flatt, A. E.: The care of minor hand injuries, ed. 4, St. Louis, 1979, The C. V. Mosby Co.
6. Gillies, H., and Millard, D. R., Jr.: The principles and art of plastic surgery, Boston, 1972, Little, Brown & Co.
7. Harris, R. W., and Houston, J. K.: Partial amputation of the hand, Can. J. Surg. **10:**431-438, Oct., 1967.
8. Kutler, W.: A new method for finger tip amputation, J.A.M.A. **133:**29, 1947.
9. Littler, J. W.: Neurovascular pedicle method of digital transposition for reconstruction of thumb, Plast. Reconstr. Surg. **12:**303, 1953.
10. Matev, I. B.: Thumb reconstruction after amputation at the petacarpophalangeal joint by bone lengthening, J. Bone Joint. Surg. **52A:**957, 1970.
11. McGregor, I. A.: Flap reconstruction in hand surgery: the evolution of presently used methods, J. Hand Surg. **4**(1):1-10, 1979.
12. Milford, L.: The hand. In Edmonson, A. S., and Crenshaw, A. H., editors: Campbell's operative orthopaedics, St. Louis, 1980, The C. V. Mosby Co.
13. Moberg, E.: Aspects of sensation in reconstructive surgery of the upper extremity, J. Bone Joint Surg. **46A:**817, 1964.
14. Murray, J. F., Carman, W., and MacKenzie, J. K.: Transmetacarpal amputation of the index finger, J. Hand Surg. **2**(6):471-481, 1977.
15. Napier, J. P.: The prehensile movements of the human hand, J. Bone Joint Surg. **38B:**902, 1956.
16. Posner, M., and Smith, Q. J.: The advancement pedicle flap for thumb injuries, J. Bone Joint Surg. **53A:**1618-1621, 1971.
17. Rank, B., Wakefield, A., and Hueston, J.: Surgery of repair as applied to hand injuries, ed. 4, New York, 1973, Churchill-Livingstone, Ltd.
18. Slocum, D. B.: Amputations of the fingers and hand, Clin. Orthop. **15:**35, 1959.

CHAPTER 11

Wrist disarticulation and below-elbow amputation

WILLIAM E. BURKHALTER
FREDERICK L. HAMPTON
JANET S. SMELTZER

SURGICAL TECHNIQUES

The below-elbow amputation is most often necessitated by trauma or its residuals. For this reason, the operative procedure, rather than being a normal amputation technique, is often debridement of a severe wound of the forearm, wrist, or hand. The wounds are untidy, and the primary consideration is careful wound management. Repeated debridements are occasionally necessary. There is no level of election, and all viable tissue should be preserved. Bone and muscle should not be shortened simply to obtain wound closure.

Split-thickness grafts, preferably using a mesh technique, are an excellent method of obtaining closure. Mesh grafts adhere well to irregular surfaces, and their natural drainage improves the overall success rate (Fig. 11-1). Wear qualities of the split-thickness graft with or without mesh are satisfactory for the upper limb amputee (Fig. 11-2).

WRIST DISARTICULATION

As previously described a formal disarticulation is rarely performed. In the elective technique, however, only the most prominent portions of radial and ulnar styloid processes are removed. Ideally, the residual limb should have adequate soft tissue for closure, and palmar skin is preferred. It is not necessary to remove cartilage from the articular surfaces. It is essential to avoid injury to the distal radial ulnar joint. Skin flaps are created in the usual manner down to the deep fascia, which should then be divided at the site of proximal skin-level retraction. Because of its long subcutaneous course, the superficial branch of the radial nerve is particularly prone to troublesome neuroma formation. It is important to identify this structure, isolate it, and section it in a manner that allows proximal retraction beneath the brachioradialis muscle. The muscle and tendon units should be divided and preserved for use in stabilization. A specific search should be made for the radial and ulnar arteries, as well as the volar and dorsal interosseous vessels. These should be securely ligated using accepted techniques. The nerves should be divided under slight tension so that they are allowed to retract into the soft tissues of the stump.

In elective cases of disarticulation in which adequate skin coverage is available, dorsal and volar tendons should be stabilized distally under physiological tension. Noting and marking the resting length prior to division will help determine the ideal tension for myodesis. This stabilization adds to the proprioceptive sensation of the stump, as well as maintains muscle function. This

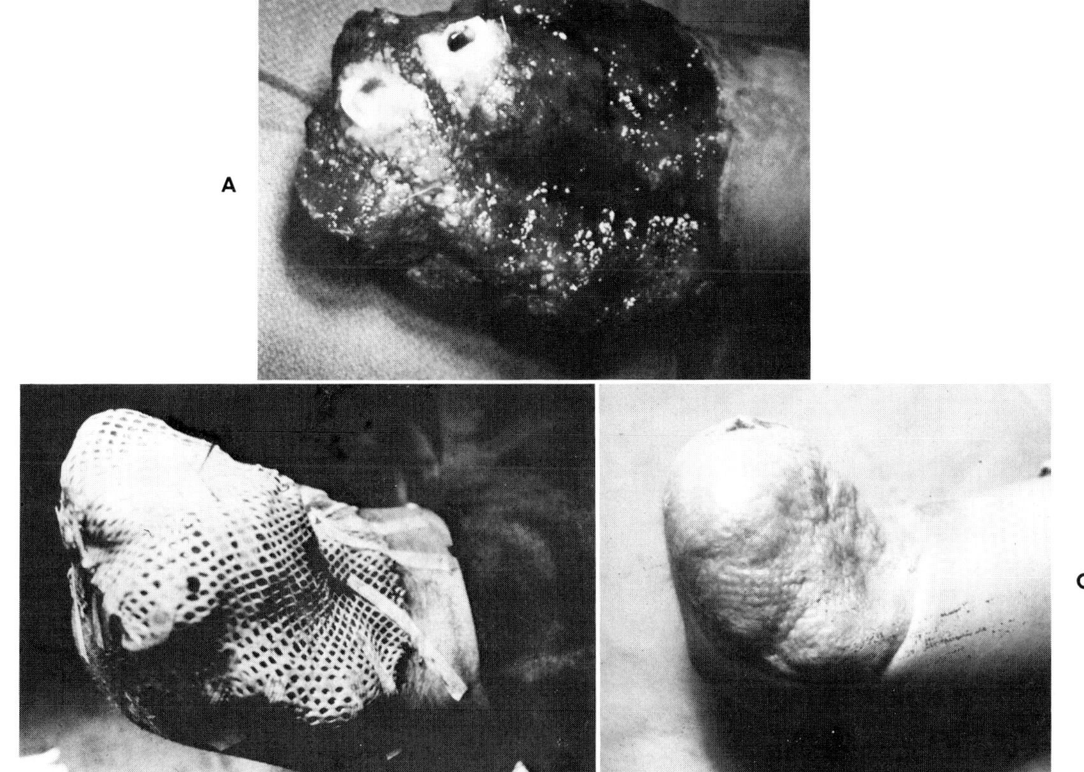

Fig. 11-1. A, Traumatic, short below-elbow amputation with circumferential loss of skin secondary to shark attack. **B,** After two debridements, meshed skin grafts were applied and held in place with paper tapes. **C,** Note condition of stump 4 weeks after injury.

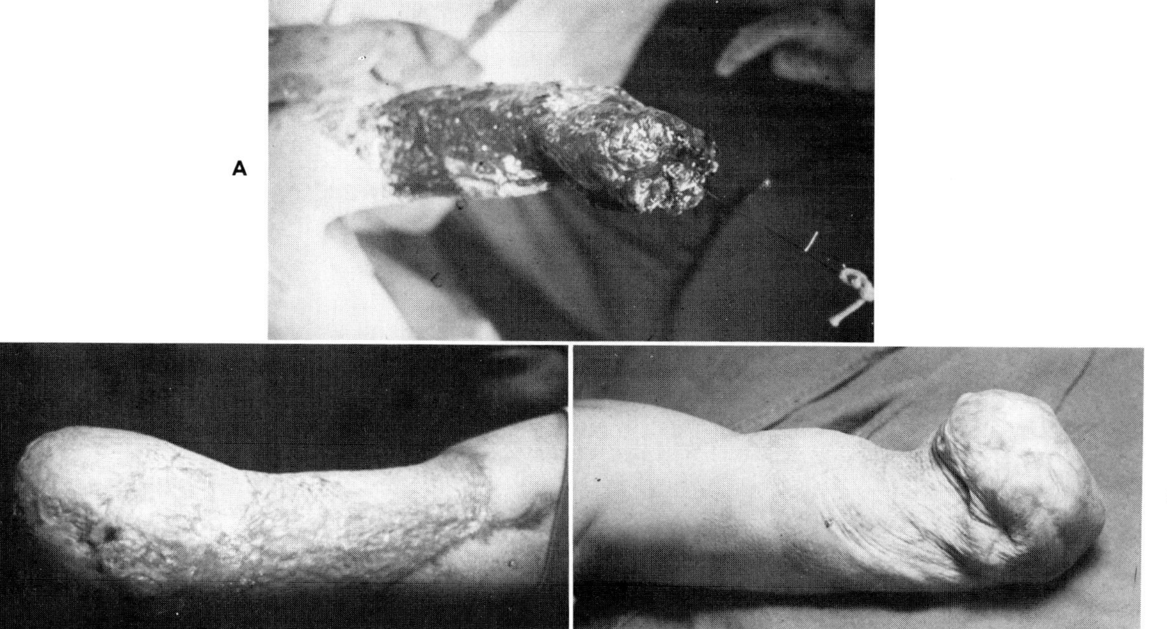

Fig. 11-2. A, Avulsing wound with short below-elbow amputation with circumferential skin loss to middle third of arm. **B,** Closure with meshed split-thickness skin graft. **C,** After 1 year note quality of graft and range of elbow. No revision or placement of split-thickness graft was necessary.

is especially useful for myoelectric prosthetic applications.

FOREARM AMPUTATIONS

Amputations through the forearms should be accomplished at the most distal effective level consistent with adequate skin coverage. Management of the skin flap, muscle, nerves, and other tissues follows the basic principles previously stated (Fig. 11-3). Both bones are usually cut at the same level, unless operative findings dictate otherwise. The sharp bone edges are carefully rounded. Distal muscle stabilization is most important in the forearm and can be accomplished by suturing opposing muscle groups across the end of the stump or by suturing the muscle directly to the bone. If care has been taken to obtain hemostasis, it is seldom necessary to use drains.

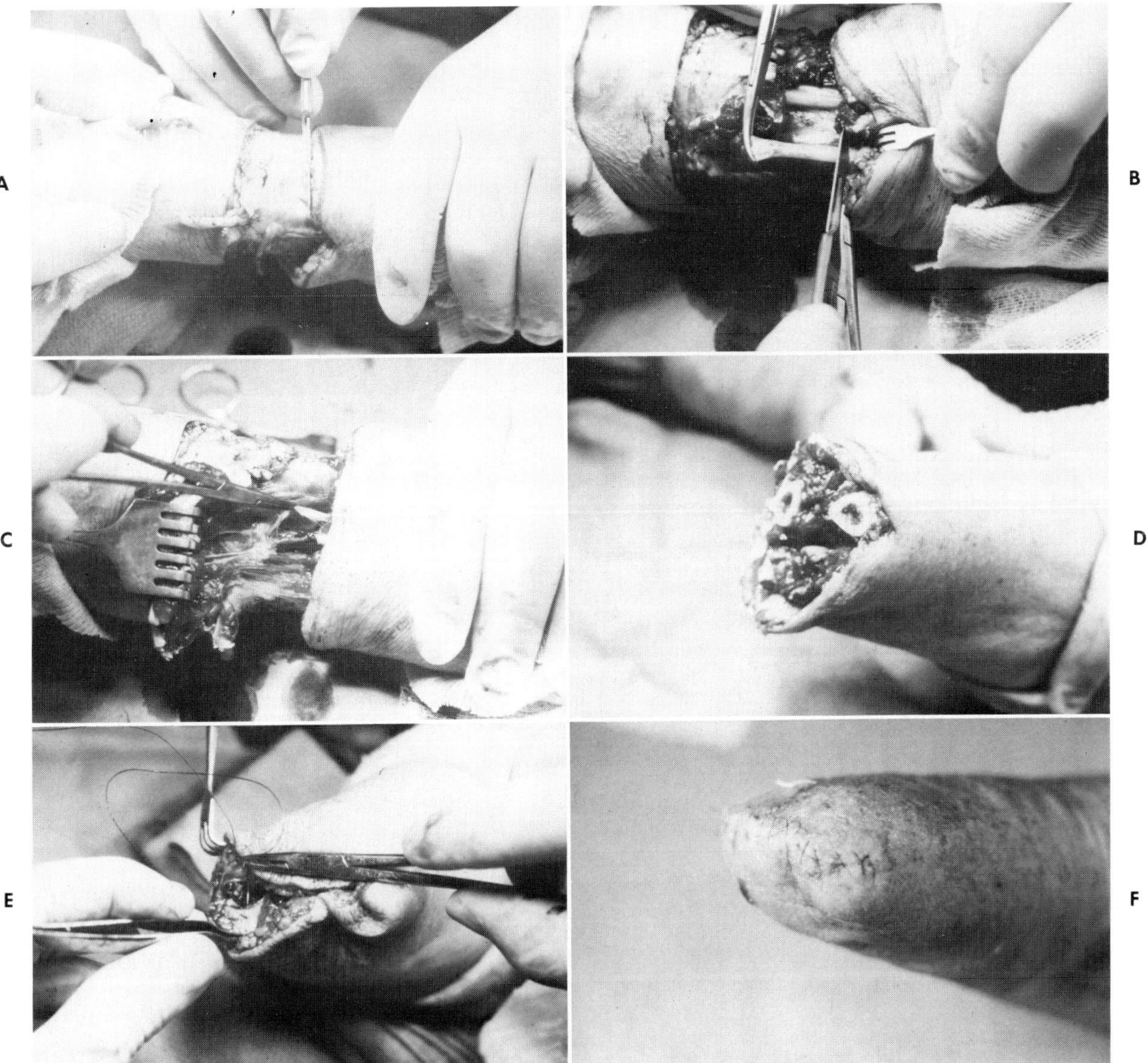

Fig. 11-3. Steps of elective below-elbow amputation. **A,** Skin is allowed to retract and is pulled proximally. Note that fascial and deeper incision is made at proximal skin line. **B,** Nerves are divided under some tension. **C,** Search must be made for both volar and dorsal interosseous arteries. **D** and **E,** With proper initial incisions, closure of deep structures with normal tension and without redundancy is possible. **F,** Stump after 5 days in rigid dressing. There is minimal swelling, and wound is nonreactive.

In very short below-elbow amputation, a functional lengthening of the stump may be accomplished by dividing the biceps tendon. This will allow for a closer fitting of the volar socket flange for more stable prosthetic use. The brachialis muscle provides sufficient strength for active flexion of the elbow.

PREPROSTHETIC MANAGEMENT

Preprosthetic management of either the wrist disarticulation or the below-elbow amputee begins immediately after the operative procedure. Where wounds are closed, immediate surgical fitting is appropriate. A rigid plaster dressing is applied over a sterile stump sock. Elasticized plaster, supported with conventional plaster, gives the most comforting fit. Elasticized plaster should be applied to conform to the stump rather than compress it. Initially the cast should extend above the elbow, with this joint in midposition. A shoulder harness, cable housing, and terminal device can be added, allowing the patient early use of the stump as a helper. If after a few days there is but minimal discomfort in the stump, and the fit about the forearm is satisfactory, the above-elbow portion of the cast can be trimmed into a Muenster configuration, so that flexion and extension of the elbow is possible (Fig. 11-4). This allows considerably more use of the terminal device, and at this time the patient may start with occupational therapy. As shrinkage of the stump occurs, the cast loosens, and the plaster may be changed. Serial Muenster casts can be used as the shrinking process continues.

As an alternative, a temporary prosthesis fabricated from Orthoplast or other plastic material can be employed. Velcro straps and stump socks can be used to vary the fit. The same harness and terminal device can be used as on the initial plaster of Paris fitting. With this technique, prosthetic training can be continued while wound healing and maturation of the soft tissues occur.

If temporary prostheses are available for training, elastomer foam inserts can be molded and used as a filler between the patient's stump and the temporary prosthesis (Fig. 11-5). This foam insert offers a gentle, continuous compression for the stump, while allowing use of a prosthesis that is similar to the anticipated permanent device. As stump shrinkage occurs, more elastomer may be added, or additional stump socks may be used. This elastomer filler technique is particularly valuable when secondary healing areas proximal to the actual amputation site are present or where there are recently applied split-thickness grafts. With open wounds, only light dressings are necessary, which allows the amputee to change the own dressings, wash and dry the wound areas, and then to reapply the elastomer filler.

During immediate or early postsurgical fitting and during early prosthetic training with a temporary device, emphasis should be placed on improving strength and range of motion in all joints of the limb. Using the prosthesis as a helper to the normal hand should be encouraged and strictly one-handed activity avoided.

Lack of sensation or the use of very thin split-thickness grafts requires extra care. Special interfaces may be necessary to avoid friction or excessive pressure. The length of the stump, range

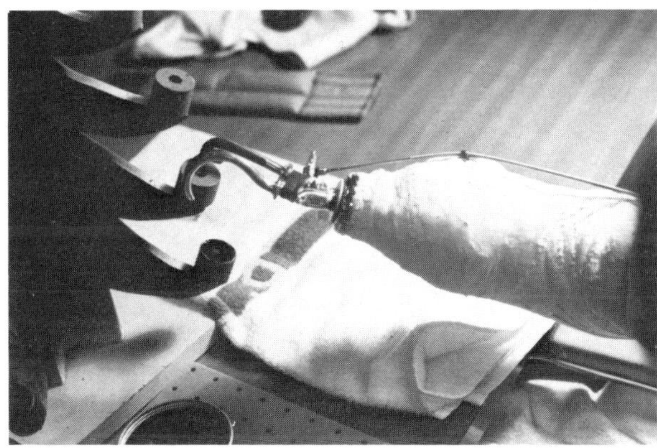

Fig. 11-4. Below-elbow amputee with immediate posturgical fitting using plaster of Paris Muenster-type cast as socket. Five days postoperatively patient begins early training.

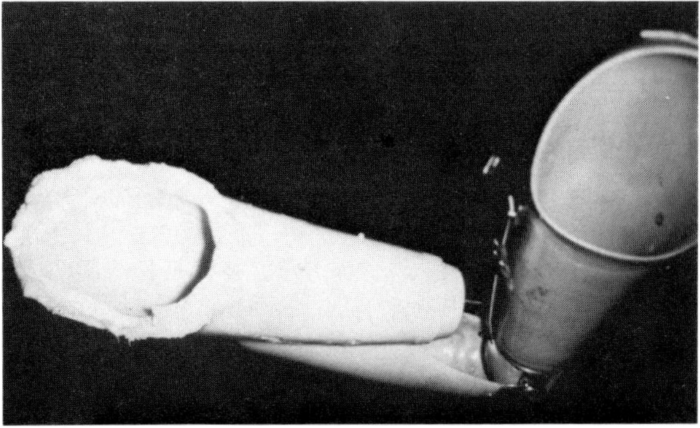

Fig. 11-5. Elastomer foam liner can be used as filler insert for below-elbow and above-knee practice prostheses. This offers gentle compression of soft tissues, much as would stump wrapping, plus protection and immobilization of soft tissues. It can be removed for stump hygiene.

of motion, and strength of proximal musculature are all important to successful prosthetic wear and function.

When myoelectric prosthesis control systems are planned, the electrodes can be incorporated in the immediate postoperative fitting or in the temporary prosthesis.

PROSTHETIC MANAGEMENT

Prosthetic management in the upper limb amputee depends on the following factors:

1. Length of the residual arm
2. Strength of the musculature
3. Range of motion available
4. Occupation of the patient
5. Functional and cosmetic requirements of the amputee
6. Availability of prosthetic maintenance

These considerations will have been discussed by the clinic team during the initial phase of patient evaluation and preprosthetic management. This information must be available to the team since it will influence the prosthetic prescription and the system used.

Wrist disarticulation

In wrist disarticulation and its homologue (stumps with 80% to 100% of normal lateral humeral epicondyle to radial styloid length), the amputee retains the ability to pronate and supinate the forearm. The socket is fabricated to use this motion. A screwdriver shape that transmits forearm rotation to the socket can be obtained by carefully molding or flattening the area in the distal third of the radius and ulna. In true wrist disarticulation, flaring of the distal stump around the styloid processes can be used for suspension of the socket, eliminating the need for additional harnessing. The posterior trim line does not contain the olecranon, and the circular proximal section of the socket permits pronation and supination of the prosthesis. Approximately 50% of residual forearm rotation can be transmitted to the prosthesis. An anterior trim line 5 to 10 cm (2 to 4 inches) distal to the cubital crease should permit a full 135 degrees of elbow flexion. Flexible elbow hinges with a posterior cross strap will permit forearm rotation with a simple triceps pad providing the reaction point for the control cable.

When the suspension is inherent in the socket configuration, as in a wrist disarticulation prosthesis, a figure-of-nine harness may be employed. For the long below-elbow stump (between 55% to 80% of epicondyle to styloid length), the prosthesis uses a figure-of-eight harness to provide both suspension and control of the terminal device.

In prescribing the terminal device the person's vocation or avocation is usually the major consideration. Bilateral activity requiring manual dexterity calls for the standard hook. For socially oriented vocations, a functional or cosmetic hand may be preferred. In a long below-elbow amputation, the available space between the socket and terminal device permits installation of a quick-change wrist unit so that both terminal devices may be used interchangeably.

Below-elbow amputation

The short below-elbow amputee (35% to 55% of the epicondyle to styloid length) has lost the function of pronation and supination. In addition, assistance may be required for torsional stability at the elbow against rotational stress to the prosthesis. Rigid elbow hinges may be used for this purpose.

As an alternative, suspension of the prosthesis may be enhanced by the configuration of the socket. The Muenster socket or its modifications accomplish suspension by enclosing the olecranon and humeral condyles. This improves suspension of the prosthesis, but may limit to some extent the range of flexion and extension of the elbow. Pronation and supination are not expected in the Muenster socket.

For the heavy-duty user, the single-axis rigid hinge may be used. A polycentric hinge, however, will provide extra clearance for the tissues at the anterior trim line during flexion of the elbow. A triceps half cuff and a figure-of-eight harness are required for this type of application. A constant friction or a quick-change wrist unit may be used.

In the case of the bilateral amputee, consideration should be given to the use of a flexion wrist unit on one side. A wrist rotator to provide pronation and supination may occasionally be advantageous. The hook is the preferred terminal device. The weight of a functional or cosmetic hand may be detrimental to its use with a high-level amputation.

In the very short below-elbow amputee (0% to 35% of epicondyle to styloid length), the short residual forearm requires a socket designed to retain the stump, while permitting a useful range of elbow flexion and extension. For heavy-duty use, the self-suspending socket that encases the olecranon and humeral condyles, trimmed anteriorly in a V configuration to provide clearance for the biceps tendon, is used. Limitation of elbow flexion requires preflexion of the Muenster forearm.

The limited range of flexion inherent in this length of amputation can also be increased by using a split-socket design with step-up hinge. Although this design can significantly increase the available flexion, it requires a proportional increase in force.

When the residual forearm is too short to power or stabilize the prosthesis in elbow flexion, a figure-of-eight harness with an above-elbow lift and control cable may be employed. If at least 30 degrees of flexion and 140 newtons of force are available, a single-axis, stump-activated locking hinge may be used. Extension of the stump unlocks the elbow joint. A half cuff with supporting billets stabilizes the elbow on the upper arm.

A variety of powered systems have increased the prosthetic armamentarium for upper limb amputees. Myoelectric systems, whether controlled by a switch or neuromuscular impulse, have many advantages for the below-elbow amputee. The system eliminates the use of a harness for suspension and control and provides excellent cosmesis and function. The terminal device is presently limited to a hand, the action of which is proportionally controlled by the myoelectric impulses.

Endoskeletal systems with soft covering add a further capacity to fulfill special needs. These systems may be passive cosmetic restorations or functional systems.

All alternatives must be considered to ensure the correct prescription for each individual's needs. However, the vast majority of prostheses for upper limb amputees still use standard and conventional components that are activated by body-powered control systems.

PROSTHETIC TRAINING

Patient evaluation and preprosthetic management

It is important for the medical team to assess and, if possible, correct any physical or psychological problem that the patient may have before prosthetic fitting to ensure maximum efficiency at the initiation of training. The patient must be given a realistic view of the future with a prosthetic device. It should be made clear at the outset that the training program may be long and sometimes frustrating, but the reward can be significant.

For the amputee there is not only the loss of functional ability, but a distressing change in body concept or self-image. Many have a difficult time adjusting to this loss. The early use of a prosthesis as a replacement may be helpful in this readjustment. During the period between amputation and prosthetic fitting the therapist should be active in the following treatment areas:

1. Psychological support
2. Maintenance or increase in range of motion of the proximal joints
3. Increasing strength in the remaining musculature
4. Stump shrinkage
5. Helping the patient adapt to the activities of daily living and providing the necessary self-help aids
6. Developing coordination and dexterity of the remaining intact limb
7. Realistically assessing the present and future capabilities of the patient

Psychological support. Psychological support of the patient is necessary throughout the entire period of care. The amputee's perception of himself will have a great influence on the training and use of the prosthesis. Since the therapist has considerable contact with the patient, he or she can help answer questions the patient may have, allay apprehensions, and assist in making the psychological adjustment to an artificial limb less traumatic.

Maintenance of joint range of motion. Successful use of a prosthesis requires good function of the proximal joints. These joints should be taken through a range of motion daily as soon after amputation as possible. Positioning the stump to prevent joint contractures is an important consideration in early aftercare.

Muscle strengthening. Once the desired range of motion has been achieved, exercise to strengthen the remaining musculature should be initiated. In the unilateral amputee, the opposite limb must not be neglected in the program. In addition to general limb strengthening, exercises should specifically include elevation of the shoulders and abduction of the scapulae, both active and resistive.

Stump shrinkage. To ready the stump for prosthetic measurement and fabrication, stump wrapping may be prescribed to promote shrinkage, prevent edema, and provide contouring. If used, the therapist should handle this responsibility at first, but later, the patient or a member of the family should be taught the technique. Reapplication of the elastic bandages should be carried out at least four or five times a day, and at bedtime if the process is to be completed rapidly. Elastic stump shrinkers often prove to be more efficacious.

Rigid dressings and immediate postsurgical fittings, whenever feasible, are advised in upper limb amputations. This technique eliminates the necessity of wrapping and also discourages the development of exclusively one-handed function.

Activities of daily living. In the interim between amputation and prosthetic fitting, the unilateral amputee learns to function as a one-handed individual. If the dominant limb is intact, this causes few problems. Usually all that is required is learning new methods for normally two-handed tasks such as buttoning a shirt or tying a shoe. If the nondominant limb is intact, however, changing dominance for activities may present some problems until the amputee becomes adept at using what was formerly as assisting hand as the primary working hand.

Stump hygiene should be stressed during this period of concern for independence in self-care. The stump should be bathed and dried thoroughly each day; special care is taken to wash in the folds of the skin. The patient must inspect the stump frequently for any skin disorder.

Improving one-handed dexterity. The amputee who has lost the dominant limb will have to work at gaining the speed and dexterity lost through amputation. In addition to normal daily activities, the therapist should provide the patient with a variety of hand activities designed to increase fine motor skills.

Assessing capabilities. During the preprosthetic period the medical team can usually determine to a large extent how the patient will accept the prosthesis. Attitudes held by the patient before exposure to the artificial limb are a major influence over later acceptance, performance, and use. The therapist can provide valuable information regarding the patient's interests and possible work alternatives. Assuring the patient of potential for independence and transition back into a home and work environment may favorably influence these attitudes.

PROSTHETIC EVALUATION AND TRAINING

Prosthetic checkout

Prosthetic checkout is a method whereby the fit, function, comfort, and cosmesis of the prosthesis are evaluated. This procedure ensures that, before the amputee begins training, the equipment is at maximum efficiency, and interruptions of the training program for prosthetic adjustments can be minimized. Any items found on the checkout not to comply with standards should be reported to the prosthetist for prompt adjustment. The equipment needed for this procedure includes a goniometer, spring scale, hook adapters, marker pencil, ruler, tape measure, a block of wood 5 cm × 1 cm × 1.5 cm, and adhesive tape.

Conformance of the prosthesis to the prescription, workmanship, and cosmesis are factors to be considered. The correct length of the prosthesis places the tip of the terminal device opposite the thumb tip on the remaining limb. A Muenster socket may give an illusion of length discrepancy due to its preflexion. The true length can be measured by having the amputee stand with his back against the wall, with both elbows touching the wall and flexed to 90 degrees.

The procedures for functional checkout of a below-elbow prosthesis follow. A simple checklist can be prepared.

Range of motion

Stump rotation. In wrist disarticulation and long, well-formed, below-elbow stumps, approximately 50% of the residual pronation and supination of the stump should be transmitted to the prosthesis. Short stumps retain little measurable motion, and, in the Muenster socket, rotation is not expected. Loss of expected range of rotation may be due to the following:

1. An inadequately fitting socket
2. An improper proximal trim line
3. Presence of rigid elbow hinges

Elbow motion. Flexion and extension of the prosthesis should approach 80% to 90% of the range present in the residual limb, except in very short stumps and with the Muenster socket. If this standard is not met it may be due to the following:

1. Improper trim line not accommodating the biceps tendon in flexion or too proximal a trim line anteriorly
2. Improper placement or alignment of rigid hinges

Terminal device opening and closing. With the fingers of the hook directed medially, the terminal device is opened manually to its fullest extent, and the gap measured. The active opening, using the control cable with the elbow flexed to 90 degrees, is then measured. This should equal the manual opening. The opening with the terminal device at the level of the waist is then measured and should be at least 70% of the manual opening. Discrepancies in any of these measurements may be due to the following:

1. Improper harnessing
2. Limitation in control motion
3. Incorrect placement of retainers or crossbar assembly
4. Sharp bends in the cable housing
5. Too long a cable housing

Control system efficiency. This measurement determines the amount of force lost between the terminal device and harness. To make this determination, a 1.5-cm width wood block is placed between the fingers of the terminal device. The cable is disconnected from the hook, and a spring scale applied. A gradually increasing pull on the scale will release the wooden block, and the force at this point is noted and recorded. The test should be performed with the prosthesis in place on the patient, and the elbow flexed at 90 degrees, with the pull applied in the line of the normal cable pull. The cable is then reattached to the terminal device, but disconnected from the harness in back. An adapter is hooked to the T bar of the control cable, and the spring scale used to pull along the line of the control cable posteriorly. Again, the force required to open the terminal device to release the wood block is noted. The efficiency is then computed:

$$\frac{\text{Force at terminal device}}{\text{Force at harness}} \times 100 = \text{Percentage of efficiency}$$

The efficiency should be 80% or greater for a single-cable system. If efficiency is less, the problem might be one or more of the following:

1. Sharp bends in the cable housing (kinking)
2. Kinked or frayed cable
3. Improper placement of the retainer or crossbar assembly

Stability. To test the stability of the prosthesis and harnessing, the prosthesis is held vertically at the side with the elbow extended. The spring scale is hooked over the terminal device. At the top of the socket, the stump sock is marked with a marking pencil. By pulling straight down on the scale until it reads 20 kg, the top of the sock will be pulled away from the pencil mark. This pull should not cause the prosthesis to slip on the stump more than 2.5 cm and should not cause failure of any part of the prosthesis or harness. With the Muenster application the slipping should not exceed 1 cm. Interference with stability may be due to one or more of the following:

1. Weak harnessing or stitching
2. Axillary loop discomfort or inadequate padding
3. The V strap suspending the prosthesis attached either too far anteriorly or posteriorly

Compression test. To test comfort and fit, the patient is asked to stand with his back against a wall and flex the elbow to 90 degrees. The examiner pushes with considerable force on the end of the prosthesis, as though trying to push it further onto the stump. This should produce no pain or discomfort.

Training

In the unilateral amputee the prosthesis will generally be used to assist the remaining limb, allowing a portion of lost function to be regained. The prosthetic device, however, is still far from duplicating the lost part, and the patient must be aware of its functional limitations. In contrast to the bilateral amputee, the unilateral patient does not entirely depend on the prosthesis. The prosthesis will be used according to the patient's motivation and specific functional needs. The training period consists of an orientation to the prosthesis and its controls and use training, which initially emphasizes activities of daily living.

Orientation. During the preprosthetic phase, the amputee was introduced to the prosthesis and learned something of its function. Now the introduction should be repeated and the patient specifically instructed in the correct terminology and function of each component part. This understanding will aid the patient in recognizing new problems that may arise and will allow him to communicate these to the therapist or prosthetist. General instruction in the care of the prosthesis should be covered at this time.

The next step in the training process is instruction for donning and doffing the prosthesis. Several methods can be used; the patient should be shown all available methods so as to choose the easiest one.

Controls training. After this initial instruction the amputee is ready to begin learning the basic motions of operation. The therapist manually takes the amputee through each required motion so that he can see and feel the motion being performed. The patient then repeats the same motion independently.

For the below-elbow amputee, this training is concentrated on operation of the terminal device. Forearm and elbow control require no special training. The basic motion for terminal device opening is forward flexion of the humerus with some assistance from biscapular abduction. The shoulder on the amputated side should not flex more than is necessary to produce a natural, smooth, reaching-out motion. The shoulder on the opposite side acts as a stabilizer. This control motion should be repeated by the patient until it is mastered at various positions near the mouth, chest, and waist.

Use training. Once the amputee has learned the mechanics of the prosthesis and to use it efficiently, he is ready for training in purposeful activity. The therapist should present the amputee with many different kinds of activities to help solve new problems that inevitably arise in the patient's own life situation.

Before attempting any activity, prepositioning of the terminal device is essential. Instruction and practice in this prepositioning is necessary. It will allow the amputee to approach an object correctly and to avoid unnecessary and awkward body movements.

Prehension is the final phase of control training before practice in daily activities is started. Drills in the approach, grasp, and release of various sizes of objects and different types of material are used. The amputee is taught to grasp objects with adequate pressure control on the terminal device. The patient may be presented with a sponge rubber cube, wooden block, cotton ball, paper cup, or even an ice-cream cone. The amputee should soon develop a harness feedback, so that the tension can be relaxed sufficiently on the control cable to avoid crushing a paper cup or an ice-cream cone. Control training may be considered complete when the patient has maximum control of the terminal device in space. He should be able to operate the prosthesis efficiently with few, if any, awkward body movements.

Time standards based on experience are useful in evaluating controls and use training. The amputee should not, however, be made to work against standards set by others during the training process. Each patient is an individual with special problems and needs.

Activities of daily living training. Once basic operations are learned, these techniques are applied to practice activities of daily living. The amputee should gain confidence in using the prosthesis in a wide range of activities that are meaningful and important. Although the prosthesis can be useful in many activities, it must be remembered that sensation in that limb is greatly impaired. The amputee must rely on vision and hearing to a far greater degree than the nonamputee. Observations of activities such as putting on a coat or a shirt where the prosthesis is behind the back will confirm this fact.

Initially the activities of most importance for the amputee are feeding and dressing. For the unilateral amputee this independence is not difficult to achieve. Since a prosthesis is not needed to achieve basic independence, the activities chosen for him should require the use of two hands. Cutting food with a knife and fork or tying shoelaces are examples. As the patient attempts, performs, and succeeds in these activities, he becomes more willing to accept and use the prosthesis and can rely on it.

After training in feeding, dressing, and grooming is completed, progression to specialized activities such as communication skills, which involve use of the telephone or typewriter, can be made. Homemaking, vocational, and recreational interests should be encouraged, and the activities associated with these interests should be emphasized in the training process.

When the therapist and the patient believe that a good foundation for independence has been established, initial prosthetic training can be considered complete. As the amputee uses the prosthesis on a daily basis, he will refine what has been taught and, in addition, will often invent his own methods for accomplishing additional tasks required for independent function.

The patient may, however, encounter some simple but necessary task at home that is not covered in the initial training process, with which he has difficulty. If the therapist can be present at follow-up visits, it will be helpful if these specific task problems are solicited from the patient. Solutions can be worked out and practiced in review therapy sessions if necessary, and frustrations avoided.

SUGGESTED READINGS

Anderson, M., Bechtol, C. O., and Sollers, R.: Clinical prosthetics for physicians and therapists, Springfield, Ill., 1959, Charles C Thomas, Publisher.

Santschi, W. R.: Manual of upper extremity prosthetics, Department of Engineering, Los Angeles, 1958, University of California.

Trombley, C., and Scott, A.: Occupational therapy for physical dysfunction, Medfield, Mass., 1975, Fleetwood Publishing Co.

Wellerson, T. L.: A manual for occupational therapists on the rehabilitation of upper extremity amputees, New York, 1958, American Occupational Therapists Association.

CHAPTER 12

Elbow disarticulation and above-elbow amputation

WILLIAM E. BURKHALTER
FREDERICK L. HAMPTON
JANET S. SMELTZER

SURGICAL CONSIDERATIONS

Elbow disarticulation

Elbow disarticulation is preferable to an above-elbow amputation if there is a choice, since suspension capabilities and rotational stability are much better. If possible, anteroposterior flaps should be made because the medial skin is thin and wears poorly. Muscle stabilization should be routinely performed as in wrist disarticulation. Bone prominences should be contoured to prevent later pressure areas in the socket. Sufficient condylar bone should be allowed to remain in order to retain the qualities of rotational stability and suspension previously mentioned. Major arteries are doubly ligated, and nerves are isolated and allowed to retract after ligation and section. It is difficult to obtain adequate hemostasis, as with other major joint disarticulations, therefore drains are a virtual necessity to prevent hematoma and resultant breakdown of skin edges. When rigid dressings are used in an elbow disarticulation or a higher level of amputation, the use of a shoulder harness for suspension is necessary, but is more difficult to apply than in the below-elbow case.

Above-elbow amputation

As a basic principle, the lowest level surgically compatible with the disease process or with tissue viability should be sought. A very short above-elbow amputation is much preferred to shoulder disarticulation regardless of the usefulness of the residual limb. The added surface contour provided by the retained head improves both cosmesis and prosthetic restoration. It is particularly important, however, to recognize that the deltoid tuberosity is the lowest level at which shoulder joint control is effective.

Amputations at or above the elbow can be managed in the immediate postoperative period similarly to more distal amputations with the use of rigid dressings. With closed wounds, a light dressing, is applied, and a long sterile stump sock rolled to the shoulder level. The axillary edge of the sock is split longitudinally, and the opened sock is then rolled proximally to the neck and again split to go on either side of the neck. These ends can then be tied about the neck to aid in suspension of the rigid dressing. Elastic plaster is then applied, extending beyond the acromion, immediately beneath the elastic plaster. The elastic plaster is then reinforced with conventional plaster of Paris bandages. This rigid dressing controls edema and immobilizes the considerable musculature in the arm and may reduce postoperative pain. As tenderness decreases postoperatively, the plaster of Paris shoulder cap should be trimmed to allow a greater range of motion.

PROSTHETIC CONSIDERATIONS

Elbow disarticulation

Although the configuration of the residual limb provides a means for suspension and control of rotation of the prosthesis, the bulbous distal end inhibits donning of the prosthesis and may require a specifically designed socket. This may be an expandable type with a flexible inner wall that allows passage of the bulbous end, yet provides supracondylar suspension. Another method of obtaining the same goals is by the use of a prosthesis with a removable panel. In all prostheses, the lateral proximal trim line should allow full abduction of the arm without impingement on the acromion.

The length of the residual limb requires the use of outside locking hinges with a cable-operated alternating lock. The forearm is of rigid exoskeletal design. A variety of wrist units is available, depending on the requirements of the amputee: a quick disconnect for use of a hook or hand, an oval wrist for cosmetic value, or a flexion wrist unit.

The choice of a terminal device should be determined by the needs and desires of the amputee. A figure-of-eight harness, split-cable housing, and dual control provide for elbow flexion and terminal device operation.

Above-elbow amputation

The standard above-elbow residual limb is 50% to 80% of the acromion to lateral humeral epicondyle length. The usual socket has a closed end with lateral proximal trim lines that allow abduction of the arm without displacement of the prosthesis. A positive-locking elbow with outside cable exit is incorporated. The forearm may be of exoskeletal or endoskeletal design. A dual control system with a figure-of-eight above-elbow harness provides for elbow flexion and terminal device operation. The wrist unit and the terminal device prescribed depend on the patient's needs and desires.

The short above-elbow residual limb is 30% to 50% of acromion to epicondyle length. The closed-end, total-contact socket should have anterior and posterior wings sufficient to prevent rotation, but not to interfere with flexion and abduction. A positive-locking elbow with a lift assist for ease of elbow flexion is recommended. The forearm and wrist unit requirements are the same as in the standard above-elbow limb. The weight of a functional hand may contraindicate its use as a terminal device for the short above-elbow amputee.

The dual control system with an above-elbow, figure-of-eight harness may be used. For heavy lifting, a chest-strap harness with a shoulder saddle is indicated.

The humeral neck level indicates 0% to 30% of acromion to epicondyle length. Use of a shoulder-bearing socket that extends approximately 4 cm or more over the shoulder provides additional stability in suspension of the prosthesis. The anterior and posterior flanges of the socket provide some control of rotation. A positive-locking elbow may require a chin nudge control to effect locking and unlocking. An elbow lift assist may be useful. The remainder of the prescription is the same as for the short above-elbow prostheses.

CONSIDERATIONS FOR THE THERAPIST

Patient evaluation and preprosthetic management

The evaluation of the patient with an elbow disarticulation or above-elbow amputation takes into consideration all areas discussed in Chapter 11. The preprosthetic training program is much the same as for other upper limb amputees with several additions.

Care must be taken to emphasize the control motions necessary to operate the above-elbow prosthesis and incorporate them in the range of motion and strengthening exercises.

For the above-elbow amputee, flexion of the humerus is the source of power for both forearm flexion and prehension. This must be developed so as to provide the amputee with adequate muscle power through a full range of motion. Humeral extension and abduction and scapular depression are control motions for locking and unlocking the elbow and must also be developed using active and active resistive exercises.

Stump shrinkage is also necessary in the preprosthetic phase, especially for the above-elbow amputee, to ensure that the residual limb is ready for prosthetic fitting.

PROSTHESIS EVALUATION AND TRAINING

Prosthetic checkout

In addition to the items discussed in Chapter 11 for the below-elbow prosthetic checkout, several checks are useful in all but the very short above-elbow amputees.

Placement. Placement of the prosthetic elbow should not be more than 2.5 cm below the normal elbow. The angle of flexion of the elbow with the cable relaxed should be no more than 10 degrees when the prosthetic arm is relaxed.

Range of motion with prosthesis on. With the prosthesis on, the above-elbow amputee should have 90 degrees of elbow flexion, 90 degrees of abduction, 45 degrees of rotation, and 30 degrees of extension at the shoulder. If these standards are not met, the causes may include the following:

1. Limited shoulder motion
2. Too short a stump
3. Improper harnessing
4. Arm retainer below level of stump
5. Improper socket fit

Manually move the forearm section through its complete arc of motion to determine the passive range of elbow flexion. This should measure 135 degrees. The patient should then be able to actively flex the elbow through the same range.

Stump flexion required to fully flex elbow. The patient is asked to completely flex the elbow. The amount of flexion of the humerus to accomplish this without using ipsilateral scapular abduction or contralateral shoulder motion is measured. The amount of shoulder flexion required should not exceed 45 degrees. If more than 45 degrees is needed to flex the forearm, it may be due to the following:

1. Improper harnessing
2. An excessively high retainer
3. Elbow lift tab too distal

Force required to flex forearm. The terminal device is taped closed, and the elbow unit unlocked. The spring scale is attached to the control cable. The therapist or patient then holds the prosthetic forearm at 90 degrees of flexion. The therapist pulls along the normal line of the cable with the scale, gradually releasing the forearm until it remains flexed at 90 degrees. The pull is increased along the line of the cable until further flexion of the forearm is noticed. If the force necessary exceeds 4.5 kg, it may be due to the following:

1. Incorrect length or proximal position of the lift tab
2. Kinking or malalignment of the cable
3. Loose harnessing, allowing full extension of the elbow

Live lift. The terminal device is taped closed. The elbow is flexed to 90 degrees and unlocked. The spring scale is hooked over the prosthesis at a distance of 30 cm from the elbow center. The therapist pulls straight down on the scale while the amputee resists the pull. The scale is read when the elbow extends beyond 90 degrees. The amputee should be able to resist a force of at least 1.5 kg at 30 cm from the elbow center. If the amputee is unable to resist the force it may be due to the following:

1. Anterior distal socket discomfort
2. A lift tab too short and/or too close to the elbow unit
3. Retainer below the level of the stump

Socket rotation stability. The elbow is flexed to 90 degrees and locked. The scale is hooked over the prosthesis at a distance of 30 cm from the center of the elbow. The amputee is asked to resist the pull of the scale as it is pulled mediolaterally. The amputee should be able to withstand 1 to 1.5 kg of pull at 30 cm in both directions. If not, it may be due to the following:

1. A loose turntable
2. Poor socket fit
3. Loose harnessing suspension
4. A poorly suspended or too low trim line

Prosthetic training

The prosthetic training period for the elbow disarticulation or above-elbow amputee follows the same general steps as outlined for the below-elbow amputee in Chapter 11.

Controls training for this level amputee is more difficult, since the amputee must now concentrate on lcoking the prosthetic elbow before being able to use the terminal device. Training with a dual control (elbow-locking) above-elbow prosthesis should not be attempted prior to age 3.

When the elbow is unlocked, the basic humeral flexion control motion produces flexion of the forearm section of the prosthesis. The shoulder on the amputation side should not flex more than is necessary for a smooth movement. The opposite shoulder acts as a stabilizer. This exercise should be repeated by the amputee until the speed of movement and the angle of flexion are smooth and controlled. As a precaution while learning this motion, the amputee's face should be protected from the terminal device by his or the therapist's hand. Elbow extension is achieved by slowly bringing the shoulder back to its starting position. The next control motion taught is that for locking and unlocking the elbow. This motion is a combination of shoulder extension, abduction, and scapular depression. Practice this motion with the elbow extended until the lock clicks.

Once the locking/unlocking of the elbow can be accomplished smoothly with the elbow extended, the amputee can be taught to flex the elbow and maintain tension on the cable while the elbow lock is used. To unlock the elbow, the amputee repeats this procedure, allowing the forearm to return smoothly to the starting position. When the elbow is locked, additional humeral flexion will then open the terminal device. This motion should be practiced at the various positions, including the mouth and waist.

For the terminal device to be operated closer to the body, rotation of the prosthetic forearm is necessary. To do this, the amputee is instructed to first flex the elbow to 90 degrees and then manually rotate the turntable medially or laterally. Use and active daily living training is virtually the same as described in the previous chapter.

SUGGESTED READINGS

Anderson, M., Bechtol, C. O., and Sollers, R.: Clinical prosthetics for physicians and therapists, Springfield, Ill., 1959, Charles C Thomas, Publisher.

Santschi, W. R.: Manual of upper extremity prosthetics, Department of Engineering, Los Angeles, 1958, University of California.

Trombley, C., and Scott, A.: Occupational therapy for physical dysfunction, Medfield, Mass., 1975, Fleetwood Publishing Co.

Wellerson, T. L.: A manual for occupational therapists on the rehabilitation of upper extremity amputees, New York, 1958, American Occupational Therapists Association.

CHAPTER 13

Shoulder disarticulation and forequarter amputation

WILLIAM E. BURKHALTER
FREDERICK L. HAMPTON
JANET S. SMELTZER

Planning for the management of a shoulder disarticulation or a forequarter amputation patient revolves around concern as to whether or not the patient will be a functional user of a prothetic device after it has been fitted. In these patients, immediate postsurgical fitting has little advantage. The muscle groups are short, and the region of the amputation is largely tendinous, so there is only minimal shrinkage. The instability of freshly cut muscle is not terribly uncomfortable at this level, and so immediate postsurgical fitting is generally not indicated for pain control. This area does, however, tolerate a split-thickness skin graft very well. Despite the bony prominences about the acromion and clavicle, split-thickness graft coverage here generally gives adequate cover for later prosthetic needs.

SURGICAL PROCEDURE

Shoulder disarticulation

The skin incision begins at the coracoid process and follows the border of the deltoid muscle distally, then again proximally to the posterior axillary fold. The two ends of the incision are joined through the axilla. The deltopectoral groove is identified, the cephalic vein divided, and the pectoralis major and deltoid muscles are divided at their insertion and retracted. The neurovascular bundle is found between the coracobrachialis and the short head of the biceps. The axillary vessels are doubly ligated and divided, and the median, ulnar, musculocutaneous, and radial nerves severed. All vessels and nerves are allowed to retract beneath the pectoralis minor muscle.

The muscles crossing the shoulder joint are now divided. The coracobrachialis and short head biceps are severed near their origin on the coracoid and the deltoid divided at its inserion on the humerus. The deltoid is reflected proximally to expose the capsule and the insertion of the rotator tendons. By externally and internally rotating the humerus, the posterior and anterior capsule and muscles are exposed and divided. The long head biceps is divided near its origin. Incision of the inferior capsule completes the dissection.

The cut ends of all muscles are placed in the glenoid, and sutured to fill the cavity. The deltoid muscle is sutured to the inferior glenoid. A drain is placed deep to the deltoid muscle, and the wound closed.

Forequarter amputation

The usual indication for forequarter amputation is a malignant neoplasm in and about the shoulder. Basically, there are two formal approaches to the operative procedure, depending on whether the subclavian vessels are approached anteriorly by preliminary osteotomy of the clavicle, or posteriorly, as one of the last steps through the muscles that attach the scapula to the chest wall. We prefer the posterior approach because of technical ease and associated decrease in blood loss.

A skin incision, extending along the vertebral border of the scapula from its tip, up over the acromion, and then medially along the clavicle, is common to both. The other portion of the skin incision extends from the tip of the scapula along its axillary border, thrugh the axilla into the deltopectoral groove anteriorly, and then communicates with the clavicle incision at the medial third of the clavicle.

Using the posterior approach, the muscles holding the scapula to the chest wall are divided along its vertebral border; the trapezius, lattisimus dorsi, levator scapulae, and rhomboids are initially divided. Then, as the scapula rotates slightly anterior, it is possible to divide the serratus anterior and the omohyoid, allowing the scapula and the arm to rotate forward when the clavicle is divided in its middle third. After severing the most posterior brachial plexus roots and divisions, the subclavian artery and vein can be readily identified, doubly ligated, and divided. A section of the pectoralis major and minor tendons then frees the humerus and scapula from the chest wall. Since there are no muscles to suture, loose closure of the skin and subcutaneous tissue is all that is required. No drains are needed. A massive supporting dressing is applied to the flaps to keep them against the chest wall. Usually within a few days it is possible to fabricate a Silastic foam shoulder cap, which is held in place by a strap about the chest. This offers improved fit of clothes and, in general, uniform compression against the wound and the flaps.

PROSTHETIC SYSTEMS AND PRESCRIPTION

Patient evaluation and preprosthetic management

As the level of the amputation becomes progressively higher, the remaining musculature to be used for prosthetic control becomes correspondingly less. However, these remaining functional parts should be put through a rigorous exercise program to ensure that all available motions are optimal for whatever control is feasible.

For the shoulder disarticulation amputee, the motion producing forearm flexion and the terminal device control will be scapular abduction on the amputated side. If an axilla loop is to be used on the nonamputated side, biscapular abduction can be used. Flexion and extension of the shoulder complex on the nonamputated side can be used to assist in flexion of the elbow and terminal device operation. The therapist should plan the exercise program to emphasize elevation and depression of the shoulder on the amputated side for the amputee to lock and unlock the elbow.

For the forequarter amputee, developing maximum range of motion and strength in the remaining shoulder girdle and maximum chest expansion are essential. Both will be required to operate controls if functional prosthetic wear is to be accomplished.

Prosthetic systems

Shoulder disarticulation. During evaluation of the shoulder disarticulation patient, it is generally possible for the clinic team to determine prosthetic acceptance and a specific system most likely to ensure cosmesis and function.

The socket may be of solid construction or a frame construction. The shoulder joint should permit passive flexion and abduction. Because weight and cosmesis are a consideration, a modular endoskeletal upper limb system should be considered for the shoulder disarticulation amputee. In fact, it is at this level that these sys-

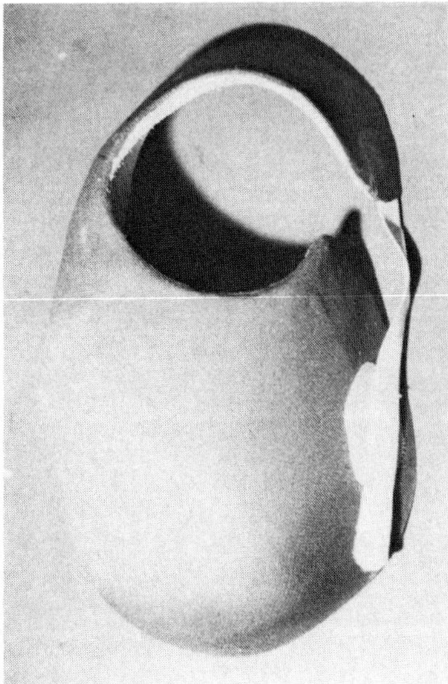

Fig. 13-1. Cosmetic shoulder restoration for forequarter amputation. Modular concept with soft outer cover. This system should serve as patient management tool in determining if additional prosthetic prescription is warranted. Another purpose of this system is to restore body image as a whole and provide cosmesis under clothing.

tems have maximum application, with a weight reduction of approximately 40% and improved cosmesis.

For functional use, a positive-locking elbow with internal cable exit and a lift assembly should be used. The dual control system (one cable, two functions) is normally used. Exceptional cases may require a triple control system. Where insufficient chest expansion precludes the use of a chest strap for locking the elbow, a nudge control is recommended. A perineal strap or waist belt, in conjunction with shoulder elevation, is functional, but the gross movement and discomfort to the amputee minimizes its use.

Forequarter amputation. The interscapulothoracic amputee differs in that the surgical area frequently is extremely sensitive to pressure. The prosthetic socket must be bulkier and less cosmetic than that used for shoulder disarticulation in order to afford suspension and control. The preferred management of this patient involves an initial prosthetic fitting with cosmetic shoulder restoration, using unicellular foams and thermoplastics, since the weight involved is minimal (Fig. 13-1). This prosthesis need not extend to the sound side for suspension; carefully designed webbing should be adequate. Use of this system will prove invaluable in determining the patient's capabilities to tolerate a prosthesis.

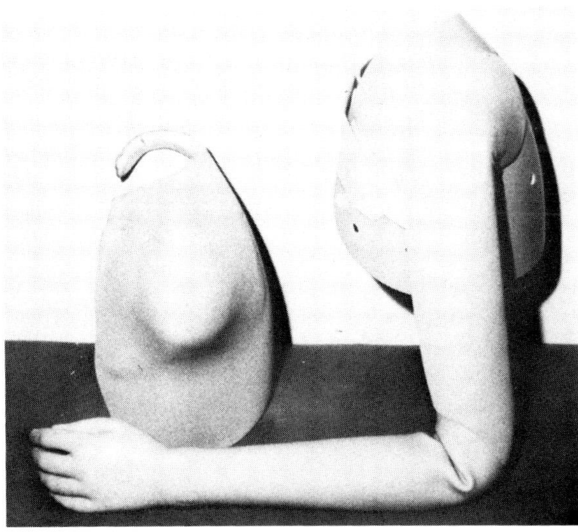

Fig. 13-2. Cosmetic forequarter prosthesis. Modular soft exterior prosthesis. Modular soft exterior with passive shoulder, elbow joints, and hand. Elbow may be positioned in flexion as desired and locked. Hand may be positioned but is nonfunctional. Single strap provides adequate suspension for this lightweight system.

Should prosthetic tolerance be established but with doubtful motor sources available to operate a standard prosthesis, a nonfunctional endoskeletal modular system should be considered (Fig. 13-2). This affords the advantage of light weight and improved cosmesis, a mechanical elbow joint that may be passively positioned, and realistic gloved hand that may be pronated and supinated. The shoulder bulk head in any forequarter or shoulder disarticulation prosthesis should always allow sufficient abduction and adduction to ease donning and doffing of clothing. The shoulder joint should also allow a full range of flexion and extension. A friction or ratchet shoulder joint will provide this range of motion and allow prepositioning. The system may also be designed with a functional cable and harness, controlled elbow and/or terminal device. Although this prosthesis is more cosmetic with its soft outer shell, it generally results in a lower efficiency rating than the standard type.

The interscapulothoracic or forequarter prosthesis differs from a shoulder disarticulation prosthesis in the configuration of the socket, which extends across to the opposite shoulder encircling the neck for suspension. The function of the socket is threefold:

1. Cosmetic restoration of contour for the missing shoulder
2. Provision of point of attachment for the shoulder joint
3. A means of suspension for the prosthesis

The highest possible efficiency should be accomplished by forearm lift assists and teflon-lined cable housings.

It has been our experience that the majority of forequarter amputees reject the prosthesis for a variety of reasons. The functional advantages appear to be outweighed by the difficulty of operation and the inconvenience of wearing the prosthesis. A protective shoulder restoration that allows normal wearing of clothes and affords protection to the amputation site seems to be more desired and acceptable. A custom-made, soft foam restoration held by a chest strap provides these functions in a comfortable. acceptable manner.

External power. External power is an important consideration for prosthetic management at these higher levels of amputation. Because the range of motion available is often limited, the functional value of a body-powered prosthesis for the patient is questionable. The electric-switch control system offers an advantage in that only 1 cm of excursion is required to activate the switch

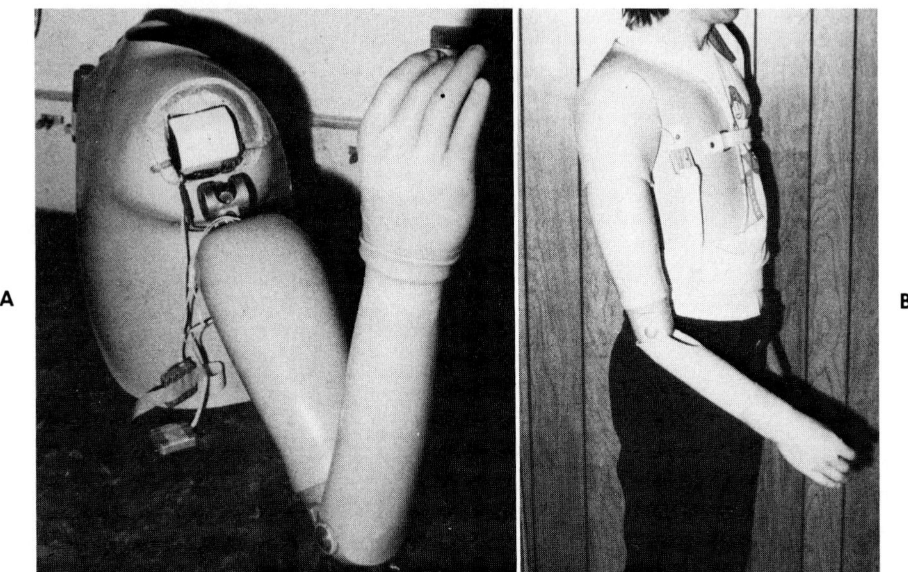

Fig. 13-3. Externally powered forequarter prosthesis. **A,** Two electric switches are designed into system. Anterior switch located in deltopectoral groove controls mechanical elbow and uses shoulder elevation and/or lateral trunk bending. Switch posteriorly controls scapular abduction. Each motion is distinct and therefore unlikely to interfere with each other. **B,** Shoulder bulkhead allows full range of motion. Battery pack is located just proximal to shoulder joint where its weight will be of least significance.

and accomplish many desired functions (Fig. 13-3). In the switch for the electric elbow, the first position is without tension being applied; this will maintain the elbow in any angle of flexion or extension. The first active position provides extension, and pressure on the switch must be maintained to achieve the desired angle.

The next position is neutral, and the elbow stops and locks. The second active position will flex the elbow to the desired angle. The fifth or final position is also neutral, which stops and locks the unit. The elbow is capable of 1 kg live lift and develops a static force in flexion of approximately 100 inch pounds.

The electric-switch controlled hand is generally operated in a similar manner. To date, no electric terminal hook is widely available for patient use. Myoelectric control for wrist disarticulation and below-elbow amputees has reached the stage where components are readily available, and systems are quite reliable. It is hoped that with ongoing research and development, external power will realize its greatest potential for these higher levels of amputation.

One of the more feasible approaches for a high-level amputee uses an electric elbow with a soft forearm shell in conjunction with a standard cable-controlled device. Aluminum terminal device hooks should always be prescribed for shoulder disarticulation and forequarter amputees to minimize the effect of distal weight. This approach does not require the complex motions needed to operate a manual elbow lock. Fabrication of the basic system is generally standard in nature. It is the approach to cabling, electric-switch placement, and control system design that challenges the prosthetist's creativity.

PROSTHETIC TRAINING

When body-powered prostheses are used, the sequence for the training of this level of amputee follows that of the above-elbow amputee. However, additional specific guidelines for basic control motions should be followed.

Forearm control

In shoulder disarticulation, elbow flexion is accomplished by means of scapular abduction. When training the amputee, the therapist manually flexes the forearm to 90 degrees and then calls attention to the cable slack. The amputee then brings his shoulder forward to take up the cable slack. To lower the forearm, the patient returns his shoulder to the starting position.

Elbow lock control

Shoulder elevation is used to control the elbow lock. The therapist manually unlocks the elbow unit. The amputee elevates the shoulder until the lock operates and then relaxes. After this motion has become smooth and controlled, the amputee must learn to combine forearm flexion and the elbow lock operation. The therapist unlocks the elbow and has the amputee flex the forearm to approximately 90 degrees and, while maintaining that flexion, elevate the shoulder to lock the elbow. The amputee then learns to reverse the procedure by unlocking the elbow and smoothly returning the forearm to the starting position.

Terminal device operation

When the elbow is locked, biscapular abduction operates the terminal device. The therapist now has the amputee go through the sequence of flexing the forearm, locking the elbow, and using biscapular abduction, opening the terminal device.

• • •

Training for prosthetic use and activities for daily living are the same as outlined for the below-elbow and above-elbow amputees in Chapters 11 and 12.

Donning and doffing the prosthesis

There are many ways to don and doff the prosthesis. The therapist and patient must develop the technique for each individual.

SUGGESTED READINGS

Anderson, M., Bechtol, C. O., and Sollers, R.: Clinical prosthetics for physicians and therapists, Springfield, Ill., 1959, Charles C Thomas, Publisher.

Santschi, W. R.: Manual of upper extremity prosthetics, Department of Engineering, Los Angeles, 1958, University of California.

Trombley, C., and Scott, A.: Occupational therapy for physical dysfunction, Medfield, Mass., 1975, Fleetwood Publishing Co.

Wellerson, T. L.: A manual for occupational therapists on the rehabilitation of upper extremity amputees, New York, 1958, American Occupational Therapists Association.

CHAPTER 14

The bilateral upper limb amputee

H. RICHARD LEHNEIS
RUTH DICKEY

This chapter is concerned with the unique problems presented by the bilateral upper limb amputee. Although it is generally recognized that the unilateral upper limb amputee uses a prosthesis as an assist and the sound limb for sensory feedback and fine manipulatory activities, the bilateral amputee does not have such a choice. As such, the general principles, preprosthetic training, prosthetic fitting and components, and prosthetic training for the bilateral upper limb amputee differ distinctly from those recognized in managing the unilateral upper limb amputee.

GENERAL PRINCIPLES

The basic objective of prosthetic management of the bilateral upper limb amputee is to provide the patient with maximum function of the prostheses and residual limbs to be independent in the activities of daily living. Throughout this chapter activities of daily living will be used in the broadest sense to include all aspects of functional skills from self-care to vocational pursuits.

To achieve these goals, independence in donning and doffing the prostheses is a necessity. This requires appropriate harnessing, preferably through interconnecting of the harness systems of both prostheses, and a socket design that enhances ease of donning and doffing.

Components

The need for maximizing the range of motion must be met by choosing appropriate components and socket designs and alignment. Generally, bilateral wrist-flexion units are a must, particularly if independence in personal hygiene is to be expected.

The choice of the terminal device should be, with few exceptions, a prosthetic hook. New amputees rarely appreciate the functional advantages of a prosthetic hook over a prosthetic hand. In these circumstances, it must be explained to the amputee that a prosthetic hook is not an attempt to duplicate the form or function of a hand, since it obviously does not look or function like a hand. Rather, the prosthetic hook represents an efficient, built-in tool, containing several functions of commonly used tools (e.g., pliers, tweezers). Once the amputee recognizes and appreciates that the hook is not just a poor replacement of a hand, but a tool, often the acceptance of a prosthetic hook becomes somewhat easier.

A major problem, unique to the bilateral upper limb amputee, is sensory loss once fitted with prostheses. Whenever possible, fitting and socket configuration for these amputees should be such that the prosthesis can be partially removed for sensory feedback through the residual limb and then reapplied. For example, in a prosthesis with a stump-activated elbow-lock control, the socket may be open ended to expose the distal portion of the residual limb for such purposes. To preserve maximum sensory feedback function, it is of utmost importance that the patient be trained not only with the prosthesis but in the use of the residual limbs for as many activities as possible. Although not very popular in this country, the Krukenberg amputation should always be considered as an alternative, particularly for blind amputees.

A final, general consideration relates to the strength and safety of prostheses for bilateral amputees. It should be appreciated that the bilateral amputee does not possess the choice a unilateral amputee possesses, that is, using the sound limb for most activities and a prosthesis as an assist. Practically *all* activities must be performed with the prostheses; thus wear and tear on joints and cables are far greater than for the unilateral amputee. This makes it especially important to provide the greatest degree of reliability and safety through proper choice of strength of material and components in the construction of the prosthesis.

The overall aim of training for the bilateral upper limb amputee is to provide the maximum degree of independence in all activities of daily living, both with and without prosthetic equipment. The final selection of all equipment for the bilateral amputee, both prosthetic and specially adapted or selected equipment, is based on total needs. Those needs are related to medical status, both diagnosis and prognosis, age, sex, intellectual and psychological functioning, social and cultural values, economic status, and general goals.

PREPROSTHETIC MANAGEMENT

Preprosthetic management should include all aspects of care preparatory to, but not directly related to, the use of prosthetic equipment. The crucial role of this preparatory phase should be strongly emphasized from both the physical and psychological points of view. From this phase important information will be derived that is necessary for prosthetic prescription as well as patient readiness. The two main areas of management to be discussed are postoperative therapy, which deals with physical care of the residual limb and residual motions, and preprosthetic evaluation, which will establish a baseline of the amputee's current functional level.

Postoperative therapy

Postoperative therapy, begun as soon as possible after surgery, is directed toward the care of the residual limbs and the strengthening of residual motions, which will be used to control the prostheses and substitute for lost motions. Postoperative treatment is carried out by the occupational and physical therapist.

Maximum active range of motion should be achieved in all remaining joints of the upper limbs to provide adequate excursion for operation of prosthetic equipment. In addition, all bilateral upper limb amputees will need maximum active range of motion of the trunk and lower limbs, particularly at the hip, for flexion and external rotation. For each level of amputation there will be specific exercises related to the parts of the upper limbs to be used for excursion of the prosthetic equipment. For the forequarter amputee, exercises for range concentrate on posture, thoracic mobility, and trunk range. For the shoulder disarticulation amputee, scapular mobility is most crucial. The above-elbow amputee requires maximum shoulder mobility, and the below-elbow amputee requires maximum elbow range and, if possible, maximum forearm rotation. Maintaining and/or increasing range for forearm rotation is vitally important because supination and pronation motions are extremely difficult to incorporate in the prosthesis.

Strengthening is necessary for those motions which are required to power and stabilize prosthetic devices. A total body strengthening program is also indicated to provide the amputee with adequate strength to function without prosthetic devices. Both isotonic and isometric exercises can be used effectively. Isotonic exercises can be in the form of progressive resistive exercises or manual assistance. Proprioceptive neuromuscular facilitation is a particularly effective approach, enabling the therapist to work in diagonal planes, vary the amount of resistance, and key into specific areas of weakness. Isometric exercises are effective in maintaining muscle bulk for stabilization of the arm in the socket of the prosthesis. The stability of the prosthesis depends on both the bulk of the stabilizing musculature and the amputee's ability to voluntarily vary stump configuration. The above-elbow amputee depends on the external rotators and biceps for the stabilization necessary to prevent the prostheses from rotating internally during shoulder flexion and abduction. For the below-elbow amputee the muscles of supination and pronation are effective stabilizers.[2,4]

Massage of the residual limbs improves circulation, reduces edema, keeps the skin mobile, prevents adhesions, and begins the toughening process necessary to protect the limb during use. This technique reduces the amputee's fear of having the residual limbs handled.[3,7]

Maximum shrinkage should occur before fitting

the socket. Although shrinkage varies with all amputees, from 2 to 3 months to 1 year or more, with an adequate postoperative program fitting can usually be considered after 2 to 3 months.[3] Elastic shrinkers and techniques using elastic bandages have been found to be successful for shrinking and shaping.[2] The elastic shrinker provides the most consistent pressure; however, caution must be taken so that the shrinker does not slide down the arm producing a tourniquet effect. On short above-elbow amputations, suspension systems are sometimes required for the shrinker to remain in place. If supervision is inadequate, this is the safest method.[3] The use of an elastic bandage wrapping offers the therapist more control over both pressure and shaping. Wrapping techniques for the short above-elbow limb frequently require use of the opposite axilla. A conical shape is preferred for the above-elbow amputation and a screwdriver shape for below the elbow. The latter preserves maximum use of residual rotation. Again, care must be taken in wrapping so as not to produce proximal pressure, which would impair desired shaping, increase edema, and reduce circulation. Residual limb shrinkage, using a plaster of Paris bandage, has also been reported effective when dealing with fatty or edematous stumps. With this method the plaster bandage is applied and suspended from a conventional harness. As shrinkage occurs, new bandages are applied.[7]

Most amputees have phantom sensation, the sensation of the presence of their missing limbs. The hands are usually felt more distinctly and over a longer period of time. Usually the sensation diminishes within a year and generally does not interfere with training.

Phantom pain is felt as cramping, burning, or lancinating. Cramping is frequently relieved by massage, vibration, or electrical stimulation. Burning pain, although uncommon, often requires drug intervention. Much treatment has been unsuccessful. Lancinating pain is most frequently caused by a neuroma and is sometimes treated by cold, vibration, or electrical stimulation. Surgical removal of the neuroma may be required.[3]

Immediate or early postoperative fitting

Immediate postoperative fitting of the upper limb amputee has come about as a result of the success of this kind of fitting for the lower limb amputee. Results of both immediate fitting (application of a rigid surgical dressing with a terminal device at the time of surgery or in the immediate postoperative period when the sutures are still in place) and early fitting (application after suture removal)[2] of the prosthetic equip-

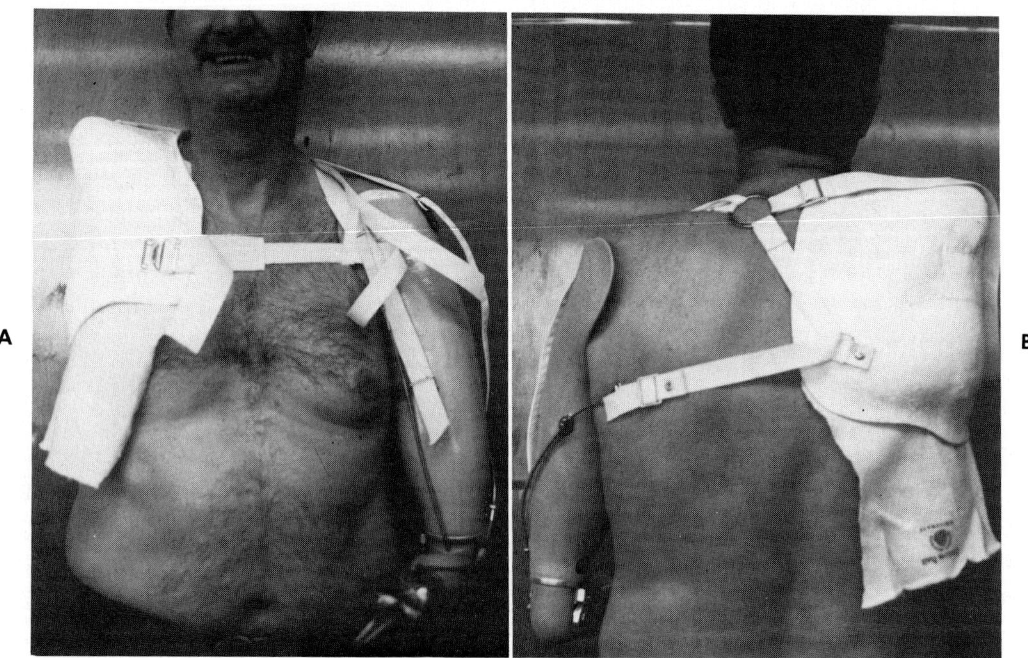

Fig. 14-1. Front view (**A**) and rear view (**B**) of patient fitted with one functional prosthesis and test socket, allowing earlier independence in activities of daily living.

ment have been similar to those for lower limb amputees: (1) reduction in postoperative pain, (2) more rapid prosthetic use (and thereby less dependency for some activities of daily living), (3) good psychological adjustment, (4) reduced postsurgical edema, (5) more rapid limb desensitization, and (6) rapid healing.[1-3,6,8] Overall hospitalization time is often significantly reduced.

In both techniques, the amputee has the terminal device mounted in the plaster of Paris socket, and the harness system is adjustable for individual needs. As shrinkage occurs, a new socket is fabricated. The difference between the fittings is that the immediate fitting is not removable, whereas the early fitting socket is. With these techniques the training process precedes the fitting of permanent prosthetic equipment. Proponents of these techniques believe that this facilitates the usual necessary adjustments in the harnessing system and design of the trial prosthesis. Also, the amputee learns early the components of the prosthesis and how to use them in activities of daily living, rather than initially using adapted devices and then having to change or modify the process when the permanent equipment is delivered.[1]

Another reason for using these early fitting techniques is to counteract the high rejection rate of prosthetic equipment use noted in the unilateral amputee. The longer he relies only on the sound arm for accomplishing functional activities, the less likely the amputee is to make good functional use of the prosthesis.[5]

The most obvious candidates for immediate or early fitting are bilateral upper limb amputees. This group is the most profoundly dependent in all activities. The sooner some of this dependency can be reduced, the sooner they are relieved of some of their frustration and fear of uselessness. Even the fitting of one limb can be of significant help, especially in allowing some independence for self-care such as eating and toileting (Fig. 14-1).

Early performance of activities of daily living

A program to give the bilateral amputee some degree of independence in activities of daily living should always be initiated early. This can be done in two ways: (1) by beginning to do some activities with the remaining limbs (both upper residual limbs and lower limbs) and (2) by the use of adaptive equipment. This begins to introduce the problem-solving process and decreases feelings of inadequacy and dependency. Principles of special device application are given in the discussion on training (Chapter 29).

Preprosthetic evaluation

It is vital to have a coordinated total team effort in the rehabilitation of the bilateral amputee, beginning with the postoperative period and throughout the rehabilitation program. The professional team should consist of the surgeon or physiatrist, prosthetist, rehabilitation nurse, occupational and physical therapists, psychologist, social worker, and vocational counselor. Equally important members of this team are the amputee family, and friends. All the members are required for their particular expertise in providing physical care, equipment, training, future planning, and follow-up. The contributions of both the prosthetist and occupational therapist are specifically discussed in relation to the equipment, treatment, and training in the remainder of this chapter.

Preprosthetic evaluation is completed prior to the prescription of the prosthetic equipment. It provides an updated account of the amputee's physical and psychological status and gives information that helps determine further therapy needed and helps make the proper choice of prosthetic equipment. The occupational therapy preprosthetic evaluation includes the following data:

I. Demographic
II. Diagnostic
   A. Diagnosis
   B. Date and etiology of amputations
   C. Date of most recent surgical procedures
   D. Dominance
III. Physical status
   A. Body mobility and awareness
   B. Passive range of motion
   C. Manual muscle strength (with emphasis on musculature to be used as control motions for prosthetic equipment)
   D. Functional motion strength (which tests motions of the body taking into specific consideration the combinations of muscular action in functional positions)[11]
   E. General coordination
   F. Endurance
IV. Residual limb descriptors
   A. Classification of amputation levels
   B. Limb shapes
   C. Limb volume measurements. Note the method of shrinkage used, and date, if applicable, of its discontinuation
   D. Skin condition

V. Sensory status
  A. Phantom limb pain
  B. Phantom limb sensation (with description of how the missing limbs are perceived)
  C. Tactile sensibility (emphasizing areas that will be in contact with the harness or socket)
  D. Position sense
VI. Current status of activities of daily living
  A. Information on level of activities of daily living independence using prior prosthetic equipment, if applicable
  B. Extent of use of residual motions for substitution of missing limbs, including specific foot usage
  C. Self-care (eating, dressing, grooming, personal hygiene)
  D. Communication skills
  E. Vocational status
  F. Leisure time activities
  G. Social skills
VII. Equipment expectations
  A. Functional
  B. Cosmetic
VIII. Recommendations
  A. Type of prosthesis
  B. Type of adaptive devices for activities of daily living with and without prosthetic equipment
  C. Prefitting therapy (recommendations, which can in most instances be carried out concurrently with the fabrication of the prosthesis)
    1. Maximum range of motion of joints through the body to provide for activities that require skilled motions of the head, neck, trunk, and lower limbs. Wherever possible, hypermobility is of advantage, especially at the hips
    2. General conditioning to strengthen all functional body motions and increase endurance and body mobility
    3. General body mechanics program and balancing exercises
    4. Postural exercises in instances where the amputee's habitual posture would decrease efficient use of prosthetic equipment
    5. Shrinkage and shaping techniques
    6. Foot usage techniques (in our experience, some degree of foot usage has been necessary for independence for all levels of bilateral amputees)
    7. Activities of daily living without prosthetic equipment
  D. Recommendations for further evaluation
  E. Training time anticipated (Although this may be difficult to estimate completely, it is sometimes necessary for coverage purposes. It has been our experience that training time varies greatly for each amputee and depends very much on individual complications encountered during training. The least amount of time experienced for training was 1 month, and the most was 5 months.)

PROSTHETIC FITTING AND COMPONENTS

The bilateral below-elbow amputee

In general, all below-elbow sockets for bilateral amputees should be designed so as to enhance easy donning and doffing, as well as to permit maximum range of residual motion. It is for this reason that the Muenster socket is contraindicated.

For wrist disarticulation and the long and medium-length below-elbow amputation, a conventional socket is indicated with a sufficiently low anterior trim line to permit full range of elbow flexion. Particular attention should be paid to an intimate interface between the residual limb and the socket to take full advantage of any residual pronation and supination. A screwdriver-shape cross section in the distal area will permit most efficient transmission of residual pronation and supination to the prosthesis. Flexible elbow hinges attached to the triceps pad are required for socket suspension, and to permit pronation and supination.

For shorter amputation levels without residual pronation and supination, a socket that encompasses the medial and lateral epicondyles is indicated so that any force applied mediolaterally to the prosthesis will not cause displacement of the socket or at least minimize displacement on the residual limb. Depending on the anticipated activity of the patient, the socket is either connected to flexible hinges and a triceps pad or metal elbow hinges, either of the single or polycentric type, that are attached to a half cuff. This will reduce socket displacement on the residual limb to a minimum when external loads are applied to the prosthetic forearm. The choice of which elbow hinge to use depends on the residual limb level and the activity of the patient and working environment. Functionally, the shorter the residual limb, the greater the indication for a polycentric elbow hinge so that prosthetic and anatomical joint congruity can be approached as closely as possible. On the other hand, polycentric hinges are more likely to require frequent maintenance, particularly in certain industrial environments, whereas the single-pivot hinge is sturdier and requires less maintenance.

For the very short below-elbow amputation, a

split socket with the elbow hinges attached to the half cuff is indicated. Although this results in a reduction of force that can be transmitted to the forearm, it is deemed far more important to provide full range of motion. It is, however, possible to increase the forearm lift force by using a split housing so that shoulder flexion and/or scapular abduction help to flex the forearm. In this instance, the residual limb is simply used to stabilize the forearm in the desired degree of elbow flexion. Very short residual below-elbow limbs with limited range of motion and/or hypersensitive areas may be fitted with a stump-activated elbow lock that uses the residual limb to trip a lever, which locks or unlocks an external elbow lock hinge. A preferred way of using the stump-activated elbow lock is to adapt the locking lever to a U-shaped configuration that may fit in pressure-tolerant areas, thus avoiding any sensitive areas. A further advantage is that it exposes a larger residual limb area for sensory feedback, especially when the forearm is flexed.

As previously discussed, for the greatest degree of universality of function a hook terminal device is preferred over a prosthetic hand, although a prosthetic hand may be used interchangeably for certain social activities or professions. The choice of a prosthetic hook should be considered in accordance with those described in Chapter 9, Section III.

The type of wrist component indicated depends on residual limb length. For wrist disarticulation and medium or long below-elbow amputations, a built-in wrist flexion unit may be used. The axis of rotation of the wrist flexion unit should be aligned so that it forms a 45-degree angle with the elbow flexion axis when placed on the prosthetic forearm in the medial-volar quadrant. For high-level below-elbow amputations, when there is no residual pronation or supination, a separate Sierra wrist flexion unit should be installed on a constant friction wrist. This permits variable angulations of the wrist flexion unit in the constant friction wrist. When the patient's elbow flexion range is limited, the wrist flexion unit should be installed directly distal to the end of the residual limb. This increases the radius of the flexion arc described by the terminal device in the various flexion positions of the flexion unit, thus increasing the effective range of operation of the terminal device in space. This is especially important for activities near the body midline, such as personal hygiene.

In general, the forearm of all below-elbow prostheses, but especially for the bilateral amputee, should be aligned with regard to the socket in such a way that it favors an alignment that brings the terminal device closer to the center of the body and forward and upward. The forward-upward alignment maybe as much as 30 degrees, simulating normal elbow flexion alignment in the sagittal plane. The inward (toward the center) alignment should be as much as cosmetically possible. Particular attention should be paid to the very short below-elbow residual limbs because such limbs accentuate the normal carrying angle in the frontal plane. Thus a forearm aligned coincident with the center of a very short residual limb would fall way short in bringing the terminal device toward the center of the body and thus would greatly diminish the function of the prosthesis, particularly with regard to personal hygiene.

Harnessing for the bilateral below-elbow amputee is rather simple. Both prostheses are interconnected by running the control attachment strap to the front support strap of the opposite prosthesis. They are sewn together in the center line of the back or they may run to a center ring. This arrangement assures independent use of each prosthesis.

The bilateral above-elbow amputee

The medium or long above-elbow residual limb may be fitted best with a low lateral socket wall such as developed by McLaurin. The anterior and posterior wings of the socket should extend sufficiently to stabilize the prosthesis against axial rotation. Angulation osteotomy of the humerus, as developed by Marquardt, gives the best rotational control is achieved. Internal or external rotation is thus transferred most effectively to the prosthesis. In this case, the socket proximal trim line can be considerably shorter than in the conventional design. Shorter amputation levels must be fitted with more conventional socket designs. The shorter the amputation level, the higher the socket trim line must extend, particularly the posterior and anterior wings. This is necessary to provide adequate control against longitudinal rotation as well as to provide suspension.

As previously discussed, if wrist flexion units are used, they should be of the Sierra type. The built-in wrist flexion unit does not provide sufficient range of motion for the same reason described for the short below-elbow unit. The choice of a terminal device should be determined in accordance with the characteristics described for each type in Chapter 9, Section IV. Conventional elbow joints with alternating locks and a friction-controlled turntable for internal-external rotation are standard components to be used. A humeral rotation lock may be indicated when positive locking of internal and external rotation of the elbow and forearm on the humeral section is required for certain vocational and avocational tasks. Although most levels of above-elbow amputations may be fitted with prostheses with dual control cables, the short and very short above-elbow prosthesis may require a cable excursion recovery unit. This unit is designed to take up the slack produced in the cable after the elbow is flexed and locked, so that the same excursion used to provide elbow flexion can also be used after the elbow is locked to provide control of the terminal device.

Normally, no deviation from standard alignment is necessary; however, when excursion is limited, alignment of the forearm and wrist unit similar to that described for the below-elbow amputee will enhance function. Another alignment consideration is for those amputees who are wheelchair bound. In this case, the length and alignment of the humeral section should be such as to be compatible with the armrests of the wheelchair. In all other cases, whenever the length of the residual limb permits, the humeral section should be lengthened and the forearm section shortened, while retaining the overall desired length. This shortens the distal lever arm, bringing the center of gravity of the forearm closer to the elbow, and thus reduces the force required to flex the elbow. Such a differential in forearm length from the normal is approximately 3 to 4 cm. Any further reduction of the forearm length would diminish the ability of the patient to reach all facial and head areas.

The principle of harnessing the bilateral above-elbow is similar to that described for the bilateral below-elbow, that is, the control attachment strap of one prosthesis is connected to or serves as the front suspension strap of the contralateral prosthesis, thus assuring independence of control. The elbow control strap and the lateral suspension straps are attached in the conventional manner.

Bilateral shoulder disarticulation

One should appreciate that today this amputation level is best served by the use of externally energized prostheses, such as a myoelectric or switch-controlled electric elbow or terminal device. Only conventional, nonpowered means of prosthetics management for the bilateral shoulder disarticulation amputee are discussed here, since externally energized prostheses are not universally available. Furthermore, some clinicians and amputees are willing to sacrifice a certain amount of function as a trade-off for the simplicity and lighter weight afforded by conventional prostheses.

If the patient is to be fitted with functional prostheses bilaterally, the conventional shoulder disarticulation socket configuration is indicated. If, however, only one side is to be fitted with a functional prosthesis, and the contralateral side is to be used as an anchor for harnessing, a much smaller socket configuration on the control side may suffice. A common problem in this situation is upward migration of the socket on the control side. This may be reduced by either a waist belt or a perineal strap. If so desired, a cosmetic prosthesis may also be attached to the control socket.

Indications for the various components are the same as described for the bilateral above-elbow amputee. Additionally, however, an excursion amplifier cable control system is often required for patients who have sufficient strength but reduced excursion to achieve full range of elbow flexion and terminal device operation. This may be preferable or used in lieu of the cable excursion recovery unit because it is simpler and does not require any special modification to the elbow mechanism, as is necessary with the cable recovery unit. Various passive, free, or friction-controlled shoulder joints are available. Those which provide motion about at least a shoulder abduction axis are indicated. If, additionally, a shoulder flexion joint is used, it must have a 180-degree extension stop to prevent shoulder hyperextension during operation of the cable control system.

Others

Other than the shoulder joint, alignment of the bilateral shoulder disarticulation prosthesis is identical to that described for the bilateral above-elbow amputee. Alignment of the shoulder joint should be such that the flexion axis is skewed internally with respect to the frontal plane; that is, it should form an angle of 30 degrees with respect to the sagittal plane.

Control harnessing for functional bilateral shoulder disarticulation amputees requires great care. The control attachment straps should be attached somewhat superior to the posteroinferior border of the socket, so that they cross each other at an angle; otherwise they may get caught on one another during operation. Furthermore, inadvertent operation may result, the closer the control attachment straps approach a horizontal matching alignment. An elastic cross-back strap connecting the posteroinferior corners of the socket and a nonelastic chest strap are required to stabilize the sockets against each other and to provide an intimate interface between the socket and the patient. The front support straps are also attached to the posteroinferior corners of the socket. If excursion and/or strength are inadequate to provide full range of motion, unilateral or bilateral perineal straps may be used, since they will provide the necessary strength and excursion capability. Elbow lock control is provided either through the attachment of the elbow lock control cable to a waist belt, which allows shoulder elevation to alternately lock or unlock the elbow, or a nudge control unit.

Bilateral forequarter amputees are best managed prosthetically through the use of external energy, which is described in Chapter 9. If, however, such technology is not available in the patient's environment, some function may be obtained through the fitting of conventionally controlled prostheses through the use of perineal straps and nudge controls for the elbow locks.

Mixed bilateral upper limb amputation levels must be treated by combining the fitting principles described for the various levels of amputation.

PROSTHETIC TRAINING

As previously stated, the overall aim of prosthetic training for the adult bilateral upper limb amputee is to provide the maximum degree of independence in all activities of daily living, both with and without prosthetic equipment. The bilateral upper limb amputee depends significantly more on prosthetic and other assistive/adaptive devices and the ability to skillfully use residual body parts and motions. Therefore a framework for skill acquisition is recommended. In following such a framework, there is no intent to force the amputee into a rigid premeditated program. On the contrary, it has proven to be a highly successful means of teaching the basic skills of prosthetic control, as well as providing a logical means of meeting the specific needs of each amputee. Although a certain amount of trial and error is necessary, a framework reduces unnecessary frustration, time, and energy. Both the amputee and therapist have clear guidelines for monitoring progress and establishing ongoing goals.

The training period provides time for ongoing evaluation of prescribed prosthetic and assistive devices from a mechanical and functional point of view. A sound liaison between the prosthetist and occupational therapist permits exchange of information about functional performance with the prosthesis, and allows time for revisions, if necessary. Reevaluation by the entire team should occur periodically.

Mention should be made of the importance of a positive working relationship between the amputee and the therapist. Training for the upper limb amputee requires the best possible collaboration of trainer skill and ingenuity and amputee motivation and ingenuity. The therapist must identify those interests and needs which will create motivation to learn in the amputee. The therapist's ability to motivate the amputee directly and to explain the importance of training related to individual needs is crucial for building successful cooperation.[3] For the adult, motivation usually depends on one or more of the following: a desire for independence in activities of daily living; cosmesis, especially related to social and/or vocational activities; securing or returning to employment; and participation in leisure time activities.[9]

The therapist must have full knowledge of current prosthetic equipment, control motions of operation, and mechanical and functional characteristics of components. This should be combined with a sound background in upper limb anatomy and kinesiology. Much of the actual training is identical to that of the unilateral amputee, and the therapist should be familiar with those principles and techniques. Also necessary are skills in practical problem solving and a knowledge of factors that affect learning.[9]

The amputee should continue a general conditioning program concurrent with any other treatment and prosthetic training. The general conditioning program should continue until such time as the use of prosthetic and other equipment and the use of residual body motions for daily needs can maintain that same conditioning. If the amputee is largely accomplishing the functional activities of dressing, grooming, personal hygiene, and eating, those needs are probably being met.

Training process

The process described includes four areas of training necessary for the transmission of basic information, acquisition of the skills of prosthetics operation, and methods to deal with special needs. Only the process itself will be defined and outlined; no attempt will be made to provide step-by-step instruction in the techniques themselves.

The four areas of training are orientation and initial checkout, controls training, skills training, and functional activity.

Orientation and initial checkout. A clear explanation of the amputee's training needs should be given, goals should be identified and/or reviewed, cooperation elicited, and mutual goals set. As a result of the fitting sessions during fabrication of the prostheses, the amputee is often somewhat familiar with the equipment before beginning training. The therapist, however, should not assume this.

Since much of the training will be difficult and sometimes frustrating, the need for maximum-functioning prosthetic equipment is increased. Therefore an initial checkout of the equipment for fit and function is completed at the time of delivery to ensure maximum comfort and mechanical operation. The checkout of fit includes evaluation of optimum harnessing system placement and socket comfort and fit. Mechanical function checkout evaluates range of motion, cable system operation, control system efficiency, wrist and wrist flexion unit operation, and terminal device operation. Factors are more often identified during the training process since they relate to the kinds and amounts of stress each amputee develops in using the equipment. Any changes that might increase mechanical function should be completed before proceeding with prosthetic training. Checkout of an informal nature should be an innate and ongoing part of the training. Major changes, of course, require more formalized checkout.

Instruction in the nomenclature of the equipment is begun during the orientation and frequently reviewed so that the amputee becomes familiar with the specific terminology necessary for discussion of the equipment. This will ultimately be most important when making appointments for adjustments or repairs. Instruction is also accomplished in the dos and don'ts of physical care of the prostheses. Often the terminology and care instruction can be given together.

Instruction in skin care provides the amputee with information regarding the need for and the kind of protection from the prostheses and harnessing system the skin will require to prevent irritation and pressure. This includes residual limb and skin hygiene and padding requirements for protection and perspiration absorption. Areas of potential pressure and irritation are defined. Direction for general visual examination of the residual limbs and other potential areas of irritation are given to all amputees, as well as specific directions for situations in which sensory impairments prohibit total feedback.

Written instructions referring to specific needs are provided, along with pictures (line drawings) illustrating nomenclature, skin care, and prosthetic equipment. Both written and verbal data should be provided in a language that is easily understood. This may require the use of an interpreter for trainees whose preferred language differs from that of the clinician.

Controls training. Controls training entails teaching methods of donning and doffing the prostheses and the control motions required for prosthetic equipment operation. This phase of training, although closely connected to an often combined with skills training, is treated separately for the bilateral amputee. This is because he typically needs to learn the more complicated control motions associated with either cross controlling harnessing systems or two control systems necessitated by mixed levels of amputations.[6] Full concentration is given to teaching necessary body control motions with minimal exaggerated motion and energy expenditure. Auditory and visual cues substitute for loss of or limitation in availability of sensory feedback (Chapter 17).

Below-elbow amputees. Donning and doffing are accomplished using one of two methods: either over the head or coat application. Removal is accomplished so as to place the prostheses in position for redonning.

Controls training for terminal device operation in space requires shoulder flexion and scapular abduction for both single and dual control systems. Passive prepositioning is needed for control of the wrist unit and wrist flexion unit.

Above-elbow amputees. Donning and doffing are accomplished by a modified method using additional support and stabilization under the elbow. Doffing again places the prostheses in position for redonning.

Controls training for terminal device operation and control of elbow motion and elbow mechanism is shoulder flexion and scapular abduction. For elbow lock it is shoulder depression, extension, and abduction in a dual control system. Terminal device operation in space requires skillful use of the elbow locking-unlocking mechanism, a control often requiring increased practice for skill, reliability, and efficiency. Auditory feedback can be specifically helpful in the training for use of the elbow lock mechanism. Passive prepositioning is needed for wrist rotation, wrist flexion, and elbow rotation.

Shoulder disarticulation and forequarter ampu-

tees. Donning and doffing require a supporting surface for stabilization both when positioning the thorax in the prostheses and while fastening the chest strap. External adaptations are frequently required for attaching the strap because of the size, weight, and reduced reaching range of the prostheses. Doffing requires a support surface to stabilize for chest-strap release and for placement for redonning as previously described.

Control motions for the shoulder disarticulation for terminal device operation and control of elbow motion is scapular abduction. Elbow mechanism control with a waist strap is scapular elevation, with a perineal strap, trunk elevation, or with a chin nudge. Passive prepositioning is needed for wrist rotation, wrist flexion, elbow rotation, and shoulder motions.

Forequarter prostheses offer such little functional replacement that external power becomes necessary (Chapter 9).

The time necessary to learn control motions varies significantly from individual to individual. Some learn the controls in the first few minutes after donning the prostheses, whereas others require concentrated practice. Progression to skills training does require a general degree of reliable terminal device operation, elbow control, and prepositioning ability with minimal energy expenditure and exaggerated use of either the body or prostheses. The refining of these motions can be accomplished as training proceeds. Ultimately the decision to move into that phase is made by the therapist.[6]

Skills training. The criterion for skillful use of the prostheses is to achieve as near normal function as can replicate normal limbs doing similar activity.[9] The third phase of training incorporates the amputee's previously learned control motions, skill, and functional understanding of the prostheses with the principles of proper prepositioning and object stability. This can be accomplished using training devices geared for increased difficulty and specific skill acquisition. Practice focus changes from concentration on the control motions themselves to control motions for purposeful static and dynamic positioning, prehension, and manipulation. The use of training devices allows this practice while separating achievement of quality performance from the completion of functional activity. Very often the amputee attaches too much initial importance to the skilled accomplishment of functional tasks and when unable to meet those expectations feels defeated and discouraged. The use of training devices permits sequential building and mastering of skills for easier transition to functional tasks.

Correct terminal device prepositioning is the key to successful use for functional activity. For the bilateral amputee this requires passive positioning of both the wrist unit for supination and pronation and the wrist flexion unit allowing positioning close to the body for self-care. Prepositioning is accomplished using the body, other ob-

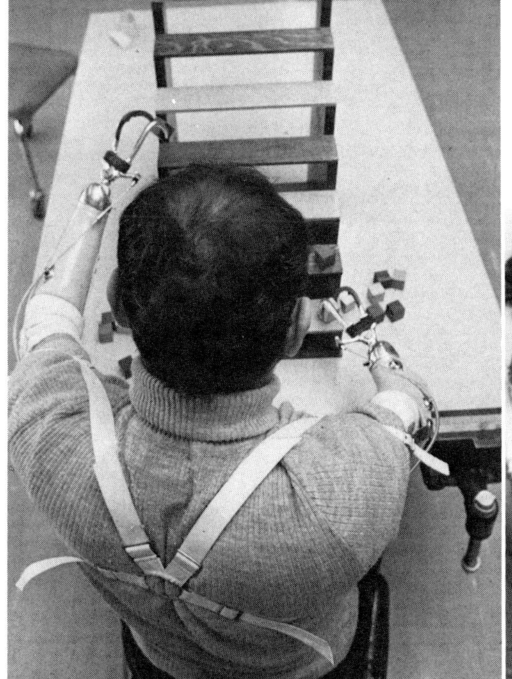

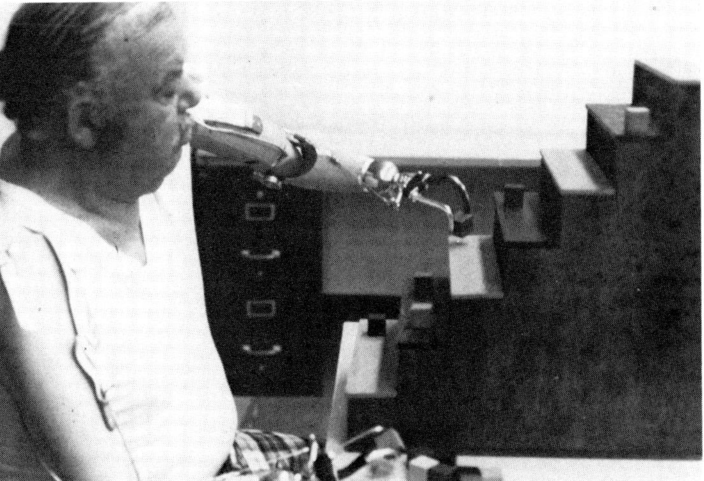

Fig. 14-2. Skill training exercise directed toward teaching bilateral upper limb amputee adjustment of body position to prevent inadvertent overflow between harnessing systems.

jects in the environment, or with the opposite prosthesis. The number and kind of drills used is specific to individual need. Most drills are directed initially toward learning the principles of approach, grasp, and release.

For the majority of bilateral amputees, the prostheses are interconnected by their harness systems so that motion in one system produces motion in the other. Specific training is directed toward adjustment of body position to prevent inadvertent overflow between systems (Fig. 14-2). The importance of this is most obviously seen in the use of one prosthesis in a static holding position while using the other dynamically.[9]

Dominance is usually established in the limb with the most residual motion. Unless there are complications, in limbs of equal length dominance remains with the preferred limb. An exception to this may be the individual with exceptional skill who chooses to use a much shorter, but preferred limb, rather than to change dominance. Choice of dominance is usually made when the amputee is performing activities without the prostheses; however, if no preference is shown, the skills training usually establishes dominance.

Functional activity. The beginning of the bonding of skillful prosthetic control with functional activity is based on the readiness of the amputee. General guidelines for determination of readiness can be established by observing how skillfully the principles of use are applied, the normalization of body motions, the time necessary to complete a task, and the amount of energy being expended.[9] Also to be considered in making this determination is noting when the control motion execution is more automatic and secondary in the amputee's concentration. The therapist's skillful choice between devices for learning skills versus those for learning functional tasks helps the amputee view progress more clearly and decreases frustration.

Functional training in activities of daily living can begin soon after basic skills have been achieved. Alternation between both types of activities bonds the functional task and skills more quickly, principally by permitting immediate feedback. Although functional training in activities of daily living has been going on concurrently in alternative forms, the initiation of these activities with prosthetic equipment focuses anew the importance of considering the needs and goals of the individual.

Certainly, it would be impossible in a training period to accomplish all the activities that would be needed by the amputee from that day forth; however, with bilateral amputees, it is often necessary to cover more of the actual activities, especially those requiring special techniques or adaptive equipment. Tasks that most notably decrease the amputee's dependence on others for personal care should be initiated first. The following list includes a general order of the sequence and areas of focus for activities of daily living:

1. *Self care.* Eating, grooming, dressing, bathing, and personal hygiene.
2. *Communication skills.* Writing, telephone use, operation of recording devices, handling books, magazines, papers, etc., typing, and general office skills.
3. *Homemaking.* Cooking, cleaning, washing, ironing, general housekeeping chores, and baby care.
4. *Social skills and avocational interests.* Evaluation of the pursuit of former interests and exploration of new interests. Social skills that relate to the individual's life-style and interests.
5. *Prevocational and vocational exploration.* Evaluation of skills in relation to previous work and/or exploration of new vocational possibilities. As skills improve, the vocational counselor will be able to more accurately assist in this phase. Follow-up as relates to the job may be necessary for adaptations and/or general work setup.
6. *Mobility.* Driving and the use of public transportation.

The use of a checklist is recommended to ensure that all areas of necessary and desired training have been covered. A final checkout on completion of training provides discharge information on equipment, fit, and function. It is recommended that a final checkout accompany the summary of final function, special devices provided, and recommendations for follow-up.

Special devices

Almost without exception, all bilateral upper limb amputees require some special selection of existing equipment and/or the adaptation of devices to meet their needs, both with and without prosthetic devices. Training would be incomplete without a more specific discussion of the role of assistive/adaptive equipment.*

*Assistive/adaptive equipment is "a special device which assists in the performance of self/care, work or play/leisure activities or physical exercise." (From American Occupational Therapy Association official glossary, Jan., 1976.)

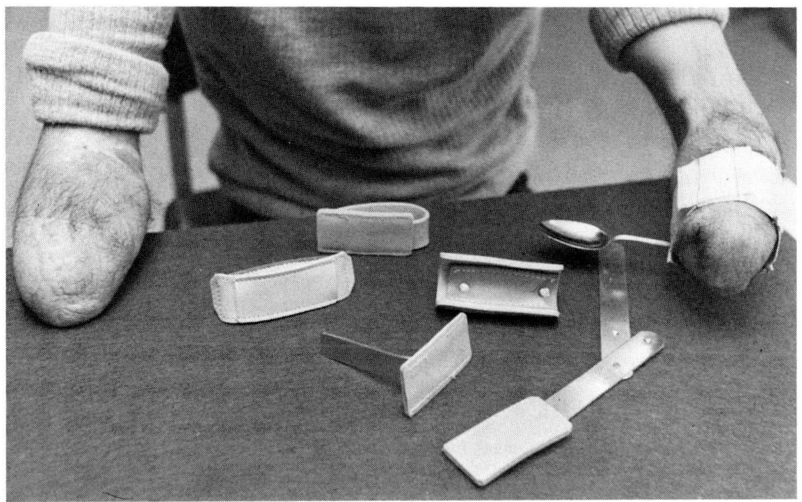

Fig. 14-3. Universal component system used to substitute for partial or complete loss of hand and arm function. (Components designed by the Occupational Therapy Department, Institute of Rehabilitation Medicine, New York University Medical Center, New York.)

Assistive/adaptive equipment is provided with the same basic considerations as previously discussed for the selection of prosthetic equipment, covering medical, psychological-intellectual, social, and economic status. Over the years the old trial and error methods have given way to more sophisticated application of devices due to advances in the following areas:

1. Evaluation techniques used to analyze motions both of normal activities and individual function
2. Increases in technical development of devices, both mechanical and electronic
3. Increased availability of commercial devices to meet varied needs
4. Increased sophistication of materials used in device construction[10]

With regard to all of these considerations, the occupational therapist must have knowledge and skill in the following areas as they relate to device application and construction:

1. Evaluation is conducted in two ways: (1) by the analysis of normal motions and forces involved in activities of daily living and (2) the evaluation of individual limitations through a functional motion test. Thus by knowing the motions required for a specific task it is possible to take into account individual limitations and determine what activities will require assistance and/or substitution.[11]

2. Awareness of commercially available equipment, both adapted or specifically suited to meet individual needs. Prefabricated equipment or component systems frequently save significant time and money for the patient and allow the therapist time to devote to other problem-solving needs that cannot be met by commercially constructed devices. Fig. 14-3 shows parts of the Universal component system that can substitute for loss of hand function.

3. A knowledge of how to design, construct, and fit adapted devices for individual needs. This is necessary when commercial devices are either unavailable or too costly. Training the patient in the use of special devices requires knowledge of the mechanical operation of the device itself and control motions required by the patient. The therapist must also be skilled in troubleshooting and problem solving.

4. Finally, the therapist must be able to estimate potential for device use based on psychological and social factors.[12]

All of these areas apply to devices in general. For the bilateral amputee, the therapist must apply the principles both with and without prosthetic equipment. This requires the therapist to be fully aware of the functional abilities of both the individual and the prostheses.

The principles of motion economy and energy conservation apply to the execution of all activity for environmental organization and individual task setup. A good general guideline to follow is an arrangement whereby maximum independence is achieved with the least amount of time, number of steps, energy expended, and equipment necessary.

The use of electronic technology in rehabilitation has added another dimension in devices to increase independence for the very severely disabled amputee through systems devoted to environmental control. Through these environmental control systems it becomes possible to operate various appliances (lights, telephone, alarm systems, intercom, television, electric bed controls, door locks and openers, drapery pulls, etc.) in a living or work area by using residual control motions to operate sensitive microswitches, pneumatic switches, or voice-actuated controls.

REFERENCES

1. Bailey, R. B.: An upper extremity training arm, Am. J. Occup. Ther. **24:5**, 357, 1970.
2. Bender, L. F.: Prostheses and rehabilitation after arm amputation, Springfield, Ill., 1974, Charles C Thomas, Publisher.
3. Friedman, L. W.: Rehabilitation of amputees. In Licht, S., editor: Rehabilitation and medicine, New Haven, Conn., 1968, S. Licht, Publisher.
4. Gullickson, G., Jr.: Exercise for amputees. In Licht, S., editor: Therapeutic exercise, New Haven, Conn., 1961, S. Licht, Publisher.
5. Laughlin, E., Stanford, J. W., and Phelps, M.: Immediate postsurgical prosthetics fitting of a bilateral below elbow amputee, a report, Artif. Limbs **12**:17, 1968.
6. Reyburn, T. V.: A method of early prosthetics training for upper-extremity amputees, Artif. Limbs **15**(2):1, 1971.
7. Santschi, W. R., and Winston, M. P., editors: Manual of upper extremity prosthetics, Los Angeles, 1958, University of California School of Medicine.
8. Sarmiento, A., McCollough, N. C., III, Williams, E. M., and Sinclair, W. F.: Immediate postsurgical prosthesis fitting in the management of upper extremity amputees, Artif. Limbs **12**(1):14, 1968.
9. Upper-extremity prosthetics, New York, 1971, New York University, Post-Graduate Medical School, Prosthetics and Orthotics.
10. Zimmerman, M. E.: The role of special equipment in the rehabilitation of the injured spinal cord. In Cull, J. G., and Nardy, R. E., editors: Physical medicine and rehabilitation approaches in spinal cord injury, Springfield, Ill., 1977. Charles C Thomas, Publisher.
11. Zimmerman, M. E.: The functional motion test as an evaluation tool for patients with lower motor neuron disturbances, Am. J. Occup. Ther. **23**(9):1, 1969.
12. Zimmerman, M. E.: Analysis of adapted equipment. Part II, Am. J. Occup. Ther. **11:4**, 1957.

CHAPTER 15

Special procedures in upper limb amputation surgery

ALFRED E. KRITTER

The wide variation of disability in upper extremity amputees depends on many factors, including the level of amputation, multimembral involvement, age, trainability, and general medical status. Common to all these patients is sensory feedback impairment that is so remarkable that it is the "eye of the blind and the voice of the mute."[3] Thus treatment of the upper extremity amputee is highly variable and must be individualized to obtain maximum function.

Surgery to the upper limb basically falls into two categories: direct, as in partial hand amputation, or indirect, as when removing a deterrent to prosthetic fitting. This is not to say that the patient is made to fit the prosthesis, but rather the stump is improved. In the present state of the art of prosthetics surgery to improve the stump can provide a better marriage of the patient and prosthesis.

Conversion surgery in upper limb deficiencies is of necessity when performed in the very young. Whenever surgery is contemplated, it is essential and axiomatic that the history of the patient's deficiency is well documented. Several deficiencies and/or anomalies lend themselves to early intervention: syndactyly, a partial hand, and resection of the biceps tendon in the very short below-elbow amputee to permit prosthetic accommodation.

IMMEDIATE POSTSURGICAL FITTING

Immediate postsurgical fitting is really not a special procedure in upper extremity amputees but is mentioned here to encourage and popularize its use. Immediate postsurgical fitting is appropriate in a patient with an acquired amputation because it reduces postoperative pain, prevents edema, decreases phantom sensation, and increases acceptance of the prosthesis.[1,2,5,6] If the patient's wound requires delayed closure because of possible contamination, or devitalized tissue, a delayed postsurgical fitting can be done safely at the time of the delayed closure of the stump. Burkhalter[1] has shown that, despite extensive wounds, early postsurgical fitting did not delay the wound healing. Early fitting prevents the patient from developing one-handedness and brings a final fitting with the definitive prosthesis much earlier than with the soft dressing technique (Fig. 15-1) (Chapter 14).

KRUKENBERG TECHNIQUE

Probably the most specialized procedure, which for years had great popularity in Europe but very limited acceptance in the United States, is the Krukenberg, or "lobster-claw," operation. In this procedure, the radius and ulna are separated to effect a pinch activity with an antenna for good sensory feedback. Great manipulative skills can be developed in a well-functioning Krukenberg limb. When the Krukenberg operation is combined with an adequate prosthesis on the contralateral side, effective bimanual function is obtained. The sensory feedback and manipulative ability provided by the Krukenberg forearm increase the effectiveness of the prosthesis because

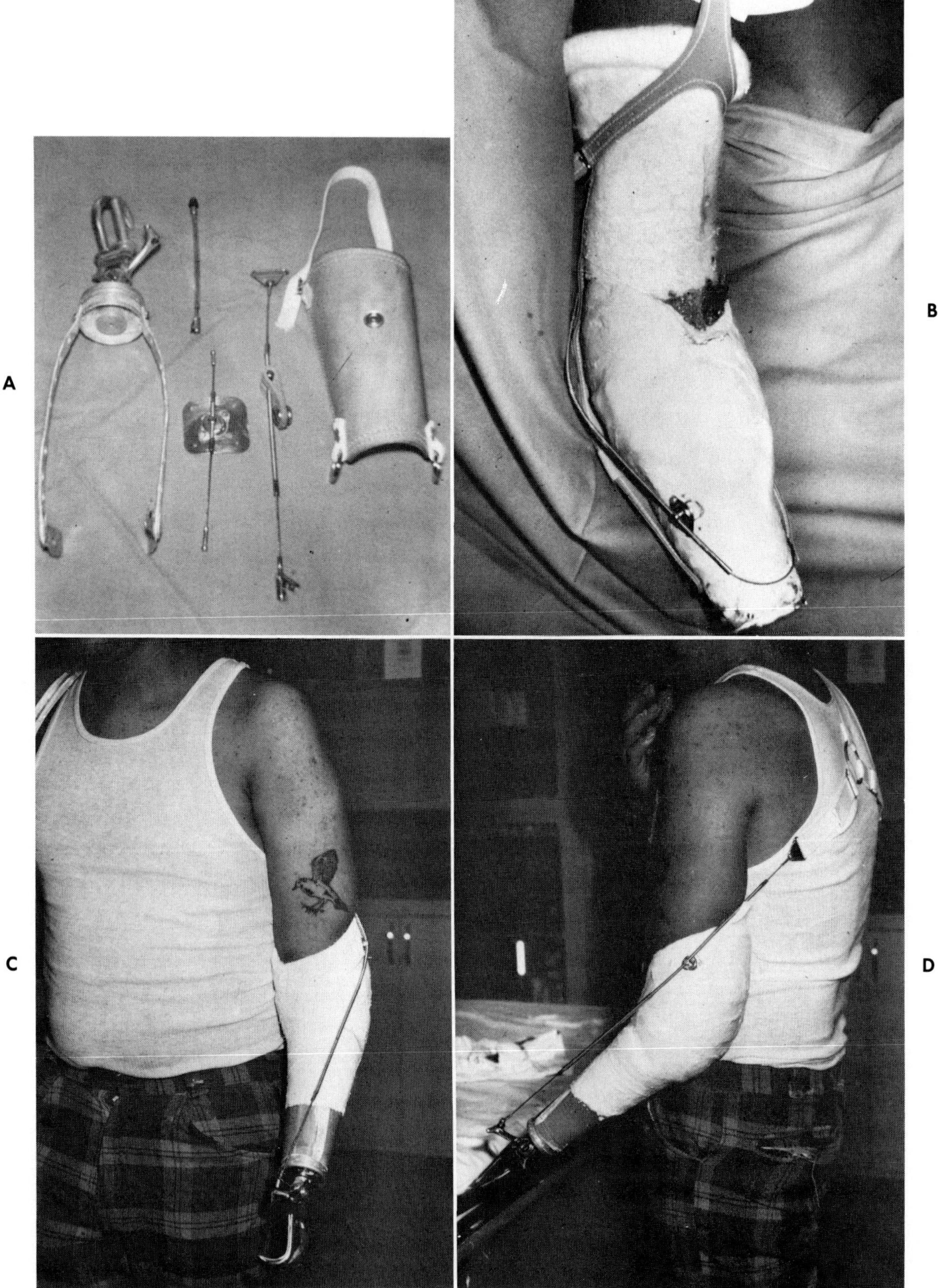

Fig. 15-1. Case 1. This 27-year-old white male had traumatic amputation at mid forearm, and open flap technique was used with delayed closure 10 days after amputation. At delayed closure of forearm amputation, myofascioplasty was performed and immediate postsurgical prosthesis was fit. Cast was changed after 2 weeks, and stump socks added as shrinkage occurred, and final definitive prosthesis was fitted at 6 weeks after closure of amputation. **A,** Prosthetic components needed for below-elbow immediate postsurgical fitting. **B,** Immediate postsurgical fitting at time of surgery. **C** and **D,** Front and side view of patient at cast change 2 weeks after closure of amputation.

the forearm can preposition objects for the prosthetic side (Fig. 15-2).[4]

Presently the major indication for this procedure is in the bilateral long below-elbow amputee with the added disability of blindness. The inability of the sightless to use a prosthesis will persist until adequate biofeedback becomes an accomplished fact. The addition of a pinch with sensation inherent in the Krukenberg technique offers the blind a degree of independence.

The major factor in rejection of the Krukenberg operation is the noncosmetic appearance and, to some, repulsiveness of the limb. This condition can be ameliorated by overfitting the limb with a standard prosthesis for special situations in which the appearance might keep the amputee from normal activity.

Surgical technique

Swanson's[8] technique, with or without minor variations, probably is the most accepted procedure for the Krukenberg operation. It is essential that approximately 15 to 18 cm of forearm stump be present to obtain adequate limb function. If the residual limb is shorter, insufficient spread of the two rays negates its functional capacity. The procedure separates the radius and ulna, with the radius as the working arm against the ulna, much the same as using a pair of chopsticks. The flexor incision is made slightly to the radial side of the center, and the dorsal incision is made slightly to the ulnar side of the center. The muscles and tendons are divided between the radial and ulnar rays equally. Care is taken to avoid disturbing the pronator teres, since this muscle is one of the strongest adductors of the radius for this procedure. The interosseous membrane must be carefully incised throughout its length along its ulnar attachment, with care taken to preserve the vessels and nerves. If the stump is too bulky to permit wound closure, portions of the pronator quadratus, flexor digitorum profundus, and flexor pollicis longus muscle body can be removed, but sufficient muscle coverage of the rays for adequate vascularity and warmth must be retained.

According to Swanson,[8] children with bilateral amputations find a Krukenberg constructed limb much more useful than a mechanical prosthesis and that the appearance of the limb after surgery

A

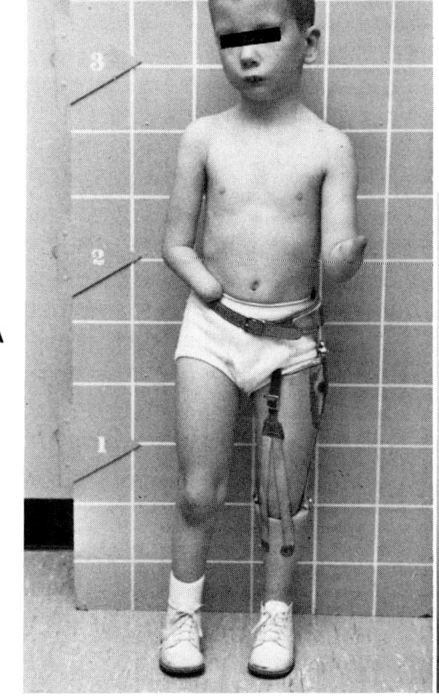

B

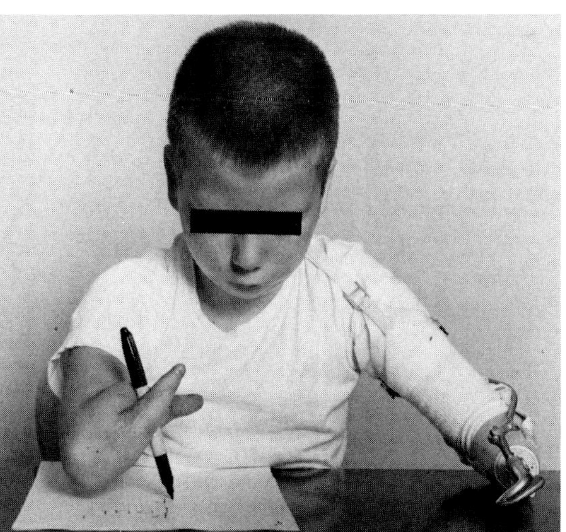

Fig. 15-2. Case 2. **A,** This 9-year-old white male is congenital trimembral amputee with bilateral short below-elbow amputations and short left below-knee amputation. Patient wore bilateral upper extremity prostheses and left below-knee prosthesis. Krukenberg operation was done on dominant side, and patient has obtained good function for primary activities, such as dressing, eating, and schoolwork, using prosthetic fitting on left as assistive device. Outside home he is able to function with bilateral prostheses, since Krukenberg forearm does not hinder prosthetic fitting.[4] **B,** After Krukenberg operation on dominant right forearm with conventional below-elbow prosthetic fitting on left.

has not been distressing. His observations on appearance and acceptance are not shared by all.

AMPUTATION AND SHOULDER FUSION IN THE FLAIL UPPER EXTREMITY

In the tragic incidence of brachial plexus avulsion that produces a flail shoulder, arm, forearm, and hand, which is usually anesthetic from the elbow distally, amputation through the humerus, 9 cm above the olecranon process, combined with a shoulder fusion is a worthwhile procedure.[9] After complete evaluation shows conclusively that a satisfactory return of function is not possible, these patients should be encouraged to consider this method of treatment. Convincing the patient and/or family to have this flail, anesthetic cumbersome extremity amputated is often difficult or impossible. The results of amputation with shoulder fusion are much better when done within 2 years after the injury, since these patients may develop single-handedness, which could become irreversible.

Because there usually is good thoracoscapular muscle control in these injuries, shoulder fusion effectively provides a good powerful humerothoracic pinch and excellent sensory feedback, since there usually is normal sensation of the chest cage and arm. It is then possible to prosthetically fit the patient as an above-elbow amputee rather than a shoulder disarticulation and have an effective humeral segment, powered by the scapulothoracic musculature. Thus the patient is able to wear and use a prosthesis with satisfactory function. The shoulder should be fused in not more than 25% of forward flexion and 25% of abduction to the vertebral scapular border (Fig. 15-3).

KINEPLASTY

The direct coupling of a motor-skeletal structure of the human body for suspension and activation of a prosthesis has been the utopian desire of all surgeons who have studied the problems of the amputee. Kineplasty, which uses masses of movable soft tissue or muscle-tendon structures, is the sole successful surgical procedure in our armentarium at present.

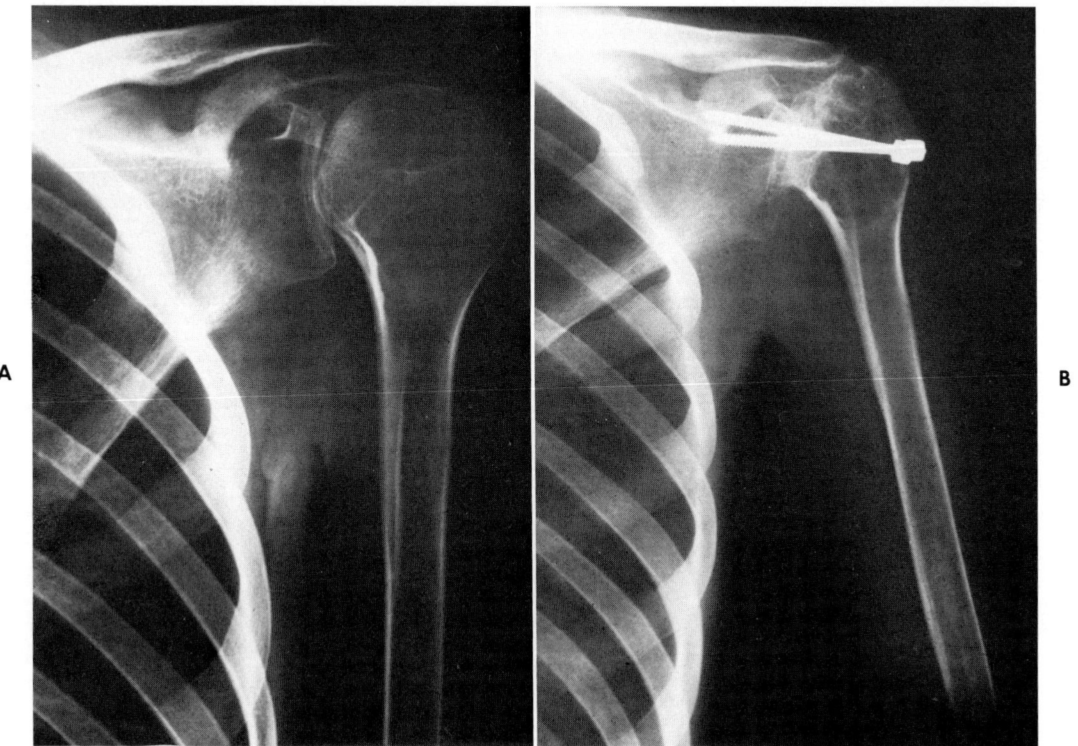

Fig. 15-3. Case 3. This 20-year-old white male had complete brachial plexus avulsion resulting in flail anesthetic left upper extremity. Amputation 9 cm proximal to olecranon process and shoulder fusion was performed. **A,** Anteroposterior preoperative roentgenogram of flail shoulder. Note osteoporosis of disuse. **B,** Anteroposterior roentgenogram of flail shoulder fused at 25 degrees of abduction and 25 degrees of forward flexion.

Kineplasty remains a controversial subject with its proponents and detractors. Interest in this subject dates to the latter part of the nineteenth century when Vanghetti reported his research efforts with various animals. Numerous other researchers have expanded on his theories. After the many successful reported cases of kineplasty from Germany and South America after World War II, there was a renewed interest in this procedure in the United States.

Virtually all the accessible muscles of the shoulder girdle, arm, and forearm have at some time or another been used as motor sources. Forearm flexors and extensors and triceps tunnels have been uniformly unsuccessful. Only 50% of all pectoral kineplasties resulted in a reasonable degree of success; however, biceps kineplasty has about a 70% success rate in properly selected cases.

Advantages

Some of the advantages of kineplasty are (1) elimination of harnessing, especially in cases of extensive scarring and tenderness about the shoulder, (2) discriminatory grasp and a degree of sensory feedback, resulting from the direct coupling of the muscle to the terminal devices, and (3) an increase in excursion power in cases in which body power sources are inadequate.

Disadvantages

Kineplasty is contraindicated for virtually all children. The immaturity of the skeleton causes tunnel migration with growth, and the resultant distortion negates continued use to maturity. Women in general do not accept the cosmetic appearance of the kineplastic tunnel on the residual limb. In bilateral limb deficiency this procedure is contraindicated, since the application of the prostheses is virtually impossible.

The surgical technique of Spittler[7] is the most commonly used, but will not be detailed in this section, since it is found in standard texts.

REFERENCES

1. Burkhalter, W. E., Mayfield, G., and Carmona, L. S.: The upper extremity amputee. Early and immediate post-surgical prosthetic fitting, J. Bone Joint Surg. **58A:**46-51, Jan., 1976.
2. Jacobs, R. R., and Brady, W. M.: Early postsurgical fitting in upper extremity amputation, J. Trauma **15**(11):966-968, 1975.
3. Kessler, H. H.: Rehabilitation of the amputee, Clin. Orthop. **12:**74-95, 1958.
4. Kritter, A. E.: The bilateral upper extremity amputee, Orthop. Clin. North Am. **3:**2, 1972.
5. Loughlin, E., Stanford, J. W., III, and Phelps, M.: Immediate postsurgical prosthetic fitting of a bilateral below-elbow amputee: a report, Artif. Limbs **12:**1-24, 1968.
6. Sarmiento, A., McCollough, N. C., III, and Williams, E. M.: Immediate postsurgical prosthetic fitting in the management of upper-extremity amputees, Artif. Limbs **12:**1-24, 1968.
7. Spittler, A. W., and Fletcher, M. J.: Technique of kineplasty surgery and prosthetic appliances for kineplasty, American Academy of Orthopaedic Surgeons Instructional Course Lectures, vol. 10, Ann Arbor, Mich., 1953, J. W. Edwards.
8. Swanson, A. B.: The Krukenburg in the juvenile amputee, J. Bone Joint Surg. **46A:**1540-1548, 1964.
9. Yeomans, P. M.: Brachial plexus injuries: treatment of the flail arm, J. Bone Joint Surg. **43B:**493-500, 1961.

CHAPTER 16

Prostheses and assistive devices for special activities

JAY D. SHEARER
MARTIN L. BUCKNER
JOHN H. BOWKER

In the present state of the art in prosthetics it is impossible to provide the amputee with a limb that will perfectly meet the wide range of needs met by the natural limb it is meant to replace. The limitations imposed by standard upper limb prostheses and terminal devices have led to the design of prostheses and assistive devices for specific activities.

This approach, however, has inherent limitations in that it would be unrealistic to require a specific terminal device for each activity of daily living. A terminal device that will meet most needs and hold ordinary tools is preferred by most amputees. It is only when the amputee has a very specific goal, which is only made feasible by the use of a special prosthesis or assistive device, that this concept becomes practical. This criterion is most often met in recreational pursuits.

Inclusion of the disabled in sports and recreational activities serves a fundamental role in demonstrating to both a skeptical society and handicapped individuals their capability to achieve recognition and personal success. A diversified program of recreation activities will enable the patient to develop prosthetic awareness skills in a pleasurable manner that is often not associated with "therapy." Participation in informal, as well as organized, sports, in which the amputee can easily be viewed as and feel like a vital contributor to group goals, will also help to allay the pressures of social acceptance. Rehabilitation can be considered successful when the appliance is accepted as a necessary extension of the patient's body.

For a given activity, the unilateral amputee may be able to use the regular prosthesis with a standard terminal device or may select an interchangeable terminal device designed for a specific activity. A standard prosthesis may also be used with an activity-specific assistive device. The amputee may actually find it easier to dispense with the prosthesis altogether for certain of the activities to be described. The bilateral upper limb amputee has less choice but can be quite effective in recreation if the residual limbs have sufficient strength and mobility.

Sports activities for the upper limb amputee may be grouped into those requiring closed or open skills. Activities such as swimming, bowling, and golf are performed in a relatively stable environment and require closed skills. If the environment is highly unpredictable and constantly changing, the amputee needs open skills so as to adjust to and/or regulate the environment.[15]

Catching, batting, or stroking moving objects in baseball, tennis, or hockey call for the use of open skills. The implications for activity selection with respect to the upper limb amputee would suggest initial instruction in closed skills in which repetition of the same movement pattern is essential for success. After proficiency is achieved with use of the prosthesis, open activities requiring flexibility and reaction to a constantly changing environment can be gradually introduced.

Activities should be designed to achieve a variety of beneficial effects in terms of increasing strength, maintaining joint flexibility, and enhancing tolerance to the prosthesis. In addition, those activities enjoyed prior to the amputation stand a greater chance of stimulating patient interest. At all times, the safety of the patient and those with whom he participates is a primary consideration.

HORSEBACK RIDING

Upper limb amputees, unilateral or bilateral, can readily be taught equestrian skills. A quiet, well-trained horse is essential, especially during the early stages of developing balance and learning methods of reining.

The upper limb amputee will depend greatly on use of the legs for maintaining balance and controlling the horse. Initially, the horse is controlled on a long strap or lunge by the instructor, with the amputee bracing his legs against the hand holds of a vaulting girth/vaulting surcingle. If the saddle is used, the surcingle is removed, and the rider can use the hand hold placed on the pommel of the English saddle as an additional holding place.

In most cases, the unilateral amputee can be taught to use reins in the usual fashion. The beginning rider, however, may benefit from one of several devices[3,6] that alleviate the problem of reins slipping from the grip of the terminal device and also allow rapid shortening or lengthening of the reins. An example would be the looped rein, which has three leather loops stitched on either side approximately 15 cm apart.

Other rein modifications are available to the amputee who prefers to use the intact limb only, as in the case of a short, weak residual above-elbow limb. An example would be the rein bar[9,10] developed by the University of Virginia Children's Rehabilitation Center. The middle of the bar is held by the unaffected hand, while radial and ulnar deviation of the wrist control the direction of the horse through the leverage of the bar, simulating two hands on the reins (Fig. 16-1).

Bilateral upper limb amputees may control the horse with prostheses or may elect to use reins attached to the stirrups, using the legs to guide or stop the horse.[11] For reasons of safety, the horse must be specifically trained for this type of reining. At no time should any device be added to the student or horse that would impede movement or a free fall from the horse.

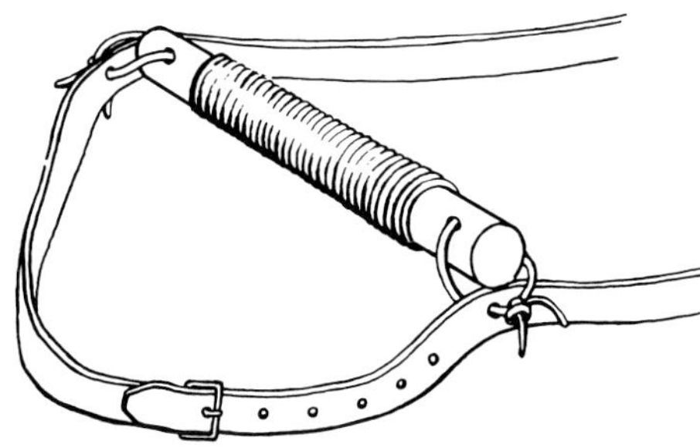

Fig. 16-1. Rein bar. (From Larkins, C.: Inter-Clin. Info. Bull. **9**(7):4-11, April, 1970.)

FISHING

Several assistive devices are available to help the upper limb amputee cast and retrieve, allowing successful participation in the pleasures and rewards provided by sport fishing.

The unilateral amputee who wishes to use the prosthesis in fishing may either hold the rod in the hand and wind the reel with the terminal device or may hold the rod in the terminal device and wind with the hand. A more secure hold on the rod may be obtained by use of a special terminal device,[16] which connects the rod directly to the wrist unit of the prosthesis (Fig. 16-2).

There are also three devices available that do not require use of a prosthesis. The Garcia Handi-Gear,* a light aluminum harness, has a holding

*Garcia Corp., 110 Charlotte Place, Englewood Cliffs, N.J., 07632.

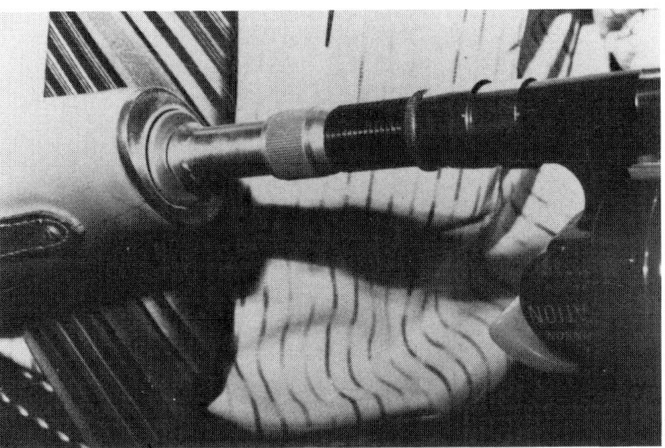

Fig. 16-2. Fishing rod directly connected to standard below-elbow prosthesis by means of special terminal device. (From Sabolich, L. J.: Inter-Clin. Info. Bull. **12**(2):13-15, Nov., 1972.)

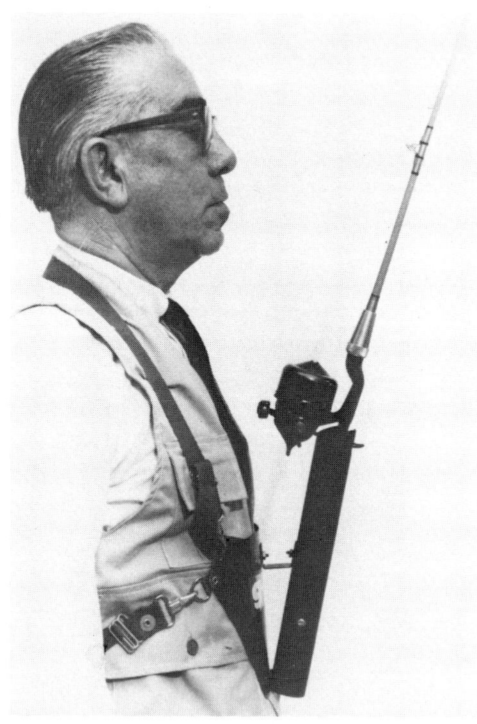

Fig. 16-3. Garcia Handi-Gear, lightweight aluminum harness for one-handed fishing. (From Adams, R. C., Daniel, A. N., and Rullman, L.: Games, sports and exercises for the physically handicapped, Philadelphia, 1975, Lea & Febiger.)

tube into which the rod butt is inserted after casting. A light twist locks the rod trigger into place for fish fighting, as well as normal retrieval (Fig. 16-3). The Dodgen Spare Hand Fishing Belt* is easily put on and operated by one hand, either right or left. The fishing rod handle is glued into a special thermoplastic rod handle that engages on the prong extending from the belt. An automatic locking device secures the rod in any position while working bait or playing the fish. When ready for the next cast, the amputee lightly squeezes the handle to release the rod in the proper grasp for casting (Fig. 16-4). An adapted fishing pole for blind, bilateral below-elbow amputees has been developed at St. Dunstan's in London. It is operated entirely without prostheses (Fig. 16-5).

The fishing stool, originally designed for the hemiplegic fisherman, will also work well for the elderly, less mobile upper limb amputee. The stool provides a stable seat, with a hinged socket for inserting the rod butt. There is storage in the stool for equipment and a work surface for knot tying and baiting.[5]

SWIMMING

One of the great attractions of swimming for upper limb amputees is that it can be readily ac-

*Roy Dodgen Shop, Blue Eye, Mo., 65611.

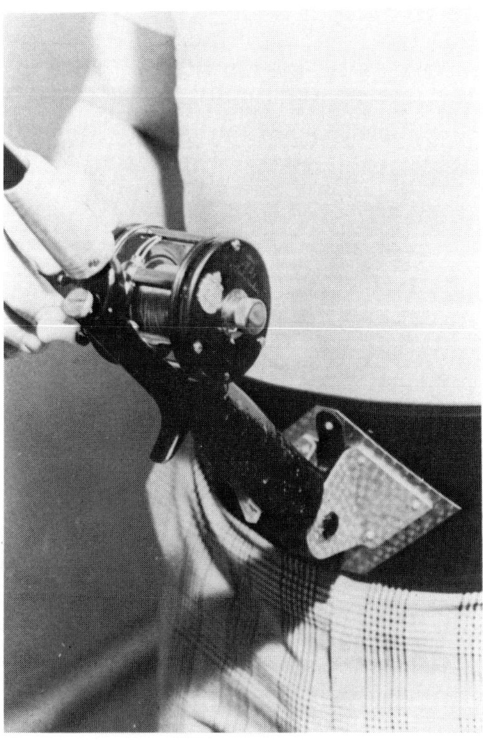

Fig. 16-4. Dodgen Spare Hand fishing belt. (Courtesy Roy Dodgen Shop, Blue Eye, Mo.)

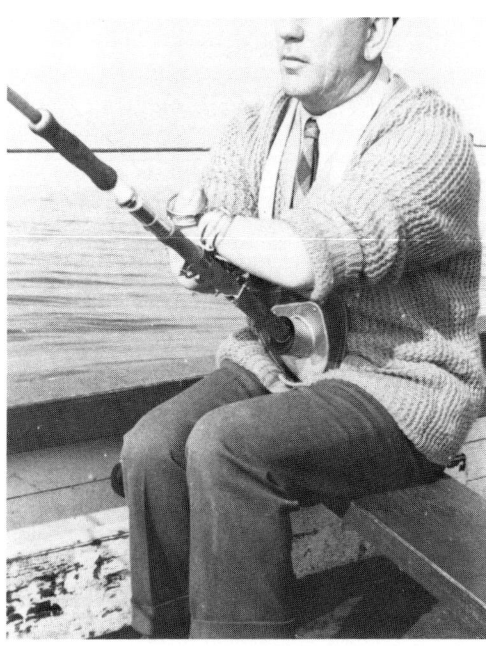

Fig. 16-5. Adapted fishing pole for blind, bilateral below-elbow amputees. (Courtesy St. Dunstan's, London, England.)

complished without any appliances. However, it may require minor adaptations of stroke technique. The four components of all swimming strokes, arm action, leg action, body position, and breathing, must be considered individually in order for the amputee to develop a style that is both functional and comfortable.

Because of self-consciousness, many amputees hesitate to actively employ their residual limbs while swimming. However, mobility and strength of even a short residual limb can often be improved by swimming. A psychological benefit, in terms of positive body image, accrues as the amputee begins to look on the residual limb as a valuable aid to swimming. Upper limb amputees can perform the back crawl, elementary backstroke, sidestroke, breaststroke, and front crawl, using adaptations of basic techniques taught the able-bodied swimmer.

Except for the crawl, kicking action provides the main propelling force. It also provides lateral stability as the swimmer with a unilateral upper limb amputation progresses through the water. The whip kick, employed in the elementary backstroke and breaststroke, and the scissors kick, used in the sidestroke, produce the most efficient forward progression.

Extensive movement exploration is recommended to enable each amputee to discover the floating and swimming position best for him. Good postural alignment must be stressed to maintain a streamlined body position. The loss of a limb causes displacement of the center of gravity and center of buoyancy to the intact side. Thus the individual who has lost a right arm has a tendency to roll to the left, where the weight of the body is centered.[17] Modification of the angle and extent of underwater pull often is required to progress in a straight course. The backstroke with the face above water provides security initially for exploration of body positions. Bilateral upper limb amputees may have some initial difficulty recovering from this position. They are aided in recovering the upright position, however, by their lowered center of buoyancy, which compensates somewhat for rotary forces normally supplied by arm action. The sidestroke, swum with the intact arm below, is a good resting stroke for swimming longer distances.

A regular breathing pattern is essential to efficient swimming technique, particularly as the swimmer seeks to increase range. Rotary breathing in the front crawl is easiest when the head rolls to inhale on the side of the unaffected limb during the press phase.[2] Bilateral upper limb amputees have greater difficulty in raising the head above water while swimming prone and must compensate by increased extension of the trunk. Swimming several strokes underwater before raising the head to breathe may alleviate this difficulty.

BOWLING

Bowling is an excellent activity for the upper limb amputee due to the availability of facilities on a year-round basis. Because of the relatively small expenditure of energy required, it may be continued long after more strenuous activities have been abandoned. Bowling fits into the category of individual sports in which the participant proceeds and learns at his own rate and competes to improve the performance. Immediate knowledge of results provides reinforcement to the bowler and incentive to improve on his skills. In addition, bowling is generally performed in a social setting.

Unilateral upper limb amputees generally can bowl with little or no difficulty by using the intact limb to deliver the ball. The bowler can use the prosthesis to assist in holding the ball above the waist at the recommended starting position. The prosthesis also assists in the development of balance and coordination during the approach and delivery.[1]

A terminal device* has been designed for the

*Hosmer/Dorrance Corp., 562 Division St., P.O. Box 37, Campbell, Calif. 95008.

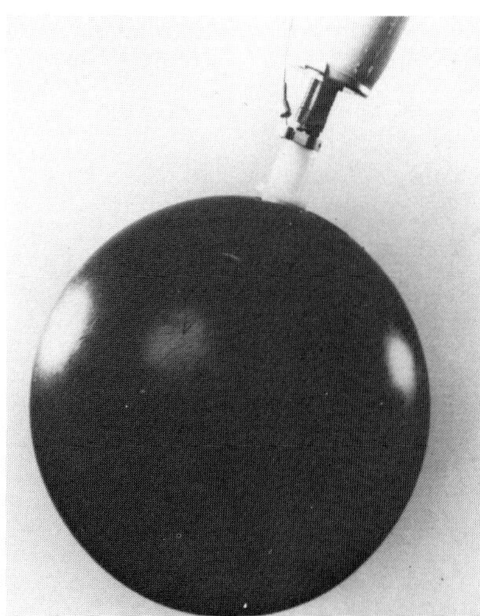

Fig. 16-6. Special bowling terminal device inserted in bowling ball. (Courtesy Hosmer/Dorrance Corp., Campbell, Calif.)

bilateral upper limb amputee or the unilateral amputee who chooses to use the prosthesis to deliver the ball. A neoprene expansion sleeve at the end of this device is under constant spring compression, which causes it to expand. When the control cable pulls on the "finger," the sleeve is stretched, causing it to elongate and release its grip on the finger hole of the ball. The releasing action is the same one used to open a conventional terminal device and is an essentially natural action in bowling (Fig. 16-6).

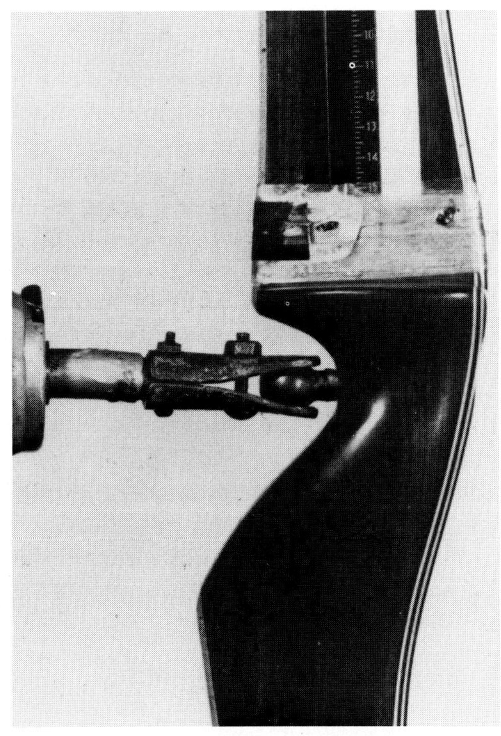

Fig. 16-7. Bow attached to regular prosthesis by use of quick-disconnect wrist unit. (From Bender, L. F.: Prostheses and rehabilitation after arm amputation, Springfield, Ill., 1974, Charles C Thomas, Publisher.)

A suction cup assistive device, enabling bilateral arm amputees to compete in duckpin bowling was designed at Sunnybrook Hospital in Toronto. The assist is attached to the prosthesis, and movement of the terminal device releases the ball.[8]

ARCHERY

Archery is an ideal sport for the upper limb amputee for several reasons. It has considerable therapeutic value in developing the muscles of the upper limbs and trunk. For example, the deltoids on both sides support the arms in a horizontal position, the biceps draw the bowstring, and the triceps hold the bow in position. Also, it offers great variety in application, with the amount of exercise determined by increasing the pull weight of the bow and by shooting greater distances.[7] It is an ideal sport in that amputees can compete with able-bodied people on equal terms.

Several options are open to the upper limb amputee who wishes to take up archery. The unilateral below-elbow amputee may attach the bow to the regular prosthesis using a ball-joint unit attached to a Fletcher-Motis adapter[4] (Fig. 16-7). Alternatively, a special prosthesis may be used. This is fitted with a forked length of metal tubing to which the bow is strapped (Fig. 16-8).

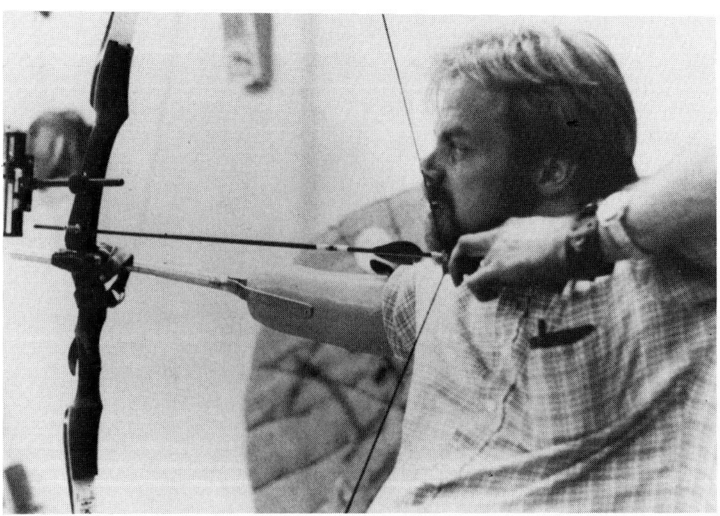

Fig. 16-8. Bow strapped to special archery prosthesis with forked metal extension.

In either case, the bowstring is pulled and released by the archer's normal hand.

The below-elbow amputee may use a wooden release assist, with the "hook" fingers fitted into grooves in the device. The bowstring is hooked by the tip of the device, while the archer draws the bow. A slight rotation of the prosthesis releases the string and arrow at full draw. It is advisable to use a pair of small rubber arrow nocks to hold the arrow on the string.[1]

A device designed for one-handed use is also available. It consists of a release device strapped to the archer's chest, with a cable extending from the release to a caliper attached at the grip of the bow. The bowstring is set in the release device and the arrow positioned. The archer extends the bow arm drawing the string anchored at the chest. When full draw is reached and aiming has been accomplished in the normal manner, a slow pressure on the caliper releases the bowstring, putting the arrow in flight toward the target.[7]

GOLF

Golf* can be played proficiently by the unilateral upper limb amputee by controlling the club and swing with one arm. The prosthesis is used as a support, while the unaffected arm establishes the control and acceleration necessary in the swing.

The backhand swing is the most effective in producing distance and control for the golfer with a unilateral arm amputation.[13] A right-handed club is used with an unaffected left arm and a left-handed club with an unaffected right arm. The backhand swing uses the serape effect, which refers to the structure in which the muscles surrounding the rib cage cross obliquely, making the backhand stronger and more accurate.

A universal joint terminal device with a sleeve designed to fit the butt of the club has been used by below-elbow amputees to provide stability throughout the swing (Fig. 16-9).

The bilateral upper limb amputee can enjoy miniature golf by obtaining clubhead control, using the hook fingers to securely hold the grip and shaft. The dominant side is held low on the shaft (cross-handed style) to swing the clubhead on a direct line to the hole.

BASEBALL

Baseball, historically known as America's favorite pastime, has long been a favorite of upper limb amputees. Peer and adult pressure exerted during childhood has led many to try their skills on the baseball field. In addition, the ready availability of baseball programs and facilities makes the sport very accessible to all age groups.

The unilateral upper limb amputee who chooses not to wear a prosthesis can field the ball with the glove, then quickly place glove and ball under the opposite residual limb, enabling him to retrieve the ball for the throw. For the unilateral below-elbow amputee who wishes to use a prosthesis, a baseball glove attachment permits wearing the glove while freeing the intact arm for throwing. The glove is secured to the two fingers of the device, which provide the necessary gripping action (Fig. 16-10). In the interest of safety, it is advisable to use a lightweight plastic ball while learning the art of fielding.

Batting can be accomplished without a prosthesis by anchoring the grip of the bat against the body while power is applied with the intact arm. Alternatively, one-armed batters can grip the butt of the handle with their prosthesis, again applying power for the swing with the intact arm.

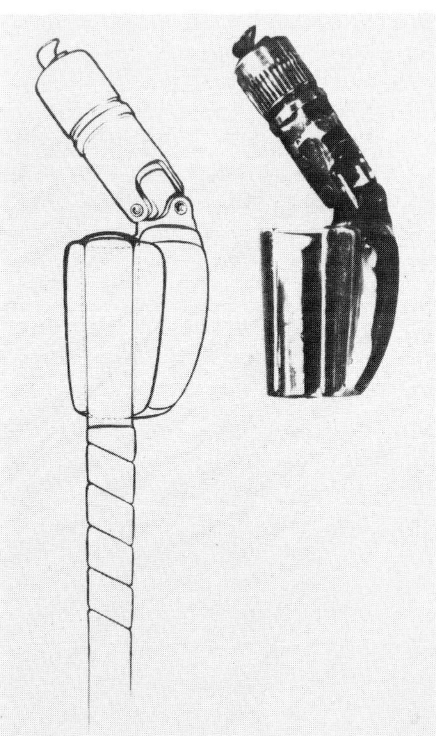

Fig. 16-9. Universal joint terminal device with sleeve holding butt of golf club. (From Bender, L. F.: Prostheses and rehabilitation after arm amputation, Springfield, Ill., 1974, Charles C Thomas, Publisher.)

*For further information, contact D. Owens, Circle E Farms, Rt. 1, Box 54, Davell, S.C. 29040.

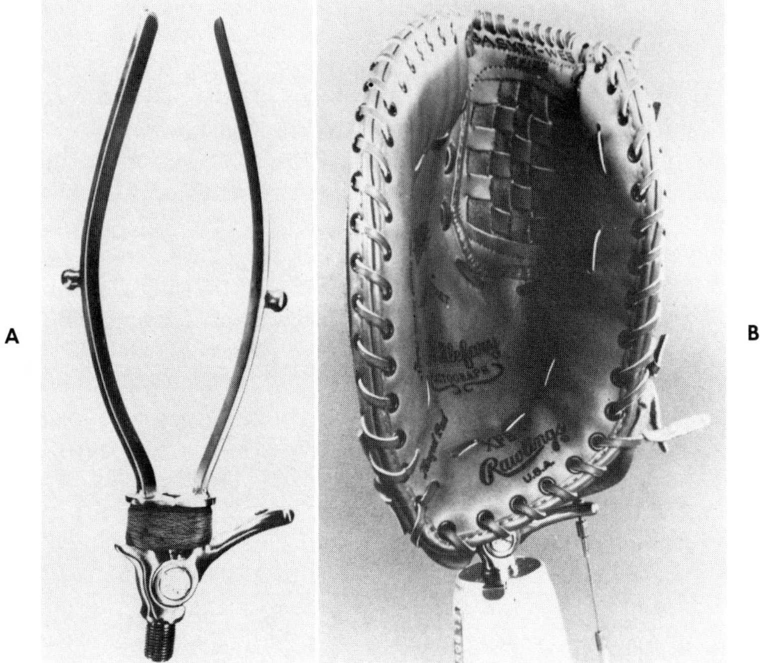

Fig. 16-10. A, Special terminal device for holding baseball glove. **B,** Glove in place on special terminal device. (Courtesy Hosmer/Dorrance Corp., Campbell, Calif.)

HOCKEY

Hockey can be played by the unilateral upper limb amputee employing a standard prosthesis. The stick can be grasped directly by the terminal device or inserted into a hole in the handle. Alternatively, the fingers of the terminal device may be converted to a pair of closed loops by welding an additional piece of metal to each. This has the advantage of better protecting the other players from the prosthesis. Stauffer developed a special device that enabled a boy with bilateral phocomelia to become a skilled forward in his local team.[14]

SKIING

The approach to skiing* for the upper limb amputee developed by the Winter Park, Colorado, Amputee Ski Program will be briefly described.[12]

The amputee begins training with shorter, more maneuverable skis, progressing to longer skis as skill allows. Because upper limb segments that allow subtle weight shifts for steering are lost, the upper limb amputee is taught to steer with the feet and legs.

Skiing technique, especially as related to trunk rotation, is impaired by loss of an upper limb. For this reason, amputees are encouraged to use their prostheses with poles, if at all feasible. This is especially true for above-elbow amputees, since the combination of prosthesis and pole restores balance and prevents nonsynchronous rotation of the shoulders. A minimum length of 20 cm (8 inches) at the above-elbow level is needed to use a prosthesis with a pole, although many at that level elect to do without. None are taught to go entirely without poles, since at least one pole is needed as an assist in getting up after falls and in walking over flat terrain.

Amputees should use a regular ski pole with a loop strap. This is firmly attached to the hook terminal device by forming a figure of eight with the loop about the hook. It is set in the same attitude as the pole held in the remaining hand. The firm fixation allows efficient use of the pole and also prevents its uncontrolled swinging, which could cause injury to the skier. Bilateral above-elbow and below-elbow amputees should place a mitten on the above-elbow terminal device to prevent self-injury during a fall.

Precautions must be taken to keep the residual limb warm, particularly when skiing with the prosthesis, because of rapid heat transfer. On

*For further information contact Hal O'Leary, Box 313, Winter Park, Colo. 80482.

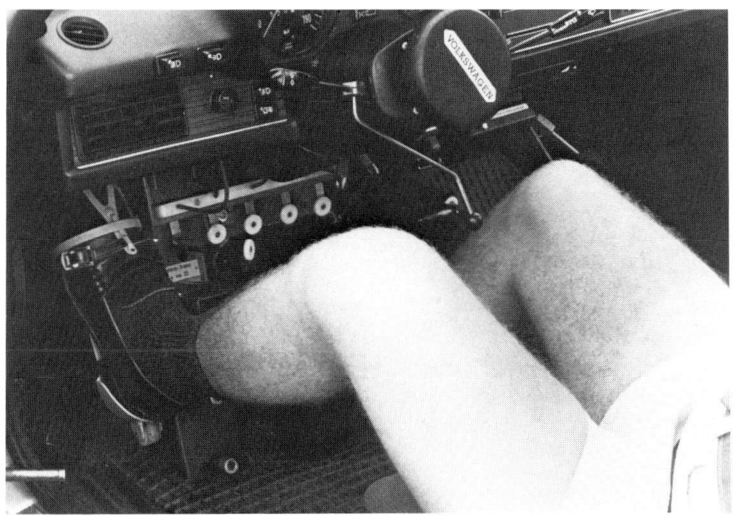

Fig. 16-11. "System Franz." Note steering plate for left foot and multiple accessory controls by right knee. (Courtesy Veterans Administration Prosthetics Center, New York.)

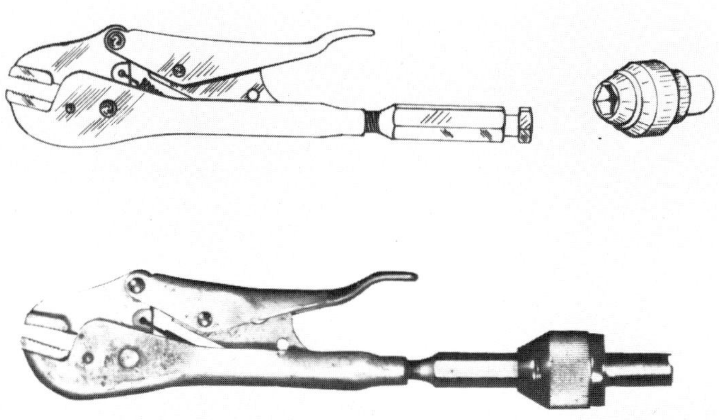

Fig. 16-12. Vise-grip pliers fitted to Fletcher-Motis wrist unit. (From Bender, L. F.: Prostheses and rehabilitation after arm amputation, Springfield, Ill., 1974, Charles C Thomas, Publisher.)

excessively cold days, the amputee should take frequent warming stops, during which the prosthesis is removed, and the skin inspected for frostbite.

DRIVING

A number of devices designed to assist the upper limb amputee in automobile driving are either commercially available or undergoing evaluation. The simplest is a ring, attached to the rim of the steering wheel, which is grasped by the standard hook terminal device.

A second type, the Malden-Care Joystick Steering Unit, is currently in use on some small British cars. It has steering function only, but has the advantages of easy adaptation to foot or hand steering, depending on the impairment, and immediate return to normal steering function at the flick of a switch.

The Kope Foot Steering Control System also has steering function alone. It is custom fabricated and adapted to passenger sedans. The driver is required to have near normal function and mobility of both lower limbs, but none of the upper limbs. The foot steering control consists of a floor-mounted round plate, installed perpendicular to the steering column. A chain-sprocket arrangement couples the foot control and steering mechanism in a 1:1 ratio. A pivotal attachment on the periphery of the foot control plate provides a place for the left shoe of the handicapped driver. Vehicle steering is therefore controlled by angular displacement of the foot control plate.

The "System Franz," designed by a bilateral upper limb amputee in Heidelberg for a compact car, is the most complete currently available. Steering is accomplished by moving the left foot, attached to a foot plate by a bicycle toe clip, forward and backward on a roller at the heel (Fig. 16-11). The remainder of normal driving functions, including braking, acceleration, shifting, and signaling, are performed with the right lower limb. The system can be easily removed and the steering wheel replaced in just a few minutes.

VOCATIONAL AIDS

In certain jobs involving repetitive manual tasks, tools adapted to fit a quick-disconnect wrist unit can be most useful (Fig. 16-12). Examples of known successful users include a machinist and a gunsmith. A set of tools commercially available includes a hammer, hacksaw, vise-grip pliers, screwdriver, and drive ratchet.*

We hope that the information presented in this chapter will provide impetus to further development of this area in three specific ways. The first is more widespread involvement of amputees in recreational activities through their own initiative and with the assistance of those skilled in the field of therapeutic recreation. Second, through knowledge of sports technology and biomechanics, the therapist, working with a skilled coach and/or, interested parent, can often devise adaptations of the amputee's style, thereby eliminating the need for special prosthetic devices or, in some cases, any prosthesis at all.

Third, the development and marketing of more useful special prostheses and assistive devices for those who need them should be encouraged. The ingenious amputee should bring ideas to a skilled and equally ingenious prosthetist for cooperative development.

*Wright & Filippis, Inc., 19326 Woodward Ave., Detroit, Mich. 48203.

REFERENCES

1. Adams, R. C., Daniel, A. N., and Rullman, L.: Games, sports and exercises for the physically handicapped, Philadelphia, 1975, Lea & Febiger.
2. American National Red Cross: Swimming for the handicapped (instructor's manual), ARC 1092, 1960, American National Red Cross.
3. Bauer, J. J.: Riding for rehabilitation: a guide for handicapped riders and their instructors, Toronto, 1972, Canadian Stage and Arts Publications Ltd.
4. Bender, L. F.: Prostheses and rehabilitation after arm amputation, Springfield, Ill., 1974, Charles C Thomas, Publisher.
5. Crewe, R. A.: Fishing for the hemiplegic, Occup. Ther. **38:** 195, Sept., 1975.
6. Davies, J. A.: The reins of life, London, 1967, J. A. Allen & Co.
7. Guttmann, L.: Textbook of sports for the disabled, Aylesbury, England, 1976, H. M. & M. Publishers, Ltd.
8. Kay, H. W., Lewis, S. L., and Stewart, W. A.: A bowling device for bilateral arm amputees, Inter-Clin. Info. Bull. **9**(7):13-16, April, 1970.
9. Kuhlthau, L.: Equitation for amputees, Inter-Clin. Info. Bull. **10**(5):9-12, Feb., 1971.
10. Larkins, C.: Horsemanship for the physically handicapped, Inter-Clin. Info. Bull. **9**(7):4-11, April, 1970.
11. McCowan, L. L.: It is ability that counts, Olivet, Mich., 1972, The Olivet College Press.
12. O'Leary, H.: Personal communication, 1979.
13. Owens, D.: Personal communication, 1979.
14. Redford, J. B.: Prostheses for hockey-playing upper limb amputees, Inter-Clin. Info. Bull. **14**(6):11-15, June, 1975.
15. Robb, M. D.: The dynamics of motor-skill acquisition, Englewood Cliffs, N.J., 1972, Prentice-Hall, Inc.
16. Sabolich, L. J.: An adapted fishing rod for arm amputees, Inter-Clin. Info. Bull. **12**(2):13-15, Nov., 1972.
17. Sherrill, C.: Adapted physical education and recreation: a multidisciplinary approach, Dubuque, Iowa, 1976, Wm. C. Brown Co., Publishers.

CHAPTER 17

Research trends in upper limb prosthetics

EDWARD PEIZER

For many years major portions of available research resources were applied to clearly defined, relatively singular goals. Thus during the 10-year period after World War II, we saw the results of a concentrated research effort: the use of synthetics for sockets and harnesses, a family of terminal devices, including special-function hooks, a range of mechanical hands, including the APRL automatic locking voluntary closing hand with three-jaw chuck grasp, two-position thumb, and cosmetic cover. During this period there also emerged from the development laboratories, wrist flexion units, quick-disconnect wrists, permitting convenient interchange of hands and hooks, devices to reduce the force and/or excursion requirements to flex the elbow, and ingenious harnessing methods to enable shoulder disarticulation amputees to flex and lock elbows and to operate terminal devices effectively but with relatively obtrusive body motions.[44] From approximately 1955 to 1970 research efforts in upper extremity prosthetics became more highly organized under guidelines established by the Committee on Prosthetics Research and Development of the NAS—National Research Council.[15,60,62] Through one subcommittee on research and another on development, efforts were focused on identifying the requirements for and developing externally powered components, as opposed to body powered, components. During this period a new array of prostheses with components powered by compressed gas and electrohydraulic and electrical systems were developed. Despite the sustained and heavy stress placed on these devices and the relatively large number of powered elbows, hands, and hooks developed, very few reached the commercial market. In this country the VAPC* elbow and the Veterans Administration Northwestern University (VA/NU) myoelectric hand currently manufactured by Fidelity Electronics, Ltd., of Chicago, Illinois, and the Myobock System manufactured by the Otto Bock Orthopedic Industries, Inc., Duderstadt, Germany, are commercially available. Other elbows and hands, such as those developed by Viennatone, Variety Village, and some others, may also be used to a minor extent. Thus some six or seven previously developed electric elbows and perhaps an equal number of powered hands developed between 1955 to 1970 did not satisfy needs sufficiently to warrant their transition into commercial production.

Since 1970, research trends in upper extremity prosthetics have not been so clearly defined. Perhaps after 15 years of intensive work in this field, a pause was needed to reassess requirements and seek new directions. Since 1970, prosthetics research and development resources expanded to

*As of July 1, 1980, the name Veterans Administration Prosthetics Center was changed to Veterans Administration Rehabilitation Engineering Center (VAREC).

meet the needs of other individuals: lower extremity amputees, paraplegics, hemiplegics, quadriplegics, and persons with other disabilities began to receive increasing attention. Spreading the available resources has tended to mask current research trends.

Nevertheless we can identify several areas of emphasis in research and development in upper limb prosthetics. Work now seems to be concentrated on the following:

1. Cosmesis
2. Sockets
3. External power
4. Myoelectric control systems
5. Sensory feedback
6. Medical manipulators

COSMESIS

The cosmetic treatment of artificial limbs has always preoccupied researchers. In certain patients, the restoration of appearance is as important as the restoration of function. Everyone is aware of upper extremity amputees who refuse to wear prostheses and prefer an empty sleeve to what they consider an unsightly hook. Strangely, the need for adequate cosmesis in the generally covered portions of the prosthesis, such as the socket or harness, is just as strong as it is for the visible portion of the prosthesis, the terminal device. Adequate prosthetic treatment requires acceptable levels of function, appearance, and some restoration of the body image.[13,54,61] The psychological basis of cosmetic acceptability is complex, with its roots in the altered body image of the amputee, his self-perception,[17] and self-esteem. Thus one amputee will cheerfully wear a chrome-plated hook and abjure the use of a functional or cosmetic hand because he is not "shamed" by the loss and has no desire to hide it by an obviously artificial replacement. Many will not use a hook and prefer either a functional hand or, in some cases, a highly customized cosmetic hand matching to the fullest extent possible the sound hand. To a lesser degree these needs and variations in taste extend to socket shapes, colors, and the noise made by prosthetic mechanisms. Over the years there has emerged a definable trend toward improved cosmesis. The concept of cosmesis, however, has been broadened to include not only the fidelity with which an artificial limb or component matches a natural limb, the general aesthetic quality of a mechanical device, but also includes the element of natural "feel" in being resilient and capable of operation by more natural, less obtrusive control movements.

The Children's Amputee Prosthetic Program (CAPP), University of California, Los Angeles, activated terminal device (Sumida hook) features one conventionally shaped finger and one broad finger containing resilient inserts designed to offer a large contact surface for grasping irregularly shaped objects. As shown in Fig. 17-1, little attention was given to appearance, and the hook represented an attempt to maximize function. The Sumida "parrot" hook for children is a clear attempt to improve the appearance of the hook,

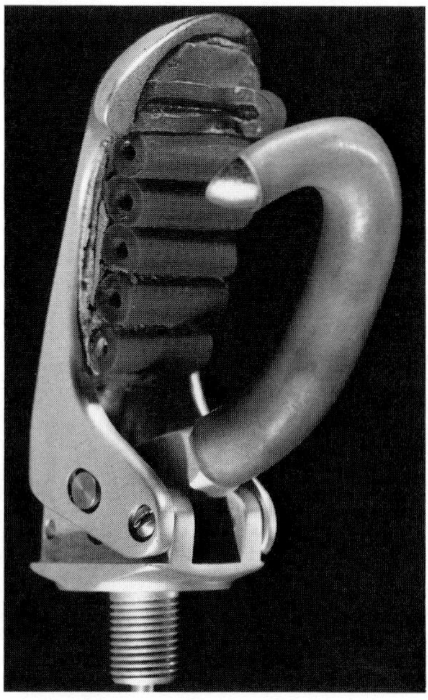

Fig. 17-1. CAPP terminal device.

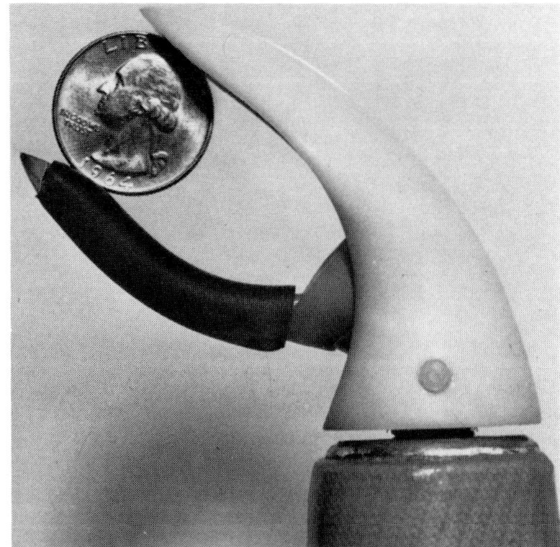

Fig. 17-2. CAPP Sumida "parrot" terminal device.

while retaining some elements of palmar prehension (Fig. 17-2).

Improving the kinematic cosmesis, that is, the naturalness of appearance during movement, was one of the major objectives in the development of the VAPC and other hybrid above-elbow prostheses, as well as of the myoelectrically controlled, self-suspended, self-contained below-elbow prostheses. The VAPC above-elbow prosthesis consists of a conventional above-elbow socket, forearm, wrist unit, and terminal device. The electric elbow, however, permits the elimination of the elbow lock control strap. This substantially reduced the highly overt shoulder abduction/extension motion required to lock and unlock the conventional elbow. The 30 to 45 degrees of shoulder abduction and extension required to operate the conventional elbow is completely eliminated with the electric elbow, since it locks automatically when it is not flexed or extending. Moreover, the 5 to 7.5 cm (2 to 3 inches) of shoulder flexion required to flex the mechanical elbow is reduced to less than 1.3 cm (½ inch) of excursion to actuate the switch of the electric elbow (Fig. 17-3). In the below-elbow prosthesis equipped with an electrically powered hand, the 5 to 7.5 cm of shoulder flexion required to open or close the terminal device is reduced again to less than 1.3 cm when an electric terminal device is used (Fig. 17-4). The VAPC electric hand and elbow system take advantage of their small excursion requirements and the internal packaging of all components to improve the overall appearance of a prosthesis (Fig. 17-5).

Rubin and Gearhardt[52] developed a cosmetic cover for an otherwise conventional metal hook (Fig. 17-6). It consisted of a glovelike cosmetic hand cover that could be readily slipped on and off a hook. It could be pocketed by the wearer

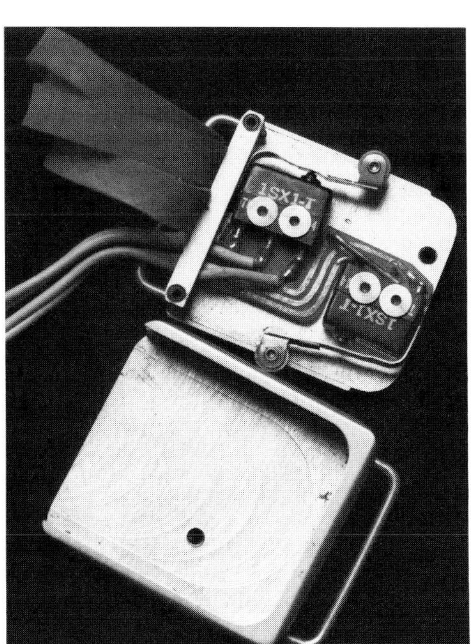

Fig. 17-3. VAPC electric control switch.

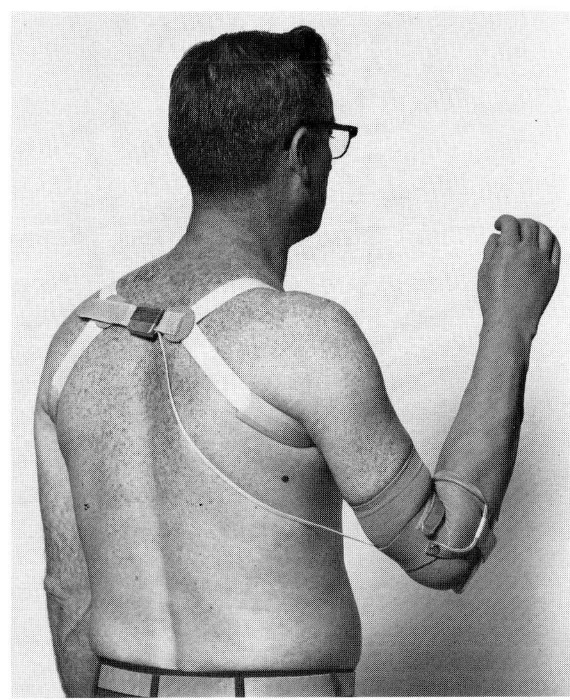

Fig. 17-4. Below-elbow prosthesis with electric hand and switch.

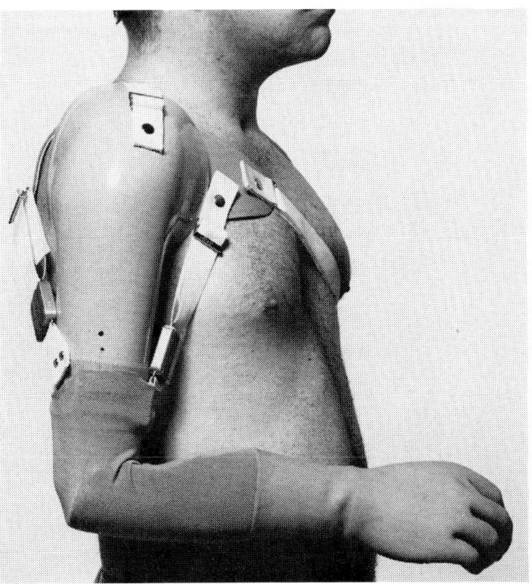

Fig. 17-5. VAPC electric hand and elbow system.

when not in use. The hook is actually fitted into the middle finger of the five-finger cosmetic glove covering the metallic hook. This device has been available since 1971 but has not come into wide use.

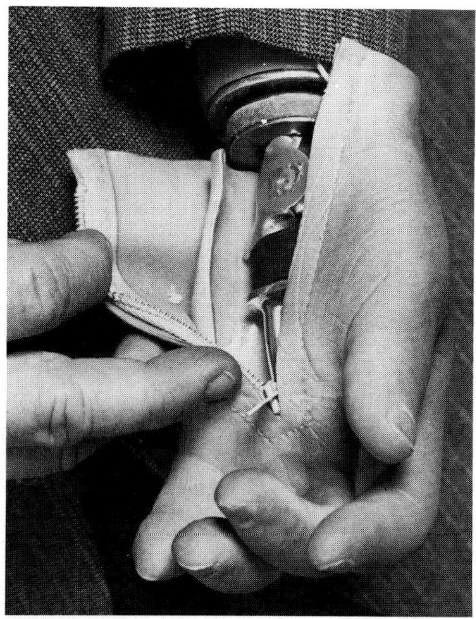

Fig. 17-6. Cosmetic hand cover for conventional hook.

A more recent development is the soft cosmetic forearm, a plastic foam skeletal-type forearm. Oval shaped at the proximal end, the forearm has a smooth profile and fairs smoothly into wrist and elbow. It is especially designed for use with the VAPC electric elbow, although it can be used with the conventional elbow as well. The entire unit consists of a stamped aluminum saddle welded to an aluminum tube that is ordered to length and equipped with a wrist fitting that matches the standard 1.3- to 51-cm (1/2- to 20-inch) United National Fine (UNF) thread. It is approximately half the weight of the conventional plastic laminated forearm. The soft forearm is a cosmetic improvement from four standpoints: (1) it is shaped more naturally, (2) it is soft and resilient to the touch, (3) it can be colored or covered with materials that more closely match the wearer's skin, and (4) it reduces the noise amplified by the hard shell of the electric elbow or that is generated when it is struck against a hard object (Fig. 17-7).

The self-contained upper extremity prosthesis (Fig. 17-8), coupled with a self-suspension system, provides several advantages to the amputee. The most obvious is the relief from what is generally an annoying harness and control cable. Gross body motions are no longer required for control.

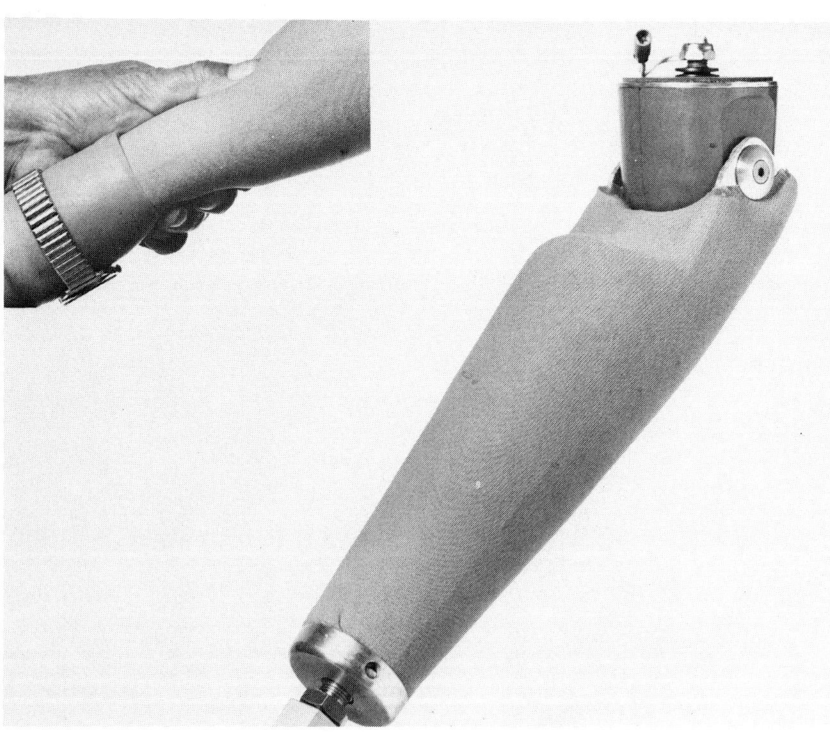

Fig. 17-7. Soft cosmetic forearm.

The self-contained prosthesis is easier to keep clean and easier to don or remove. This may now be accomplished without removing garments, makes possible more natural movement of the limb, and contributes to improved general comfort and appearance of the wearer.

The most recent research and perhaps the most modern approach to faithful replication of the appearance and texture of the human limb has been conducted by Leonard[35] at the George Washington University Medical Center. This research is directed toward the development of high-strength translucent latex for use in improved cosmetic gloves for amputees (Fig. 17-9). This material resists oxidation and irreversible staining by water and oil-soluble substances. New materials and procedures might replace the current Veterans Administration cosmetic glove materials and those fabrication techniques which use PVC polymers, plasticizers, and stabilizers dissolved in volatile organic solvents. Present systems have several drawbacks: they require a long time to make gloves that do not have either the desired stain resistance or desirable mechanical properties.

SOCKETS

Modern socket design began with the development of the Muenster or Hepp-Kuhn concept for eliminating external harnessing for upper extremity prostheses (Fig. 17-10). The fundamental procedure was to form the socket snugly around the olecranon and the epicondyles of the forearm in such a way that the socket wall "pinched" the soft tissue of the antecubital portion of the arm and the bony prominences with sufficient force to remain in place under substantial distal loading. With well-formed and otherwise uncomplicated stumps, this kind of socket could frequently be fitted without external harnessing; in certain cases, however, epicondyle straps or other auxiliary harnessing was required.

"Self-suspension" in this manner offers the advantage of eliminating the sometimes uncomfortable harnesses and control cables. The limb is also free to move more naturally, improving the general cosmetic effect. The Muenster-type socket, as described in studies from New York University,[1] has disadvantages that affect the use and function of a myoelectric system. The standard Muenster-type socket may limit the range of flexion and extension and therefore decrease the total function of the system.

Childress and Billock[6] at Northwestern University further refined the original concept. The Muenster-type socket was retained on the stump principally by opposing forces generated between the anteroposterior proximal edges of the socket opening. The socket has to be maneuvered over and around the olecranon to withdraw the stump. The relatively high anterior wall required to maintain the narrow anteroposterior dimension sometimes prevented full flexion of the elbow. Childress and Billock believed that this problem could be solved without sacrificing the stability of the socket by designing it to fit higher and more

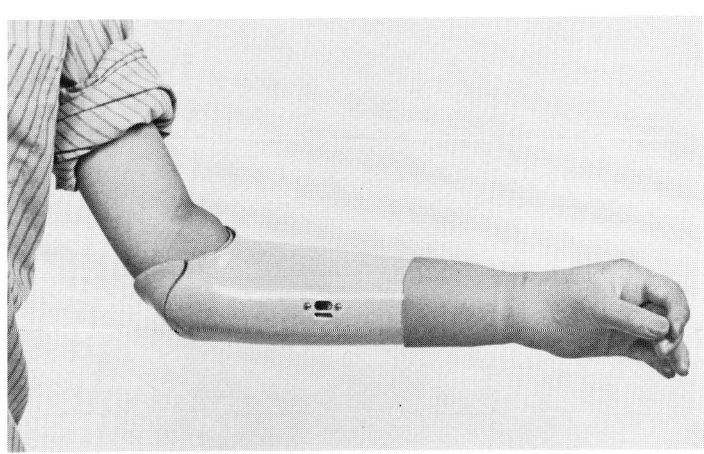

Fig. 17-8. Self-contained, self-suspended below-elbow prosthesis.

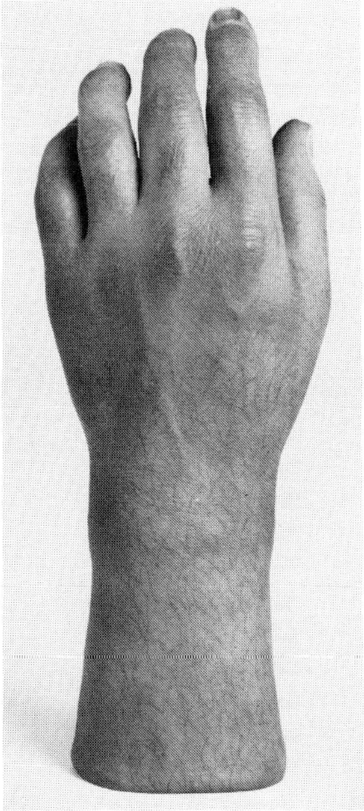

Fig. 17-9. Cosmetic glove.

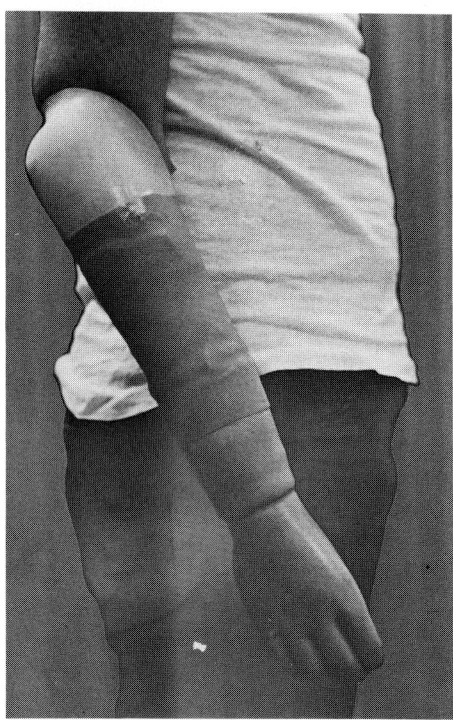

Fig. 17-10. Hepp-Kuhn socket.

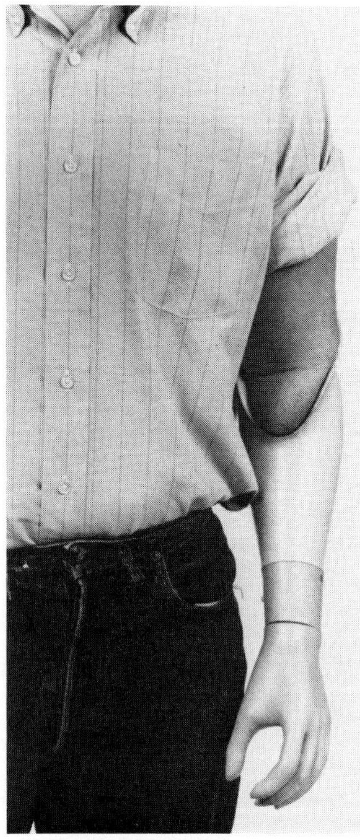

Fig. 17-11. Northwestern University self-suspended socket (Courtesy Veterans Administration Prosthetics Center, New York.)

intimately over the epicondyles. The greater lateral rigidity prevents the withdrawal of the stump. This permitted trimming the anterior proximal edge of the socket lower to eliminate the restriction sometimes imposed on elbow flexion by the original Muenster socket (Fig. 17-11).

The anteroposterior corner of the socket trim line is the point at which the humeral condyles enter the socket. The trim line must be 0.3 cm (1/8 inch) smaller than the measured mediolateral dimension of the condyles in this area to allow the condyles to pass into the socket with only slight expansion of the socket. If the mediolateral dimension is too small, the condyles will not pass into the socket, and if it is too large, the suspension will not be adequate. Suspension is also affected by the flexibility of the finished socket. The best results have been obtained with a 70% rigid and a 30% flexible mixture of polyester resin.

The humeral condyles may be rather tender during the first few days after the initial fitting. Tenderness may also develop in the tissues of the antecubital fold. This tenderness should diminish as the stump builds up a tolerance of the socket. It is therefore advisable to build up this tolerance gradually and not overuse the prosthesis during the first week or so after the initial fitting. Experience has shown that amputees may initially have some difficulty in donning the prosthesis. This problem disappears quickly as they gain experience in putting it on.

In some cases the proximal mediolateral measurement of the cast in the area above the condyles will be too small even before the cast is modified. Generally this occurs with atrophied or thin stumps because of the contour of the arm above the medial condyle. In this case the cast must be built up on the medial side and plaster removed on the lateral side so that each side is 0.2 cm (1/16 inch) medial to the apex of the condyle.

The original Muenster socket and the Northwestern modified Muenster socket or special variants of them are prescription choices and are considered developed items.

The current trend of research has remained in the area of self-suspension: mainly efforts to suspend sockets for higher level amputation by suction, friction, and by percutaneous bone attachments. At Northwestern University, Billock[3] designed an atmospheric-pressure suspension socket. This socket was constructed with a soft, clinging, rubberlike sleeve inside a rigid shell. This inner sleeve was fastened distally, and as the prosthesis was loaded and the stump started to withdraw, the inner sleeve tightened around the stump preventing further motion. Although the same principle is often applied in above-knee sockets, it still remains experimental for upper extremity sockets and has not become part of the general treatment procedure.

The ultimate prosthetic attachment is being sought in techniques for attaching sockets directly to the bones of the stump. It would be advantageous to attach and detach an above-elbow socket by means of an appropriate external fastener attached to the bone and brought out through the skin on the distal end of the stump. Obviously the long-term acceptance of foreign materials is a primary obstacle but nevertheless a great deal of work has been done at Rancho Los Amigos Hospital,[40] Downey, California, and at the Southwest Research Institute, San Antonio, Texas.[24]

Malgaigne,[36] in 1845 to 1850, was the first to use external fixation of fractures, involving both attachment to bone and penetration of the skin. Two parallel overlapping plates were attached by a screw. The plates were then forced to bring the hooks toward each other, attempting to close the gap in the patella.

Early in this century Steinmann[64] of Bern, Switzerland, reported in a series of papers in Switzerland and Germany a method of driving a steel nail through skin and bone (e.g., tibia) to permit skeletal traction on a fracture. This method is still successfully used, with the pin left in place for months.

Fully buried implants for the head of the femur, the head plus the neck and trochanter area, and the total hip joint have been developed in great profusion in the last 20 years.

During and just after World War II there were independent attempts in Germany and the United States at direct attachment of a below-knee prosthesis to the tibia. Dümmer,[14] a general surgeon in Pinneberg, Germany, experimented at first with sheep and eventually fitted four humans in May 1946 (Fig. 17-12). Cutler and Blodgett[12] at Harvard University also studied below-knee skeletal attachment.

In the Harvard University project experiments were conducted with a total of eighteen dogs. Stainless steel or cobalt-chromium alloy (Vitallium) fracture plates were applied to the amputated foreleg bones of dogs. In some cases, Vitallium lag screws were inserted in the medullary canal (Fig. 17-13). Their final report asserts that Vitallium attached to the bone is well tolerated, but that motion of the metal against the bone is probably the chief factor in bony degradation and that any prosthesis must be free of such motion.

Esslinger[16] began experiments on animals around 1956. Initially he tried skeletal attach-

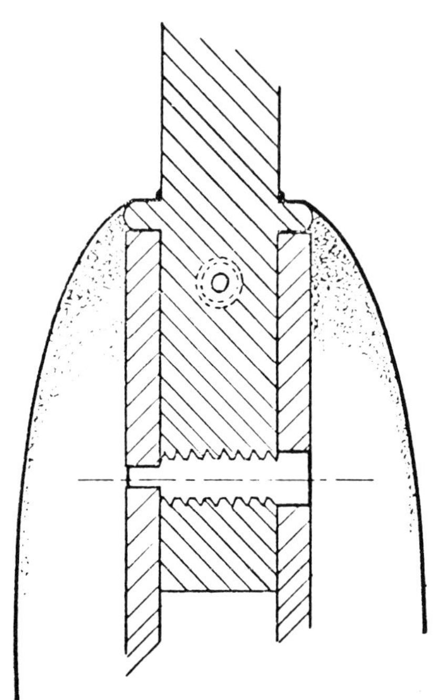

Fig. 17-12. Early method of external fixation of fractures.

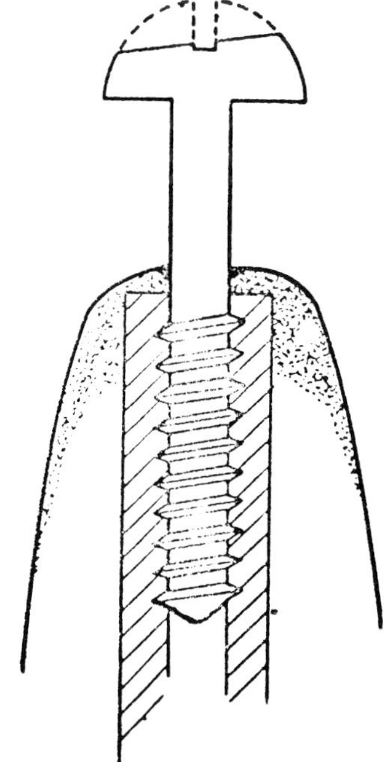

Fig. 17-13. Cobalt-chromium alloy (Vitallium) lag screw.

ments on dogs, achieving his best result on the first case. In some cases, the prosthesis became loose in the medullary canal, and there was gross infection, but the skin remained attached and supported the prosthesis during swing phase. Esslinger also studied plugging of the medullary canal in a two-step operation. He inserted a threaded plug into the medullary canal with a distal attachment device, closed the wound, and waited for thorough healing and development of firm adherence between the plug and bone. Then, in a second stage, he reopened the stump, attached the prosthesis to the plug, and tried to create an infection-resistant interface between the prosthesis and the skin, presumably by a subcuticular perforated collar. Esslinger experimented with several types of plugs to increase the tolerance to end-weight bearing. His work with room-temperature-vulcanizing silicone rubber led Swanson et al.,[65] to develop a heat-cured silicone plug that has been used successfully to increase tolerance to end-weight bearing of a number of human amputees.

Hall et al.[27] experimented with Dacron velour backed with silicone rubber as a skin interface. He wrapped the velour around a metal prosthesis, which allowed the skin to grow into the velour loops, thus providing a chemomechanical bond. Mooney et al.[41] initially experimented with several types of animals, then fitted the right humerus of a human trilateral amputee (high above-elbow amputation, hip disarticulation, and below-knee amputation). The skin grew into the Dacron velour wrapped around a load-bearing shaft. For some months the seal and the overall structure appeared successful, but eventually seepage occurred, the shaft was accidentally loaded during falls, and finally the prosthesis was removed. Mooney et al. have continued to study various semiburied implants, finding best success with vitreous carbon buttons. They believe an implant must allow epithelial downgrowth to a level of about 4 mm.

Mooney selected Cerosium because it was the only ceramic material that had undergone extensive laboratory and clinical testing. But it was necessary to increase its strength by prestressing—a process used for many years to increase the strength of ceramics. Their device was a prestressed ceramic tube, divided into two main parts: a partially tapered ceramic member with a distal nylon velour cuff, and a threaded stressing rod with permanently attached proximal and distal nuts (Fig. 17-14). A distal offset provides attachment for the velour cuff without increasing the overall diameter of the prosthesis.

In April, 1968, the first surgical procedure to implant this prosthetic device was performed at Rancho Los Amigos Hospital, Downey, California. The patient was a 26-year-old triple amputee (left below-knee amputation, right hip disarticulation, and right proximal humerus amputation). A square recess, approximately the same size as the proximal square nut of the prosthesis, was cut in the superior portion of the humeral head. The implant was driven down the medullary canal of the humeral segment with the square nut of the device seating itself in the prepared squared recess. The flap of bone from the humerus was replaced, and the shoulder incision closed. Distally

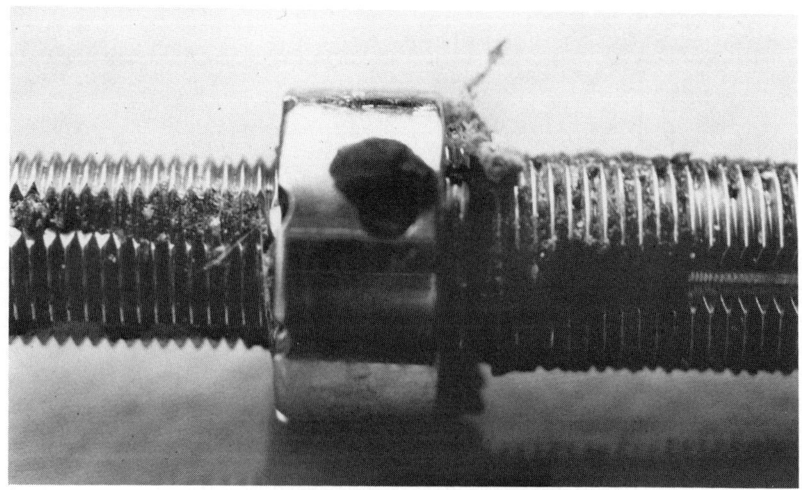

Fig. 17-14. Threaded stressing rod.

the skin was sutured firmly around the velour cuff. A sterile dressing was placed on the shoulder and stump incisions, and the protruding end of the prosthesis was covered with a mound of fluffed gauze. The patient tolerated the procedure well and experienced no difficulty in the immediate postoperative period. Several weeks after the operation the patient began an exercise program to build strength in the remaining musculature of the stump. Approximately 2 months after surgery, an upper extremity artificial limb was fitted to the skeletal attachment by a specially designed snap-on device. The patient controlled the prosthesis in the standard manner. The limb is removed nightly.

This prosthetic device was initially successful from the standpoint of providing a bond between bone and the prosthesis so that the functional use of a limb prosthesis was available to the patient. Nonetheless, as time passed (8 months), gradual drainage at the skin interface resulted in progressive low-grade inflammation about the prosthesis, and eventually the prosthesis had to be removed.

Other approaches were taken with (1) composite carbon; (2) vitreous carbon, both smooth and grooved annularly; and (3) graphite-vitreous carbon. However, vitreous carbon appeared to be the best candidate for bone implant material, being well accepted by all tissue, with no evidence of toxicity related to it.

To date no clinically useful results have been achieved. Two problems have to be solved before percutaneous attachment of a prosthesis to a bone is clinically feasible. First, a successful, long-term bond between bone and the prosthetic device must be achieved, and second, a drainage-free perforation of the skin by prosthetic material must be available. The rationale for the skeletal prosthetic bond has been described as the achievement of a close bond between bone and inert materials so that excessive stress concentrations at any living site are avoided. Although porous ceramics at one time were thought necessary to achieve this, the view has changed to that of an appropriately designed device which allows direct bone apposition without any presence of fibrous interface. Vitreous carbon has been demonstrated by Mooney to allow such direct bone apposition and to present respectable resistance to shear when implanted into bone tissue.

Hall et al.,[26] discussing skin interfacing, point out that no other aspect of this work deserves or has received, more attention. The skin is the body's first line of defense against microbial invasion. In the presence of percutaneous foreign material it becomes even more important to maintain the integrity of the skin. Metals, plastics, and ceramics have been tried, including solids, textiles, and foams. No ideal material has yet been found, although vitreous carbon, Dacron, and nylon velour fabrics bonded to a solid surface to form impervious laminates have offered the most suitable solutions thus far.

As regards bone interfacing, numerous investigators have found various types of porous ceramics with satisfactory qualities that allow new bone ingrowth into the porous structure of the material.[29,33] Other investigators have pointed out that adhesion of bone to a solid nonporous surface is also possible.[7,28] Sintered metals that create a porous surface have also been used for application in this area.[5,46] Surface ingrowth, however, appears quite different and often disturbed when presented with a dynamic load.

Hall[25] is working with goats to develop a permanently attached artificial limb. Goats selected for surgery are isolated from the herd, an x-ray examination of the left hind leg is given, and the leg is amputated.

Initially, he used an intramedullary rod with a pedestal made of plastic. Nylon velour bonded to the pedestal's surface served to anchor the skin and new tissue ingrowth. Regardless of the composition of the intramedullary rod, the tibia was counterbored and "tailored" to fit the pedestal mortise. The mortise was designed to prevent axial rotation of the intramedullary rod.

Most of the fifty-one animals so treated walked on the prosthesis immediately after awakening from anesthesia. One animal managed to clear a 1.7-m-high (5½-ft) corral fence on the afternoon of the day of surgery. Some goats are reluctant to bear weight for several days after surgery. Why some animals show evidence of pain and others do not is somewhat puzzling.

Regardless of what material had been used for skin interfacing, the results eventually terminated in the skin retracting beyond the reach of the skin interfacing material. Best results to date have been obtained using nylon or Dacron velour as the skin interfacing material.

EXTERNAL POWER

As in every area of endeavor in which achievement is the product of motivation, neuromuscular coordination, and need, the regain of function among arm amputees using conventional prostheses can be astonishing. A well-known bilateral below-elbow amputee, using standard bilateral below-elbow prostheses with hooks, was one of the most adept users in history. Personal observation, along with thousands of others' observations, support the view that his ability to do manual tasks soon made the observer forget he was wearing prostheses. Another legendary user of prostheses had a bilateral above-elbow amputation and shoulder disarticulation. The majority of upper extremity amputees regain function in varying degrees. A small but significant number are unsuccessful, never achieving satisfactory service from their prostheses. Failure to achieve adequate performance levels was sometimes attributed to lack of motivation or to lack of neuromuscular coordination. But professional observation of amputees on the lower end of the achievement scale revealed that objects were dropped, misplaced, or could not be grasped at all. This was generally attributed to lack of sufficient closing force in a voluntary opening hook. A lack of strength on the part of the amputee prevented sufficient force from being exerted on a voluntary closing device. Backlash or other poor grasp characteristics of terminal devices were also blamed. It was clear that sockets became uncomfortable, and harnesses chafed. For bilateral amputees especially, cross talk, that is, the inability to operate one prosthesis completely independently of the other was sometimes a problem. Prostheses for above-elbow and shoulder disarticulation amputees had even a larger number of deficiencies. Operating the mechanical elbow required several other control motions, and additional harnessing resulted in a limited range of motion. All of the above problems have been cited as major reasons for the development of externally powered prosthetic components.

Early theories held that externally powered components, even those to be operated by switch-type mechanisms in the harnesses, would pro-

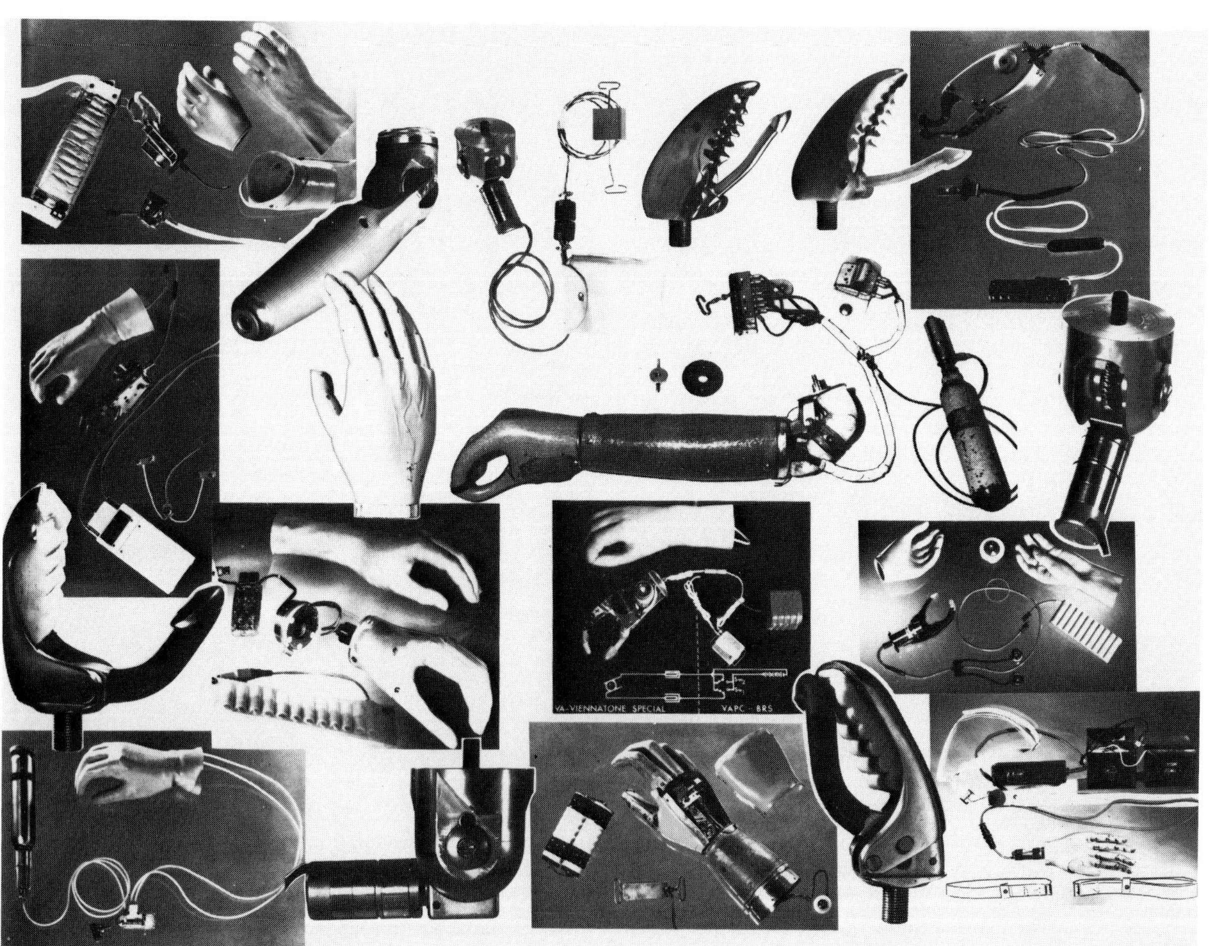

Fig. 17-15. Elbows and terminal devices developed throughout world.

vide higher pinch forces at the terminal device, permit elbow flexion without high excursion, control motions, and reduce harnessing. In addition, designers and engineers find the prospect of working on externally powered hands, hooks, elbows, and other components challenging and alluring. The use of external power for terminal devices was discussed as early as 1919 by Schlesinger.[55] Between 1965 and 1975 a number of electrical prosthetic components for the upper extremity amputee were developed here and abroad. Fig. 17-15 illustrates just a few of the terminal devices and elbows developed in the Soviet Union, Liechtenstein, United Kingdom, Canada, Italy, Germany, Japan, Sweden, and the United States. The net result of this work to date has been that none of the original electrically powered, switch-controlled components are in general use today. Available in the United States from commercial sources are the Myobock System and the VAPC System. Occasionally, externally powered prostheses of Canadian or Italian design are fitted. A complex set of factors are at the root of this situation in which extensive and expensive resources were applied without satisfactory results to date. Perhaps the most significant reasons are intrinsic, the electrically powered, switch-controlled terminal devices and elbows were heavier, noisier, and less reliable than mechanical devices. They still required harnessing, required added componentry (battery packs), and they were expensive.

It has generally been conceded that the use of externally powered components was greater in Europe than in the United States. This phenomenon was attributed to the greater centralization of fitting services in Europe as contrasted to the thousands of individual shops offering prosthetic fitting services in the United States. Education and skilled development in fitting, training, and use could be more readily accomplished in centers where the required skills could be concentrated.

In the United States and perhaps in Canada, acceptability by professional prosthetists and the medical profession is equally important as acceptability by patients. The introduction of new devices requires the support of the practitioners because amputees do not learn about them until after they have used them. Therefore education and training of prosthetists, therapists, and physicians about electrical components is an essential step to the successful introduction of new components.

It is clear that external power for below-elbow amputees is of greatest advantage when the prosthesis is entirely self-contained and self-suspended. This means that the power sources, control elements, and electrical components are encased within the forearm prostheses and not visible externally. It also means that the socket must be designed for suspension without the use of external harnessing, perhaps by the methods developed at Muenster or at Northwestern University. Prostheses of this type are more cosmetic without external impediments, more comfortable, and, perhaps, self-contained and less subject to accidents and wear and tear. A completely self-contained prosthesis implies the use of myoelectric control with the electrodes embedded in the inner wall of the prosthesis to capture and use signals of wrist extensors and flexors in controlling the terminal device. The modern externally powered prosthesis is myoelectrically controlled, miniaturized, and far more reliable than earlier versions. This has been made possible by the development of better motors, batteries and other components. Today energy is stored in Ni-Cd batteries, cylindrical, high-performance cells originally developed by the communications industry for portable transceivers and security systems. Battery voltage, and therefore the number of cells, has been reduced, with consequent reduction of size and weight and increase in efficiency and reliability. Other improvements are integrated circuits for signal processing and power transistors with lower voltage and quiescent power drains. The Myobock system now available operates on 6 V provided by Ni-Cd cells. The VAPC hand and elbow manufactured by the Fidelity Electronics, Ltd., have a seven-cell fast-charge battery system.

The trend in motor technology has been toward using "ironless" rotors, permanent magnets, shell wound systems, a class of motors with high electromechanical efficiency (85% to 90%), high power-to-weight ratios, and very fast response. Magnet technology has produced the sumarian-cobalt and other alnico alloys for microscopic motors. Electronic devices have been added to the VAPC hand that limit current flow to the motor after closing or opening to conserve energy. Other mechanical improvements are free swing at the elbow to overcome the stiff arm appearance that previously characterized electric elbows and other load releases for both elbows and hands. These mechanical features reduce malfunction, wear, and system inefficiency.

Novel power transmission systems are being

used, including eveloid gears and harmonic drives because of their high torque-to-weight ratios. Helical gears are also being used to reduce noise. In general, the performance of the electrical powered systems available in the United States, the Bock and the VAPC, has been substantially improved. They respond faster with a 30-cm/sec hand closing velocity. They provide up to 10 kg of prehension force between the fingers. They are also lighter, quieter, and self-contained in that they do not require external wiring or batteries. Among the newest developments is the work of the SVEN group[23] and others to provide articulated fingers to improve the quality of prehension.

The VAPC electric hook is interchangeable with the VAPC electric hand. Using the basic housing of the hand as applicable, the hooks will meet the following functional performance specifications (Fig. 17-16):

1. The opening-closing time is less than 500 msec
2. The opening distance is 15 cm (6 inches)
3. The maximum closing force is up to 7 kg (15½ pounds)

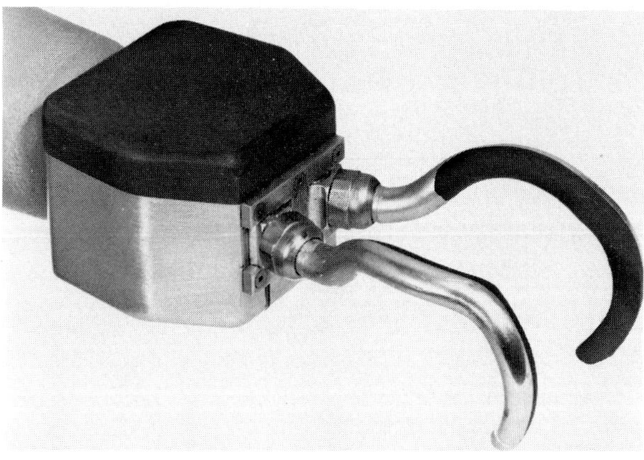

Fig. 17-16. VAPC electric hook.

Northwestern University is developing the Synergetic Myoelectric Hook, which is also interchangeable with the VA/NU system. Powered hooks and conventional hooks offer an improved view of the object being grasped and are generally considered superior in this respect to hands. The Northwestern University Synergetic hook system consists of an electric hook controlled by a myoelectric signal and a modular wrist unit with amplifier and adjustable friction wrist. The hook meets the following functional performance specifications:

1. The opening-closing time is 450 msec
2. The opening distance is 11 cm (4¼ inches)
3. The pinch force is up to 9 kg (20 pounds)

Both the Viennatone Corporation of Vienna, Austria, and Fidelity Electronics, Ltd., of Chicago, Illinois, are experimenting with hybrid power systems that use external power for those functions (Fig. 17-17).

MYOELECTRIC CONTROL SYSTEMS

Conventional below-elbow, above-elbow, and shoulder disarticulation prostheses are generally controlled by the ingenious and reliable harness and control cable systems illustrated in Fig. 17-18. The value of these systems, developed some 35 years ago and refined to their present state perhaps 20 years ago, is often overlooked. In the laudable desire generally to improve the control of prostheses, there is a tendency to concentrate on their deficiencies rather than their advantages. From one viewpoint they are easily fitted, readily adjusted, and easily repaired. They are light, relatively cheap, and maintained without difficulty. Particularly for the below-elbow am-

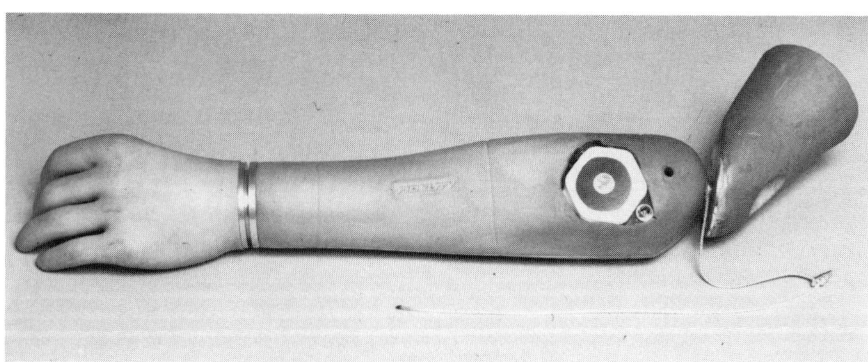

Fig. 17-17. Hybrid externally powered system.

putee and the above-elbow amputee with reasonably long stumps, they afford a high degree of effective control over the terminal device and elbow. This is especially true in younger, highly trained amputees. In addition, these systems provide a certain sensory feedback in the kinesthetic sense of tension in the muscle and harness and in the running of the cable.

From another viewpoint they are uncomfortable, particularly in the area of the axilla, and they wear out clothing, the cables being externally mounted. They cause clothing to appear lumpy. Most important, their functional value diminishes with the number of motions to be controlled. That is, they serve a below-elbow amputee controlling only a terminal device very well, but as the harness and control system also becomes more complex, as for above-elbow, shoulder disarticulation, and, particularly, bilateral amputees, their efficiency falls off. For example, if elbow flexion control and elbow lock control need to be performed bilaterally, the conventional harness becomes increasingly inadequate. Separation of control is difficult, inadvertent operation of components is more frequent, and of course, bulk and discomfort are increased.

The potential advantages of myoelectric control are manifest; they were first recognized in the mid 1940s in Germany.[48] Contraction of a muscle is accompanied by a depolarization wave across the membranes of muscle fibers. This electrical change is detectable on the surface of the skin over the muscle. Since magnitude and occurrence of the wave are related to the time and intensity of contraction, it offers an attractive control mode. For the below-elbow amputee, for example, it permits the reestablishment of a physiological relationship between muscle contraction and the function of opening and closing a terminal device. The long flexors of the wrist normally contract when the fingers are clenched (closing), and the long extensors of the wrist normally contract when the fingers are extended (opening). Other advantages of myocontrol lie in the possibility of substantially improving cosmesis. The control signals can be detected by means of electrodes located on the inner wall of the socket. The signal can be transmitted within the prosthesis to amplifiers and other internal signal processing components that drive the electric motors responsible for opening and closing the hand. This technology eliminates the need for mounting components external to the prosthesis.

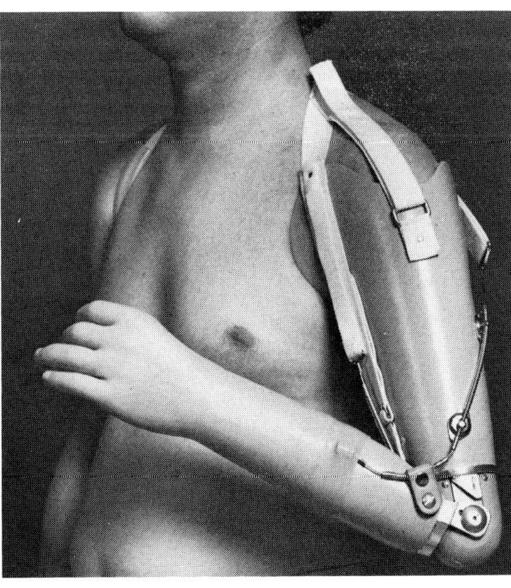

Fig. 17-18. Conventional above-elbow prosthesis and control system.

In the above-elbow amputee, the performance advantages are not so clear, although the need is greater than in the below-elbow amputee. With a sufficiently long stump, residual biceps and triceps may be used to provide control signals, but these control sites are not "physiologic" in the sense that they are not the muscle groups which normally open and close the hand. Moreover, in the short above-elbow stump, electrodes may have to be mounted outside the socket. This may cause problems related to electrode placement and retention and does not permit the fabrication of a completely self-contained unit. Thus the major advantages of myoelectric control would appear to accrue to the bilateral below-elbow amputee, principally because he has the most appropriate control sites, and to the high, bilateral above-elbow or shoulder disarticulation amputee, principally because he is served so poorly by conventional systems. It is erroneously thought that myoelectric signals provide intrinsically finer control than that achieved by the gross movements used to operate conventional prostheses. There is no evidence to indicate that performance with a prosthesis is significantly enhanced when the prosthesis is myoelectrically controlled. Perhaps most things done with conventionally controlled mechanical or electrical terminal devices and elbows are generally of a gross nature, and they are easily accomplished with conventional control systems.

In general, current research trends are aimed at exploring three types of control. Work continues along the older line with the goal of improving the detection of myoelectric activity on the surface of the skin and using it more effectively to control a terminal device or flex and extend an elbow. In effect this approach is an extension of the normal physiological signal and is best applied in a below-elbow prosthesis, using the wrist flexor for hand closing and the extensor for hand opening.

A second type of control system is being explored with a view toward improving prosthetic control for above-elbow and shoulder disarticulation patients. This differs from the direct type of control just described in that secondary or even tertiary information is used for control of terminal devices and elbows. An above-elbow amputee no longer has the long wrist flexors and extensors, and therefore signals from other muscles must be used to operate the terminal device. Normal motion of limbs is usually accomplished by primary muscles that actually move the limb segments. The efficient function of the primary movers is mediated by other individual muscles or groups of muscles that either neutralize unwanted movement in other limb segments or stabilize limb or body segments while the desired limb motion takes place. Thus the contraction of secondary muscles (those which do not directly move a limb segment) produces a myoelectric signal that controls the desired prosthetic function. Flexion of the elbow, for example, normally accomplished by the biceps, also depends on stabilization of the scapula by the trapezius and other muscles. In the absence of the biceps group, one might detect secondary myoelectric signals in the trapezius while attempting "elbow flexion" and use them to control an electric elbow. Using multiple signals from sources remote from the primary movers of a joint and comparing them to a stored predetermined pattern is known as "pattern recognition."

A third trend in research on control systems is to use myoelectric signals from even more remote, but available, sources. This is generally considered "nonphysiological," since it requires learning new neuromuscular skills. Previously used neural pathways are ignored, and new pathways are developed by training. The learning generally consists of developing the ability independently to contract one or more muscles at will. Sometimes normal movement of the eyes, eyebrows, or masseter muscles of the jaw is used.

The most common type of nonmechanical control for upper limb prostheses is direct myoelectric control using the muscles that previously performed a given function to operate the analogous function in the prosthesis. Thus long flexors and extensors of the forearm are used to open and close hands and hooks. Biceps and triceps are used to flex and extend elbows. Although users can reach a training level that reduces the control to a subconscious level, the function does require two separate muscles to control one prosthetic function. Opening the hand may be looked on as simply a repositioning function to enable the hand to close again. This view is somewhat at variance with the conventional concept that opening is release of an object, a coequal function with grasp. The difference is academic, the point at issue being that two separate muscles are required to either open or close a hand or to flex and extend an elbow. Early models of the Bock, Viennatone, and Instituto Nazionale per l'Assicurazione contro gli Infortuni sul Lavoro (INAIL) hand used a simple threshold detection system (the so-called bang-bang or on/off system). The VA/NU hand is operated by the myopulse proportional system developed by Childress. In the older systems the pinch force between the fingers was indirectly related to the duration of the signal; generally, the longer the closing motor ran, the harder the fingers pinched. Newer systems, such as the Bock, operate on a proportional system in which the forces exerted between the fingers are proportional to the magnitude of the myoelectric control signal.

In addition to myoelectric control, attempts have been made to use neurosignals to control prosthetic devices. Stein[63] in Canada has studied the utility of detecting nerve signals by means of microminiature platinum electrodes to control the VA/NU hand. Stein has implanted the electrodes directly on the radial nerve, obtaining a potentially superior signal, since the spatial and temporal delays attendant on detecting surface signals are avoided. Wileman et al.,[70] have addressed the problem of simplifying the transcutaneous passage of leads by connecting the implanted electrodes to vitreous carbon buttons implanted permanently through the skin. Corresponding leads from a terminal device are connected to the external portion of the implanted carbon buttons, and either myoelectric or neuroelectric signals are obtained from the permanently implanted electrode that may be used to operate the prosthetic device.

Interpreting myoelectric signals from secondary or higher order muscle groups and relating them to their former physiological function have been attempted successfully by several laboratories and are clearly a research trend. Jacobsen[30] of the University of Utah is developing a system to reestablish the relationship between residual muscle groups and the forces they apply. His main objective is to relate these forces to the torques generated by a prosthesis. This requires equations of motion for the arm, its torque, and a multiple electromyogram (EMG) array. Jacobsen's laboratory also developed a commercially available, high impedance myopreamplifier to reduce unwanted electrode effects.

Graupe,[20] currently associated with the Veterans Administration in Chicago and the Illinois Institute of Technology, developed the Auto Regressive Moving Average (ARMA) mathematical technique for interpreting for multiple myocontrol signals. His aim is to obtain a relatively large number of control functions (output) from a small number of control signals (input). Signals from two muscles, the biceps and triceps, when analyzed with a microprocessor-based system, could control two functions, elbow flexion-extension and hand prehension-opening, with the user still feeling the system as a physiological entity.

Wirta et al.[71] of Moss Rehabilitation Hospital, Philadelphia, participated in the development of a control system based on a synergy pattern-recognition concept. The sampled muscle set is similar to that used by the group at Utah, but the Moss group establishes a pattern employing time selection and a waiting coefficient to determine which function is desired as opposed to the vector equations used in Utah.

Mason[38] of the Veterans Administration Prosthetics Center developed an antagonist compensating proportional control system, which uses the bicep signal alone to determine the elbow velocity with the EMG related to the elbow function as it would be in a normal person with a torque load in the hand. None of the extended interpretive physiological systems are currently available; work still continues in many laboratories here and abroad, and a trend is clearly evident.

Nonphysiological related signals have also been successfully used to control upper extremity myoprostheses. A significant number of EMG level and rate of change control systems have been fitted by Schmidl[56] at INAIL. These systems use available EMG signals provided the patient can be trained independently and volitionally to activate the muscle. The signals can control the INAIL hand, wrist, and elbow. Parker and Scott[44] of the University of New Brunswick have used three-level detection and time-domain manipulation to control bidirectional functions, particularly of the hand from a singular EMG site. They are presently interested in five-level detection to permit control of two devices from one signal source. Childress of Northwestern University has established muscle space by relating two muscles on orthogonal axes and then partitioning the space so generated. They then use this space to control two devices with the appropriate no-function zone.

SENSORY FEEDBACK

Improving control of a prosthesis has been a challenge for many years. "Sensory feedback" has often been cited as an important element of prosthetic control. Sensory feedback refers to tactile information or other sensations related to position, force, and speed of elements of the prosthesis. The function of the normal hand depends on sensory feedback. In addition to information regarding imminent injury, calibration of force of grasp and pinch, recognition of the shape of an object, and knowledge of the position of the hand in space all contribute largely to the dexterity that we take for granted.

With conventional prostheses for upper limb

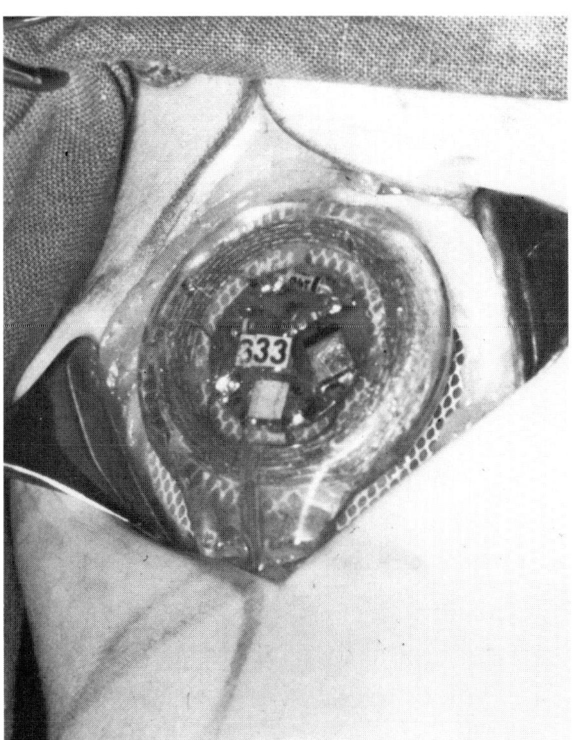

Fig. 17-19. Implanted receiver unit.

amputees, much of this information is obtained principally by visual observation and the remainder through contact pressure changes between the stump and socket and between the skin and harness. In mechanical voluntary closing terminal devices sensory feedback is related to force applied between the fingers, which is proportional to the force the wearer applies to close the terminal device.

Biceps kineplasty used with a voluntary closing hook provides similar information, since pressure between the fingers could be calibrated by interpretation of pressure changes between the surface of the tunnel and pin. Kineplasties have not been widely accepted in the United States, however, because of the difficulty in maintaining the skin in good condition within the depths of the tunnel.

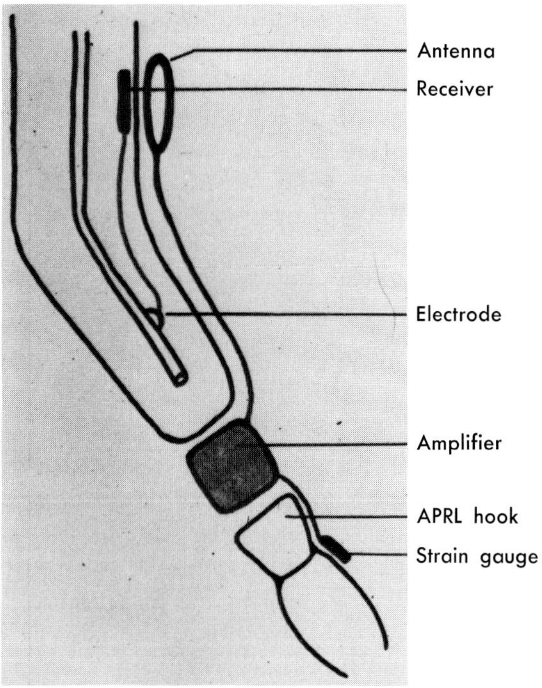

Fig. 17-20. Sensory feedback system.

Clippinger et al.[8] describe efforts to improve control of prostheses by taking advantage of miniaturization of electric circuits and components and the development of small electrical devices that can be implanted in the human body. They implanted an induction-powered radio receiver/ pulse generator for motor stimulation of the peroneal nerve in hemiplegic patients. They believed that this type of system could be used to produce sensory stimulation from the terminal device of a prosthesis in the following situations:

1. If the electrode were placed on the median nerve to provide a mental image of the peripheral cutaneous distribution of that nerve—the thumb, index, long, and half the ring finger
2. If sufficient voltage were used to produce a stimulus, but not at a painful level
3. If a transducer in the terminal device were capable of varying frequency related to activity
4. If the entire system, including the amplifier, transmitter, and power source, were small enough to fit within the prosthesis to avoid external wires and battery packs
5. If the system were sufficiently durable to withstand normal use of an amputation prosthesis
6. If the design were such that the patient would don and adjust it with one hand

Clippinger et al. used an implant designed by Avery Laboratories (Fig. 17-19). It was an inductively coupled radiofrequency receiver, measuring 2.9 cm in diameter and 0.9 cm in thickness. It was tuned to 2.05 MHz. Their implant is

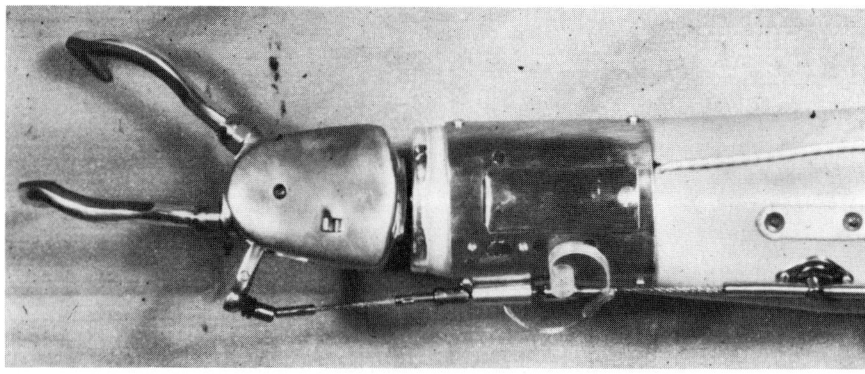

Fig. 17-21. Type II prosthesis with APRL hook.

embedded in biocompatible epoxy and encased in Silastic. A Silastic sheet skirt incorporating Dacron mesh is attached. The skirt was used to suture the unit to the fascia to prevent migration. The output of the implant was a capacity-coupled pulse, producing a zero net direct current flow in the nerve at rates and amplitudes that are determined by the external transmitter.

Fig. 17-20 illustrates the feedback system. The first patients were below-elbow amputees to minimize the mechanical problems of prosthetic use. The implant was placed subcutaneously in the medial aspect of the distal arm, away from interference from any part of the prosthesis. The prosthesis was activated in a conventional manner using a figure-of-eight harness and cable control. An APRL hook (Fig. 17-21) with the locking cam removed was used to force the amputee to "hold on" to an object. It was believed that this was a normal function and that removal of the cam would eliminate the additional force and subsequent pressure increase necessary to unlock the hook.

In all, some fifteen patients, ten below-elbow and five above-elbow amputees, were fitted. Early results suggested that the concept was correct; nerve stimulation with resulting appropriate interpretation and mental image can be obtained by use of an implanted induction-powered nerve stimulator and at voltage levels that are comfortable.

Prior and Lyman,[47] at the University of California, Los Angeles, Biotechnology Laboratory, have been investigating the effectiveness of supplying electrocutaneous sensory feedback as an aid in controlling upper limb prostheses. They designed several different electrocutaneous sensory feedback systems. They also studied methods of encoding sensory feedback parameters with single and multiple electrodes. They compared bipolar and monopolar stimulation and studied the importance of a reference signal to feedback effectiveness. Other investigations were conducted of undesired interaction between myoelectric control and electrocutaneous feedback when used simultaneously in an arm prosthesis.

Three different sensory feedback systems were developed for a 2 degree-of-freedom (DOF) (hand and elbow), proportionally controlled, externally energized prosthesis with grasp-force and hand-opening feedback (Figs. 17-22 and 17-23).

Various coding schemes were selected by means of a sixteen pin dual in-line package (DIP) plug on the electronics circuit board. The hand is a standard VA/NU myoelectric hand with strain gauges, power supply, signal amplifier, and a finger-position potentiometer installed by the Veterans Administration Prosthetics Center (Fig. 17-24).

Myoelectrically controlled hands suffer from a reduced amount of sensory feedback available to the patient as compared with even the small amount of feedback available in conventional cable-operated prostheses. When grasping objects with a myoelectrically controlled hand, visual feedback is the dominant mode. Electrocutaneous sensory feedback from the hand can be expected to improve function, but unfortunately another problem arises with the use of simultaneous myoelectric control and electrocutaneous feedback-interaction between the two. To date, this problem has not been adequately investigated, although some research has been done. Kaplan[32] and Rohland[49,50] employed separate electrode sites for control and stimulation and various filtering schemes as a solution to the interaction problem. Scott[58] described the use of time-sharing and gain-control principles to enable a myoelectric control unit and a sensory feedback stimulator to function from a common set of electrodes. Carl Mason of the VAPC is investigating modifications of the VA/NU hand EMG amplifier circuits to achieve (1) rapid recovery from input overload transients from the stimulator and (2) filtering of stimulator frequency components.

Other research was carried out by Schmidl[57] to increase the gripping speed of artificial hands. The artificial hands he used had gripping speeds of 8 to 12 cm/sec, the highest speed that can be managed by on/off controls. Higher gripping speeds require proportional control speed. In addition, a sensory feedback device was designed for the location of close objects by sightless persons without hands.

Control signals with considerable information content must be originated by the patient to execute the complex motions desired of an upper limb prosthesis or orthosis. As the level of dysfunction becomes more proximal, the complexity of the amputee's control task increases.

Supplemental sensory feedback systems usually contain electronic transducers (strain gauges, potentiometers, etc.) installed at key points in the artificial limb. In addition, a signal-conditioning and display-driving electronics package and an information display interfaced to the amputee are required. Any type of visual, auditory, and/or tactile displays can be used, but both visual and au-

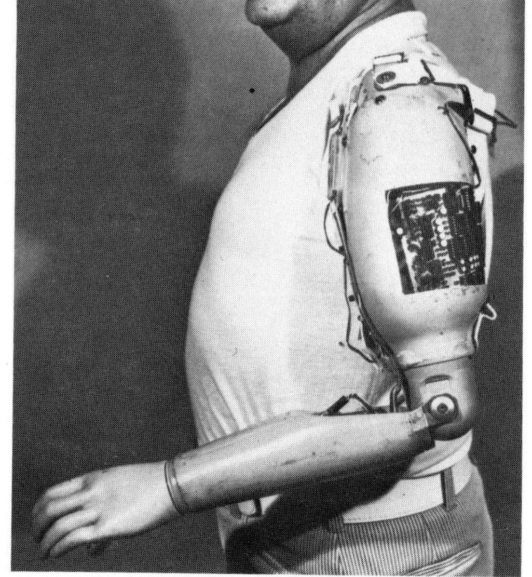

Fig. 17-22. Experimental prosthesis.

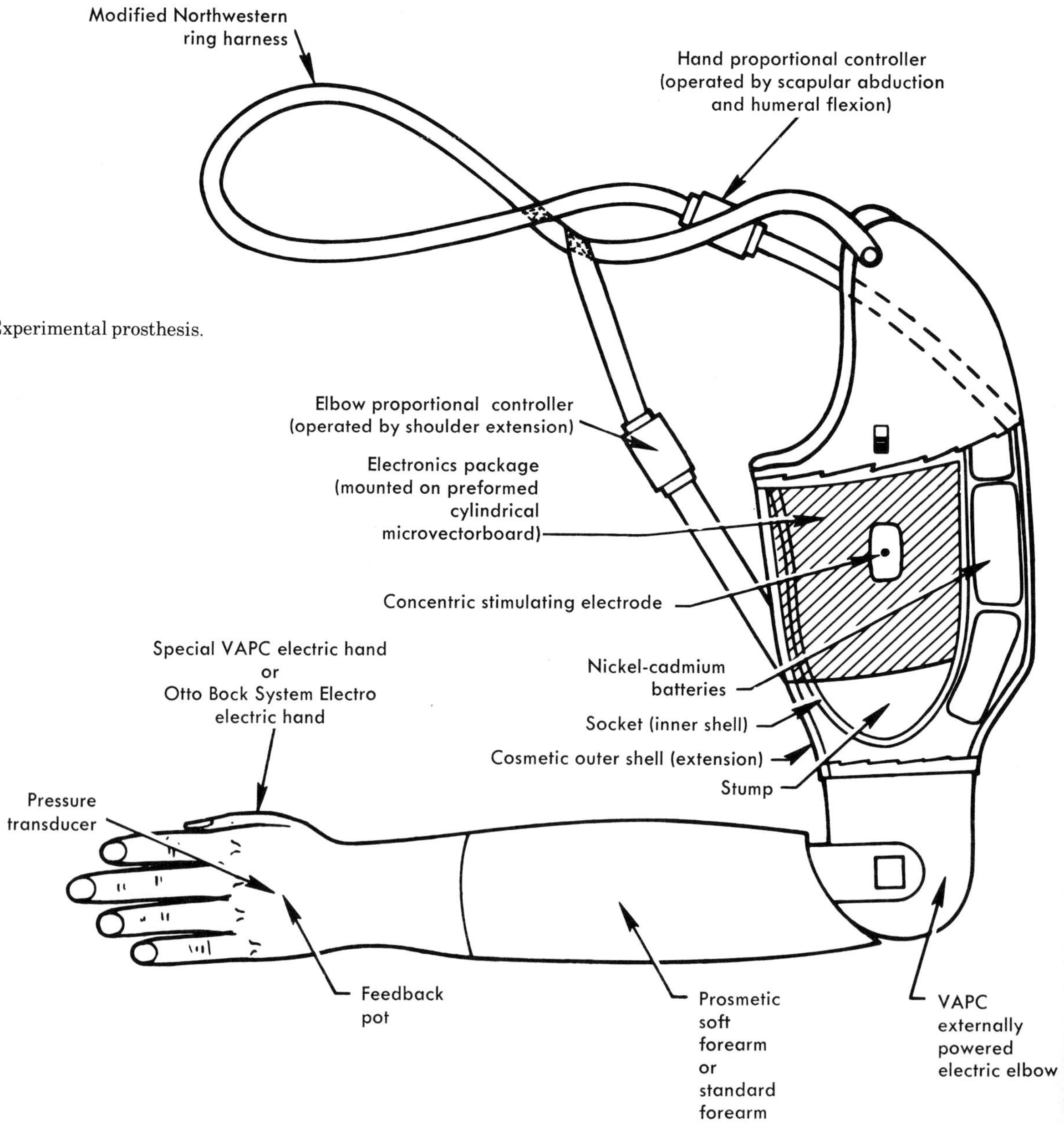

Fig. 17-23. Experimental prosthesis.

Modified Northwestern ring harness

Hand proportional controller (operated by scapular abduction and humeral flexion)

Elbow proportional controller (operated by shoulder extension)

Electronics package (mounted on preformed cylindrical microvectorboard)

Concentric stimulating electrode

Special VAPC electric hand or Otto Bock System Electro electric hand

Nickel-cadmium batteries

Socket (inner shell)

Cosmetic outer shell (extension)

Stump

Pressure transducer

Feedback pot

Prosmetic soft forearm or standard forearm

VAPC externally powered electric elbow

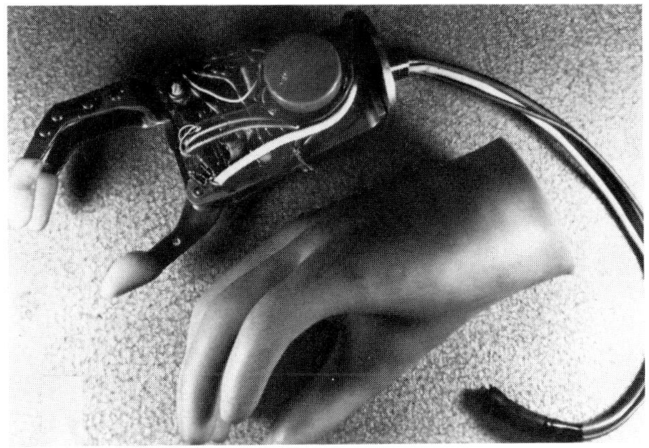

Fig. 17-24. Special VAPC electric hand.

ditory displays tend to be conspicuous, drawing further attention to an already self-conscious individual. A better approach might be to use some sort of silent and unobtrusive tactile display, preferably contained within the prosthesis.

Drawbacks, however, exist. Tactile displays must be properly designed to be effective. If electrocutaneous stimulation is employed, pain and skin irritation can result from improper design. Also, the rate of information transfer possible with a tactile display is typically orders of magnitude lower than with either a visual or auditory display.

These drawbacks are not insurmountable, and solutions appear to exist using available technology. For example, Saunders[53] and Collins and Madey[9] have largely resolved the problem of painful stimuli. The problem of low information transfer rates still persists, although rates adequate for artificial limb applications have been achieved.

The VAPC provided a special myoelectric hand, complete with strain gauges, to measure grasp force and a potentiometer to measure hand opening. Originally it was planned to incorporate two stimulation electrodes into the prosthesis, one to be used to indicate grasp force and the other hand opening. Both electrodes were to use pulse width or rate modulation or a combination of the two. However, the results of subject testing indicated that the choice of codes should be carefully considered.

The following system requirements should be met by any myoelectric hand–stimulated sensory feedback prosthesis to be clinically practical. The stimulated sensory feedback system should be completely contained within the prosthesis and must not degrade cosmetic appearance. The only exception would be the placement of stimulation electrodes on the upper arm if, and only if, the use of a large number of electrodes can promise a dramatic increase in function for the amputee. Most amputees who prefer a myoelectric hand do so because it is more cosmetic and easier to don and doff than a conventional harness and cable-operated prosthesis. Thus any stimulated sensory feedback system that degrades cosmesis or is not completely contained within the prosthesis should be avoided. Since containment of the stimulated sensory feedback system within the forearm and hand is important, miniaturization of electronic circuitry is required. If simple circuit designs using relatively few components prove adequate, conventional printed circuit board construction techniques will suffice. If this is not the case, custom hybrid circuits will be required.

The space available for the amputee's stump must not be reduced by more than 5 cm (2 inches). A complaint by some prosthetists is that only those amputees with medium to short stumps can use the VA/NU hand. Approximately 20 cm (8 inches) are required from the distal end of the prosthesis to the electrode connector bulkhead. Increases in this depth should therefore not exceed 5 cm (2 inches) after the stimulated sensory feedback system is added, or few amputees will be able to wear the prosthesis. Complete containment of the electronic components in the hand is required if midlength amputees are to wear the prosthesis.

The stimulator(s) must not interfere with the myoelectric control system. The goal is isolation of the myoelectric amplifier input and the stimulator common ground points. Three methods of isolating the grounds are under investigation:

1. Transformer coupling of the stimulator output pulse to the stimulation electrode
2. Use of a low-voltage (12 V to 12 V) DC-to-DC converter to power the stimulated sensory feedback circuitry
3. A separate stimulated sensory feedback battery pack

The operating time for each battery charge must not be substantially reduced by the addition of the stimulated sensory feedback system. An estimate is that the total stimulated sensory feedback system should consume no more than 10 mA at 12 V continuous (25 mA during movements) if powered from the 12-V, 225-mAh battery supplied with the hand, or no more than 36 mW if powered from a separate stimulated sensory feedback battery pack. The stimulated sensory feedback system must function properly throughout a typical battery discharge cycle. This requires that all stimulation parameters be insensitive to normal battery voltage changes. Critical circuits must therefore possess good supply-voltage rejection, or a voltage regulator must be incorporated into the design. Proper operation must be maintained for all anticipated temperature conditions. The system should operate at least from 10° to 38° C (50° to 100° F) and from −1.1° to 49° C (30° to 120° F), if possible. Temperature sensitivity of the stimulation parameters as measured at the electrodes should be 10% or less over the minimum temperature range. The weight of the stimulated sensory feedback system should not exceed 227 g (8 ounces), and 113 g (4 ounces) or less is preferred. Codes chosen for the stimulated sensory feedback system must require no more than a minimal conscious effort by the amputee to decode the sensory feedback information. Code in this instance refers to the relationship between variations in a parameter of the prosthesis (e.g., grasp force) and variations in the stimulation that is applied to the amputee (e.g., pulse rate, width amplitude changes). Also, how the amputee perceives changes in the stimulation is part of the code (e.g., "the buzz is faster, therefore I know that the hand is more widely opened").

MEDICAL MANIPULATORS

The tetraplegic patient whose spinal cord has been traumatized at a level that prevents use of the arms and hands has the greatest need for remote control of objects in the environment. Trauma of the spinal cord is a catastrophic event in which treatment requires saving the patient's life and salvaging all residual limb function, a course that invokes the full range of medical and paramedical skills available. Many patients with high-level lesions live their lives in bed with their energies directed toward simply staying alive and maintaining reasonable hygiene. Once they are medically stabilized, these patients have two fundamental requirements—mobility and manipulation. The problem of locomotion for such patients has had a great deal of recent attention, particularly in the variety of newly developed powered wheelchairs, some of which recline, rotate, or enable the user to stand up. Some are controlled by movements of the chin, negative and positive intraoral pressures, and other more exotic control systems employing eye movements and spoken speech.

Manipulation in the sense of the ability to move objects or operate devices has also been advanced, giving quadriplegics independent access to music, television, reading material, telephones, food, and recreational devices. This increased capability, developed primarily during the past 5 years, has resulted from the use of so-called environmental controls. The "POSSUM" was the first environmental control system. It was designed by Maling[37] of Aylesbury, England. Since then, the number of such devices has proliferated (Fig. 17-25). In general all of them enable a user to turn on and off switches to control a variety of electrical devices, such as televisions and radios. The most recent advances in this area of technology include physically decoupling the patient from the device by using radio links between the switch operated or the breath pressure control employed by the user and the appliance to be controlled. Another recent improvement is the use of devices that recognize spoken speech to permit the user to "speak" to devices to turn them on or adjust them. Environmental control development can be considered a fait accompli. Some six to ten systems of various types are available commercially, and their use is increasing.

However, many highly important functions cannot be performed by relatively simple on/off systems because they require multidimensional displacement of an object in space. The three-dimensional orientation of a user, the three-dimensional orientation, and the three-dimensional location in space of an object to be "manipulated" must be considered simultaneously when a person rolls up to a table in a wheelchair, picks an object off the table, carries it to another place, and releases it. To accomplish tasks of this type, adaptations of industrial manipulators are now being considered.

Some of the earliest work on manipulator development was performed by Goertz et al.[18,19] at the Argonne National Laboratories, Argonne, Illinois. Goertz designed a bilateral master/slave control manipulator for work with radioactive materials. A similar master/slave control approach was used by Mosher and Wendel[42,43] in the General Electric Company "Handyman." This unit, like Goertz's, incorporated force feedback for improved operator performance. The concept was expanded from initiation of human manipulation to its augmentation in a combination pedipulator/manipulator exoskeleton by the General Electric group.

The concept of a basically anthropomorphic

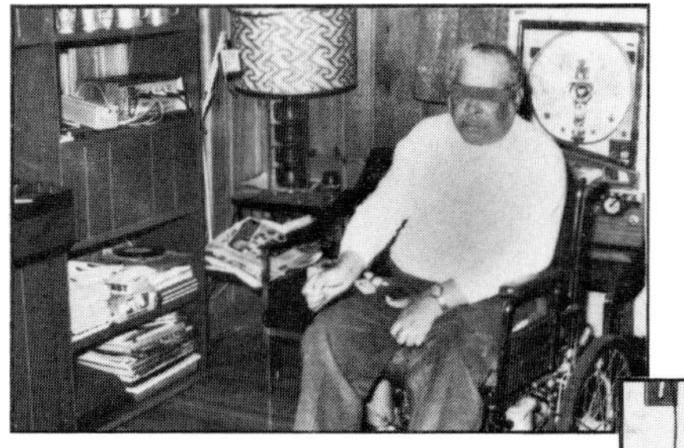

Fig. 17-25. Montage of three environmental control systems.

design for a general purpose manipulator has become fairly well established. The primary benefit of such a system design is the ease of master/slave control, in which the manipulator becomes an analog of the operator's arm. Anthropomorphic designs are thought to benefit from kinematic similarity to human motion and the resultant control compatibility. The multiple articulations required for "reach around" capability are also inherent in anthropomorphic designs.

The limited control capability of the disabled operator breaks the loop required for master/slave control. As Roth[51] states, there is no a priori reason to construct a manipulative device that is kinematically identical to the human limb. It should be noted that the anthropomorphic designs previously discussed are extremely reduced kinematic replications of the human arm and hand manipulative ability. The most complex of the manipulators has 8 DOF, as compared with the human range of 42 DOF.

The design requirements for industrial and medical manipulators are quite different. Industrial manipulators usually are computer controlled to perform predetermined tasks. They can also be designed in a master/slave arrangement in which the normal human operator can provide a manipulator with a huge amount of control information in the form of position, velocity, and acceleration of shoulder, elbow, wrist, and finger joints. In this case the manipulator needs only to be designed to duplicate to the required scale the control information provided by the operator.

A quadriplegic person is not capable of providing the manipulator with a great deal of control information; he can only command it by breathing in a code of puffs and sucks, one- or two-dimensional movements of the head, myoelectric signals in the active muscles of the face and neck, movements of the tongue and eye, or by the spoken word. Each of these control modes and the mechanical configuration of the manipulator itself are a terra incognita; no one really knows the relative merits of extensible, jointed, anthropomorphic, or other design configurations for the mechanical portion of the manipulator. No one is certain how best to build a manipulator to enable a person to pick food up and feed himself, select a book or other reading material, position it to be read in bed or in a wheelchair and return it to its place, shave, wash, comb hair, play games, write, answer a phone, type, and otherwise perform a variety of functions that require a higher form of control than simple on/off switching.

During the past several years some ten to twelve medical manipulators in different configurations have been designed and are now gradually being evaluated. The earliest known version, the Rancho Golden Arm, was developed some 15 years ago at Rancho Los Amigos Hospital in Downey, California. A number of factors contributed to the slow development in this area. The need for medical manipulators is not firmly established because during the past 10 to 15 years substantial improvements have been made in orthotic devices and the previously cited environmental controls that have come into use. Another retarding factor is the high expense associated with the design and development of such complex devices and, perhaps equally important, the absence of an adequately objective method of evaluating them.[4,66] Generally accepted methods of evaluation are crucial to development to provide a rational basis for the direction of research, design, and further development. In the last 5 years particularly, a clear-cut, strong trend has been generated to develop evaluation methods and to build medical manipulators and control systems.

Table 1. Motor voltage measurements of Rancho Los Amigos remote manipulator*

Motion	*Voltage unloaded (V)*	*Voltage with load (V)*
Wrist		
Flexion	12.16	12.17
Extension	12.02	11.85
Wrist rotation	11.0	10.78
Elbow		
Flexion	11.57	11.87
Extension	11.86	11.25
Humeral rotation		
Clockwise	11.35	11.35
Counterclockwise	11.80	11.80
Shoulder rotation		
Flexion	11.78	11.64
Extension	11.30	9.60
Horizontal shoulder versus gravity		
Down	11.9	11.9
Up	11.30	9.60

*From Rancho Los Amigos Hospital, Downey, Calif.

With a Veterans Administration contract, Corker et al.[10] at the University of California, Los Angeles, have developed a standardized protocol to make evaluation data on manipulators compatible, comparable, and additive. This is the first evaluation technique for manipulators that permits the valid comparison of several systems and therefore provides the only suitable basis for prescriptive judgments. Corker states that the patient/manipulator system consists of the following two interactive subsystems:

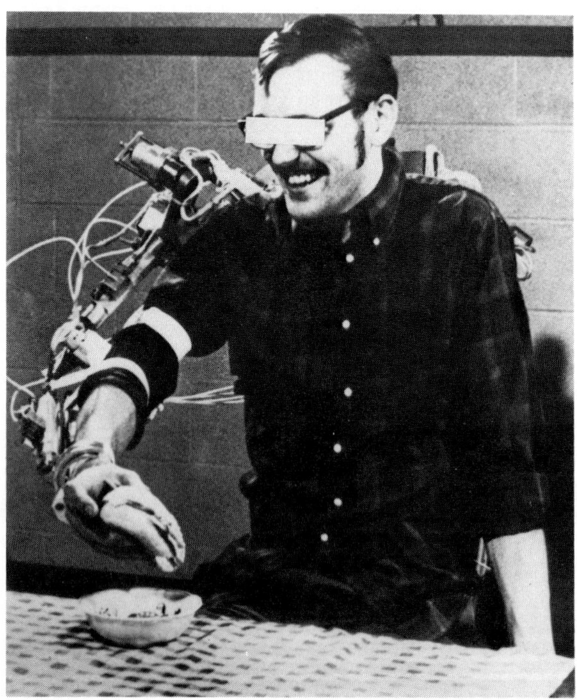

Fig. 17-26. Case Institute powered orthosis.

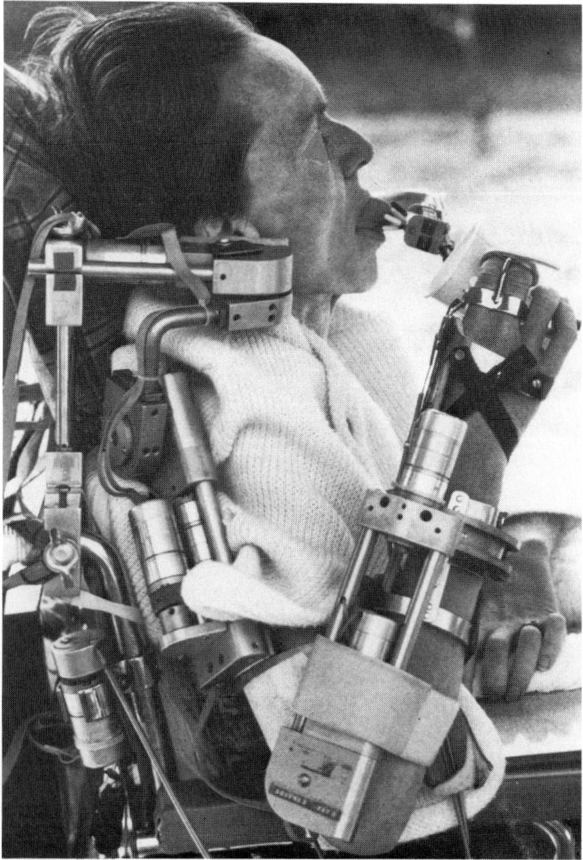

Fig. 17-27. Rancho Golden Arm and tongue switches.

1. The manipulator/effector subsystem, which is made up of the manipulator hardware and its mountings
2. The control subsystem, which is composed of the components that transduce the operator's physical control motions or signals, the control logic, including aiding or processing elements, and those components which drive the system

Evaluation at the University of California, Los Angeles, Biotechnology Laboratory is directed toward specification of the general principles applicable to manipulator design and toward characterization of those situations which call for individual consideration in prescription of manipulator systems. Because of the complexity of manipulator systems, the selectivity of the patient population, and the multiplicity of factors, as well as the nature of the practical situation in dealing with extremely disabled patients, the evaluations are conducted in a "semi-case study" style using etiologically varied patients.[21] After performance tests are conducted to familiarize the patient with the machine and to determine the range of the patient's control abilities, he is provided a manipulator system, and his activity will be monitored with unobstrusive integrated circuit counters. The long-term aspect of monitoring surmounts some of the problems of novelty effect produced by the increased attention paid the patient.

The manipulator as an intimate interface between humans and machines has had effects not only on the patient's functional ability, but also in the patient's attitude toward himself and rehabilitation. There is no doubt that the evaluation procedure represents a considerable novelty effect in the lives of the participants, who are all chronic care clinic patients and as such lead very routine existences. The introduction of the manipulator and tests into that system will cause an increase in motivation and interest in something new. This novelty effect should be circumvented by a long-term monitoring system to record machine use when the machine is available to the patient on a 24-hour basis.

It has been reported through the staff psychologists that patients experience a considerable elevation in mood and self-concept from participation in the project. As the tests and practice are conducted in the ward setting, the participant receives considerable attention from staff and other patients. It can be tentatively concluded that a large ancillary benefit of the medical manipulator is its positive influence on other aspects of rehabilitation. The patients report a sense of usefulness in contributing to a study that may ultimately benefit others. There is a strong psy-

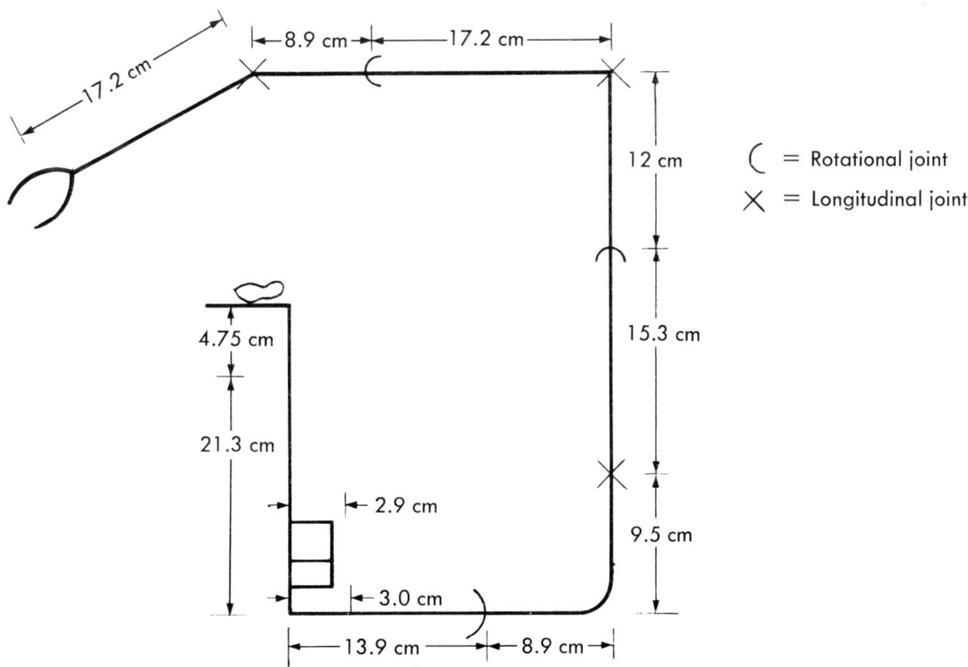

Fig. 17-28. Performance parameters of Rancho remote manipulator.

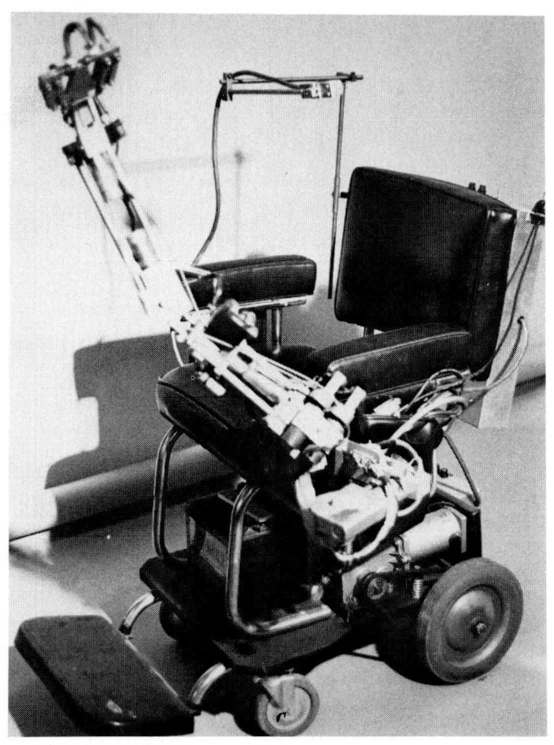

Fig. 17-29. General Teleoperator manipulator mounted on wheelchair.

chological benefit in the attempt to provide new procedures for rehabilitation.

All the known configurations of manipulators are being or will be evaluated at the University of California, Los Angeles, by Corker and his group. Included among them are telescoping systems, articulated systems that are more or less related to prosthetic designs, wheelchair-mounted units, and table-mounted units, some with special table-top environments. At the same time several kinds of controls are being evaluated, including those which depend on force and motion of the body, intraoral pressures, reflected light controlled by eyeball motion, voice recognition, and some hybrids employing several of these controls.

Rancho Los Amigos remote manipulator (Golden Arm). The Rancho Los Amigos Remote Manipulator (Golden Arm) has a design configuration (Table 1) similar to the Case Institute powered orthotic brace (Fig. 17-26). It is a 7-DOF manipulator with a kinematic range similar to the human arm. The manipulator is controlled through a bank of seven bidirectional "bang-

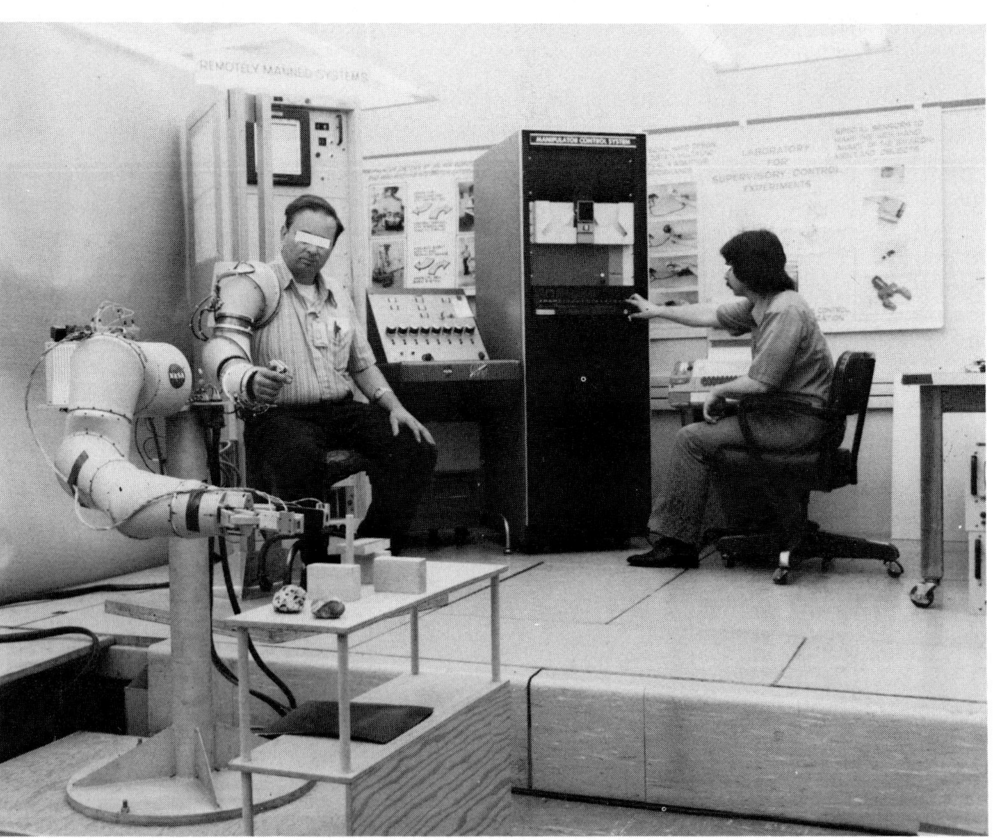

Fig. 17-30. NASA/Ames manipulator.

bang" tongue switches (Fig. 17-27). The functional details of its performance include speed of motion, force developed, torque, and ranges of motion for seven elements of the manipulator. These parameters are described for prehension, wrist extension, flexion and rotation, elbow flexion, and humeral and shoulder rotation (Fig. 17-28).

General Teleoperators, Inc., remote controlled manipulator. General Teleoperators, Inc., Downey, California, has adapted a similar manipulator for wheelchair mounting (Fig. 17-29). This provides a mobile mount with the possibility of control by telemetry. Remote control permits handling objects at a distance from a patient's bed or chair. The control problem however is far more difficult. Vision, the primary source of feedback control, is reduced as the range increases. Presently, the quadriplegic only has available chin control, breath control, light-beam control, or voice control.

NASA manipulators. Anthropomorphic articulated arms have also been developed at the Jet Propulsion Laboratories in Pasadena, California. The NASA/Ames arm is an 8-DOF arm originally designed for master/slave control (Fig. 17-30). The 7-DOF NASA/CURV arm employs a multilinkage design with basically anthropomorphic kinematics[68] (Fig. 17-31). These arms are not used clinically; they are used in the development of control dynamics and in interactive sensor control technology.[2] "Aiding" may be incorporated to reduce the operator control burden of an anthropomorphic design in a structured work environment.

Applied Physics Laboratory (APL), Johns Hopkins manipulator. The APL manipulator and worktable combines a 5-DOF anthropomorphic design on a sliding track with a structured work environment. Seamone et al.[59] use the stability of the work area to allow preprogrammed computer control of certain fixed trajectories and/or repetitive action. It employs a novel dual-mode chin controller to enable a person to control both a wheelchair and the table-mounted manipulator.

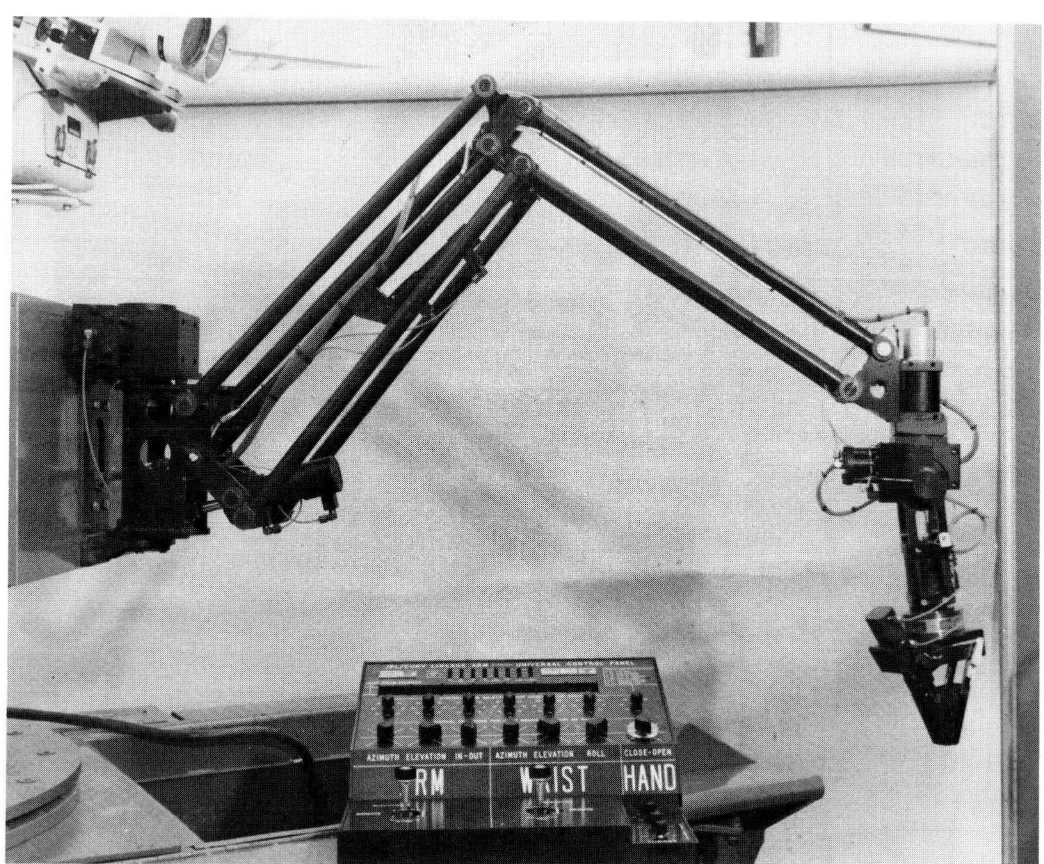

Fig. 17-31. NASA/CURV linkage arm.

To use this chin controller for robotic arm control after driving the wheelchair in front of the robotic arm/worktable system, the user lifts the chin control lever momentarily to switch control from the wheelchair motors to an optical link located on one arm of the wheelchair. This frequency modulation optical link transmits pulse and proportional signals from the chin controller to operate all of the manual modes and programmed sequences of the robotic arm. When the quadriplegic desires to leave this worktable area, he need only to momentarily lift the chin controller lever with

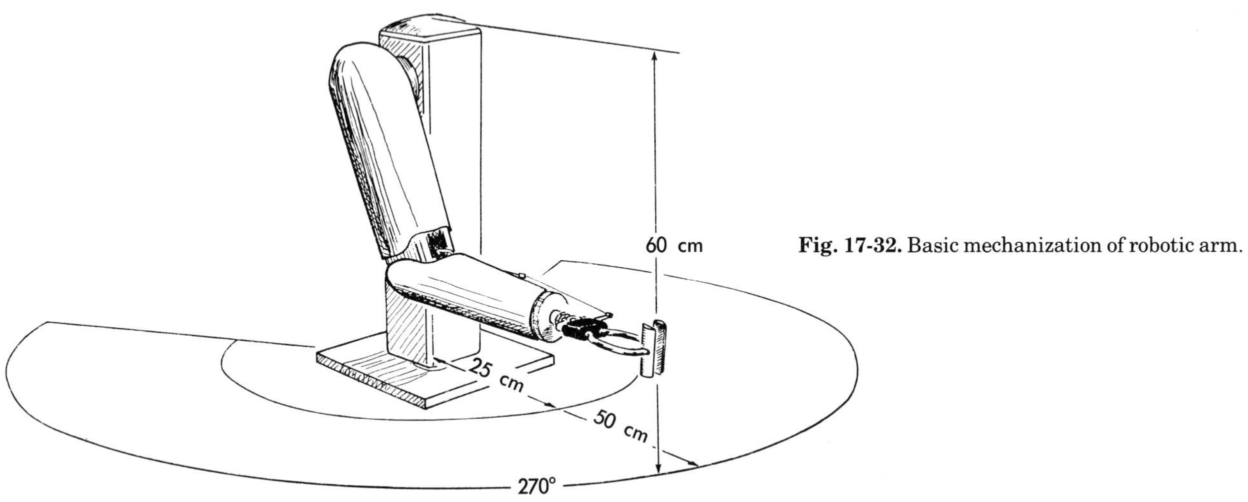

Fig. 17-32. Basic mechanization of robotic arm.

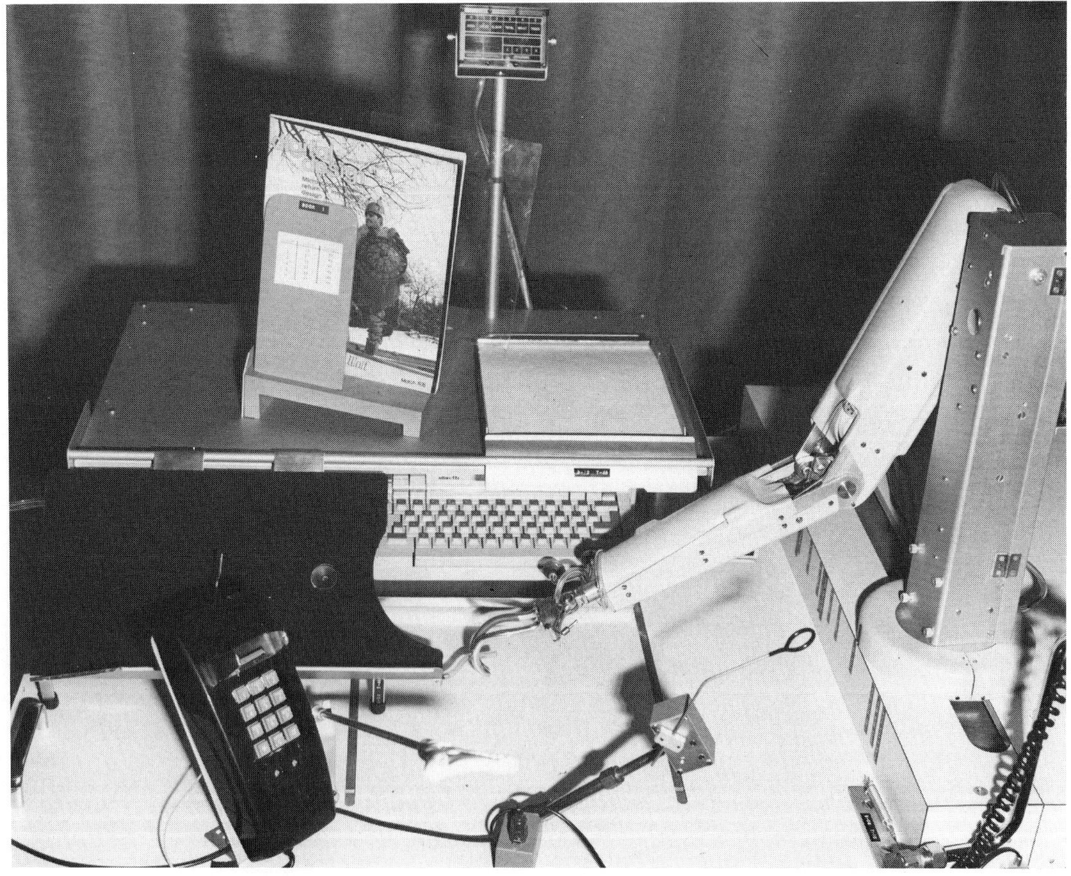

Fig. 17-33. Clinical testing of APL manipulator.

his chin to return the control to the wheelchair motors. Many of the components of a powered shoulder prosthesis are used in the robotic arm. A schematic diagram of the basic mechanization of the robotic arm is shown in Fig. 17-32. Its 5 DOF include hook grasping, wrist pronation-supination, elbow flexion, shoulder flexion-extension with parallelogram motion of the forearm, and shoulder turntable. The unit is mounted on a motorized track to allow linear motion of 75 cm along one axis of the worktable.

A microprocessor has been incorporated in the latest model of the robotic arm to control manual and semiautomated motions. The microcomputer is commanded by the user from the chin controller and provides feedback to the user by a light-emitting diode display panel. Programming of desired automatic motion sequences is accomplished with a functional keyboard.

The robotic arm has 6 degrees of motive freedom. Motive power comes from three motors located in the upper arm, support column, and translocation table. The upper arm motor activates shoulder, elbow, and wrist motion, whereas the support column motor activates column rotation and the terminal device. Except for the translation table, the motors actuate cable-driven–spring-return mechanisms. All axes of motion are normally held in discrete positions with a solenoid-actuated lock mechanism.

The layout of the worktable has been arranged to minimize the effort required to carry out practical tasks. The worktable top is 86 cm by 152 cm and may be placed on a stationary table for operation from a wheelchair or may be placed on a mobile cart for over-the-bed use. Placement of components and special tools on this worktable makes maximum use of the quadriplegic's capabilities with a mouthstick. The table arrangement for the latest model undergoing clinical testing is shown in Fig. 17-33.

The typewriter is mounted in a thin flat cart to allow the robotic arm to move it into or out of range of the user. A semiautomatic programmed sequence moves the typewriter into position and places the paper into the typewriter. The actual typing is accomplished by use of a mouthstick. This concept takes full advantage of the individ-

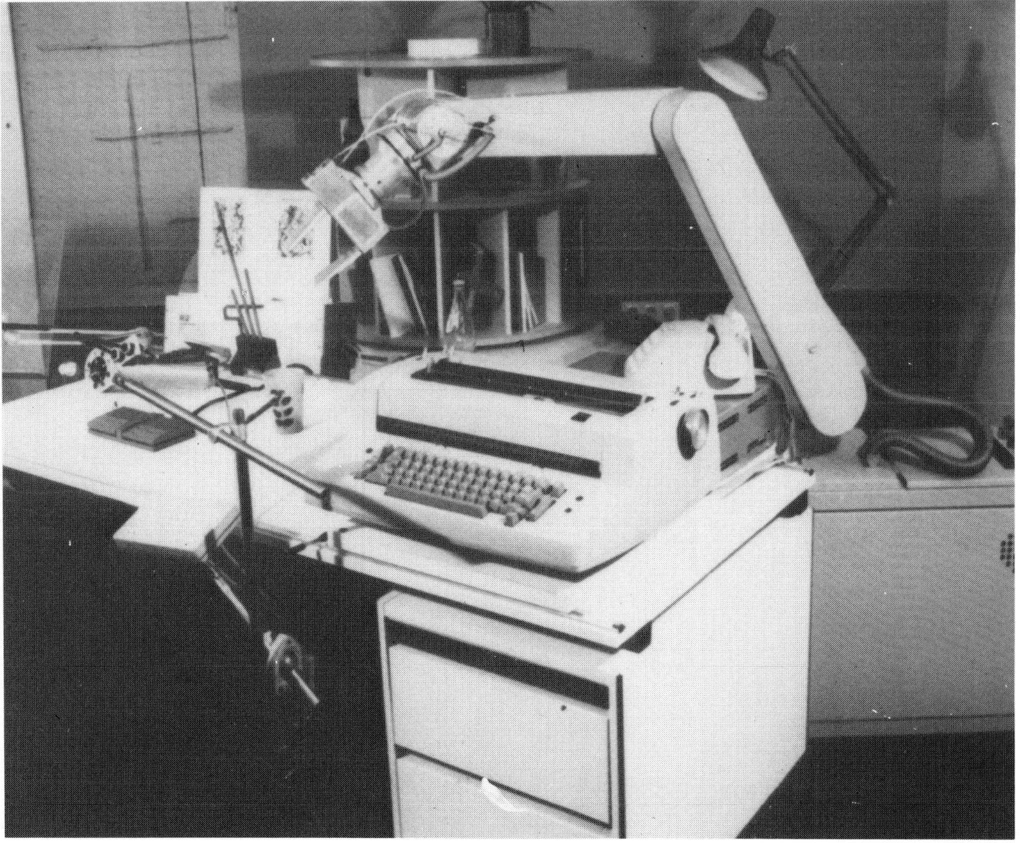

Fig. 17-34. Heidelberg manipulator.

ual's training and skill with the mouthstick. Similarly, magazines and other reading materials are placed in a reading rack for easy accessibility by the robotic arm. Again, an automatic programmed sequence is used to accomplish picking up the reading material and placing it on the rack for reading. Only the book selection portion is done with manual control. The mouthstick is used to turn the pages, a technique commonly employed in rehabilitation centers for retraining quadriplegics.

A touchtone telephone with a touch pad located on the handset is used on this worktable. A programmed sequence will pick up the phone and bring it to the quadriplegic or hold it in front of him for touchtone dialing. Tasks such as these require minimal inputs to perform somewhat complicated mechanical functions. The user can always stop the motions during the programmed sequences by simply pulsing the microswitch to revert to manual control.

Heidelberg manipulator. Another structured environment and manipulator system has been developed by the Heidelberg group, headed by Roesler (Fig. 17-34). This 6-DOF semianthropomorphic manipulator system is designed to work interactively with a special purpose work environment. The manipulator itself is kinematically similar to the human arm. Its range in the selected degrees of freedom is larger than the corresponding human range.

Spartacus manipulator. The design of medi-

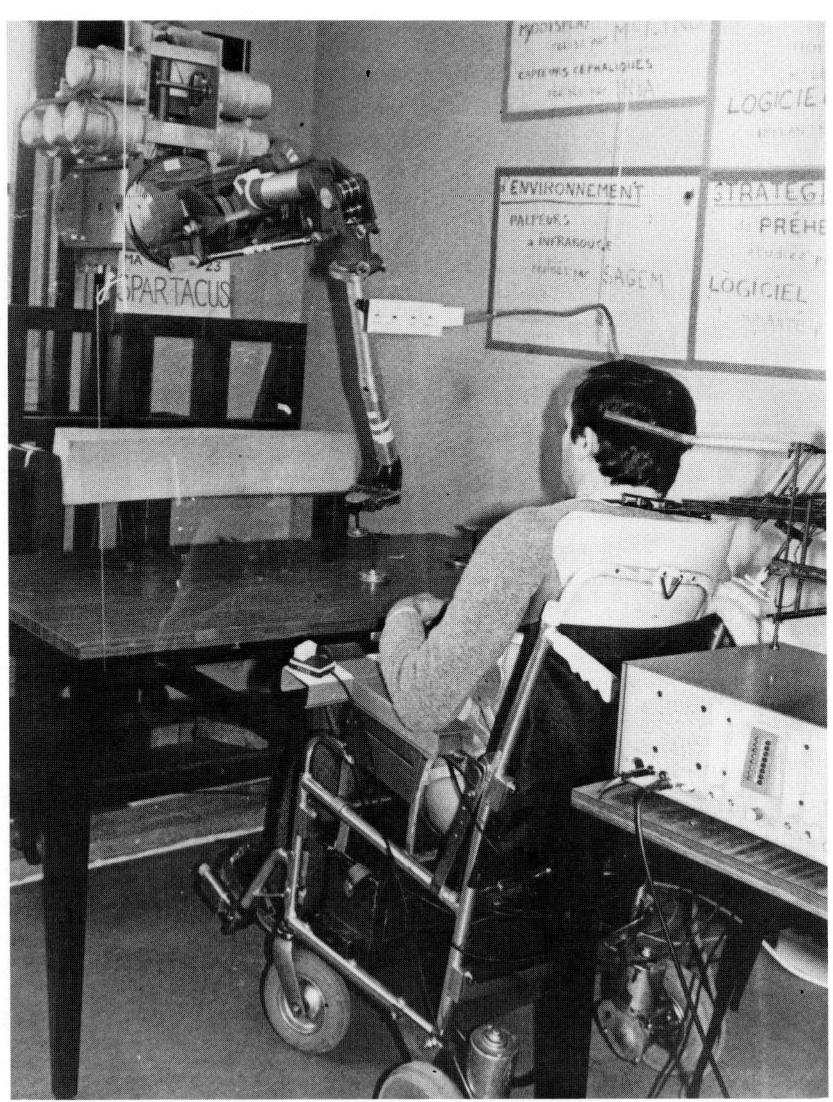

Fig. 17-35. Spartacus 7-DOF manipulator.

cal manipulators has also moved away from the orthotic and prosthetic idea in which a user "wears" the device. Some developers are exploring the commercially available manipulators for rehabilitation purposes. The potential benefits of such commercially useful manipulators are a reduction of cost, an availability of maintenance, and a broad user base to support development. The Spartacus Project in France employs a 7-DOF manipulator (Fig. 17-35), the CEA, LaClahene,

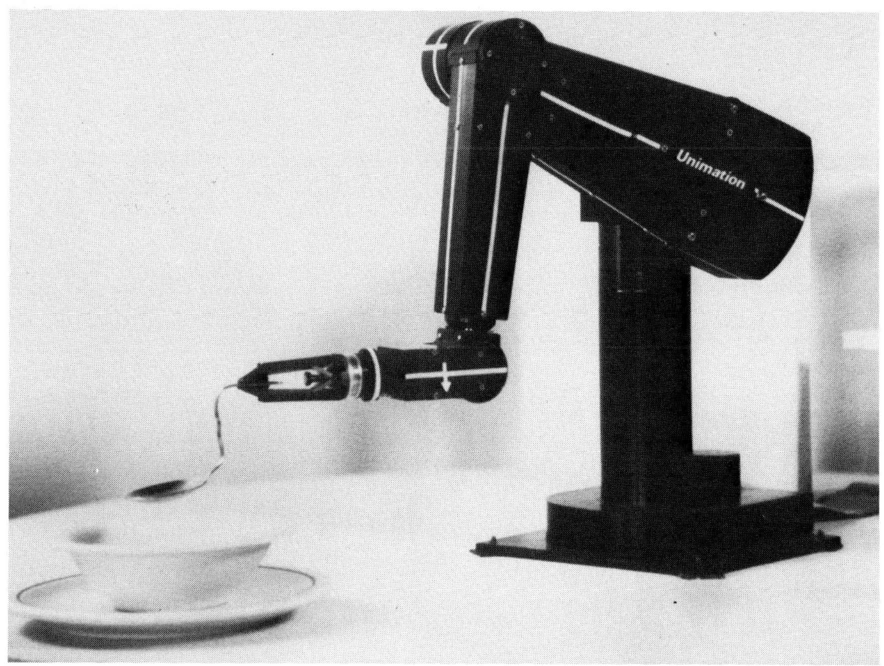

Fig. 17-36. Unimation model 250 electric arm.

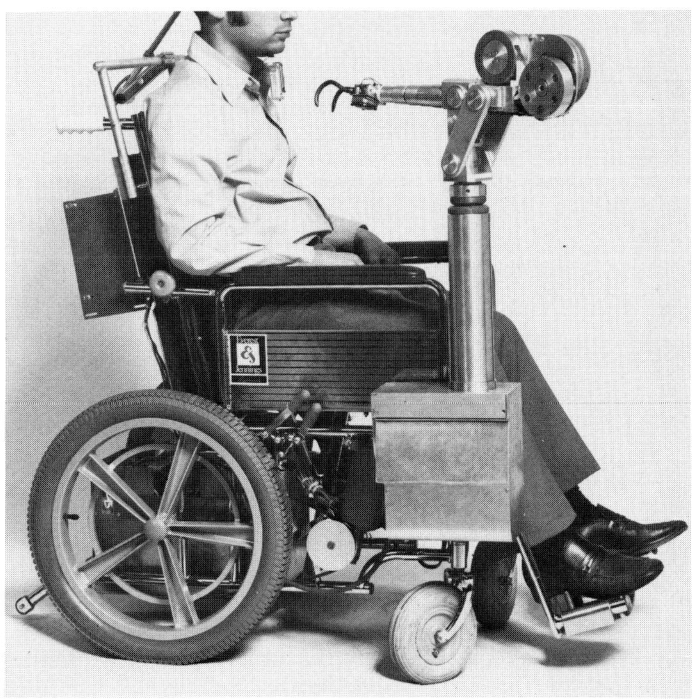

Fig. 17-37. VAPC manipulator.

Massachusetts, used by the French Atomic Energy Commission.[22]

Unimation model 250 electric arm. Leifer et al.[34] report the adaptation to clinical use of the commercially fabricated 7-DOF Unimation model 250 electric arm (Fig. 17-36). The manipulator has been designed for computer control. It is a "smart robotic arm" in that it can remember position.

VAPC manipulator. Mason[39] has developed an extensible medical manipulator system (Fig. 17-37). The system has 8 DOF, and the wheelchair on which it is mounted is driven by the manipulator control system. The manipulator provides 3 DOF to determine the location of the end effector (terminal device). The end effector provides an additional 3 DOF, opening and closing the fingers, rotation of the wrist, and flexion-extension of the wrist. The VAPC manipulator (Fig. 17-37) is controlled by a pound per square inch (psi) or logarithmic expansion interpretation of the force applied by the user's head (Fig. 17-38). This form of control reduces the intellectual de-

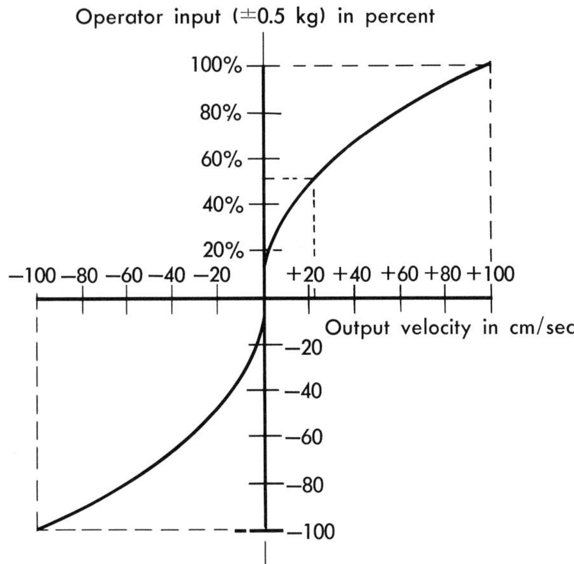

Fig. 17-38. VAPC manipulator operator input-output relation.

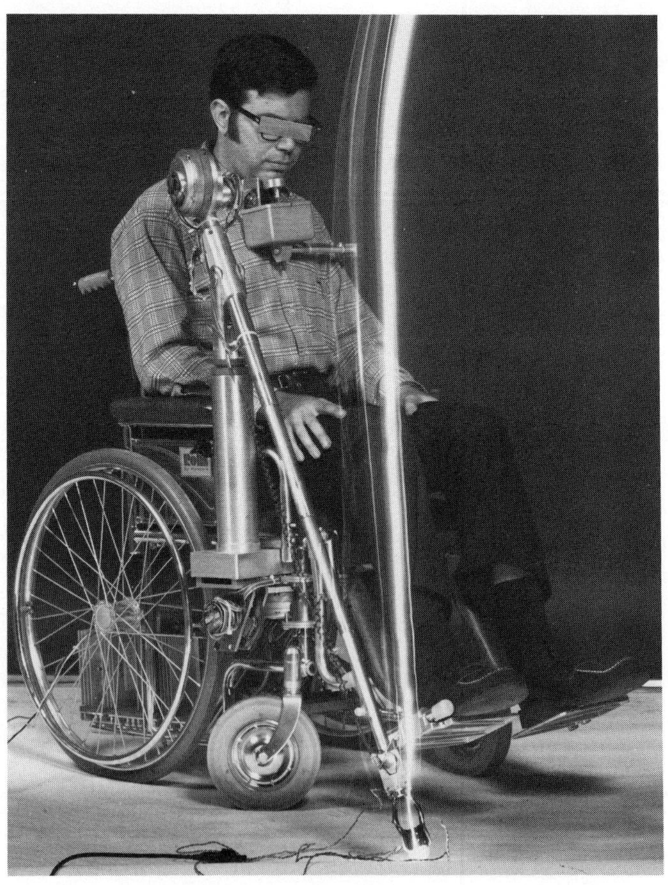

Fig. 17-39. Control of terminal device of VAPC manipulator.

mand on the operator (Fig. 17-39). Velocity of the end point and velocity and force of the effector were chosen as the control variables to have both a no-input, no-output situation (dead man), a large field of fine control, and a dead zone for inputs below the control threshold of the operator. This control system provides stable position with no oscillation.

In this system, the operator provides direct commands required to move the manipulator up or down, right or left, or in or out (Figs. 17-40 and 17-41). This is similar to the chin-controlled wheelchair, in which the chin operates the system in proportional Cartesian coordinates. Conversion from Cartesian inputs to spherical servopower drive for endpoint Cartesian control makes the operation for the user easier, but the design significantly more complex.

Visual feedback in the form of projected symbolic images informs the user of the status of the system (Fig. 17-42). Feedback in the form of resistance to chin motion informs the user of input force or position. Control is exercised over eight variables—elevation velocity, mediolateral velocity, anteroposterior velocity, wheelchair velocity and direction, terminal device prehension, rotation, and orientation attitudes. Simultaneously, control of several variables is based on an analysis of simple daily living activity, such as taking food from a table to the user's mouth and returning to the table. The automatic sequencing of one variable servomechanism after another provides "aiding." A zone of safety was established to limit the system's velocity to a safe rate near the user.

Being extensible and spherically coordinated, the system presents a small visual image providing visual feedback. It does not require a large clearance area. Extensible spherical systems require only three drive elements to determine position, and there is only one solution to the mathematical description of the location: a unique solution to three simultaneous equations. The system requires a high ratio of extended length to retracted length for a full sphere of operation and good visibility. Low-inertia pancake-printed circuit motors with built-in gear reduction and feedback tachometers are used for economical reasons.

The VAPC manipulator is wheelchair mounted on the notion that it is potentially more useful to the operator. A mobile system can be used in a fixed location, but the reverse is not necessarily true. Mounting the manipulator on a wheelchair does not compromise functions or accessibility to the chair.

The terminal device is a three-jaw chuck ar-

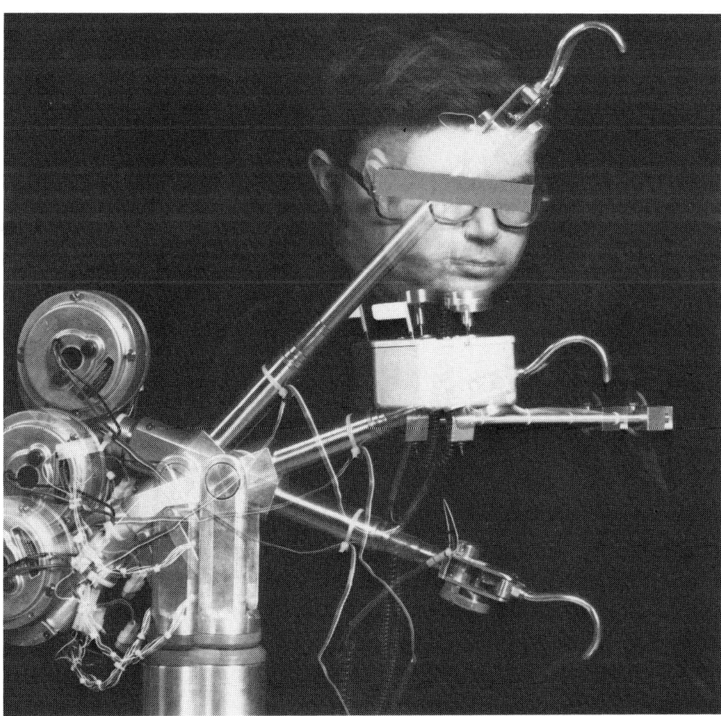

Fig. 17-40. Control motion, up and down.

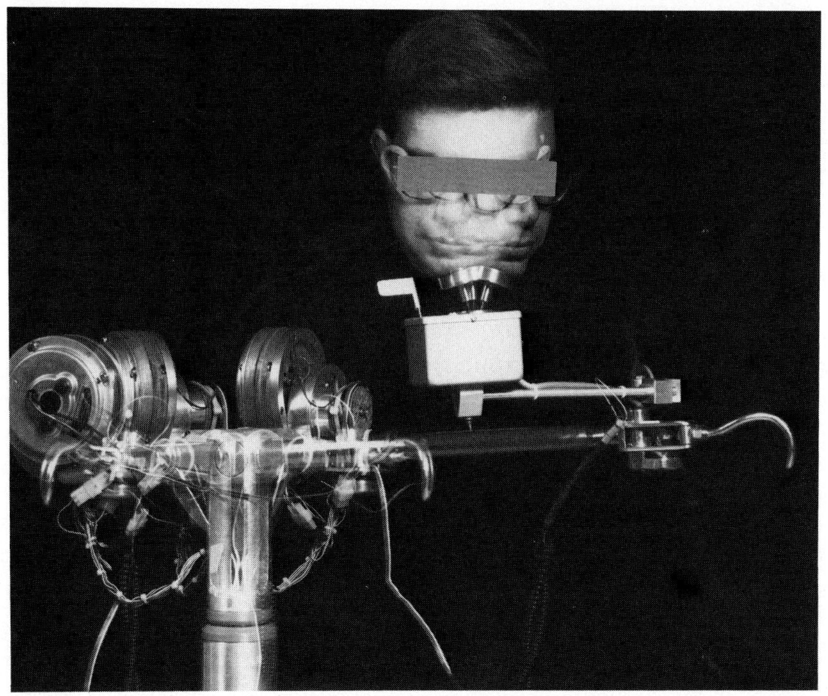

Fig. 17-41. Control motion, right and left.

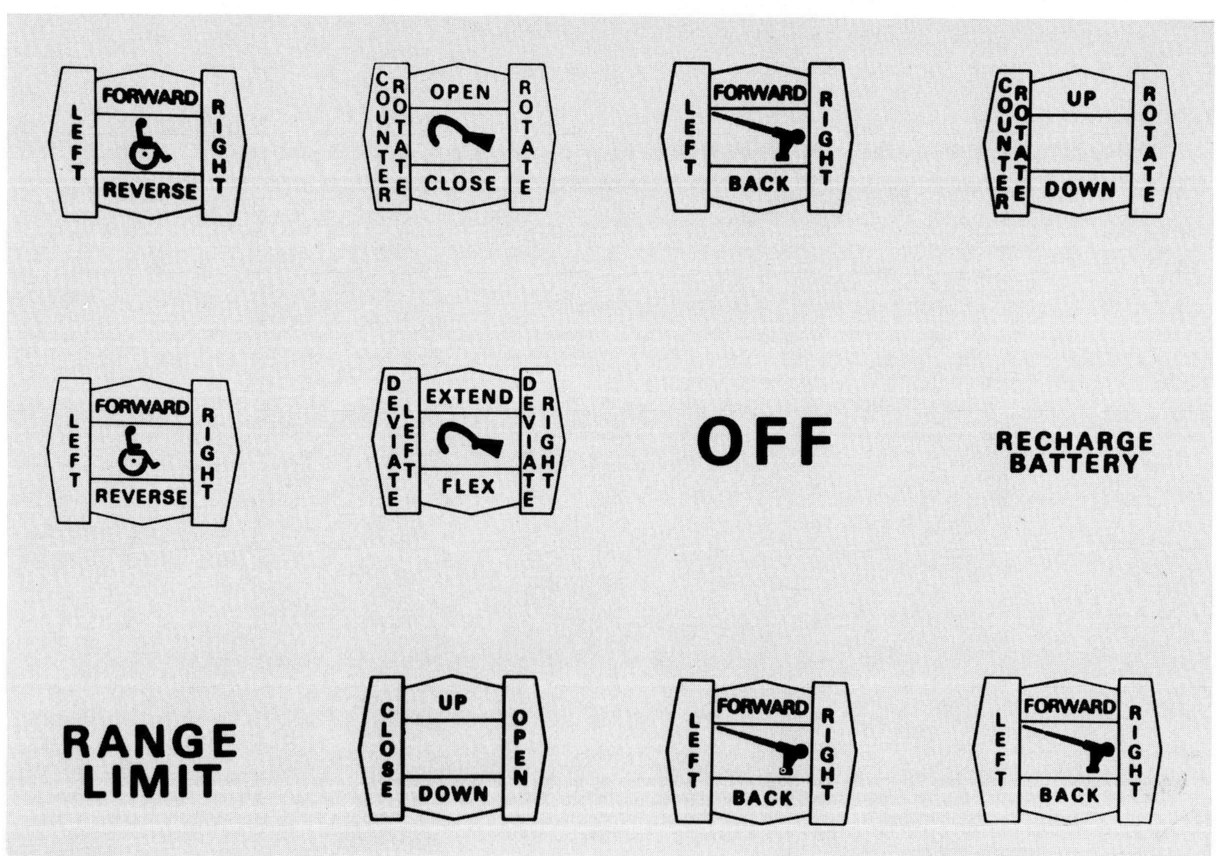

Fig. 17-42. Symbolic images inform user.

rangement. Powered prosthetic hooks (Fig. 17-43) with strain-gauge prehension feedback and potentiometer position feedback were used.

The manipulator extension-retraction of the VAPC is controlled by an internal constant-force spring. The elevation of the system is controlled by a motor drive located in the base. Linkages reduce the high loads on the gearing and provide an output force of 2 kg. The rotational drive is a pinion-spur gear system. The entire system mounts on any standard powered wheelchair (Everest and Jennings model 32P) and weighs just over 20 kg. The Gould 105 amp/hour batteries and the electronics add about 50 kg.

The control system is a coordinate-converting operational amplifier manifold (Fig. 17-44) as follows:

$$\frac{\partial \theta}{\partial t} = \frac{\sin\theta - y\cos\theta}{R\cos\theta}$$

$$\frac{\partial \theta}{\partial t} = \frac{(x\cos\theta + y\sin\theta)\sin\alpha - z\cos\alpha}{R}$$

$$\frac{\partial R}{\partial t} = (x\cos\theta + \sin\theta - z)\sin\alpha$$

The nonlinear functions are generated with diodes used as function generators for the opera-

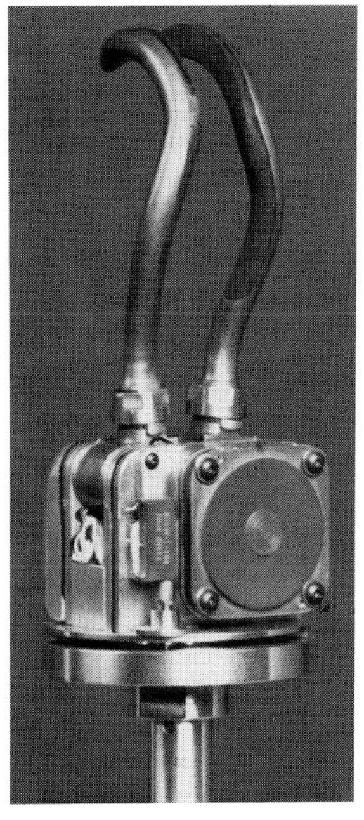

Fig. 17-43. Powered hook with position and prehension feedback.

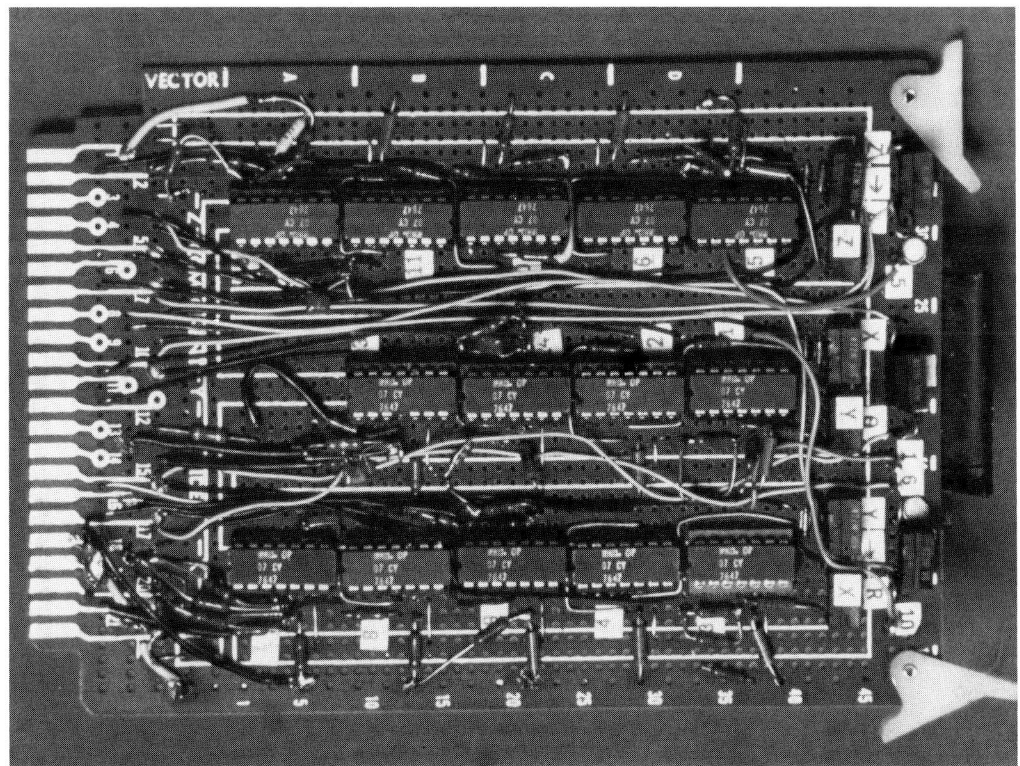

Fig. 17-44. Operational amplifier.

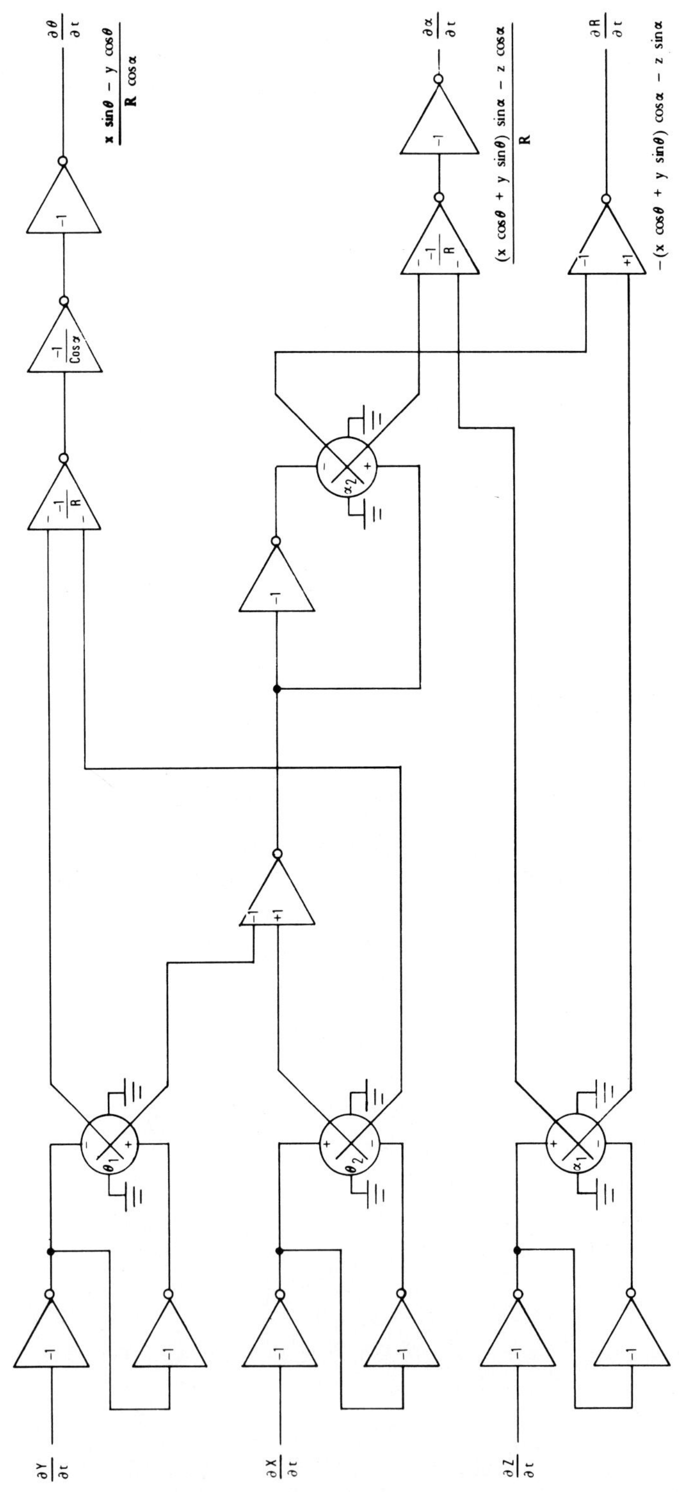

Fig. 17-45. Schematic amplifier.

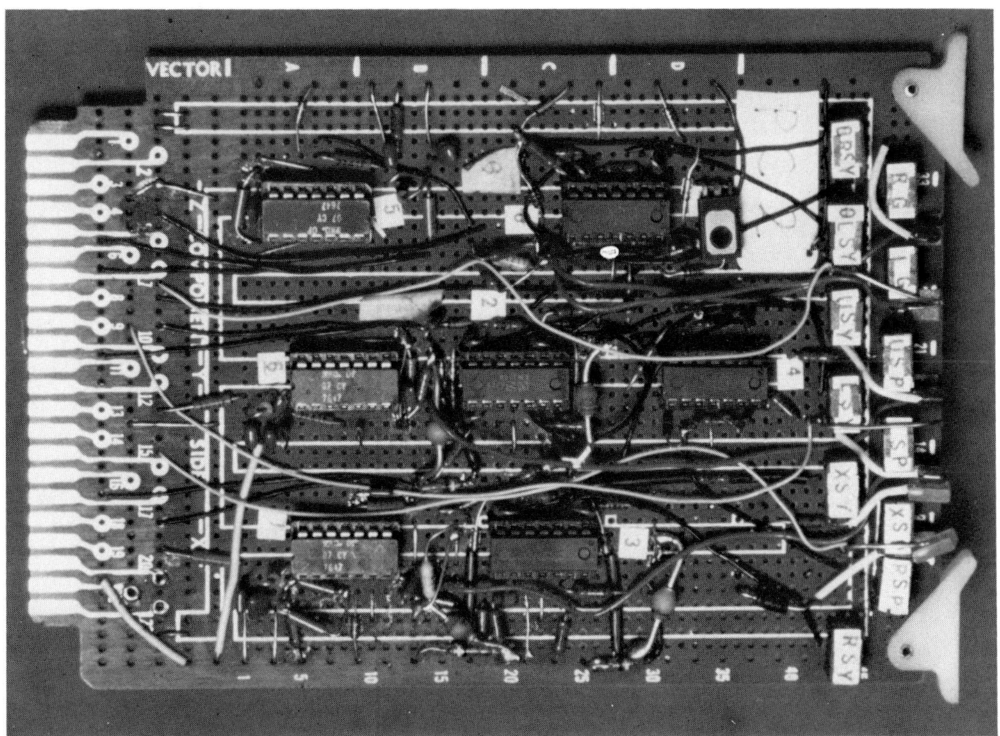

Fig. 17-46. Operation amplifier used to solve equations.

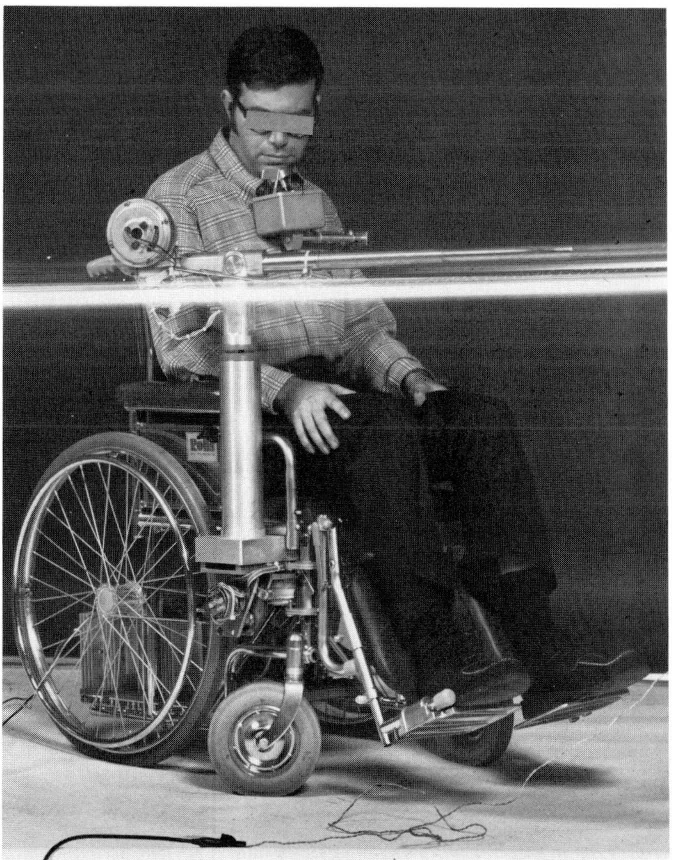

Fig. 17-47. VAPC manipulator sphere of function.

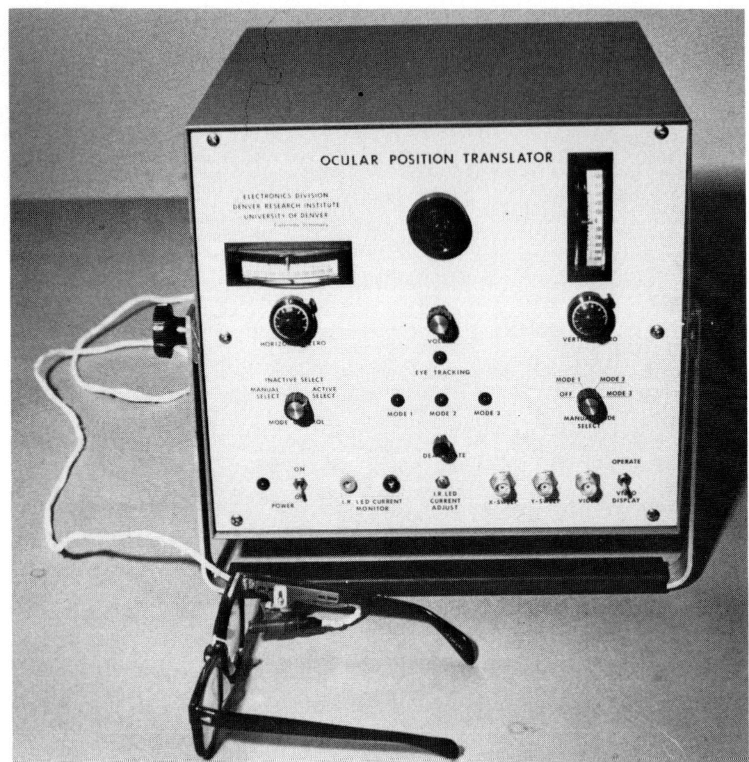

Fig. 17-48. University of Denver ocular control unit.

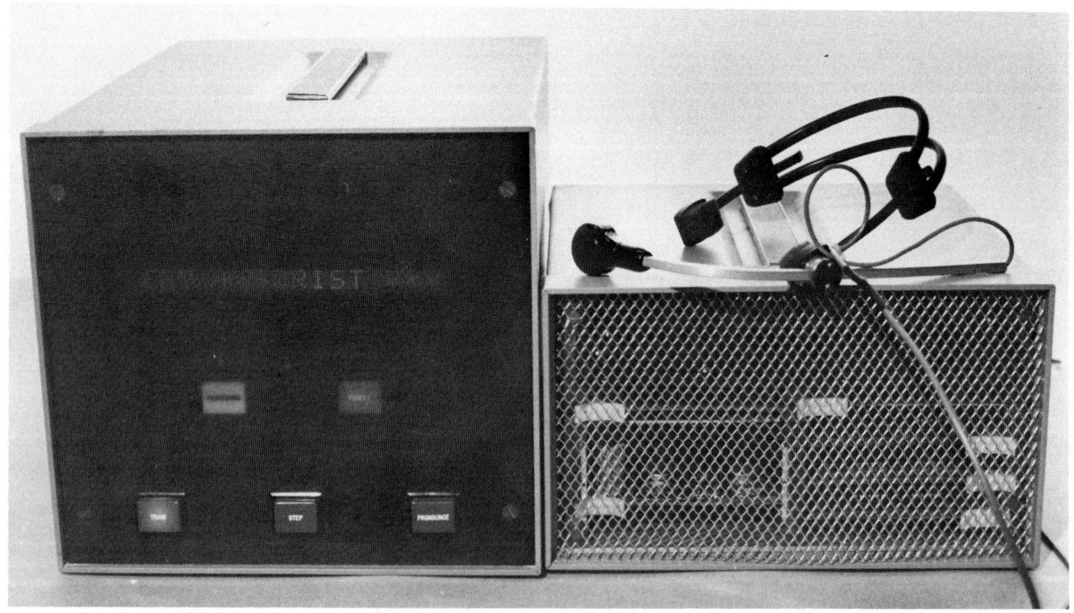

Fig. 17-49. Voice control system developed at University of California, Santa Barbara.

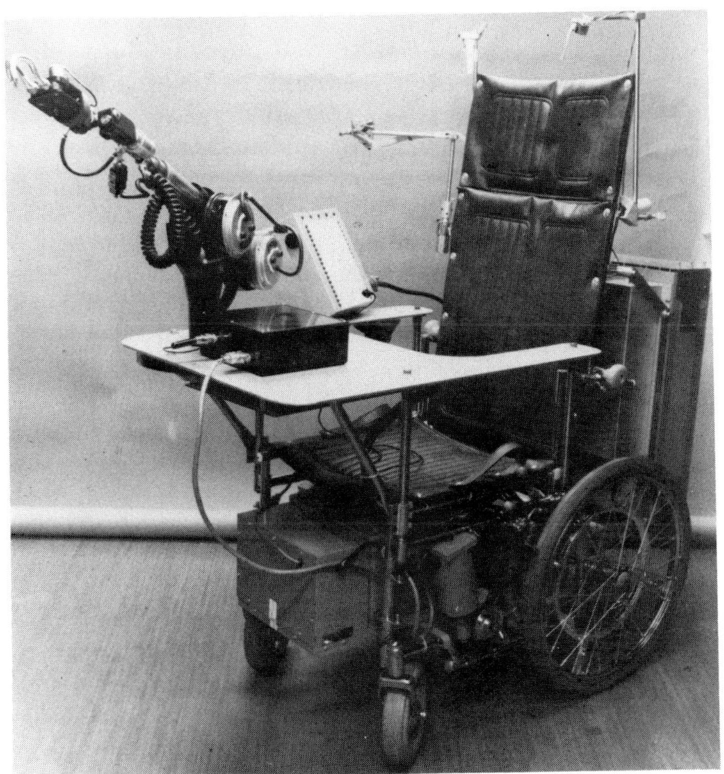

Fig. 17-50. NASA/JPL manipulator mounted on wheelchair.

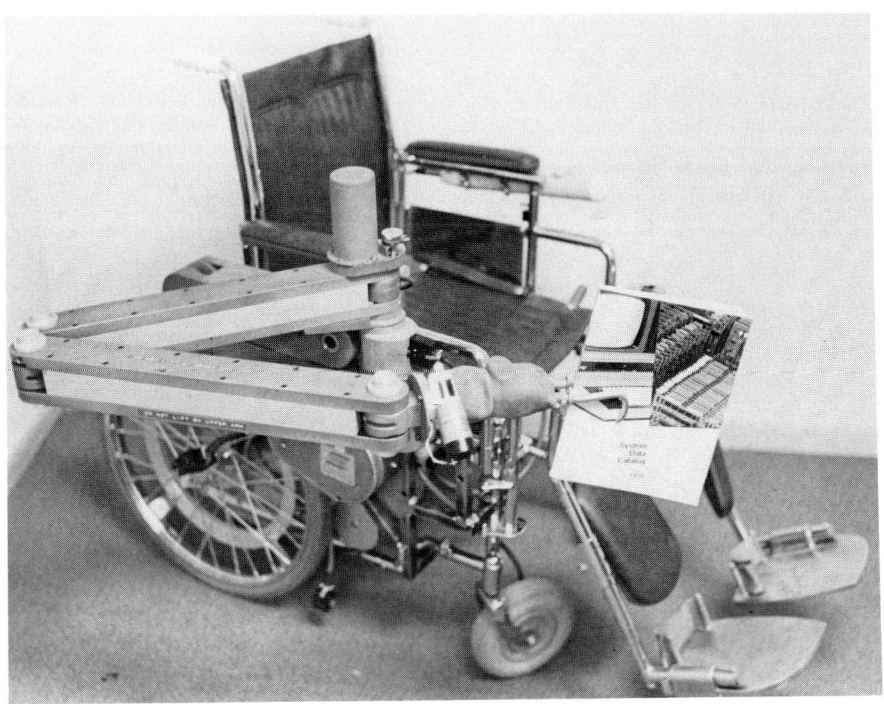

Fig. 17-51. SPAR manipulator.

tional amplifier (Fig. 17-45). Compilations, coordinate conversion, and equation solving are done with operation amplifiers and nonlinear feedback elements. This permits sine and cosine multiplication and division (Fig. 17-46).

The manipulator sphere of function is 2½ m in diameter (floor to ceiling) (Fig. 17-47). It can lift a 2-kg load anywhere in the sphere. It can retract to within 25 cm of its origin. It can pull in excess of 12 kg. Velocity varies between 1 m/sec and 1 mm/sec. The prehension range is from ½ to 7 kg. The linear error in any major chord translation is less than 1% (2½ cm). The system can operate all day (16 hours) on a battery charge.

Further developments. Several adaptations of Mason's design[39] are under evaluation in the University of California, Los Angeles, Biotechnology Laboratory. General Teleoperators has built three telescoping manipulators. One has been interfaced with the Denver Research Institute, University of Denver, Ocular Control Unit (Fig. 17-48). Another is controlled by voice command through a microprocessor voice control system developed at the University of California, Santa Barbara, by Roemer's group (Fig. 17-49). The third General Teleoperators version of the VAPC telescoping manipulator is controlled by a proportional joystick. NASA/JPL has provided an additional approach, in which, using the advantages of the telescoping design, they have mounted the manipulator on a wheelchair controlled by a voice recognition system (Fig. 17-50). The SPAR manipulator (Fig. 17-51) is being tested at the University of Virginia. The wrist unit was made at the University of Virginia, and the two-fingered hook was designed at Northwestern University and loaned by them through the courtesy of the Veterans Administration.

SUMMARY

Understanding the nature and course of research trends at a particular time presents a paradox. By its nature, a field of research is often arcane, and it is difficult to identify the individual threads in its fabric. Another associated phenomenon is the emergence simultaneously, or at close intervals, of a spate of research in the same new area. Ideas come to fruition simultaneously in different places because workers in that field become aware of their developments at about the same time. This has been the case in the field of research dealing with upper extremity prosthetics. Clear-cut trends were easy to identify as the field grew apace for some 20 years.

At this writing no single predominant focus of research characterizes the field. Instead, some six areas of improvement in upper extremity prosthetics are being attended to with sufficient intensity to warrant calling them research trends: cosmesis, socket design, the use of external power sources, myoelectric control for powered components, sensory feedback, and medical manipulators. Research in cosmesis is generally aimed at more lifelike replication of human limbs with respect to color, shape, texture, and noise reduction. The emphasis in research on sockets is placed on eliminating bulky and uncomfortable harnessing. Lighter, cheaper, quieter, and more efficient electrical power systems are being sought through research efforts. Interest still remains high in studying ways to maximize the benefits of myoelectric control. Sensory feedback has been established as a desideratum and is receiving appropriate research attention. Work in the new area of medical manipulators seems to be converging on two concepts: the third arm, or mobile directly controlled manipulator, and the more specialized fixed manipulator designed for use in a special tabletop environment.

REFERENCES

1. A fabrication manual for the "Münster-type" below elbow prosthesis, Prosthetic and Orthotic Studies, New York, 1965, New York University.
2. Bejczy, A.: Sensor systems for automatic grasping and object handling. International Conference on Telemanipulators for the Physically Handicapped, Rocquencourt, France, September, 1978.
3. Billock, J.: Northwestern University supracondylar suspension technique for below-elbow amputations, Orthot. Prosthet. **26**(4):16-23, Dec., 1972.
4. Bruet, J.: Twelve activity of daily living scales, Phys. Ther. **49:**857-862, 1969.
5. Cameron, H., Pilliar, R., and Macnab, I.: Porous Vitallium in implant surgery, J. Biomed. Mater. Res. **8**(5):238, 1974.
6. Childress, D. S., and Billock, J. N.: Self-containment and self-suspension of externally powered prostheses for the forearm, Bull. Prosthet. Res. **10-14:**4-21, Fall, 1970.
7. Clark, A. et al.: Surface chemical analysis of bioglass orthopedic implants, Symposium on Materials for Reconstructive Surgery, Clemson, S.C., 1974, Clemson University.
8. Clippinger, F. W., Avery, R., and Titus, B.: A sensory feedback system for an upper-limb amputation prosthesis, Bull. Prosthet. Res. **10-22:**247-258, Fall, 1974.
9. Collins, C., and Madey, J.: Tactile sensory replacement, Proceedings of the San Diego Biomedical Symposium **13:**15-16, 1974.
10. Corker, K., Lyman, J. H., and Sheredos, S.: A preliminary evaluation of remote medical manipulators, Bull. Prosthet. Res. **10-32:**107-134, Fall, 1979.
11. Corliss, W. R., and Johnsen, E. G.: Teleoperators controls, Washington, D.C., December, 1968, NASA Office of Technology Utilization, NASA SP-5070.

12. Cutler, E., and Blodgett, J. B.: Skeletal attachment of prosthesis for the leg (final report of Harvard University). Contract OEM cmr-214, Washington, D.C., May 1, 1945, Committee on Medical Research of the Office of Scientific Research and Development.
13. Dembo, T., Leviton, G., and Wright, B.: Adjustment to misfortune—a problem of social rehabilitation, Artif. Limbs **3**:4-62, 1956.
14. Dümmer, G.: Personal interview, during which he described experiments on sixty attachments, provided newspaper clippings of May, 1946, and displayed examples of prostheses, August 30, 1954, Pinneberg, West Germany.
15. Eighth Workshop Panel on Upper Extremity Prosthetics of the Subcommittee on Design and Development, Washington, D.C., 1970, National Academy of Sciences—National Research Council.
16. Esslinger, J. O.: A basic study in semi-buried implants and osseous attachment for application to amputation prosthetic fitting, Bull. Prosthet. Res. **10-13**:219-225, Spring, 1970.
17. Fishman, S.: Self-concept and adjustment to leg prosthesis (Doctoral dissertation), New York, 1949, Columbia University.
18. Goertz, R. et al.: ANL Mark E4A electric master/slave manipulator. Conference on Remote Systems Technology, Hinsdale, Ill., 1966, American Nuclear Society.
19. Goertz, R., and Thompson, W.: Electronically controlled manipulator, Nucleonics **12**(11):46-47, 1954.
20. Graupe, D. Beex, A. A. M., Monlux, W. J., and Magnussen, I.: A multifunctional prosthesis control system based on time series identification of EMG signals using microprocessors, Bull. Prosthet. Res. **10-27**:4-16, Spring, 1977.
21. Groth, H. et al.: Rationale and methodology for the evaluation of upper extremity prosthetic systems. Technical Note No. 27, Los Angeles, 1963, University of California Biotechnology Laboratory.
22. Guittet, J. et al.: A telemanipulator for the handicapped. Proceedings of the Third International Rehabilitation Medicine Association, Basel, Switzerland, 1978.
23. Hägg, G., and Spets, K.: SVEN Project I electrically controlled hand prosthesis, Stockholm, June, 1973, The Research Institute of the Swedish National Defence.
24. Hall, C. W.: Permanently attached artificial limbs, Veterans Administration Contractors Report, Bull. Prosthet. Res. **10-24**:243-249, Fall, 1975.
25. Hall, C. W.: Permanently attached artificial limbs, Veterans Administration Contractors Report, Bull. Prosthet. Res. **10-27**:165-168, Spring, 1977.
26. Hall, C. W., Cox, P., and Mallow, W.: Skeletal extension development: criteria for future designs, Bull. Prosthet. Res. **10-25**:69-94, Spring, 1976.
27. Hall, C. W., Liotta, D., O'Neal, R. M., Adams, J. G., and DeBakely, M. E.: Medical application of the velour fabrics, Ann. N. Y. Acad. Sci. **146**(1):314-324, Jan. 8, 1968.
28. Hench, L. et al.: Interfacial behavior of ceramic implants, National Bureau of Standards Special Publication 415, 1975.
29. Hulbert, S. et al.: Bone segmental replacement—the interface problem. International Symposium on Biomaterials, 1973.
30. Jacobsen, S. C., and Knutt, D.: A preliminary report on the Utah Arm, Salt Lake City, 1973, University of Utah.
31. Johnsen, E. G., and Corliss, W. R.: Teleoperators and human augmentation, Washington, D.C., December, 1967, NASA Office of Technology Utilization, NASA SP-5047.
32. Kaplan, J.: Augmented myo-sensation—a preliminary study (Masters thesis), Evanston, Ill., 1971, Northwestern University.
33. Klawitter, J.: A basic investigation of bone growth into a porous ceramic material (Doctoral thesis), Clemson, S.C., 1970, Clemson University.
34. Leifer, L., Roth, B., Kelly, D., Sachs, J., and Perkash, I.: Robotic aids for the severely disabled needs assessment. International Conference on Telemanipulators for the Physically Handicapped, Rocquencourt, France, Sept. 4-6, 1978, pp. 19-34.
35. Leonard, F.: Improved cosmetic gloves for the upper extremity amputee. Quarterly Progress Report, Washington, D.C., 1978, George Washington University.
36. Malgaigne, J.: A treatise on fractures. Packard, J. H., translator: Philadelphia, 1859, J. B. Lippincott Co.
37. Maling, R.: Control systems—concept and development (POSSUM). In Copeland, K., editor: Aids for the severely handicapped, New York, 1974, Grune & Stratton, pp. 22-30.
38. Mason, C. P.: Practical problems in myoelectric control of prosthesis, Bull. Prosthet. Res. **10-13**:39-45, Spring, 1970.
39. Mason, C., and Peizer, E.: Medical manipulators for quadriplegics. International Conference on Telemanipulators for the Physically Handicapped, Rocquencourt, France, 1978, pp. 309-312.
40. Mooney, V., Hartmann, D., McNeal, D., and Benson, J.: The use of pure carbon for permanent percutaneous electrical connector systems, Arch. Surg. **108**:148-153, 1974.
41. Mooney, V., Predecki, P., Renning, J., and Gray, J.: Skeletal extension of limb prosthetic attachment—problems in tissue reaction, J. Biomed Mater. Res. Sym. **2**(part 1):143-159, 1971.
42. Mosher, R.: Handyman to hardiman, Society of Automotive Engineering Paper 670088, 1967.
43. Mosher, R., and Wendell, B.: Force-reflecting electrohydraulic servomanipulator, Electro-Technology, December, 1960.
44. Parker, P. A., and Scott, R. N.: Myoelectric signal processing. In Scott, R. N. et al., editors: Myoelectric control systems. Progress report no. 11. Fredericton, New Brunswick, Canada, November, 1971, University of New Brunswick Bioengineering Institute, pp. 9-12.
45. Peizer, E., and Pirrello, T.: Principles and practice in upper extremity prostheses, Orthop. Clin. North Am. **3**(2):397-417, July, 1972.
46. Pilliar, R. M., Cameron, H., and Macnab, I.: Porous surface layered prosthetic devices, Biomed. Eng. **10**(4):126-131, April, 1975.
47. Prior, R. E., and Lyman, J.: Electrocutaneous feedback for artificial limbs. Summary progress report (February 1, 1974 through July 31, 1975), Bull. Prosthet. Res. **10-24**: 3-37, Fall, 1975.
48. Reiter, R.: Eine neue Elektrokunsthand Grenzgebiete der Medizin, **1**(4):133-135, 1948.
49. Rohland, T.: Sensory feedback system for a myoelectrically controlled arm prosthesis (Masters thesis), New Brunswick, Canada, 1972, University of New Brunswick.
50. Rohland, T.: Sensory feedback in upper limb prosthetic system, Inter-Clin. Info. Bull. **8**(9):1-4, 1974.

51. Roth, B. et al.: On the design of computer controlled manipulators. International Symposium on Theory and Practice of Robots and Manipulators, Amsterdam, Netherlands, 1974.
52. Rubin, G., and Gearhart, D.: Cosmetic hand cover for a hook, Bull. Prosthet. Res. **10-17**:83-87, Spring, 1972.
53. Saunders, F.: Electrocutaneous display. In Geldard, F., editor: Conference on vibrotactile communication, Austin, Texas, 1974, The Psychonomic Society.
54. Schilder, P.: The image and appearance of the human body, New York, 1950, International Universities Press, Inc.
55. Schlesinger, G.: Der Mechanische Aulband der Künstlinchen Glieder. In Ersatzglieder und Arbeitshilfen, Berlin, 1919, Julius Springer, pp. 407-410.
56. Schmidl, H.: The I.N.A.I.L. experience fitting upper-limb dysmelia patients with myoelectric control, Bull. Prosthet. Res. **10-27**:17-42, Spring, 1977.
57. Schmidl, H.: The importance of information feedback in prosthetics for the upper limbs, Prosthet. Orthot. Int. **1**:21-24, 1977.
58. Scott, R. N.: Myoelectric control systems. Progress report no. 13. Fredericton, New Brunswick, Canada, June, 1974, University of New Brunswick Bioengineering Institute.
59. Seamone, W., Schmeisser, G., and Schneider, W.: A microprocessor controlled robotic arm/worktable system with wheelchair chin-controller compatibility. International Conference on Telemanipulators for the Physically Handicapped, Rocquencourt, France, Sept. 4-6, 1978, pp. 51-62.
60. Seventh Workshop Panel in Upper Extremity Prosthetics of the Subcommittee in Design and Development, Washington, D.C., 1969, Committee on Prosthetics Research and Development, National Academy of Sciences—National Research Council.
61. Siller, J., and Peizer, E.: Some problems of the amputee child in school, Education **78**(3):1-7, Nov., 1957.
62. Sixth Workshop Panel on Upper Extremity Prosthetic Components of the Subcommittee on Design and Development, Washington, D.C., 1968, Committee on Prosthetics Research and Development, National Academy of Sciences—National Research Council.
63. Stein, R. et al.: Regeneration electrode units: implants for recording from a single peripheral nerve fiber in freely moving animals, Science **183**:4124, 1974.
64. Steinmann, F.: Z Orthop. Chirurg. **29**(96), 1911.
65. Swanson, A., Hotchkiss, B., and Meadows, V.: Improving end-bearing characteristics of lower extremity amputation stumps, Orthop. Prosth. Appl. J. **21**(1):23-26, March, 1967.
66. Taylor, D.: Goals for quadriplegic and paraplegic patients, Am. J. Occup. Ther. **28**:1, Jan., 1974.
67. Taylor, H.: The development of two wheelchair manipulator systems. International Conference on Telemanipulators for the Physically Handicapped, Rocquencourt, France, Sept. 4-6, 1978, pp. 117-131.
68. Ulrich, R.: NUC manipulators. Ocean Technology Department contributions to IEEE, Ocean Environment Conference, San Diego, September, 1971, Naval Undersea Center.
69. Vertut, J.: Contribution to analyze manipulator morphology coverage and dexterity. International Symposium on the Theory and Practice of Robots and Manipulators, Amsterdam, Netherlands, 1974.
70. Wileman, W., Mooney, V., McNeal, D., and Reswick, J.: Surgically implanted peripheral neuroelectric stimulation: two year experience at Rancho Los Amigos Hospital.
71. Wirta, R., Taylor, D., and Finley, F.: Pattern recognition arm prosthesis: an historical perspective, Philadelphia, 1977, Rehabilitation Engineering Center, Moss Rehabilitation Hospital.

PART THREE

The lower limb

CHAPTER 18

Kinesiology and functional characteristics of the lower limb

JOHN H. BOWKER

Each person's unique pattern of walking represents his solution to the problem of how to get from one place to another with minimum effort, adequate stability, and acceptable appearance. The inability to walk with reasonable facility and stand with adequate security are the principal handicaps of individuals with lower limb incapacities. Restoration of these deficiencies as completely as possible is the first goal of lower limb rehabilitation.

The importance of fully understanding the elements of the rehabilitation process cannot be overestimated, including prosthetics engineering and design, surgical procedures, prosthetic prescription practice, and training in the use of these devices. If functional substitutes for missing limb segments are to be prescribed, then it is obvious that complete comprehension of the elements of normal gait is essential.

Because of the large number of handicapped individuals with malfunctioning lower limbs, a research team combining the talents of electrical and mechanical engineers, physicians, physiologists, orthotists, and prosthetists was assembled under the Advisory Committee on Artificial Limbs, National Research Council, at the University of California, Berkeley, during World War II. The report of this group provides an "analysis of the magnitudes, directions and rates of change of translations, rotations and forces in the lower limb and pelvis with respect to three coordinate axes in space." By capitalizing on work already accomplished, proceeding with innovative techniques, and combining their multiple talents, the team was able to obtain findings that comprise the cornerstone of our knowledge of human gait.

THE GAIT CYCLE*

The gait cycle is confined to the movement of the body below the level of the umbilicus, although we recognize that trunk sway, arm swing, and head motion play on extremely important role in normal gait. For ready comprehension, the human locomotor system is reduced to its simplest possible form: a series of articulated sticks assembled to resemble the limb segments of man, stripped of muscles, but moving with the same pattern in response to the many forces involved. These forces are gravity acting on the body mass, counteractions of the floor, muscular effort generated within the limb segments, and resultant forces from the potential and kinetic energy developed in this moving mass. The movements of the limb segments have been arrested, as by a camera, at certain constantly recurring critical incidents in the gait cycle to allow study of the activity and relationships of the segments in

*Remainder of chapter from Bowker, J. H., and Hall, C. B.: Normal human gait. In American Academy of Orthopaedic Surgeons: Atlas of orthotics: biomechanical principles and application, St. Louis, 1975, The C. V. Mosby Co.

normal walking as compared to altered patterns created in abnormal locomotion.

Viewed from the side, stroboscopic photographs of suitably marked thigh, leg, and foot segments resemble articulated sticks moving through space, allowing the viewer to focus attention on one limb at a time. It can be seen that the limb repeats its movements for each step, progressing through a sequence of standing on the ground followed by swinging through the air. By convention, the start of a complete gait cycle is that instant at which the swing-limb heel strikes the gound. Following a progression of events, the cycle ends when that particular heel again strikes the gound. Hence heel strike indicates both 0% and 100% of the gait cycle.

Careful review of still photographs taken sequentially throughout the gait cycle reveals certain generally accepted divisions and events. The gait cycle is seen to consist of two phases. *Stance,* which comprises 60% of the entire cycle, is followed by *swing*, the remaining 40%. The résulting overlap of phases, when both limbs are weight bearing, is *double stance.* The two phases are subdivided into periods by events known as *critical incidents* (Fig. 18-1).

Stance phase implies support of the body weight. The stance limb assumes increasing amounts of this weight transferred from its mate soon after *heel strike,* the first critical incident. This first 15% period of the gait cycle, known by the same term, heel strike, terminates at *foot-flat,* the second critical incident. It is followed by that period between 15% and 30% known as *midstance.* During this period the person is balanced on the stance limb, and his body continues to move forward to the critical incident of *heel-off,* terminating the midstance period and initiating the push-off period. The mass of the body is now on the downhill portion of its undulating path, adding potential energy by its movement as it falls through the next 25% of the cycle known as *push-off.* This starts with the initial critical incident of heel-off, which is an interval of single limb support, and continues to *knee bend,* where the stance knee is seen to bend as hip and knee flexion prepare the limb for the swing phase. At this time 55% of the entire gait cycle has been completed.

Shortly before knee bend, the opposite limb has completed its swing phase, contacted the ground and started to prepare for the transfer of weight to the new stance limb. This shift of weight from the old stance limb has prompted many individuals working in the orthotic and prosthetic fields to consider the true stance phase terminated at about this time (55%) even though the "original" stance foot is still in contact with the ground. Careful consideration of all factors, however, suggests that it is best to retain the older designation while recognizing that the original stance limb is supporting a rapidly decreasing portion of the body weight during the final 10% of stance phase. The final 5% of stance phase, known as *acceleration,* extends from knee bend at 55% to the final critical incident of toe-off, marking the completion of stance phase and the beginning of the swing phase at 60% of the full gait cycle.

The *swing phase,* occupying the last 40% of the cycle, is divided into three periods: initial swing, midswing, and deceleration. The first 10% of swing phase is known as *initial swing* and begins with the critical incident of *toe-off* and continues

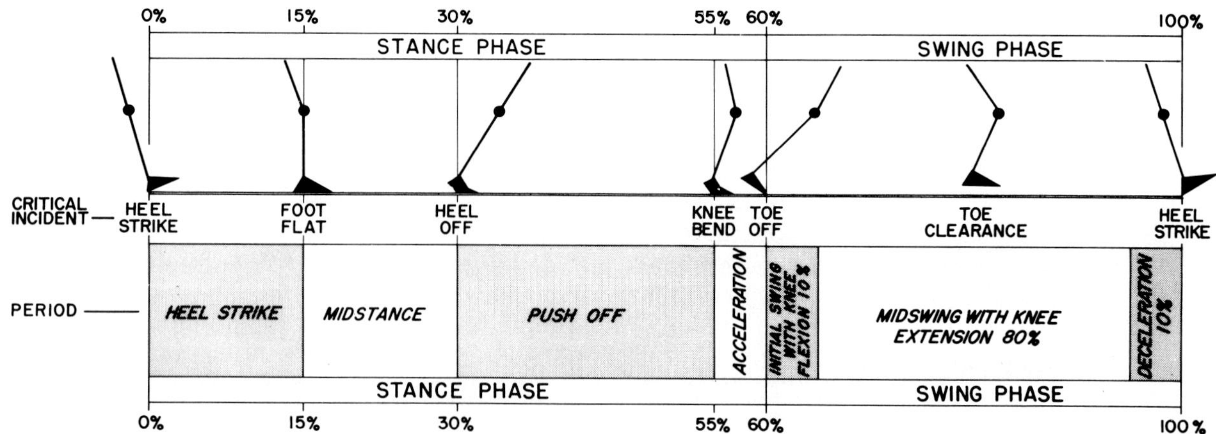

Fig. 18-1. Analysis of single stride. (From Bowker, J. H., and Hall, C. B.: Normal human gait, Chapter 7. In The American Academy of Orthopaedic Surgeons: Atlas of orthotics: biochemical principles and application, St. Louis, 1975, The C. V. Mosby Co.)

as the foot rises in an arc responding to flexion of the knee and continued forward motion of the limb well started by hip flexion in the stance acceleration period. *Midswing,* which represents 80% of swing phase, begins as the swing limb passes its stance counterpart, the knee extends, and the path of the foot reverses to fall in a forward swinging arc. During this period, the foot is actively dorsiflexed by the anterior leg muscles to avoid stubbing the toe at the bottom of the pendulum swing (toe clearance). During the final 10% of swing phase, *deceleration* occurs. The rapidly moving swing limb, now out in front of the body, is smoothly braked by gravity and the limb musculature to conclude the full sequence at 100% of the gait cycle with ground contact at *heel strike.*

It is evident that the foot is in contact with the ground through 60% of the cycle and is swinging forward in the air to pass its stationary mate during 40% of the cycle. It is also obvious that an overlap of stance phases must occur if each foot is to have ground contact for 60%. Observation reveals that the swing foot hits the ground before the opposite stance foot is lifted. The period during which both feet are weight bearing is termed "double stance." It is of greatest duration when a person walks slowly and is of least duration when the person moves rapidly. Double stance must occur with each sequence; should the swing foot fail to contact the ground prior to the departure of the stance foot at toe-off, the individual will momentarily have both feet off the ground at the same time and will be trotting, leaping, or running. The striding, energy-conserving gait of man is characterized by this double-stance phase in the walking pattern.

The cycle is continually repeated, with feet alternating as the individual walks over level ground. It is important to recognize that this sequence is observed only in normal limbs moving over level surfaces at a normal walking speed. Ramps, inclines, stairs, or uneven ground, and jogging or running will sharply alter this smooth, repetitious cadence.

The energy requirements of stance phase result from muscular activity of (1) the hamstrings and gluteus maximus, in decelerating the swing limb through the last milliseconds prior to heel strike and their continued activity as hip stabilizers during the initial part of stance; (2) the quadriceps femoris, in stabilizing the knee and absorbing shock by eccentrically contracting to allow the knee to flex under increasing loading; (3) the anterior leg muscles, in eccentrically contracting to absorb the shock of heel strike and thereafter to lower the forefooot to foot-flat; (4) the paraspinous and trunk musculature, in balancing the torso at foot-flat; (5) the contraction of the triceps surae through most of the stance phase; and (6) the contraction of the hip abductors to stabilize the pelvis throughout the stance phase.

Analysis of muscle function during swing reveals that (1) hip flexors initiate acceleration of the stance limb and continue to provide support throughout swing; (2) knee extensors dampen knee flexion to prevent excess heel rise after toe-off; (3) knee flexors aid in lifting the toe from the ground; (4) foot dorsiflexors elevate the forefoot during swing to prevent toe stubbing; (5) hip extensors decelerate the swing limb prior to heel strike; and (6) hamstrings decelerate both knee extension and hip flexion.

To understand the effect of the articulated lower limb on the moving mass of the human body, we shall use a well-understood, constantly employed reference point used to study bodies in motion – the center of gravity (CG). The center of gravity of a body, volume, area, or line is that point at which it would be perfectly balanced in any position. In the upright human, the center of gravity lies just anterior to the second sacral vertebra within the true pelvis. Seen from the front, this is just above the symphysis pubis; from the side, just above the tip of the greater trochanter. By studying the reactions of the CG to certain situations, we can often predict or analyze what the body as a whole is doing. By substituting the CG as an entity for the complex form of the trunk with limbs attached, the human figure can be reduced to a lump much as the complex thigh and leg were reduced to the sticks employed to analyze a single forward stride. Using the concept of a single mass moving in space, the laws of physics can then be applied to understand some of the peculiarities of human gait.

Newton's first law of motion states that a body set in motion will continue in a straight line until compelled by impressed force to alter its path. However, Newton's first law of motion in itself is not so important in studying walking and what it costs to walk as is this corollary. A body in motion following a crooked path has numerous impressed forces acting to alter its pathway, at an increased cost of energy consumption. Thus the study of a CG path moving in space provides some comprehension of energy expenditure. Human CG movement may be effectively recorded on a photograph produced by an open-shuttered still camera in a darkened room exposed to a pinpoint source of light marking the CG while the person walks. Such photographs taken from the side, above, and in front of the subject will produce a streak of light, wavering across the film. From the side, matching the vertical rise and fall of the CG, this streak describes a sine wave rising and falling a total of only 5 cm (2 inches). The summit of this rise appears at midstance when balanced on one limb and the low point when both feet are on the ground in the double-stance phase. Thus, as a person walks, he rises and falls a total of 5 cm (2 inches) with each step. The energy expenditure is proportional to the person's weight and is measurable in foot-pounds of work. In addition to rising 5 cm (2 inches) when balanced on one foot in midstance, the body moves laterally over that foot to place the CG in true balance while the person is on one limb. On taking the next step, he moves to the opposite side, and the light streak on the photograph taken from above shows the total lateral shift of the human CG from left to right to again be approximately 5 cm (2 inches). An individual moving with a limp might have a drop in CG of a full 10 cm (4 inches) instead of 5 cm (2 inches) and shift to the side 10 cm (4 inches) at a greatly increased cost in energy. It becomes apparent, therefore, that a limp is not only cosmetically undesirable but functionally demands a much higher expenditure of energy than does a smooth, normal gait, and it follows that everything possible must be done to eliminate the limp from the gait of a prosthesis wearer.

BASIC DETERMINANTS OF GAIT

With the conviction that man, for all his complexity, is a structure capable of undergoing mechanical analysis, an attempt was made to devise a mechanical model for more exact engineering studies of gait. A simple pylon of average limb length was fitted with a nonarticulated foot. Instead of the sine-wave pattern of the human with its energy-conserving, smooth reversal from stance to swing phases, the tracing of the CG path was a series of connected arcs with sharp reversal points. The arc described by the moving CG at the tip of the artificial greater trochanter, given an average stride length, was found to produce a 7.5-cm (3-inch) vertical displacement from heel strike to midstance. The 7.5-cm (3-inch) CG shift of the model would produce a 50% greater expenditure of energy in elevating the body weight with each step than normal. To identify the critical features in human gait that differ from the mechanical model, a detailed study was made of thousands of enlarged prints from high-speed motion pictures of individuals walking while fitted with identifying targets to show translatory and rotary motion of the several limb segments. The elements of human lower-limb function that account for the smooth sinusoidal CG path with vertical and horizontal displacement of only 5 cm (2 inches) have become known as the basic determinants of gait.

There are six determinants, but they apply only if the individual is walking across a level surface at normal speed. The effect of arm swing, shoulder rotation, trunk flexion and extension, and head bob all contribute to the final molding of the human pattern of gait, but they do not affect the path of the center of gravity.

First determinant of gait – pelvic rotation (Fig. 18-2)

The pelvis (Latin, 'a basin') can be pictured as a bowl supported by two legs. At the start of double stance with the swing foot at heel strike and the stance foot at heel-off, the pelvis is supported by a bipod, forming an isosceles triangle, the apex of which establishes the CG height from the ground, and the sides of which intersect the plane of the floor at a given angle. The center of gravity of the bowl is at the lowest point of its undulating path. Photographs taken by overhead cameras of living people reveal that the pelvis rotates in the horizontal plane 4 degrees forward with the swing limb and 4 degrees to the rear with the stance limb, thereby spreading apart the apex of the isosceles triangle, propping up the leaning bipod legs, and consequently elevating the center of gravity 0.95 cm (3/8 inch). By horizontal pelvic rotation alone, the theoretical 7.5-cm (3-inch) amplitude of CG displacement had now been cut by 0.95 cm (3/8 inch) to 6.7 cm (2 5/8 inches) total.

Second determinant of gait – pelvic tilt (Fig. 18-3)

Study of gait photographs taken in front and to the rear of the walking person reveal that the pelvis normally tilts down 5 degrees from the stance limb at midstance. This lowers the CG in the center of the pelvis and also lowers the hip joint on the swing side. The person is therefore required to flex the knee of the swing limb to prevent toe stub during swing. The lowering of the CG at the crest of the summit has been found to be about 0.5 cm (3/16 inch), reducing the amplitude of vertical displacement from (6.7 to 6.2 cm (2 5/8 to 2 7/16 inches).

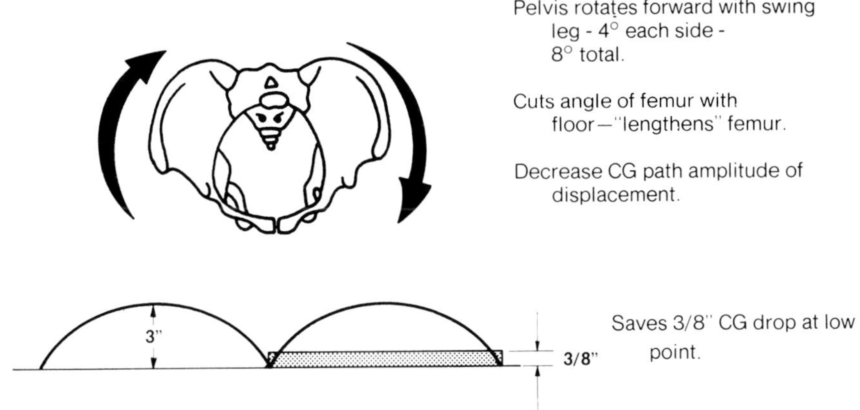

Fig. 18-2. First determinant of gait—pelvic rotation. (Courtesy University of California, Los Angeles, Prosthetics-Orthotics Education Program, Los Angeles, Calif.)

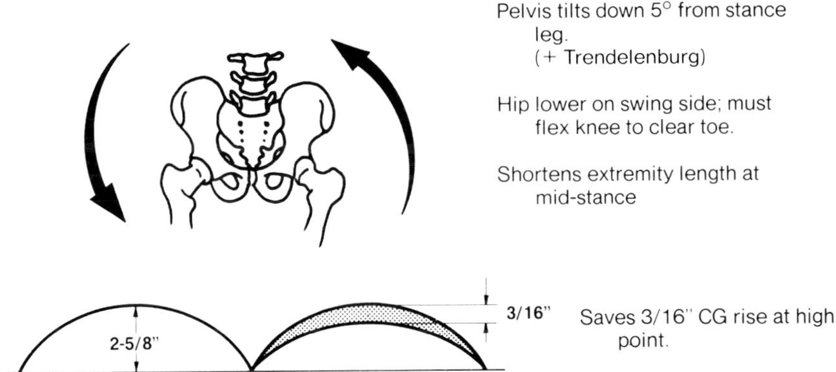

Fig. 18-3. Second determinant of gait—pelvic tilt. (Courtesy University of California, Los Angeles, Prosthetics-Orthotics Education Program, Los Angeles, Calif.)

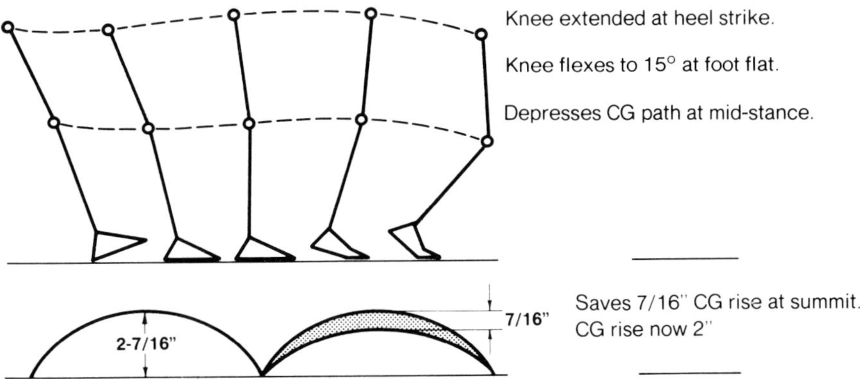

Fig. 18-4. Third determinant of gait—knee flexion after heel strike. (Courtesy University of California, Los Angeles, Prosthetics-Orthotics Education Program, Los Angeles, Calif.)

Third determinant of gait—knee flexion after heel strike (Fig. 18-4)

The mechanical model, a pylon with a nonarticulated foot, would seem an adequate reproduction of the normal limb during the stance phase up to the point of knee bend. However, careful review of published data reveals that the human knee is flexed twice within the gait cycle. It first begins to flex in response to heel strike, serving to absorb shock under the control of the eccentrically contracting quadriceps femoris until foot-flat. This first knee flexion also allows a diminution in the rise of the CG summit by 1.1 cm (7/16 inch), resulting in the final CG amplitude of displacement of 5 cm (2 inches). The knee then progressively extends to assist stretching the triceps surae, in prepartion for heel-off. Shortly thereafter, the knee flexes again to lift the toe from the ground.

A summation of the first three determinants of gait reveals that pelvic rotation, pelvic tilt, and knee flexion after heel strike together provide the 2.5-cm (1-inch) reduction of the mechanical model's 7.5-cm (3-inch) vertical amplitude of CG displacement to the 5-cm (2-inch) total seen in the normal human lower limb. However, they do not reproduce the center of gravity's smooth, undulating sine-wave path. Further actions are necessary to avoid an abrupt direction change at the low point with a corresponding acute energy expenditure. These actions are found in the next two determinants.

Fourth determinant of gait—foot and ankle motion (Fig. 18-5)

In producing the desired CG reversal pattern it is best to consider the fourth determinant, foot and ankle motion, and the fifth determinant, knee motion, as being intimately related.

The center of rotation of the ankle joint, roughly a point on the axis connecting the tips of the medial and lateral malleoli, rises and falls over a small but definite arc formed by the lever arm of the calcaneus from heel strike to foot-flat. At heel

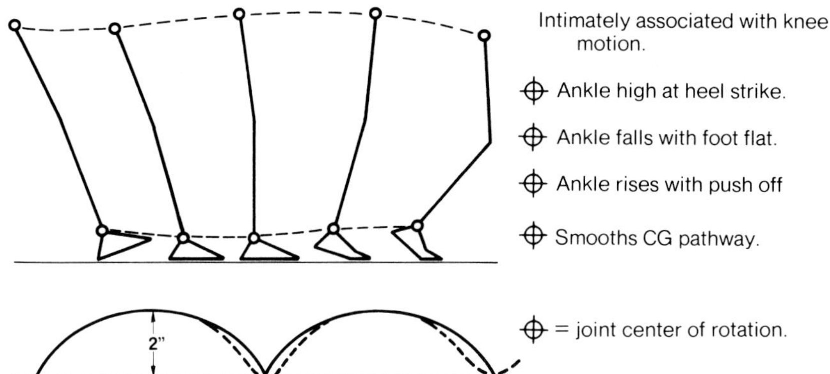

Fig. 18-5. Fourth determinant of gait—foot and ankle motion. (Courtesy University of California, Los Angeles, Prosthetics-Orthotics Education Program, Los Angeles, Calif.)

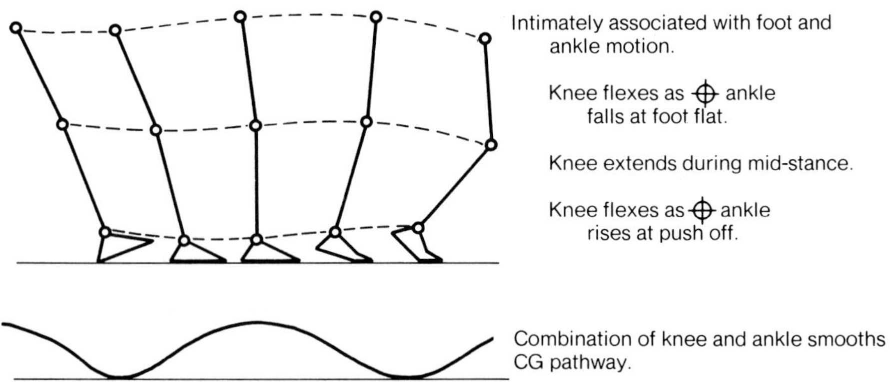

Fig. 18-6. Fifth determinant of gait—knee motion. (Courtesy University of California, Los Angeles Prosthetics-Orthotics Education Program, Los Angeles, Calif.)

strike, the ankle center is elevated, whereas through midstance the foot is flat on the ground and the center of rotation remains at a fixed height. Soon after midstance, however, the heel lifts from the ground, causing the center of rotation of the ankle to rise again, and the total effect is to round off the sharp reversal of the CG at its low point.

Fifth determinant of gait—knee motion (Fig. 18-6)

As previously mentioned knee motion is intimately associated with the fourth determinant, foot and ankle motion. The interplay serves to achieve the final baseline reversal pattern of the CG path. For convenience, one may consider the joint center of rotation to be a point on the axis connecting the greatest prominences of the femoral condyles, recognizing that the knee actually has a moving center of rotation. In response to heel strike, the knee begins to flex and, as previously noted, the ankle center of rotation falls until the foot reaches the foot-flat position. Then the knee reverses its action to one of extension while the ankle level remains stationary. During this period of time the limb has become progressively more vertical. The concurrent knee and ankle actions serve to produce further smoothing of the body's CG path that otherwise would have included an abrupt reversal point. With heel-off, the ankle rises and compensates for the accompanying loss in limb verticality. Further heel rise is counterbalanced by accompanying knee flexion; so the CG level change is again smoothed.

The combination of these five determinants—pelvic rotation, pelvic tilt, knee flexion after heel strike, foot and ankle motion, and knee motion—results in a smooth, undulating CG path with its 5-cm (2-inch) amplitude of vertical displacement. The final determinant is concerned with lateral movement of the center of gravity.

Sixth determinant of gait—lateral pelvic motion (Fig. 18-7)

In order to balance on one foot, it is not sufficient to simply raise the other. By so doing a person will immediately fall to the unsupported side. To remain upright, he must shift his body to the side of the supporting foot, bringing his CG directly over the support point to establish equilibrium.

In a similar fashion, man's alternating bipedal gait demands that the CG be shifted over the stance foot for balance while the swing limb is being carried forward. It has been said that walking is a series of falls and recoveries, allowing one to move along the line of progression.

The CG is in the center of the pelvis just anterior to the second sacral vertebra. Some 10 to 12.5 cm (4 or 5 inches) to either side lie the hip sockets. Fortunately, the femoral and tibial axes do not drop vertically from the hip joints. Instead, the femoral shafts are adducted in varus and the tibial shafts are vertically aligned in valgus at the knee joint. This effectively narrows the base of support so that, to be sufficiently secure, one must move the CG only 2.5 cm (1 inch) laterally toward the stance foot.

This action is reversed when weight is transferred to the other foot, resulting in a total CG displacement of 5 cm (2 inches) per gait cycle. The trunk is not completely centered over the support foot by this displacement. Instead a mixture of momentum and displacement is used for security. As lateral momentum abates, and the trunk tends to fall toward the other side, that limb is already preparing to accept body weight.

The final combination of all six determinants—pelvic rotation, pelvic tilt, knee flexion after heel strike, foot and ankle motion, knee motion, and lateral pelvic motion—allows the CG to rise and fall as well as to move from side to side within a 5-cm (2-inch) square box, thus providing a person with efficient and unique gait.

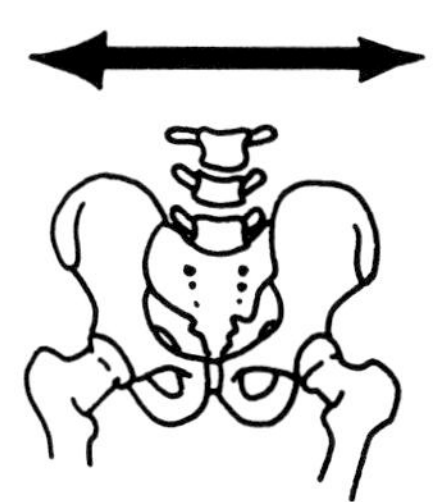

Fig. 18-7. Sixth determinant of gait—lateral pelvic motion. (Courtesy University of California, Los Angeles, Prosthetics-Orthotics Education Program, Los Angeles, Calif.)

AXIAL ROTATION OF LEG SEGMENTS

Viewed from above, the anatomic components of the lower limb do not swing forward and backward, well aligned in the sagittal plane. Actually, there is considerable rotation of the various segments of the limbs about their long axes.

In general, there is a progressive, serial internal rotation of the lower limb that starts in swing phase and progresses to foot-flat, followed by an abrupt reversal of direction into external rotation as the foot prepares to leave the ground. At the conclusion of swing phase, the hip, with the pelvis swung forward on this side, is in relative external rotation. At heel strike, with the foot in neutral rotation, the tibia rotates internally to align the ankle with the foot. This motion occurs in the subtalar joint. Rotational forces are reversed as foot-flat is completed, after which strong external rotation occurs against the still fixed foot. This brings the foot into the last vestiges of internal rotation to stabilize it during push-off. The moment the foot leaves the ground, it is externally rotated and the limb prepares for heel strike by again internally rotating.

The pelvis rotates forward 4 degrees during swing and backward 4 degrees with stance, producing a total pelvic rotation of 8 degrees. At the same time, the swing femur externally rotates about 5 degrees as the stance femur internally rotates 3 to 4 degrees, giving a total femoral rotation of 8 to 9 degrees during the full gait cycle. The tibia rotates a total of 9 degrees on the femur.

MUSCLE ACTIVITY IN GAIT CYCLE

For simplification of initial analysis, the lower limb has been considered a structure of articulated skeletal levers operating in space without sources of power. Muscles are now added, grouped about the joints as primary flexors, extensors, abductors, adductors, and internal or external rotators. Some span only one joint, whereas others cross two or more. Some may act as flexors in one limb position while serving as abductors or external rotators in another.

In general, muscles accelerate, decelerate, or stabilize limb segments. They may act, therefore, while contracting, lengthening, or remaining the same length. For the most part their function during walking will require short periods of activity and allow longer periods of relaxation during each individual complete single stride. The pendulum-like action of the limb and momentum perform great service in the movement of the limb or its components.

Motors

As motors, muscles perform work in a mechanical sense, lifting, moving, pushing, or twisting a certain mass with a certain force for a certain distance, allowing the calculation of work performed. Muscles use concentric contraction in this type of activity. Concentric contraction implies a shortening of the distance between the origin and the insertion of the muscle. The force exerted can be readily measured.

Shock absorbers

Absorption of shock by deceleration of a moving limb segment is possibly the major function of the great bulk of muscles in the lower limb while walking. This function is performed by eccentric contraction, which allows the distance between the origin and the insertion of the muscle to progressively increase. Contrary to the concept that a muscle is at rest while being lengthened, these muscles are performing significant work while being elongated, since they are resisting the passive forces that tend to create motion in an opposite direction.

Stabilizers

As stabilizers, muscles perform work in a biologic sense. They serve basically as guy wires to hold a limb in a certain fixed position by locking the joints. They move no mass through no distance, and the mechanical evaluation of their function is difficult. Isometric contraction is used for this function, and the muscle, although working hard, does not shorten the distance between its origin and insertion. These muscles perform increasing magnitudes of work without visible motion as the load supported increases.

Measurement of muscle activity

The most accurate measurement of muscle activity remains the wire electromyograph even though it records only the electrical signals brought by the motor nerves from the brain and tells us little about the actual force, amplitude, or type of contraction of the muscles themselves. The electromyograph is extremely useful in the determination of when a particular muscle is being signaled by the brain to contract, but the recording of this signal cannot tell us whether this muscle is requested to contract concentrically, eccentrically, or isometrically. For that reason the analysis of the following electromyograph taken of each muscle during a single stride is quite revealing. The chart itself has been ar-

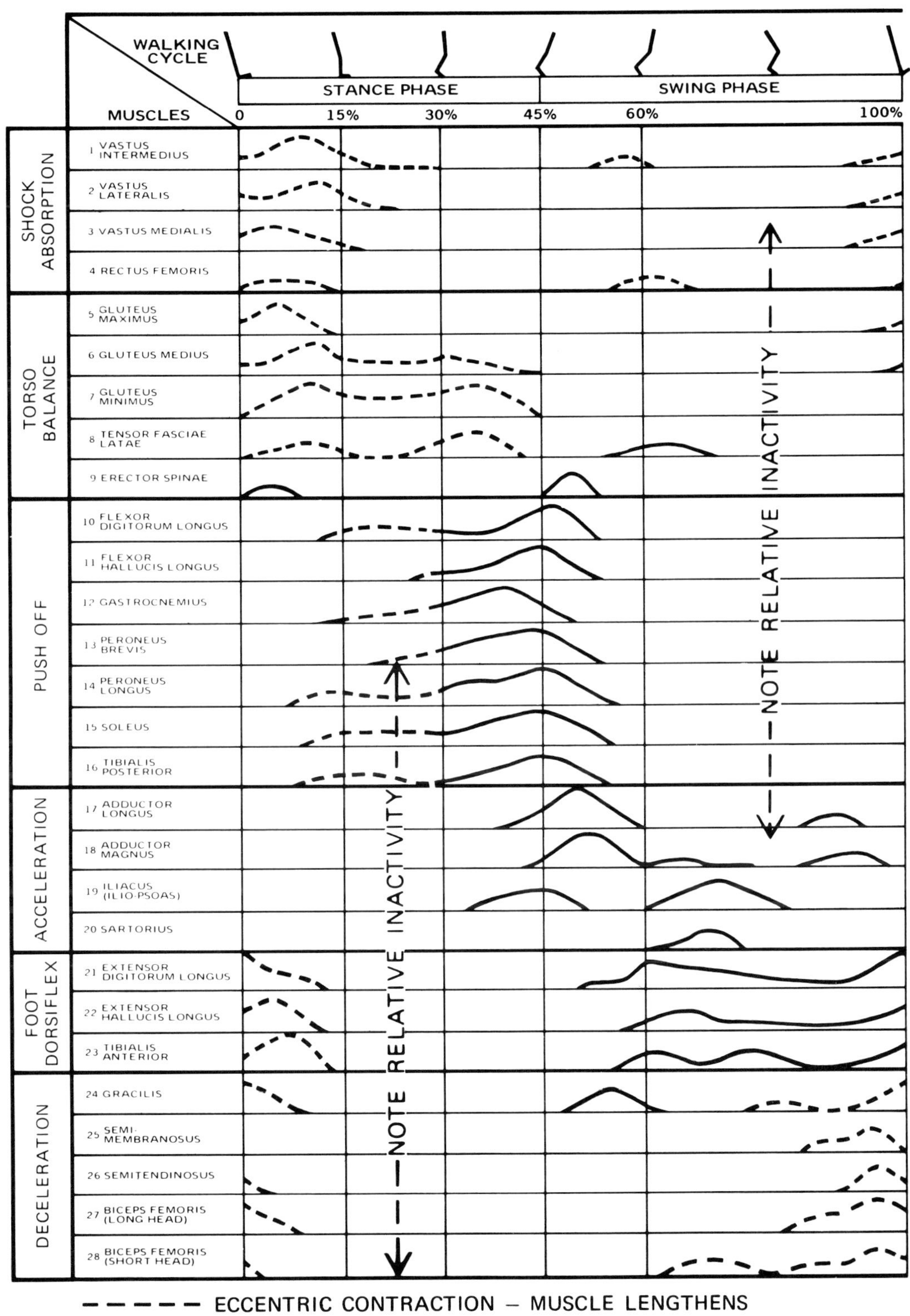

Fig. 18-8. Electromyograph of lower limb during walking. (Courtesy Dr. Charles O. Bechtol, Los Angeles, Calif.)

ranged to follow the usual single-stride sequence with muscles grouped, as much as possible, to show their major effect on the limb segment. They are chronologically arranged in the order of their appearance as the stride progresses. The curves of their electrical potential have been altered to identify concentric or eccentric contraction.

Electromyograph of lower limb during walking (Fig. 18-8)

A muscle active at heel strike is the quadriceps femoris, which is found to be in full contraction at the start of the stance phase, showing good activity potential. It is contracting eccentrically, lengthening to act as a shock absorber by allowing controlled flexion of the knee to 15 degrees by foot-flat. The duration of quadriceps activity is extremely brief, originating in the last 10% of the swing phase to stabilize the knee and ceasing at the end of the initial 15% of stance. The rectus and vastus intermedius portions fire again briefly after toe-off to dampen excess heel flexion, again contracting eccentrically.

The muscles that make up the hip abductor, pelvis balancer, and torso supporter groups begin activity at heel strike and complete their function by heel-off. Like the quadriceps, these muscles are contracting eccentrically, allowing the pelvis to drop 5 degrees into a Trendelenburg sign from the stance hip. The small tensor fasciae latae contracts concentrically after toe-off to slightly abduct the limb in initial swing, placing it in a better position to initiate hip flexion.

The next set of muscles to become active is the triceps surae and posterior tibial group. During initial firing just after foot-flat they are stretched in eccentric contraction to stabilize the tibia and permit knee extension. Near the end of midstance, they contract concentrically to return the ankle from 10 degrees of dorsiflexion to neutral. It is a moot point as to whether they are actually shortening or isometrically holding. Regardless of interpretation, the force demands on the soleus and gastrocnemius are high. Some investigators believe that these muscles primarily act to lock the ankle, with heel rise and the registered push-off force resulting from the anterior angulation of the tibia combined with the body mass being far forward of the supporting foot.

The hip accelerators, which are fairly massive muscles, contract concentrically. The iliacus begins its action in terminal stance and continues into early swing, while the other flexors, which include sartorius, gracilis, adductor longus, and tensor fasciae latae, trade off throughout swing.

The foot dorsiflexors are made up of the three principal anterior leg muscles. They contract eccentrically after heel strike to allow smooth descent of the forefoot to the ground. Their concentric contraction in swing phase is minor and of low magnitude, simply providing enough force to dorsiflex the unloaded foot to prevent toe stub.

The hamstrings are in the last stages of eccentric contraction at the time of heel strike and rapidly assume a rest phase until they again eccentrically contract in the last stages of swing to decelerate the swing limb just prior to heel strike. Their brief action at initial contact is essential for limb stability. During initial swing, the short head of the biceps contracts to flex the knee and allow toe clearance.

In summary, a number of interesting observations can be made. The first is that the electromyogram cannot tell us whether muscles are contracting, lengthening, or isometrically stabilizing. The recordings are all identical.

The second finding is that the three really massive muscle groups of the lower limbs—the gluteals, the quadriceps and the soleus—all contract eccentrically during normal walking over level ground.

The third finding, derived by observation of the amount of muscle activity during the midstance period, while a person is theoretically supporting all his mass in the upright position, is that muscle activity is recorded only in the ankle plantar flexors. This would appear to be a state of equilibrium with conservation of energy for the more proximal muscles.

The fourth finding of interest is derived by similarly checking midswing, at which time the mass of the limb is being moved through the greatest distance at the greatest velocity. Although considerable muscle activity occurs at initial swing, during midswing only scattered muscle activity is found. The conservation of energy is remarkable and possibly further substantiates the extreme efficiency that man has developed in locomotion patterns. The smooth sinusoidal path of his CG is shown to be an efficient design for elevating and depressing body weight. From a mechanical standpoint the drop of the CG down the slope from midstance to double stance will be exactly balanced by the rise from that point to again achieve midstance on the summit of the opposite slope. The kinetic energy lost in descending this slope is equal to the potential energy gained by achieving the summit. Even with this saving, man uses approximately 38% of his energy-producing capacity in level walking at 3 miles per hour.

REACTIONS BETWEEN FOOT AND FLOOR

The foregoing demonstrates the pattern of the production and the application of forces within the body. These power systems may or may not result in efficient locomotion, depending on the factors of gravity and friction.

Without gravity, ground contact is undependable and adequate functional stabilization of the foot for acceleration and deceleration would be absent. The magnitude, direction, and extent of these factors can be measured by a force plate, a complex device on which a person may stand or walk. The plate will measure the amount and direction of the forces of vertical loading, fore and aft shear, medial and lateral shear, and internal and external torque. Vertical force is shown to increase steadily from heel strike to foot-flat, exceeding body weight momentarily as the descending mass of the CG loads the new stance foot. A subpeak representing 60% of body weight occurs immediately after heel strike, well before the maximum at foot-flat. It has been suggested that the heel-strike phase be divided into two subphases, initial contact and contact response, eliminating the term "heel strike" completely, since many handicapped individuals, such as spastics with their equinus gait, never strike the heel at any time. Through midstance the vertical loading may drop below the body weight as the CG passes over the summit with the vertical forces rising again as the forces of heel-off are added. Heel-off, for the same lack of descriptive accuracy in other than normal gaits, might well be termed "terminal stance." Vertical loading drops rapidly in the final stages of stance as the opposite foot contacts the floor and assumes the support of the falling CG mass.

Fore and aft shear recordings demonstrate a forward peak immediately after heel strike. This is quickly reversed as the foot pushes back on the floor with the acceptance of body weight as the CG climbs to its summit on the stance leg, after which the falling mass again pushes backward on the foot after heel-off with a resultant thrust to the rear by the push-off foot.

Lateral and medial shear recordings reveal the initial adducting forces secondary to the swing foot striking the ground, followed by a shift to lateral pressure as the CG applies a bending moment to the hip joint resisted by the hip abductors. The effect of the pelvic stabilizing group returns to near equilibrium as the CG comes directly above the support foot through midstance. With heel-off, the CG is shifting to the opposite side in its 5 cm (2-inch) lateral excursion, and the lateral forces rise as a result through the push-off phase.

SUMMARY

This brief introduction to the study of normal gait should assist in the initial understanding of the basics of how humans walk. It is in no way intended to be an exhaustive or authoritative treatise on any aspect of gait technology. It is intended to stimulate students in the many specialties concerned with the care of the handicapped to seek the excellent technical material published by their respective professions.

SUGGESTED READINGS

Inman, V. T.: Conservation of energy in ambulation, Bull. Prosthet. Res. **10-9:**26-35, Spring, 1968.

Murray, M. P., Drought, A. B., and Kory, R. C.: Walking patterns of normal men, J. Bone Joint Surg. **46A**(2):335-360, March, 1964.

Peizer, E., and Wright, D. W.: Human locomotion. In Murdock, G.: editor: Prosthetic and orthotic practice, London, 1969, Edward Arnold, Ltd.

Peizer, E., Wright, D. W., and Mason, C.: Human locomotion, Bull. Prosthet. Res. **10-12:**48-105, Fall, 1969.

Saunders, J. B. deC. M., Inman, V. T., and Eberhart, H. D.: The major determinants in normal and pathological gait, J. Bone Joint Surg. **35A**(3):543-558, July, 1953.

Sutherland, D. H.: An electromyographic study of the plantar flexors of the ankle in normal walking on the level, J. Bone Joint Surg. **48A**(1):66-71, Jan., 1966.

CHAPTER 19

Principles of amputation surgery in the lower limb

ERNEST M. BURGESS

Legs allow us to stand and move about, supporting the superimposed body against gravity. During stationary and moving body attitudes, the lower limbs must provide stability. Stability supersedes mobility in functional priority. The above-knee amputee can move about successfully using a simple rigid peg device; the same amputee with an articulated prosthesis lacking knee alignment stability will frequently fall, thus demonstrating the priority of weight-bearing stability over motion. With the amputee, stable support is directly related to the length and strength of the residual limb and the position of remaining joints. Conservation of residual limb length, retention of muscle strength, and the absence of joint contractures enhance rehabilitation. The amputation is performed consistent with these facts.

Proprioception, the conscious and unconscious sense of position and movement, is as important as providing mechanical support. Sensory data are transmitted to the central nervous system for conscious and subconscious processing, then transmitted back to the motion organs, the muscles, for purposeful use. Since the mechanical properties of support, stability, and motion are so evident in lower limb function, it is easy to overlook the completely correlative and necessary role of sensory input.

Nature has wisely provided the energy-saving features of alignment stability in lower limbs. Minimal muscular effort is needed to allow stable upright stance when the CG is critically placed to employ the restraining nature of the appropriate ligaments about the hip, knee, ankle, and foot. Even the slightest shift in the CG to alter alignment stability will, however, recruit compensatory muscle activity throughout the entire lower limb and, in fact, the trunk and upper limbs as well. Continuous sensory information as to position in space allows immediate accommodation of force moments so that people can stand and move about economically and without falling.

The foot with its articulated lever arms is the platform on which people stand. Since this platform is reduced in size or eliminated by amputation, the size of the stabilizing foot surface area is reduced or eliminated. Loss of muscle power to the foot either by section of the tendons of the leg muscles acting on the ankle and foot or by loss of intrinsic muscles will unbalance or eliminate control of the ankle and foot joints.

Absence of one or all of the lesser toes results in very little functional loss, except in unusual foot attitudes such as toe stance. Loss of the first toe is of considerably more consequence. Not only is platform surface reduced, but also a powerful lever arm has been removed, resulting in important loss of strength and balance.

Forefoot and midfoot amputations are useful especially when the foot functions in an acceptable plantigrade attitude and is painless (Fig. 19-

1). If the residual portion of the foot adopts a fixed position of equinus, valgus, or varus alone or in combination, walking and running may be painful and difficult. An inclined platform surface, as with a midfoot amputation in equinus, is obviously less effective than in neutral weight-bearing position. Resulting high areas of pressure concentration, even on good plantar skin, often cause pain, skin breakdown, and difficult prosthetic fit.

Amputations at this level may require muscle rebalancing with or without joint arthrodesis. Arthrodesis, however, which would be used to place the foot in a neutral weight-bearing attitude, eliminates accommodating and compensatory joint movement that may actually be more functionally available in a prosthetic substitute, thus somewhat diminishing the value of the more distal amputation level.

The value of muscle stabilization in all amputations through the lower limb is well established. Appropriate tendon transfer rebalancing in the foot provides the twofold benefit of motor control and prevention of contractures. When the positive factors for muscle stabilization are present and can be done without undue risk to wound healing, they should be carried out at midfoot and hindfoot level.

Transmetatarsal and ray amputations are quite often useful for ischemia, especially in diabetics. Amputation through the midfoot and hindfoot is usually the result of trauma. Conservation of length alone in the midfoot area is not justified unless the attributes of stability, absence of pain, pressure-tolerant skin, and a useful range of joint motion are achieved. All amputations of the foot, including the Syme amputation, use plantar skin to cover the weight-bearing surface. This skin is particularly adapted to pressure and when properly placed with no underlying firm prominences, the skin will allow full weight bearing. (Grafted skin is unsuited to full weight bearing.) The anesthetic foot, including feet with plantar skin graft coverage, often breaks down and becomes infected. Amputation at a higher level may be necessary.

Amputations through the foot, including the Syme amputation, all allow end-bearing weight. The Syme amputation is included, since its distal weight-bearing surface is covered with heel skin physiologically adapted to sustain pressure (Fig. 19-2). The bilateral Syme amputee can be compared to the person standing on both heels. Instability is related both to the reduced size of the support platform and to the inability to compensate to force changes by shifting the weight-bearing contour of the reduced platform surface through muscular action across the joints of the foot. The Syme prosthesis restores platform surface and is designed to accommodate to some degree for shifting of body weight. This is particularly true when a SACH type foot is used.

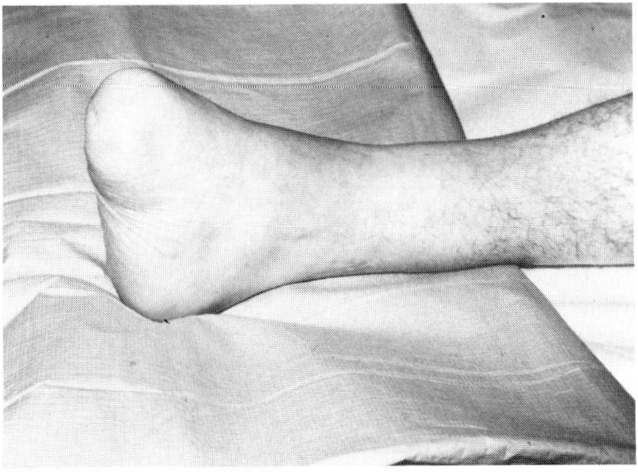

Fig. 19-1. Forefoot amputation proximal to metatarsals. Full active ankle dorsiflexion retained.

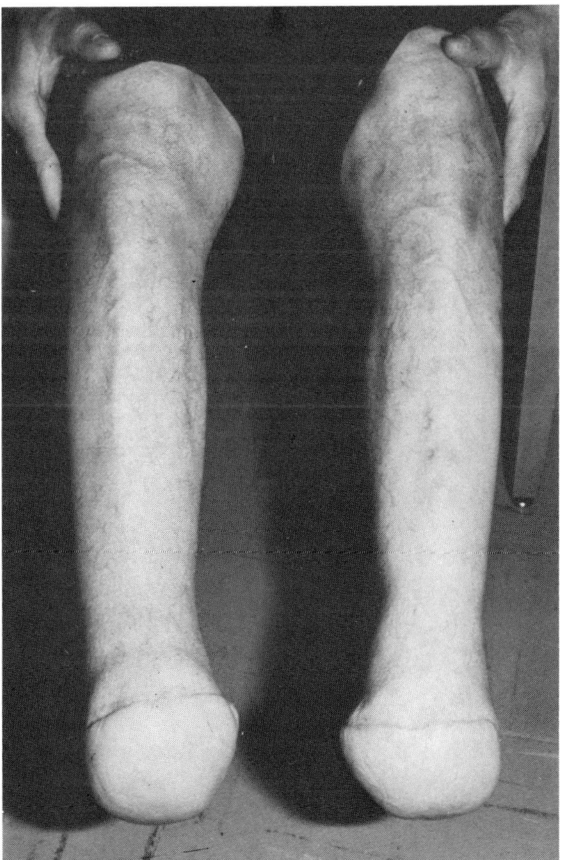

Fig. 19-2. Bilateral Syme amputation, classical technique.

AMPUTATIONS THROUGH THE LOWER LIMB PROXIMAL TO THE ANKLE JOINT

Conservation is the central theme of major lower limb amputation surgery. Maximum limb length is achieved consistent with surgical circumstances that allow proper skin, muscle, and other soft tissue management. The residual limb is covered with healthy, nonadherent, nontender, well-vascularized skin, either local or by skin graft. Nerves are sectioned with a sharp instrument and allowed to retract away from pressure-sensitive areas. The larger nerves are ligated to control bleeding. Adequate hemostasis, preferably by small ligature, is axiomatic. Muscles are stabilized distally under physiological tension. Bone ends are carefully rounded, not simply beveled, whenever surgically possible. Location of the skin incision and subsequent scar is determined by the anatomical circumstances present. Modern lower limb prostheses all are designed to provide distal contact and as much terminal weight bearing as possible. Since only the skin on the sole of the foot, the anterior aspect of the proximal tibia, including the patellar tendon area, and the ischial tuberosities normally tolerate superimposed body weight in standing, kneeling, and sitting respectively, skin not normally designed for continuous weight bearing will most often be used at the site of wound closure.

Skin covering any portion of the leg can tolerate pressure with varying degrees of efficiency, depending on its quality, location, and the presence or absence of underlying firm prominent body tissue. Increased skin tolerance to pressure is a normally occuring condition. The calluses on the working person's hand attest to this principle. Since it is desirable to design the lower limb amputation for partial end-weight bearing and placement of the skin scar with adequate subcutaneous tissue and deep soft tissue coverage between the skin and bone, precise care in rounding sectioned bone ends to remove prominences, ridges, and sharp edges then becomes essential. Careless surgical management of these tissues imposes pressure, shear, and stress interface moments, which can cause pain, dermatitis, and skin breakdown. Adherent scars over areas subjected to pressure result in similar difficulties. A well-placed and well-healed split-thickness skin graft over smooth underlying tissue can be entirely satisfactory in contrast to normal skin lying over a sharp bony prominence. The amputation is a plastic and reconstructive procedure. The surgeon is reconstructing a terminal motor and sensory end organ. When surgeons performing amputations accept this principle as the standard of success with skin management, then and only then will the amputee achieve maximum function.

Elective sites of leg amputation are largely eliminated when the principles of amputation just outlined are followed (Figs. 19-3 to 19-6). However, in the lower limb three levels are generally unsatisfactory for anatomical and prosthetic reasons. The first of these is the lower two fifths of the leg proximal to the ankle joint. The added

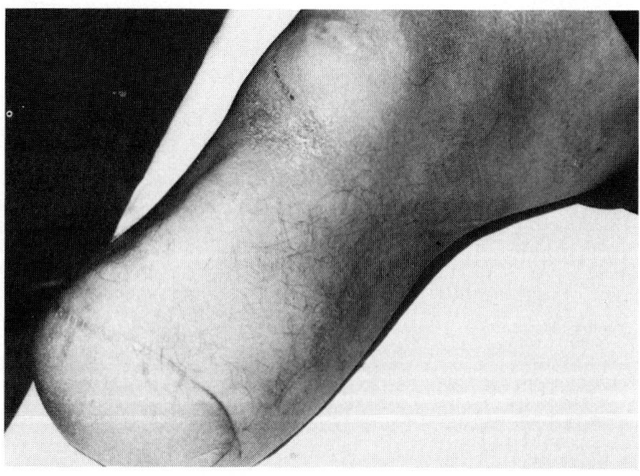

Fig. 19-3. Standard posterior flap below-knee amputation.

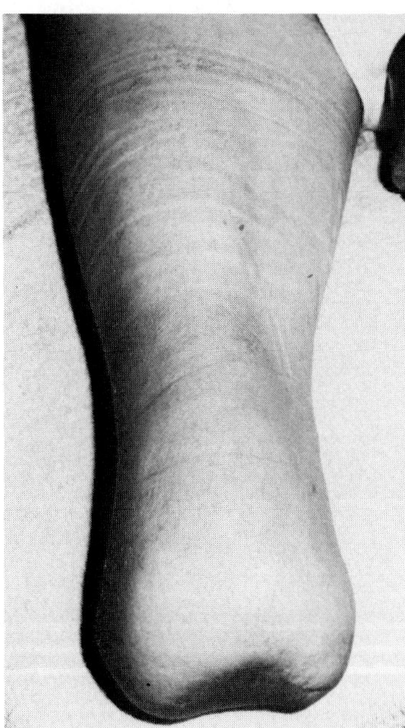

Fig. 19-4. Knee disarticulation, Burgess osteoplastic technique.

length of the lever arm at this level is outweighed in importance by difficulties in good skin and soft tissue management, since here the tibia and fibula are both subcutaneous. The conventional below-knee prosthesis is difficult to shape and contour in a cosmetic manner with amputations at this level. Modular limbs do not circumvent this cosmetic difficulty.

The second unsatisfactory level is the very short below-knee amputation proximal to the tibial tubercle. Knee extension strength is lost, and the knee becomes valueless. The added length creates difficulties in prosthetic fit as compared to a knee disarticulation. Knee flexion contractures are the rule. What then is the shortest remaining length of tibia permissible in the below-knee amputation? When active knee extension is present and the knee can be flexed through a range of 45 degrees or more, the residual limb can be comfortably fit with an effective prosthesis if surgery is performed not less than 3 cm below the tibial tubercle. Above this level most patients will be better served by knee disarticulation. Bilateral amputees may be the exception, especially when the surgeon and prosthetist innovate as with a bent-knee prosthesis.

The very high above-knee amputation is the third relatively undesirable site. When transection is just a short distance below the lesser trochanter, the limb tends to develop excessive flexion and abduction at the hip joint. Socket fit may become a difficult problem. This can be circumvented by releasing the deformity through flexor and abductor muscle release at the hip. Many surgeons prefer to leave a short segment of femur rather than amputate at the hip disarticulation level. Consultation with the prosthetist and an overall review of the patient's functional capacity will assist in deciding whether or not to leave a short residual section of femur rather than disarticulate the hip.

The principle of muscle stabilization has been emphasized throughout this book. Muscles form the major soft tissue mass in the extremity. Retention of muscle mass and function is fundamental to good amputation surgery. Anatomical circumstances will vary with every amputation, and the elderly ischemic patient for whom wound healing is critical may be best served by simple fascial closure. Also, muscle stabilization may not be possible in the scarred limb, in the presence of paralytic disease, in the presence of infection with open surgery, and with delayed healing, as well as other circumstances. Muscle stabilization with consequent improved residual limb muscle function is the goal, however, to be achieved consistent with good surgical judgment. This is especially true at amputation levels where muscle mass is large, such as through the thigh.

Few professional experiences are more satisfying to a surgeon than to participate in the rehabilitation of a high school student with limb loss due to trauma or neoplasm who can engage actively in sports or the elderly dysvascular amputee who can walk unassisted and is freed from an institutional setting to the warmth of a home environment.

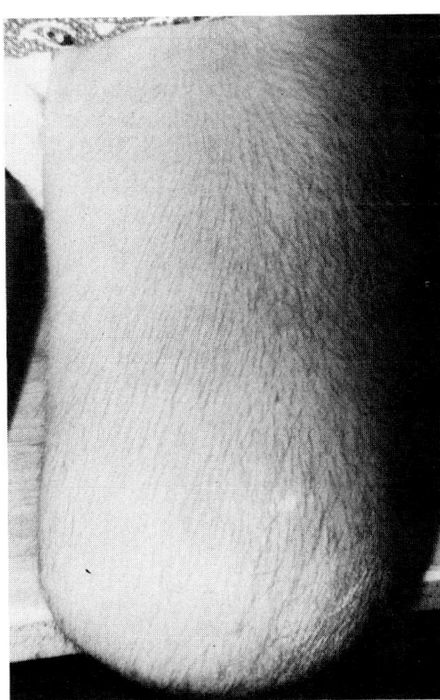

Fig. 19-5. Above-knee amputation, muscle stabilized.

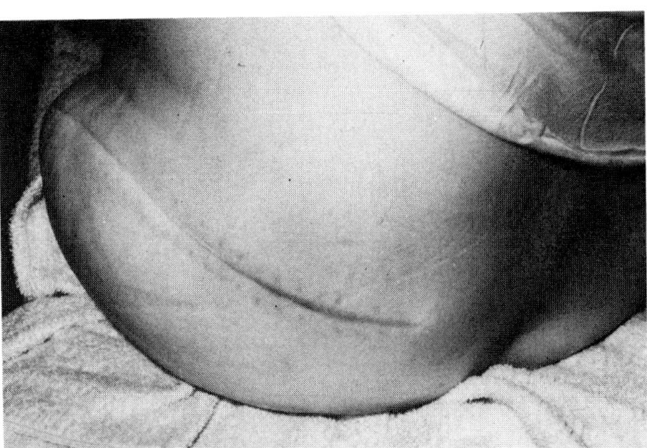

Fig. 19-6. Hemipelvectomy.

More than 80% of all amputations carried out in the Western world are through the lower limb. Attentive to the principles of modern amputation surgery, armed with a knowledge of prostheses, and working as leader of the amputee health care team, the surgeon is richly rewarded in human terms for his contribution.

SUGGESTED READINGS

Burgess, E. M.: The stabilization of muscles in lower extremity amputation, J. Bone Joint Surg. **50A:**1486-1487, 1968.

Burgess, E. M.: Immediate postsurgical prosthetic fitting: a system of amputee management, Phys. Ther. **51:**139-143, Feb., 1971.

Burgess, E. M.: Major amputation. In Nora, P. F., editor: Operative surgery: principles and techniques, Philadelphia, 1972, Lea & Febiger.

Burgess, E. M.: Above-knee amputation, Surg. Tech. Ill. **3**(3): 23-28, Summer, 1978.

Burgess, E. M.: Below-knee amputation, Surg. Tech. Ill. **3**(3): 59-67, Summer, 1978.

Burgess, E. M., Romano, R. L., and Zettl, J. H.: The management of lower extremity amputations, Publication TR 10-6, Washington, D.C., 1969, Veterans Administration.

Edmondson, A. S., and Crenshaw, A. H., editors: Campbell's operative orthopaedics, ed. 6, St. Louis, 1980, The C. V. Mosby Co.

Holloway, G. A., and Burgess, E. M.: Cutaneous blood flow and its relation to healing of below knee amputation, Surg. Gynecol. Obstet. **146:**750-756, 1978.

Kegel, B., Carpenter, M. L., and Burgess, E. M.: A survey of lower limb amputees: prostheses, phantom sensations, and psychosocial aspects, Bull. Prosthet. Res., BPR 10-27, Spring, 1977, pp. 43-60.

Kegel, B., Carpenter, M. L., and Burgess, E. M.: Capabilities of lower extremity amputees, Arch. Phys. Med. Rehabil. **59:** 109-120, March, 1978.

Little, J. M.: Successful amputation—by whose standards? Am. Heart J. **90**(6):806-807, Dec., 1975.

Murdoch, G.: Amputation surgery in the lower extremity, Prosthet. Orthot. Int. **1:**72-83, Aug., 1977.

Muslin, H., Hofstra, J., and Levine, R.: On psychologic amputation, Orthop. Rev. **6**(3):37-40, March, 1977.

Slocum, D. B.: An atlas of amputations, St. Louis, 1959, The C. V. Mosby Co.

CHAPTER 20

Lower limb prosthetic systems

ANTHONY STAROS
BERT GORALNIK

INTRODUCTION TO THE LOWER LIMB SYSTEM

A prosthesis is essential if wide-ranging upright mobility is to be restored to those who have suffered the loss of a lower limb. An artificial leg is basically a component array with functions and appearance simulating the anatomical parts lost. Since leg design depends on the geometrical relationship between these components and the interface with the amputee, the prosthetic socket, its alignment on the limb, and the means employed to provide suspension are therefore the most significant elements in limb design.

Amputation above the knee means that up to three major joints could be missing: the hip and/or the knee and the foot-ankle joint system. The below-knee amputee suffers the loss of the foot-ankle joint alone. For both groups, the functions of the joint replacements are critical but only insofar as they are a part of a total system, with the socket and suspension.

Therefore discussion of the prosthetic joints for lower limb prostheses takes place in that context. The functions of the prosthetic joints, knees, ankles, feet, and special rotators, relate directly to the use of the rest of the system. Similarly the relation of the socket and suspension of the joints helps determine the function of the joints and thus of the entire system.

SOCKET AND SUSPENSION DESIGN

Terminology

The interface between the amputee and artificial limb is the surface between the residual limb or stump and the socket.

residual limb The limb remaining after amputation, traced to the next proximal joint or referred in the joint of a disarticulation. In most cases, the joint is used in the name as in the below-knee limb, above-knee limb, or hip disarticulation residual limb.

socket The prosthesis component designed to provide a comfortable and functional control and weight-bearing pressure distribution over the stump.

end-bearing socket A socket designed to support a substantial amount of body weight on its distal surface.

hard socket A socket of rigid material whose entire inner surface is unlined.

nontotal-contact socket A socket designed to provide contact with some, but not all, surfaces of the limb.

open-end socket A socket designed with an airspace or chamber beneath the residual limb.

patellar tendon–bearing socket A below-knee limb socket designed to provide some weight support in the area of the patellar tendon as well as (primarily) in other weight-support areas below the knee, such as the medial tibial flare.

quadrilateral socket An above-knee limb socket that is essentially a four-sided configuration designed to minimize rotation of the prosthesis and distribute pressure on weight-supporting areas.

soft end A socket of rigid material having a resilient pad of foam or other yielding substance distally.

soft socket A socket whose inner surface is lined with a resilient material.

suction socket An essentially airtight socket held to the limb by external atmospheric pressure as the internal socket pressure decreases when the prosthesis is lifted from the ground.

total-contact socket A socket designed to maintain contact with the entire residual limb surface.

Design requirements

To provide the weight support and control so essential for standing and walking, the socket cannot be simply an inverted replica of the shape of the remaining limb. It must be designed rather precisely to accommodate the pressures developed between the limb and prosthesis under dynamic as well as static conditions.

A principal function of the residual limb, is to function as the lever to power and control the prosthesis; this it does through the socket. The more intimate and accurately defined the socket and the more precise the fit to the residual limb, the more efficient will be the force transfer. Moreover, the greater the surface area in contact between the residual limb and the socket, the better the feedback and thus the better the control of the prosthesis. For these reasons, *total contact* for all sockets is the most desirable.

Prosthetic socket design consists of four major interrelated considerations: support, control, suspension, and alignment.

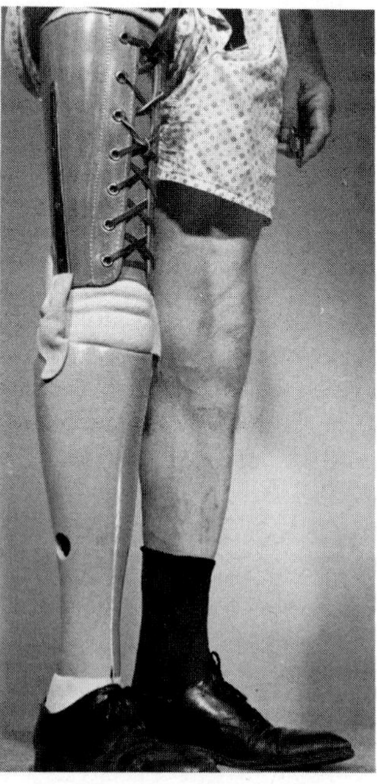

Fig. 20-1. Below-knee prosthesis with thigh corset.

Support in a socket is provided through the distribution of pressures on residual limb tissues in relation to those tissues which are pressure sensitive or pressure tolerant.

Soft materials *may* be used to accommodate pressure-sensitive areas, but pressure distribution for sensitive areas must be based on socket contouring that distributes limb contact pressures evenly as far as possible by putting the maximum loads in areas which can tolerate them.

Control depends on the pressures generated between the residual limb and the socket surface with different considerations applying (1) during the support (or stance) phase of walking and (2) during the swing phase.

During the support phase the body must be stabilized over the prosthesis by forces applied by the residual limb to the socket; the socket must be designed so that these forces are comfortably accommodated, providing stability with a minimum of lateral motion. The total-contact socket best fills these requirements.

In swing phase, full limb-to-socket contact is required to provide control over the prosthesis that is necessary when it is elevated off the walking surface. Relative motion must be minimized. For this reason a total-contact socket assuring close fit throughout the gait cycle is needed.

Suspension can be provided in any one or in a combination of five basic types: mechanical joint-corset system, gluteal-ischial weight-bearing thigh corset, suspension belt, suction socket, and socket contouring.

Mechanical joints with thigh corset or pelvic corset (belt). This kind of suspension system spans the knee or hip joint. The mechanical joint or joints must be placed carefully to minimize conflicting motion with the body joint. Since the suspensory forces and directional control provided by this system reduce the requirements of the socket itself, maintaining an intimate fit between the limb and socket becomes less critical. Actually a looser fit may be required to allow for stump-to-socket displacements caused by the differences in joint kinematics. Limb socks must be used with this kind of suspension. Thigh corsets may also provide some additional weight support, relieving the socket pressures to various extents (Fig. 20-1).

The gluteal-ischial weight-bearing thigh corset. The gluteal-ischial weight-bearing thigh corset used with below-knee prostheses is an adjustable system providing a means for controlling the direction of swing and providing some weight support.

The ischial weight-bearing thigh corset is usually fabricated of heavy molding leather, a material sufficiently rigid to maintain a quadrilateral shape in accordance with biomechanical principles of weight support in the thigh region. This shape is preferred, since weight is borne high above the knee joint, as in above-knee prostheses, with check lacers required to prevent genu recurvatum (hyperextension). Corset eyelets should be evenly spaced.

Suspension belt. Suspension belts, usually the below-knee cuff suspension and the Silesian bandage, are designed to encircle the body immediately above the joint just proximal to the amputation. They have no fixed mechanical joints but are connected to the socket by a flexible link. Their role is purely that of suspension. Suction may be employed as a supplementary suspension aid.

The suction socket. The suction socket is an essentially airtight socket held to the residual limb by the difference between atmospheric pressure and the internal socket pressure. The internal pressure is lowered below atmospheric pressure when the prosthesis, while off the ground, tends to pull away from the residual limb. In the suction socket design with a distal chamber, air remains beneath the residual limb. This type of suspension should be avoided because it frequently causes edema.

Preferred is the total-contact suction socket with no airspace next to the stump's surface. The face of the air-expulsion suction valve is positioned in the socket wall near the limb end, flush with the inner socket surface, thereby maintaining a smooth unbroken interface. *The total-contact support of the entire residual limb surface prevents the formation of edema.*

The socket-contour suspension system. The socket-contour suspension system uses socket shape to hold the socket to the residual limb. Usually, the condyles or portions of the condyles remaining in the stump (as in Syme's amputation) supply good suspension when accurately fitted into a socket. The condyles superior to the residual limb, such as those of the knee in below-knee amputations, are also frequently used for suspension. For these situations, the socket is carefully contoured over these bony protuberances.

The socket-contour suspension system is accurate and dependable, providing good suspension, control, and excellent sensory channels. Although this design is most often used with a limb sock, it may be used without one.

Alignment refers to the angular and linear position of the socket in relation to the knee and foot. Particularly important in *angular* alignment is that the socket is in a position in which the amputee can gain the best control with what remains of muscle capability. *Linear* alignment must be adjusted to position the socket over the prosthetic knee to achieve proper balance and/or to obtain the maximum function from the prosthetic components.

The total-contact principle

The fitting of all lower limb amputees typically employs a plastic socket. For the above-knee amputee, it is one with a quadrilateral shape, gluteal-ischial bearing, and support along the lateral aspect of the limb.[6] For the below-knee amputee, the socket uses patellar tendon and medial tibial flare support. Both types of fittings are based on anatomical and biomechanical considerations to yield the proper pressures in the socket-limb interface.

Not only at these two most common amputation levels, but for all lower limb prostheses, the best clinical results in artificial limb fittings have been obtained with a socket that provides relatively gentle, usually low-pressure contact with the entire surface of the stump. However, this could involve support of a significant proportion of body weight on the distal tissues, depending on the capability of the residual limb.

Edema may often be observed on amputees using sockets without total contact primarily because of limitations in limb circulation, which is aggravated by tight proximal fittings. Not only is distal edema likely from such proximal constrictions combined with no support of distal tissues, but also from the disturbing "bell-clapper" action of the residual limb within the socket; a "false joint," in effect, can result. Dermatological problems due to excessive pressures in the proximal socket region frequently result.

Although gluteal-ischial bearing and support on the medial tibial flare and the patellar tendon are the major sources of body support in total-contact above-knee and below-knee prostheses, a slight pressure uniformly distributed over the distal part of the limb will result in some support through these tissues. This relatively uniform contact pressure of low magnitude contains and thus stabilizes the distal tissues, balancing to some extent the hydrostatic pressure within the limb, preventing edema. This additional contact, although only providing a small portion of body support, allows a looser fit proximally. Greater comfort and better gait result, since constriction and its associated problem with circulation will be eliminated, false-joint action reduced, and control and sensation improved because of the larger interface between the residual limb and prosthesis, permitting better perception of any residual motion of the distal end of the tibia or femur within the socket.

The possibility of using a check socket made of wax or plaster-of-Paris bandage formed over the modified plaster-of-Paris replica of the residual limb to assure the adequacy of the total-contact fit should not be overlooked. Small holes are made in the wall of the socket to check contact in critical areas.

Another type of check socket, the transparent type molded from a strong plastic, can also be used to evaluate fit, especially for patients with whom problems have been experienced. The use of the transparent plastic provides a relatively inexpensive and expeditious means for a direct visual assessment of the total-contact fit of the socket with respect to the residual limb. X-ray examinations can be avoided. Because direct observation of the residual limb–socket interface under static and dynamic conditions is possible, some of the obstacles to optimum fit and training, such as residual limb pain and skin breakdown, are substantially reduced. The plastics commonly used are polycarbonate and polypropylene (Fig. 20-2).

These check sockets are of course of the hard contact types; nevertheless, following the fit check, the prosthetist can still use a soft end in the definitive plastic socket.

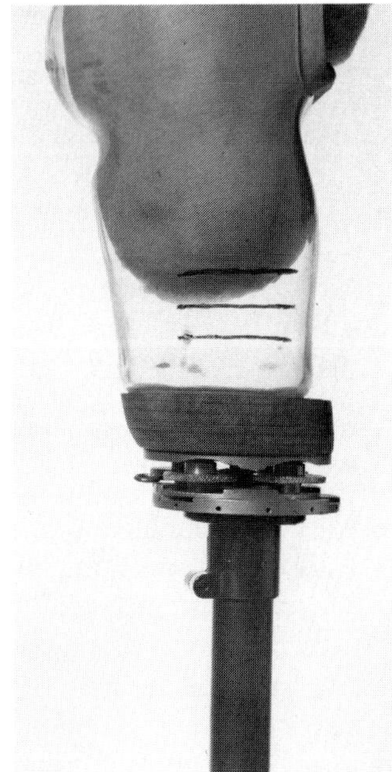

Fig. 20-2. Polycarbonate below-knee check socket.

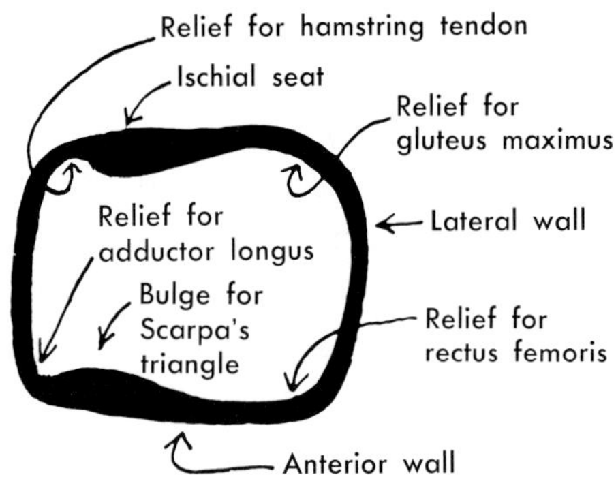

Fig. 20-3. Schematic of above-knee quadrilateral socket.

The above-knee prosthetic socket (total-contact gluteal-ischial bearing quadrilateral design)

Regardless of the method used for achieving total contact for the above-knee amputee, the gluteal-ischial bearing component of support is the primary mechanism for weight transfer and horizontal stabilization of the limb and body. Such support can only be achieved by pressure in the proximal limb region of magnitude sufficient to provide adequate horizontal and vertical stabilization of the limb. The pressures of total contact in the distal limb regional also provide some support and stabilization, but they are relatively small in magnitude. It is necessary that the socket design and shape and therefore the method of fabrication include a gradual change of the pressures from higher in the proximal region to significantly lower in the distal region. Otherwise, sharp pressure gradients will result, possibly causing, by choking and shearing, a number of limb tissue difficulties.

Fig. 20-3 illustrates a top view of the quadrilateral socket. The inner contour of the socket differs significantly from the relaxed contour of the amputee's thigh. The difference in contour is a deliberate modification made to achieve a certain type of pressure distribution.[1]

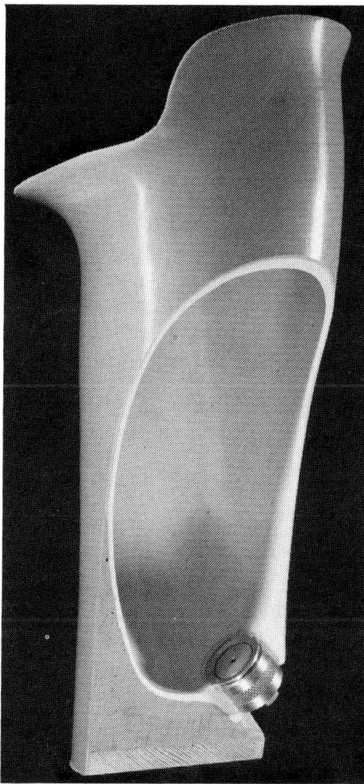

Fig. 20-4. Cutaway of plastic laminate total-contact above-knee socket (hard end) with total-contact suction socket valve.

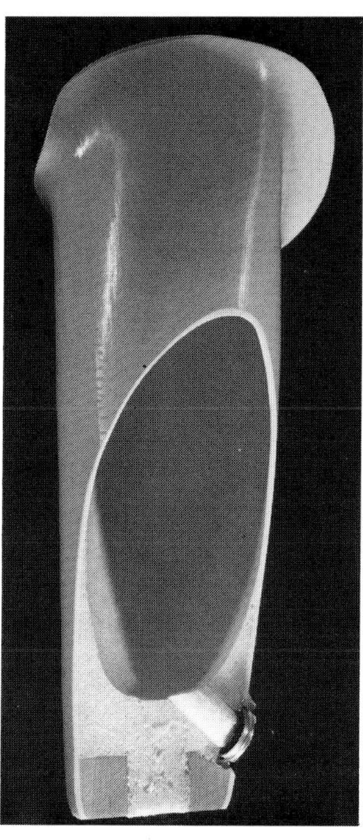

Fig. 20-5. Cutaway of plastic laminate total-contact above-knee socket with soft end.

The quadrilateral socket has reliefs (concavities) and bulges (convexities) on its inner surface. Reliefs are hollowed-out areas to reduce pressure on relatively firm tissues, such as tendons, contracting muscles, and bony prominences. Bulges are inward directed contours of the socket wall to press on soft, pressure-tolerant areas of the residual limb so that these areas will take higher pressures and thereby their appropriate share of the load.

Distortion of the residual limb and of the wrap cast while it hardens yields the desired quadrilateral contour of the socket. With reasonable accuracy, the volume assumed by the plaster-of-Paris wrap cast after distortion is the same as before distortion, that is, the normal volume of the residual limb. Modifications to the stump replica taken from this cast are made primarily to achieve final contours for support and stabilization.

The prosthetist usually has a plastic laminate total-contact socket formed over the modified plaster-of-Paris replica of the residual limb. A total-contact valve must be employed (Fig. 20-4).

A soft, total-contact socket (Fig. 20-5) can be achieved by placing foam in the distal end of the socket. Regular suction socket valves may be used in these "soft-end" sockets, since a cylindrical foam cap, formed to fit on the valve, will provide the necessary continuity of the interior distal socket surface.

Biomechanics of an above-knee socket

Anterior wall of the above-knee socket. With an ischial seat provided in a socket, the anterior wall of the socket must be relatively high to maintain the ischial tuberosity in its proper place on the ischial seat. Since the weight line passes anterior to the ischial seat, the pelvis tends to rotate downward and forward, with the tuberosity tending to slide off the ischial seat. A posteriorly directed counterforce applied high enough is necessary to generate a moment to prevent this. The required counterforce is provided by the anterior wall of the socket. A low anterior wall might provide sufficient counterforce, but because of the smaller moment arm, this force would be of limited effectiveness in resisting the tendency of the pelvis to rotate downward and forward. In contrast, an anterior wall that is 5 to 7.5 cm (2 to 2½ inches) higher than the posterior wall provides a much more effective stabilizing moment. The high anterior wall also provides more area over which to distribute the force required.

However, there is a limit to the height of the anterior wall. The wearer of the prosthesis must be able to flex his hip to slightly more than 90 degrees to sit comfortably. If the anterior wall is too high, the brim of the socket wall impinges on the abdomen, causing discomfort when the wearer is seated.

Lateral wall. During the swing phase of *normal* walking, the pelvis tends to drop slightly on the unsupported side. This tendency is primarily opposed by the opposite gluteus medius.

In Fig. 20-6, the weight line through the center of the body falls medial to the hip joint. A moment, equal to the product of the weight (W) and the perpendicular distance (D_W) from the hip joint to the line of action of the weight, tends to make the pelvis drop to the unsupported side. A moment in the opposite direction resists this tendency. This countermoment is equal to the product of the force developed by the gluteus medius (F_g) and the perpendicular distance (D_W) from the hip joint to the line of action of the force.

But with the above-knee amputee, support to prevent pelvis drop must be provided by the prosthesis. The lateral wall of the socket is therefore designed to provide stabilization of the pelvis by holding the femur in the position where the gluteus medius is at rest length, its maximum force position.

The lateral wall thus provides the counterforce, directly helping to stabilize the pelvis. In Fig. 20-7, the line of action of the weight passes medial to the support point (S), which is located near the ischial seat. When the intact limb is in swing phase, the pelvis will tend to drop to the unsupported side. Any slight dropping of the pelvis to the unsupported side will tend to rotate the residual limb, but as long as the gluteus medius stabilizes the hip joint and maintains the femur in a relatively fixed position with respect to the pelvis, forces will be generated by the lateral wall on the stump to stabilize the stump and the pelvis. If the lateral wall of the socket is adequately shaped and fitted, it will exert these resisting counterforces over the broadest possible area of the lateral aspect of the stump.

Assume that F_1 represents the net effect of these forces acting at a perpendicular distance (D) from the support point. The magnitude of the total counterforce necessary to stabilize the pelvis is $\frac{WD_W}{D_f}$, in which the W equals that portion of the body weight supported by the prosthesis, D_W is the perpendicular distance from the support point to the line of action of the weight, and D_f is the perpendicular distance from the support point to the line of action of F_L.

Prescription criteria. There are essentially no special contraindications to use of the total-

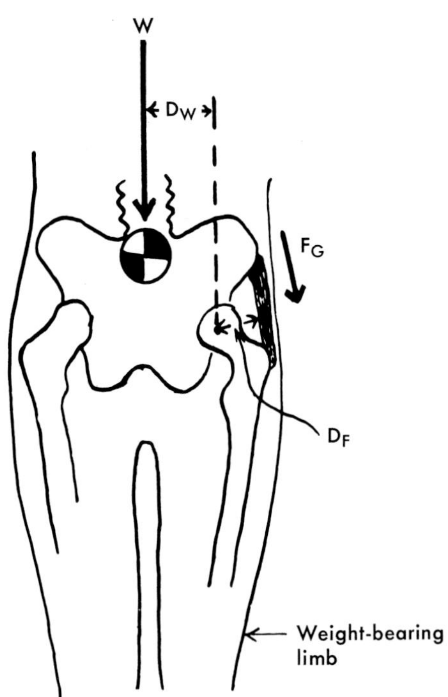

Fig. 20-6. Schematic depicting weight line falling medial to hip joint on normal person.

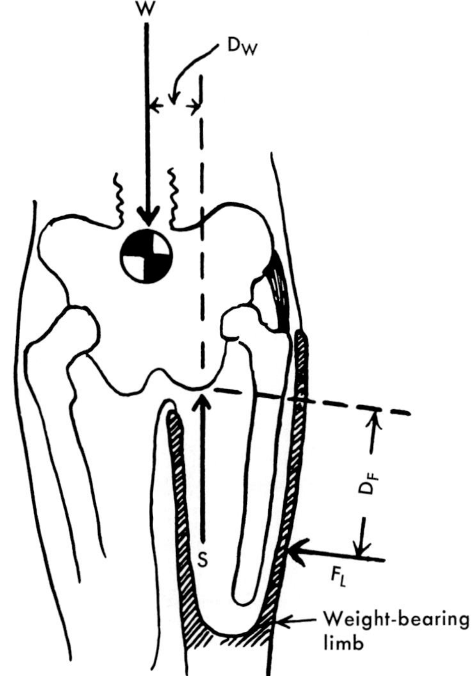

Fig. 20-7. Line of action of weight passing medial to ischial seat on prosthesis.

contact above-knee socket other than those which apply to other types of lower limb prostheses. A draining osteomyelitis, of course, would contraindicate any prosthesis. Total contact might not be adequate for an amputee with a flabby residual limb and little muscle strength. Limbs with painful neuromas, particularly those caught in scars, might not be suitable for total contact or at least would require special local relief.

It would seem appropriate to use hard total-contact sockets most generally for the softer bulkier residual limb in which there is room for the femur or tibia to move with minimal resistance.

The center of rotation of the femur in the anteroposterior plane during the stance phase is at the acetabulum; this obviously is not at the same point as the center of rotation of the prosthesis (including the socket), which is at or near the ischium. Therefore a displacement of the femur with respect to the socket wall will take place. In a fleshy limb, such relative motion can be accommodated by displacement of the soft tissues. In a firm limb, however, painful impingement of the femur against the limb end and the socket may result; therefore soft-end sockets might be advantageously employed.

The clinician should recognize that soft-end designs, besides offering a soft bottom to allow long bone displacements without painful impingements or to provide relief for highly sensitive limb areas, might also permit the achievement of total-contact through the swing phase, as well as in the stance phase, with a minimal increase in contact pressure. Depending, of course, on the adequacy of the suspension mechanism, normal pumping of the limb tissues within the hard-end socket may result in excessive pressures during stance phase, especially if the socket design were made to assure total contact during the swing phase.

Above-knee total-contact sockets commonly employ suction suspension with no limb sock used by the amputee. Nevertheless, an auxiliary suspension, such as a Silesian belt, can be added. A total-contact socket can also be made for an amputee needing a pelvic joint and waist belt. If a limb sock is to be used, the prosthetist can allow for sock thickness during the casting process.

Suspension systems for above-knee prostheses that do not use suction are usually of two extremes, the flexible webbing type of Silesian belt or the rigid, steel pelvic joint and band with an attached belt. Both designs have their uses, but excessive numbers of repairs are needed with the pelvic joint and band.

The Veterans Administration Prosthetics Cen-

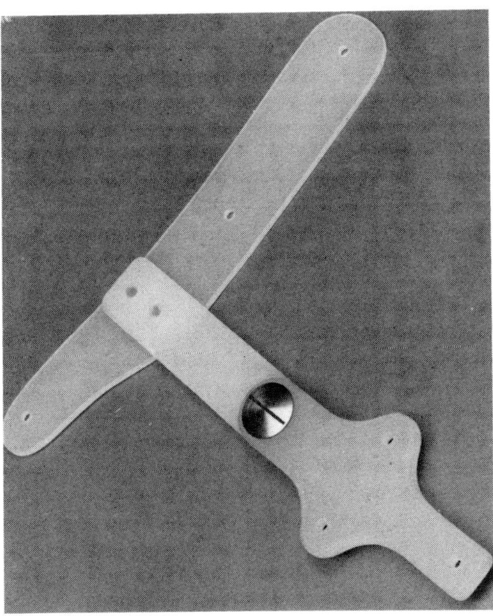

Fig. 20-8. VAPC polypropylene hip joint and band.

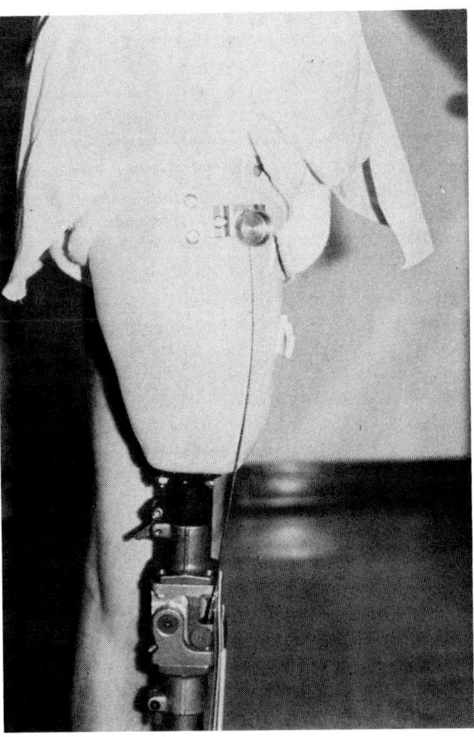

Fig. 20-9. Rancho adjustable above-knee polypropylene socket.

ter* had been using a thin, flexible spring-steel pelvic joint and band combination for many years, but the frequency of breakage, noise, and binding at the joint continued to be high. A new design (Fig. 20-8) is made of 6-mm (1/4-inch) polypropylene using a stainless steel bolt. The employment of nyliner bearings ensures long wear and smooth operation. The band is fabricated from a 3-mm (1/8-inch) thick polypropylene sheet. The joint and band can be shaped readily with a heat gun and attached to the socket wall with rivets.

A new system for management of the above-knee geriatric patient has been developed at Rancho Los Amigos Hospital using a polypropylene adjustable socket, an endoskeletal structure, and a manual locking knee. The design shown in Fig. 20-9 uses polypropylene. By this means and by the use of the endoskeletal structure, a prosthesis weight of about 50% of the conventional wood exoskeletal designs can be achieved. The prosthesis, however, is designed for light duty; extremely active patients would not be served well by its use.

The adjustable socket is marketed with a manual locking knee to provide knee stability. The patient's gait is less cosmetic than with an unlocked knee, but the elimination of knee buckling is a major safety asset. The socket can be tightened or loosened to allow for volume changes or to adjust weight-bearing and suspension pressures.

The below-knee prosthetic (PTB) socket

The other major total-contact socket is that used with the below-knee prosthesis; this socket is best known as the PTB socket.

In 1957 the University of California Biomechanics Laboratories (in Berkeley and San Francisco) held a symposium on below-knee prosthetics, which resulted in synthesis of the many concepts of prosthetic fitting then prevalent. The result was the PTB below-knee prosthesis (Fig. 20-10) described in a manual published by the University of California with an explanation of the biomechanical principles of this concept of weight bearing and control.

The upper portion of the shank of the PTB prosthesis usually consists of a molded plastic laminate socket, which provides an intimate, total-contact fit over the entire area of the residual limb. In most cases a thigh corset and side joints are not used with this prosthesis, which has usually been constructed with a shank of wood covered by a plastic laminate that provides reinforcement.

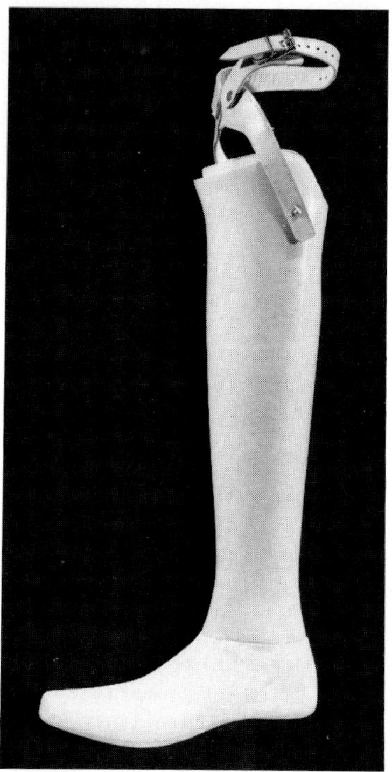

Fig. 20-10. PTB prosthesis.

A special lightweight prosthesis for the below-knee amputee has been designed by personnel of the Moss Rehabilitation Hospital/Temple University in Philadelphia. The prosthesis, including both socket and shank as shown in Fig. 20-11, is fabricated primarily from polypropylene. It uses a lightweight suspension strap.

This major reduction in prosthesis weight appears advantageous to both the active, young below-knee amputee and the infirm geriatric amputee. Aside from energy savings, fewer suspension problems are encountered, and prosthesis control also appears improved. Fig. 20-12 represents the Rancho polypropylene design.

The socket is shaped so that a substantial amount of weight is borne on the patellar tendon and the medial flare of the tibia. The sides of the socket are also made high enough (approximately 75 mm [2 1/2 inches] above the midpatellar tendon) to gain stability against side loading. A soft insert that fits intimately in the socket is often used with this type of prosthesis.

*As of July 1, 1980, the name Veterans Administration Prosthetics Center was changed to Veterans Administration Rehabilitation Engineering Center (VAREC).

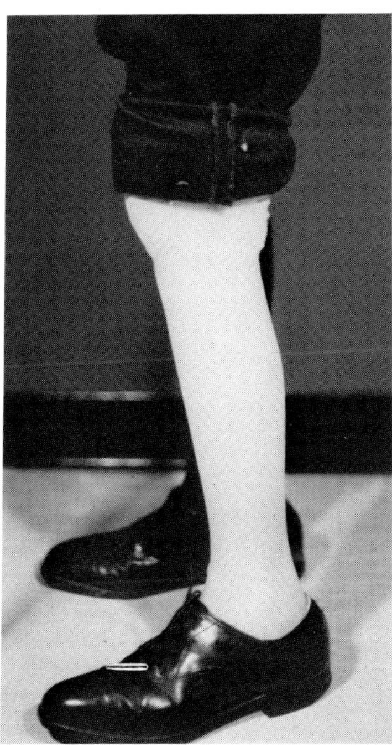

Fig. 20-11. Moss Ultralight below-knee polypropylene prosthesis.

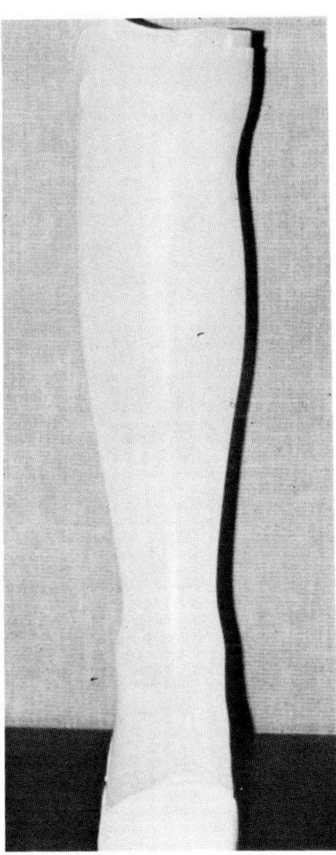

Fig. 20-12. Rancho below-knee polypropylene prosthesis.

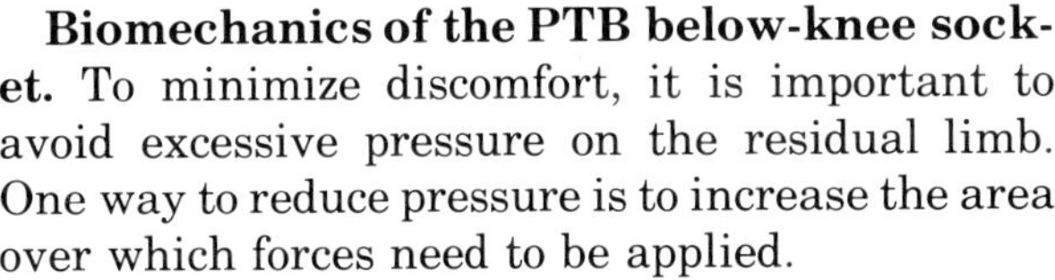

Biomechanics of the PTB below-knee socket. To minimize discomfort, it is important to avoid excessive pressure on the residual limb. One way to reduce pressure is to increase the area over which forces need to be applied.

The typical PTB prosthesis for the below-knee amputee has an inward protuberance that fits under the patellar tendon and an inward contour that slants under the medial flare of the tibia. The posterior wall bulges inward slightly, and the lateral wall is shaped to provide firm pressure on the distal half of the residual limb. Reliefs in the socket are usually provided for pressure-sensitive areas at the anterior distal aspect of the residual limb, over the crest of the tibia, and over the head of the fibula.

Although the supporting area for the patellar tendon is not steeply inclined, it still has a slight downward and backward slope. The residual limb, supported on this area, tends to slide downward and backward. To prevent this, an anteriorly directed counterforce is required. The anteriorly directed force is applied by the posterior wall of the prosthesis, which should be relatively high to provide as much area as possible over which to distribute the force, but it must not be so high that it interferes with sitting comfort. It is not enough for the posterior wall to match the posterior aspect of the residual limb. The posterior wall of the socket must be flattened or even have an inward bulge so that the tissues with which it is in contact are under moderate, controlled compression. If the posterior wall (or popliteal bulge) does not produce sufficient pressure on the soft tissues posteriorly, then the anterior aspect of the stump tends to "fall off" the patella tendon – bearing shelf. As a result, the stump will migrate distally and result in end bearing that is painful.

An inward contour of the socket in the area of the medial flare of the tibia can provide an effective weight-bearing area. To maintain the residual limb on this inclined medial limb surface, a force must be applied by the socket. The major part of this force will be applied to the distal half or distal third of the residual limb.

If the downward forces applied by the residual limb to the prosthesis and the opposing counterforce applied by the ground were acting along the same straight line as shown in Fig. 20-13, there would be no tendency for the socket to change the angular relationship with respect to the residual limb. But such is not the case.

Fig. 20-14 shows the results of the forces applied to the prosthesis from above and the ground reaction from below. These opposing forces, which are not collinear, tend to rotate the prosthesis in a counterclockwise direction. This rotation must be resisted by forces applied to the socket by the residual limb, resulting in a clockwise moment. The clockwise moment is produced by a force couple, with one force applied to the proximal medial aspect of the socket and the other applied to the distolateral aspect of the socket. The distance between these forces must be maximized to prevent excessive pressures on the residual limb.

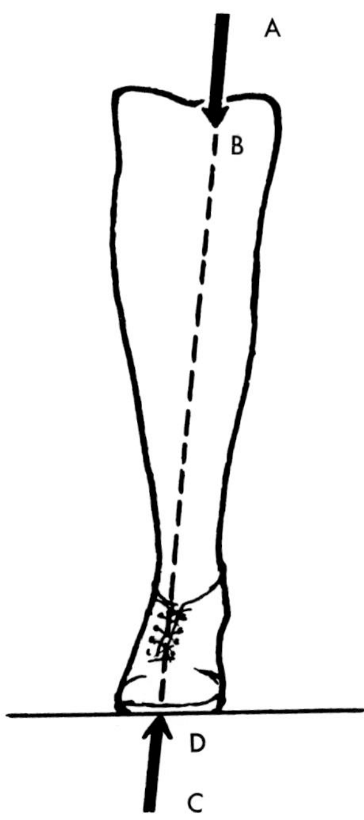

Fig. 20-13. Theoretical force applied to prosthesis by amputee and collinear ground reaction.

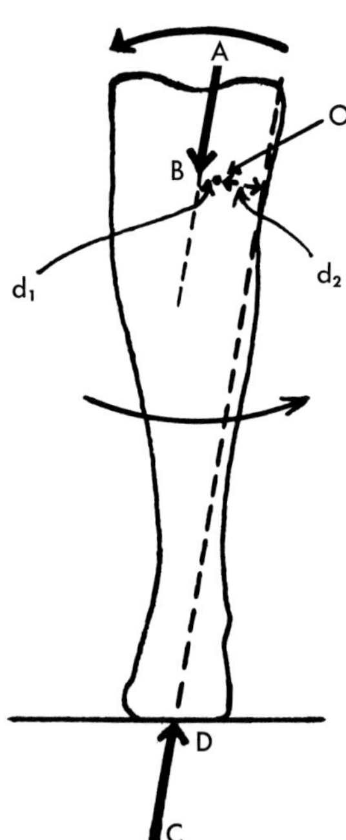

Fig. 20-14. Forces and moments actually applied to prosthesis by amputee.

Critical considerations in fitting the PTB. The PTB socket as a total-contact design helps to avoid edema and provides better sensory feedback to the wearer because of the greater area of contact between the residual limb and the socket.

In 1965 Foort reviewed the critical factors in PTB socket shaping and offered key points about the weight-bearing concepts, particularly the shape of the brim (Fig. 20-15). Clinicians should continually refer to the key points raised by Foort[3]:

1. Posterior pressure needed to balance the posteriorly directed force against the patellar tendon by the weight-bearing bar of the socket must be provided by the posterior and posteromedial aspects of the tibial condyles and the overlying tendinous structures, as well as by the popliteal area of the stump.

2. The posterior and posteromedial aspects of the tibial condyles and the overlying tendinous structure are important weight-bearing surfaces of the stump.

3. The back brim of the socket should be formed into a broad, flared surface against which the hamstring tendons can rest when the amputee sits.

4. To achieve mediolateral stability of the

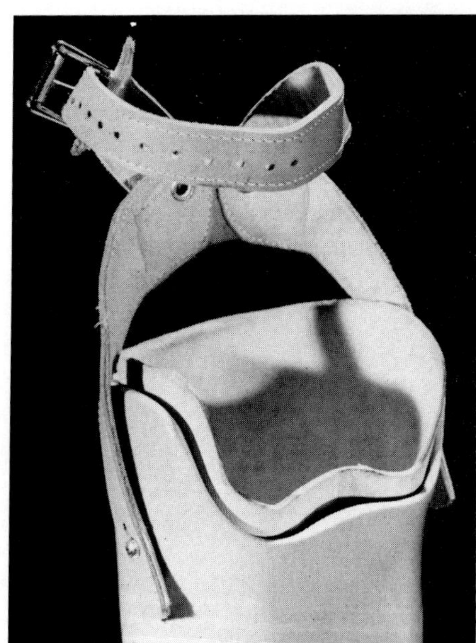

Fig. 20-15. Shape of proximal PTB brim.

stump in the socket, the socket should fit securely against either side of the tibial crest and against the medial and lateral surfaces of the knee joint.

5. The socket should be placed over the foot so that there is little tendency for the prosthesis to tilt medially or laterally on the residual limb as the amputee walks.

6. The socket should support distal tissues with sufficient pressures to aid venous and lymphatic return without pressing against the bone end.

7. The foot should be applied and aligned to give a smooth rolling action as the amputee walks, as though the foot were a segment of the wheel rim.

8. Tissues that are snugly pressed in a socket will shrink until pressures are reduced to suitable levels.

Variants of the PTB. The variants in PTB design are of two kinds: (1) socket designs to improve distal pressure and weight-bearing control or to improve the environment around the residual limb and (2) mechanisms for improvement in suspension and knee stabilization.

Fig. 20-16 shows the major variations in PTB prosthesis design. Included are the "conventional" PTB, with a liner and a cuff suspension; air-cushion variants; and variations possible for suspension and knee control.

The variants do not affect the fundamental principles of PTB fitting, which should involve careful planning of pressure distribution on the proximal weight-bearing areas of the below-knee limb and *provision for total contact.*

The PTB with a hard socket and soft-end will offer advantages to the patient in that retention of fit will probably be maintained longer. A liner will deteriorate quite rapidly due to perspiration and will compress and take on a permanent set, which may require modifications earlier than necessary. However, adjustments by the addition of pads are probably easier with a liner than with a hard socket, although hard sockets too can be adjusted by the addition of pads. This process involves more time.

Soft ends for PTB sockets are best done by foaming them in place to assure total contact. Carving distal pads is not recommended because this method is not as errorproof as the foaming-in-place process.

The PTB air-cushion socket will assure ade-

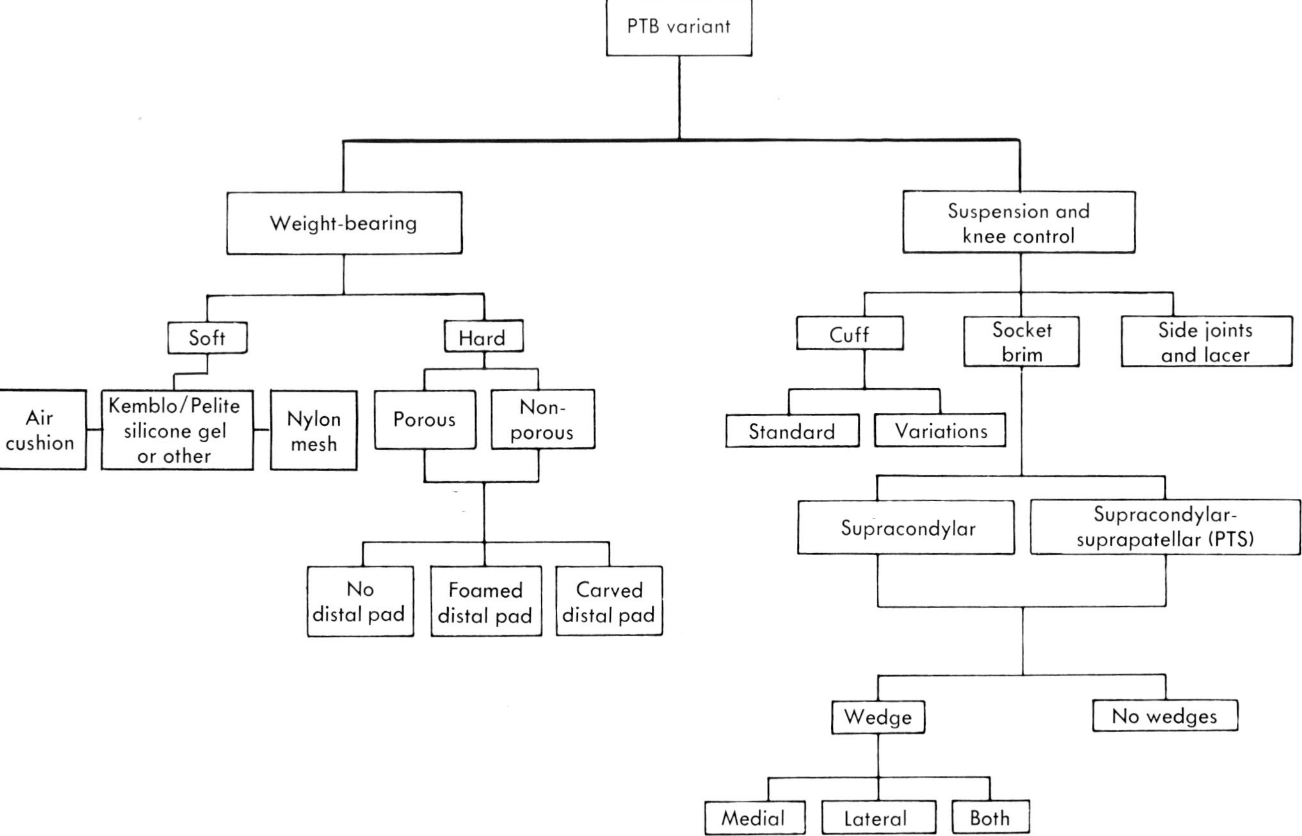

Fig. 20-16. Variations of PTB prosthesis. (From Veterans Administration Program Guide, Prosthetic and Sensory Aids Service, Washington D.C, April, 1970.)

quate pressure on the distal portion of the limb, minimizing the risk of edema. The elastic sleeve that will displace longitudinally under weight bearing will tend to minimize abrasive skin damage, which might occur with the residual limb in contact with a rigid socket wall.

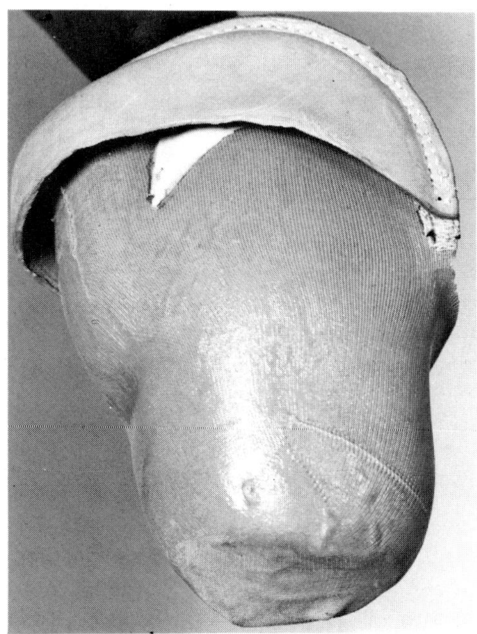

Fig. 20-17. Porous flexible insert.

The air-cushion socket also offers a possibility for higher distal loading, when feasible. Increasing the distal pressure will decrease the need for the more constrictive proximal loading and thus benefit circulation. The higher distal pressure will maintain total contact with slight limb volume changes.

When an amputee using a total-contact PTB prosthesis or one of its variations perspires excessively, the residual limb will become immersed in a pool of fluid, a condition which not only causes discomfort but also constitutes a potential cause of skin maceration and breakdown.

The PTB without a liner will permit the employment of a porous socket wall that should only be used *when severe perspiration problems make it absolutely necessary* and when the prosthetist has obtained the required skill. A porous, flexible insert (Fig. 20-17) is another possible remedy for this problem. Total contact can be maintained while allowing for escape of the fluid from the residual limb-socket interface.

The cuff suspension strap of the PTB, if properly designed and fitted, provides an adequate suspension mechanism for many patients. This design, however, with the strap over the patella, may in certain cases cause difficulty either in not reducing piston action sufficiently or in restrict-

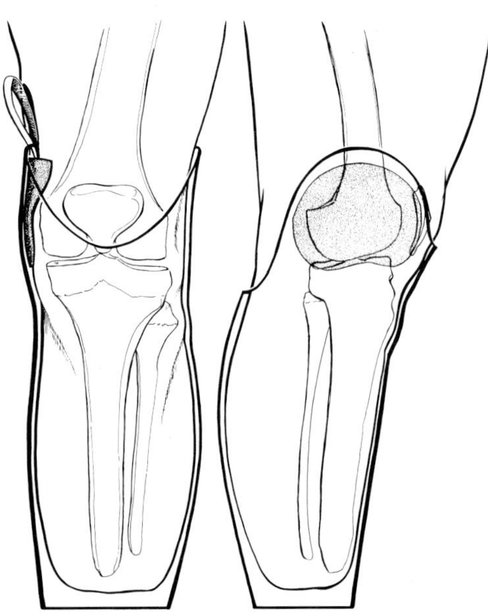

Fig. 20-18. PTB socket with supracondylar suspension employing medial wedge.

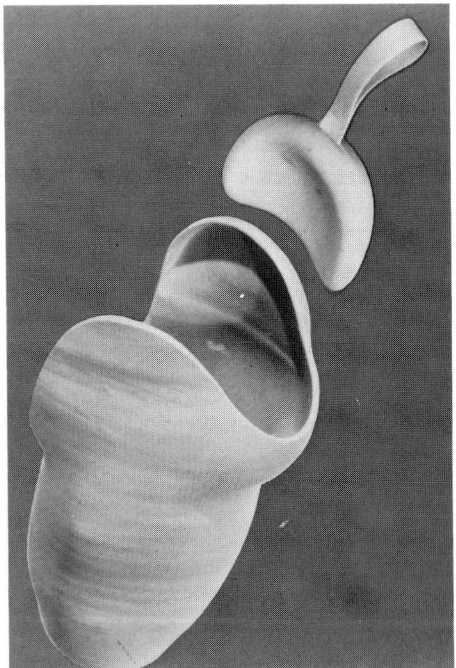

Fig. 20-19. Medial wedge and supracondylar socket.

ing circulation. Often with short residual limbs the strap may be found to be inadequate, forcing a clinician to prescribe the sidebars and lacer suspension. Mediolateral instability of the knee is a special problem that may be solved with the use of metal joints and or thigh lacer.

For most cases, the PTB has allowed the elimination of the sidebar and lacer suspension with its restrictive effects. But when below-knee limbs are not able to take full weight bearing, the use of a thigh lacer may be indicated to assist in that function. When used, the guidelines offered by Gardner and Clippinger[5] should be followed.

The supracondylar suspension system employs high medial and lateral socket walls to encompass fully the medial and lateral aspects of the femoral condyles. If these proximal extensions were flexible enough, the prosthesis could easily be donned by expanding the extensions and then allowing them to retract over the condyles. Since the laminate used in the socket walls is generally not that flexible and no liner is normally used in the socket, the supracondylar suspension of the PTB uses a prefabricated wedge of a flexible material, which can be inserted between the socket and the medial condyles to obtain a locking fit over that condyle (Figs. 20-18 and 20-19). The wedge has to be carefully fitted with special attention given to the construction of its seat in the medial socket wall. Properly fitted over the condyles, the wedge provides very adequate suspension. The amputee removes the prosthesis by first removing the wedge and then putting the wedge back after donning the limb. With this type of suspension, there is probably less restriction to knee flexion in comparison to the circumferential strap, and mediolateral stabilization of the knee is provided. Significant in the fitting of this device is the care that must be taken in measuring the mediolateral dimension over the condyles.

A description of the supracondylar suspension is given by Fillauer.[2] This design has sometimes been called the condylar clip, the KBM, or the STP, but the terminology recommended is PTB-SC, with the addition of the letters SC for supracondylar. Table 2 presents the recommended abbreviated terminology for this and other variants.

Another variant, sometimes called the PTS but preferably the PTB-SC/SP (supracondylar/suprapatellar PTB), employs high mediolateral walls to encompass the condyles as well as a high anterior wall coming up and over the patella, as described by Marschall and Nitschke.[8] This suspension (Fig. 20-20) was also designed to eliminate the cuff suspension strap and normally is used with a liner, unlike the supracondylar design previously described. The compressibility of the liner allows the limb to pass the close-fitting proximal brim and achieve full entry into the socket. The anterior brim line is brought into direct contact with the quadriceps tendon with a properly designed flare. The anterior fitting provides the main support function.

For certain cases the SC/SP design can be fitted without the liner, but wedges must be employed to permit entry and removal of the socket, as suggested by Marschall and Nitschke. The high walls of this type of socket may take some of the weight

Table 2. Terminology of PTB variants

	*Weight-bearing interface features**				*Suspension and knee control design*				
	Hard end	*Soft end*	*Liner*	*Air cushion*	*Thigh lacer*	*Cuff*	*Wedges*	*High mediolateral wall*	*High anterior wall*
Conventional PTB or PTB cuff (lined)			X			X			
PTB thigh lacer (lined)			X		X				
PTB cuff (hard)	X					X			
PTB cuff (soft)		X				X			
PTB cuff (AC)				X		X			
PTB-SC (hard)	X						X	X	
PTB-SC (soft)		X					X	X	
PTB-SC (AC)				X			X	X	
PTB-SC/SP (lined)			X					X	X
PTB-SC/SP (soft)		X					X	X	X
PTB-SC/SP (AC)				X			X	X	X

*Terminology system: PTB-suspension (weight-bearing feature); AC, air cushion; SC, supracondylar; SP, suprapatellar.

Table 3. Guidelines for clinical employment of PTB variants as compared to PTB conventional suspension with liner and cuff

	Weight bearing	*Suspension*	*Knee control and stabilization*	*Cosmesis*	*Process*
Conventional PTB cuff (lined)	Liner will compress; leather liner deteriorates with perspiration; easiest to modify	May cause constriction; may limit knee flexion; may not prevent piston action	Minimally provided	Poor around knee	Probably easiest to make and fit, except liner consumes significant amount of time
PTB thigh lacer (lined)	Liner will compress; leather liner deteriorates with perspiration; easiest to modify; some weight can be taken on lacer	May limit knee rotation and increase piston action due to location of axes	Mediolateral stabilization and against hyperextension	Poor around knee and above	Liner consumes time; lacer and side joint fitting and alignment increase difficulty and time; probably needs reduced PTB shelf due to piston action
PTB cuff (hard)	Extremely difficult to fit and adjust to provide total contact	Same as conventional PTB	Same as conventional PTB	Same as conventional PTB	More difficult to fit; no liner saves time
PTB cuff (soft)	More difficult to fit and adjust than lined socket; soft end assures total contact temporarily	Same as conventional PTB	Same as conventional PTB	Same as conventional PTB	More difficult to fit; foam end easier to make than liner
PTB cuff (AC)	Air cushion assures total contact longer; increased distal bearing possible; very difficult to adjust for shrinkage	Same as conventional PTB	Same as conventional PTB	Same as conventional PTB	More difficult to make and fit

PTB-SC (hard)	Extremely difficult to fit and adjust to maintain total contact	Very good; will not cause constriction or limit knee rotation	Mediolateral stabilization	Improved around knee, except may be bulky medially	More difficult in fitting and assuring proper mediolateral for wedge and construction of wedge seat; no liner saves time
PTP-SC (soft)	More difficult to fit and adjust than lined socket; soft end assures total contact temporarily	Very good; will not cause constriction or limit knee rotation	Mediolateral stabilization	Improved around knee, except may be bulky medially	More difficult in fitting and assuring proper mediolateral for wedge and construction of wedge seat; foam end easier to make than liner
PTB-SC (AC)	Air cushion assures total contact longer; increased distal bearing possible; very difficult to adjust for shrinkage	Very good; will not cause constriction or limit knee rotation	Mediolateral stabilization	Improved around knee, except may be bulky medially	More difficult to fit, both for distal press, control and wedge location including mediolateral control
PTB-SC/SP (lined)	Liner will compress; leather liners deteriorate with perspiration; easiest to modify	Excellent but may cause restriction in knee flexion	Mediolateral stabilization and against hyperextension	Improved around knee, except may be bulky generally	Difficult to fit; care needed for anterior brim
PTB-SC/SP (soft)	More difficult to fit and adjust than lined socket; soft end assures total contact temporarily	Excellent but may cause restriction in knee flexion	Mediolateral stabilization and against hyperextension	Improved around knee	Difficult to fit; care needed for anterior brim; foam end easier to make than liner
PTB-SC/SP (AC)	Air cushion assures total contact longer; increased distal bearing possible; very difficult to adjust for shrinkage	Excellent but may cause restriction in knee flexion	Mediolateral stabilization and against hyperextension	Improved around knee, except may be bulky generally	Difficult to fit; care needed for anterior brim

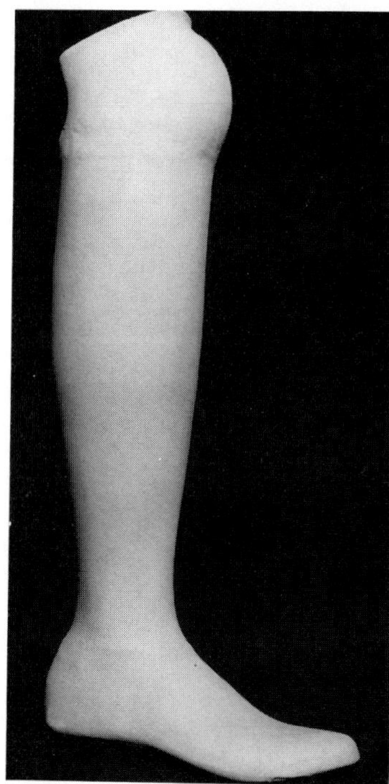

Fig. 20-20. PTB prosthesis with supracondylar/suprapatellar suspension.

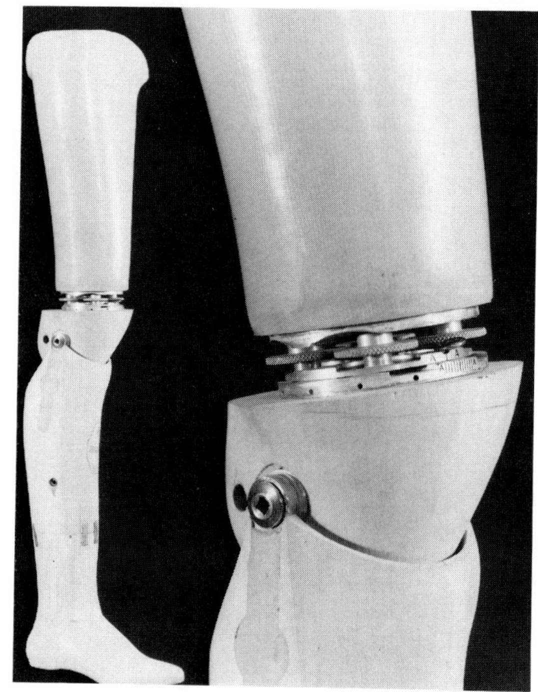

Fig. 20-21. Staros-Gardner alignment coupling.

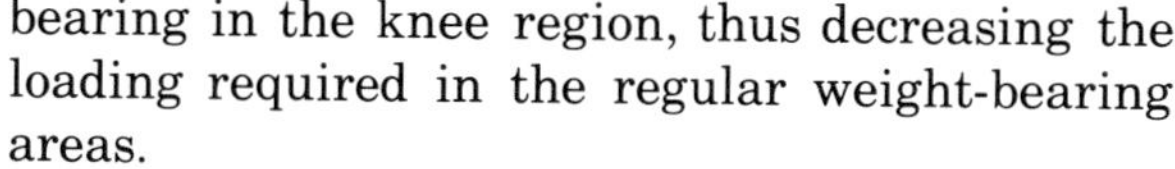

bearing in the knee region, thus decreasing the loading required in the regular weight-bearing areas.

The PTB-SC/SP also provides mediolateral stabilization of the knee, as well as a stabilization in the sagittal plane, especially at pushoff. Consequently, it will reduce any tendency of the knee to go into hyperextension.

This socket offers an improved suspension but is obviously more difficult to fit than a conventional PTB socket. The proximal brim appears somewhat bulky and in some cases may restrict extreme flexion as would be required in kneeling. The PTB-SC/SP does offer a variant of the PTB socket that may be employed for short residual limbs, particularly when the anatomical knees are unstable. Hamontree, Tyo, and Smith[7] indicated on the basis of ninety seven fittings the success that can be achieved with this design for patients they normally could not have fitted with a PTB prosthesis.

Even with this array of suspension aids developed for below-knee prostheses, friction and shear between the amputees' residual limb and prosthesis still remain a problem. Aids such as fork straps, thigh lacers, condylar straps, condylar wedges, and suction with valves have all been used with good results, but the rubber sleeve suspension developed at the University of Michigan deserves some mention. The rubber sleeve is applied so that it extends over the proximal portion of the prosthesis onto the patient's thigh in such a manner that a negative pressure can be developed in the socket.

Clinical employment of the PTB and its variants: prescription guides. There is the possibility of combined PTB variants, for example, by altering the design for weight bearing in the distal socket through the use of an air cushion and by the use of a suspension variant such as a supracondylar wedge or the SC/SP system.

Table 2, a summary of the terminology of the presently used PTB variants, shows combined variants. Table 3 gives some of the guidelines for employment of all the PTB variants.

Sockets for other lower limb amputation levels

After lower limb amputation a patient suffers not only the loss of proprioception from full ground contact but also loss of joint control that is essential in weight support and ambulation. When standing on a prosthesis, the amputee must depend on mechanical control to lock the various joints of the artificial limb into a stable weight-bearing structure and then to free them for func-

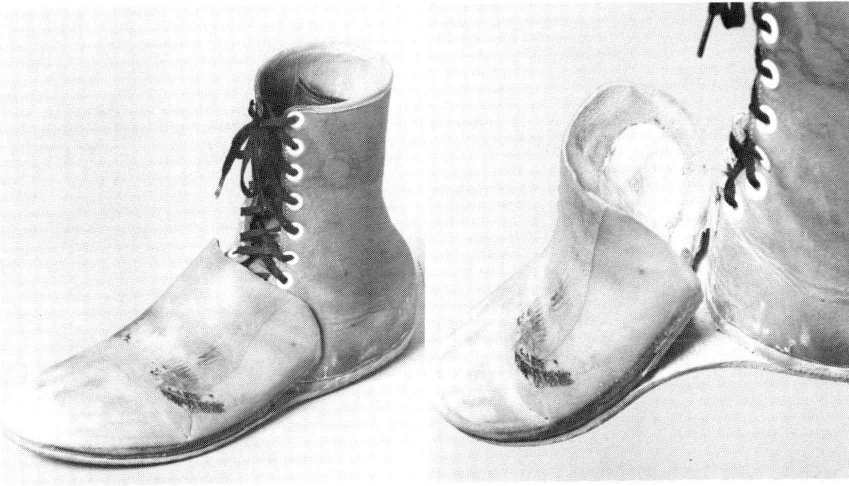

Fig. 20-22. Early Chopart design.

tion. The degree of difficulty in this control increases at the higher amputation levels. Patients suffering amputation through the foot, for example, have relatively few prosthetic problems if the remnant of the foot is capable of weight support. The only challenge is the reestablishment or simulation of the functions of the joints removed.

All sockets, other than those of the Syme and partial-foot prostheses, must be fitted and aligned in the prosthesis by means of an adjustable alignment device during walking trials (Fig. 20-21). In this way, an amputee's gait can be evaluated for control over stability, swing-phase initiation, general appearance, and overall efficiency.

The above-knee and below-knee socket designs already described represent the most common lower limb prosthetic systems used. But the total-contact principles described for them also apply to all other lower limb socket designs. Similarly, the prescription criteria for these two major lower limb systems can be used for all other sockets.

Although prostheses are classified by levels of amputation, many variations in socket design and construction are used within each group. Described are the other major types of lower limb prostheses, the sockets used with them, and other types of prosthetic support structures. Included are the partial foot, Syme, bent-knee, through-knee, and hip disarticulation prostheses.

Partial foot prosthesis. Early Chopart sockets (Fig. 20-22) were cumbersome designs fashioned of heavy leather laced tightly around the patient's shank; the ankle was immobilized.

Recent designs use features and materials developed for orthotics such as in the polypropylene and polyethylene ankle-foot orthoses. A device such as the Ortholene functional prosthesis (Fig. 20-23), although fabricated of flexible plastic, provides stability and control by means of its contour. This thermoplastic polyethylene structure not only permits plantar flexion when weight is applied to the shoe heel, but also provides a yielding resistance late in stance. The flexible characteristic of the structure also forms an effective toe

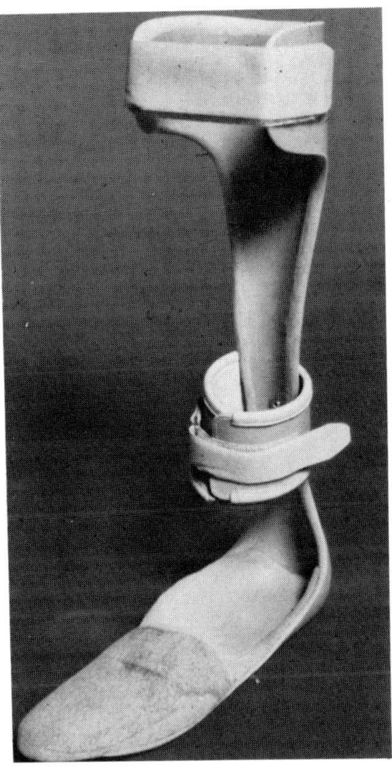

Fig. 20-23. Ortholene prosthesis designed for partial foot.

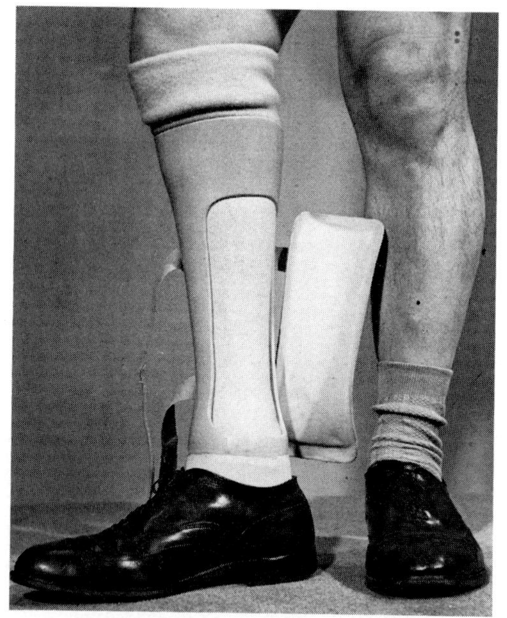

Fig. 20-24. Medial opening Syme prosthesis.

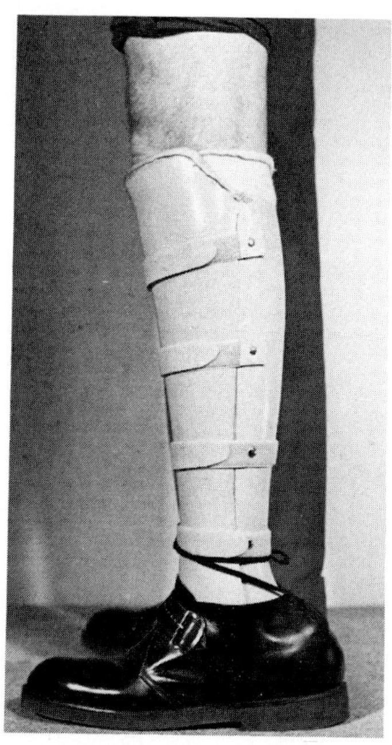

Fig. 20-25. Posterior opening Syme (Canadian type) prosthesis.

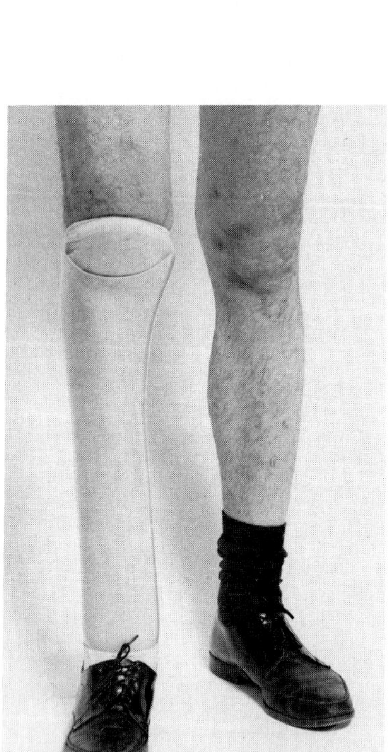

Fig. 20-26. Closed Syme prosthesis.

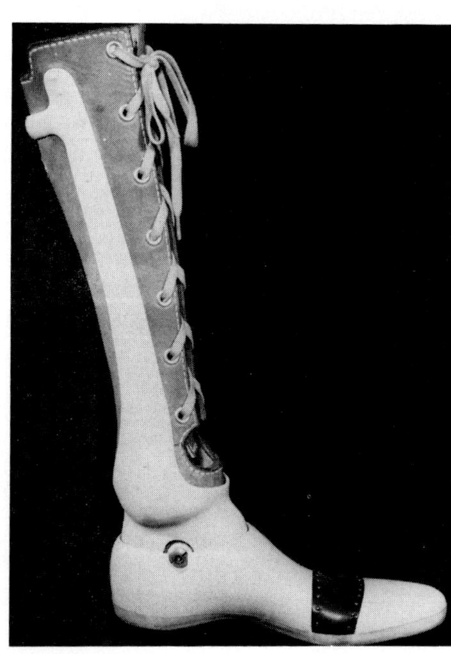

Fig. 20-27. Early Syme prosthesis with leather socket.

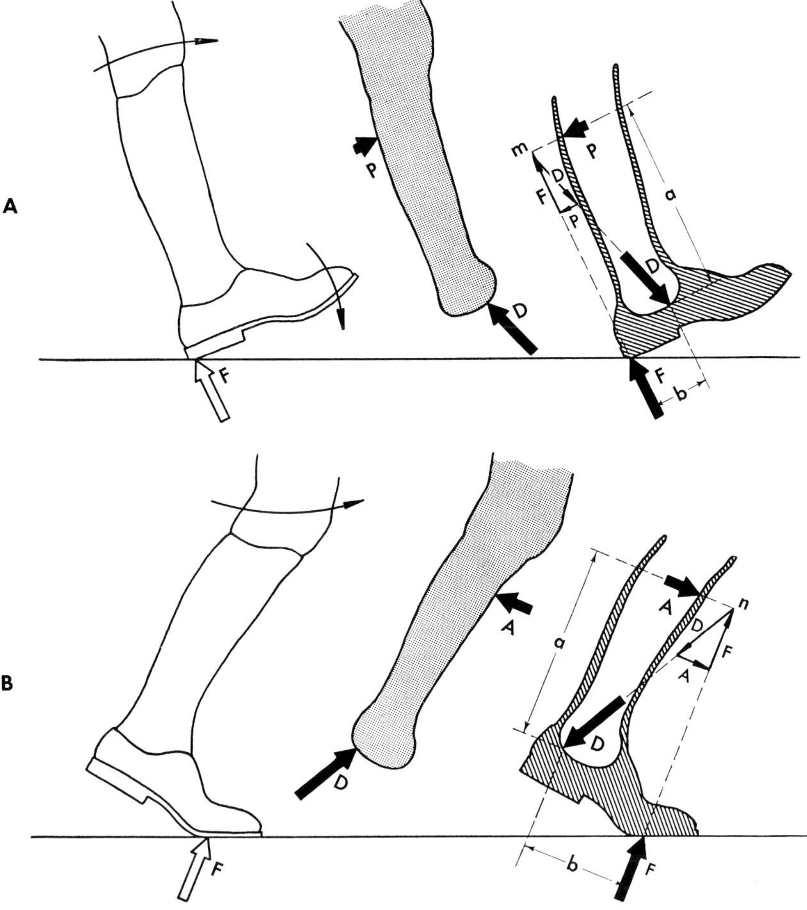

Fig. 20-28. Forces that develop as Syme amputee rolls over ball of foot during push-off. **A,** Shock absorption. **B,** Push-off. If force system is to be in equilibrium, path of forces *P*, *D*, and *F* must intersect prosthesis.

spring at push-off, enabling the patient to walk with a near normal gait.

Syme prosthesis. There are basically three variations in modern Syme prostheses: the VAPC version with a medial opening (Fig. 20-24), the Canadian type with a posterior opening (Fig. 20-25), and the closed, contoured soft wall (Fig. 20-26). All are designed for the same purpose: to accommodate the typical, bulbous-ended limb resulting from the transmalleolar or Syme (complete tarsal) amputation.

By flattening the end of the socket, the prosthetist can permit a fair degree of body weight to be carried on the distal end of the stump after a Syme amputation; nevertheless, typically a large portion of body weight is borne on more proximal surfaces with the most proximal portion of the socket usually having special contouring under the tibial condyles and patellar tendon, like in the below-knee prosthesis. This proximal support also provides an extended moment arm, yielding leverage for the forces applied in the anteroposterior plane during the stance phase.

Since the end of the Syme limb is much larger in circumference than the segment immediately above it, various socket designs are employed to facilitate insertion of the limb into the socket. Early Syme prostheses were made of leather and steel, with a molded leather socket opened anteriorly and secured to the limb with a lacer (Fig. 20-27). The socket usually terminated below the knee at the inferior border of the patella. No special provisions were available for distribution of weight on the proximal flares of the tibial condyles. Peripheral weight bearing was provided by tightening the lacer along the crest of the tibia, thereby embracing the entire portion of the limb below the knee.

The modern plastic sockets cited, especially the "closed" version, are preferred over this earlier metal and leather design. The enclosed proximal portion of the VAPC socket and the closed socket permit more effective contouring and provide better proximal weight-bearing areas for patients who cannot tolerate end bearing. If an opening is needed, the medial opening leaves intact the material of the posterior distal socket, which resists the high forces applied to this area while walking.

The biomechanics of the Syme prosthesis. Analysis of the distribution of contact pressures between stump and socket at various times during the stance phase is useful in the design of a socket that will be comfortable for the amputee. Since pressure distribution varies during each of the two subphases of stance, shock absorption to rollover and rollover to push-off, each must be analyzed separately.

Shock absorption to rollover. Assuming that body weight is supported at the distal end of the residual limb, it can be seen from Fig. 20-28 that during shock absorption the major forces between the residual limb and socket occur in the anterodistal and posteroproximal areas. During rollover, the need for posteroproximal pressure decreases, and the contact pressure at the end of the residual limb shifts toward the center of that area.

Rollover to push-off. Fig. 20-28 also shows the force system that develops as the Syme amputee rolls over the ball of the foot, terminating in push-off. At the instant shown, the hip joint is being used to help flex the knee against the force acting upward on the ball of the foot. A posterodistal and an anteroproximal contact force between the residual limb and socket are seen to be necessary to resist the floor reaction against the ball of the foot. It is essential that the anteroproximal force against the tibia be kept as far from the floor as possible. Shortening of this distance will result in an increased inclination of the line of action of the posterodistal force, in effect, a transfer of the force away from areas surgically prepared for end bearing.

Since some change in the inclination of the distal residual limb socket force is unavoidable, it must be anticipated during the fitting procedure. If the line of the floor reaction is kept in a particular position relative to the knee, the amputee can use some voluntary control in shifting the distal contact point. Moreover, the anteroproximal force at push-off will be several times the posteroproximal force at heel contact. For this reason, the prosthesis must be strong enough to resist the large bending moment in the ankle region during push-off.

To satisfy the requirements of a comfortable transmission of functional residual limb and socket contact forces, the socket must provide the following features:

1. Comfortable support of the body weight on the distal end of the residual limb or on the proximal part of the socket brim or both.
2. Firm support against the anteroproximal surface of the leg at the time of push-off. Careful fitting against the wedgelike medial and lateral surfaces of the tibia can satisfy this requirement.
3. Similar support against the posterior surface of the leg at the time of heel contact. This requirement can be satisfied by pressure in the region of the gastrocnemius. Here the main interest is to prevent lost motion between the socket and residual limb as the reaction point shifts from the posterior to the anterior surface of the leg.
4. Provision for shifting the center of pressure against the distal end of the residual limb, as indicated by the force analysis. If a cuplike receptacle is provided for the residual limb end, it must extend around and up the sides of the bulbous limb far enough to prevent relative motion between the residual limb and socket in the anteroposterior direction. It is particularly important to provide for the horizontal component of the force against the posterodistal region of the residual limb during push-off.
5. Adequate stabilization against the torques about the long axis of the leg. A three-point stabilization against the medial and lateral flares at the anteroproximal margin of the tibia and a flattening of the posteroproximal contour can be highly effective in providing the necessary torque resistance.

Bent-knee prosthesis. The "bent-knee" prosthesis (Fig. 20-29), although fitted to a below-knee amputation, is essentially a knee disarticulation (partial-thigh) prosthesis, since prosthetic *knee* function must be provided. Prostheses of this type are usually used for very short and/or very weak stumps. A full thigh socket is also required. Unfortunately, the available prosthetic devices for the knee are poor.

The conventional bent-knee prosthesis has a foot and shank with side joints mounted medially and laterally in the upper part of the shank. These provide the external knee axes around the socket of the bent-knee limb. Directional guid-

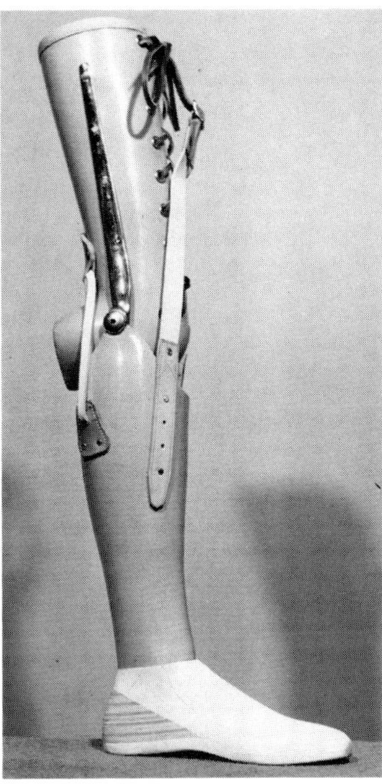

Fig. 20-29. Bent-knee prosthesis.

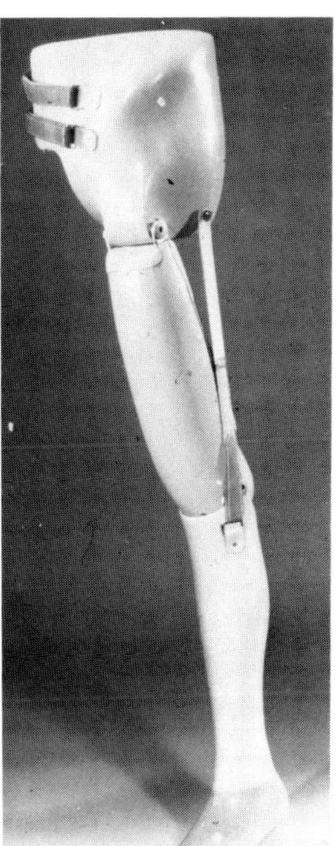

Fig. 20-30. Hip disarticulation prosthesis.

ance to knee flexion and extension is provided by these external joints, but swing-control functions are limited to the small amount of friction in the joints. The socket is usually fabricated of molded leather or a plastic laminate to form a receptacle for the amputated limb, which is placed in a kneeling position. Suspension is often achieved by means of pelvic joints and belts, occasionally using roller cords to control abduction and rotation.

The bent-knee prosthesis is used in cases in which scar tissue and other physiological factors preclude the use of the below-knee prosthesis, such as when the anatomical knee joint cannot be extended sufficiently to fit a below-knee socket.

Through-knee (complete-leg) prosthesis. In the past, through-knee prostheses consisted of a foot and shank with side joints mounted externally in the upper shank to provide a center of knee rotation at a level approximating the natural one. These joints controlled knee flexion and extension but without adequate resistance. Resistance against flexion was therefore provided by an elastic fork or kick strap. In some recent designs, hydraulic or pneumatic systems are used to provide resistance to both flexion and extension.

The current "modern" prosthesis uses a polycentric system mounted in the shank below the natural knee level. The kinematics of this design project the functional knee axis to near the normal level and provide a better appearing limb in the seated position.

Total-contact sockets are used but with a variation. The through-knee limb can tolerate substantial distal weight bearing, far more than shorter above-knee limbs. The sockets, fabricated of molding leather or laminated plastic, provide for a large amount of distal bearing.

The supracondylar amputation at this general level yields a more conical stump, but even this limb shape is capable of bearing large amounts of weight on the distal end. Contractures, which are often seen in above-knee amputation limbs, are seldom present in the through-knee limb.

Hip disarticulation prosthesis. Hip disarticulation leaves little or no residual limb. Therefore the socket must encapsulate a major portion of the pelvis and lower trunk on the amputated side. The socket thus must be designed to provide a cradle or "seat" independently constructed from the thigh of the prosthesis. Suspension is provided by a waist belt, fabricated either separately or as an integral part of the socket.

This prosthesis consists of a foot, knee-shank assembly, thigh section, and socket (Fig. 20-30). A major difference between the two major designs for such prostheses, the Canadian and the "tilting table," is based on the mechanical hip joint location. In the preferred version, the Canadian design shown in Fig. 20-30, the hip joint is placed in front of and below the anatomical hip joint to permit an unrestricted 100 degrees of hip flexion. The single-axis knee joint is set in a position of mechanical stability. An elastic strap from behind the hip joint to the shank with attachment below and ahead of the knee limits the forward swing of the thigh and assures full-knee extension. Gait with this type of prosthesis, allowing for both hip and knee motion, is superior to that of the "tilting-table," which employs a locked hip joint located in line laterally with the normal anatomical axis of the hip joint.

The principal advantages of the Canadian socket, therefore, are the greater functional control provided and, to a lesser extent, the materials used in its fabrication.

Biomechanics of the Canadian hip disarticulation prosthesis. The biomechanical analysis of the Canadian hip-disarticulation prosthesis can be based primarily on an evaluation of the residual limb and socket forces required to support the torso in the stance phase.

Fig. 20-31, with its free body diagrams of the hip disarticulation prosthesis and the amputee's torso, shows the force system acting on the artificial limb and, in turn, on the body of the amputee. If the body weight and gluteal-ischial-support forces were the only two forces acting on the torso, the body would have a tendency to rotate about the point of support and to drop toward the unsupported normal side. This tendency is counteracted by the moment of the couple formed by the two mediolateral forces H and S. For moment equilibrium, taking the summation of moments about point 2 equal to 0, $W \times b = H \times a$, or $H = \frac{b}{a}W$. Thus the magnitude of reaction against the normal hip, or tension in the waistband, or both, can be reduced by increasing the distance a. Moving the concentration of lateral forces on the residual limb to a lower level by alteration of fit is practical only within certain limits. Too low a position would result in shear forces along the bottom of the residual limb and considerable relative motion between the residual limb and socket. It is also apparent that, due to the limitations on increasing dimension a, the lateral forces H and S are of the same order of magnitude as the vertical forces W and I, since dimensions a and b would be approximately equal.[4]

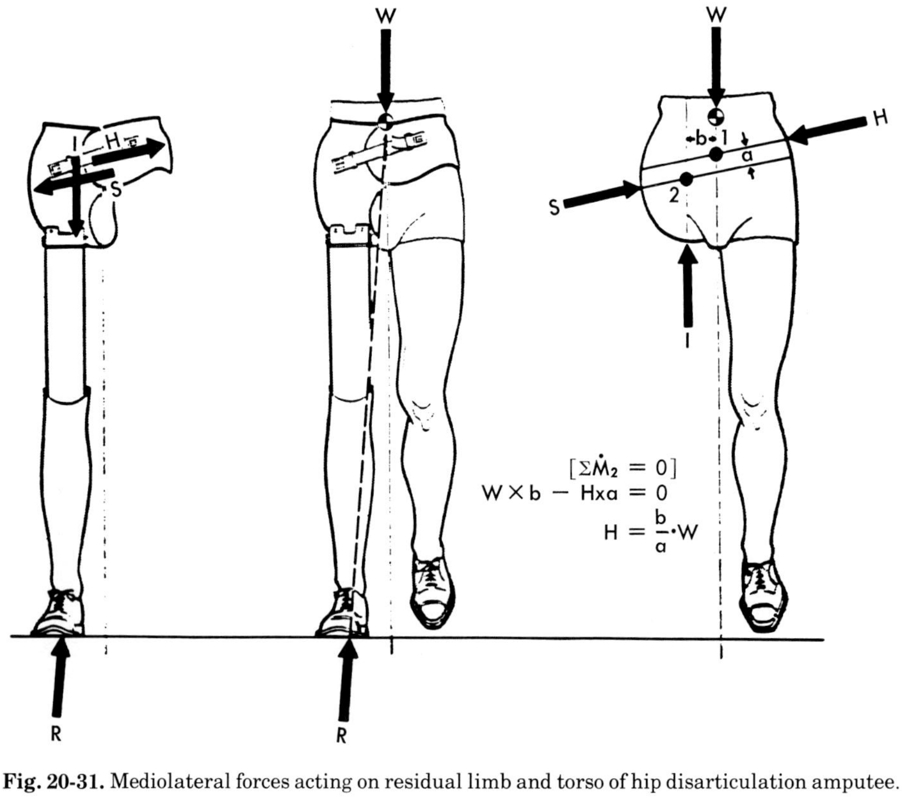

Fig. 20-31. Mediolateral forces acting on residual limb and torso of hip disarticulation amputee.

Temporary sockets. After appropriate postsurgical treatment with a rigid dressing or controlled environment, possibly with a form of an early ambulation device, there still may be doubt about the ability of an amputee to use an artificial limb. Prescription of a permanent prosthesis may yield little benefit and would be a costly, unnecessary expenditure. Moreover, physical changes brought about by the first use of a prosthesis may require tiresome revisions to the permanent prosthesis.

It is reasonable therefore to provide simple, temporary prostheses that can be used early in the rehabilitation process to evaluate an amputee, as well as to provide early ambulation for conditioning purposes. To be valuable, fitting and the use of a temporary prosthesis must be performed as soon as it is physiologically feasible.

Temporary prostheses are therefore fitted for several reasons. An evaluation of an amputee's ability to cope with the problems of using a prosthesis may be obtained, and the early ambulation obtainable accelerates residual limb conditioning. Training in gait can be initiated sooner than would be the case if a temporary limb were not used. A temporary prosthesis is indicated in these situations because of its immediate availability, as well as its simplicity and economy in comparison to a permanent prosthesis.

Nevertheless, arbitrary socket shapes should not be provided for these first prosthetic trials. The socket should have the biomechanical shape that will be provided in the permanent prosthesis. Inadequate alignment and socket shape in the temporary prosthesis, besides confusing any evaluation of the amputee's physical abilities, may cause the development of poor gait habits, which will be difficult to overcome in the use of the permanent device.

In fitting a socket for a temporary prosthesis, the socket shape should be based on accepted concepts as developed from biomechanical considerations of the stump-to-socket relationship. Adequate alignment determinations should, as nearly as possible, be made for temporary prosthesis use.

PROSTHETIC KNEES

General discussion

The prosthetic knee provides controlled absorption of knee motion in a prosthesis for a person who has suffered a lower limb amputation and has need for either a functional substitute for the knee (through-knee, above-knee, and hip disartic-

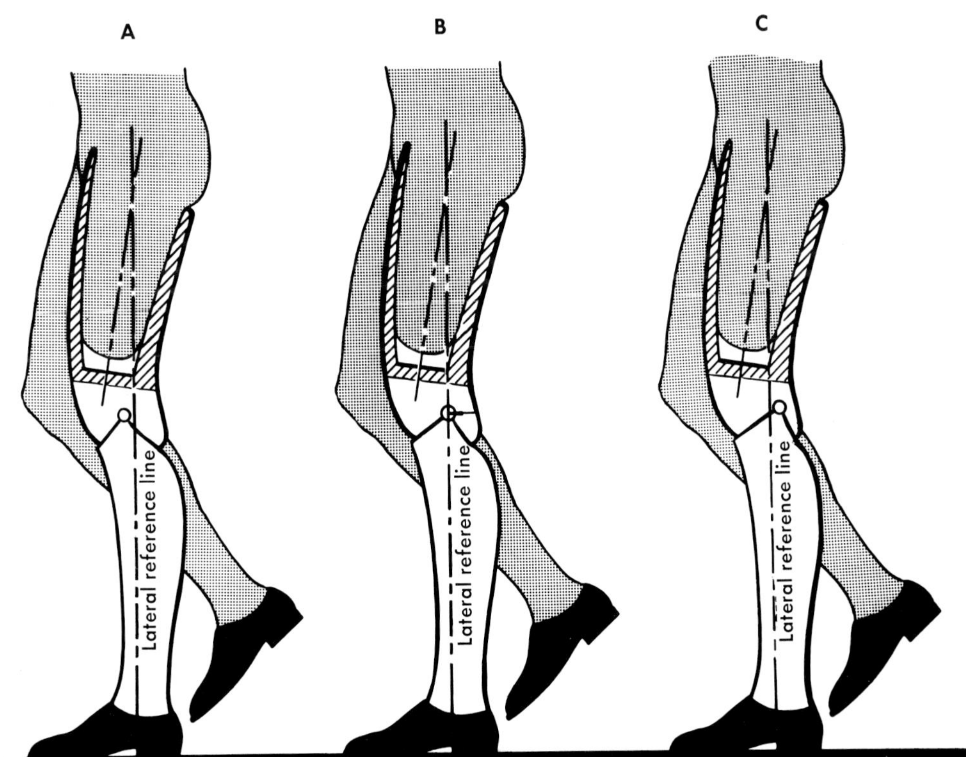

Fig. 20-32. TKA (trochanter-knee-ankle) line. **A,** Knee axis placed anterior to TKA line. **B,** Knee axis placed exactly on TKA line. **C,** Knee axis posterior to TKA line.

ulation) or needs some form of directional or stabilizing control (in some below-knee cases). Some devices perform these functions by mechanical friction, others by resistance to fluid flow. The simple side joints for the below-knee amputee who needs them are unidirectional and thus provide control by this means. The swing-control component of a knee mechanism for through-knee, above-knee, and hip disarticulation patients therefore is the mechanical analog of the quadriceps and hamstring muscles acting to dampen the swing of the knee at the extremes of flexion and extension. Since the joints for a below-knee amputee are relatively simple, most of the discussion here covers the more complex knee systems for through-knee, above-knee, and hip disarticulation amputees.

"Alignment stability" is a key element in prosthetic fitting (Fig. 20-32). By reference to "TKA," that is, a vertical line in the sagittal plane through the trochanter, knee, and ankle (static), the prosthetist strategically shifts the position of the socket with respect to the knee center to maintain stability in late stance and to take advantage of certain special features of particular knee mechanisms. For example, with a single-axis mechanical friction knee the prosthetist aligns the socket forward of the knee to assure that the body weight will be transmitted through the prosthesis along a line falling anterior to the knee center in late stance. However, this is done at the expense of impeding, to some extent, the initiation of swing. With the special stance-phase control features of the Mauch S-N-S the prosthetist aligns the socket so that body weight is transmitted through the prosthesis along a line falling posterior to the knee center to take advantage of the high resistance to knee flexion in stance. High resistance makes it unnecessary to use alignment stability to prevent knee buckling and, at the same time, facilitates initiation of swing phase.

Understanding these relationships and taking advantage of the special features of knee mechanisms for the benefit of the patient is necessary for successful prosthetic fitting. The highest level of prosthetic treatment the clinic team can provide the patient rests on selecting the specific knee mechanism whose features are most closely matched to the patient's needs.

Knee mechanisms for above-knee prostheses include a large number of devices ranging from very simple single-axis knees to increasingly complex components that control the character of knee rotation in various ways. The simpler devices permit a range of motion about the knee to meet the requirements of swing phase, sitting, and kneeling, but furnish no other functions or controls. Other, more sophisticated, mechanisms control the character and timing of swing and stance phase stability. Despite the variety of functions and features afforded by these mechanisms, it is possible to classify them on the basis of certain primary functions: (1) knee rotation, (2) resistance to knee rotation in swing phase and/or in stance phase, and (3) extension aid. All other functions are considered accessory features.

Terminology

To describe the variety of knee functions in a meaningful way, the following terms of reference to knee functions have been standardized:

adjustable resistance The capacity for presetting the magnitude of knee rotation resistance at one of many prescribed levels.

alignment Proper use of the major components of an above-knee prosthesis socket, knee, and foot-ankle assembly requires that they be joined in a particular relationship. The foot must remain flat on the floor when standing or during midstance. The body weight carried by the socket must project slightly anterior to the knee joint so that standing can be effected without excessive hip extension. Knee flexion must be initiated smoothly. This basic relationship is commonly referred to as TKA alignment, which is the preliminary alignment step in the fabrication of all aboveknee prostheses. Prescribed variations from basic TKA alignment are made in relation to anatomical anomalies and the special functions of various knee mechanisms.

cadence response Resistance to knee rotation at any preset resistance level varies as a function of *angular velocity*.

constant resistance The characteristic resistance pattern provided by a swing-control mechanism in which its magnitude remains relatively constant throughout the swing phase independent of angular velocity or time.

correlated knee and ankle A mechanism in which knee and ankle motion are coupled; the motion of one is accompanied by motion of the other.

extension aids Devices that provide a force to facilitate active negative rotation of the knee (extension). They may be internally, that is, integral components of the knee mechanism, or externally applied devices.

independent adjustment of resistance to flexion/extension The capacity for altering the ratio of the resistance to positive or negative rotation.

knee lock A mechanism that prevents rotation at the

joint in stance phase. Automatic knee locks operate cyclically under the control of applied loads, inertia, or other forces to prevent positive knee rotation (flexion). Manual knee locks are noncyclical in that, once engaged, they prevent knee rotation until disengaged manually.

knee moment The product of the force tending to produce knee rotation and the perpendicular distance from the line of action of that force to the center of knee rotation.

knee rotation Knee rotation is the angular motion about the knee joint or relative motion between the thigh and shank. Flexion or positive rotation is that portion of knee rotation in which the angle inside the joint formed by the knee block and the shank is diminishing. Extension or negative rotation refers to motion in which the angle is increasing.

locus The path of a point or curve moving according to some law, that is, the path followed by the instantaneous axis of rotation of a polycentric knee through the cycle from full extension to full flexion.

polycentric joint A mechanism whose instantaneous center of rotation displaces posteriorly to decrease positive knee moment (flexion) during stance phase or proximally to decrease the hip extension moment required to prevent knee flexion.

stance phase The portion of the gait cycle in which any part of the extremity is in contact with the ground.

swing phase Swing phase is the portion of the gait cycle in which the reference leg is not in contact with the ground.

swing phase controls Devices that provide resistance to control angular velocity and/or acceleration of knee rotation. Included are mechanical and fluid resistance mechanisms.

variable resistance Resistance to knee rotation varies as a function of *angular position* of knee rotation.

yielding resistance in stance phase A higher degree of resistance to positive knee rotation than normally available, designed to reduce the rate of knee rotation under load.

Classification

Since knee mechanisms provide control over swing phase, stance phase, or both, it is simple to classify those which control either swing or stance on the basis of the type of control they offer. Classification of units providing both swing-phase and stance-phase control is difficult because a particular unit may embody highly sophisticated swing controls and very simple stance controls or the reverse. The other function, extension aid, must also be considered. The following classification has been developed to include all the major classes and types of knee mechanisms.[9]

Class 1. Class 1 includes knee mechanisms that provide "free knee rotation." This type of knee rotation is resisted solely by friction inherent in the bolt and bushing assembly. They do not permit adjustment of the magnitude or phase (time pattern) or resistance (Fig. 20-33). Accessory features include (internal) or permit inclusion (external) of an extension aid whose force is adjustable. The extension aid produces moments of different magnitudes in flexion and extension.

Other accessories, such as stability controls consisting of manual knee locks or polycentric joints, may be featured. Two units fall into this category: the Otto Bock 3P24 knee with manual lock and the Polymatic knee with a polycentric knee joint to control stance phase (Fig. 20-34).

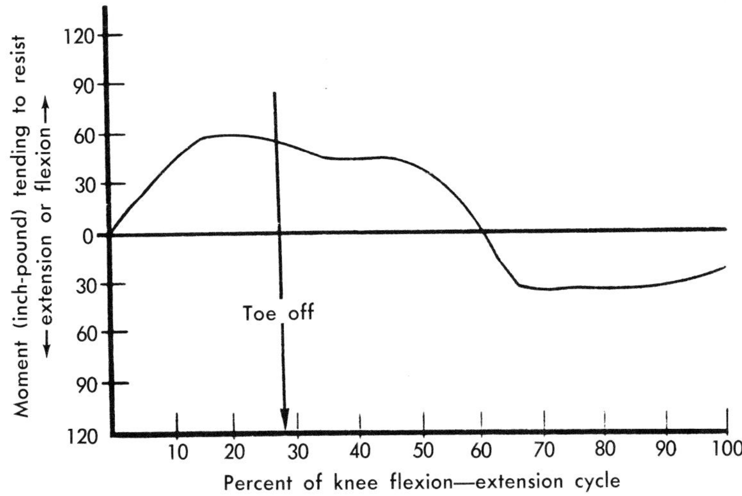

Fig. 20-33. Class 1, free knee constant resistance.

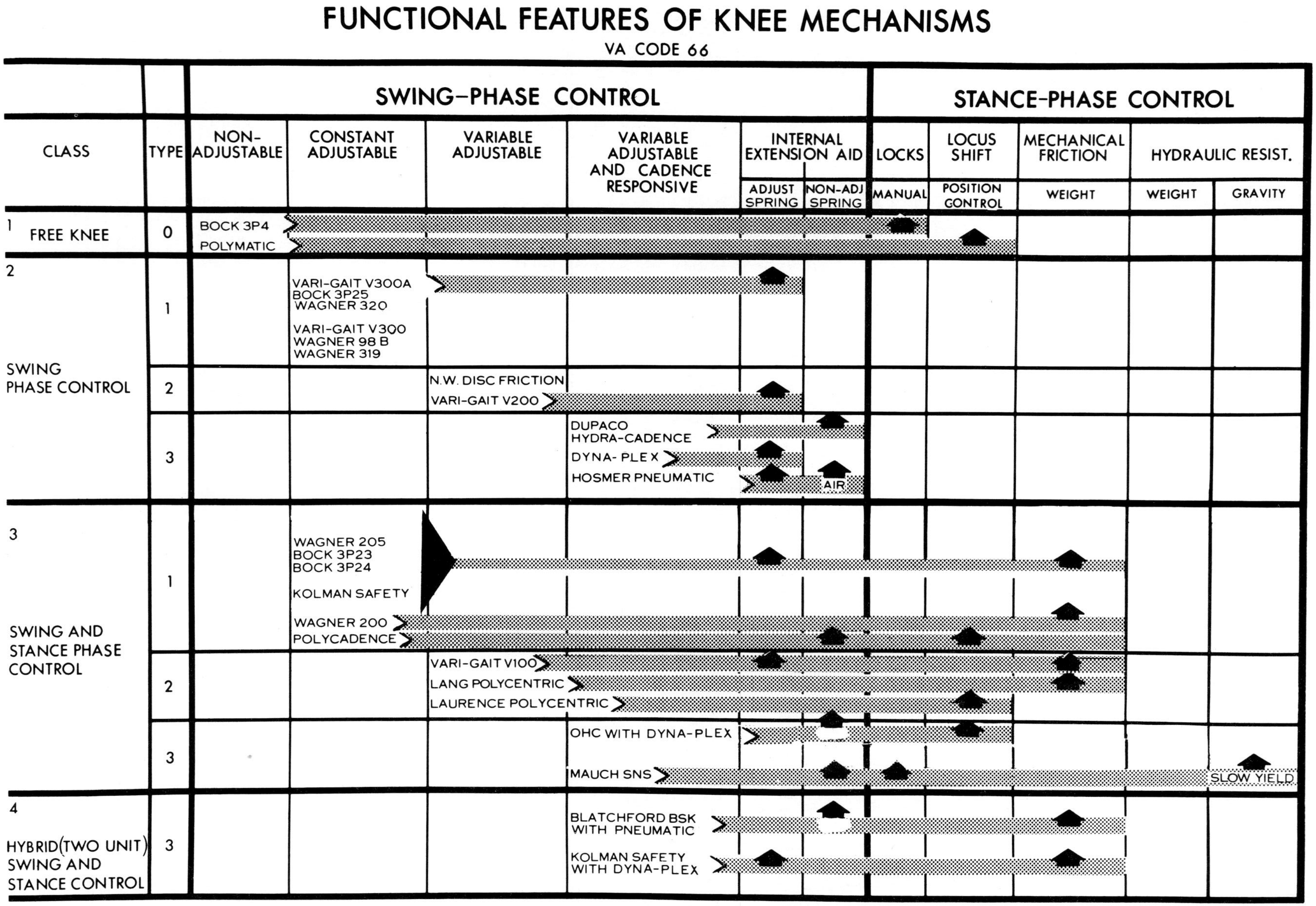

FUNCTIONAL FEATURES OF KNEE MECHANISMS

VA CODE 66

CLASS	TYPE	SWING-PHASE CONTROL: NON-ADJUSTABLE	CONSTANT ADJUSTABLE	VARIABLE ADJUSTABLE	VARIABLE ADJUSTABLE AND CADENCE RESPONSIVE	INTERNAL EXTENSION AID: ADJUST SPRING	INTERNAL EXTENSION AID: NON-ADJ SPRING	STANCE-PHASE CONTROL: LOCKS: MANUAL	LOCUS SHIFT: POSITION CONTROL	MECHANICAL FRICTION: WEIGHT	HYDRAULIC RESIST.: WEIGHT	HYDRAULIC RESIST.: GRAVITY
1 FREE KNEE	0	BOCK 3P4 POLYMATIC										
2 SWING PHASE CONTROL	1		VARI-GAIT V300A BOCK 3P25 WAGNER 320 VARI-GAIT V300 WAGNER 98 B WAGNER 319									
	2			N.W. DISC FRICTION VARI-GAIT V200								
	3				DUPACO HYDRA-CADENCE DYNA-PLEX HOSMER PNEUMATIC		AIR					
3 SWING AND STANCE PHASE CONTROL	1		WAGNER 205 BOCK 3P23 BOCK 3P24 KOLMAN SAFETY WAGNER 200 POLYCADENCE									
	2			VARI-GAIT V100 LANG POLYCENTRIC LAURENCE POLYCENTRIC								
	3				OHC WITH DYNA-PLEX MAUCH SNS							SLOW YIELD
4 HYBRID (TWO UNIT) SWING AND STANCE CONTROL	3				BLATCHFORD BSK WITH PNEUMATIC KOLMAN SAFETY WITH DYNA-PLEX							

Fig. 20-34. Functional features of knee mechanisms.

Accessories common with class 1 knee mechanisms

Extension aids. Extension aids are of the internal or external type. The stick control usually pivots at its proximal end about an axis 2.5 cm (1 inch) posterior and slightly below the level of the knee axis. The stick is made of fiber or wood and is approximately 18 to 20 cm (7 to 8 inches) long. The distal end inserts into a leather or plastic pocket suspended from the back of the upper shank by means of elastic straps or springs. Both the shank and knee are padded in the area of contact with the stick to provide damping and an extension stop as the stick is forced against the posterior wall of the shank by the knee moving into maximum extension. The stick control being suspended in elastic also acts as an extension aid. The elastic straps are placed under increasing tension as the knee is flexed toward 90 degrees. From full extension to 90 degrees of knee flexion, the tension on the elastic strap increases, casuing a higher extension moment. Beyond 90 degrees of knee flexion, the upper pivot of the stick passes forward of the knee axis, and the shank is drawn into full flexion by the elastic straps. This permits sitting with the knee fully flexed.

The two basic types of external extension aids are (1) an adjustable anterior or elastic webbing strap attached to the upper anterior wall of the shank, passing anterior to the knee and attached on the socket, and (2) an elastic strap passing through the roller portion of a knee extension stop through the socket wall anteriorly and fixed to the anterior socket wall or pelvic belt. This strap acts as an extension aid (kick strap), similar in function to that of the stick control. However, when flexed 90 degrees or more, the anterior elastic strap does not produce flexion force as does the stick type.

Extension stops. The metal knee stop is fixed about the knee axis and attached posteriorly at the top of the shank. The extension control extends anterior to the knee axis and stops the motion of the knee at full extension. The knee area of contact with the metal stop is padded with rubber or felt to dampen the impact.

Mechanical locks. The bilateral above-knee amputee and the unilateral amputee with an extremely short residual limb occasionally require more stability than that provided by the knee unit and the alignment of the prosthesis. New amputees learning to stand on their first prosthesis, and elderly, weaker patients may require manual knee locks. These locks are usually designed as a bar or rod that passes through the knee anteriorly from above the axis to a point below the axis. When the rod is manually elevated or depressed, it engages a slot or hole located in the shank, thereby locking the knee. The most advanced locks are spring loaded to lock automatically after a person rises from a seated to a standing position.

Class 2. Included in class 2 are knees whose rotation is controlled by special mechanical or fluid resistance mechanisms that permit adjustment of resistance to knee rotation. All such units include a knee extension aid that is adjustable. They may include other accessory features. This class consists of three different types of knee mechanisms.

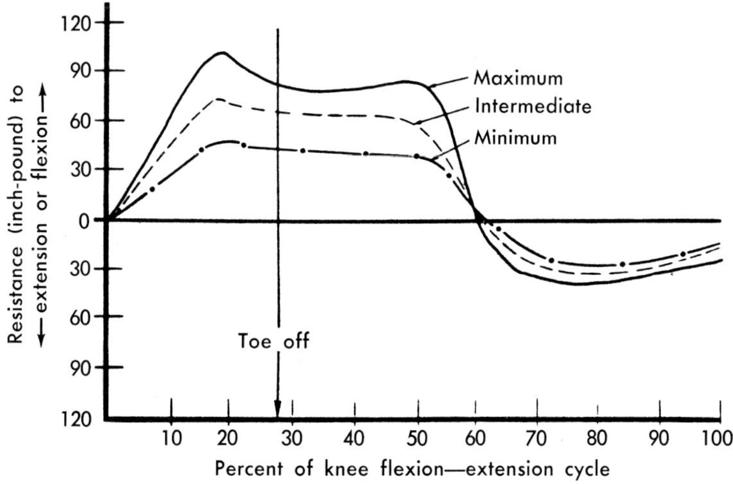

Fig. 20-35. Class 2, type 1, adjustable resistance (constant).

Type 1. These units permit adjustment of the magnitude of resistance to knee rotation. They provide constant resistance at any setting; their resistances at any setting do not change significantly during the swing phase (Fig. 20-35). They do not provide variable resistance or cadence response. There is no resistance change in relation to either angular position of the knee or to walking cadence. Some of the units in this category are the Standard Wood, Standard Metal, Vari-Gait V300, and Wagner 98.

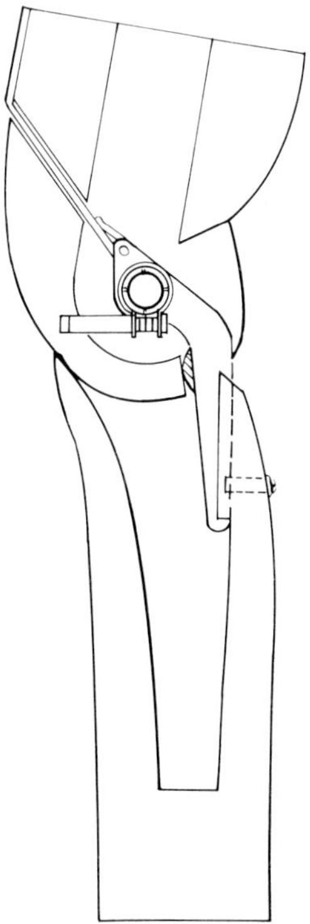

Fig. 20-36. Constant adjustable friction arrangement.

Swing-phase control in these single-axis mechanical knees is usually achieved by means of friction devices acting on the knee bolt. Typical of these devices are dual screw arrangements that wedge or compress a section of fiber or other material against the surface of the knee bolt (Fig. 20-36). This type of friction is called "constant adjustable friction."

Type 2. These units also permit adjustment of the magnitude of resistance to knee rotation. They also provide variable resistance. The magnitude of resistance varies with angular position of knee rotation at any given resistance setting (Fig. 20-37). They do not provide cadence response.

Type 2 units are the Northwestern University Disc Friction Unit and the Vari-Gait V200. Variable resistance in these units may be controlled by increments or decrements in frictional force. This is accomplished in some units by concentrically mounted friction discs or by eccentric bearing surfaces whose functional resistance varies during swing phase.

Type 3. These knees permit adjustment of the magnitude of resistance, provide variable resistance, and are also cadence responsive. Resistance at any setting varies with walking cadence or knee angular velocity. Devices in this category provide the most sophisticated control of swing phase in their class. All these devices are fluid piston/cylinder arrangements; some are pneumatic and others are hydraulic.

FLUID KNEE CONTROL. The major advantages of

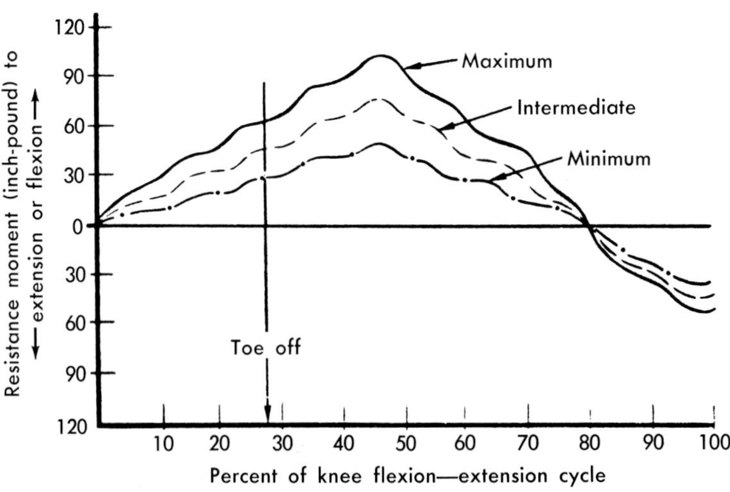

Fig. 20-37. Class 2, type 2, adjustable resistance (variable).

fluid knee mechanisms are better gait, quiet and smooth operation, versatility in adapting to different speeds of walking, and, in some cases, better performance on inclines and stairs. Since resistance to turbulent fluid flow is proportional to the square of the fluid velocity, all such systems are inherently cadence responsive (Fig. 20-38). Units depending on mechanical friction are not inherently cadence responsive because frictional force depends on the coefficients of friction of the two mating surfaces and the force clamping the two surfaces together. With both of these values fixed in a particular design, frictional forces are not closely correlated with flexion-extension velocities. However, mechanical resistance knee controls can be designed to preprogram a particular resistance pattern, but they are not as versatile as fluid systems.

A common fallacy is the notion that fluid units are inherently more energy consuming than mechanical frictional devices. Actually, the amount of energy required for starting, swinging, and stopping the motion of the shank depends on the resistance to be overcome. A mechanical friction knee and a fluid resistance device will require exactly the same amount of energy, provided that their mass moments on inertia and resistance settings are equal. The idea that fluid resistance units require more energy is probably based on the fact that they are capable of operating at higher resistance settings than most mechanical friction units, a distinct advantage for many, particularly for vigorous patients with long residual limbs. Two other advantages characterize the fluid resistance systems. Under ordinary circumstances, resistance levels, once set, need not be frequently readjusted, whereas mechanical friction units are constantly subject to wear of the surfaces in contact and need more frequent adjustments. Fluid resistance mechanisms are also inherently more stable, that is, they do not collapse (a form of very rapid knee flexion), since resistance is increased with the velocity of fluid flow. This enables prosthetists to align hydraulic units with the vertical projection of the body weight passing closer to the knee center, a procedure that improves the initiation of flexion in walking.

Class 3. Class 3 includes mechanisms that control knee rotation during both swing phase and stance phase by mehcanical friction, by shifting the effective center of knee rotation, or by fluid resistance devices. Class 3 mechanisms can be divided into three types.

Type 1 units permit adjustment of the magnitude of resistance to knee rotation, but they do not provide variable resistance or cadence response. *Type 2* units permit adjustment of the magnitude of resistance to knee rotation and provide variable resistance, but they are not cadence responsive. *Type 3* units permit adjustment of the magnitude of resistance to knee rotation, provide variable resistance, and are also cadence responsive.

Swing phase in types 1, 2, and 3 in all class 3 units is controlled in the same way as in class 2 units, types 1, 2, and 3, respectively. However, stance phase is controlled in a variety of ways.

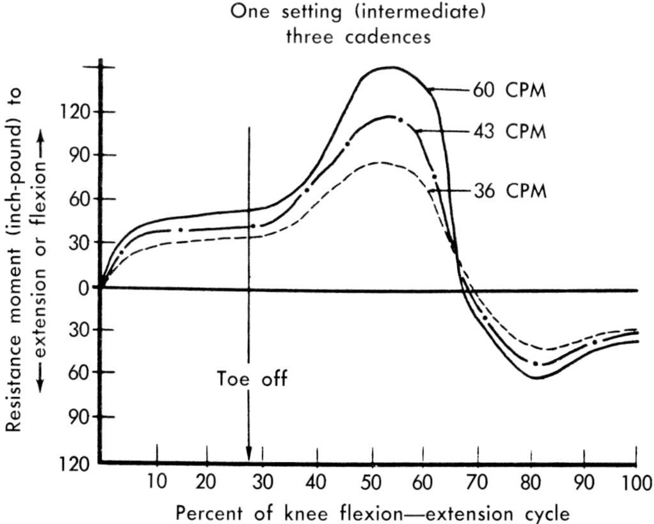

Fig. 20-38. Class 2, type 3, cadence responsive resistance.

Stance-control methods. The different methods employed to control stance phase have created a certain amount of confusion due to basic similarities and differences among them. Stance control includes manual locks, hydraulic locks, yielding resistance devices, polycentric linkages, and friction brakes. Despite the variations in their designs and in descriptions supplied by their distributors, all of these units fall into three basic categories, depending on the fundamental physical principle on which they operate: mechanical friction, changing locus of rotation, or fluid resistance.

MECHANICAL FRICTION (IN TYPES 1 AND 2). Some knee mechanisms resist flexion in stance phase by the application of mechanical friction: Friction between the two surfaces is substantially increased during stance phase. The increase in friction may be accomplished by contact between two mating surfaces with high coefficients of friction or by a system similar to a brake drum. This group includes all devices that depend on wedging, or rubbing together of components, or on tightening a friction band about a drum. All stance-control units operating on the friction principle depend on the body weight applied during stance phase either to compress a spring and bring bearing surfaces in contact (Otto Bock 3P24, or 3P23) or to tighten a belt about a drum (Blatchford BSK). A biaxial arrangement is often used when the proximal axis, which is the center of rotation during swing phase, is linked to another point of rotation on the shank. As weight is applied, the link rotates a few degrees about its lower center of rotation, causing the upper center of rotation to descend, placing the bearing surfaces in contact, and increasing the resistance to rotation in stance phase (Fig. 20-39).

These stance controls might be considered polycentric devices, since their effective center of rotation is displaced downward to bring into play the stance-phase friction mechanism. However, defining them in these terms serves no useful purpose, since the "polycentricity" is incidental to the function.

SHIFTING LOCUS (CAN APPLY TO TYPES 1, 2, AND 3). A second group of stance-phase controls depends on displacing the center of rotation to a more proximal and posterior position in stance phase than it occupies in swing phase. This may have two significant effects: (1) with the center of rotation moved backward, an extension moment about the knee is generated during most of stance phase; (2) if the device is properly aligned, the hip extension force required to stabilize the knee is reduced when the knee center is raised.

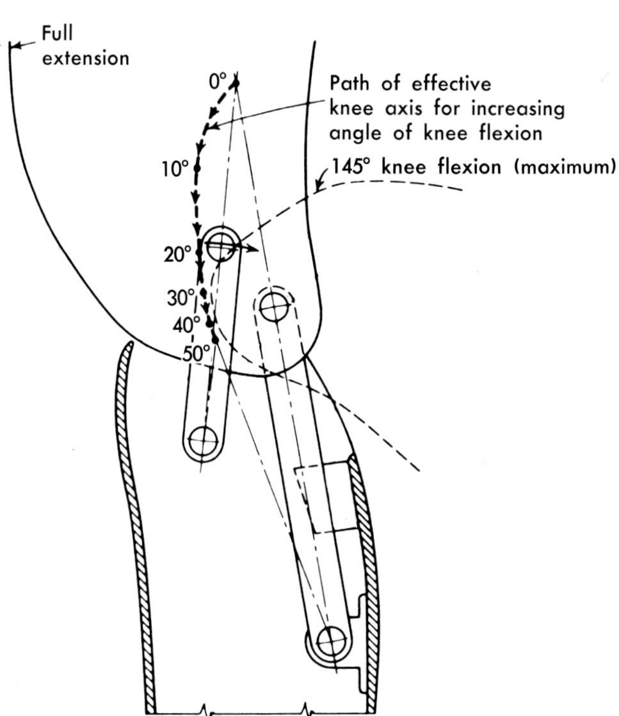

Fig. 20-39. Increased resistance to rotation in stance phase.

This is commonly accomplished by means of four (or more) bar linkages whose instantaneous centers of rotation are shifted strategically. In some, an extension moment is generated about the knee when it is extended or even when it is flexed several degrees. In another approach, the instantaneous knee center ascends in stance phase, enabling a patient to maintain knee stability with less forcible extension of the hip. All of these units depend on the angular position of the knee to displace the center of rotation and are therefore not weight controlled as are the friction devices. They are properly called polycentric devices because their function depends on the shifting center of rotation.

FLUID RESISTANCE (TYPE 3 ONLY). A third group of stance-control units depends on relatively high resistance to fluid flow to stabilize the knee in stance phase. The units are designed with valves that increase the resistance to piston displacement. One such mechanism is controlled by application of the patient's weight to block the flow of fluid completely and effectively lock the knee. The heel of the foot contains a wobble plate connected by a rod to the valve that ordinarily controls swing phase. When weight is applied to the heel, the valve is closed and acts as a hydraulic lock in stance phase. It unlocks when weight is taken off the heel and controls swing phase as adjusted.

Another type is controlled by gravity, which causes a pendulum to rotate, depending on the angle of the unit with respect to the horizontal plane. The pendulum is released when a hyperextension moment about the knee is generated. When the leg is advanced and placed on the ground at an angle in the beginning of stance phase, the pendulum rotates and closes orifices through which the fluid normally flows in swing phase, sharply increasing resistance to knee rotation. In this unit, however, the flow is not completely blocked and a certain amount is permitted to "leak" past the valve, providing a high, although yielding, resistance. The leak rate and hence the rate of yielding under various loads can be adjusted. As the patient proceeds from heel contact to midstance and begins to generate a hyperextension moment about the knee, the pendulum rotates in the opposite direction, opening the valve to its swing-phase setting, permitting the desired transition into swing phase, and exercising the required control over knee flexion-extension.

Following are several types of class 3 swing-control and stance-control units:

Type 1. In addition to adjustment of resistance magnitudes in these units, stance phase is controlled by friction generated under weight bearing. Examples of knees that fall into this category are shown in Fig. 20-34.

Except for one or two infrequently seen "physiological" knees that are not designed with conventional knee bolts, all of these systems rotate about a single axis during swing phase. Body weight applied as stance phase begins causes the spring-mounted knee block to descend and engage two friction surfaces to increase resistance to flexion during stance phase. However, knee flexion before sufficient weight is borne to engage the braking may result in buckling. The knee must be stably aligned posterior to the TKA line to support the portion of body weight applied before the braking occurs. Also included in this type are units that provide adjustment of resistance in swing phase, but that depend on a shifting center of rotation for stability in stance phase.

Type 2. These units permit adjustment of the magnitude of resistance to rotation and provide variable resistance, but they are not cadence responsive. Some units of this type are also designed to control stance phase by increasing friction between mating knee surfaces under weight bearing. In other units of this type, stance-phase control is accomplished by means of displacement of the center of knee rotation to produce an extension rather than a flexion moment in stance phase or to raise the effective knee center.

Type 3. Units of this type (1) permit adjustment of the resistance to knee rotation, (2) provide variable resistance, and (3) are cadence responsive. Stance-phase control is also effected by means of fluid resistance. The Henschke-Mauch S-N-S is an example of this type.

The Mauch S-N-S hydraulic system is a multi-orifice swing-control mechanism that offers the amputee a high degree of control. It provides independent adjustment of flexion-extension resistance. In stance phase, resistance to flexion is increased when the device is not perpendicular to the ground in early stance phase, stabilizing the knee against flexion during this period. Shortly after midstance, after a hyperextension moment has been generated about the knee, the resistance control valve is opened, and the unit is free to flex. Although the stance-phase control stabilizes the knee, it is not of the "locking type"; the knee actually yields at a slow rate under high moments. This is particularly effective in stair and hill descent. The Mauch S-N-S hydraulic system also features a manual locking device that locks the knee against flexion but permits extension.

Another knee system that falls into the class 3, type 3 is the OHC knee disarticulation prosthesis. The system permits adjustment of the magnitude of resistance to knee rotation and provides variable resistance.

To reduce the effects or eliminate the disadvantages at the knee disarticulation level, the prosthetics-orthotics research department at the Orthopedic Hospital in Copenhagen developed a polycentric knee based on a four-bar linkage with a built-in swing control, presently a hydraulic damper.

Not only is the amputee offered the established advantages of both a polycentric knee and good swing control, it has also been possible, by locating the knee mechanism immediately below the socket, to obtain significant improvements in cosmesis, of particular importance to young female amputees.

Class 4 (hybrids). Included in this class are "hybrid" knee systems that consist of two separate components—one to control swing phase and another one to control stance phase. They usually combine mechanical friction stance controls with fluid swing controls. Either of the two components may be used alone. Two such systems have been demonstrated and are presently in use on a small scale.

1. One system is the combination of the Blatchford BSK, described in class 3, type 1, and the Blatchford pneumatic knee, described in class 2, type 3 mechanisms. In this system the patient depends on the BSK for stance control as described previously, and the Blatchford pneumatic knee controls swing phase.
2. The Kolman knee, described in class 3, type 1, has been combined with the Dyna-Plex (class 2, type 3) to provide both swing and stance control.

Requirements of knee mechanisms

Regardless of class or type, all knee mechanisms should meet the following general requirements:

1. The knee-shank assembly should readily attach to above-knee sockets and should receive prosthetic feet conveniently.
2. The knee must be durable, safe, relatively lightweight, and of good workmanship.
3. A range of sizes should be available.
4. All knee mechanisms should provide smooth rotation through a range of not less than 120 degrees measured from a position in which the long axes of the knee block and shank are aligned vertically through the knee center (180 degrees).
5. Extension aids should provide a force of sufficient magnitude to measurably decrease the resistance to negative knee rotation. The peak moment should occur in the last 20 degrees of negative knee rotation. The magnitude of the extension moment should be readily adjustable.
6. The lower limit of the range of resistance to knee rotation should be not less than 30% above the minimum setting for each unit.
7. The magnitude of resistance to knee rotation should vary with angular knee velocity or cadence in class 2, type 3, and class 3, type 3 units.

Prescription of prosthetic knee mechanisms

The ultimate purpose of an above-knee prosthesis is to restore the capacity to walk in a reasonably normal manner. The knee-control mechanism must be considered the functional heart of the above-knee prosthesis. No knee mechanism can restore any semblance of normal walking in the absence of other components, nor can it function effectively without a well-fitted, comfortable socket, proper alignment, and properly selected foot-ankle mechanism. However, the functions of the socket are to provide comfortable, nontissue-damaging weight bearing; a mechanical link to and suspension for the knee and foot; and sensory feedback to the stump about the behavior of the knee and foot. The foot-ankle-shank assembly also provides support and contributes to the normality of walking. Nevertheless, the major element in simulating normal gait is control of the knee flexion-extension cycle and stability in early stance. These are the principal functions of knee mechanisms.

Prescription rationale. Clinicians prescribing a prosthesis for a recent amputee and/or for a very experienced amputee are frequently told that the patient prefers a particular knee mechanism. The preference may be based on experience with the knee mechanism or, in the case of the new amputee, on hearsay about its virtues. Simply acceding to the patient's request may indeed satisfy him, particularly if the prescribing clinic team's rationale is based on the question: "How can we satisfy the patient?" or "Which set of components, socket, knee, foot-ankle assembly, will satisfy the patient?" Although a strong patient preference is a dominating factor, the information contained in this chapter provides a more effective rationale that takes the form of the following question: "What is best for the patient?" "What is best for the patient" usually turns out to be adherence to the basic prescription considerations.

Basic prescription considerations

Alignment. All patients with above-knee amputations should be fitted with the least stable alignment consistent with required security to provide maximum control over the prosthesis by minimizing the effort required to initiate swing phase. Alignment stability must be thought of as a component of the prosthesis just as though it were a piece of hardware. The more alignment stability built into the prosthesis, the more gait is compromised, although security may be increased. The first step in prescription is to consider the selection of the most appropriate knee mechanism, which is to say, the one that will require the least alignment stability. The degree of alignment stability required in any case is deter-

Table 4. Prescription related to stump and activity level

	Activity level		
	High, versatile	*Fairly active*	*Relatively inactive*
	Fast walker Walks long distances Uses stairs Walks on hills and uneven ground Alignment stability is insufficient for uneven terrain and other activities	Fast walker Mostly level ground Walks long distances Minimum alignment stability is adequate for level walking	Slow hesitant walker Short distances Needs stability rather than fine swing control
Stump			
Long (50% of femur remaining)	Prescription No. 1: quadrilateral total-contact suction socket; classes 3 and 4 knees; SACH foot for general use; multiaxis foot for special activities and sports	Prescription No. 2: quadrilateral total-contact suction socket; class 2 knees; SACH foot for general use; multiaxis foot for special activities and sports	Prescription No. 3: quadrilateral total-contact; nonsuction suspension; Class 1 knees; single-axis foot for maximum stability
Medium (between 30% and 50% of femur remaining, of stump is strong, consider it long)	Prescription No. 1	Prescription No. 2	Prescription No. 3
Short (less than 30% of femur remaining)	Prescription No. 1: nonsuction suspension	Prescription No. 2	Prescription No. 3
Bilateral and/or others involvements affecting balance	Prescription No. 1:	Not indicated	Prescription No. 3
Prescription advantages	Knee mechanisms provide best adjustable variable cadence response and extension aid and best nonweight dependent stance control Socket provides best control of knee mechanism, better weight distribution, better feedback Foot provides lightweight is prefabricated standardized, and has minimal maintenance	Knee mechanisms provide good swing control, cadence response, use alignment stability for level walking, and have adjustable extensions aid. Socket provides best control of knee mechanism, better weight distribution, and better feedback Foot provides lightweight is prefabricated standardized, and has minimal maintenance	Knee mechanisms provide positive lock-in stance phase, are light-weight, and low maintenance Socket provides good control of prosthesis, good weight distribution, and feed back Foot provides maximum stability and adjustability of resistance to plantar and dorsiflexion

mined by two factors: (1) the length and strength of the residual limb and (2) the type of knee mechanism to be used.

In general, residual limb length and strength are highly correlated; short residual limbs are usually weaker than medium length residual limbs, which in turn are weaker than long residual limbs. Because they have more residual muscle masses, longer residual limbs are stronger. The effective strength of long residual limbs is increased due to their advantage in mechanical leverage. With exactly the same muscular forces available, a longer residual limb will exert a greater extension moment than a shorter residual limb. Moreover, long residual limbs have greater surface areas in contact with the socket, resulting more in positive control and better feedback.

As shown in Table 4 it may be too much to expect that patients with short above-knee stumps can be fitted with a "trigger" alignment, that is, the least alignment stability. All the units listed in Fig. 20-34, class 3, type 1; class 3, type 2; and all the class 4 knee mechanisms will permit the patient with a short residual limb to be fitted with moderate knee stability. The choice is quite wide, and the best knee mechanism for the patient with a short residual limb can be selected from within this group on the basis of additional criteria.

Stance control. It is preferable to control stance phase by weight bearing or by shifting the locus of the knee to a more stable or controllable position when the knee is extended. Polycentric knee mechanisms are more dependable stance-phase controls but in general are somewhat heavier than the weight-control types; on the other hand, their swing characteristics may be inferior. Polycentrics generally provide more positive stance control. The choice, then, lies in balancing the stability needs against the mobility needs.

Extension aid. Certain units in these categories have internal extension aids, whereas others require external elastic band–type extension aids (Fig. 20-40). In general, internal extension aids of the spring type, although adjustable, do not provide high extension aid forces. The external extension aids of the elastic band–type are uncosmetic, wear rapidly, and may interfere with clothing. But they are adjustable by the patient and provide higher forces than are available from springs. The order of preference, therefore, should be (1) external elastic extension aids in which high extension forces are necessary as, for example, in the patient with a short residual limb whose activity pattern requires taking very short steps for lengthy periods and who still tolerates the cosmetic compromise; (2) internal adjustable spring extension aids in which high forces are not required as, for example, patients with medium and long residual limbs who do not work in confined areas and for whom external straps are not desirable. The last choice in almost any case is for the nonadjustable internal spring type.

Suction suspension has the advantage of eliminating external belts and straps, although putting on and taking off the prosthesis may be more difficult, especially for old or infirm patients.

APPLICATION OF EXTENSION AIDS	
INTERNAL ADJUSTABLE	1. PERMITS KNEELING AND SITTING WITH KNEE RELAXED. 2. CAN BE ADJUSTED TO SUPPORT THE SHANK IN HORIZONTAL EXTENSION FOR DRIVING. 3. INTERNALLY CONCEALED FOR BEST COSMESIS. 4. MAINTAINS ADJUSTMENT FOR LONG PERIODS OF TIME. 5. LOW MAINTENANCE.
EXTERNAL ADJUSTABLE	1. DOES NOT RELAX WHEN SITTING OR KNEELING. 2. CAN BE ADJUSTED TO SUPPORT THE SHANK IN HORIZONTAL EXTENSION FOR DRIVING. 3. INEXPENSIVE AND OF SIMPLE DESIGN. 4. REQUIRES CONSTANT RE-ADJUSTMENT. 5. POOR COSMESIS. 6. HIGH MAINTENANCE.
INTERNAL ADJUSTABLE	1. PROVIDES LOW EXTENSION FORCE. 2. PROVIDES GOOD COSMESIS. 3. LOW MAINTENANCE 4. PERMITS KNEELING AND SITTING WITH KNEE RELAXED.

Fig. 20-40. Application of extension aids.

Use of the total-contact suction socket reinforces the principle of fitting with the least alignment stability possible. Minimum alignment stability requires greater control over the prosthesis, an advantage of total-contact sockets. The more sophisticated knee mechanisms, including highly functional stance controls, also require finer control by the residual limb. To prescribe a Mauch S-N-S, for example, with an open-end plug-fit socket and pelvic belt is to deny the patient the kind of control needed to take advantage of the features of this unit. There is no recorded basis whatsoever for prescribing anything but total-contact above-knee sockets. There may be several reasons for prescribing nonsuction suspension in the form of Silesian bandages or even a pelvic belt, but total-contact sockets are still indicated.

If, for reasons such as patient preference, the clinic team prescribes an open-end, plug-fit socket, it makes little sense to couple this component with the sophisticated knee mechanisms in class 2, type 3; class 3, type 3; or class 4.

Control of a prosthesis depends on contact between the residual limb and the socket during all phases of walking. It is essential that the greatest possible limb surface area is firmly in contact with the socket at all times. Accurately fitted total-contact sockets are required for best results. Regardless of the sophistication of the knee mechanism, its value is not available to the patient *unless it is used with a socket that permits the patient to employ the features it offers.*

Variations from basic prescriptions

Short residual limbs. If for any reason the best knee mechanism (class 3, type 1; class 3, type 2; or class 4) for the patient with a short residual limb cannot be prescribed, the clinic team must recognize that the next most appropriate knee mechanisms for this patient, class 2, types 1, 2, or 3, can only be fitted at a cost of increasing alignment stability. This means that the selection of class 2 units without integral stance-phase control components will require that the prosthesis be aligned in a relatively stable position to reduce the effort required of the patient to stabilize his knee in early stance. Moreover, the secondary consequence of stable alignment is increasing difficulty in initiating swing phase.

Medium length residual limbs. It is generally quite possible to align the prosthesis for a patient with a medium length residual limb with minimal alignment stability by prescribing knee mechanisms of class 3, types 2 and 3, or class 4.

The other factors previously mentioned in relation to the patient with the short residual limb (type of stance-phase control, type of extension aid, etc.) deserve the same consideration for the patient with the medium residual limb. If for any reason such as patient preference, prejudice, or cost, it becomes necessary to prescribe other units, it must be recognized that the second choice group, consisting of class 2, types 2 and 3; and class 4, can only be fitted with increased alignment stability. In addition, patients with uncomplicated residual limbs of medium length and strength can use more sophisticated swing controls to better advantage. Class 3, type 1, and class 2, type 1 units do not provide as much functional versatility.

Long residual limbs. Patients with long residual limbs might be considered to have the least need for stance-phase control because their long, strong residual limbs can readily generate muscular forces to stabilize the knee in early stance, even in the absence of mechanical stance controls. These patients, however, are likely to be more vigorouswalkers than the others and can benefit most from the sophisticated swing-control systems. In addition, they are more likely to be users of stairs and to walk on uneven terrain and down hills, activities in which stance-phase control mechanisms would be most advantageous. The prescription choice for these patients resides in class 3, types 2 and 3, and class 4 to obtain all the advantages of (1) the most versatile swing-phase pattern, (2) stance control to reduce the hazard of walking on nonlevel surfaces, and (3) minimum alignment stability. Apart from all secondary criteria mentioned in relation to patients with short and medium length limb remnants, an additional criterion must be considered for the patient with the long stump. The knee center to floor dimension must be considered to determine which of the available class 3 and class 4 units can be fitted—excessively long residual limbs may not permit fitting of certain units.

Residual limb condition. Residual limb surface conditions may cause difficulties in fitting. Conditions that cause pain or sensitivity must be considered in prescription. Painful scars, neuromata, or other skin conditions on the posterior aspect of the stump, for example, may make it difficult or impossible for the patient to extend his hip with sufficient force to stabilize the knee in early stance. Apart from medical/surgical solutions, the most obvious and least effective method of dealing with this problem is to increase alignment stability in the hope of reducing the hip extension force the patient is required to apply. A better solution is to prescribe a knee mechanism that provides stance control and a foot-ankle assembly that provides minimal resistance to plantar flexion to reduce any tendency toward knee instability.

A more severe problem is pain in the area of the ischial tuberosity. An intimately fitted total-contact socket will do much to relieve the pressure in the painful area. A common site of pain is the lateral distal aspect of the residual limb due to impingement of the sharp end of the femur against soft tissue. In this case, a well-fitted total-contact socket and proper mediolateral alignment can often relieve the problem. A sound skin without blemishes and with nonadherent scars is considered most desirable for prosthetic fitting.

Other physical impairments. In the presence of other physical impairments, prescription criteria often change radically. The use of braces, additional amputations of either the upper or lower limbs, and blindness are factors that require serious consideration.

Patients in a clinic for prescription of an above-knee prosthesis who also have upper extremity amputations cannot be prescribed a suction socket because of difficulty in donning. A nonsuction socket will require either a Silesian or pelvic band, a fact that need not influence the choice of knee mechanism. Obtaining the full function available in a class 2, types 2 or 3, class 3, or class 4 knee mechanism depends on the control afforded by intimate stump-socket contact and not on the type of suspension.

If a patient wears a brace on one side and is being prescribed an above-knee prosthesis, the clinic team's concern should be more for stability and reduced energy consumption than for aesthetic swing characteristics. For these patients, class 3, types 1 and 2 knee mechanisms should be combined with total-contact suction sockets.

The blind above-knee patient has no visual feedback to cue him about the behavior of the limb. He depends on noise and proprioceptive feedback to control the prosthesis and should be prescribed one of the polycentric units.

Level of activity. A patient's anticipated or actual level of activity is a critical factor influencing the prescription of knee-control systems. Many patients are content only to stand and walk sufficiently to care for their personal needs, whereas others compete with nonamputees in all daily activities, including sports. The demands made on the prosthesis may vary from sedentary wearers with poor strength to very active wearers with excellent strength. The more active wearers usually require the highest degree of knee swing control, whereas the more sedentary wearers may not. Stance-control features can be of benefit to both.

Maintenance. Prosthetic knee systems are designed to withstand long periods of use with minimal wear or malfunction. However, the more complex mechanisms, due partly to the numbers of components and moving parts, tend to require more care and periodic preventive maintenance than the simpler systems. This care must be given by a competent, qualified technician. Thus the cost and convenience of maintenance are important factors to consider. The system should be chosen according to the distance the patient lives from the nearest qualified limb facility and the patient in a heavy-duty occupation. For patients living in remote areas with long travel times involved, the clinic team should consider a compromise in favor of low-maintenance components.

Cost. The cost of the unit should ordinarily not be a consideration, except in situations in which two or more devices of absolutely equal function are being considered.

Cosmesis. Cosmesis does not consist of appearance features alone. Weight, texture, noise-free function, as well as color and shape, are important. Until recently, cosmetic requirements were being met by the generally anthropomorphic shape of socket, shank, and foot, and by reasonably homogeneous coloration. Demands for improved cosmesis have led to the development of new unitized cosmetic leg covers that (1) cover the entire limb, including the knee, without impairing its function; (2) are shaped to approximate the contours of the sound leg; (3) are soft, resilient foam, reducing noise and impact; (4) feel more lifelike.

FOOT-ANKLE SYSTEMS AND ROTATORS

There are three functional classifications for foot-ankle systems.

Class I includes foot-ankle assemblies principally designed to provide motion in the anteroposterior plane in simulation of plantar flexion and dorsiflexion of the ankle and extension of the toes.

Class II includes foot-ankle assemblies principally designed to provide motions in both anteroposterior and frontal planes simulating plantar flexion and dorsiflexion and inversion and eversion.

Class III includes foot-ankle assemblies principally designed to provide motion in three planes, simulating plantar flexion, dorsiflexion, inversion and eversion, and transverse rotation of the ankle.

Foot-ankle systems are designed primarily to absorb impact on heel-contact, at the same time permitting plantar flexion, improving knee stability for the above-knee amputee during the early part of the stance phase. The ankle is usually blocked against dorsiflexion to improve knee stability during the latter portion of the stance phase, as well as to prevent drop-off of the body center of gravity at the end of the stance phase. Lateral motion and transverse rotation in class III devices and toe pickup in the special Hydra-Cadence system are also available. Although their use is not widespread, these functions are desirable for special activities.

A main factor in achieving good gait for the below-knee amputee is near-normal knee flexion. With a class I single-axis ankle, an excessively soft heel bumper will allow the prosthetic foot to plantar flex too rapidly, and thus the foot will slap against the floor. This early floor contact also decreases the amount of knee flexion.

The SACH foot, a class II system, with a soft heel will also reduce the amount of knee flexion because the knee can only flex readily after the heel cushion has been fully compressed. A soft heel is thus a hindrance to an active below-knee amputee.

Multiaxis foot-ankle (class III) assemblies should be considered for extremely active patients or for those who often engage in special activities such as dancing and sports. These types of foot-ankle assemblies offer no more function than either the SACH or the properly "tuned" single-axis foot in ordinary walking activities when the only concerns are knee stability and knee flexion.

The positive effects of a well-fitted total-contact socket and a knee mechanism aligned with the least possible alignment stability can be lost by the improper selection of a foot. The more the prosthesis is "triggered" toward instability, the more necessary it is to have a dependable and sophisticated stance-control knee mechanism; it also is necessary to provide a low plantar-flexion resistance. Unnecessarily high resistance to plantar flexion will reduce the knee stability in early stance phase.

Presently, the choice of foot-ankle assemblies remains between class I feet with single-axis ankles and the classes II and III multiaxis foot-ankle assemblies, including the SACH foot. For the patient without complications, regardless of residual limb length, the SACH foot is preferred because it permits the selection of a sufficiently soft plantar-flexion resistance, is available in a full range of sizes, and is readily attached to the shank. The molded SACH foot has no open sections, and the combination of a proper keel length and the resiliency of the toe provide an adequate control of rollover in late stance. In fact, stability in late stance phase is principally a function of the rollover characteristics of the foot and has little to do with the function of the knee.

However, patients who have been prescribed

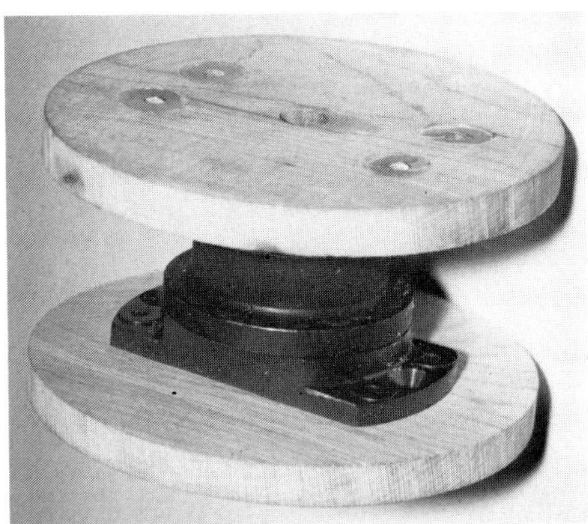

Fig. 20-41. USMC Star rotator.

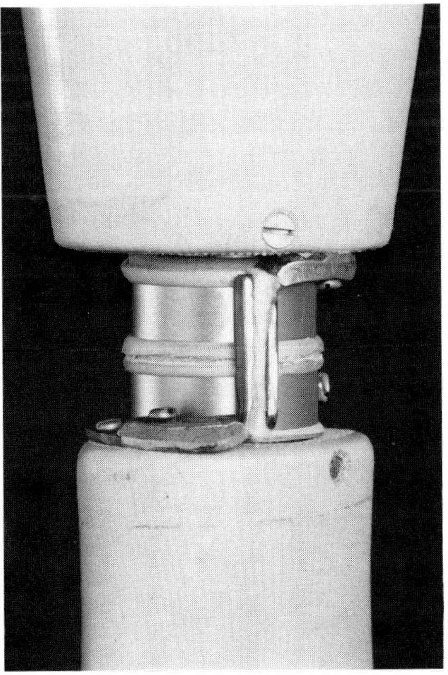

Fig. 20-42. Weber-Watkins rotator.

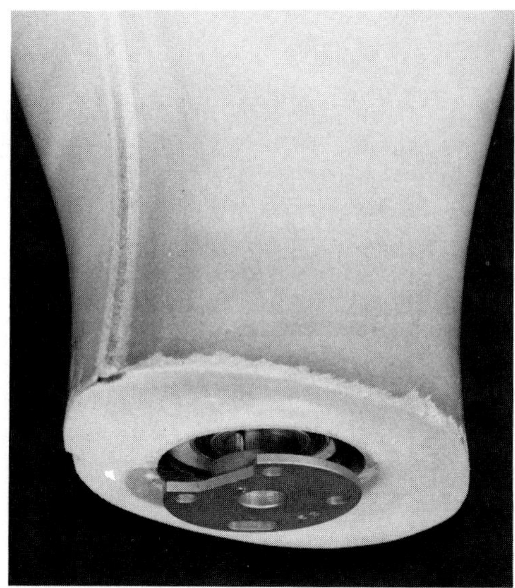

Fig. 20-43. Hosmer rotator.

any of the class 2 knees (without stance-phase control features) may require finer adjustment of the resistance and ranges of motion in the foot-ankle assembly than is readily achievable in the SACH foot. In the absence of integral stance-control features in the knee, the patient must depend on alignment ability and the plantar-flexion function of the foot and ankle. Cases of this type might be more adequately served by a single-axis foot, which the prosthetist "customizes" for the patient by appropriate variations in the selection of the plantar-flexion resistance and in the adjustment of the permissible dorsiflexion range. Accurate alignment and adjustment of the foot can allow better knee control in the initiation of flexion by permitting a more unstable knee alignment even in the absence of a knee mechanism with stance-control features.

Pelvic and tibial rotation are dynamic factors of walking that often produce serious problems for the amputee. Gait analysis studies have shown that the greater the restriction of axial rotation, the greater the shear stresses between the residual limb and socket. In an effort to minimize these shear stresses, rotators or torque absorbers have been developed for use in above-knee and below-knee prostheses. Essentially, these devices provide a means of controlling axial rotation within the prosthesis during the weight-bearing (stance) phase of walking. This is of special value to the amputee in compensating for both pelvic rotation and tibial rotation. Unilateral amputees, who are active walkers and experience a high degree of shear stress, may benefit significantly from torque absorption devices (Figs. 20-41 to 20-43). This is especially true for amputees engaged in sports; an outstanding example of this is golfing.

ACKNOWLEDGMENTS

Much of this chapter has been taken from material that we and our colleagues have previously written for the Veterans Administration. Mr. Henry Gardner, formerly of the Veterans Administration Prosthetic Center, contributed some of the material on sockets, and Dr. Edward Peizer organized a large portion of the material on knee mechanisms. We are indebted to them and to Mr. Berdsell Franklin and Mr. John Beagles of the Veterans Administration Prosthetics Center, who provided the illustrations. Special thanks to Ms. Linda Mattocks for her secretarial support throughout this project.

REFERENCES

1. Anderson, M., Bray, J., Hennessy, C., and Sollers, R.: Prosthetic principles: above-knee amputations, Springfield, Ill., 1960, Charles C Thomas, Publisher.
2. Fillauer, C.: Supracondylar wedge suspension of the PTB prosthesis, Orthot. Prosthet. **22:**(2)39-44, June, 1968.
3. Foort, J.: The patellar-tendon-bearing prosthesis for below-knee amputees: a review of technique and criteria, Artif. Limbs **9**(1):4-13, Spring, 1965.
4. Foort, J., and Radcliff, C. W.: The Canadian type hip disarticulation prosthesis, Berkeley, Calif., 1956, Prosthetic Devices Research Project Institute of Engineering Research, University of California.
5. Gardner, H., and Clippinger, F.: The location of prosthetic and orthotic knee joints, Artif. Limbs **13:**31-35, Fall, 1969.
6. The geriatric amputee, Publication 919, Committee on Prosthetics Research and Development, Washington, D.C., National Academy of Sciences – National Research Council, pp. 95-116.
7. Hamontree, S. E., Tyo, H. J., and Smith, S.: Twenty months' experience with the "PTS," Orthot. Prosthet. **22**(1): 33-30, March, 1968.
8. Marschall, K., and Nitschke, R.: Principles of the patellar tendon supra condylar prosthesis, Orthot. Prosthet. Appl. J. **21**(1):33-38, March, 1967.
9. Program guide G-7 for the selection and application of knee mechanisms, Washington, D.C., Dec., 1976, Veterans Administration Prosthetics Center.

CHAPTER 21

Partial foot amputations

Section I

Surgical procedures

F. WILLIAM WAGNER, JR.

Vascular disease and trauma are the major causes of lower limb amputations. Neoplasms, congenital and acquired deformities, and infection account for relatively fewer cases. In recent years, an increasing number of young people have been suffering trauma severe enough to require amputation. Occasionally, foot deformities from previous trauma, infections, and congenital anomalies may require amputation through the foot. In the immature skeleton, disarticulation is the procedure of choice, whenever possible, to accommodate the problems of continued growth.

LEVEL SELECTION

Most authorities agree that all length possible should be saved in the forefoot. Innervated plantar skin should cover all weight-bearing surfaces. An occasional patient has been able to bear weight on pedicle flaps over bony prominences, but split-thickness grafts on weight-bearing surfaces usually break down with continued pressure.[2]

Loss of toes, either partial or complete, leads to little disability in the elderly and can usually be compensated for with simple shoe corrections. Transmetatarsal amputations can be fitted with sole stiffeners and toe fillers with minor apparent loss of function during stance and walking on level surfaces. Lisfranc disarticulations do well only if invertor and evertor muscle power is well balanced, and there is no tendency to talipes equinus. Chopart amputations in general have not done well, especially if they are posttraumatic and there is much scarring or skin grafting. With few exceptions, then, the general consensus is that amputation of the foot is most satisfactory when performed distal to the tarsometatarsal joints. The next higher level of choice may be the Syme amputation or ankle disarticulation.[3,4]

Level selection in dysvascular patients (arteriosclerosis, diabetes) has frequently been difficult.[11] Oscillometry, arteriography, plethysmography, ergometry, fluorescein tests, histamine wheal, and similar procedures all have had their adherents and detractors. However, with all of these tests, *clinical judgment* still remains a most important part of level selection. Three recent diagnostic procedures have increased the accuracy of level selection:

1. Radioactive xenon has been used to measure skin blood flow. The greatest correlation between blood flow of various tissues and success of amputation level has been with skin flow. Radioactive xenon (Xe 133) is injected into the skin or placed on the skin under a sealed cover glass. Decay in radioactivity is based on capillary pickup and dispersion of the material. There appears to be fewer artifacts with the noninjection method. Sufficient blood supply to sustain an amputation is present if the flow is over 0.6 ml/100 g tissue/min in one study[9] and 1.5 ml/100 g tissue/min in another study.[6]

2. Appearance of bleeding at the skin level after release of the thigh tourniquet has been timed. When the most distal skin bleeds within 3 minutes after release of the tourniquet, there is 80-85% successful healing of the amputation incision. If bleeding is prolonged beyond 3 minutes, the

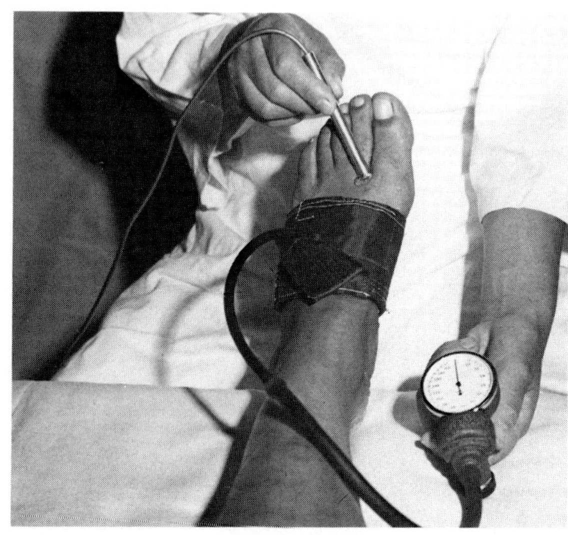

Fig. 21-1. Doppler probe placed over arteries to first and second toes below the sphygmomanometer cuff placed at midfoot. Signal of 9 or 10 MHz is better for smaller vessels.

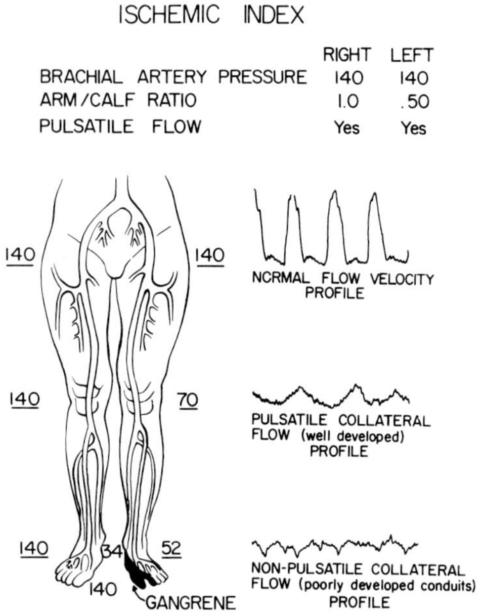

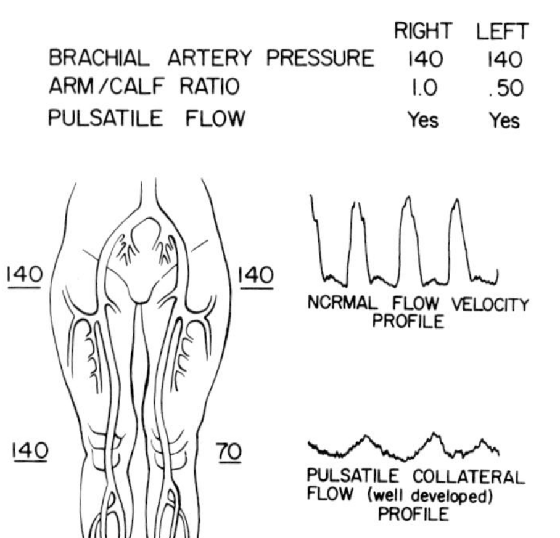

Fig. 21-2. Pulse signal can indicate degree of collateral circulation by pulsatility. Ischemic index is computed by dividing lower extremity pressure by brachial artery pressure. Satisfactory healing is predicted if index is over 0.45 in diabetics and over 0.35 in nondiabetics.

ISCHEMIC INDEX OF .45 OR GREATER
WITH PULSATILE FLOW

Level of Amputation	Total	Ratio 0.45+ Puls. Flow	Healed	Failures	Healing Rates	
Above knee	21	18	18	0		
Through knee	10	10	10	0		
Below knee	29	26	24	2		
Syme's	46	37	34	3	93.2%	
Ray and Mid-tarsal	15	13	11	2		93.3%
Toes	15	13	12	1		
Mid-tarsal Op.	17	17	16	1	94.1%	

Fig. 21-3. Results in 134 consecutive diabetic patients with ischemic index over 0.45 with pulsatile flow. Selection of level was 93.3% accurate as indicated by healing rate.

next higher level should be tested.[12] The tourniquet is not used if there have been previous vascular surgical procedures in the limb.

3. Transcutaneous ultrasound has been coupled with the Doppler effect to provide an instrument that acts as a sensitive stethoscope or flow detector. Systolic blood pressure can be measured when the pulse cannot be palpated or heard with the ordinary stethoscope.[5,12,13] For this purpose the instrument does not need to be directional, and several relatively inexpensive portable machines are available. The smaller the vessel to be measured, the higher the frequency of the signal should be. Frequencies at 9 to 10 MHz are recommended for the foot and toes (Fig. 21-1). As recommended by the American Heart Association, the cuff width should be 120% of the diameter of the extremity at the level being measured. Thus four different cuff sizes are the usual number for a satisfactory complete examination of a lower limb. The major vascular tree can be mapped with the instrument and areas of lessened flow and zero flow determined and marked on a chart. Collateral circulation can be mapped in a similar manner (Fig. 21-2). Pulsation of the flow can be determined. Systolic pressures are measured from the groin to the toes at the upper thigh, midthigh, knee, calf, ankle, foot, and toe level. An ischemic index is calculated for each level by dividing the systolic pressure by the brachial artery pressure. For example, the systolic pressure may be 120 mm at the arm and at the thigh, 90 mm at the calf, 60 mm at the ankle, and 20 mm at midfoot. The ischemic index would be 1 at the arm and thigh, 0.75 at the calf, 0.50 at the ankle, and 0.17 at midfoot. A Syme amputation is indicated if the skin of the heel pad is intact.

Study of a series of diabetic lower extremity amputations has shown over 93.3% successful healing when the ischemic index was over 0.45 at the level of amputation (Fig. 21-3). Similar results are obtained in nondiabetics if the ischemic index is over 0.35. This study is now being extended with transcutaneous pO_2 analysis in a search for further noninvasive indicators of healing potential in the dysvascular limb and its surgical flaps.

If the ischemic index is insufficient for local healing, a consultation is obtained from the Vascular Surgery Service. Successful revascularization procedures, such as endarterectomy, profundaplasty, or bypass procedures can aid in the local healing of a lesion, allow local surgical procedures to be performed, or may allow amputations to be performed at a low enough level to save the knee.

SURGERY

Anesthesia

All types of anesthesia are used. Individual selection is made from preference of the patient, coexisting medical problems, and preferences of the anesthetist and surgeon. Intravenous regional anesthesia with a two-level tourniquet is excellent and appears to interfere least with the patient's general condition. A contraindication to the use of the tourniquet would be recent vascular surgery. Over 2000 thiopental (Pentothal) induction and inhalation anesthetics have been administered at Rancho Los Amigos Hospital for diabetic and dysvascular patients with no intraoperative deaths. Hospital mortality has been less than 1% in the Syme and foot amputation procedures.

Open versus closed techniques

All open wounds are eventually infected even if with nonpathogenic bacteria. A paradox thus is created in leaving an amputation open when performed for severe infection.[1] Removal of the major amount of infected or gangrenous tissue by amputation usually leaves a number of bacteria behind in the surrounding cellulitis and lymphangitis. This usually can be controlled by the body's own defense mechanisms with the aid of appropriate antibiotics. Kritter[7] has developed a technique for irrigating wounds of this type. His technique has done away with open amputation in foot patients at Rancho Los Amigos Hospital. A small plastic catheter is drawn into the wound through a separate stab incision (Fig. 21-8). The wound is closed over the catheter relatively loosely and slowly irrigated with an appropriate antibiotic solution for 72 to 96 hours. The fluid dilutes the hematoma and aids in the removal of blood clots and debris between the sutures. Care must be taken with nephrotoxic and ototoxic antibiotics so that total amounts given do not exceed allowable limits. In a recent personal communication, Kritter states that he is now irrigating the wounds of his patients without antibiotics and believes that the irrigating effect appears to be the more important.

SPECIFIC SURGICAL TECHNIQUES

Partial toe amputation

Toes can be excised from the tip to the base through any type of incision, provided the flaps have adequate base for length. Flaps must close

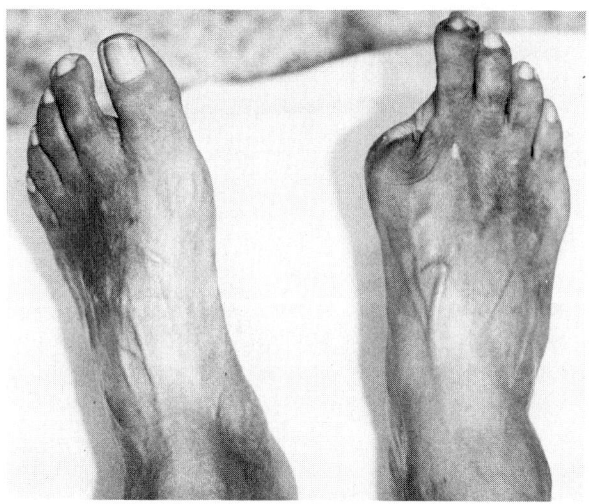

Fig. 21-4. Amputation of great toe through base of proximal phalanx. Mobile pad aids in protection of metatarsal head. No orthosis is necessary.

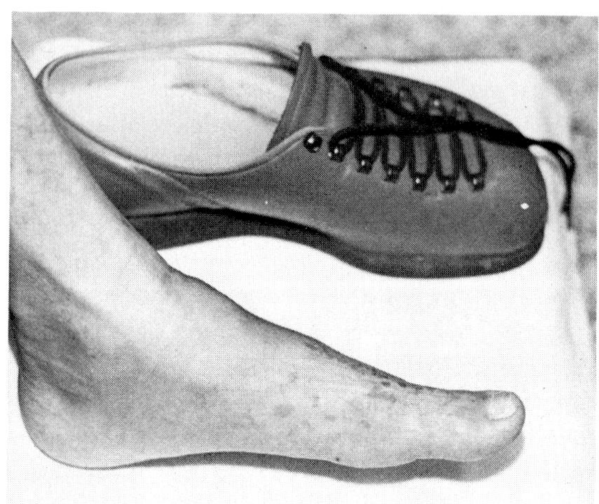

Fig. 21-5. Amputation of lateral toes and rays. Plastazote filler in extra depth shoe aids in shoe stability.

without tension. They may be side-to-side flaps, long dorsal flaps, long plantar flaps, fishmouth, or any combination. With the great toe, it is desirable to keep enough of the base of the proximal phalanx to preserve the attachment of the short flexor and extensor tendons. The mobile pad remaining appears to offer more protection to the skin under the first metatarsal head (Fig. 21-4). In the lesser toes, this does not seem to be as important, except in the fifth toe.

Toe disarticulation

If sufficient viable skin is not present to allow a partial toe amputation, a disarticulation at the metatarsal phalangeal joint is quite satisfactory. Metatarsal head pressure can become more pronounced, and fixation of the long extensor tendon to the dorsal joint capsule aids in elevation of the metatarsal head. A longer plantar flap provides more durable skin coverage. Articular cartilage is resistant to infection and need not be arbitrarily removed.

Metatarsal ray resection

Third, fourth, and fifth metatarsal ray resections have been quite successful and leave a functional partial foot. With the use of the ischemic index obtained by transcutaneous Doppler ultrasound, the success rate has improved. Complete removal of infected and necrotic tissue is important. Enough bone must be removed so that flaps may be closed without tension. For single second, third, or fourth toe and ray, a pie-shaped wedge is removed. This closes well and leaves a symmetrical foot. On occasion, all of the lateral rays have been removed, leaving the great toe and first metatarsal (Fig. 21-5). This leaves a functional foot that can give a better gait than a transmetatarsal amputation.The wounds in metatarsal ray resections are irrigated with antibiotic solutions when removal has been done for infection and with Ringer's lactate solution or similar fluid when the wound has been noninfected.

Transmetatarsal amputation

This amputation may be performed for deformity resulting from trauma to the toes, loss of tissue, and infection or gangrene due to frostbite, diabetes, arteriosclerosis, scleroderma, Buerger's disease, and similar conditions. McKittrick and Pederson outlined the indications for transmetatarsal amputation in the diabetic in 1949.[8,10] They remain as true today as they were then. Gangrene must be limited to the toes and should not involve the web space. The infection should be controlled. The incision should not extend through hypoesthetic areas or through infected areas. The patient should be free of pain. Palpable foot pulses are not necessary, but there should be no dependent rubor. Venous filling should be less than 25 seconds. To these we have added the transcutaneous Doppler ultrasound index. Healing has occurred in over 93% of the diabetics when the ratio was over 0.45 and nondiabetics when it was over 0.35.

Technique. A slightly curved incision is made

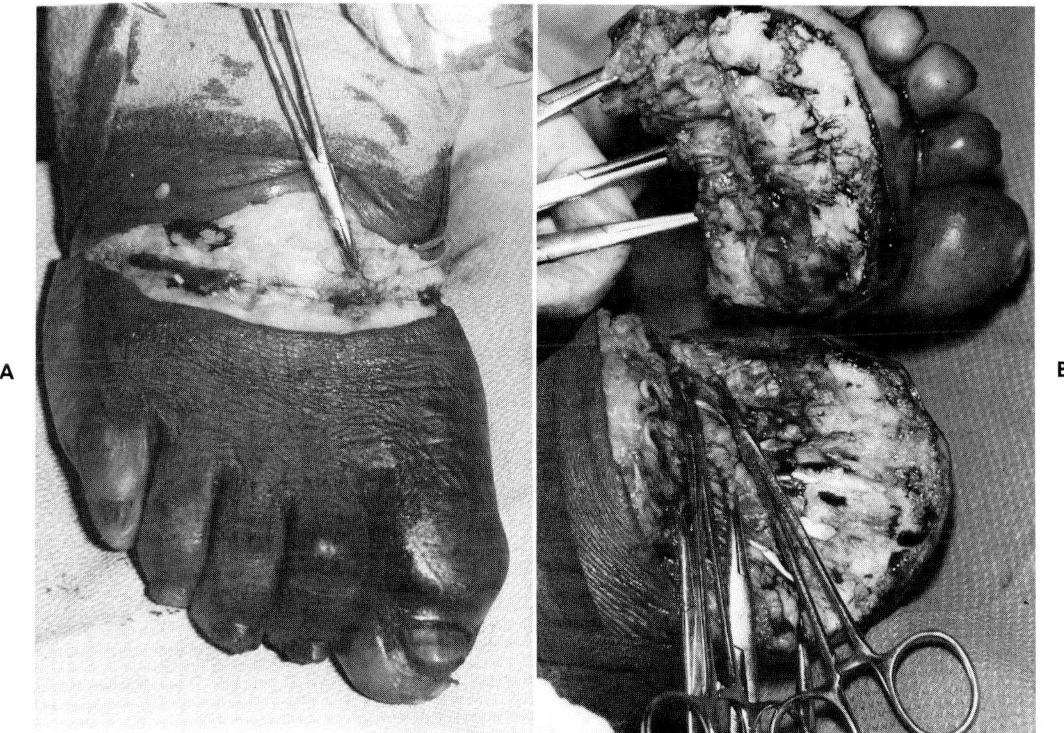

Fig. 21-6. A, Dorsal incision for transmetatarsal amputation performed for infected diabetic gangrene. **B,** Plantar incision for transmetatarsal amputation.

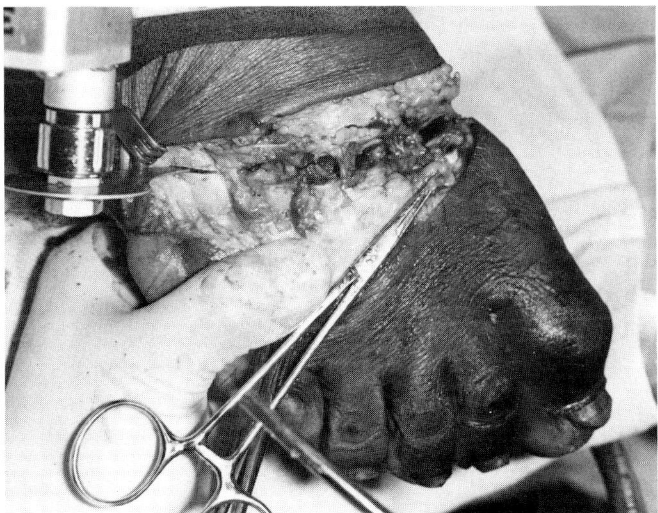

Fig. 21-7. Metatarsals are sectioned at level of dorsal skin incision. Lateral bevel of osteotomy prevents later pressure point.

dorsally across the metatarsal necks to the midpoint of the foot on either side. From there it extends distally and curves plantarward to the sole and then across just proximal to the toe crease (Fig. 21-6). No tissue planes are dissected. The metatarsals are cut on the dorsum at the level of the incision. All inferior edges are rounded, and the medio lateral edges of the first and fifth are beveled (Fig. 21-7). The toes are then separated by beveling the soft tissue under the metatarsal

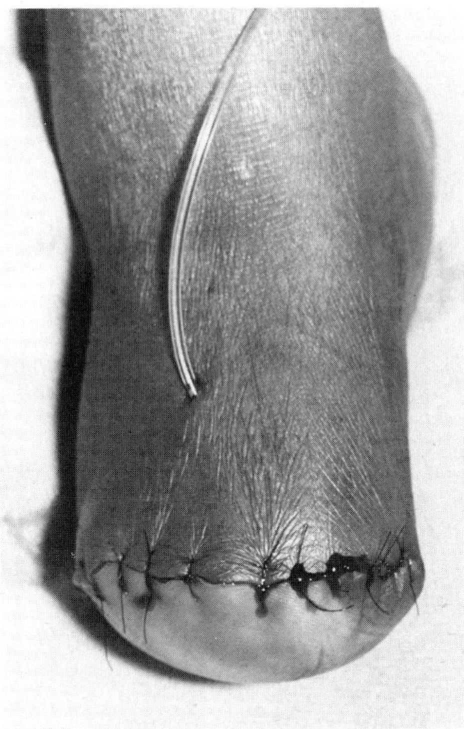

Fig. 21-8. Irrigation fluid exits between sutures. Skin closure is with nylon or similar nonabsorbable suture.

heads down to the distal skin edge. The tendons are pulled down, divided, and allowed to retract. Pinpoint electrocoagulation and fine absorbable ligatures are used for hemostasis. The skin is closed over an irrigation tube that is removed in 48 to 72 hours (Fig. 21-8). Ambulation is begun in a walking cast in approximately 10 days.

Chopart, Lisfranc, Vasconcelos, Pirogoff, and Boyd amputations

As stated earlier, these levels have not been successful in most patients with ischemia and diabetes. An occasional long-term successful case may be found in an amputation clinic, but a much higher percentage have had to be converted to the Syme or below-knee amputation. Ulcerations tend to occur over the pressure points, resulting from the progressive equinus position of the stump. Most Chopart amputations result from severe trauma, and some of these have had split-thickness skin grafts over the weight-bearing area. The greatest number of these grafts have broken down with everyday use. Fixation of the extensor tendons to the dorsum of the foot can sometimes aid in the salvage of such a stump. However, fixation of the extensor tendons in the presence of infection frequently fails. The requirements of bony union in the Boyd, Pirogoff, and Vasconcelos procedures can add the further complication of a painful nonunion.

POSTOPERATIVE CARE

Kritter's[7] irrigation system is used in all cases of infection and in all areas with open bleeding bone. It is used in disarticulations if there is a cavity. Irrigating fluid is run through at approximately 500 ml/24 hours. The tube is removed in 48 to 72 hours, and the tip is cut aseptically and sent to the laboratory for culture and sensitivity studies. This step aids in the selection of proper antibiotics if residual bacteria should be present. Soft dressings are used until the irrigation system is discontinued. Short leg casts are then applied. Ambulation is started within 24 hours in nondiabetic patients and within 10 days for diabetics. The cast is continued for 2 to 6 weeks. A shoe constructed of Plastazote provides a forgiving surface that protects the healing wound. Regular shoe wear is begun when the wound is mature.

Section II

Prosthetic and orthotic management

THOMAS LUNSFORD

Very few partial foot amputations distal to the transmetatarsal joints require prosthetic devices to increase function. Cosmetic partial feet with toes and even painted nails have been fabricated for wear in sandals and open shoes. Little function is derived from such a prosthesis. Occasionally, patients relate that it helps stabilize the shoe on the foot. Transmission of force through a cuff or similar device at the heel or ankle is usually not possible, and attachment must be at the calf through metal sidebars or plastic shells if the force of transmission is to be effective. At the Lisfranc and Chopart levels, an ankle-foot orthosis (AFO) will add to gait function.

PROSTHETIC AND ORTHOTIC SYSTEMS

Regular shoes

Toe fillers. Toe fillers are usually not needed for single toe loss. With loss of the first toe and a portion of the metatarsal, a toe block can aid in keeping the metatarsal elevated. Plastazote, mi-

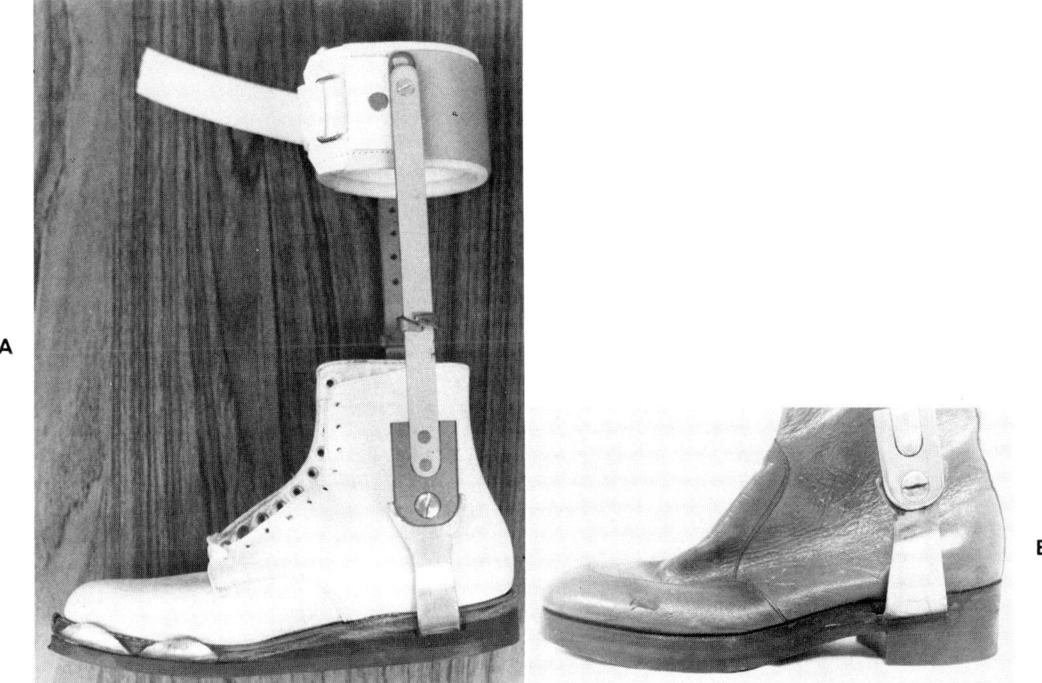

Fig. 21-9. A, Conventional double sidebar AFO for Chopart or Lisfranc amputation in child who is unable to keep standard shoe on residual foot. **B,** Conventional metal AFO for short residual foot.

crocellular rubber, room temperature – vulcanizer foam, and similar materials can be used. Many patients make their own fillers with cotton, foam rubber, and other easily obtainable materials. If roll-off is lost in a regular shoe, thickening of the sole and rocker bottom contouring can restore this motion.

If the amputation has been at the transmetatarsal, Lisfranc, or Chopart level, the shoe may be fitted with a definitive orthosis if the patient lacks roll-off. The orthosis may be of double sidebar or polypropylene construction (Figs. 21-9 to 21-12).

Biomechanical purpose

1. To prevent anterior migration of the foot
2. To provide resistance to creasing of the shoe vamp
3. To provide shoe-size symmetry

Fabrication and materials. Many materials can be used, including Plastazote, Kemblo, cork, leather, Silastic and sponge, and microcellular rubbers. A plaster positive mold is made from a plaster bandage impression of the residual foot. The orthosis is formed between the plaster model and a pattern of the shoe insole and toe box. A soft interface is provided, and the orthosis may be removable or cemented into the shoe.

Special foot appliances. Partial foot loss at the transmetatarsal level can lead to imbalance in eversion and/or eversion and equinus. UCBL foot orthoses can be lengthened to the toe area to provide a sole stiffener as well as everting or inverting stability (Fig. 21-10).

Ankle-foot orthoses. Amputees with loss at the Lisfranc and Chopart levels (Fig. 21-11) can obtain a better gait if ankle stability and forefoot leverage are provided by an AFO (Fig. 21-12). The orthosis can be of standard double sidebar construction with calf band, stirrup, and adjustable ankle joint (Fig. 21-9). However, the vacuum-formed plastic AFO is steadily replacing the conventional metal orthosis as greater experience is gained. The orthosis is lighter, provides foot support, and may be worn with regular footwear (Fig. 21-13).

Fabrication. A cast is made from a standard plaster impression of the leg, ankle, and foot. Thermoplastic (e.g., polypropylene) is vacuum formed over the cast. The degree of ankle motion is controlled by the placement of the trim line with respect to the malleoli and the thickness of plastic used. Greater motion is permitted by trimming posterior to the malleoli; less motion is permitted by trimming anterior to the malleoli.

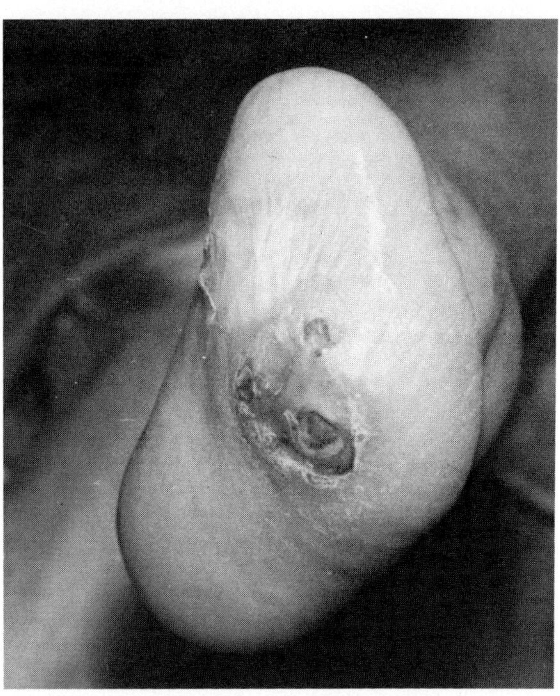

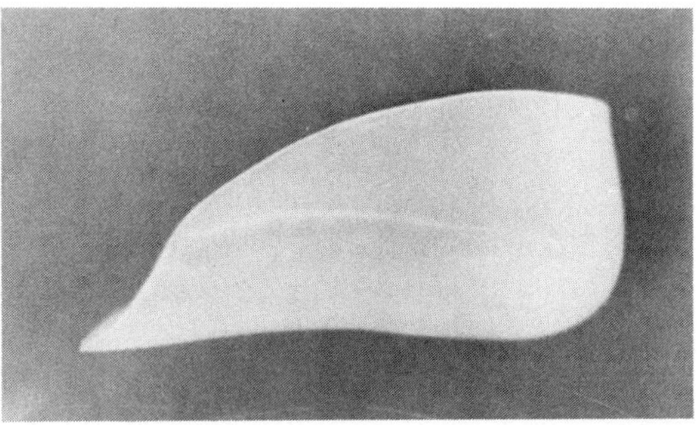

Fig. 21-10. Orthosis for transmetatarsal amputation fabricated of polypropylene vacuum formed over plaster cast.

Fig. 21-11. Lisfranc amputation with typical pressure area. This is difficult to control with orthoses. Patient recently requested Syme amputation after several episodes of healing and breakdown.

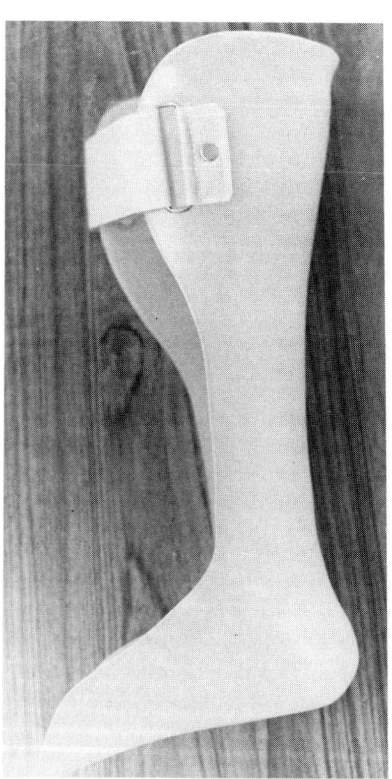

Fig. 21-12. Polypropylene AFO. Degree of stiffness can be controlled by location of trim line and material thickness.

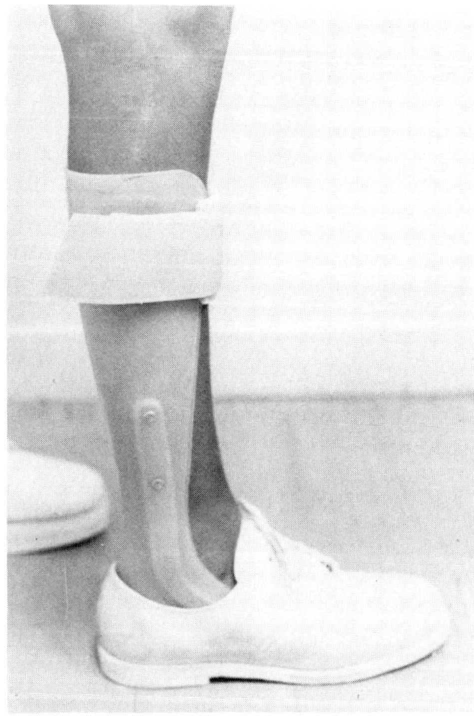

Fig. 21-13. Orthosis in nurse's shoe. Note stiffener along lateral edge.

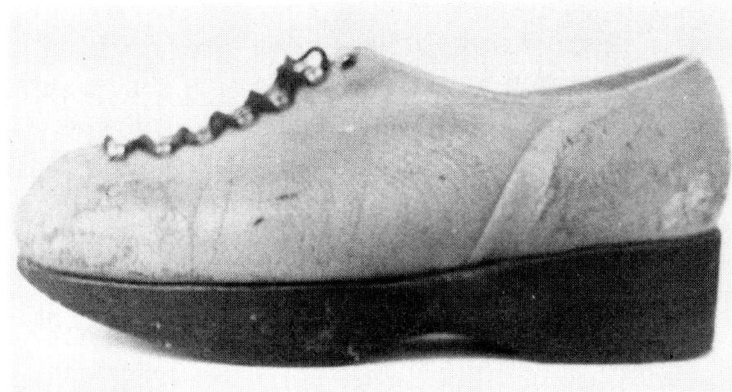

Fig. 21-14. Rocker bottom added to extra deep shoe to aid in roll-off and unweighting of metatarsal and toe areas.

The proximal edge is 2 cm distal to the fibular neck to avoid peroneal nerve insult. The orthosis is held on the leg with Velcro straps or standard straps and buckles.

Variations. Edema can be controlled with the addition of an anterior panel and several straps. Increased rigidity is afforded by corrugations and the anterior panel. If further rigidity is needed, anterior struts or recessed metal sidebars can be added. As rigidity increases, the need for a rocker bottom shoe increases to simulate ankle motion through the shape of the sole. Pressure areas and plantar ulcers at the tip of a transmetatarsal amputation can be relieved with a combination of AFO, rocker bottom sole, and Plastazote or similar inserts.

Biomechanical purposes

1. To reproduce the lever arm of the normal foot for pressure transmission in stance phase
2. To provide mediolateral stability to the shortened midfoot

Special shoes

Sole stiffeners. The shortened lever arm of an amputated foot can lead to instability in a regular shoe. The lack of the distal foot allows greater bending of the sole of the shoe, which tends to concentrate pressure at the end of the amputated bones. Stiffness of the sole can increase the lever arm, but usually at the expense of extra pressure at the tip of the stump. Thickening of the sole and contouring to a rocker can relieve this pressure by distributing the floor reaction force over a greater area and longer time (Fig. 21-14).

Biomechanical purposes

1. To prevent bending of the sole so that floor reaction is not concentrated at the metatarsal heads
2. To provide a lever arm to control the torque produced by body weight

Fabrication. Sole stiffeners may be used externally, between the inner and outer sole, or inside the shoe. An external sole may be constructed of a lightweight rigid material such as alder wood. Occasionally, an extra layer of sole leather is sufficient in a child's shoe. A flat or corrugated metal shank may be placed between the insole and outsole. Inside the shoe a UCBL plastic orthosis can be extended beyond the metatarsal head area. The motion lost by stiffening the sole is reproduced by contouring it to a rocker bottom shape.

Rocker bottoms. The contoured sole has been used for many years. Its shape can be seen in the illustrations for shoes and orthoses in most of the older catalogs and manuals. Gait clinics are now providing closer analysis of forces and moment arms. The rocker bottom shoe is now being studied in separate gait clinics at Rancho Los Amigos Hospital under the direction of Dr. Jacquelin Perry. Several classes of patients are benefiting from having a rocker contour to the sole. The biomechanical purposes and construction differ slightly with each problem presented by the patients.

Biomechanical purposes

1. Patients with motor loss, such as those with multiple sclerosis, poliomyelitis, meningomyelocele, and direct nerve pressure or severence, can benefit from a sole contour that replaces motion no longer supplied by the patient's own motor power. With the apex of the rocker placed approximately 3 cm proximal to the metatarsal head area, a passive knee flexion moment is produced at terminal stance that prepares the limb for swing phase toe clearance.
2. Patients with fused ankles, pantalar fusions, and stiff forefoot segments lack dorsiflexion movement. A rocker bottom with the apex just proximal to the metatarsophalangeal joint and a smooth curvature terminating in a 2.5-cm toe clearance can reproduce 25 to 30 degrees of combined ankle and subtalar motion.
3. Patients with plantar ulcers, hypersensitive feet, anesthetic feet, and partial amputations can derive relief of pressure at the ulcerated or hypersensitive area. The rocker bottom reduces the time that body weight is concentrated at any specific point. Thus plantar surface floor reaction is distributed

over a wider area of the foot. Heat-formed insoles of foamed polyethylene also help distribute the body weight (Fig. 21-15).

4. Patients with deformities, such as forefoot equinus, ankle equinus, depressed metatarsal heads, and claw toes, require a higher heel and longer radius on the sole to reproduce their ankle motion. The heel must be higher and the sole thinner to accommodate the equinus contour of the foot. Rocking begins at or just proximal to the metatarsal head line. If the problem is unilateral, a similar shoe must be provided for the contralateral foot so that a leg length discrepancy does not result from the higher heel. The thickness and contour of this sole more closely approximates that of the wooden Danish clog (Fig. 21-16). Care must be taken that the contour is smooth and that there is no straight portion of the curve at the end that would give a "bump" just before toe-off.

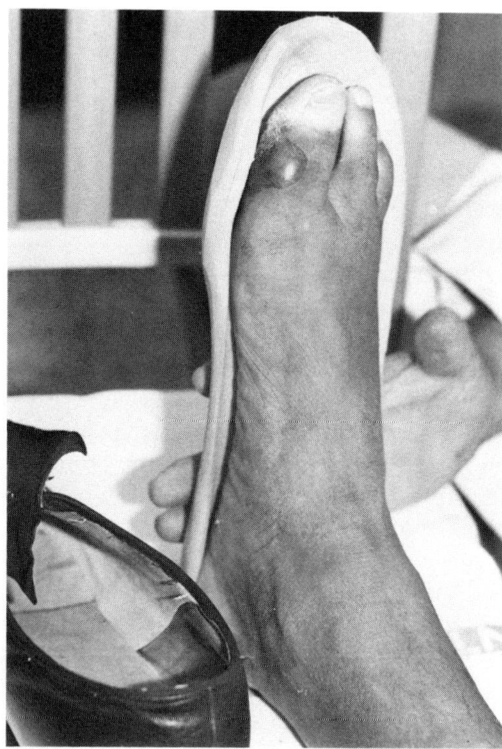

Fig. 21-15. Heat-formed polyethylene (Plastazote) insert for distribution of weight. Fourth and fifth phalanges and metatarsals have been amputated.

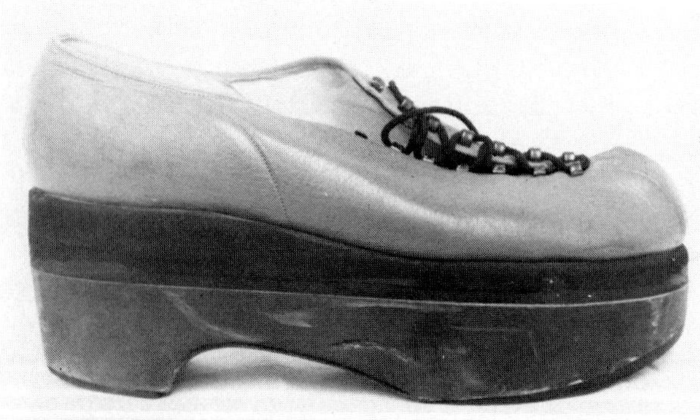

Fig. 21-16. Rocker bottom shoe with greater heel height for equinus problems and leg length discrepancies.

CLINICAL EVALUATION

Gait analysis can provide clues as to the proper orthosis or shoe correction needed. Knee, hip, and trunk deformities may also be present in a patient with an amputation of the foot or ankle. Mild to moderate equinus deformities of the ankle can render the finest prostheses, orthoses, or shoe corrections virtually unusable if these deformities are not recognized. Not infrequently, grinding a gently rounded contour on the sole will change a gait significantly and solve a pressure problem on the sole or tip of a stump. After prosthetic or orthotic fitting, reevaluation in the gait clinic may be necessary if the patient has not obtained the gait predicted by the team. At times, the grinding of a few millimeters from the distal end of the rocker may make a spectacular difference in gait. The average patient with a partial foot amputation will require little gait training unless other parts of the body are involved. The patient is instructed in donning, doffing, cleansing of the orthosis, care of the skin, and in actual orthosis use. Fit and alignment must be tested dynamically as an essential part of the delivery by the prosthetist or orthotist. Reevaluation after a period of use is essential.

REFERENCES

1. Ecker, M. D., and Jacobs, B. S.: Lower extremity amputations in diabetic patients, Diabetes **19:**189, 1970.
2. Harris, W. R., and Silverstein, E. A.: Partial amputations of the foot: a follow-up study, Can. J. Surg. **7:**6, 1964.
3. Hulnick, A., Highsmith, C., and Boutin, F. J.: Amputations for failure in reconstructive surgery, J. Bone Joint Surg. **31A:**639, 1949.
4. Hunter, G. A.: Results of minor foot amputations for ischemia of the lower extremity in diabetics and non-diabetics, Can. J. Surg. **18:**273, 1975.
5. Kazamas, T. M., Gander, M. P., and Franklin, D. L.: Blood pressure measurements with Doppler ultrasound flowmeter, J. Appl. Physiol. **30:**585, 1971.

6. Kostuik, J. P., Wood, D., Hornby, R., Feingold, S., and Matthews, V.: The measurement of skin blood flow in peripheral vascular disease by epicutaneous application of $xenon_{133}$, J. Bone Joint Surg. **58A:**833, 1976.
7. Kritter, A. E.: A technique for salvage of the infected diabetic gangrenous foot, Orthop. Clin. North Am. **4:**21, 1973.
8. McKittrick, L. S., McKittrick, J. B., and Risley, T. S.: Transmetatarsal amputation for infection of gangrene in patients with diabetes mellitus, Ann. Surg. **130:**826, 1949.
9. Moore, W. S.: Determination of amputation level measurement of skin blood flow with $xenon_{133}$, Arch. Surg. **107:**798, 1973.
10. Pedersen, H. E.: The problem of the geriatric amputee, Artif. Limbs **12**(2):i-iii, Autumn, 1968.
11. Romano, R. L., and Burgess, E. M.: Level selection in lower extremity amputations, Clin. Orthop. **74:**177, 1971.
12. Wagner, F. W., Jr.: Amputations of the foot and ankle: current status, Clin. Orthop. **122:**62, 1977.
13. Yao, S. T., Hobbs, J. T., and Irvine, W. T.: Ankle systolic pressure measurements in arterial disease affecting the lower extremities, Br. J. Surg. **56:**676, 1969.

CHAPTER 22

The Syme amputation

Section I

Surgical procedures

F. WILLIAM WAGNER, JR.

James Syme was Clinical Professor of Surgery at the University of Edinburgh from 1833 to 1869. He first performed his amputation at the ankle in 1842, which was prior to the use of anesthesia and antisepsis. He listed three advantages as compared to the below-knee level: "(1) The risk to life will be smaller, (2) a more comfortable stump will be afforded, (3) the limb will be more seemly and useful for progressive motion."[17]

With the advent of antibiotics, anesthesia, and blood transfusions, the first advantage is no longer as important. However, experience with over 500 Syme amputations at Los Angeles County, University of Southern California Medical Center and Rancho Los Amigos Hospital has shown the second and third advantages to be as true today as 137 years ago. Review of the literature shows mixed acceptance of this amputation. Alldredge and Thompson[1] stated that it should never be performed in patients with diabetes, peripheral vascular disease, or neurotrophic foot problems. However, they believed that good results could be obtained in most other patients with proper selection of cases and proper surgical techniques. Sarmiento[13] reported 50% revision to a higher level in Syme amputations in diabetic and dysvascular patients. McKeever[10] related satisfactory experience in a large series of military amputees. "For a male, the Syme amputation is the best possible amputation stump in the lower limb." Most authors report satisfactory experience with the procedure and conclude that the stump is ideally suited for weight bearing and lasts virtually the life of the patient when surgery has been performed properly.[2,3,8,9,11] Several authors believed it was not a good amputation for women because of their aversion to the appearance of the prosthesis. Hunter[7] and Shelswell[14] concluded that Syme amputations should not be performed in a pulseless foot. There are a few references to its use in the dysvascular patient and most of these are small series.[4,9,12,18] Srinivasin[16] reported twenty cases performed for leprosy and points out that a Syme stump can last with proper care even in an insensitive foot.

THE CLASSICAL SYME AMPUTATION

Harris[5,6] of Toronto has published two erudite articles that describe the history, development, and technique of the Syme amputation. Except for trauma or a congenital defect that might dictate the selection of different flaps, no deviation is recommended.

Indications

The classical one-stage Syme amputation is indicated in all circumstances in which this level is the most distal effective amputation that will heal primarily. It is generally not used in patients with infection or ischemia. For infection the two-stage Syme procedure is preferred. Trauma about the foot, congenital anomalies, tumors, and deformities that necessitate amputation of the foot are best treated by the Syme amputation.[1,2,5,6,8,9,14,20] Since modern Syme prostheses are comfortable, durable, and cosmetically acceptable, this level is equally useful in men and women. Healthy plantar heel skin is a necessary prerequisite for the Syme amputation. In recent years the Syme level has gained popularity and assumed a justifiable and important place in major amputations through the lower extremity.

Technique

The incision (Fig. 22-1) begins at the tips of the malleoli, goes up across the ankle joint and then straight down across the sole. The anterior tendons are pulled down, divided, and allowed to retract. Arteries are transfixed and large veins ligated. Small vessels are electrocoagulated. The mediolateral collateral ligaments are divided at their insertion into the body of the talus, allowing it to dislocate (Fig. 22-2). Care must be taken on the medial side not to damage the posterior tibial nerve and artery. Dissection of the os calcis is started subperiosteally on the dorsal and lateral surfaces (Fig. 22-3). This allows gradual exposure of the flexor hallucis longus tendon, which is just lateral to the artery and nerves and aids in their protection. The continued subperiosteal dissection medially pushes the vital structures from the body of the os calcis. Division of the Achilles tendon must be done carefully so that the posterior skin is not buttonholed. Continued stripping of the os calcis distally completes the removal of the foot. The tourniquet is released and hemostasis secured. Mediolateral tendons are pulled down, divided, and allowed to retract. Opinion is divided as to the need to remove the plantar muscles. At Rancho Los Amigos Hospital they are left in place.

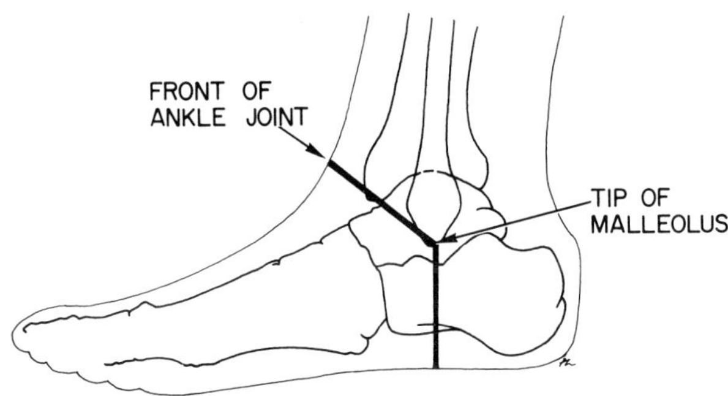

Fig. 22-1. Incisions for classic Syme amputation start at tips of malleoli. Upper arm goes directly across ankle joint. Lower arm goes directly across sole.

The malleoli and about 1 cm of the anteroposterior tibia are exposed subperiosteally. Transection of the tibia and fibula are performed at right angles to the long axis of the weight-bearing line. The weight-bearing surface thus becomes parallel to the floor. To obtain the broadest surface, the cut is made so that the dome of the plafond is left with about 1.5 cm of cartilage (Fig. 22-4). The heel flap is now folded up into place for measurements, and the bones are palpated through the soft tissue. Any possible pressure points are smoothed with rongeurs. If the flap is too large, a full-thickness wedge is removed from the distal edge. On rare occasions bone must be removed to allow closure without tension. No attempts should be made to trim the dog ears, since the vascular supply to the flaps might be endangered.

Migration of an imperfectly anchored flap has been a problem. Various methods have been de-

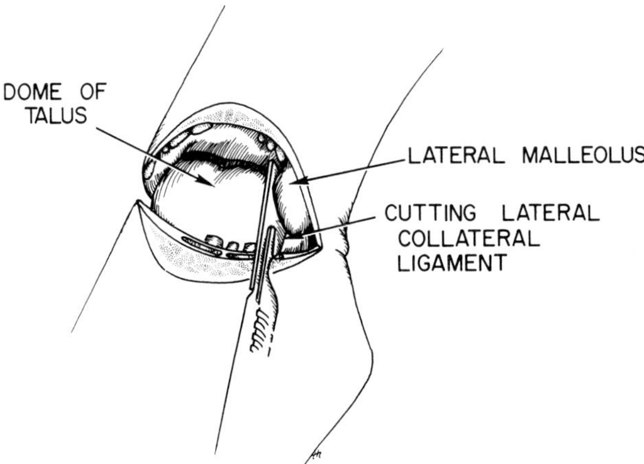

Fig. 22-2. Medial and lateral collateral ligaments are divided, allowing talus to dislocate. (See also Figs. 22-8 and 22-9.) Care must be taken not to cut posterior tibial nerve and artery on medial side.

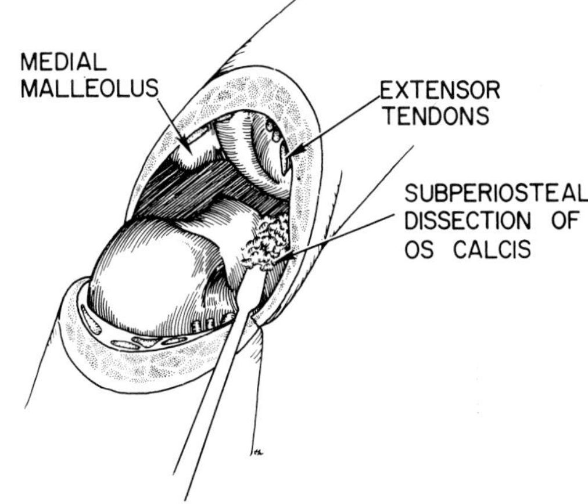

Fig. 22-3. Subperiosteal dissection of os calcis begins on lateral and dorsal surfaces. Septa of heel pad are not cut through. Intact septa maintain hydraulic effect of enclosed fat.

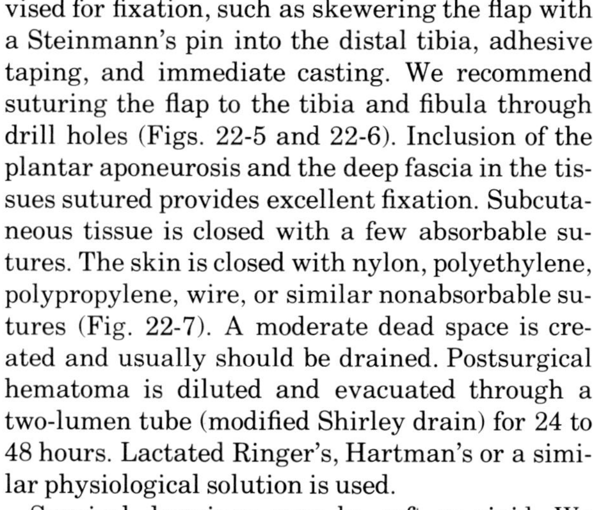
vised for fixation, such as skewering the flap with a Steinmann's pin into the distal tibia, adhesive taping, and immediate casting. We recommend suturing the flap to the tibia and fibula through drill holes (Figs. 22-5 and 22-6). Inclusion of the plantar aponeurosis and the deep fascia in the tissues sutured provides excellent fixation. Subcutaneous tissue is closed with a few absorbable sutures. The skin is closed with nylon, polyethylene, polypropylene, wire, or similar nonabsorbable sutures (Fig. 22-7). A moderate dead space is created and usually should be drained. Postsurgical hematoma is diluted and evacuated through a two-lumen tube (modified Shirley drain) for 24 to 48 hours. Lactated Ringer's, Hartman's or a similar physiological solution is used.

Surgical dressings may be soft or rigid. We have found no advantage to immediate ambulation and have allowed 7 to 10 days healing before applying a weight-bearing plaster.

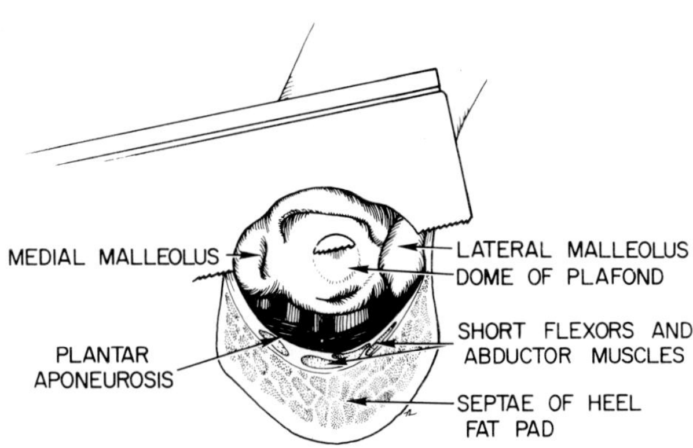

Fig. 22-4. Care must be taken to cut tibia at right angles to weight-bearing line of leg. Cut must be low enough to leave flare of tibia, which is important in suspension of prosthesis.

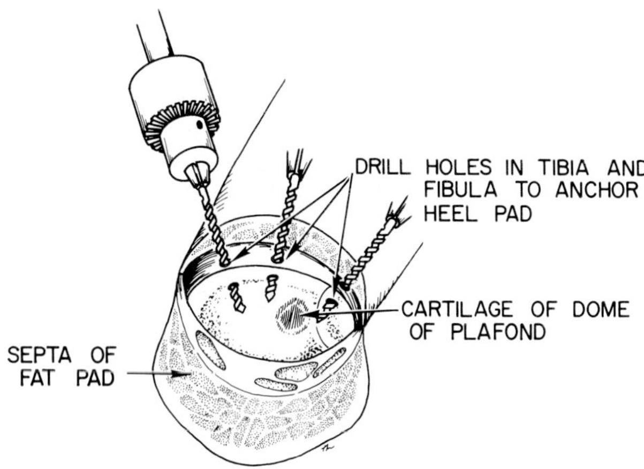

Fig. 22-5. Drill holes are made around periphery of tibia and fibula to anchor heel pad.

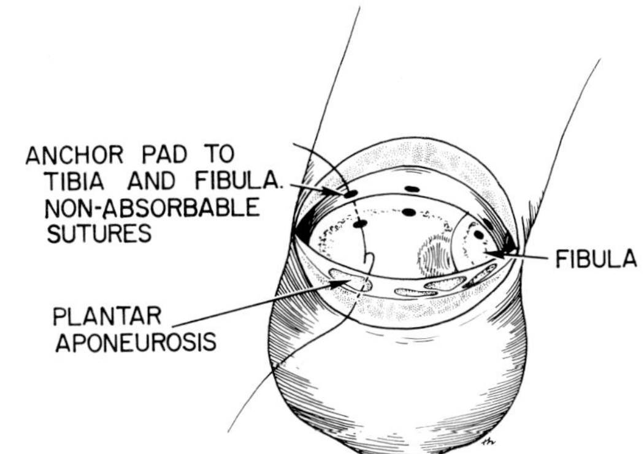

Fig. 22-6. Nonabsorbable sutures are placed through drill holes and into plantar aponeurosis and other fascial structures of heel pad.

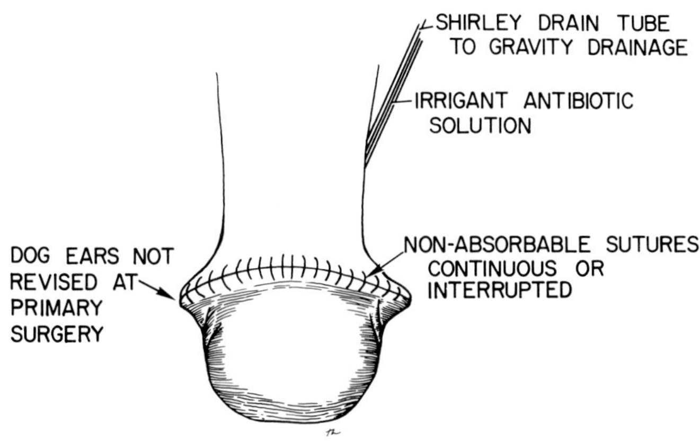

Fig. 22-7. Closed stump with irrigation system to remove hematoma and debris. Dog ears are not trimmed because posterior blood supply to flap may be disturbed.

THE TWO-STAGE PROCEDURE

The Syme amputation frequently failed in dysvascular and infected patients. The superior function at the Syme level pushed the search for a method to allow its use in infected patients. Spittler et al.[15] related their experience with Hulnick's two-stage procedure at Walter Reed Hospital. The infected forefoot was removed through disarticulation at the ankle. Virtually 100% of these patients healed, and the definitive amputation was performed 6 to 8 weeks later.

This technique was first adapted to the diabetic foot at the Los Angeles County General Hospital in 1954 and at Rancho Los Angeles Hospital in 1969. Experience, improvement of technique, and refinement of clinical indications gradually led to a 70% success rate. In 1970, a post-tourniquet reaction time was added. If the distal skin bled within 3 minutes, the healing rate was around 80%.

Present indications

The Syme amputation performed in two stages is indicated in patients who have gangrene or infection of the forefoot, are not suitable for a transmetatarsal amputation, and have not responded to medical treatment or distal surgical care. The ischemic index should be 0.45 or higher in the diabetic and 0.35 in others. The patient should be a prosthetic candidate. The heel pad should be intact. There should be no gross pus at the amputation site.

With the use of the ischemic index derived through transcutaneous Doppler ultrasound, the success rate now approximates 95% (Chapter 21).

First stage

Technique. To allow slightly longer skin flaps to cover the malleoli, the incisions are started 1 cm distal and 1 cm anterior to the tip of the malleoli (Fig. 22-8, *A*). The inferior incision courses directly down and across the sole, cutting all layers to the bone. The superior incision goes obliquely across the ankle joint. No planes are dissected. The tendons are pulled down, cut off, and allowed to retract. The dorsalis pedis artery is ligated with a transfixing suture. The joint is entered across the dorsum of the talar neck. The mediolateral collateral ligaments are divided alternately, allowing the talus to be dislocated (Fig. 22-8, *B*). Care must be taken not to cut blindly along the medial malleolus because the neurovascular bundle may be damaged at this point (Fig. 22-9). Subperiosteal dissection is started on the superolateral surfaces of the os calcis. A bone hook is driven into the body of the talus for trac-

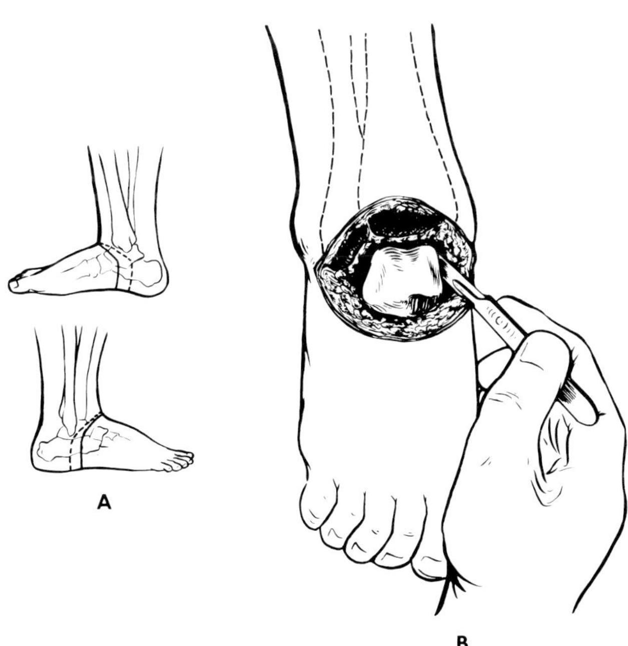

Fig. 22-8. A, Incision for two-stage technique is 1 to 1.5 cm more distal than classical Syme amputation to allow for volume of malleoli. **B,** Collateral ligaments are divided side to side to allow talus to dislocate distally.

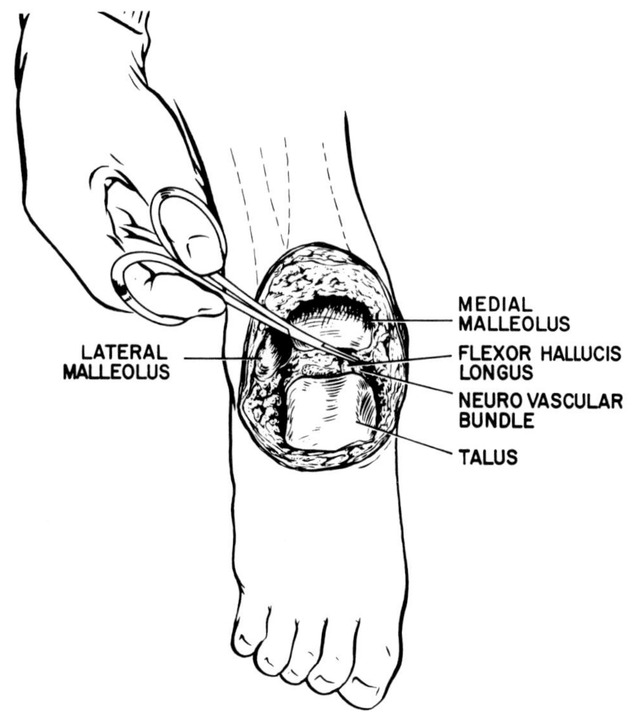

Fig. 22-9. Scalpel must not be pushed in too far on medial side. Exposure of flexor hallucis longus identifies lateral limit of neurovascular bundle and aids in its protection.

tion on the ligaments and control of the foot during dissection (Fig. 22-10). Direct vision of the neurovascular bundle allows transection distal to the division into mediolateral plantar branches. Continued dissection distally allows medial retraction of the bundle and medial dissection of the os calcis. Care must be taken with division of the Achilles tendon at its attachment to the os calcis where it is virtually subcutaneous (Fig. 22-11). Penetration of the skin has led to failure of the amputation. Division of the plantar aponeurosis and subperiosteal dissection of the os calcis medially complete the excision of the forefoot.

The tourniquet is released at this point, and timing is started. Larger arterial bleeders are transfixed. Larger veins are ligated. Smaller vessels are coagulated. Bleeding is then assessed. If the most distal skin does not bleed within 3 minutes, serious consideration should be given to going to the next higher level. If there is no bleeding in the flap distally at 5 minutes, then the Syme procedure should be abandoned and the amputation carried out at the below-knee level. A Shirley drain is modified for irrigation and gravity drainage. The air filter is removed, and an intravenous tubing set is attached. The tip of the drainage tube is cut on a bevel. A forceps is pushed through the soft tissue under the posterior tibiofibular ligament, then out posteriorly along the fibula and through a stab wound about 10 cm above the ankle joint. The tube is then drawn into the cavity (Fig. 22-12). Irrigation is started with 1 L of Ringer's lactate solution with 50,000 units of bacitracin and 500,000 units of Polymyxin per 24 hours.

Closure. The heel pad is tested by folding it against the malleoli and plafond. If it is excessive in length, skin and tissue should be removed until it closes with little or no tension. On occasion, the pad may shift medially or laterally due to a fascial band pressing against one or the other of the malleoli. Division of the band and incision of the fat pad to provide a "nest" for the malleolus will hold the pad centered. Deep fascia over the anterior tibia and the remnants of the collateral ligament are sutured to the deep fascia of the sole. A few subcutaneous sutures will level the skin edges. The skin is closed with nylon, polypropylene, or similar suture (Fig. 22-13). A compression dressing of fluffs is contoured over the stump and wrapped in place with bias-cut stockinette.

Drainage from the Shirley tube is collected in a urine bag or similar container. Every 2 to 3 hours the exit tube is clamped for 5 minutes to distend

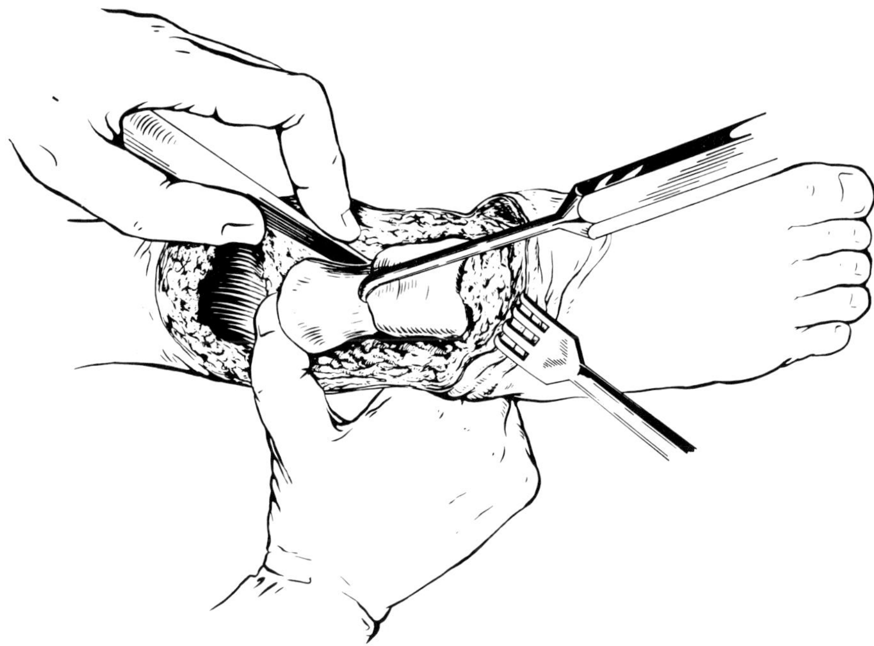

Fig. 22-10. Subperiosteal dissection of os calcis preserves fibrous septa of fat pad and hydraulic mechanism of heel in weight bearing. Bone hook aids in traction and control of foot during surgery.

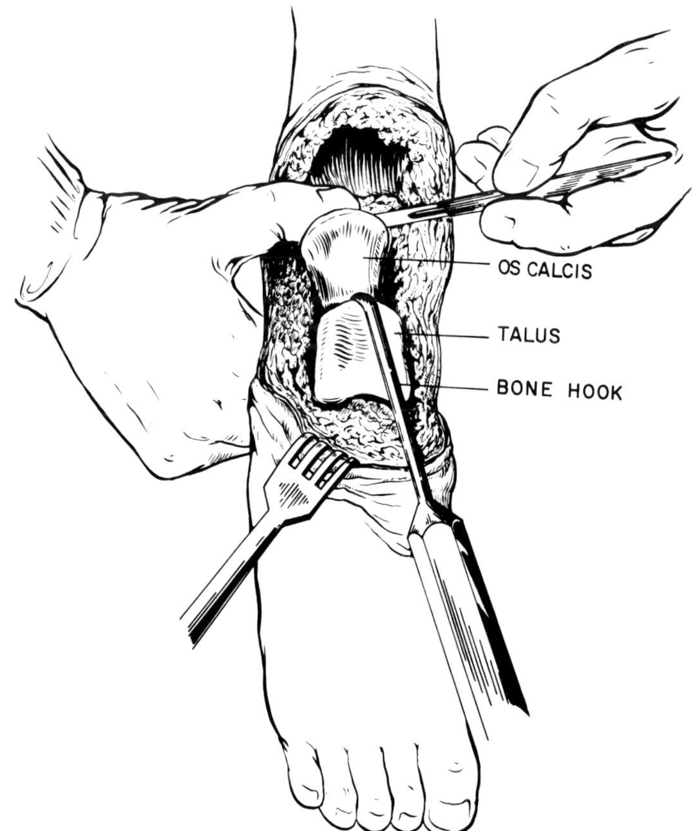

Fig. 22-11. Care must be taken not to buttonhole skin when dividing Achilles tendon, which is almost subcutaneous at this point.

the cavity with irrigating fluid. Irrigation is continued for 48 to 72 hours, depending on the degree of preoperative infection. The postoperative clinical course is also watched, and if there is fever or signs of local infection, the irrigation is continued. On occasion the system has been left in place for 7 to 14 days. On removal, the tip is cut off aseptically and sent for culture and sensitivity studies. Systemic antibiotics are continued according to preoperative cultures for 1 week, un-

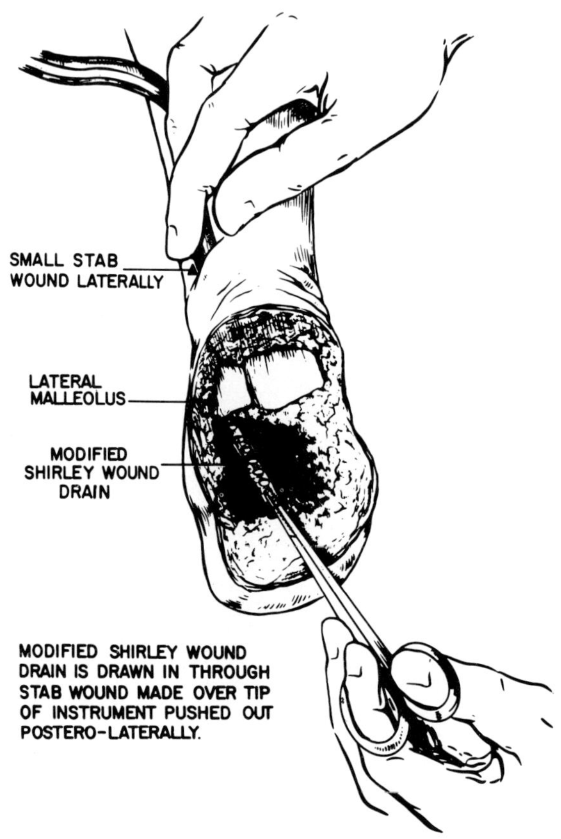

Fig. 22-12. Irrigation drainage of large residual cavity is with two-lumen Shirley sump drain. No suction is used; drainage is to gravity collection system. Irrigation is through tube normally used for allowing air to enter when used as abdominal drain. An antibiotic solution is used if the foot has been infected.

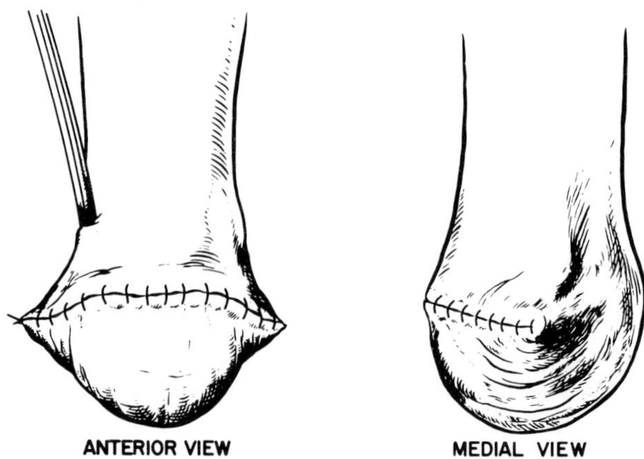

Fig. 22-13. No attempt is made to tailor dog ears at closure of first stage. Further posterior dissection narrows base of flap and jeopardizes its circulation.

less the clinical course or late culture shows the presence of bacteria.

On removal of the tubing the stump is wrapped in plaster. Care must be taken not to fold the dog ears and create pressure areas. Two fairly thick pieces of felt with holes cut in for the malleoli work well to protect them. When the patient is clinically stable, crutch ambulation is allowed. Weight bearing is begun for those who have a firm heel pad, good skin turgor, and no signs of residual infection. About 50% of the patients are weight bearing after the first stage, while awaiting the second stage.

Second stage

Healing is usually secure enough at 6 weeks to perform the definitive amputation. Occasionally, a week or more in a walking cast is needed. An occasional patient will be infected and will require debridement and removal of the malleoli to allow closure over an irrigation system. If healing does not occur rapidly, a below-knee amputation is performed.

Technique. Two elliptical incisions are made over the malleoli to remove the dog ears (Fig. 22-14). The amount of tissue removed should be equal to the volume of the malleolus. Care must

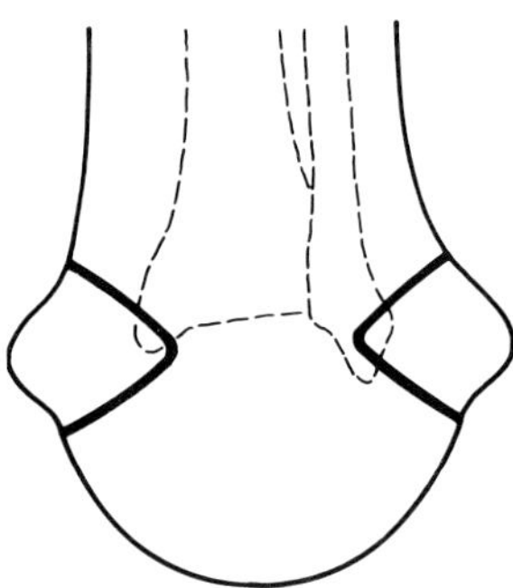

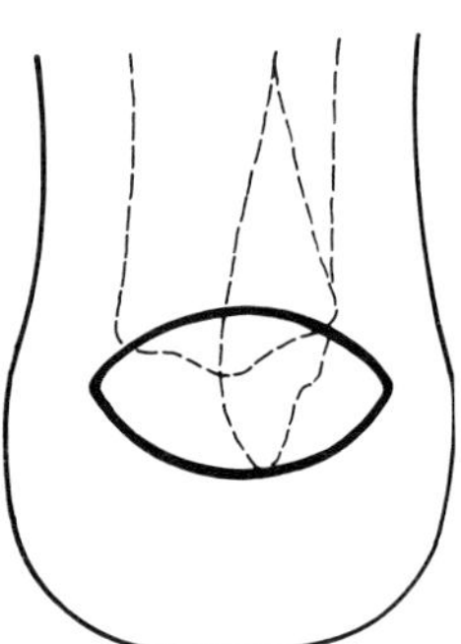

Fig. 22-14. Second-stage Syme amputation. Elliptical incision removes tissue equal in volume to bone removed.

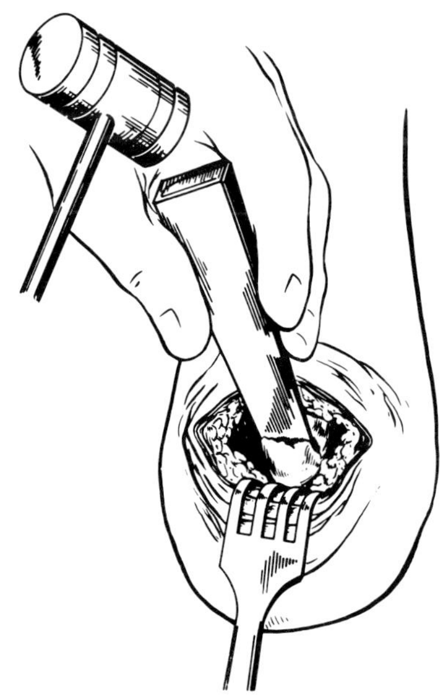

Fig. 22-15. Second-stage Syme amputation. Malleoli are removed flush with joint surface. Central cartilage is not disturbed.

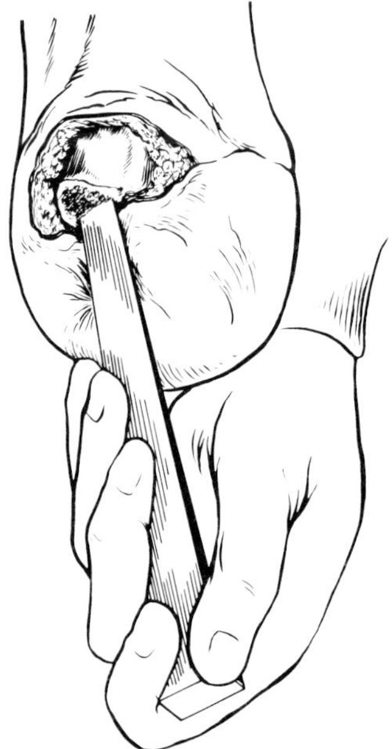

Fig. 22-16. Second-stage Syme amputation. Flare of tibia and fibula removed to narrow stump, remove potential pressure point, and flatten sides.

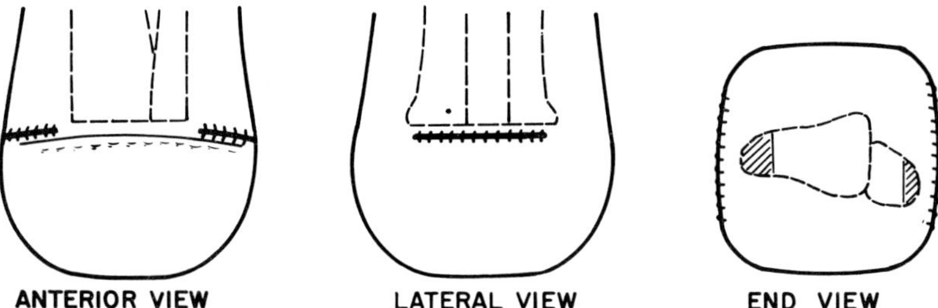

Fig. 22-17. Second-stage Syme amputation. Removal of malleoli and distal flare through lateral and medial incisions.

be taken on the posteromedial aspect not to damage the posterior tibial nerve and artery. Close dissection around the medial malleolus will protect the neurovascular bundle. After subperiosteal dissection, the malleoli are cut flush with the joint surface (Fig. 22-15). The fat pad is partially adherent to the central cartilage that is left intact.

The malleoli are dissected subperiosteally to approximately 3 cm above the joint line. The flare is then removed parallel with the shaft (Fig. 22-16). This leaves the anterior and posterior flares for suspension and a moderate narrowing and flattening of the sides of the stump (Fig. 22-17). Closure is important in that the pad must be anchored to bone. The deep fascia of the sole is clamped to the periosteum, and the pad is tested. If it is too loose, soft tissue must be removed from the ellipses until the pad is tight. It is then sutured through two drill holes in the tibia and fibula as well as to the periosteum. A few subcutaneous sutures level the skin, which is closed with nonabsorbable suture. Soft dressings are used for a few days and then replaced with plaster. Weight bearing is begun at 10 to 12 days.

POSTOPERATIVE CARE

On discharge from the hospital, the patient is usually independent in a walking cast. He is observed in the outpatient clinic, and casts are changed at 2-week intervals. The warning is given to stop weight bearing and to return immediately if any pistoning should occur due to stump shrinkage. At about 8 weeks the stump has matured, and the first prosthesis is fabricated. The plaster cast has been an invaluable aid as it mobilizes the patient, aids in the musculovenous pump action of the leg, protects the healing wound, and controls and maintains apposition of the heel pad.

The Gait Laboratory, under the direction of Dr. Perry, has performed function tests that show the Syme amputee to have greater stride length, faster cadence (Fig. 22-18), greater velocity, and to consume less oxygen per meter traveled (Fig. 22-19) than patients with more proximal amputations.[19]

> On these grounds, I think amputation of the ankle joint may be advantageously introduced into the practice of surgery. I regret having cut off many limbs that might have been saved by it, and shall be glad if what has been here said in its favour encourages others to its performance.
>
> James Syme, 1843

Section II

Prosthetic management

RICHARD VONER

Amputation at the ankle has challenged the prosthetist since the procedure was first introduced by Syme in 1842. Surgical modifications have been introduced to make the stump neater and less bulky, allow more room for the ankle joint, and produce a more cosmetic prosthesis.

A satisfactory end-bearing Syme limb demands a prosthesis with the following characteristics:

1. Transmission of body loads
2. Light enough to wear comfortably
3. Ability to supply the equivalent of foot and ankle function
4. Lengthening of the limb to adjust for loss of the talus and os calcis
5. Distribution of the high forces developed in the ankle area
6. Provision of rotary stability about the long axis
7. Provision of shock absorption
8. Suspension during swing phase

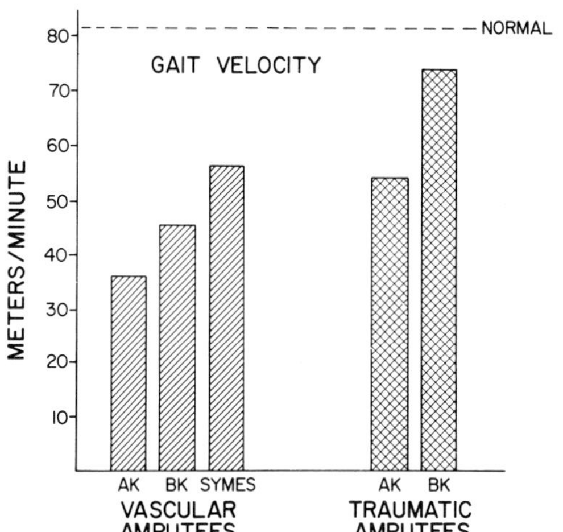

Fig. 22-18. Gait analysis of dysvascular amputees contrasted with young traumatic amputees. Syme amputation superior to below-knee and above-knee levels in gait velocity. Young traumatic amputees show value of saving knee by their superior function with below-knee level.

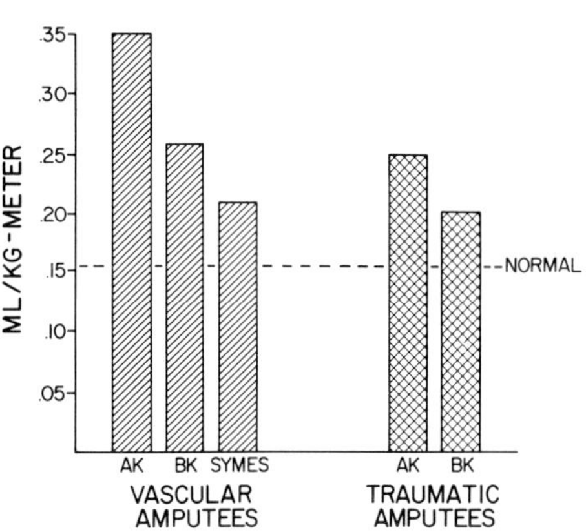

Fig. 22-19. Oxygen consumption per meter walked is true net energy cost and is excellent comparison of gait efficiency of various amputation levels.

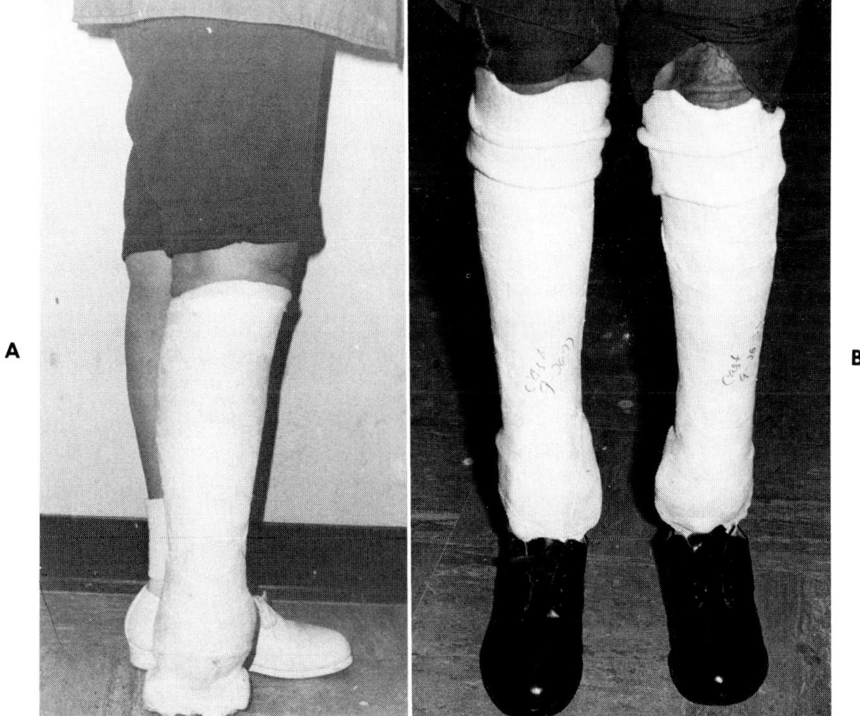

Fig. 22-20. A, Total-contact cast with walking heel for early ambulation. Cast extends to PTB area to aid in control of rotation. Cast is trimmed lower in popliteal space to allow adequate knee flexion. Suspension is obtained from distal tibiofibular flares. Walking heel height is adjusted to correct leg length discrepancy. It is used in selected cases after stage one and in most cases after stage two. B, Casts for bilateral Syme amputees are fitted with prosthetic feet to assist in anteroposterior and mediolateral balance.

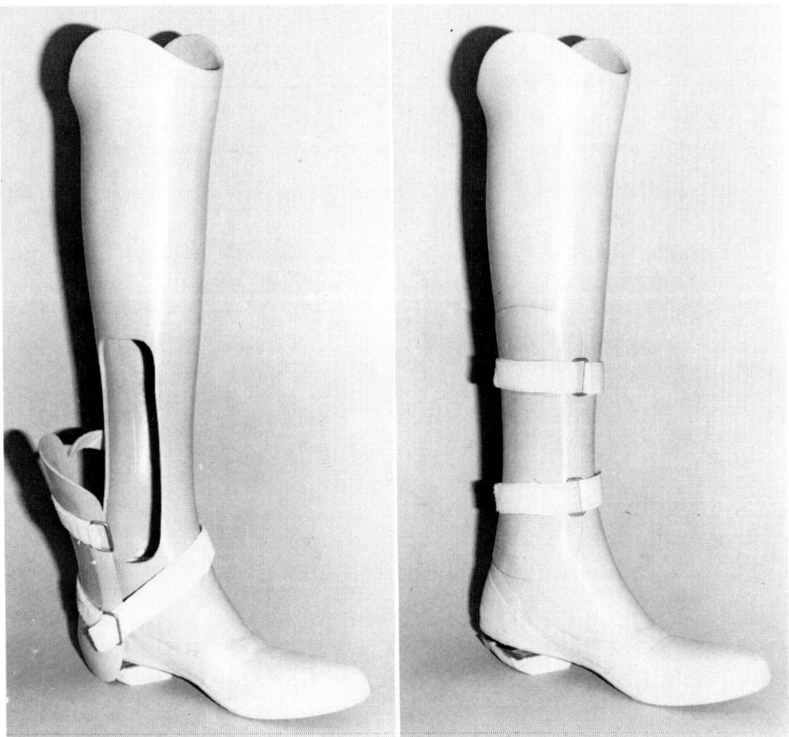

Fig. 22-21. Canadian-type Syme prosthesis as modified by Veterans Administration Prosthetic Center.

9. Readily donned without requiring multiple noncosmetic, difficult fasteners
10. Adjustability to relieve pressure along a sensitive scar line
11. Cosmesis

Despite the advantages provided by the long lever arm of the essentially intact tibia and fibula and the virtually full end-bearing capabilities of the heel pad, multiple problems still exist in the design of the "ideal" prosthesis. Reports in the literature of "new prosthetic approaches" attest to the fact that the final perfect prosthesis has not yet been designed.[1,3,4,5,7,8,9]

In addition to producing the artificial limb, the prosthetist may aid in postoperative management by applying walking casts. These protect the tissues during the healing phase and hasten contouring of the stump (Fig. 22-20).

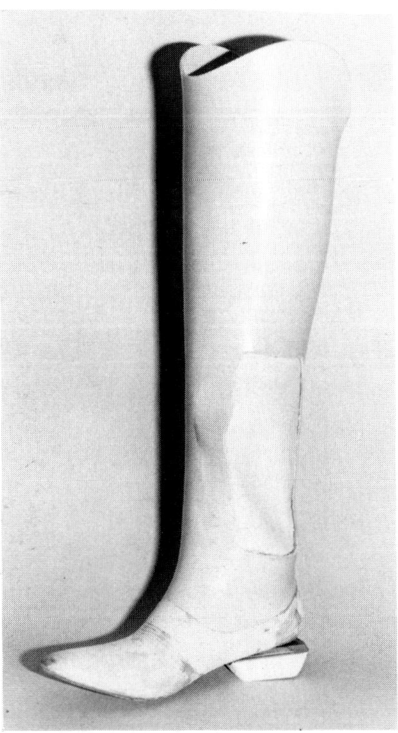

Fig. 22-22. Modification of medial-opening Syme prosthesis, which incorporates panel of expandable rubber. This allows expansion during donning and retraction for suspension about flare of distal tibia. Removable window is thus eliminated.

SOLUTIONS TO PROBLEMS INHERENT IN THE DESIGN AND MANUFACTURE OF SYME PROSTHESES

Weight and bulkiness

Until 1940, the usual prosthesis was a leather socket reinforced with steel straps and with an anterior tongue and lacer.[10] The ankle was frequently a single-axis joint with bumpers. Early use of polyester-fiberglass laminate with an opening for entry of the residual limb materially reduced bulkiness. However, to increase the strength of the socket, it was necessary to substitute epoxy resins for the polyesters before adequate strength was obtained. A prosthesis of this type was developed and is being used by the Canadian Department of Veteran Affairs.[1,10] It is commonly called the "Canadian Syme prosthesis" (Fig. 22-21).

Reproduction of ankle joint motion

Articulated joints and compressive members were unsuccessful due to space limitations. Decreased space also limits the degree of shock absorption that can be afforded the Syme amputee with the SACH foot. The volume of shock-absorbing material is increased by eliminating the ankle joint and using the greatest possible volume of sponge rubber cushion. In the SACH foot, the contour of the inferior surface and the radius at the end of the keel provide a substitute for motion at the end of push-off or roll-off.[2,3]

Provision for donning

Provision for donning is necessary to allow the bulbous distal end to pass the narrow shank portion of the prosthesis.

Following are some of the methods of providing the different diameters:

1. Older prostheses had an anteriorly opening corset that could be laced.[10]
2. Plastic prostheses have windows either medially, posteriorly, or posteromedially (Fig. 22-22).[1,3,10]
3. Closed double-wall prostheses with flexible inner walls allow expansion so that the bulbous end is inserted past the expandable portion.[4] The elasticity is sufficient to close about the end and provide suspension (Fig. 22-23, *A* and *C*). A double wall with an elastic panel also provides enough expansion (Fig. 22-23, *B*).
4. A flexible inner socket of Kemblo rubber, Silastic foam, or similar material bridges the narrow portion of the stump above the heel pad and maintains a total-contact, stump-socket wall relationship (Fig. 22-24).

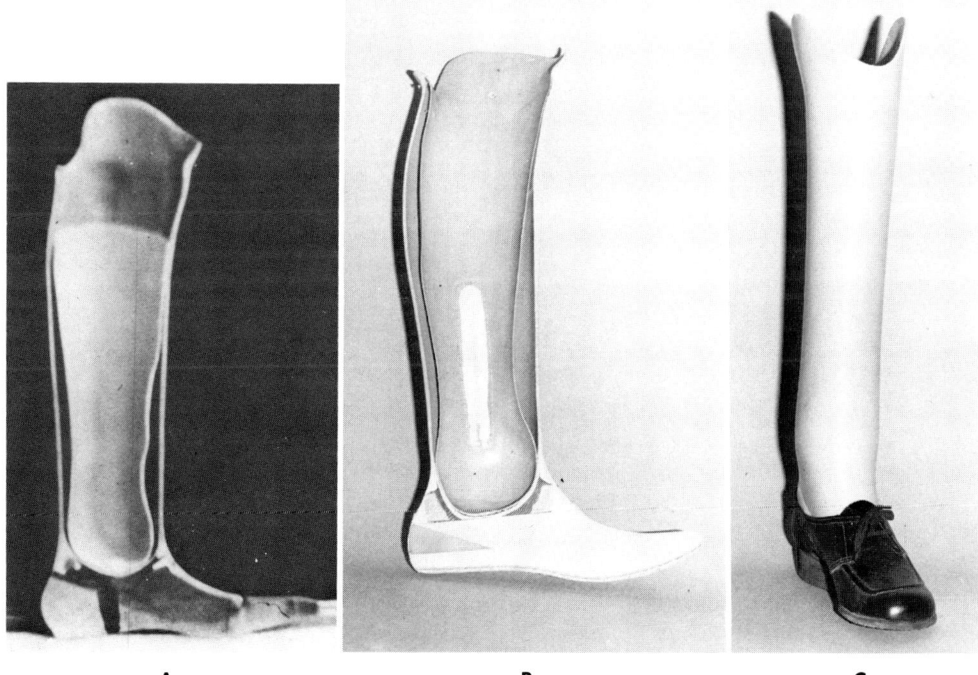

Fig. 22-23. A, Double-wall prosthesis with elastic liner has advantage of requiring no window and thus no buckles, straps, or other devices. Greater strength is possible with less material, and there is also smoother cosmetic finish while total-contact suspension is still maintained. **B,** Double-wall elastic panel type of prosthesis also eliminates removable window of conventional prosthesis. Elastic panels may be varied in size and width to accommodate various sizes of terminal stumps. **C,** Finished windowless prosthesis with internally expanding panel and external keel SACH foot.

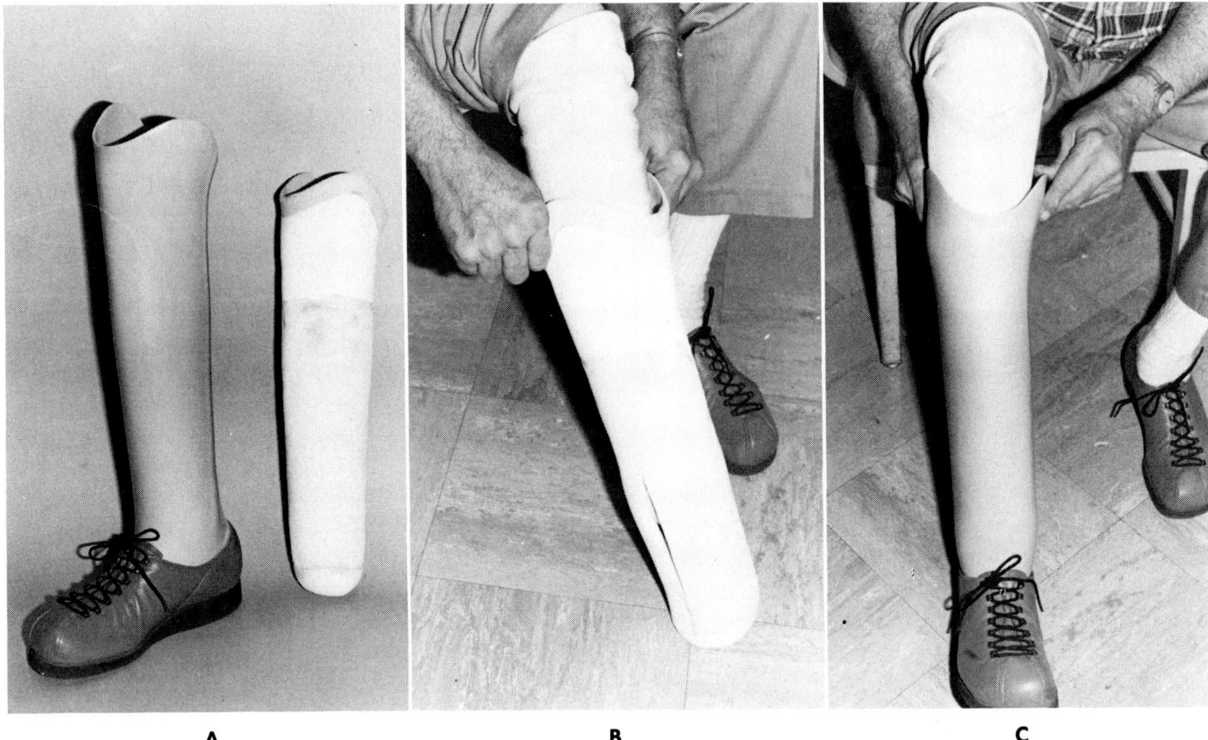

A B C

Fig. 22-24. A, Single-wall Syme prosthesis with insert that is expandable and supplies suspension through friction. **B,** Donning suspension insert. **C,** Donning single-wall prosthesis over expandable insert.

Distribution and absorption of stresses developed during stance phase

Uniform distribution of loads along the tibia is necessary during push-off or rollover. Careful molding is necessary along the tibial crest. High forces in the ankle area require sufficient material to absorb the stress. Because of the bulbous form, there will be a certain bulky appearance to any prosthesis design. There is a constant problem then between thickness requirements for strength and thinness required for appearance. Strength is most easily obtained by using high strength-to-weight ratio plastics that can be molded easily over a plaster positive model.[6]

Provision of rotary stability about the long axis

A patellar tendon–bearing shape of the proximal brim will stabilize against the mediolateral flares of the tibia. Flattening of the posterior brim adds to a triangulation effect.

Provision of pressure relief along a sensitive scar line

Direct end bearing can be reduced by proximal loading of the prosthesis along the tibial flares.[5]

Provision of suspension during swing phase

The bulbous distal end and the flare of the tibia and fibula provide sufficient surface. The contour of the distal socket must be in intimate contact with the residual limb in its most bulbous portion. If the distal end is especially narrow and has minimal flare, a suprapatellar suspension strap may be added.

Provision of shock absorption

The cushioned heel of the SACH foot is smaller than in an above-knee or below-knee prosthesis. A good share of the impact force is dissipated in the heel, but some load must be assumed by the knee, which flexes just after heel contact.[6]

Sweating in a plastic prosthesis

Porous plastic laminates have been introduced but have not proven completely satisfactory to date. Substitution of several layers of prosthetic socks may provide better moisture distribution.

Cosmesis

Plastic laminates provide a thinner wall. Air-cushion types, which require no window, and double-walled types, with an inner elastic panel, are less unsightly because they require no straps, buckles, or other outside paraphernalia for closure. However, they are thicker just above the ankle (Figs. 22-23, *C*, and 22-24, *C*).

Relief over bony prominences

The use of 0.3-cm (1/8-inch) adhesive felt patches applied before casting appears to be superior to modifications made on the male mold.

Correction of limb-length discrepancy

A thinner SACH foot must be used for the Syme amputation than that used for below-knee or above-knee amputations. Because of this, it is not always possible to use as thick a heel cushion as desired for shock absorption. In bilateral amputees, this is not a problem and such improvements as a five-way ankle may be used.

Comfortable transmission of stump-socket forces through a satisfactory socket

Socket design must provide the following:

1. Stabilization against rotary forces about the long axis. Three-point or triangular stabilization against the flares of the tibia plus a flattening across the posterior portion of the gastrocnemius will provide a good share of stability. In the two-stage method, the distal stump is squared slightly. This possibly aids in preventing rotation about the long axis.
2. Weight support can be distributed between the end of the prosthesis and the proximal portion of the socket brim. Dispersion of forces against the proximal surface of the leg at push-off can be accomplished through careful fitting against the mediolateral surfaces of the tibia.
3. Dispersion of force encountered at heel contact is accomplished through contact from the heel to the upper gastrocnemius. The cuplike contour for the stump end must extend superiorly enough to prevent motion between the socket and the stump in an anteroposterior direction.[6]

PROSTHETIC CONSIDERATIONS

Indications for each of the described types of prostheses will depend primarily on the physical characteristics of the residual limb. Most patients can be fitted with a closed double-wall prosthesis with attached flexible inner walls fabricated with expandable material. The closed rigid shell with a flexible removable inner socket may allow even earlier donning of the limb without undue difficulty. The closed prosthesis presents a much neater appearance and is particularly desirable for women.

When the amputation has a bulbous and irregular distal end, often seen in older amputees and after trauma, it may be necessary to fabricate one or more windows in the prosthetic shell to allow the terminal tissues to slide past the smaller and narrower proximal area. The prosthetist may need to innovate and deviate from standard designs in certain unusual circumstances. Almost without exception all prostheses will be fitted with the SACH foot described earlier.

Surgeons performing the Syme amputation can often simplify prosthetic considerations by careful attention to bone contour and heel-pad positioning. Improvements in design and materials have allowed amputees using old style prostheses to convert successfully to the modern limbs now available.

PHYSICAL THERAPY

The Syme amputee has usually walked in a plaster cast with a rubber heel or artificial foot prior to delivery of the definitive prosthesis. Virtually no training is required during the cast period except for occasional use of crutches or a pickup walker at the outset.

After delivery of the prosthesis, instructions are given for donning and doffing. In addition, the patient is taught stump hygiene, use of prosthetic stockings, and daily maintenance of the prosthesis. Most patients state that it will take a day or 2 to get used to the limb.

SUMMARY

Modern plastic materials and construction techniques permit manufacture of Syme prostheses, which are improved in appearance and durability, lighter in weight, free from malfunction of mechanical components, and simpler and less costly to manufacture.

REFERENCES

Surgical procedures

1. Alldredge, R. H., and Thompson, T. C.: The technique of the Syme amputation, J. Bone Joint Surg. **28**:415, 1946.
2. Baker, G. C. W., and Stableforth, P. G.: Syme's amputation. A review of sixty-seven cases, J. Bone Joint Surg. **51B**:482, 1969.
3. Catterall, R. C. F.: Syme's amputation by Joseph Lister after sixty-six years, J. Bone Joint Surg. **49B**:144, 1967.
4. Dale, G. M.: Syme's amputation for gangrene from peripheral vascular disease, Artif. Limbs **6**:44, 1961.
5. Harris, R. I.: Syme's amputation, J. Bone Joint Surg. **38B**: 614, 1956.
6. Harris, R. I.: The history and development of Syme's amputation, Artif. Limbs **6**:4, 1961.
7. Hunter, G. A.: Results of minor foot amputations for ischaemia of the lower extremity in diabetics and nondiabetics, Can. J. Surg. **18**:273, 1975.

8. Lindqvist, C., and Riska, E. B.: Chopart, Pirogoff, and Syme amputations. A survey of twenty-one cases, Acta Orthop. Scand. **37:**110, 1966.
9. Mazet, R. R.: Syme's amputation, J. Bone Joint Surg. **50A:** 1549, 1968.
10. McKeever, F. M.: A discussion of controversial points—amputation surgery, Surg. Gynecol. Obstet. **82:**495, 1946.
11. Ratliff, A. H. C.: Syme's amputation: result after forty-four years. Report of a case, J. Bone Joint Surg. **49B:**142, 1967.
12. Rosenman, L. D.: Syme amputation for ischemic disease in the foot, Am. J. Surg. **118:**194, 1969.
13. Sarmiento, A., and Warren, W. D.: Re-evaluation of lower extremity amputations, Surg. Gynecol. Obstet. **129:**799, 1969.
14. Shelswell, J. H.: Syme's amputation, Lancet **2:**1296, 1954.
15. Spittler, A. W., Brennan, J. J., and Payne, J. W.: Syme amputation performed in two stages, J. Bone Joint Surg. **36A:**37, 1954.
16. Srinivasan, J.: Syme's amputation in insensitive feet, J. Bone Joint Surg. **55A:**568, 1973.
17. Syme, J.: Amputation at the ankle joint, London Edinburgh Monthly J. Med. Sci. **2:**93, 1843.
18. Warren, R., Thayer, T. R., Achenbach, H., and Kendall, L. G.: The Syme amputation in peripheral arterial disease. A report of six cases, Surgery **37:**156, 1955.
19. Waters, R. L., Perry, J., Antonelli, D., and Hislop, H.: Energy costs of walking of amputees: the influence of level of amputation, J. Bone Joint Surg. **58A:**42, 1976.
20. Wood, W. L., Zlotsky, N., and Westin, G. W.: Congenital absence of the fibula: treatment by Syme amputation—indications and techniques, J. Bone Joint Surg. **47A:**1159, 1965.

Prosthetic management

1. Foort, J.: The Canadian type Syme prosthesis. Lower extremity amputee research project, series 11, issue 30, Berkeley, Calif., Dec., 1956, University of California, Institute of Engineering Research.
2. Gordon, E. J., and Ardizzone, J.: SACH foot prosthesis, J. Bone Joint Surg. **42A:**226, 1960.
3. Marx, H. W.: An innovation in Syme's prosthetics, Orthot. Prosthet. **23**(3):131, 1969.
4. Mazet, R. Jr.: Syme's amputation, J. Bone Joint Surg. **50A:**1549, 1968.
5. Murdoch, G.: Syme's amputation, J. Royal Coll. Surgeons Edinburgh **21**(1):15, 1975.
6. Radcliffe, C. W.: The biomechanics of the Syme prosthesis, Artif. limbs **6**(1):76, 1961.
7. Romano, R. L., Zettl, J. H., and Burgess, E. M.: The Syme's amputation: a new prosthetic approach, Inter-Clin. Info. Bull. **11**(4):1, 1972.
8. Sarmiento, A., Gilmer, R. E., Jr., and Finnieston, A.: A new surgical-prosthetic approach to the Syme's amputation. A preliminary report, Artif. Limbs **10**(1):52, 1966.
9. Warner, R., Daniel, R., and Leswing, A. L.: Another new prosthetic approach for the Syme's amputation, Inter-Clin. Info. Bull. **12**(1):7, 1972.
10. Wilson, A. B.: Prostheses for Syme's amputation, Artif. Limbs **6**(1):52, 1961.

CHAPTER 23

Below-knee amputation

NEWTON C. McCOLLOUGH, III
ANNE R. HARRIS
FREDERICK L. HAMPTON

When amputation in the lower limb becomes necessary due to trauma, tumor, or disease, the importance of saving the knee joint cannot be overemphasized. For the young person, preservation of the knee joint means preservation of a near-normal life-style with minimal physical limitations. For the elderly amputee, saving the knee joint may well mean the difference between being able to walk or being confined to a wheelchair. Studies performed to compare the energy requirements of below-knee amputees to above-knee amputees in walking have consistently shown significantly greater demands at the above-knee level.[2,12,26] Gonzalez et al.[12] have further shown that significantly less energy costs are present with a long below-knee stump as compared to a short below-knee stump. Waters et al.[26] have also demonstrated that Syme amputees require less energy expenditure in walking than do other below-knee amputees.

The feasibility of performing a below-knee amputation as opposed to a higher level amputation will be determined by tissue viability in cases of trauma and by principles of tumor surgery when dealing with neoplasms. In the case of the dysvascular patient, below-knee amputation is not only feasible but is the level of choice in most instances, as attested to by many surgeons.[3,4,6,7,8,13,17,19,25] Healing rates of 80% to 90% for below-knee amputation performed for ischemia have commonly been reported.[1,6,14,24]

There is general agreement in the literature that mortality is lower following below-knee amputation than after above-knee amputation. This fact has previously been attributed to the poorer state of health of patients requiring above-knee amputation.[21] That this is not necessarily the case has been shown by Sarmiento and Warren.[25] They reported that the mortality rate fell dramatically from 24% to 10% in two large groups of patients, the only significant difference being a complete reversal of a 2:1 ratio of above-knee amputations to below-knee amputations.

SURGICAL MANAGEMENT

Level selection

Previous "sites of election" for amputation are no longer valid in modern amputation surgery. The surgeon should attempt to save all length possible consistent with tissue viability and healing capacity. The longer the below-knee stump, the greater will be its leverage, strength, and proprioceptive qualities, and the better the amputee will walk. The energy cost of walking will be less if a longer amputation stump is provided to the amputee.[12] On the other hand, a very short below-knee stump is far superior to a knee disarticulation, and satisfactory fitting with a below-knee prosthesis can frequently be accomplished at levels as high as the tibial tuberosity.

In the case of amputation for trauma, all length should be saved, which is consistent with principles of adequate and thorough debridement and with the known level of tissue viability. The amputation should be left open, and the final level will be determined by revision at the time of delayed primary or secondary closure. Proximal revision of the amputation with sacrifice of some length may be necessary to obtain full-thickness skin coverage over the distal end. However, a split-thickness skin graft may be used for closure of the very short below-knee stump rather than revision to a higher level. Modern prosthetic methods can frequently accommodate the scarred or grafted below-knee stump with minimal compromise of function.

Selection of site of amputation in the dysvascular patient should also be at a level of tissue viability that is compatible with healing. In our own experience, as well as in the experience of others, this level almost invariably falls within the proximal half of the leg, usually at the junction of the proximal and middle thirds, although it may be as high as the tibial tuberosity. Much has been written about various techniques to determine the level of amputation compatible with healing in the dysvascular patient. These techniques include such procedures as oscillometry, plethysmography, thermography, arteriography, ultrasound,[9] and radioactive isotope measurements of skin blood flow.[18] Although all of these procedures may be helpful to a degree in the preoperative evaluation, none is as reliable an indicator of circulation as is bleeding of the skin edges at the time of surgery.[6,17]

The patient should be informed preoperatively that as much of the limb as possible will be saved, depending on the level at which adequate circulation is found at the time of surgery. The limb is then draped to an above-knee level, and the site of amputation is determined by bleeding of the skin edges at the time of incision. A transverse incision is made over the pretibial area at the intended level of amputation. If bleeding of the skin occurs here, in the area of poorest blood supply, the surgeon may be relatively certain that the skin of the medial, lateral, and posterior aspects of the leg carries sufficient circulation to proceed with the amputation at that level. If adequate bleeding does not occur at the pretibial level, progressively more proximal incisions are made to determine the amputation site. If no bleeding of the skin edges is noted as high as the level of the tibial tuberosity after 3 minutes of observation, the surgeon should proceed to an above-knee amputation, since lack of adequate circulation at this level also precludes knee disarticulation.

It should be emphasized that the presence or absence of popliteal pulses has no bearing on the determination of amputation level below the knee. Burgess et al. have demonstrated consistent healing of amputations at the below-knee level in the presence of complete occlusion of the superficial femoral artery.[6]

Occasionally, in performing a below-knee amputation for vascular disease, the surgeon encounters good skin bleeding only to find that the musculature of the anterior tibial compartment is brownish or pale gray secondary to infarction. It is not necessary in this instance to carry out an extensive debridement of the dead muscle tissues, which would be likely to require excision of the entire anterior compartment and creation of a large dead space. If the skin edges have shown good evidence of bleeding, it is probable that primary healing will ensue, and the infarcted anterior tibial compartment tissues will proceed to fibrosis. On the other hand, if liquefaction necrosis of muscle groups has occurred, debridement is necessary, since the chance of infection in these tissues is great even with adequate skin circulation.[16,23] Revision of the intended amputation level to a higher level may be necessary if necrosis is extensive and involves more than one compartment.

Contraindications to below-knee amputation

The major contraindication to below-knee amputation is inadequate circulation for healing at the most proximal level, as previously described.

A second contraindication is in the nonambulatory patient with ischemia and flexion contracture of the knee. Such patients are usually senile and bedridden and will be better served by proceeding to a knee disarticulation or an above-knee amputation.

In the ambulatory patient with a dysvascular limb and flexion contracture of the knee, below-knee amputation may or may not be contraindicated. If the flexion contracture is severe (greater than 50 degrees) and the limb is ischemic, knee disarticulation should be the procedure of choice, although a very short below-knee amputation may be fitted as a knee disarticulation with a bent-knee prosthesis. If the contracture is 50 degrees or less, a short below-knee amputation should be done, since these patients can be fitted with a below-knee prosthesis with a flexed socket and thigh corset. In the younger patient with non-ischemic disease (e.g., osteomyelitis) and knee flexion contracture, the longest below-knee amputation possible should be done. The flexion contracture may then be resolved by operative or nonoperative means at a later date.

Amputation procedures

As in amputation at any level important general principles of surgery must be adhered to if a successful outcome is to be anticipated. These principles relating to the management of bone, muscle, nerve, vessels, and skin have been thoroughly discussed in Chapter 2 and will not be further elaborated on in this chapter. It should be emphasized, however, that the below-knee level of amputation is the *critical level,* particularly in the dysvascular patient, and strict adherence to principles of tissue management in these cases may well mean the difference between saving the knee joint or doing a later revision to an above-knee level.

Following are four below-knee amputation procedures that should be a part of the armamentarium of every amputation surgeon:

1. Equal anterior and posterior myocutaneous flaps
2. Long posterior myocutaneous flap
3. Equal medial and lateral flaps (sagittal incision)
4. Osteomyoplasty

All of these procedures should employ the principle of myoplasty so that the flaps formed are actually *myocutaneous* flaps with no dissection between tissue planes. There are indications and contraindications for each of these procedures, and the surgeon must determine the best procedure for the individual situation.

Generally, equal anterior and posterior flaps may be used routinely for the below-knee amputation. When the problem of ischemia exists, it may be desirable to use the long posterior flap operation, described by Ghormley[11] and popularized by Burgess,[5] which takes advantage of the superior posterior blood supply and eliminates the poorly vascularized anterior flap. The long posterior flap, however, necessitates some sacrifice in stump length, therefore it is not the procedure of choice in the absence of ischemia. The operation using medial and lateral flaps described by Persson[22] is also designed to eliminate the poorly vascularized anterior flap in ischemic cases. It may also be indicated when a recent longitudinal incision from failed vascular reconstruction procedures compromises the long posterior flap technique, or when the posterior calf skin as well as

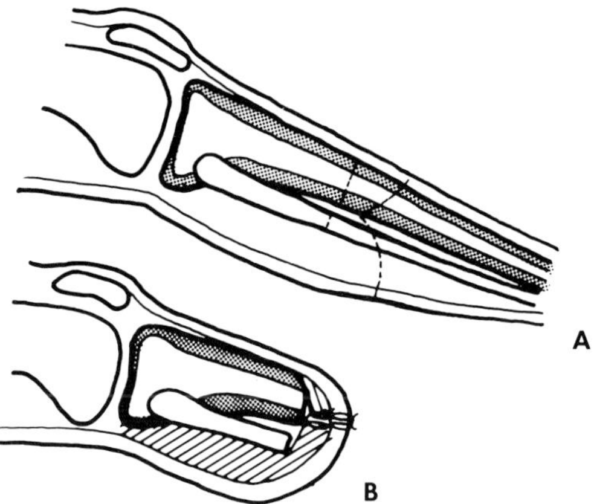

Fig. 23-1. A, Anterior and posterior flaps should be short and bone section slightly above level of flaps. **B,** Myoplastic closure with fibular cut slightly shorter than tibia.

the anterior skin is compromised. Osteomyoplasty as described by Loon[15] and originally developed by Ertl[10] is contraindicated in vascular disease, but may be indicated in young patients to provide a stronger stump with improved end bearing. This operation, advocated strongly by Murdoch[20] for routine use in younger patients, also has the disadvantage of sacrificing about 7.5 cm (3 inches) of stump length. In our opinion, it should be reserved for revisions of traumatic below-knee amputations that have occurred at the supramalleolar level.

Equal anterior and posterior myocutaneous flaps. Flaps are designed at a level thought to possess adequate vascularity for healing. Flaps in a dysvascular patient are purposely made short (Fig. 23-1, *A*), the apices of the incision being made no farther than 2.5 cm (1 inch) proximal to the end of the anterior and posterior flaps. The skin is incised first at the distal limit of the anterior flap. If adequate bleeding occurs from the skin at this level, the procedure is continued as described below. If the skin does not bleed, more proximal flaps are designed. The incision is at once carried through skin, subcutaneous tissue, fascia, and muscle around the circumference of the leg following the previously outlined flaps. Posteriorly, the incision is carried just deep to the gastrocnemius fascia, but anteriorly it is carried through the anterior tibial compartment muscles obliquely, superiorly, and posteriorly. The vessels are clamped and ligated following section. The periosteum of the tibia and fibula is incised transversely, and a periosteal elevator is used to elevate the tibial and fibular periosteum proximally with the anterior myocutaneous flap to a distance of approximately 2.5 cm (1 inch) above the apex of the previously designed flaps. At this point, the fibula is transsected with the Gigli saw. The tibia is similarly transsected at the same level, but in such a manner that the Gigli saw is pulled proximally to give a bevel as it approaches the anterior cortex. If preferred, a power saw may be used. It is most important that the soft tissues by retracted adequately to prevent injury during this stage. An amputation knife is then inserted between the ends of the divided bones, and the entire posterior compartment is divided with a cut that passes obliquely, distally, and posteriorly to merge at the previous level of incision in the gastrocnemius fascia. Vessels are clamped and ligated following section, and the posterior tibial nerve is drawn down, ligated, severed sharply with a knife, and allowed to retract. If a tourniquet has been used, it is released at this time, and meticulous hemostasis is achieved. The sharp corners of the beveled tibia are then smoothed carefully with a rasp. This is a most important part of the procedure because to have a well-healed stump break down over a sharp bony prominence is nothing short of a tragedy. The muscle and fascia of the anterior tibial compartment are then approximated to the posterior compartment musculature (Fig. 23-1, *B*). At more proximal levels, the surgeon must frequently trim out some muscle posterolaterally as well as anterolaterally to prevent a bulbous stump. After myoplastic closure, the subcutaneous tissues are then carefully approximated so that minimal tension is required on the skin sutures. The skin is then carefully approximated with a fine suture to gain accurate apposition of skin edges, which is particularly important in the dysvascular patient.

The resultant stump is one with short flaps in which no dissection has taken place between subcutaneous and muscle layers, thus preserving circulation to the skin from the deeper tissues. Because of the short flaps, there may be some tendency to formation of "dog ears," but these will atrophy readily and should not be excised.

Long posterior myocutaneous flap. This flap is designed as shown in Fig. 23-2, *A*, with the anterior incision being two thirds circumferential on each side and the lateral incision directed somewhat anteriorly and distalward to form the posterior flap. The usual level of the anterior incision is approximately 12 cm below the knee joint as described by Burgess.[6] The anterior incision passes at once through skin, subcutaneous tissue, and muscle, to bone. The tibia and fibula are sectioned with a power saw or a Gigli saw, if preferred, at the same level as the anterior incision, the fibula, being sectioned approximately 5 mm shorter than the tibia. An amputation knife is then used to section the deep posterior compartment muscles at the same level as the bone section, identifying and dealing with the neurovascular structures as they are encountered. The knife then passes in the plane between the deep posterior tibial compartment and the triceps surae muscle group distalward emerging through the gastrocsoleus group at the level of the distal posterior portion of the incision. Thus a single myocutaneous flap is formed without dissection between tissue planes. It may be necessary to excise a portion of the soleus muscle in some cases to reduce the bulk of the flap. The myocutaneous flap is then drawn anteriorly, and the gastrocsoleus muscles are sutured directly to the anterior compartment muscle and fascia and to the periosteum of the tibia medially. Any excess of skin and subcutaneous tissue is then trimmed, and the subcutaneous tissues are approximated carefully so as to reduce the tension on the skin sutures. The skin is then closed with lightweight sutures and careful approximation of skin edges. The completed amputation is diagrammed in Fig. 23-3, *B* and *C*.

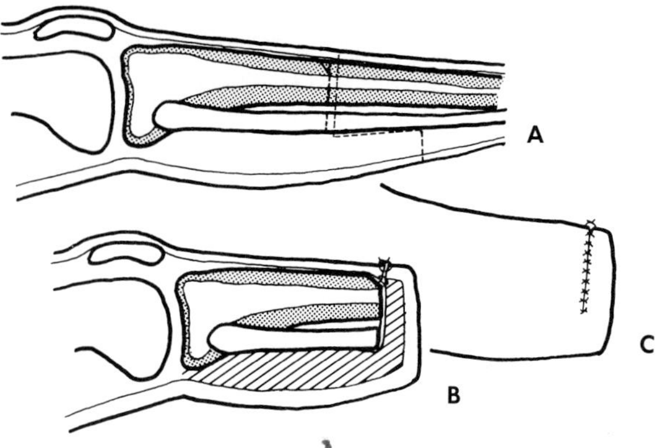

Fig. 23-2. A, Outline of skin flaps for long posterior flap amputation. **B** and **C,** Myoplastic closure using long posterior myocutaneous flap.

Equal medial and lateral flaps (sagittal incision). Medial and lateral skin flaps are outlined as illustrated in Fig. 23-3. Distance from the anterior and posterior apices of the incision to the most distal end of the flaps should not exceed 3 cm in vascular cases. The incisions are deepened through the subcutaneous tissue and muscle with

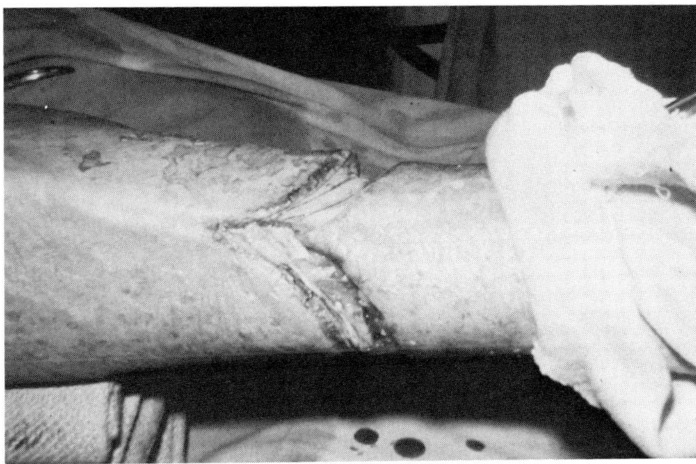

Fig. 23-3. Medial and lateral skin flaps for sagittal amputation.

no dissection between layers so as to form myocutaneous flaps. As the incision is deepened through the muscular layers, the knife is directed somewhat proximally so as to produce a beveled muscle flap. The periosteum is elevated from the tibia to a level slightly superior to the original anterior apex of the skin incision. The fibula is likewise exposed to a similar level. The tibia and fibula are then divided with a power saw, the fibula being cut slightly shorter than the tibia. The posterior portion of the medial and lateral muscular incisions can then be completed, with the surgeon identifying and dealing with the neurovascular structures as they are encountered. (Fig. 23-4). The tibia is then beveled. It is important to make a very oblique bevel, since failure to do so will result in a tibial prominence in the line of the anterior portion of the incision. Persson[22] advocates a 45-degree cut through the entire tibia, instead of a bevel on the anterior cortex. In our opinion, however, this diminishes the end-bearing circumference of the tibia by eliminating the anterior cortex, and a long oblique bevel that does not extend through the anterior cortex into the medullary canal is preferred. After hemostasis has been secured, the medial and lateral muscle flaps are sutured to each other over the cut ends of the tibia and fibula (Fig. 23-5). Subcutaneous tissues are carefully approximated so as to reduce the tension on the skin sutures, and the skin is closed with an interrupted fine suture. The completed amputation is shown in Fig. 23-6.

Osteomyoplasty. Osteomyoplasty requires the use of osteoperiosteal flaps approximately 7.5 to

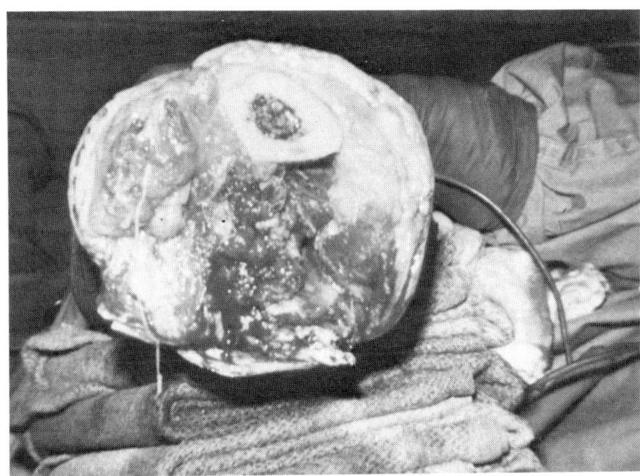

Fig. 23-4. Completed sagittal amputation showing medial and lateral myocutaneous flaps.

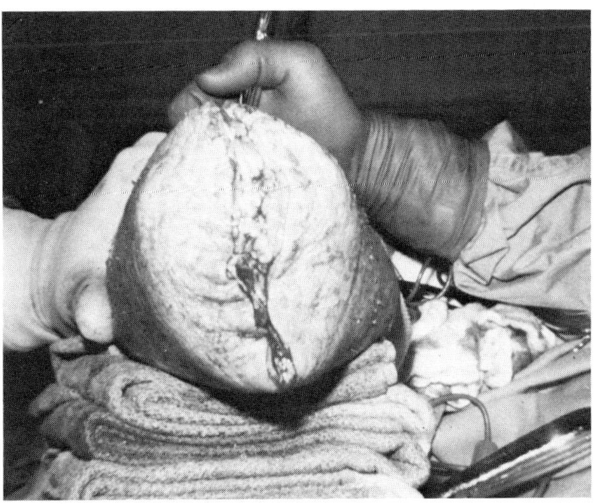

Fig. 23-5. Myoplastic closure in sagittal amputation.

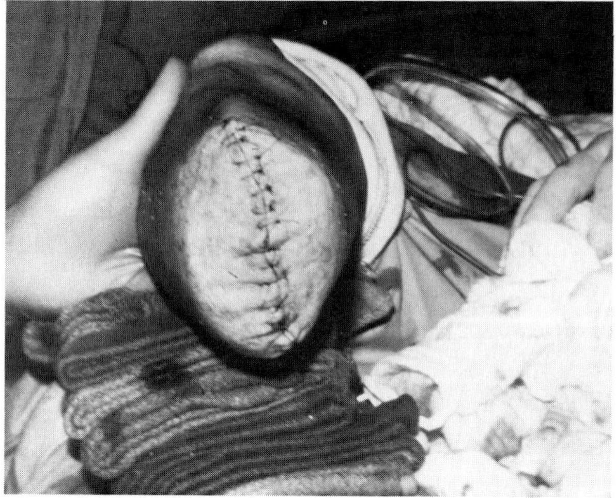

Fig. 23-6. Completed sagittal amputation.

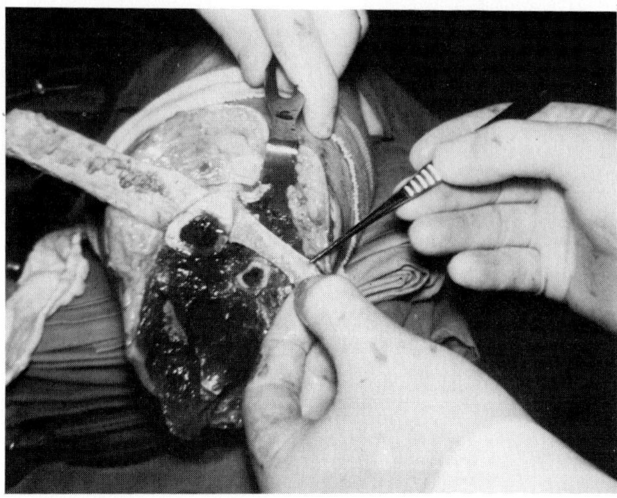

Fig. 23-7. Osteoperiosteal flaps raised from tibia for osteomyoplastic amputation.

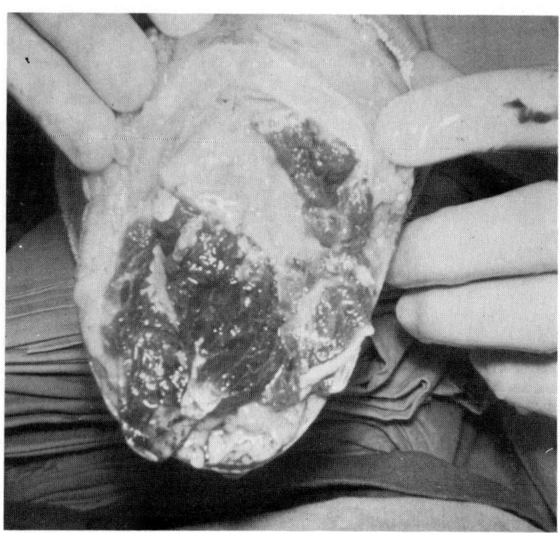

Fig. 23-8. Completed osteoperiosteal bridge between tibia and fibula.

10 (3 to 4 inches) in length, raised from the tibia distal to the level of bone section for the amputation. Therefore it should not be used in amputations in the proximal half of the leg because the sacrifice of length produces an unnecessarily short amputation stump. The procedure is also contraindicated in vascular cases, since the extra time involved and the details of technique are not well tolerated by devitalized tissues.

Conventional anterior and posterior flaps are outlined, and myocutaneous flaps are formed by avoiding dissection between the subcutaneous tissue and muscle and cutting the anterior and posterior musculature obliquely in a proximal direction. It is most important not to cut the periosteum inadvertently as the anterior incision is made. After the myocutaneous flaps have been developed down to the periosteum of the tibia and fibula, the distal musculature is stripped extraperiosteally from the tibia and fibula for a distance of approximately 10 cm (4 inches) and excised. Two osteoperiosteal flaps are then raised, one from the anteromedial aspect of the tibia and one from the lateral aspect of the tibia. These flaps should be approximately 2.5 cm (1 inch) in width, and elevation is accomplished with a very sharp osteotome to the level of intended bone section (Fig. 23-7). The tibia and fibula are then divided at a level just below the hinge of the osteoperiosteal flaps. The level of fibular section is approximately 5 mm more proximal to the level of tibial section. Nerves and vessels are dealt with appropriately and hemostasis secured, after which the lateral osteoperiosteal flap is then reflected on itself and sutured to periosteum and fascia on the medial side of the fibula. The anteromedial osteoperiosteal flap is then brought over the distal end of the tibia and fibula and sutured to the periosteum and fascia on the lateral aspect of the fibula. The two osteoperiosteal flaps are then sutured to one another, completing the periosteal tube bridging the two bones. (Fig. 23-8). The anterior and posterior muscle flaps are now sutured together, forming a myoplasty over the osteoplasty. Closure of the subcutaneous tissue and skin is then performed in routine fashion.

An osseous bridge then develops between the tibia and fibula and is usually visualized radio-

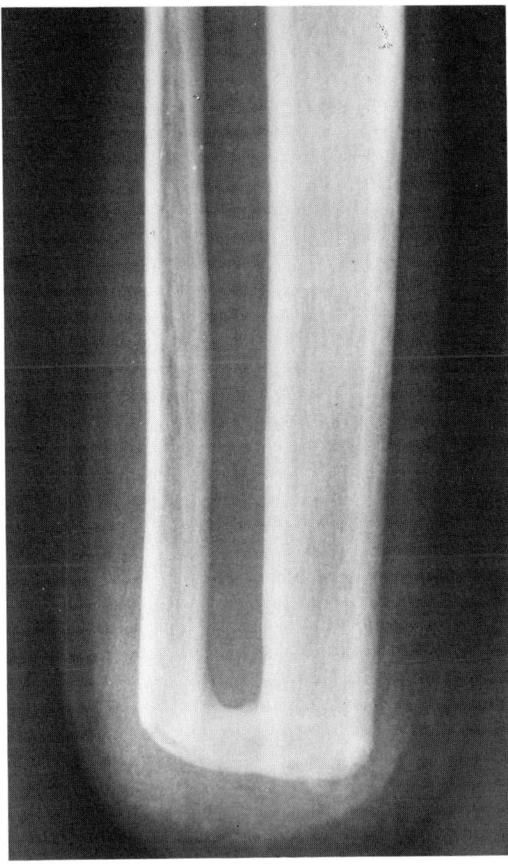

Fig. 23-9. Roentgenogram of bone bridge 5 months after osteomyoplastic amputation.

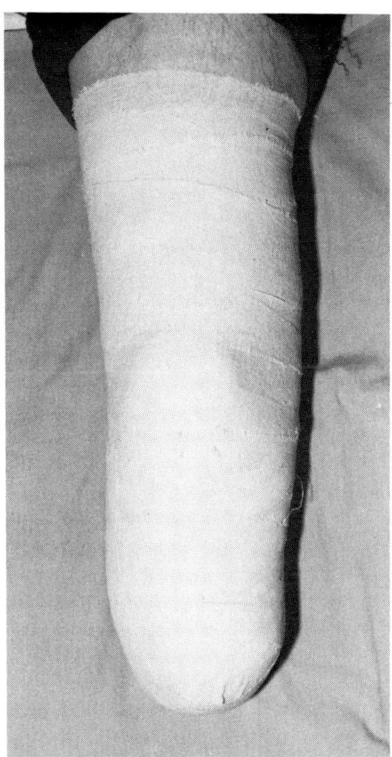

Fig. 23-10. Unna paste below-knee semirigid dressing.

graphically in 8 to 10 weeks (Fig. 23-9). The formation of the bridge is believed to stabilize the fibula and to improve the end-bearing characteristics of the below-knee amputation stump. Postoperative care in no way differs from routine postoperative care, and immediate or early prosthetic fitting may be used.

Postoperative management

After surgical wound closure, standard practice for many years has been to apply sterile soft dressings with compressive bandaging to control postoperative edema and bleeding. The residual limb is elevated with the knee extended. The dressings are changed periodically for wound inspection and adjustment of pressure from the bandages.

This long established soft tissue dressing technique has a number of signicant disadvantages. Pressure at the amputation site varies, depending on the skill of bandage application and the experience of the surgeon or therapist. Even when carefully supported in place, there is a tendency for proximal constriction to occur, producing terminal edema. Moving about and changing positions in bed cause discomfort. Reflex muscle spasm draws the knee into flexion, with loss of quadriceps tone and strength. The residual limb is painful to handle, large amounts of analgesic medication are often required, and the undesirable generalized sequelae of immobilization and sedation are harmful, especially in the elderly frightened and apprehensive patient. Change of dressing becomes a fearful and unpleasant ordeal. Pain patterns thus established can continue for months and delay rehabilitation.

Rigid dressings. Modern postsurgical management should provide a rigid dressing encompassing the operative site and the residual limb to the mid or upper thigh level with the knee in extension. A variety of rigid and semirigid dressing techniques are available, including preformed metal, fiberglass, or polymer splints. A posterior plaster of Paris splint or a bivalved circular plaster cast provides a similar degree of support. Semirigid dressings fabricated from Unna paste (Fig. 23-10) and similar materials also can be used (Fig. 23-11).

A compressible interface material is placed about the site of the amputation following sur-

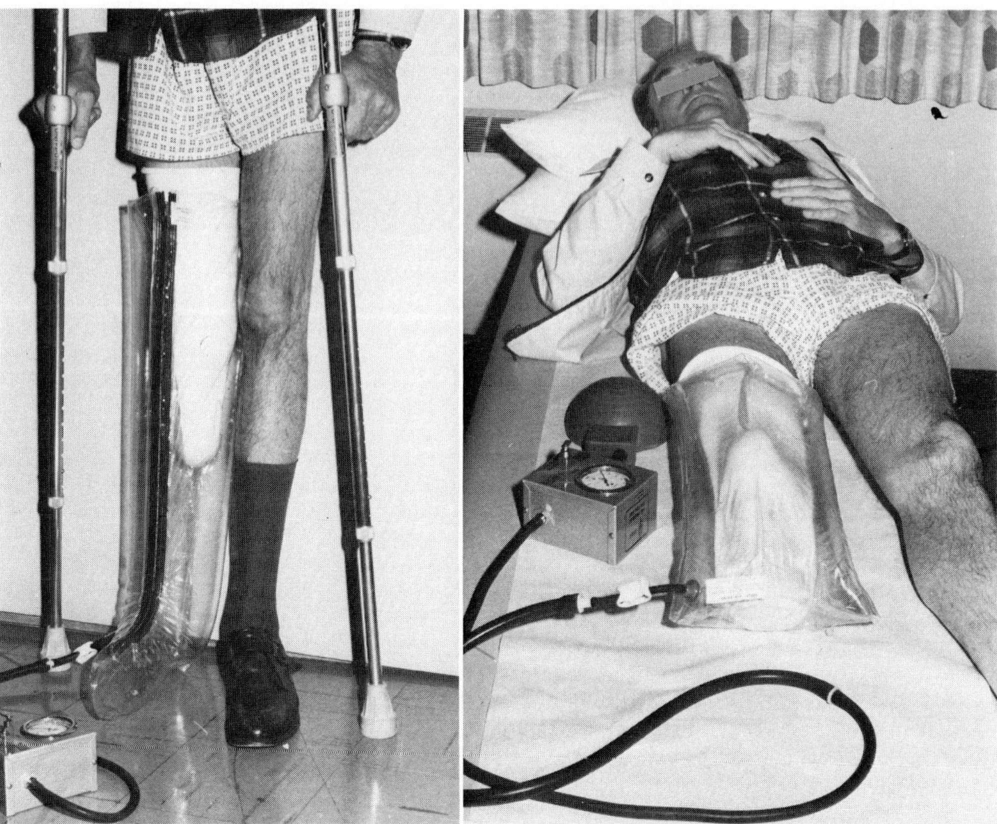

Fig. 23-11. Air splint immediate postsurgical dressing bag.

gery to maintain gentle wound pressure during early healing. This type of pressure interface, similar to that used in hand and foot surgery, can be simple fluffed gauze, lamb's wool, or a variety of other materials. Sterile reticulated polyurethane foam is an inexpensive and useful pressure dressing. Whatever material is used, it should not retain fluids or heat. The wound surface should be dry and permit the free exchange of air. For this reason, foam rubber, occlusive plastic dressings, and similar materials should not be used. Wound-healing potential is marginal in the ischemic limb. The postsurgical wound environment is particularly critical when tissue viability is poor. Optimum postsurgical wound management is mandatory under these circumstances.

The rigid dressing technique, properly applied, avoids proximal constriction and provides terminal wound support. The dressing must be properly suspended so that it does not fall away from the operative site with resulting loss of terminal pressure. Suspension can be accomplished by proper molding of the dressing about the knee and also by suspension using a light waist belt with suspensory straps attached to the dressing. This postsurgical system promotes comfort and allows the patient to move about freely in bed and up in a chair. Knee flexion contractures do not develop, and early leg exercise can be initiated with comfort.

The rigid dressings are usually left intact for a week to 10 days before being changed, unless it is necessary to remove a drain. Self-assistance and overhead trapeze and general body exercises are encouraged from the day of surgery.

Some surgeons complain that the rigid dressings prevent frequent inspection of the wound. Actually this is an advantage because frequent wound dressings do not necessarily promote healing; in fact, they may disturb the healing process. If complications develop they will be evident by both local and general physical signs and complaints.

Immediate postsurgical prosthetic fitting. The postsurgical rigid dressing can be used as an initial prosthetic socket to permit restricted early ambulation (Fig. 23-12). This system of management has been developed and popularized by

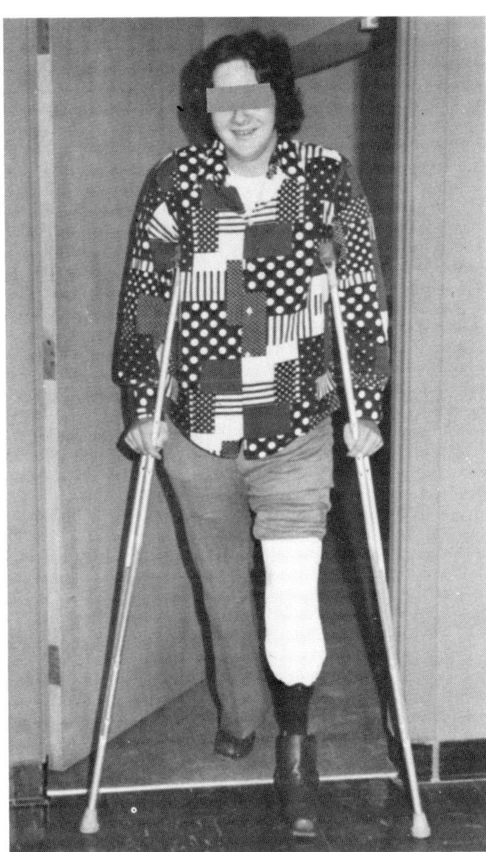

Fig. 23-12. Immediate postsurgical below-knee rigid dressing with temporary prosthetic unit.

Burgess in the United States and Weiss and Berlemont in Europe. The now-standardized below-knee technique uses a single layer of a fluid permeable sterile dressing over the wound site, such as Owens silk with a small amount of fully fluffed gauze sponges over which a sterile properly sized Orlon closed-end stump stocking is placed to the upper thigh level. A sterile polyurethane end pad is then applied. Relief pads are provided for pressure-sensitive areas along each side of the anterior tibia and over the patella, the limb is encased in an elastic plaster cast with pressure applied distally, but with care, to avoid proximal constriction as the cast is extended up to the junction of the middle of the thigh. While the plaster sets, it is contoured about the condyles of the knee to provide suspension, also suspension straps are used with a pelvic belt to properly support the cast so that it does not fall away with loss of distal wound pressure. A light temporary terminal weight-bearing device is used. This is detachable when the patient is not standing.

The immediate postsurgical fitting system provides sterility at the wound site, a rigid support with the knee in extension, appropriate pressure relationships and early limited ambulation under supervision. It presents an excellent wound healing environment, as well as the psychological benefits of an early functional device. It also allows the patient early mobility, thus avoiding generalized complications, especially in the elderly.

When this method was introduced there was undue emphasis on the early weight-bearing and walking aspects of treatment. Wound breakdown and healing failures resulted from undue early wound stress. It must be emphasized that no weight bearing or attempted ambulation should be carried out until early wound healing is assured. For that reason, especially in the geriatric patient, present management minimizes or eliminates weight bearing until the first cast change, which is usually 10 to 14 days after surgery. The well-vascularized wound, as in the case of trauma, tumors, and congenital amputations, tolerates the early light weight bearing, and these patients can begin early ambulation, often the day after surgery. Thus weight bearing must be very carefully monitored either by a balance scale system of training or an audible load-cell warning incorporated into the temporary prosthesis.

Immediate postsurgical prosthetic management has met with outstanding success at the below-knee amputation level when the surgeon adheres strictly to the recommended technique. It is particularly applicable to amputee centers in which personnel can be trained in its use and its full benefit exploited. The interest generated by the IPSP method has beneficially affected amputee rehabilitation generally and made the surgeon aware of his continuing responsibility to the rehabilitation process until maximum function has been restored.

Controlled environment treatment and related air bag pressure dressings. Since amputation surgery involves the most distal part of the limb, it allows a degree of control of the surrounding physical environment during healing that is not permissible with other extremity surgery. This is particularly true with the application of pressure. Since no tissue remains beyond the operative site, the influence of pressure on the healing wound can be localized, calibrated, and monitored without concern for viability and possible damage to more distal limb tissues.

Air and other gas mixtures are used in a closed polyvinyl transparent bag encompassing the limb

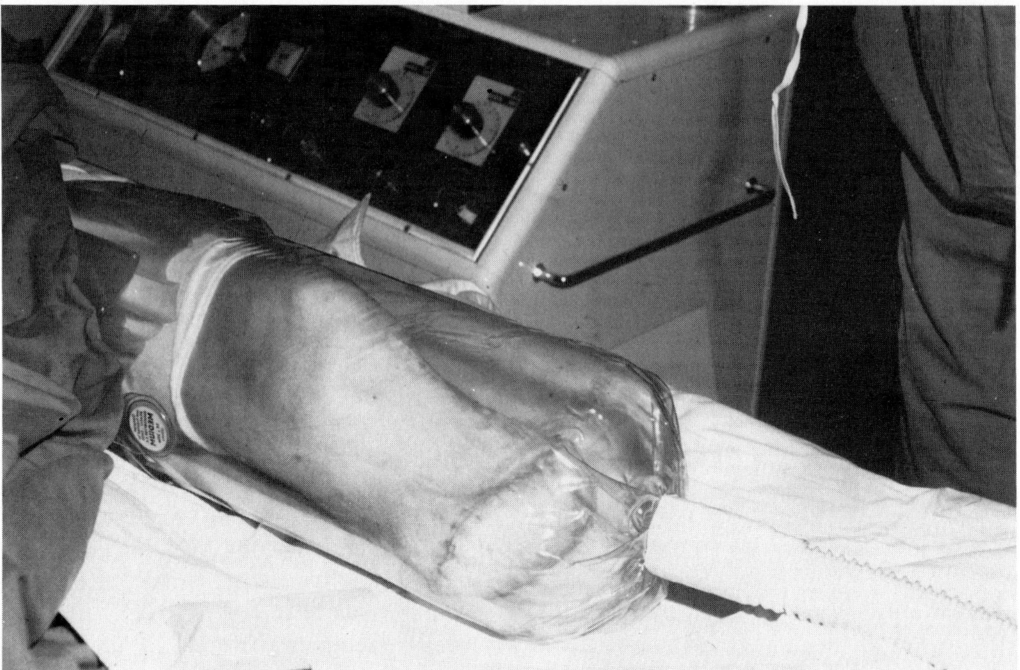

Fig. 23-13. Controlled environment treatment postsurgical system.

(Fig. 23-13). This postsurgical dressing was developed at the British Research and Development Unit, Roehamptom, England, and has been used for postsurgical amputation dressings in the United States by Burgess and his associates. In addition to controlling pressure on the amputation site, the environment also controls temperature, humidity, and sterility. The air within the bag is not static but flows through to vent proximally. The flutter-type (Hovercraft) proximal seal ensures an even amount of pressure within the bag and eliminates the possibility of proximal pressure constriction.

A number of modifications of the controlled environment treatment are commercially available. Since the operative site can be visualized and palpated through the bag without disturbing sterility, the surgeon has the added advantage of observing the wound at all times. Reports on the controlled environment treatment are encouraging and indicate that wound healing proceeds in a quiet and uneventful manner within this environment and that pain appears to be substantially reduced. The closed environment treatment for wounds is also being used for hand surgery, burns, skin grafts, extremity fractures and sprains, and a variety of other circumstances. As development and experience proceed with this system of postamputation management, it may find a wide area of use.

REHABILITATION

Preprosthetic management

Rehabilitation of the below-knee amputee should ideally be initiated preoperatively. This can have a rewarding and permanent effect on the prospective amputee both physically and emotionally.

The patient should be evaluated at this time as to functional abilities before amputation so that realistic goals can be set postoperatively. The preoperative evaluation should cover pertinent medical problems (such as previous stroke, poor cardiac status, visual difficulties, contractures, vocational history, and premorbid ambulatory status).

Preoperatively, the patient should be familiarized with the procedures and activities to be performed after amputation. Instruction should be given in proper bed and wheelchair positioning and exercises to be executed, as well as the rationale for such treatment. If possible, the patient should be taught ambulation techniques with the appropriate external support. The patient should also be introduced to the type of prosthetic device to be used postoperatively. Frank discussion should be carried out regarding the approximate level of function to be achieved, the type of prosthesis to be used, the length of time before receiving the final prosthesis, and the events that will transpire in the interim. If there is to be a period of several days before surgery, the patient should begin a maintenance program of exercises and ambulation to prevent debilitation.

After amputation, the individual should again be evaluated by the physical therapist, a preprosthetic program instituted, and intermediate goals set.

The evaluation should encompass the entire individual and his capabilities and not just the amputation site. The individual should be evaluated both in the recumbent position and dynamically as to his skill in functional activities, such as in walking and transfers. Muscle strength, endurance, balance, and coordination should be assessed. Any change from the preoperative status should be noted.

After the individual has been thoroughly evaluated, a treatment plan and goals should be set. For the purpose of this discussion, the program outlined will be for a unilateral below-knee amputee not undergoing immediate postsurgical ambulation. This technique is discussed in Chapter 3.

Treatment of the below-knee amputee should be started within 2 or 3 days after amputation. At this time a program of proper positioning, progressive exercise of all extremities, stump wrapping and conditioning, and nonweight-bearing ambulation should be initiated. This is then followed by a prosthetic period of rehabilitation. Each of these phases will be considered separately.

Proper positioning. Proper positioning is an essential part of rehabilitation of the amputee. If done properly, complications from contractures can be prevented.

While in bed, the patient should be encouraged to change position often. He should change from a prone position, with legs adducted in proper body alignment that encourages hip extension, to side and supine positions. All pillows should be removed from the bed, except for the head, approximately 2 days after surgery. The use of pillows under the stump encourages hip flexion, and in many instances the knee is kept flexed over the pillow. If the stump must be elevated, the entire stump should be kept extended. Pillows should not be kept between the legs, since this encourages abduction, which may develop into a contracture.

Proper positioning in the wheelchair should also be taught. Prolonged sitting should be discouraged. Sitting should be interspersed with periods of lying and walking. When sitting in the wheelchair the stump should be kept extended on the same plane as the hip. This can be achieved by the use of a stump board, which is inserted beneath the seat cushion of the wheelchair. The stump thus rests on the board in the extended position. The other foot should rest on a foot plate to prevent its being injured, especially in the dysvascular amputee.

Preprosthetic exercises. A program of active, passive, and resistive exercises should be started about 2 to 3 days postoperatively. These exercises should be gauged according to the individual's tolerance and progressively increased as strength and endurance increase. The entire person should be incorporated into the program in contrast to only the amputated limb. The amputee at first may have to receive bedside exercises but as soon as possible should be encouraged to visit the therapy area daily. This will provide an opportunity to see other similarly afflicted individuals in different stages of rehabilitation.

If space, time, and other logistics permit, a mat class may be developed. This is an excellent tool to develop balance, coordination, and endurance before entering the prosthetic period. It can also be carried into the prosthetic phase after some familiarity with the prosthesis is achieved.

Early stump exercises should emphasize hip and knee extension. Initially, this may consist only of quadriceps and gluteal setting exercises several times a day. As endurance and strength increase, isotonic exercises should follow. Initially, these should be executed actively and then progress to manual resistance. This in turn may be followed by a program of progressive resistive exercises using increasing weight to the limb. Some passive stretching to the hip and knee should also be incorporated into the program if the hip flexors and hamstrings are tight.

During this period resistive exercises should be given to the unaffected limbs to help maintain general body endurance, particularly in the older patient.

There are some special considerations in the below-knee amputee with regard to the management and prevention of contractures. First, passive exercises should be avoided in the painful stump. If the stump is passively stretched into extension, this increases pain and encourages the individual to hold the stump in a flexed position. Therefore active exercises or the contract-relax technique has been found to be more beneficial over a long period of time. In most instances, the painful period can be prevented by placing the stump in a bivalved above-knee rigid dressing fabricated by the prosthetist or physician. Even

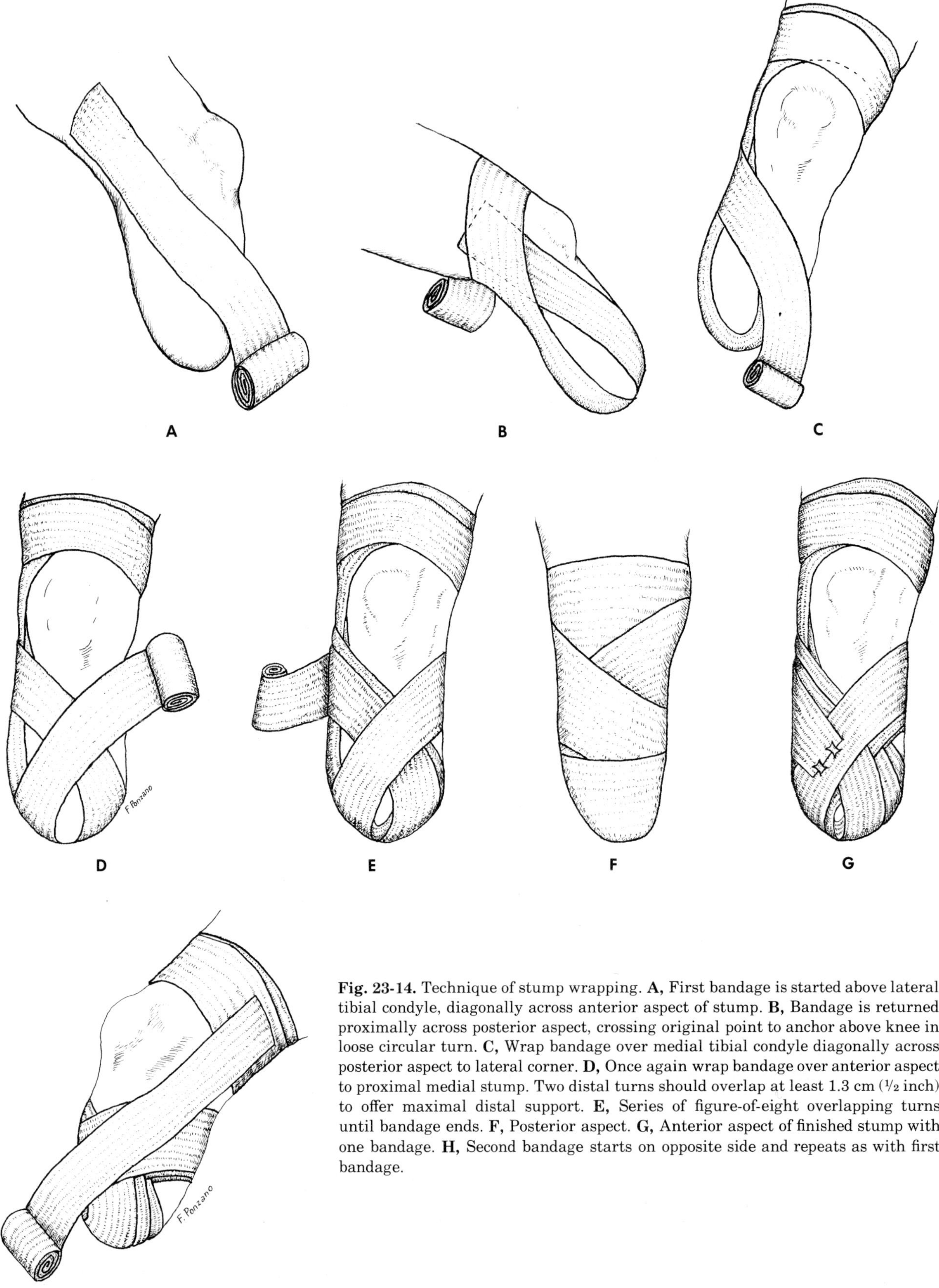

Fig. 23-14. Technique of stump wrapping. **A,** First bandage is started above lateral tibial condyle, diagonally across anterior aspect of stump. **B,** Bandage is returned proximally across posterior aspect, crossing original point to anchor above knee in loose circular turn. **C,** Wrap bandage over medial tibial condyle diagonally across posterior aspect to lateral corner. **D,** Once again wrap bandage over anterior aspect to proximal medial stump. Two distal turns should overlap at least 1.3 cm (½ inch) to offer maximal distal support. **E,** Series of figure-of-eight overlapping turns until bandage ends. **F,** Posterior aspect. **G,** Anterior aspect of finished stump with one bandage. **H,** Second bandage starts on opposite side and repeats as with first bandage.

though the stump is immobilized for a period of time, there is usually no limitation in range of motion of the knee after a week or so of exercises.

The best technique in the management of contractures is early prevention. This can be easily accomplished by giving concise instructions to the amputee and his family, as well as the entire clinical team. This must be followed by constant encouragement and reinforcement.

Posterior splinting in the prevention of contractures has not been entirely successful. The stump has a tendency to flex in the splint and often causes it to swell if not properly fabricated.

Active and resistive exercises, as previously outlined, in conjunction with early ambulation seem to be the most gratifying method in preventing and managing contractures. The constant activity of the knee and hip musculature under weight bearing in a prosthesis seems to secure the best results in correcting both knee and hip flexion contractures, should they develop.

Another very important key in managing and preventing contractures is the development of proper cooperation and motivation of the individual involved.

Stump conditioning. Proper stump shrinkage is an important part of a successful prosthetic program. It should be initiated as soon as possible to prepare the stump for prosthetic fitting.

This can be accomplished by either of two methods. The residual limb may be wrapped with elasticized bandages using a figure-of-eight technique or through the use of a stump shrinker sock. Stump shrinkers are a series of elastic bands, sewn together to form a cylinder. They can be obtained in varying sizes as the stump shrinks.

The residual limb is conditioned using one of these methods for several reasons. First, edema is reduced. Edema may be painful, thus causing the amputee to hold the limb in the flexed position and predisposing it to contractures. Second, it prepares the stump for a prosthesis by inducing stump shrinkage and the formation of a uniform clinical shape. Finally, it helps condition the residual limb to pressure, preparatory to prosthetic wear.

The technique of stump wrapping that satisfactorily accomplishes these objectives and can be easily learned by most individuals is one using a series of figure-of-eight turns. The recurrent method is also effective but difficult for some people to learn, especially the elderly. In the figure-of-eight method, two 10-cm (4-inch) elastic bandages are used to wrap the entire residual limb to above the knee. This method is illustrated in Fig. 23-14. As shown, there should be no circular turns except the two loose turns above the knee, which are used to anchor the bandage. Most of the pressure is on the distal end of the stump, progressively looser at the top, so as not to impede circulation. The bandage should feel snug, but should not cause throbbing, or a tourniquet effect may develop. To gain maximal shrinkage with this method the bandage should be changed three to four times daily.

If a stump shrinker is used to condition the stump, several sizes should be obtained. As the stump shrinks, a smaller size should be applied. Care should be taken to be sure the elastic does not roll down behind the knee and impede circulation.

The shrinker should not be left on for long periods of time without inspecting the skin for breakdown or abrasion.This method is quite effective for the individual who cannot master the technique of proper stump wrapping.

Preprosthetic ambulation. Nonweight-bearing ambulation should begin as soon as the amputee is physically able to stand. This, in most instances, is within 3 to 4 days after surgery. Early ambulation should be started in the parallel bars where the patient has maximal support and security. The period of ambulation should initially be short with frequent rest periods even if the individual feels well. As endurance increases, the duration should be progressively lengthened. The amputee should be encouraged to stand erect with the below-knee stump in the extended position. Progression should be made to the proper external support (i.e., crutches, walker) outside the parallel bars when the amputee's capabilities warrant it.

Nonweight-bearing ambulation should be taught on all surfaces (ramps, stairs, uneven ground). This is an integral part of the rehabilitation program and is often neglected. It prepares the individual for situations when the prosthesis cannot be worn, such as stump breakdown or prosthetic repair.

Prosthetic rehabilitation

The prosthetic period of rehabilitation usually starts between 2 weeks to 1 month after amputation. At this time the amputee begins ambulating with a temporary prosthesis and progresses to varying degrees of independence within his capabilities.

The recent below-knee amputee usually begins

weight-bearing ambulation in a temporary plaster prosthesis (Fig. 23-15). This is used to obtain maximal stump shrinkage and achieve early weight-bearing ambulation with a prosthetic limb. After most of the edema has diminished, a definitive prosthesis will be fabricated.

Initially, the amputee should bear partial weight on the parallel bars for short periods two to three times a day under close supervision of a therapist. This is necessary to be certain that the proper number of stump socks is worn so as to prevent stump breakdown in a rapidly shrinking stump.

A well-executed three-point gait pattern should be insisted on early to avoid developing an abnormal gait pattern that cannot be rectified later. Some of the most common gait deviations are too long a prosthetic step, premature knee flexion to avoid bearing weight on the prosthesis, and a stiff-legged gait. Some minimal balancing activities can be incorporated into the program. These include body shifting forward and back over the prosthetic device, as well as side to side.

As the amputee gains independence on the parallel bars, he should be progressed to the appropriate bilateral external support. Bilateral support with the plaster pylon is essential due to the possibility of breakage under full weight bearing. When the amputee leaves the parallel bars a walker should be avoided as often as possible, since it is difficult to obtain a gait pattern with equal stride lengths.

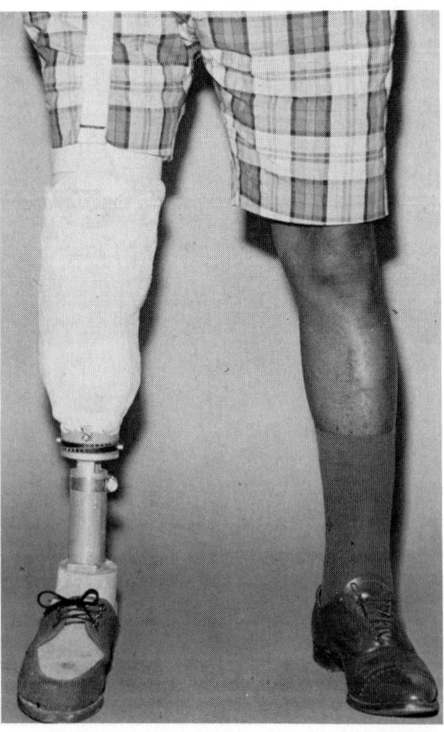

Fig. 23-15. Temporary plaster prosthesis for below-knee amputation.

After independence is gained on crutches on a level surface with the plaster prosthesis, progression should be made to stair climbing. In this activity a railing may be used initially. When ascending stairs both crutches are placed under one arm and the railing is grasped with the other hand. The amputee leads with the unaffected lower limb and brings the prosthesis up with the crutches. The crutches are always kept with the prosthetic leg. When descending the stairs, the opposite pattern is used. As balance improves, the amputee may learn to negotiate stairs using two crutches and no railing. In areas where a large number of stairs are encountered, it is usually advisable to use the railing for safety.

The next functional activity that may be attempted is negotiating a ramp. This is usually more difficult than stairs due to the limitation in dorsiflexion of the prosthetic ankle. For that reason, an unequal stride length is acceptable. When ascending an incline, the railing may or may not be used, depending on the individual's capabilities. The amputee leads with the unaffected lower extremity and then takes a shorter step with the prosthesis. When descending, the opposite pattern is again used. If the individual is unsteady he may ascend and descend the ramp in a diagonal manner to avoid knee buckling. If he has difficulty rolling over the rigid prosthesis, the below-knee amputee may have to side step up and down an incline, but this pattern is more common in the above-knee amputee.

A third functional activity is getting up from the floor. This may be accomplished in many ways. If the individual is weak he should crawl to a stationary object and pull himself up. The more agile individual should get on all four extremities. The unaffected leg is brought up under the chest with the foot flat. Both hands are placed on the normal knee. The amputee then pushes down hard on the knee, straightens the knee at the same time, and swings the prosthesis under him as he assumes the erect position.

After the stump has matured in terms of stump shrinkage a definitive prosthesis will be fabricated. At that time the amputee should be instructed in the proper use of a cane, if necessary. This usually requires little instruction for the amputee who has been walking well on a temporary plaster prosthesis. All functional activities should again be reviewed to ensure safety and independence.

Prosthetic hygiene and care

Prosthetic hygiene and care are of utmost importance in total rehabilitation of the below-knee amputee. In some instances complications could have been avoided if proper instructions were given.

Time should be spent in taking care of stump socks and the prosthesis. The socks should be changed at least every other day and more often if the individual perspires a lot. This can prevent maceration of the stump. Also, adding a small amount of powder when donning the prosthesis can cut down on perspiration and friction. The prosthesis should be cleaned every 2 days with a damp cloth and the end pad exposed to the air to dry.

The stump should also be washed with soap and water daily, preferably at night to ensure dryness. At that time the stump should be checked for red marks and abrasions. A hand mirror may be of assistance in inspecting the posterior aspect of the stump.

Finally, the remaining foot, especially in the dysvascular amputee, should be given consideration. The patient should be cautioned against cutting his own nails, particularly if he has limited vision, and taught to check between the toes and over the sole of the foot for breakdown.

Donning and doffing the prosthesis properly is essential for effective prosthetic management. The amputee should don the proper number of stump socks one at a time, being sure to avoid any wrinkles. The stump is then placed in the prosthesis holding the knee in a slightly flexed position. The stump is slowly eased into position avoiding a screwing action. The prosthesis should be entirely on before any weight is borne.

When doffing the prosthesis one hand grasps the stump sock and the other pushes the prosthesis off slowly while the knee is slightly flexed.

If a liner is worn, it should be donned first, then placed in the prosthesis. A nylon stocking placed over the outside of the liner allows it to slide into the prosthesis easier. When removing the prosthesis the liner may be removed separately or together depending on the individual's preference.

Rehabilitation of the amputee can be a very rewarding experience for the patient, as well as for all of the health care team, if carried out in an atmosphere of mutual cooperation. No aspect of the individual should be neglected, making each member of the team equally important.

PROSTHETIC SYSTEMS AND PRESCRIPTION

In the past few years, the variety of prosthetic systems available for the below-knee amputee has greatly increased. The introduction of the PTB total-contact socket resolved many of the problems in fitting the below-knee amputee and is the basis for the weight-bearing characteristics of both the hard and insert sockets of the present day. With the introduction of the supracondylar socket, the condylar strap suspension system with or without a waist belt has in many instances been replaced by a variety of condylar wedge suspension systems. These wedges may be an inherent part of an insert, or a fixed or removable wedge may be used for a hard socket.

The development of immediate postsurgical fitting procedures created a great interest in design of the pylon system of construction and provided the impetus for the endoskeletal system available today.

Although individual practice may vary to some degree, there has been a definite trend toward earlier prosthetic fitting of the below-knee amputee. In its extreme, this may mean immediate postsurgical application of a temporary prosthesis and ambulation within the first few days after surgery. This technique is generally confined to the younger more vigorous amputee in the absence of vascular disease. Early prosthetic fitting, however, using a temporary plaster prosthesis at about 2 weeks postoperatively has nearly universal application to the below-knee amputee who has ambulatory potential. Waist-belt suspension is generally used with protected weight bearing. Use of this method in combination with elastic bandaging of the stump at night provides an extremely efficient method of stump shrinkage, usually resulting in a mature stump by 4 to 8 weeks. By the time the stump is mature, and the amputee is ready for definitive prosthetic fitting, he has already undergone a significant portion of gait training.

Nomenclature

For prescription purposes, the nomenclature used to describe the prosthetic systems is as follows:

1. Open-end socket knee joints and thigh corset

Table 5. Prosthetic considerations

Type of stump	*Age of amputee*	*Socket*	*Foot*	*Construction*
Standard bulbous new	Adult	Insert	SACH	Temporary
Atrophied short below-knee	Elderly dysvascular	Insert	Litefoot SACH	Endoskeletal
Very short flex contracture	Adult	Bent-knee	SACH	Exoskeletal

2. Total-contact socket knee joint and thigh corset
3. Patellar tendon–bearing total-contact socket; condylar strap suspension
   a. Hard socket
   b. Insert
4. Supracondylar total-contact wedge suspension
   a. Hard socket
   b. Insert
5. Supracondylar-suprapatellar total-contact wedge suspension
   a. Hard socket
   b. Insert
6. Air-cushion socket
7. Bent-knee prosthesis
8. Foot components
   a. SACH foot
   b. Single-axis foot
   c. Multiaxis foot
   d. Light foot

Construction

1. Exoskeletal
2. Endoskeletal

Preprescription information

Definitive prosthetic prescription must be preceded by a thorough assessment of the amputee by the clinic team. Prosthetic prescription for the below-knee amputee depends on many factors. Preprescription information that should be obtained by the clinic team members includes:

1. New or long-term amputee
2. Length of the residual limb presented
3. Stump edema
4. Atrophied or bony stump
5. Configuration of the stump (bulbous distal end)
6. Condition of the skin
7. Flexion contractures
8. Stability of the knee joint
9. Status of the remaining leg
10. Physical and mental condition of the amputee
11. Availability of prosthetic service
12. Vocation and avocation

Prescription considerations

The prosthetic prescription may vary according to such diverse characteristics as age, sex, activity level, vocation, and type of stump. Young active adult men are usually better served by a prosthesis of exoskeletal design, and, if very active, supracondylar strap suspension may be preferred over wedge suspension. Women may require some sacrifice of durability for cosmesis, and the endoskeletal design with supracondylar-type socket and wedge suspension may be the best choice. In the older more sedentary individual regardless of sex endoskeletal design may also be preferable because of its light weight, but a supracondylar-suprapatellar type of socket can be used for more security and stability at the knee. In more humid climates, hard sockets are preferred over insert designs because of the ease of cleaning the socket. Hard sockets are also less bulky than sockets with inserts, so that cosmesis is generally better than with the insert design. Amputees who may be actively engaged in sports may prefer the added feature of a rotator unit. This unit is also useful in decreasing rotary frictional forces imposed by the socket on the stump and therefore may be indicated when scarring or other skin problems exist. The long-term amputee who has been accustomed to an open-end socket with thigh corset for many years may not accept the more modern versions of the below-knee prosthesis. The obese patient may find that wedge suspension is inadequate and that supracondylar strap suspension is too confining in flexion. For this patient a thigh corset or a waist belt may be preferred to auxiliary suspension. The prosthetic foot of choice in nearly all instances is the SACH foot because of its durability, but geographic or patient preference may dictate a single-axis or multiaxis foot.

The following prescription considerations are based on stump type and are summarized in Table 5 and p. 357.

PROSTHETIC CONSIDERATIONS

Level of amputation	*Sockets*	*Suspension*	*Foot assembly*	*Construction*
Very short below-knee	Supracondylar-suprapatellar	Medial wedge	SACH	Endoskeletal or exoskeletal
	PTB	Thigh corset or waist belt	SACH	Endoskeletal or exoskeletal
Short below-knee	Supracondylar-suprapatellar	Medial wedge	SACH	Endoskeletal or exoskeletal
	Supracondylar	Medial wedge	SACH	Endoskeletal or exoskeletal
	PTB	Supracondylar strap	SACH	Endoskeletal or exoskeletal
		Rubber sleeve		
Standard below-knee	Supracondylar	Medial wedge	SACH	Exoskeletal
	Supracondylar-suprapatellar	Medial wedge	SACH	Exoskeletal
	PTB	Supracondylar strap Rubber sleeve	SACH	Exoskeletal
Long below-knee	Supracondylar	Medial wedge	SACH	Exoskeletal

Medium to long stump. In the otherwise uncomplicated medium to long stump the supracondylar design with medial wedge suspension is a good prosthetic choice (Fig. 23-16). If, because of activity or body habitus, this type of suspension is inadequate, the PTB prosthesis with supracondylar strap may be preferred. Geographic or patient preference will dictate whether a hard socket or an insert design is to be used.

Short stump. Suspension and stability of the prosthesis on the stump become the primary considerations when fitting a short stump. The supracondylar-suprapatellar design provides good suspension in this situation and reasonably good mediolateral stability (Fig. 23-17). In the very short stump, auxiliary suspension, such as a waist belt or a thigh corset, in conjunction with the PTB design may be necessary. The slip socket, rarely used today because of its demanding fabrication, may also be used for the very short below-knee stump.

Ligamentous instability of the knee. Below-knee amputees with ligamentous instability of the knee are best managed with a PTB-type of prosthesis with the addition of a thigh corset and external knee joints (Fig. 23-18). In this way, the

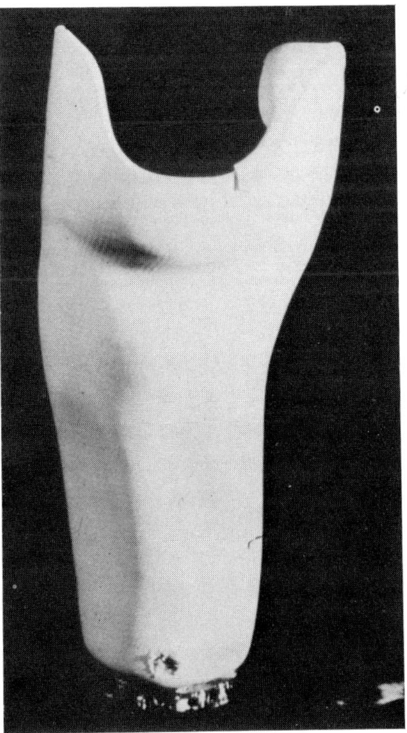

Fig. 23-16. Supracondylar socket design with soft fixed medial wedge suspension.

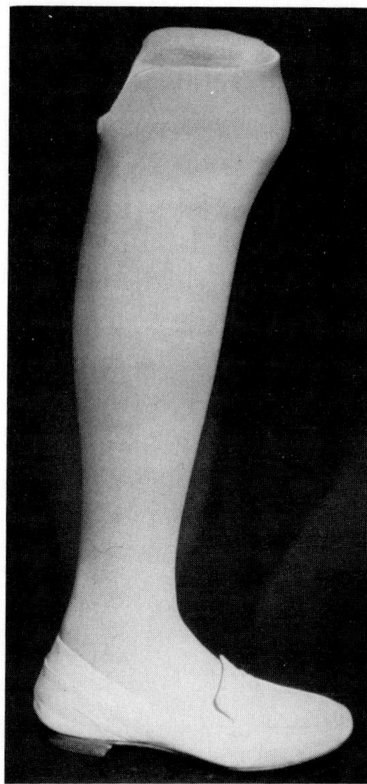

Fig. 23-17. Supracondylar-suprapatellar socket design with soft medial wedge fixed suspension.

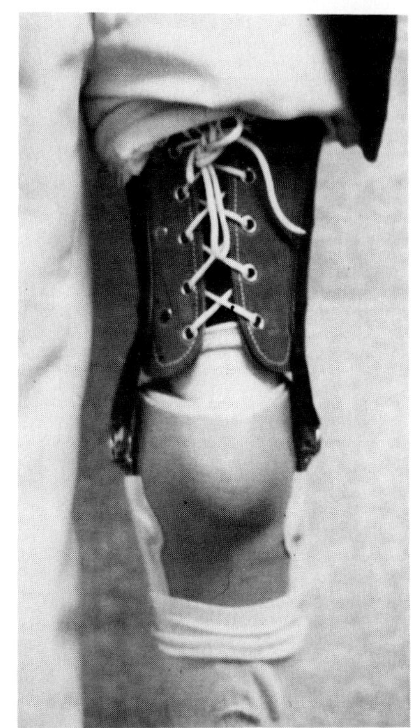

Fig. 23-18. Thigh corset attached to supracondylar-suprapatellar socket for very short below-knee stump or ligamentous instability.

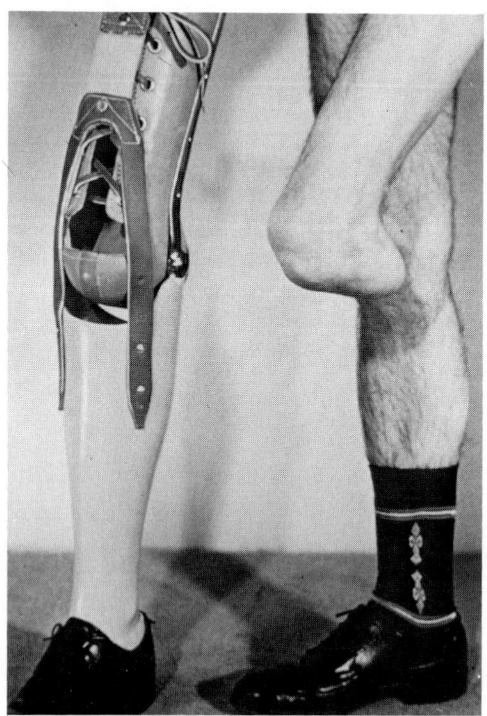

Fig. 23-19. Short below-knee amputation with knee flexion contracture fitted with bent-knee prosthesis and outside hinge joints.

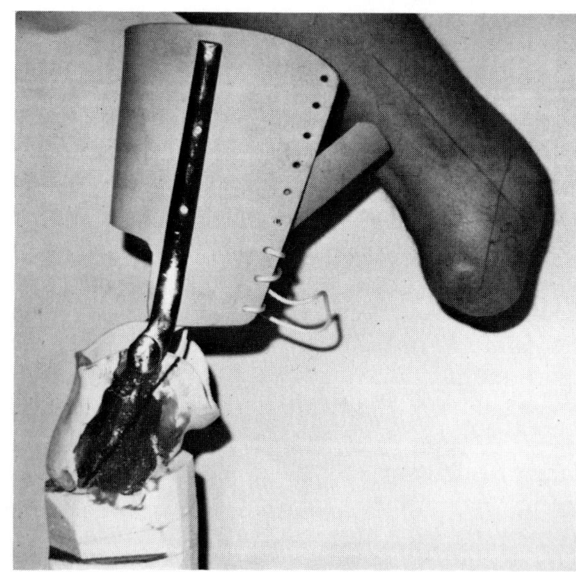

Fig. 23-20. Total-contact PTB prosthesis with thigh corset and flexion of socket to accommodate knee flexion contracture of 50 degrees.

advantages of total contact are preserved and knee stability provided. If minimal ligamentous laxity is present, it may be possible to gain the required stability by the supracondylar-suprapatellar design of the socket, which because of its high trim line provides increased mediolateral stability.

Atrophied stump. Many older amputees have generalized tissue atrophy and the mature stump may be bone with absence of subcutaneous tissue covered by fragil skin. An insert liner is indicated in this situation, using either the supracondylar-suprapatellar or PTB socket. It may be advisable to fabricate the prosthesis and insert over a 3- or 5-ply stump sock so that an additional cushioning effect is obtained.

Scarred stump. Below-knee amputations secondary to trauma may have excessive scarring present from healing by secondary intention or from the use of split-thickness grafts on a portion or all of the stump. An insert for the prosthetic socket in combination with a gel end pad may be used in this situation. If the scarring is confined to the distal end of the stump, the air-cushion socket has been of value. Additionally, one may choose to add a thigh corset to provide some unloading of the stump, and, in extreme cases, an ischial weight-bearing thigh corset can be used.

Flexion contracture. The short below-knee amputation with a flexion contracture may be managed satisfactorily with a bent-knee prosthesis (Fig. 23-19). This provides an end-bearing situation, converting the patient functionally from a below-knee amputee to a knee disarticulation amputee. In women, cosmesis is an objection to this type of prosthesis, and reamputation to a disarticulation level or an above-knee level should be considered. If the flexion contracture is less than 40 or 50 degrees in a short stump, the patient can be fitted satisfactorily with a total-contact PTB prosthesis or the supracondylar-suprapatellar design (Fig. 23-20).

Bulbous stump. A bulbous below-knee amputation stump is one in which the distal circumference is greater than the proximal circumference. This is usually due to errors in surgical technique with failure to taper muscle properly at surgery (Fig. 23-21). If the enlargement of the distal end is due primarily to muscle mass, rather than to excessive subcutaneous tissue, atrophy of the stump may be extremely prolonged. Initially such patients may be fitted with a "pull-in" socket similar to the above-knee suction socket in which the patient either wraps the stump and pulls in with

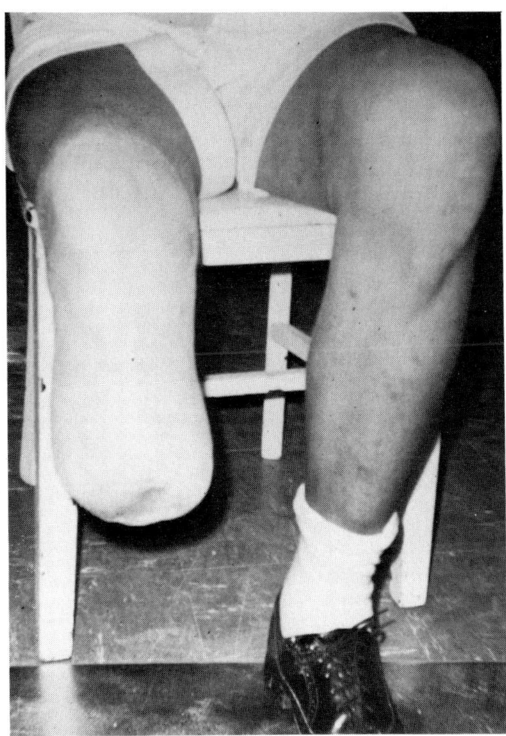

Fig. 23-21. Bulbous amputation stump due to failure of tailoring muscle bulk at time of surgery.

an elastic bandage or uses a stockinette to accomplish the same purpose. Extreme cases may require a hinged popliteal opening, using a hard socket, closing the trap door posteriorly after the stump has been inserted. Another method has been to use a popliteal wedge in combination with an insert that provides a larger diameter proximally, which is then closed using a popliteal wedge with Velcro (Fig. 23-22). The prosthesis may be left in the unfinished state until sufficient atrophy occurs to fabricate a conventional permanent prosthesis.

Volume fluctuation and edema. Patients who have borderline cardiac decompensation and patients who are undergoing chemotherapy for malignancy may have considerable fluctuation in the volume of the below-knee stump. An insert should be used for the prosthesis and this may be fabricated over a 3- or 5-ply stump sock. In this manner the patient can adjust the number of stump socks as the stump shrinks or expands, and, if the swelling becomes severe, the patient may use the prosthesis without the insert.

PROSTHETIC EVALUATION

Gait analysis is a procedure used to identify gait deviations and to determine the causes asso-

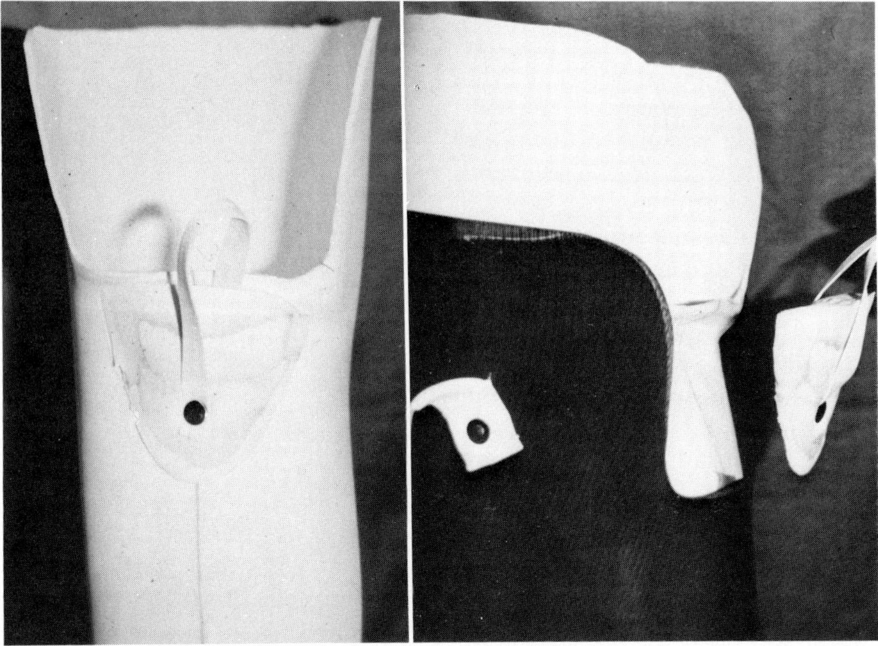

Fig. 23-22. Soft insert using removable popliteal wedge with Velcro attachment to allow entry of bulbous amputation stump.

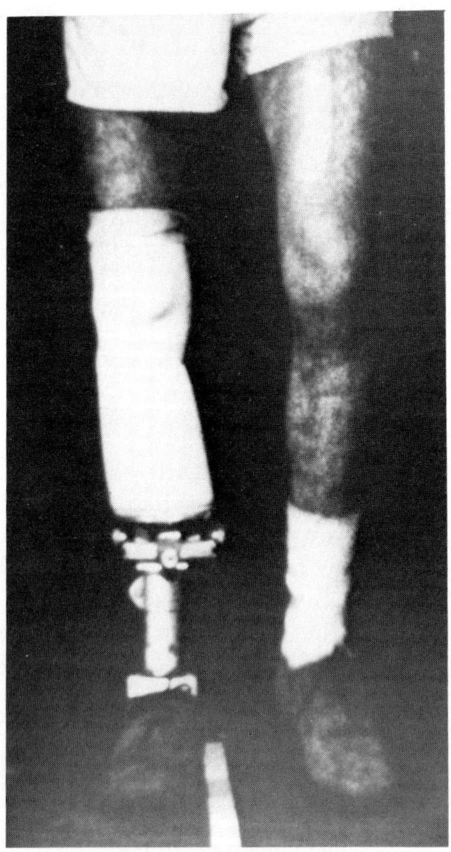

Fig. 23-23. Optimum below-knee prosthetic alignment with pylon vertical at midstance.

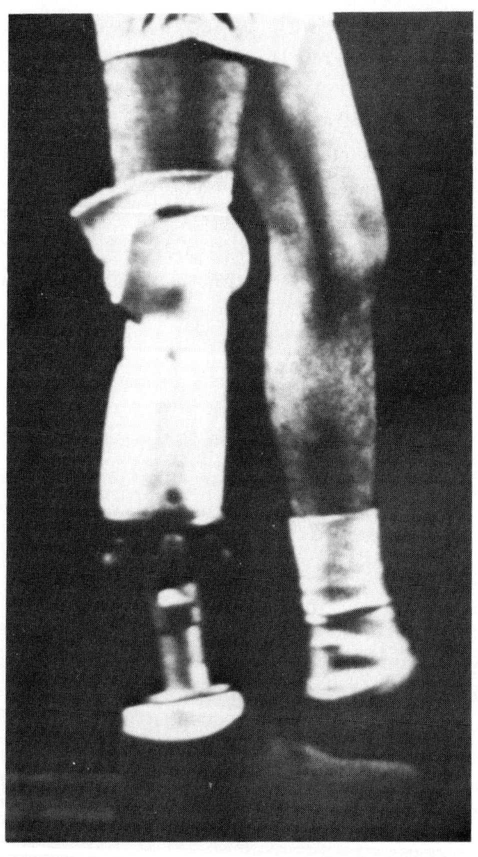

Fig. 23-24. Posterior leaning pylon, indicating anterior placement of foot, too much initial socket flexion, or too soft heel.

ciated with each deviation. To use this analytical procedure, it is necessary to have a detailed knowledge of normal human locomotion biomechanics and the prosthetic principles of fitting and alignment.

The gait pattern of the below-knee amputee depends on many factors, including the physiological age of the amputee, weight, height, coordination, balance, vision, motivation, length of the stump and its weight-bearing characteristics, musculature, presence of flexion contractures, mediolateral stability of the knee joint, and condition of the remaining lower limb.

Static alignment

For evaluation of static alignment the patient stands erect with equal weight on each leg and the leg and the feet approximately 10 cm (4 inches) apart at the heels. The prosthetic foot should be flat on the floor and the pylon vertical (Fig. 23-23). Following are some deviations that may be apparent:

1. A posterior leaning pylon, indicating too anterior placement of the foot, too much initial flexion of the socket, or a soft heel cushion (Fig. 23-24).
2. An anterior leaning pylon may indicate insufficient initial flexion of the socket, causing the amputee to move the knee forward and stand on the toe (Fig. 23-25).
3. The proximal end of a laterally leaning pylon inclines away from the midline of the body, indicating an inverted foot (Fig. 23-26).
4. The proximal end of a medially leaning pylon inclines toward the midline of the body. Weight is borne on the medial border of the shoe, indicating an everted foot (Fig. 23-27).

A common method used to verify the height of the prosthesis is by observation of the crests and the anterior superior spines of the ilium to ensure that the pelvis is level.

Another method is by observation of the spine. A piece of string held between C-7 and the coccyx will serve as a straight reference line. If one leg is

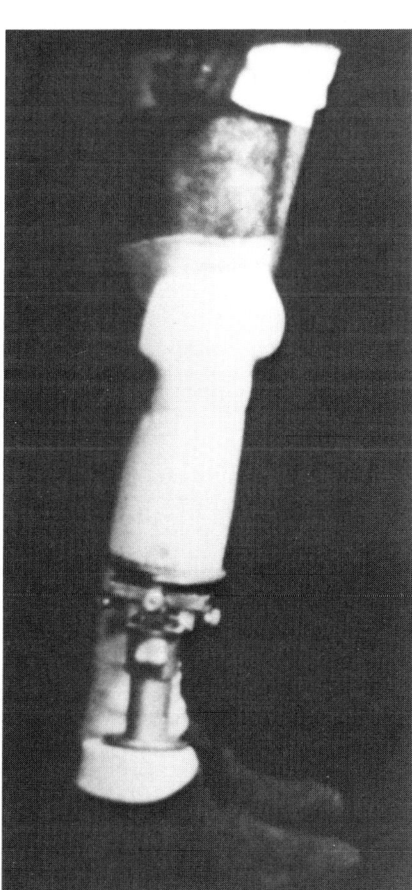

Fig. 23-25. Anterior leaning pylon, indicating insufficient initial socket flexion.

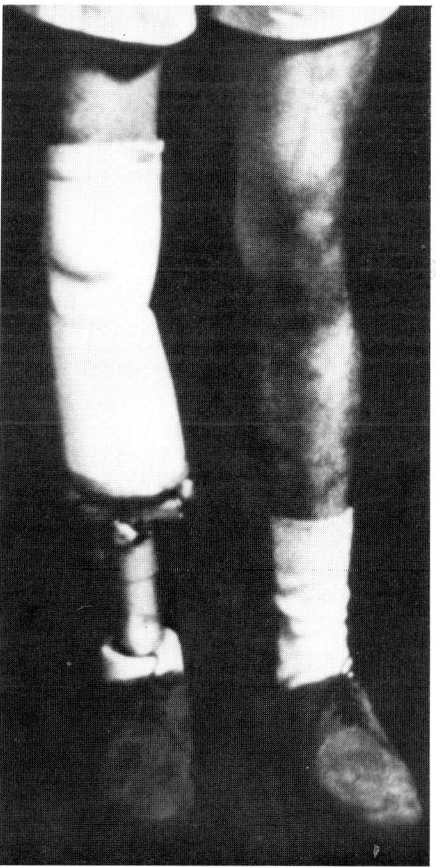

Fig. 23-26. Laterally leaning pylon, indicating inverted foot.

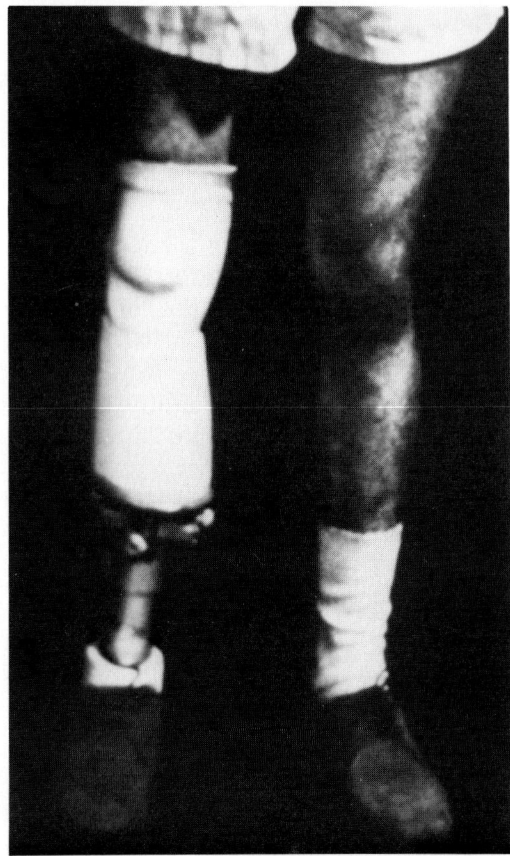

Fig. 23-27. Medial leaning pylon, indicating eversion of prosthetic foot.

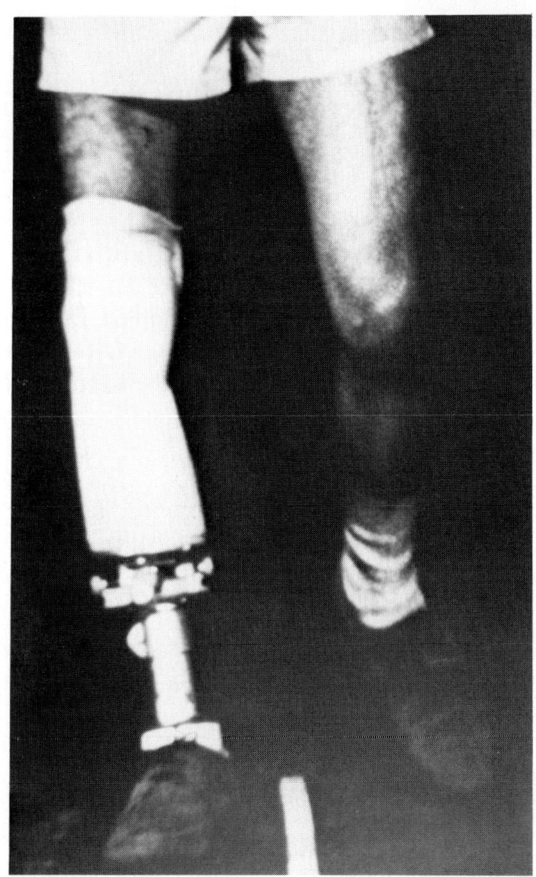

Fig. 23-28. Laterally leaning pylon, indicating mediolateral instability at midstance.

Table 6. Below-knee gait analysis

	Problems	*Cause*
Heel strike to midstance	Knee stays extended	Soft heel wedge; insufficient flexion socket; foot too plantar flexed; foot too far advanced
	Knee forced into excessive flexion	Heel wedge too hard; foot too far posterior
	Pain at anterodistal aspect of tibia	Excessive initial flex in socket
	Toe tends to rotate laterally	Foot too dorsiflexed; foot too inset or too much toe-out; hard heel wedge
Midstance	Excessive varus moment at knee (varus-produced pressure distolateral fibula)	Foot too inset
	Excessive valgus moment at knee	Foot too outset
	Excessive pressure against patella	Foot too plantar flexed; anteroposterior of socket
	Too wide walking base	Prosthesis may be too long or foot outset
	Excessive lateral trunk bending	Prosthesis may be too short
Midstance to toe-off	Drop-off: foot too dorsiflexed	Foot too posterior
	Tendency to fall to amputated side	Insufficient toe-out
	Excessive extension moment at knee	Foot too plantar flexed; anterior foot lever arm too long

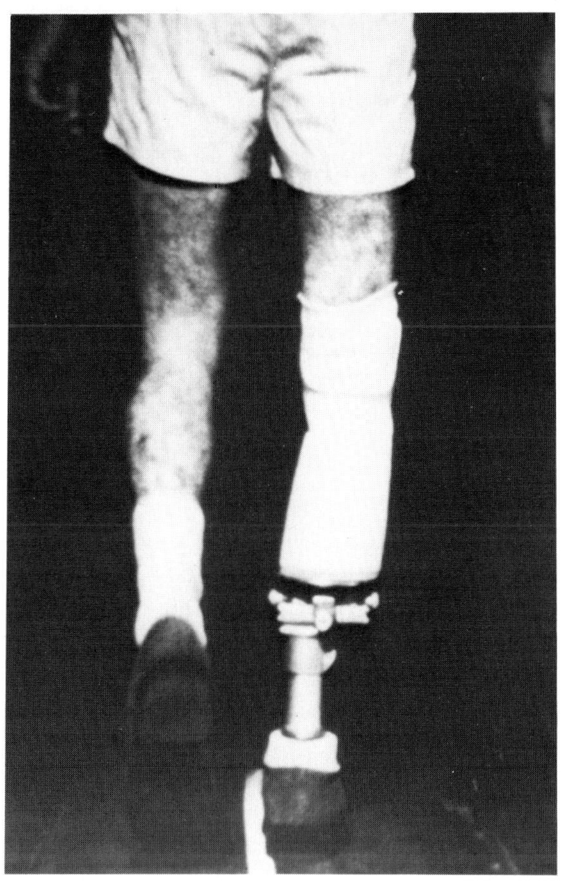

Fig. 23-29. Excessively inset foot causes too narrow-based gait.

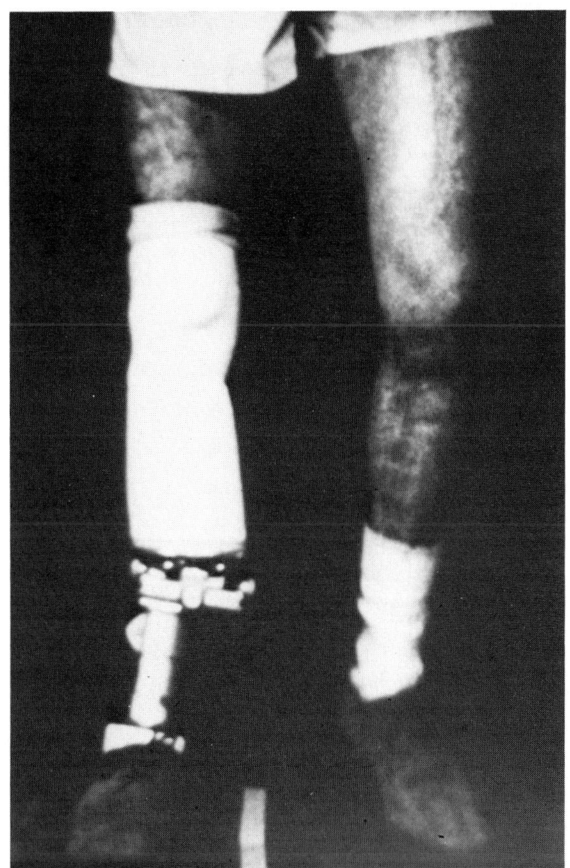

Fig. 23-30. Medial leaning pylon is accompanied by excessively wide-based gait.

short, the convexity of the spinal curve as observed from a posterior view is always to the short side. Of course, natural scoliosis precludes the use of this technique.

Dynamic alignment

Dynamic alignment is accomplished through observation of the amputee's gait from the front, back, and side views and is a necessary requisite to achieve a gait as near normal as possible. This requires a gait in which the shoulders remain level, body lean or side sway is minimal, arm swing is equal, stride length is symmetrical, and the width of the walking base is from 5 to 10 cm (2 to 4 inches) between consecutive heel strikes.

There is a smooth transition from heel strike through foot-flat to toe-off (Table 6). Any deviation from normal will produce increased energy expenditure, discomfort, and a poor gait.

Mediolateral instability. Mediolateral instability is evidenced at midstance by a laterally leaning pylon and is usually accompanied by a narrow-base gait (Fig. 23-28). The amputee tends to walk on the lateral border of the shoe, indicating an inverted foot.

A socket with a wide mediolateral dimension that provides inadequate support to the medial tibial condyle will also cause mediolateral instability and a laterally leaning pylon. This condition results in excessive pressure exerted on the proximomedial and laterodistal aspects of the stump. It will cause an excessive varus moment to occur at the knee made apparent by lateral gapping at the proximolateral brim of the socket. Eversion of the foot to correct this malalignment may require a horizontal medial adjustment to reestablish a narrow-base gait.

Narrow-base gait. A very narrow-base gait is caused by an excessively inset foot (Fig. 23-29). This deviation is evidenced by an excessive varus moment at the knee and sometimes may cause lateral rotation of the toe at heel strike. To clear

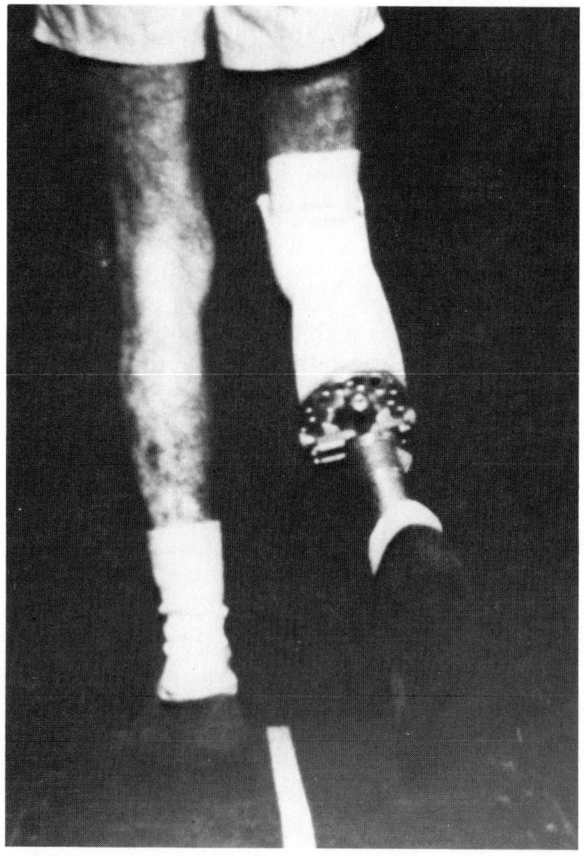

Fig. 23-31. Lateral heel whip may be due to improper placement of attachment studs for condylar cuff.

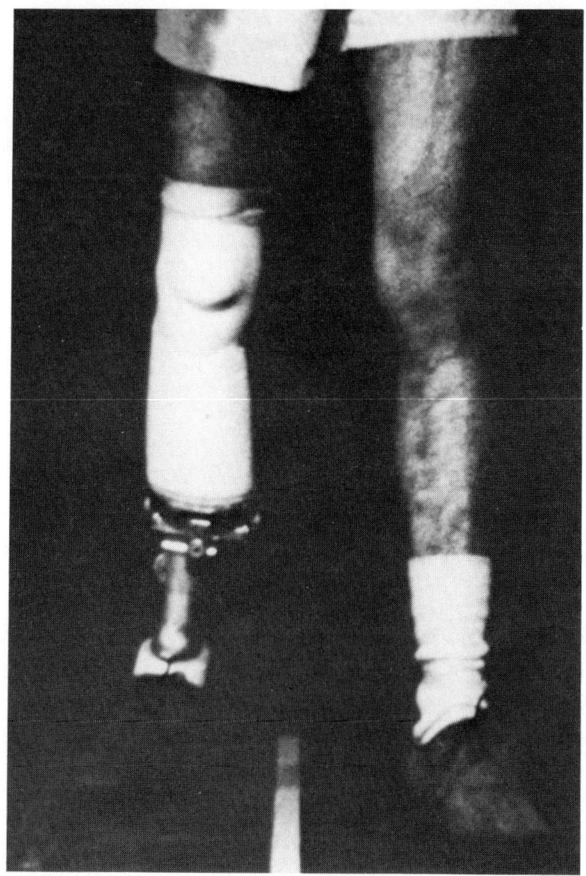

Fig. 23-32. Instability of amputee toward sound side due to excessive toe-out of prosthetic foot.

the sound leg, the amputee tends to circumduct the prosthesis during swing-through.

Wide-base gait. A medial leaning pylon is usually accompanied by a wide-base gait (Fig. 23-30). The foot is everted, and the amputee is walking on the medial border of the shoe. Pressures are exerted on the lateroproximal and mediodistal aspects of the stump. A valgus moment at the knee is sometimes evident. Increased lateral bending of the trunk and body sway are evident. Inversion of the foot will correct this malalignment, after which a horizontal adjustment may be necessary to reestablish the correct medial replacement of the foot.

Whips. Whips are not a common problem with the supracondylar below-knee socket, but are sometimes caused by improper placement of the attachment studs for the condylar cuff used for suspension of the standard PTB prosthesis. Whips are best observed from the posterior view. A lateral whip is when the heel displaces laterally at toe-off (Fig. 23-31).

The medial whip is not as apparent, but is a displacement of the foot medially from toe-off to midswing and then a lateral displacement occurs prior to heel strike.

Excessive toe-out. Imbalance of the amputee toward the sound side and excessive lateroanterior support at heel-off is caused by excessive toe-out (Fig. 23-32). A medial leaning pylon from midstance to toe-off is apparent.

The final result of the anteroposterior alignment whould be represented by a medially placed foot, which gives a normal narrow-base gait and a slight varus moment at the knee. A foot that is flat on the floor at midstance is represented by a vertical pylon. A tendency toward flexion occurs at heel strike, and there is no hypertension force acting at the proximoanterior border of the socket at heel-off or toe-off.

The lateral view is used to evaluate knee control of the prosthesis during heel strike, foot-flat, heel-off, and toe-off.

The ideal alignment produces a tendency to-

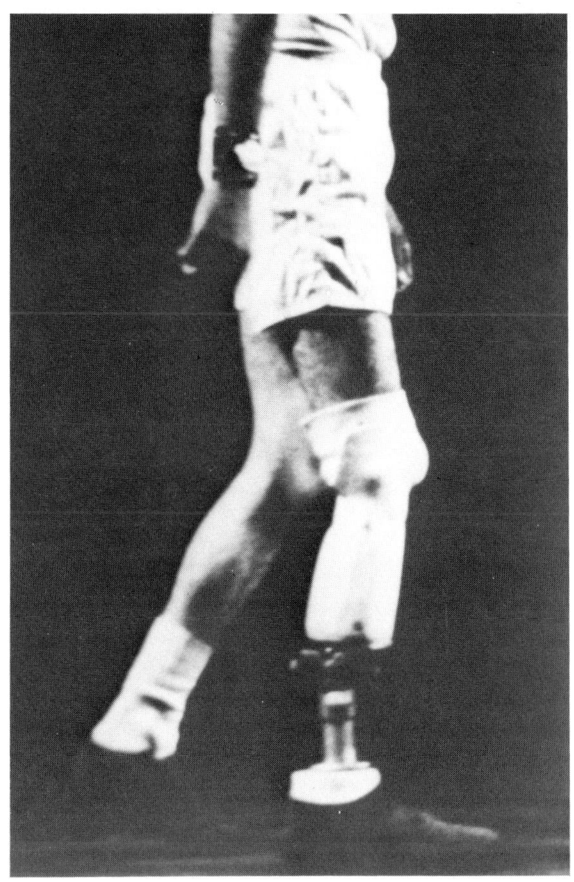
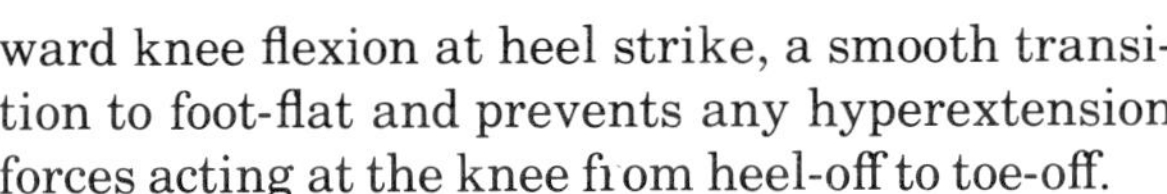

Fig. 23-33. Excessive knee flexion or instability at heel strike due to excessive posterior placement of prosthetic foot.

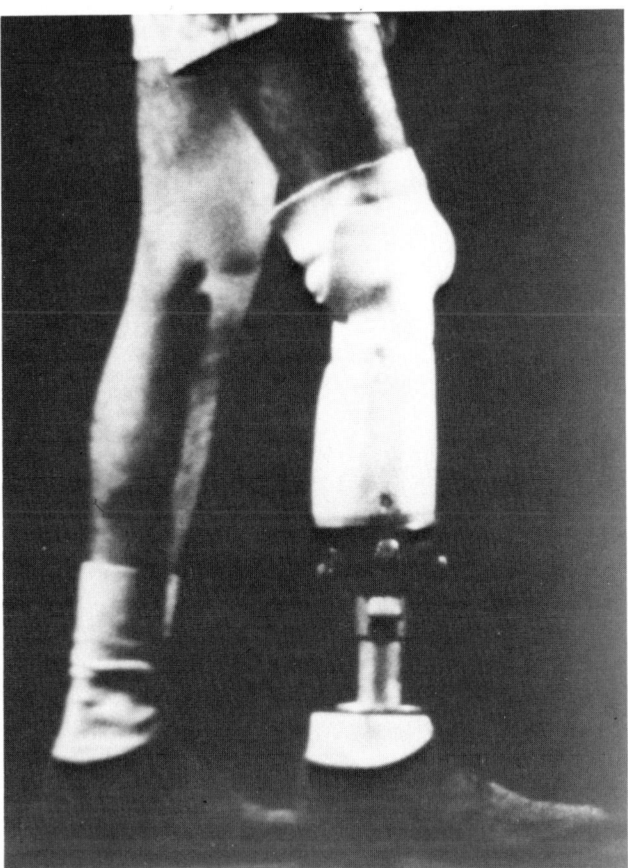

Fig. 23-34. Insufficient socket flexion can produce toe walking gait.

ward knee flexion at heel strike, a smooth transition to foot-flat and prevents any hyperextension forces acting at the knee fi om heel-off to toe-off.

Knee instability at heel strike. Knee instability at heel strike results in the knee being forced into rapid flexion, and contraction of the quadriceps to control this motion usually results in pressure and pain at the anterodistal aspect of the tibia. This is caused by a foot positioned too far posterior in relation to the socket, a heel wedge that is too hard, or a foot that is too dorsiflexed (Fig. 23-33).

Short prosthetic step. Insufficient flexion of the socket (Fig. 23-34) during bench alignment will produce a toe walking gait. No heel contact is evident. A short prosthetic step is apparent. Dorsiflexion of the foot and reestablishment of the anteroposterior placement of the foot will correct this gait deviation.

Excessive knee stability at heel strike. Excessive knee stability at heel strike is caused by the foot being positioned too far anterior in relation to the socket (Fig. 23-35). The weight line is over the heel during most of stance phase. The knee is kept fully extended at heel strike. The anterior portion of the foot provides minimal function from midstance to toe-off. A soft heel cushion may also cause this gait deviation evidenced by a posterior leaning pylon.

Knee instability at toe-off. Knee instability at toe-off creates a condition commonly known as drop-off and is caused by insufficient anterior support. It is evidenced by uncontrolled knee flexion and a rapid downward acceleration of the body prior to toe-off. This may be caused by a foot placed too far posterior to the socket, resulting in a short anterior lever arm or by an excessively dorsiflexed foot (Fig. 23-36).

Excessive knee stability from midstance to toe-off. Excessive knee stability from midstance to toe-off is caused by too much anterior resistance to rollover and is the result of too long an anterior lever arm in the foot or by a foot that is excessively plantar flexed (Fig. 23-37). Insufficient

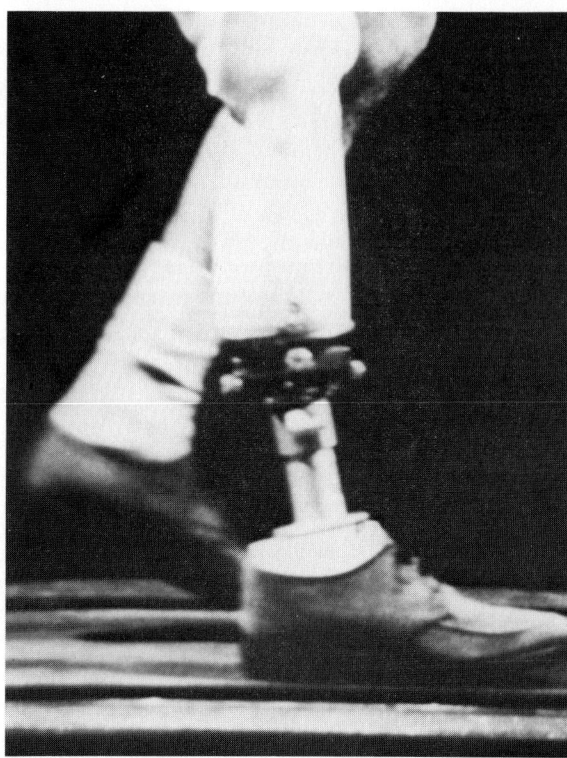

Fig. 23-35. Excessive knee stability at heel strike (hyperextension) due to excessive anterior placement of prosthetic foot.

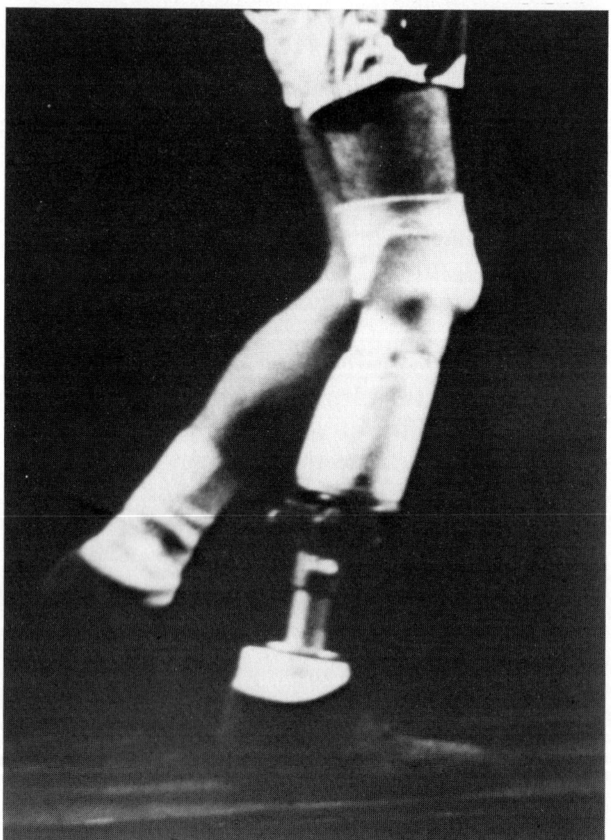

Fig. 23-36. Knee instability at toe-off (drop-off) caused by excessive posterior placement of prosthetic foot.

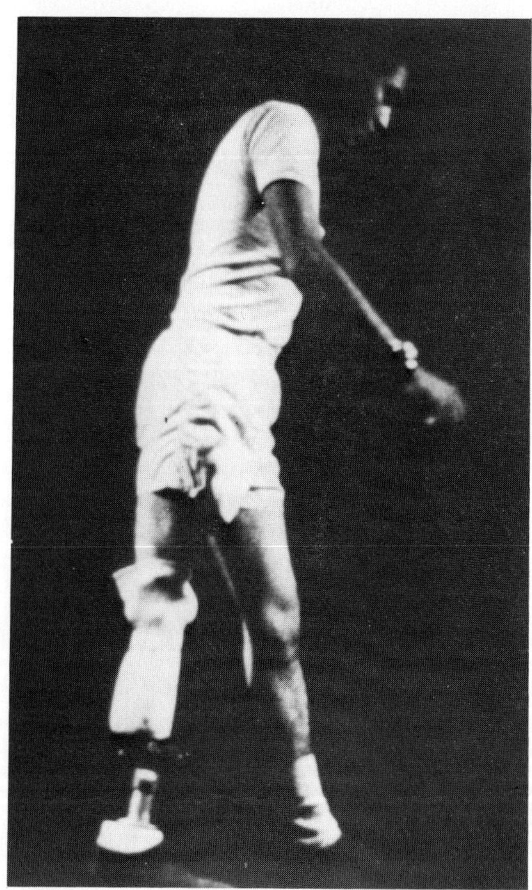

Fig. 23-37. Excessive knee stability from midstance to toe-off results from too long anterior lever arm in foot, secondary to forward placement of foot or excessively plantar flexed foot.

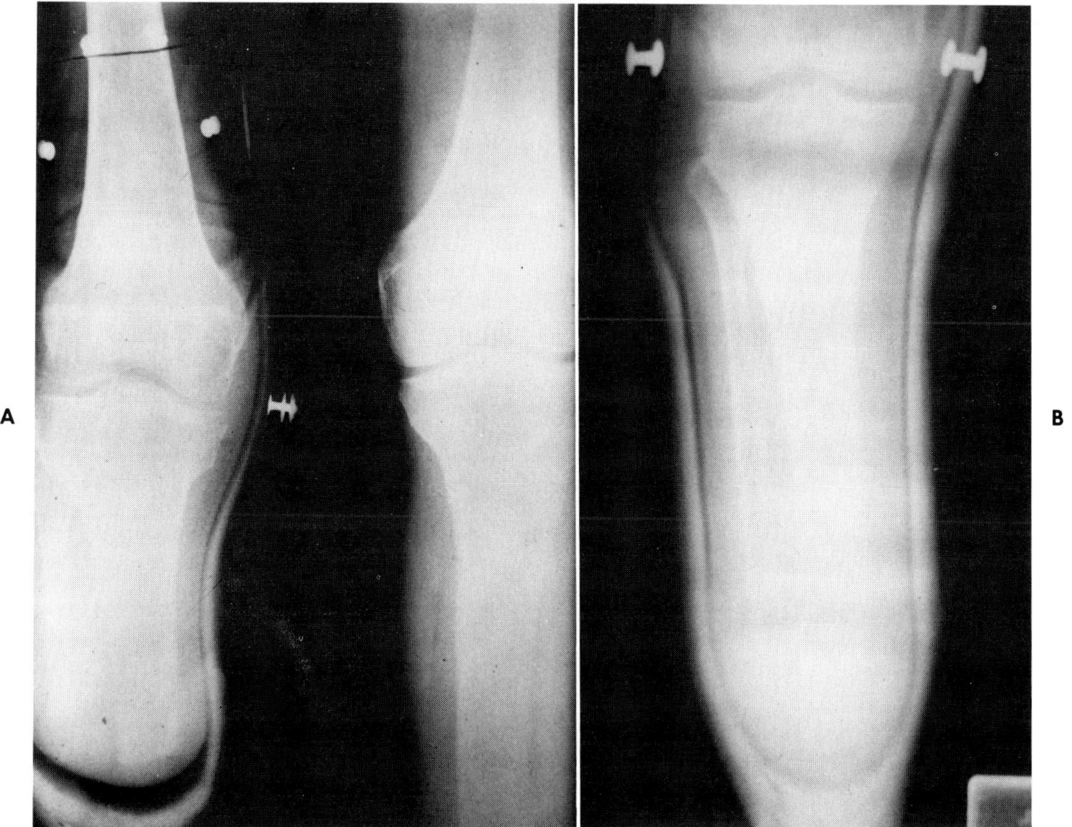

Fig. 23-38. A, Weight-bearing roentgenogram with lack of total contact distally in prosthesis. **B,** Weight-bearing roentgenogram of stump in socket demonstrating total contact.

initial flexion of the socket is a major cause of this defect. Hyperextensive forces result in a short step on the sound side. A heel wedge that is too soft allows too much plantar flexion of the foot at heel strike, causing the amputee to feel that he is climbing a hill during rollover. A tight fit of the toe section of the foot in the shoe will not allow flexion of the toe at heel-off, thereby resulting in an increased anterior resistance to rollover. One of the most common causes of this gait abnormality is the patient's selection of a shoe with a lower heel height than was initially fitted.

Toe clearance. Adequate clearance of the foot during swing-through is evaluated from the lateral view. If the toe contacts the floor during extension, it may be due to poor suspension of the prosthesis, or the prosthesis may be too long. Good suspension will help to prevent abrasions of the stump and contribute to the security of the amputee.

Checkout of the amputee seated is an important aspect of dynamic alignment. There must be no painful impingement of the hamstrings on the posterior wall with the knee in at least 90 degrees of flexion and the foot flat on the floor.

There should not be any painful pressure exerted at the anterodistal aspect of the tibia. Suspension should be adequate to retain the stump in the socket without causing pain at the femoral condyles. The proximal trim lines should be flush with the anterior surface of the thigh to enhance cosmesis.

When total-contact sockets are used, it is important that total contact between the stump and socket is maintained. The below-knee stump may continue to shrink for several months, causing loss of total contact, or excessive end bearing may also be permitted in this situation. Weight gain frequently will result in the inability to introduce the stump fully into the socket, leaving an air void with resultant loss of total contact distally. The presence or absence of distal total contact can be checked clinically by dropping a small ball of clay in the bottom of the socket and asking the amputee to walk on the prosthesis. Flattening of the clay indicates total contact. Anteroposterior and lateral radiographs are also an excellent clinical tool for evaluating total contact (Fig. 23-38). A change in the number of stump socks or modification of the prosthetic socket may be necessary to correct lack of total contact.

REFERENCES

1. Baker, W. H., Barnes, R. W., and Shuror, D. G.: The healing of below knee amputations: a comparison of soft and plaster dressings, Am. J. Surg. **133:**716-718, June, 1977.
2. Bard, G., and Ralston, H. J.: Measurement of energy expenditure during ambulation, with special reference to evaluation of assistive devices, Arch. Phys. Med. Rehab. **40:**415-420, 1959.
3. Block, M. A., and Whitehouse, F. W.: Below-knee amputation in patients with diabetes mellitus, Arch. Surg. **87:** 682, 1963.
4. Bradham, R. R., and Smoak, R. D.: Amputation of the lower extremity, Arch. Surg. **90:**60, 1965.
5. Burgess, E. M., Traub, J. E., and Wilson, A. B., Jr.: Immediate postsurgical prosthetics in the management of lower extremity amputees, Washington, D.C., 1967, Veterans Administration.
6. Burgess, E. M., Romano, R. L., Zettl, J. H., and Schrock, R. D.: Amputations of the leg for peripheral vascular insufficiency, J. Bone Joint Surg. **53A:** 874-889, July, 1971.
7. Condon, R. E., and Jordan, P. H., Jr.: Below-knee amputation for arterial insufficiency, Surg. Gynecol. Obstet. **130:** 641, 1970.
8. Cranley, J. J., Krause, R. J., Strasser, E. S., and Hafner, C. D.: Below the knee amputation for aterioscleroSis obliterans, Arch. Surg. **98:**77, 1969.
9. Dean, R. H., Yao, J. S., Thompson, R. G., and Bergan, J. J.: Predictive valve of ultrasonically derived arterial pressure in determination of amputation level, Am. J. Surg. **41:**731-737, Nov., 1975.
10. Ertl, I.: Uber amputationsstumpf, Chirurg **20:**218, 1949.
11. Ghormley, R. K.: Amputation in occlusive vascular disease. In Allen, E., and Barker, N. W., editors: Peripheral vascular diseases, Philadelphia, 1946, W. B. Saunders Co.
12. Gonzalez, E. G., Corcoran, P. J., and Reyes, R. L.: Energy expenditure in below knee amputees: correlation with stump strength, Arch. Phys. Med. Rehab. **55:**111-119, 1974.
13. Kane, W. J.: Lower limb amputations in peripheral vascular disease: factors influencing the level, Minn. Med. **51:** 179, 1968.
14. Kirg, B., McIntyre, R., and Myers, K.: Below knee amputation in peripheral arterial disease, Aust. N.Z. J. Surg. **45:**301-304, Aug., 1975.
15. Loon, H. E.: Below knee osteoplasty, Artif. Limbs **6:**86-99, 1962.
16. McCollough, N. C., III: The dysvascular amputee, Orthop. Clin. North Am. **3:**303-321, July, 1972.
17. McCollough, N. C., III, Shea, J. D., Warren, W. D., and Sarmiento, A.: The dysvascular amputee: surgery and rehabilitation, Curr. Probl. Surg., Oct., 1971.
18. Moore, W. S.: Skin blood flow and healing, Bull. Prosthet. Res., Fall, 1974, pp. 105-108.
19. Moore, W., Hall, A. D., and Wylie, E. J.: Below knee amputation for vascular insufficiency, Arch. Surg. **97:**886, 1968.
20. Murdoch, G.: Amputation surgery in the lower extremity, Prosthet. Orthot. Int. **1:**72-83, Aug., 1977.
21. Otteman, M. G., and Stahlgren, L. H.: Evaluation of factors which influence mortality and morbidity following major lower extremity amputations for arteriosclerosis, Surg. Gynecol. Obstet. **120:**1217, 1965.
22. Persson, B. M.: Sagittal incision for below knee amputation in ischemic gangrene, J. Bone Joint Surg. **56:**110-114, Feb., 1974.
23. Romano, R. L., and Burgess, E. M.: Level selection in lower extremity amputations, Clin. Orthop. **74:**177-184, Jan., 1971.
24. Sarmiento, A., May, B. J., Sinclair, W., McCollough, N. C., III, and Williams, E. M.: Lower extremity amputation: the impact of immediate post surgical prosthetic fitting, Clin. Orthop. **68:**22-31, 1970.
25. Sarmiento, A., and Warren, W. D.: A reevaluation of lower extremity amputations, Surg. Gynecol. Obstet. **129:** 799, 1969.
26. Waters, R. L., Perry, J., Antonelli, D., and Hislop, H.: Energy cost of walking amputees: the influence of level of amputation, J. Bone Joint Surg. **58A:**42-46, Jan., 1976.

CHAPTER 24

Knee disarticulation

NEWTON C. McCOLLOUGH, III
FREDERICK L. HAMPTON
ANNE R. HARRIS

Amputation by disarticulation through the knee has been a controversial procedure over the years. In the United States, its use has been confined primarily to children and young adults for tumor or traumatic conditions and has rarely been selected as a procedure for vascular disease.[2,8] In Great Britain, on the other hand, this level of amputation has been used commonly in the dysvascular patient for many years.[3,4,5,9,10]

SURGICAL CONSIDERATIONS

Knee disarticulation has certain inherent advantages and disadvantages, which account for the controversy surrounding its routine use. Advantages include the fact that it is less traumatic than amputation through bone, blood loss is minimal, a long, strong stump with excellent end-bearing quality is produced, and prosthetic suspension is facilitated by the bulbous contour of the stump end. The primary disadvantage of through-knee amputation is that relatively long flaps are necessary, and healing may be impaired in the dysvascular patient. A valid objection to the common use of this procedure in vascular disease is that a short below-knee amputation can usually be performed if sufficient soft tissue is available to cover a knee disarticulation. There is a fine line of distinction between sufficient viable skin for coverage of a short below-knee stump and sufficient viable skin for coverage of the knee disarticulation. A short below-knee stump that is otherwise unimpaired is functionally quite superior to knee disarticulation. Until relatively recently, another major disadvantage to knee disarticulation was the inability to provide the patient with a prosthesis that was functionally and cosmetically equivalent to above-knee prosthetic designs. Recent advances in prosthetic knee mechanisms and socket design now permit swing and stance phase control and cosmesis that equal available above-knee prostheses.

Indications

As a result of these recent prosthetic advances, which will be discussed subsequently, there is no longer any question that knee disarticulation should be preferred in all but the below-knee amputation. Even in the dysvascular patient, knee disarticulation is preferred to above-knee amputation, when possible, because of its superior end-bearing quality. This feature may be of great importance to an individual who is likely to become a bilateral amputee at a later date due to the disease process. Howard et al.[5] reported healing in 81% and an incidence of reamputation to a higher level of 19% in a series of ninety-three knee disarticulation procedures performed for peripheral vascular disease.

Contraindications

Knee disarticulation is contraindicated when sufficient viable skin and soft tissue remain to perform a very short below-knee amputation, unless a preexisting flexion contracture of the knee is greater than 50 degrees. The procedure is also contraindicated when there is inadequate bleeding from the skin margins after flaps have been formed by incision through the skin and subcutaneous tissues. A third contraindication to knee disarticulation is a preexisting significant hip flexion contracture, since the length of the knee disarticulation stump makes any permanent flexion contracture at the hip less tolerable from a prosthetic fitting standpoint.

Surgical procedures

The conventional knee disarticulation procedure described by Rogers[11] and later modified by Batch, Spittler, and McFaddin[1] has served well for the younger amputee whose disarticulation was for trauma, tumor, infection, or deformity. Because this technique uses a long anterior flap, it is not well suited for the dysvascular amputee. Recent modifications using a circular incision[10] or medial and lateral flaps[6] have led to a much higher success rate when the operation is performed for vascular disease. Other recent modifications by Mazet[7] and Burgess[5] have been developed to permit better prosthetic fitting, while still preserving the end-bearing qualities of the amputation stump. The following five different knee disarticulation procedures should be in the armamentarium of the amputation surgeon:

1. Conventional anterior and posterior flaps (Rogers)
2. Circular flap (Jansen)
3. Medial and lateral flaps (Kjølbe)
4. Reduction osteoplasty (Mazet)
5. Reduction osteoplasty (Burgess)

Conventional anterior and posterior flaps (Rogers). The incision for anterior and posterior flaps begins on the posteromedial aspect of the limb just proximal to the joint line and extends convexly, distally to a point 2.5 cm (1-inch) distal to the tibial tuberosity, then curving proximally to end at a point just proximal to the joint line on the posterolateral aspect of the limb. The posterior incision begins at the origin of the anterior incision and extends convexly, distally to a point 2.5 to 5 cm (1 to 2 inches) distal to the popliteal flexor crease, curving proximally to end at the other end of the anterior incision. The incisions then extend through subcutaneous tissue, down to ligamentous structures, dividing the patellar tendon at its insertion at the tibial tuberosity, and reflecting the broad anterior flap proximally with no dissection between tissue planes. Medial and lateral collateral ligaments of the knee are identified and severed, and the cruciate ligaments are severed close to the tibial attachment. The posterior capsule of the knee is then divided, and the popliteal nerves and vessels identified and dealt with. The hamstring muscles are then sectioned, leaving sufficient length for their attachment to the patellar tendon in the intracondylar notch. Heads of the gastrocnemius muscle are stripped from the posterior aspect of the femur, separating the leg from the thigh. The articular surface of the femoral condyles is not disturbed and usually the patella is left intact. The patellar tendon is then drawn posteriorly in the intracondylar notch and sutured to the cruciate ligaments and to the hamstring tendons with several interrupted sutures. The iliotibial band and the pes anserinus are sutured to the fascial part of the extensor mechanism. Skin and subcutaneous tissues are closed in routine fashion over a Penrose drain. A rigid dressing is applied. The technique for this amputation is illustrated in Fig. 24-1.

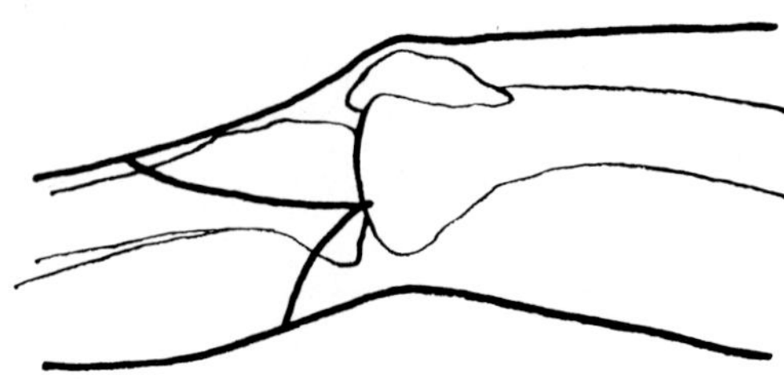

Fig. 24-1. Skin incision for conventional anteroposterior flaps. Relatively long flaps are needed to cover bulbous femoral condyles.

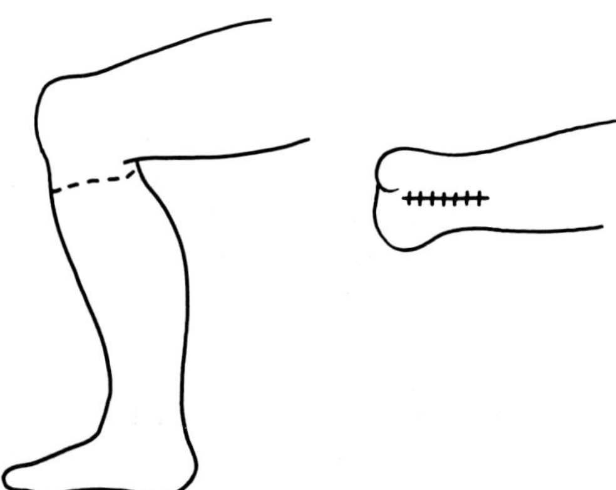

Fig. 24-2. Skin incision for circular plate of knee disarticulation. Level of incision is approximately 1.3 cm (1/2 inch) distal to tibial tuberosity, and closure may be vertical or horizontal, depending on relative ease of closure.

Circular flap (Jansen). The circular flap procedure is useful in the dysvascular patient, since no flaps are created, and healing is more satisfactory. With the patient prone on the operating table and the knee flexed to 90 degrees a circumferential circular incision is made approximately 1.3 cm (½ inch) distal to the tibial tuberosity (Fig. 24-2). Anteriorly and medially the knife passes through the soft tissues to bone; posteriorly and laterally it passes through the subcutaneous tissue and fascia to muscle. Dissection is carried to the knee joint anteriorly and medially, staying close to bone and including the patellar tendon, pes anserinus, and quadriceps expansion in the flap. Laterally the plane superficial to the anterior tibial compartment is followed to the joint level. Proximal retraction of tissues then exposes the anterior portion of the knee joint. The cruciate ligaments are divided close to the tibia, and the medial and lateral collateral ligaments are severed. Attention is then turned to the posterior aspect of the knee joint, where skin, subcutaneous tissue, and fascia are peeled upward from the underlying gastrocnemius heads or origin. The origins of this muscle are detached from the femur, and the tendon of the biceps femoris is detached from its insertion on the fibula. The popliteal vessels and nerves are identified and dealt with appropriately. The posterior capsule is divided close to the tibia, preserving its attachment to the semimembranosis tendon and the amputation is complete. The patellar tendon is sutured to the stumps of the cruciate ligament as is the biceps tendon. The remainder of the anterior muscle expansion, together with the pes anserinus, is sutured to the posterior capsule and semimembranosis. Skin and subcutaneous tissues are brought together longitudinally in line with the axis of the femur (Fig. 24-3). A rigid dressing is then applied. The healed amputation stump is shown in Figs. 24-4 and 24-5.

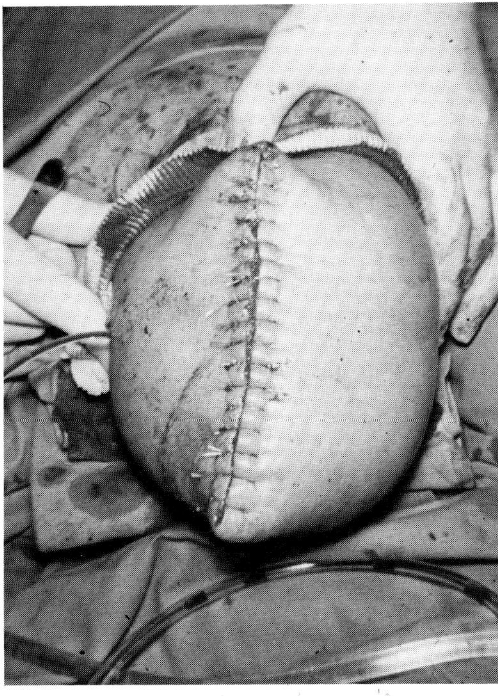

Fig. 24-3. Posterior vertical closure of circular type of knee disarticulation. (From McCollough, N. C., III, et al.: Curr. Probl. Surg., Oct., 1971.)

Medial and lateral flaps (Kjølbe). This operation is also well suited to the dysvascular patient, since the medial and lateral flaps produced are shorter than the conventional long anterior flap, and healing is more satisfactory. The patient is placed prone on the operating table, which provides easy access to both anterior and posterior aspects of the knee when the knee is flexed. The incision begins just below the tip of the patella and continues downward vertically to the upper border of the tibial tuberosity, then curves laterally for the lateral flap and medially for the inner flap, ending in the midline at the popliteal crease posteriorly at a level approximately 2.5 cm above the joint line. The lowest point of the lateral flap should be half of the anteroposterior diameter of the knee joint or about 3 cm below the upper border of the tibial tubercle. The medial flap should be 2 to 3 cm longer than the lateral flap to secure adequate covering of the larger and more prominent medial femoral condyle. The incision is carried down through skin, subcutaneous tissue, and fascia, and the flaps are raised, keeping close to the periosteal covering of bone. The patellar tendon and the medial and lateral hamstrings are divided. With the knee flexed, the lateral and medial cartilages are freed from their tibial attachment on the capsule, and the collateral ligaments of the knee are incised at the margins of the joint surfaces, leaving the menisci in contact with the femoral condyles. Cruciate ligaments are divided and the posterior capsule of the joint dissected from the tibia. The popliteal vessels and nerves are identified and dealt with appropriately. The disarticulation is completed by dividing the remaining soft tissues. The patellar tendon is sutured to the remainder of the cruciate ligaments, and the divided hamstrings may be sutured to the patellar tendon and cruciate ligaments. The patella and fat pad are left undissect-

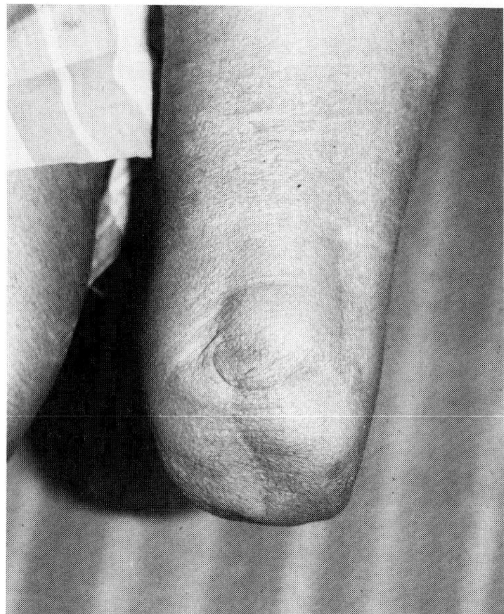

Fig. 24-4. Healed posterior vertical closure after circular type of knee disarticulation.

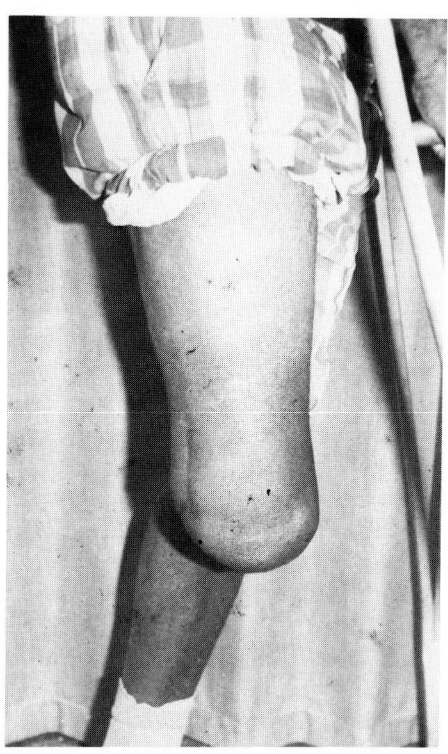

Fig. 24-5. Lateral view of knee disarticulation stump shown in Fig. 24-4.

ed and all articular cartilages left undisturbed. Routine skin and subcutaneous closure over a drain is then performed. A rigid dressing is applied. The procedure for this amputation is shown in Fig. 24-6.

Reduction osteoplasty (Mazet). Reduction osteoplasty decreases the bulk of the femoral condyles, both in the sagittal and coronal plane, to permit a more cosmetic prosthetic socket to be used. Reduction of the bulk of the condyles however reduces the inherent suspension mechanism provided by a knee disarticulation stump, so that a suction socket must be employed. This modification may be indicated when cosmesis is a major factor.

The usual fish-mouth skin incision is fashioned, making the anterior flap longer and extending 10 cm (4 inches) distal to the level of the knee joint and the posterior flap shorter, extending only about 2.5 cm (1 inch) distal to the same level. The skin and knee fascia are then reflected well proximal to the femoral condyles, and the patellar tendon is divided at the tibial tuberosity. The knee is then flexed, and the collateral and cruciate ligaments are sectioned. The posterior capsule of the knee is divided, and the popliteal vessels and nerves are identified and dealt with. The hamstring muscles are detached from their insertions,

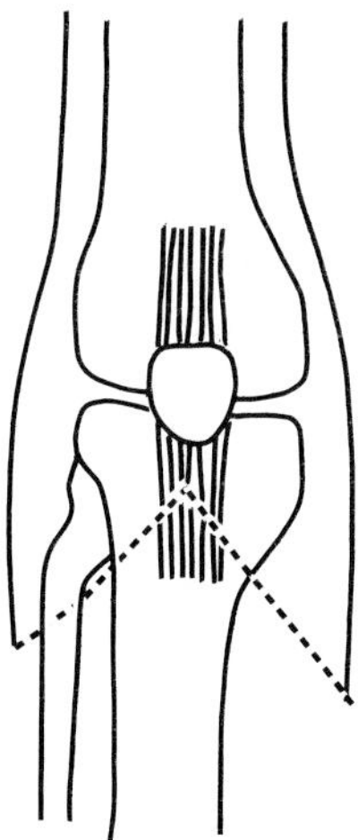

Fig. 24-6. Skin incisions for medial and lateral flap type of knee disarticulation. (From Murdoch, G. et al.: Prosthet. Orthot. Int. 1(2):72-73, 1977.)

and the leg is removed. The patella is dissected from the patellar tendon and removed. The femoral condyles are then remodeled by driving a wide osteotome vertically in a proximal direction through the medial femoral condyle to emerge at the level of the adductor tubercle. The lateral

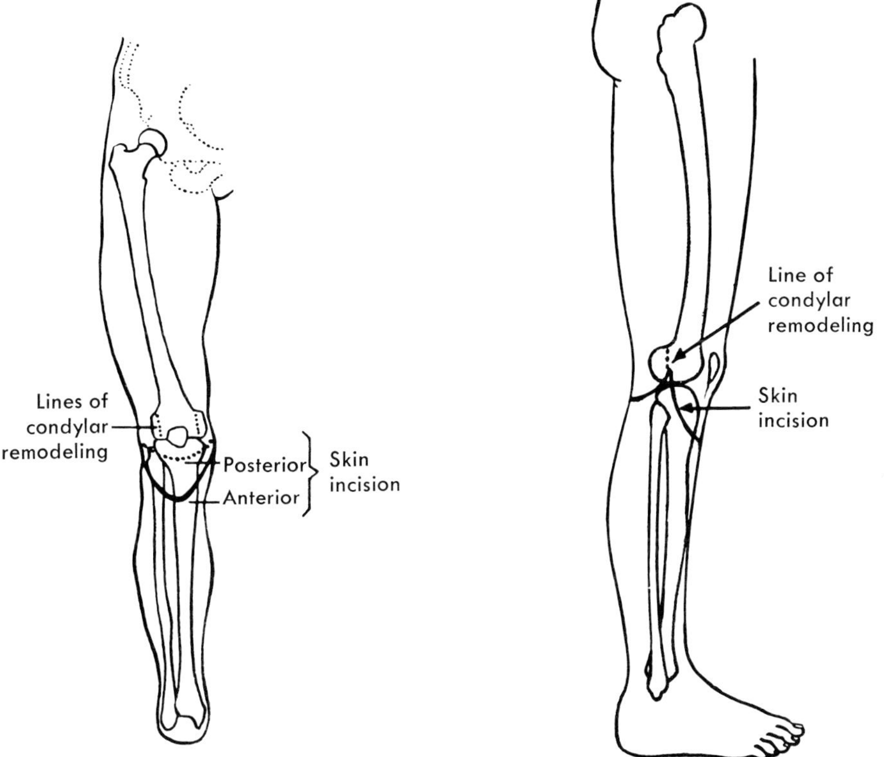

Fig. 24-7. Reduction osteoplasty advocated by Mazet. (From Mazet, R., and Hennessee, C. A.: J. Bone Joint Surg. **48A:**128, 1966.)

femoral condyle is narrowed in the same fashion. The posterior projections of both condyles are then resected by using a broad osteotome in the coronal plane. All bone edges are then smoothly rounded with a rasp, but the remaining articular cartilage not disturbed. The patellar tendon is then sutured to the hamstrings and the intercondylar notch under slight tension. Skin and subcutaneous tissues are closed routinely over drains. A rigid dressing is applied. The procedure for this amputation if diagrammed in Fig. 24-7.

Reduction osteoplasty (Burgess). The essential feature of this operation is reduction of length of the knee disarticulation stump, with preservation of end bearing so that prosthetic replacement does not make the thigh on the amputated side longer than the opposite thigh. Any of the previously mentioned skin incisions may be used, and the technical aspects of the disarticulation are similar to those described. When disarticulation has been completed, a power saw is used to make a transverse cut parallel with the floor 1.5 cm above the ends of the femoral condyles. Bone edges are then contoured carefully with a rasp. The patella is removed by a conventional patellectomy procedure, and the defect in the quadriceps mechanism is repaired with a vertical suture. The patellar tendon and the hamstrings are then sutured to each other and to the cruciate tendons in the intracondylar notch. Routine closure over drains is performed, and a postoperative rigid dressing is applied. The technique for this amputation procedure is shown in Fig. 24-8.

PROSTHETIC CONSIDERATIONS

The knee disarticulation amputee has been provided with a stump capable of providing full or partial distal weight bearing. The length of the residual limb provides an excellent lever arm for mediolateral stability and control of the prosthesis. The configuration of the distal stump may provide a means for suspension of the prosthesis and control of rotation. Flexion contractures must be avoided for cosmetic and functional reasons.

Various types of sockets are available for the knee disarticulation amputee. The molded leather socket with anterior lacing has been replaced to a large extent by the plastic quadrilateral socket. Entry for large bulbous distal end stumps may be facilitated by an expandable socket (Fig. 24-9).

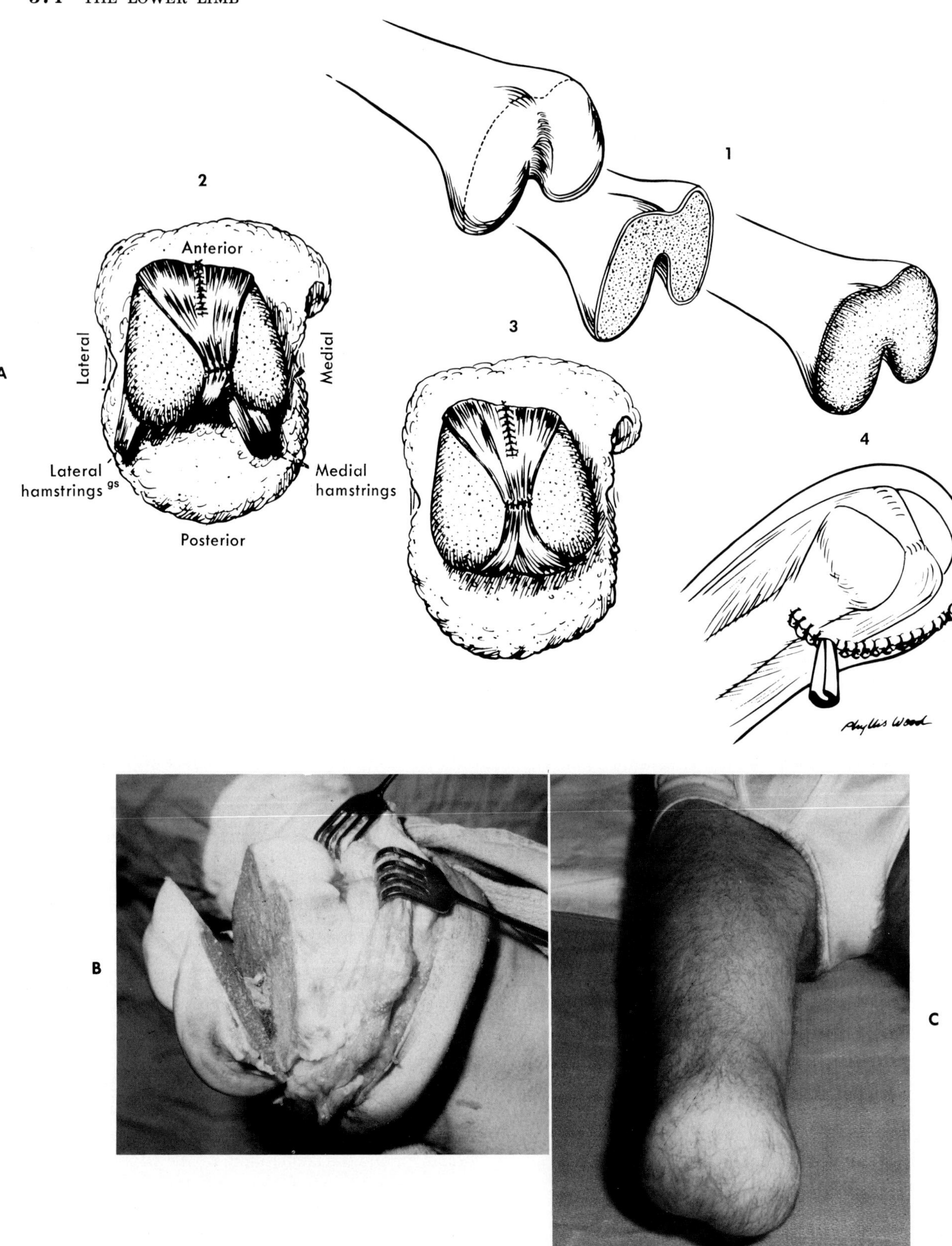

Fig. 24-8. A, Weight-bearing surface of femoral condyles illustrating bone preparation: transverse cut 1.5 cm above condylar ends and femoral margins contoured *(1)*. Muscle stabilization with patellar tendon sewn to cruciate ligaments. Biceps tendon and medial hamstrings are also sutured in intracondylar notch. One or more medial hamstrings may be stabilized. Site of patellar tendon removal and repair is shown *(2)*. Surgical closure of aponeurosis: hamstrings sutured through femoral notch to patellar tendon and cruciate ligaments *(3)*. Closed wound over drainage using classical long anterior skin flap *(4)*. **B,** Distal portion of femoral condyles removed transversely. **C,** Healed knee disarticulation residual limb. (From Burgess, E. M.: Arch. Surg. **112:**1250-1255,

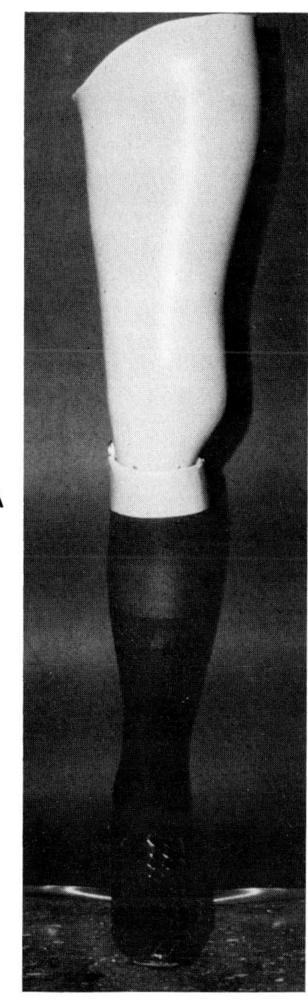

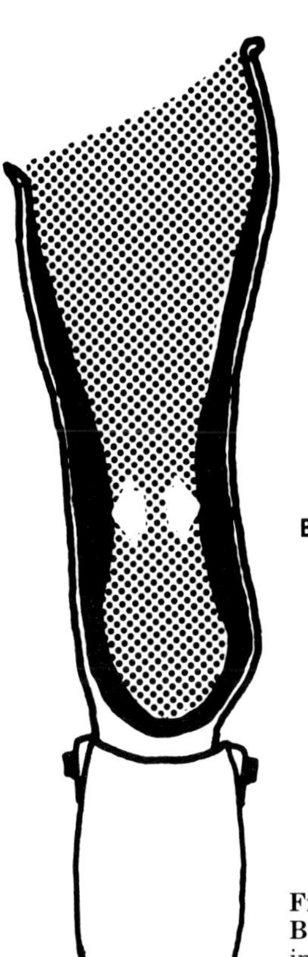

Fig. 24-9. A, Expandable socket-type knee disarticulation prosthesis. **B,** Coronal section of prosthesis, illustrating expandable nature of interwall, which also serves suspensory function above femoral condyles. (From McCollough, N. C., III, et al.: Curr. Probl. Surg., Oct., 1971.)

The characteristics of the stump will determine the distribution of weight bearing between the ischial tuberosity, the periphery, and the distal end of the stump.

Outside knee joints were commonly used with a knee disarticulation prosthesis in an attempt to maintain equal knee level height. The added width of the joints provided poor cosmesis. Swing phase control was nonexistent with outside knee joints until the introduction of a yoke with a hydraulic system (Fig. 24-10).

The polycentric knee joint (Fig. 24-11) provides swing and stance phase control. The swing phase control may be either hydraulic or mechanical, and stance phase control is through the stability of the four-bar linkage system in extension. The socket may be mounted directly to the knee joint mechanism, which is contained in the shank of the prosthesis, thus eliminating the problem of cosmesis because of stump length. A rotator may

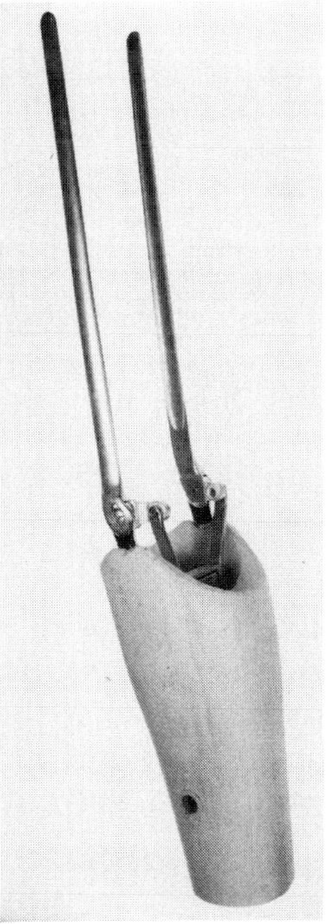

Fig. 24-10. Knee disarticulation prosthesis with outside knee joints and hydraulic swing phase mechanism.

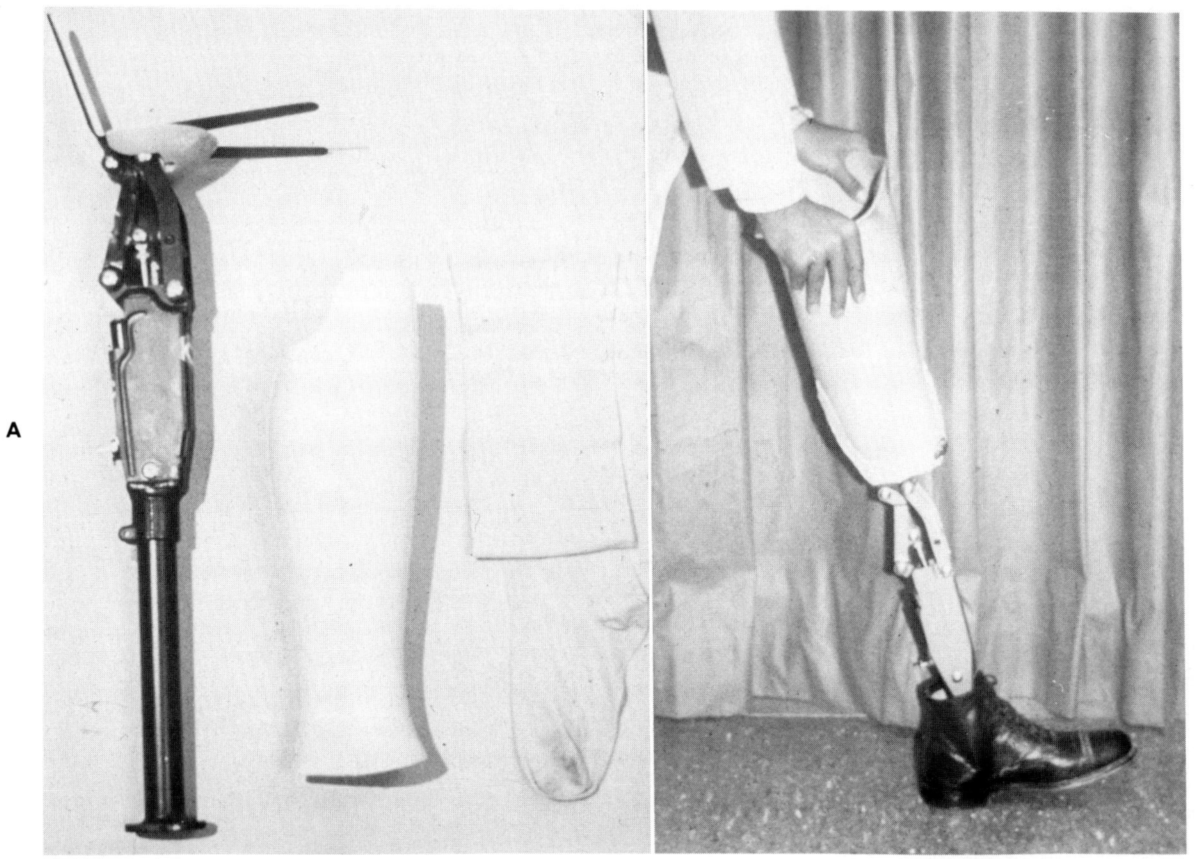

Fig. 24-11. A, Orthopaedic Hospital at Copenhagen (OHC) polycentric hydraulic knee disarticulation unit with four-bar linkage. This unit provides swing phase control through hydraulic mechanism and stance phase control through stability of four-bar linkage. Entire knee mechanism is contained within shank beneath cosmetic cover, and center of rotation is comparable to level of opposite knee joint. **B,** Demonstration of stability afforded at heel strike by four-bar linkage mechanism.

be incorporated into the system to reduce torque friction at the stump and socket interface.

Clinical evaluation of the amputee will determine the use of a SACH or articulated foot and the type of swing phase control to be included in the system.

REHABILITATION

The rehabilitation prognosis of the individual with an amputation through the knee joint is quite similar to that of one with an above-knee amputation. Some special considerations unique and important to this level of amputation will be discussed. For general exercises and gait training procedures refer to Chapter 25.

Preprosthetic management

As with an amputee, the individual should be evaluated preoperatively as to ambulatory status and general capabilities. A second evaluation should be done after amputation to note any change in status and to set realistic goals. The patient should then begin a general preprosthetic exercise program.

Careful note should be made as to the range of motion of the hip joint. In the knee disarticulation level, contractures of the hip are poorly tolerated. Therefore all precautions should be taken to prevent on from developing. If a contracture is present, it is very difficult for the amputee to lock the prosthesis, and it affects the cosmesis of the prosthesis drastically.

If the individual is well motivated and cooperative, knee disarticulation is an excellent level of amputation. The stump is well balanced, since no major muscle group is sacrificed. Therefore few abduction contractures are seen. This level also provides an end-bearing stump, which gives added proprioception in the prosthesis.

During the preprosthetic phase of rehabilitation the amputee should begin a program of general strengthening exercises to maintain endurance and prevent contractures. This is as for the above-knee amputee. The stump should be wrapped and special conditioning exercises given to build up end-bearing tolerance.

The stump should be wrapped in a spica bandage, using the same technique as for the above-knee amputee. Since the stump is long, it is very easy to choke the tissues and cause an adductor roll and bulbous end. This is often caused by the pressures being concentrated more proximally than distally. The bandage should therefore be changed three or four times daily to gain maximal shrinkage and prevent this from occurring.

Since the knee disarticulation is an end-bearing stump, tolerance to weight bearing should be initiated early so the stump gets accustomed to the pressures that will be present in the prosthesis. This may be accomplished by having the indistump, good muscular balance, and the end-bearing and proprioceptive characteristics around the stump.

Prosthetic training

Prosthetic management and gait training for a knee disarticulation patient is similar to that for the above-knee amputee. In the knee disarticulation amputee there is less difficulty learning knee control of the prosthesis due to the length of the stump, good muscular balance, and the end-bearing and proprioceptive characteristics around the stump.

Donning and doffing the prosthesis depends on the type of prosthesis fabricated. This, however, is contingent on the type of surgery performed. If the condyles are not too prominent, a suction socket is usually made if the individual is capable of pulling himself into it. Otherwise, a modified suction socket should be used with a Silesian bandage or pelvic belt. If the condyles are to be used for suspension, an expandable walled socket may be fabricated. This allows the individual merely to slip the stump into the prosthesis, which is held on by the condyles. There are also anterior opening prostheses made for this level of amputation. Their use depends on the type of surgery performed.

REFERENCES

1. Batch, J. W., Spittler, A. W., and McFaddin, J. G.: Advantages of knee disarticulation over amputations through the thigh, J. Bone Joint Surg. **36A:**921, 1954.
2. Burgess, E. M.: Disarticulation of the knee: a modified technique, Arch. Surg. **112:**1250-1255, Oct., 1977.
3. Harris, E. E.: Prosthetic management of lower limb amputation. In Modern trends in vascular surgery, London, 1970, Butterworth & Co.
4. Harding, H.: Knee disarticulation and Syme's amputation, Ann. R. Coll. Surg. Engl. **40:**235, 1967.
5. Howard, R. S., Chamberlain, J., and McPherson, A. F. S.: Through knee amputation in peripheral vascular disease, Lancet **2:**240, 1969.
6. Kjøble, J.: The surgery of the through-knee amputation. In Murdock, G., editor: Prosthetic and orthotic practice, London, 1970, Edward Arnold Publishers, Ltd.
7. Mazet, R., Jr., and Hennessy, C. A.: Knee disarticulation: a new technique and a new knee joint mechanism, J. Bone Joint Surg. **48A:**126, 1966.
8. McCollough, N. C., III: The dysvascular amputee: surgery and rehabilitation, Curr. Probl. Surg., Oct., 1971.
9. Murdoch, G.: Levels of amputation and limiting factors, Ann. R. Coll. Surg. Engl. **40:**204, 1967.
10. Murdoch, G.: Knee disarticulation amputation, Bull. Prosthet. Res., 1968.
11. Rogers, S. P.: Amputation at the knee joint, J. Bone Joint Surg. **22:**973, 1940.

CHAPTER 25

Above-knee amputations

Section I

Surgical procedures

VERT MOONEY

Above-knee amputation surgery is considered probably the least technically demanding of the various surgical approaches to the lower extremity. This concept relates to earlier classical techniques that provided simple myofascial and skin closure by layers with the primary object of obtaining wound healing. When surgery is designed to retain maximum function in the residual limb, that is, physiological amputation, the technique is precise and demanding. These circumstances prevail when the amputee is young, physically active, and needs a strong, muscle-stabilized amputation to obtain full function and control of the modern, well-designed, above-knee prosthesis.

The above-knee amputation has been the most common level of amputation in the past because it was so easily accomplished in cases of peripheral vascular disease and could more easily assure satisfactory healing. Today, because of greater understanding of the principles of site selections, potentials for rehabilitation, and improved fitting methods for amputations at lower levels, the above-knee amputation is done much less frequently, even in the presence of ischemia. Approximately 85% of above-knee amputations are secondary to vascular disease. The single greatest advance in amputation surgery during the past decade has been the statistical increase in lower (below-knee) levels of amputation for patients with ischemia. At least two thirds of all major amputations performed for lower extremity peripheral vascular disease will heal and be functional at the below-knee level. Many studies indicate below-knee healing with prosthetic rehabilitation in 75% to 80% of the patients.

Prosthetic fitting at the level of the above-knee amputee is often quite complex. Recent experience indicates that only one fourth of the geriatric patients at this level of amputation can be considered functional users. With application of the adjustable, lightweight socket and other prosthetic refinements, functional use is being elevated to about 50%. Function is defined as daily independent application of the prosthesis. This always correlates with at least short walking distance with or without external aid.

The energy demands required to return to normal ambulatory functions are considerable. Even the healthiest amputees cannot achieve normal gait in terms of velocity, cadence, or energy consumption. Near normal quality of life and physical activity can be attained, however, in younger, stronger well-motivated patients. In older age groups the energy demands are severe, frequently requiring double the amount of energy necessary for normal ambulation.

In an effort to provide the amputee as much function as possible, considerable ingenuity in the design of above-knee prosthetic systems has been required. A significant portion of this discussion concerning the above-knee amputee will be in the area of trade-offs between complex prosthetic systems and human tolerance for sophisticated devices to achieve maximum function. Prescription principles and intelligent rehabilitation measures are indispensable to maximize use capability.

LEVEL SELECTION

The length of the lever arm in the residual limb is of considerable importance. The longer the residual limb, the easier it becomes to suspend and align the prosthesis. Energy demands required of the amputee to move the prosthesis are in direct ratio to the length of the residual limb. Maximum thigh length is retained consistent with the specific circumstances presented at the time of surgery. Cosmesis has been considered a factor as the level of amputation approaches the knee joint because standard prostheses required outside hinges. The conflict between cosmesis and function as they relate to prosthetic fitting is no longer a major consideration. Modern prosthetic systems, even at knee disarticulation level, are generally acceptable in appearance. An exception might be an occasional female in whom an amputation 6.3 cm (2½ inches) short of the knee joint could provide sufficient improved cosmesis to justify this level rather than a transcondylar amputation.

At the other extreme of the problem, shortness of the limb is usually determined by limitation of vascular supply or the overriding demands of ablative tumor surgery or trauma. If a choice is available, leaving even a residual small portion of femur at the trochanteric area is advisable. This will supply additional contouring to allow enhanced prosthetic fit either as an extremely short above-knee socket or a pseudohip disarticulation prosthesis.

If no prosthetic function is anticipated in the individual, then an extremely short above-knee amputation with the bone length at or just below intertrochanteric level may result in a hip flexion contracture with subsequent erosion of the residual femur through the anterior skin of the leg. This complication is unwarranted if its potential is anticipated.

Within these guidelines above-knee amputations should be performed with maximum retention of limb length, consistent with good surgical and wound healing principles.

SURGERY

Choice of incision for the above-knee amputee can be based purely on inflammatory, vascular, and other local considerations. The fleshy characteristics of the thigh allow any orientation of incision to be comfortably tolerated within the prosthesis. When peripheral vascular disease is present physical characteristics will usually identify the potential levels of healing. Laboratory studies, including Doppler ultrasonic monitoring, skin temperature measurements, comparison of local arterial pressures with blood pressure in the upper extremity, thermography, skin oxygen level determination, and other tests of dynamic blood flow, are available. More often the level for surgery in ischemia can be determined on the basis of skin temperature and other physical examination characteristics without resorting to the more complicated laboratory tests, which are most effective in establishing limb viability and limb salvage potential below the knee.

Many above-knee amputations are required following failed vascular reconstruction. In this situation frequent practice has been to make incisions into the groin and along the medial aspect of the thigh as part of the vascular reconstruction. The incisions, particularly those at the groin level, may present significant problems in later prosthetic fitting. It is important to identify and incorporate femoral incisions into the flaps of the above-knee amputation whenever possible.

As a general rule the skin flaps are short. Long flaps compromise skin blood supply. Preliminary marking of the flaps with a pencil is appropriate. A common mistake is in making skin closure too tight. Allowance should be made for enough skin to close the cylindrical, muscle-stabilized amputation (Fig. 25-1).

Especially in the dysvascular amputee an incision through skin, subcutaneous tissue, and fascia should be accomplished with as few cuts as possible and with minimal undermining or beveling of the soft tissues. Identification of the major vessels can be easily accomplished. Control with ligature is performed.

Ligation of the sciatic and femoral nerves is routinely necessary if for no other reason than to control bleeding: arterial blood supply lingers longer within the nerves than elsewhere. No special precautions other than the ligation of the nerves under moderate traction seem warranted to avoid painful neuroma formation. As long as the nerve has been ligated short of the bone length and resides in the surrounding soft tissue, painful neuroma should not develop. The most common cause of painful neuroma is amputation associated with severe trauma and the subsequent scarring related to regrowing peripheral nerves. Thus in surgery at the above-knee level related to trauma considerable effort should be undertaken to identify the nerves and ligate them as short as possible.

The bone can be divided with a hand, power, or

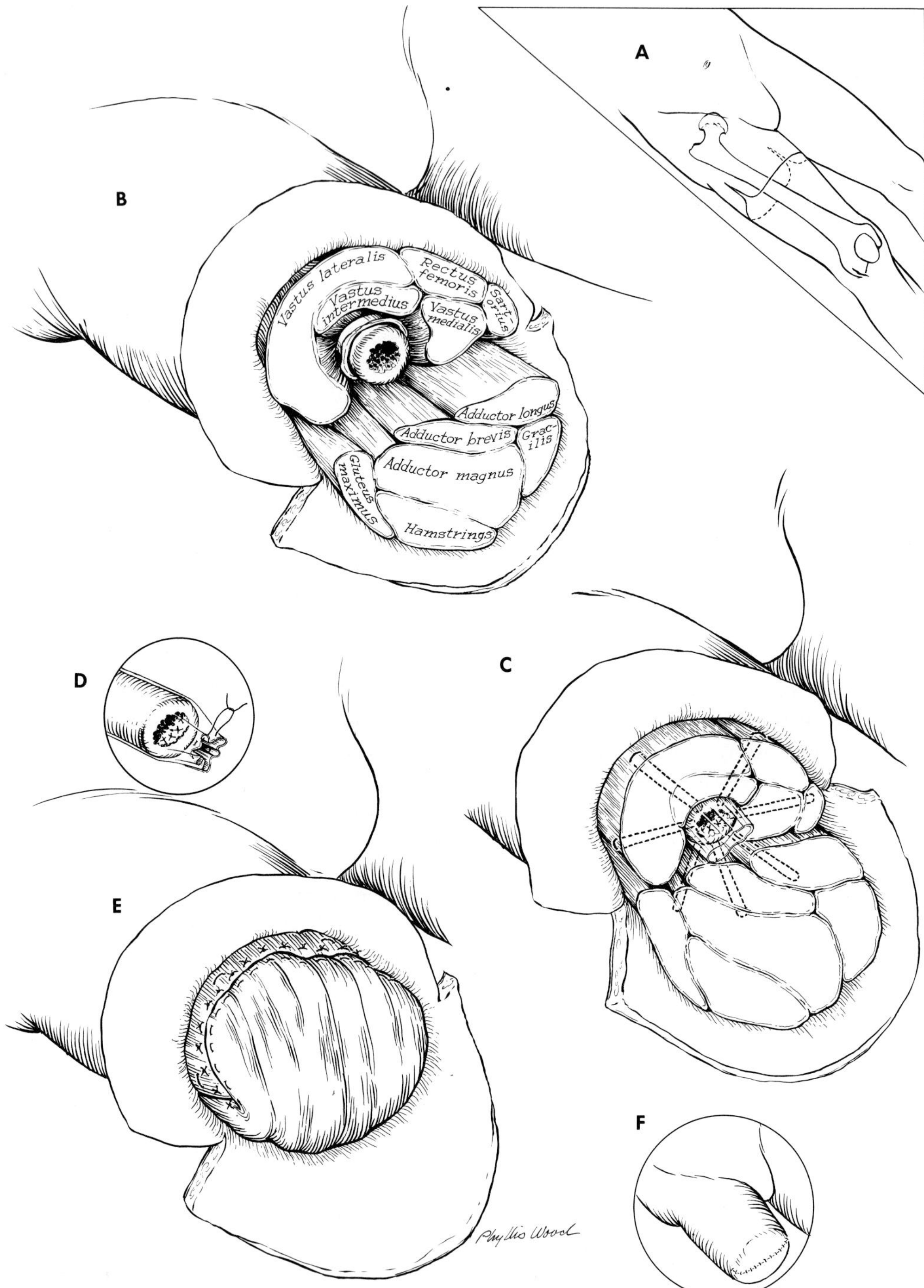

Fig. 25-1. A, Skin flaps. The more flabby the tissue, the more transverse may be the skin incisions of anteroposterior flap. Firm musculature will require more oval-shaped flaps because stump at rest will tend to have anteroposterior diameter similar to mediolateral diameter. Longest portion of flap should be about same length as radius of cross section of thigh at bone amputation level. **B,** Cross section of longer posterior musculature, which is appropriate if vascularization is available. Also, beveling of sharp edges of femur is notable with rolled back periosteum. **C,** Stabilization is of musculature with various bone-muscle stabilization sutures appropriate. Chromic gut is appropriate suture material. **D,** Purse-string closure of periosteum over end of femur. This usually is only available in young people. **E,** Closure of fascia is noted. Long posterior flap of myofascia is closed over bone end. For clarity I have separated subcutaneous tissue from fascia to demonstrate closure. However, surgically this should not be done. **F,** Cylindrical stump is demonstrated with skin suture closure. Orientation of suture closure, however, can be in any appropriate situation, depending on local skin needs. Dressing for this stump should be maintained in position by Elastiplast. Suction drain should be used if muscle ooze continues after ligation of vessels.

Gigli saw. A transverse section of the bone should be carried out and the sharp cortical bone carefully rounded, particularly the anterior and lateral areas. With simple myofascial closure the bone end routinely migrates laterally and anteriorly. It can come to lie directly under the skin, causing pain and occasional tissue necrosis. Meticulous beveling of the cortex is important.

Muscle stabilization is an absolute requirement if a strong physiological residual limb is to be obtained. Since most above-knee amputations are performed for ischemia and wound healing is the primary consideration, it may not be possible to properly stabilize the muscles to each other or to the distal femur without further compromising the healing of devitalized tissue. Simple myofascial closure can partially centralize the femur in the surrounding muscle, but careful muscle stabilization should be carried out wherever blood supply is adequate and surgical circumstances permit.

Because flexion deformity of the above-knee stump is a common complication, the techniques of muscle stabilization become important relative to hip position. The femoral flexor system is anatomically stronger than the femoral extensor system no matter which level, long or short, of the above-knee amputation is performed. On the other hand, it is desirable to have overlying quadriceps musculature defending the anterior subcutaneous tissues from potential migration and protrusion of the femoral shaft.

When dividing the musculature, the quadriceps is cut longer than the hamstrings and abductors. These muscles should be attached to one another with the hamstrings somewhat tighter than the quadriceps. The adductors are pulled down under moderate tension. Proximal adductor migration is seen in a great many poorly muscle-stabilized, above-knee amputations. Strong, active, well-stabilized adductor muscles are of great importance in satisfactory prosthetic control.

Surgical closure is routine. The Penrose drain or suction drain should be used even though minimal bleeding was present at the time of surgical closure. Skin closure with a running monofilament suture or with interrupted sutures supported by Steri-strips is routine.

Postoperative dressing. The principles of postoperative wound management have been considered elsewhere. The rigid dressing techniques, including immediate postoperative fitting, are difficult to apply at the above-knee level. Soft tissues dressings are equally difficult to maintain in proper position with the gentle compression necessary for edema control and wound support. If soft dressings are to be used, they are best held in place with strips of elasticized adhesive (Elastoplast). This material contours well and creates slight compression. The use of Ace bandages and similar materials to create figure-of-eight spica dressings tends to be self-defeating unless carefully watched and rewrapped as necessary. Such wrappings in the immediate postoperative period become entangled and loosened or too tight. Alternatives to holding the soft dressings in place are tapered stump shrinker–type stockings with belt suspension.

Rigid dressings and the immediate fitting of a temporary prosthesis have presented technical difficulties, which, in many circumstances, outweigh their possible value. Suspension is difficult even with several ingenious systems available. Elderly patients poorly tolerate the waist or over-the-shoulder mobilization.

An excellent postoperative dressing consists of Owen silk and sterile, well-fluffed gauze at the amputation site, over which an Orlon stump stocking is firmly rolled and held in place above the site of amputation on the remaining thigh and hip tissue by medical adhesive. A sterile polyurethane end pad can then be applied to allow gentle terminal pressure and a number of turns of elastic plaster carried over the soft dressings to protect the site of surgery and maintain pressure and immobilization.

A variety of new materials, including air compression systems, are now available. As these develop and become more effective and improved, immediate postoperative dressings for above-knee amputations should be available.

It is most important to permit early activity, including assisted standing, when possible. Most above-knee amputees are elderly and in poor health. The early postoperative period is fraught with medical complications. As in all phases of rehabilitation one would like to mobilize the patient as rapidly as possible, as soon as functional capabilities are available. Temporary limb fitting can be carried out when the patient has become independent in self-care and standing transfers. Once the patient has become independent in transferring and self-care he probably still is in the immature phase of limb healing. This is an ideal situation for a lightweight plastic adjustable socket to which an appropriate knee mechanism can be attached. Adjustable plastic sockets answer the need of keeping pace with changing volume and contour of the stump while being rigid enough to allow mechanical stability for suspension and knee joint attachment.

Young vigorous patients, whose amputations are the result of trauma, congenital anomalies, or neoplasms, do exceptionally well with the immediate postsurgical prosthetic fitting routine. This is particularly true in the adolescent above-knee amputee whose limb was removed for malignancy. Many of them are walking with crutches in 3 or 4 days after an above-knee amputation. The psychological, as well as the physical, benefits of the immediate postsurgical technique under these circumstances have been repeatedly demonstrated.

The above-knee amputee can significantly benefit from an environment in which there are other similar amputees going through various phases of training and therapy. He must now get used to a fairly complex piece of equipment, perform some unaccustomed physical activities, and get used to the psychological blow of having a significant segment of the body missing. More than with other levels of lower extremity amputations, clustering of amputees in the rehabilitation program greatly speeds the progress through this phase of care.

Ideally, physical and functional training of the above-knee amputee starts before the surgical care has been accomplished. Preliminary training in terms of hip extension and abductor strengthening is valuable. More important, some understanding of the posttreatment plan, meeting of the personnel involved, and even seeing the prosthesis itself, all smooth the way for more effective postsurgical care. In many areas cancer visitation programs add another dimension to this preliminary phase.

The specifics of the postoperative and postfitting training program are summarized in Fig. 25-2, the lower extremity amputee evaluation and progress form. As suggested by the scope of this form, especially in the geriatric patient, only a minor part of the physical therapy training program is focused on gait training. The majority of the time spent is related to physical and functional potentials at the highest available level.

Strength and range of the residual limb are the keys to good functional gait. Careful measurement at the beginning of training allows one to note and monitor progress. The primary method of noting ambulatory functions is the analysis of gait velocity. This function summarizes best all progress in the physical and functional training of the above-knee amputee.

Not all of the training is focused on prosthetic use. The functional use of crutches and wheelchairs is a necessary aspect for training. Certainly the very high-level above-knee amputee will find ambulatory activity less energy consuming without the prosthesis. He must be aware of this and recognize the trade-offs between prosthetic function, which returns use of the hands, and a greater rate of tiring than he has been used to in the past. Also, the energy demands of prosthetic use must be recognized, especially in the geriatric patient. The use of a wheelchair need not be considered shameful for long-distance mobilization. Often the availability of wheelchairs for the otherwise independent amputee is the difference between allowing the slower walking above-knee amputee to return to the family setting or relegating him to a nursing home.

The specifics of gait training to a certain extent are related to the specific knee mechanisms and suspension systems used. Details are usually provided by the prosthetist, depending on the characteristics of the equipment supplied. Reinforcement and coaching by the physical therapist when available is, of course, ideal. Here communication between the two individuals is necessary so that the coaching to the patient is not blurred. As the age of the patient increases, changing of any habit patterns of walking becomes progressively more impossible, and tolerance of deviation from ideal prosthetic gait should be accepted. No matter what the training, the gait patterns of the patient will generally fall into that system which costs the least energy. He thus must have sufficient hip joint range and strength. Abduction strength should be sufficient to allow stability on stance phase of gait. Alignment of the residual limb with as much adduction as feasible will give this musculature its greatest advantage. Alignment of the limb in slight flexion will give the hip extensors some advantage in extending the limb. Too much flexion in the stump, however, does not allow full extension of the prosthesis and presents a cosmetic liability with a large anterior bulge in the thigh portion. Considerations such as these supply the background for details of prosthetic prescription and recommendations.

PHYSICAL THERAPY

LOWER EXTREMITY AMPUTEE EVALUATION & PROGRESS NOTE

CHECK ONE: ☐ INITIAL ☐ INTERIM ☐ DISCHARGE

PATIENT'S NAME LAST FIRST MIDDLE	ONSET	RLAH #	UNIT	Rx AREA	AGE
DIAGNOSIS	ADM. TO P.T.	DC FROM P.T.	MOS. ON P.T.	DISCHARGED TO	

GENERAL INFORMATION:

R.T.C. DATE:

STRENGTH & R.O.M.					
UPPER EXTREMITIES	LEFT	RIGHT			
LOWER EXTREMITIES & TRUNK		LEFT		RIGHT	
		STR.	R.O.M.	STR.	R.O.M.
TRUNK	FLEXION				
	EXTENSION				
HIP	FLEXION 0-120				
	EXTENSION				
	ABDUCTION 0-45				
	ADDUCTION 0-35				
	INT. ROT. 0-45				
	EXT. ROT. 0-45				
KNEE	FLEXION 0-135				
	EXTENSION				
ANKLE	DORSI FLEX. 0-20				
	PLANT FLEX. 0-45				
	INVERSION 0-35				
	EVERSION 0-35				

COMMENTS:

SENSATION:

GAIT

Velocity______ cm/sec ______% Normal

PHYSIOLOGICAL RESPONSE:

V.C.

DESCRIPTION OF PROSTHESIS:

EQUIPMENT:

FUNCTIONAL LEVEL I-INDEPENDENT A-ASSISTED S-SUPERVISED U-UNABLE NA-NOT APPLICABLE

ACTIVITY	GRADE		EQUIPMENT USED
Rolls side to side & prone			
Sits or stands from supine			
Stands from chair			
TRANSFERS (sitting/standing)			
To & from bed			
To & from toilet			
To & from shower/tub			
To & from car			
WHEELCHAIR			
Manages brakes/footrests			
Propels - level			
Ramps - up & down			
Manages doors			
AMBULATION	$\bar{s}$ PRO	$\bar{c}$ PRO	
Puts on & removes prosth.			
____ft. smooth surface			
20 ft. rough terrain			
Up & down curbs			
Up & down stairs			
Gets up from ground			
Up & down ramp			

MAJOR PROBLEMS:

GOALS:

TREATMENT PLAN:

Frequency: Duration:

R.P.T. DATE

M.D.

76P2 RD413 (R6-79)

RANCHO LOS AMIGOS HOSPITAL
COUNTY OF LOS ANGELES • DEPARTMENT OF HEALTH SERVICES

Fig. 25-2. Lower amputee evaluation and progress form. (Courtesy Rancho Los Amigos Hospital, Downey, Calif.)

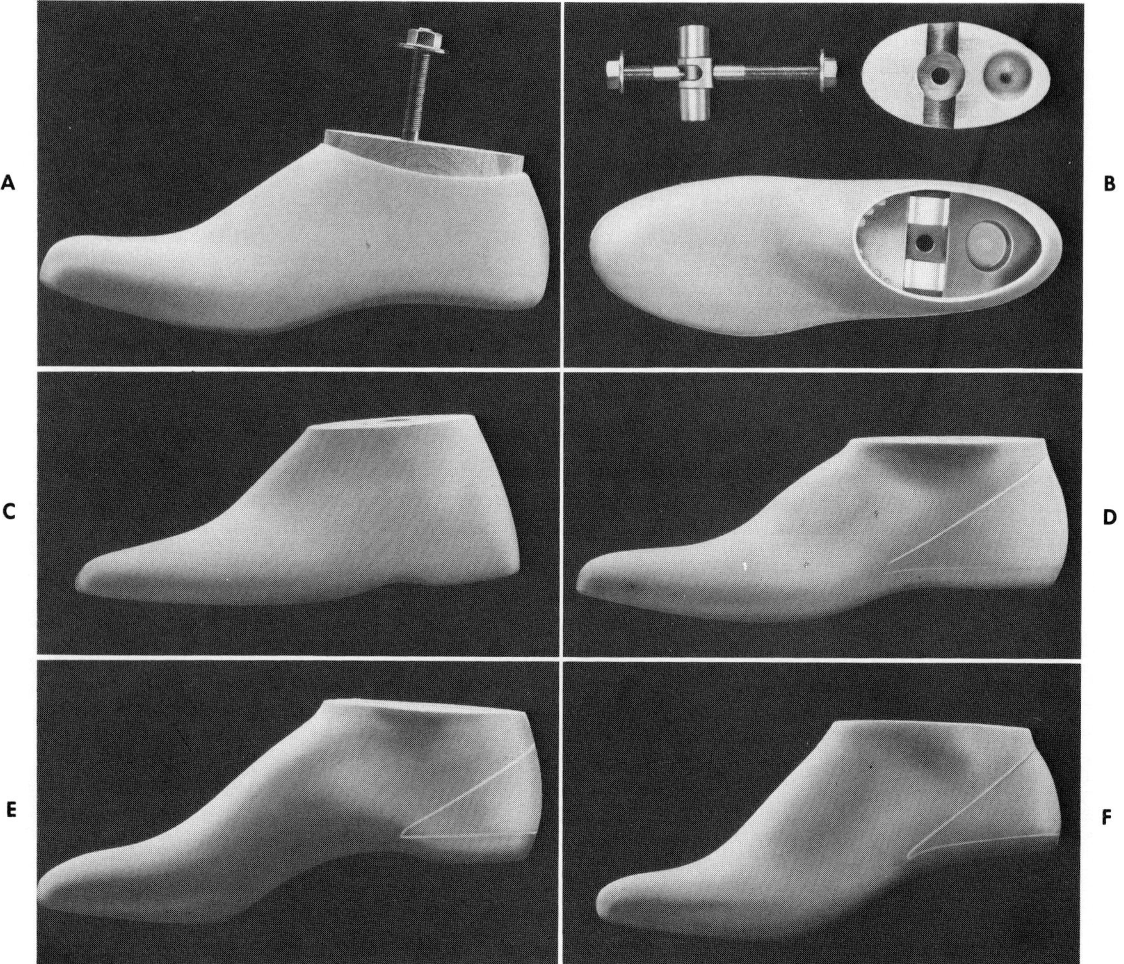

Fig. 25-3. Solid ankle, cushion heel (SACH) feet come in great number of sizes but must still require custom modification to fit each patient's shoe properly. Different heel heights are also available. **A,** Single-axis lateral view. **B,** Components of single-axis foot. **C,** Postoperative foot was designed for walking without shoes or in slippers without heel. Wide sole is provided for more stability. **D,** Men's SACH foot for regular heels. **E,** Men's high heel foot for contemporary fashion shoes and western boots. **F,** Women's feet range from 0.9-cm (3/8-inch) heel to 5.6-cm (2 1/4-inch) heel. (Courtesy Kingsley Manufacturing Co., Costa Mesa, Calif.)

Section II

Prosthetic management

VERT MOONEY
MICHAEL J. QUIGLEY

General guidelines for above-knee prostheses are given in Table 7 at the end of the chapter.

ABOVE-KNEE PROSTHETIC COMPONENTS

Prosthetic feet

Essentially four different designs of prosthetic feet are available for above-knee prostheses:

1. Solid ankle, cushioned heel (SACH)
2. Single axis
3. Multiaxis
4. Hydraulic

All prosthetic feet provide similar function. During the stance phase of gait the foot serves as a weight-bearing platform, absorbing the impact of heel strike, then plantar flexing to allow the forefoot to contact the floor smoothly and rapidly, giving the patient a solid base of support. When midstance occurs, ankle motion in the prosthetic foot is blocked, and the patient must then roll forward over the forefoot, which is solid up to the

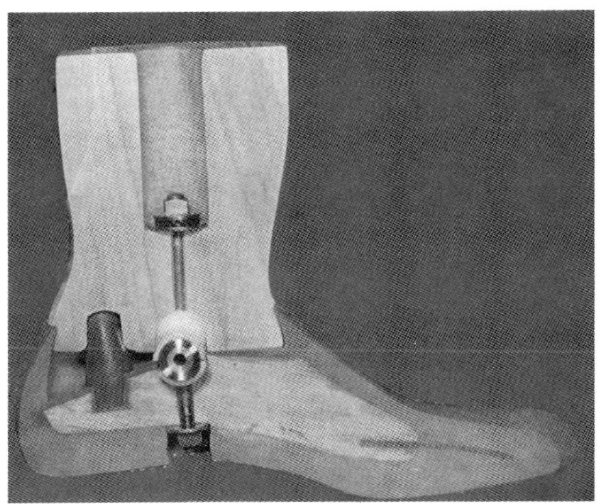

Fig. 25-4. Cutaway of single-axis foot. Note plantar flexion bumper in heel. This bumper can be adjusted for exact control of plantar flexion action. Also notice wood keel set in rubber to provide anterior stability to foot. (Courtesy Otto Bock Orthopedic Industries, Inc., Minneapolis, Minn.)

"toe break." The toe break simulates the metatarsal-phalangeal joints, allowing the patient to roll smoothly over the forefoot and the foot and shoe to bend in a natural fashion.

The major differences in the type of prosthetic feet are weight, maintenance, and the capability of providing inversion-eversion and transverse rotation functions.

SACH foot. The durability, light weight, and excellent cosmesis of the SACH foot make it the most popular of all prosthetic feet used in the United States (Fig. 25-3). The SACH foot has no actual moving parts but approximates joint motion by the compression of rubber around a solid hard wood core called the "keel." The SACH foot can be used on most types of lower extremity prostheses. It is used almost exclusively on prostheses for children, females, and patients with below-knee and Syme amputations. Its use in above-knee prostheses is somewhat more discretionary. Heel-strike stability and the necessity for coordinated knee-ankle-foot biomechanics exemplify consideration of foot-type prescription requirements for the above-knee amputee.

The durability of the SACH foot makes it particularly suitable for children, since the child's high level of activity and tendency to soil the prosthesis with dirt and water may result in breakdown of feet that have metal hinges or other mechanisms. The SACH foot is preferred for females, since it provides a very smooth contour and appearance throughout the ankle area. Most other types of feet have a visible joint line at the ankle area, which moves as the patient walks and can be noticeable.

Presently, the majority of above-knee prostheses are fitted with SACH feet. One must be aware, however, of the circumstances that contraindicate a SACH foot, such as the patient who requires the foot to plantar flex very rapidly at heel strike to increase stability by allowing the total foot to contact the floor. The prosthetic knee may be unstable if too much time is spent on the heel.

Single-axis foot. The single-axis foot differs from the SACH foot in that a metal hinge is used to provide dorsiflexion and plantar flexion (Fig. 25-4). Behind this metal ankle joint in the heel section of the foot is a rubber plantar flexion bumper insert that can be adjusted to allow the patient to plantar flex the foot very quickly at heel strike. Anterior to the metal-hinge ankle joint is a flat rubber dorsiflexion stop that prevents the foot from dorsiflexing past 90 degrees. The dorsiflexion stop can be adjusted to the precise position that permits alignment push-off, as the weight is carried forward over the anterior portion of the prosthetic foot. The single-axis foot may also have a rubber or neoprene body, which will allow it to flex at the forefoot, using the toe-break principle earlier described.

Advantages of the single-axis foot are (1) easy adjustment of plantar flexor action to allow maximum stability of the knee joint at heel strike, especially on ramps and uneven surfaces and (2) more "life," or spring, a quality that some patients enjoy, since it provides a greater range of plantar flexion mobility than the SACH foot.

Disadvantages of the single-axis foot are (1) the amount of maintenance needed for mechanical parts to control breakage, functional adjustment, and squeaking and (2) a visible joint line at the ankle, which can be seen as the foot moves up and down. This joint line is more noticeable than the smooth surfaces provided by the SACH foot, so the single-axis foot may be contraindicated for cosmetic reasons.

Multiaxis prosthetic foot. The multiaxis prosthetic foot allows plantar flexion and dorsiflexion, as well as a degree of inversion, eversion, and transverse rotation. These mechanical qualities more nearly represent normal ankle subtalar and midtarsal joint movement. The outside appearence of the multiaxis prosthetic foot is the same as the single-axis unit. However, instead of using a metal ankle joint, a solid rubber block with cables running across the ankle areas is used. This solid rubber joint allows motion in all planes. Motion is limited by contouring and changing the hardness of the rubber. The advantage of the multiaxis foot is its ability to absorb forces that are placed on the mediolateral aspect of the foot as well as a certain amount of transverse or rotary torque. This action is particularly valuable when walking on uneven terrain, since these forces would be transmitted as shear forces directly to the socket and the patient's residual limb if they were not partially absorbed at the foot level.

The disadvantages of the multiaxis foot are essentially the same as the single-axis foot, except that it typically weighs a few ounces more than the SACH or single-axis foot.

Hydraulic foot. Presently only one hydraulically controlled foot is available. A second design is being developed. The hydraulic foot available is part of a hydraulic knee and foot system known as Hydra-Cadence. The foot is linked to the knee mechanism so that when the knee flexes a few degrees the foot will dorsiflex to clear the floor during swing phase of gait. The same hydraulic cylinder used to control knee motion is also used to absorb plantar flexion forces at heel strike. This foot has the advantage that the heel height can be adjusted for use in shoes with different heel heights. No other prosthetic foot has this capability. The disadvantages of the hydraulic Hydra-Cadence foot is that it must be used with the entire system. This prosthesis is heavy and requires a greater than normal amount of maintenance.

Prosthetic knee units

A great number of prosthetic knee units are available. It is probable that as much research had been done in this one area of prosthetics as in all other areas combined. All prosthetic knee units use the patient's forward motion and hip flexion to initiate knee flexion. The amount of knee flexion obtained is limited by using a number of different mechanical hydraulic or pneumatic systems. During knee extension all prosthetic knee units tend to dampen the speed the lower leg is extending to decrease terminal impact when knee movement hits the extension stop.

All prosthetic knees must be stable during the stance phase of gait yet allow the knee to swing naturally during the swing phase of gait and allow for comfortable sitting. All prosthetic knees are designed to function with some amount of stability inherent in the alignment of the knee units in relation to the patient's line of weight

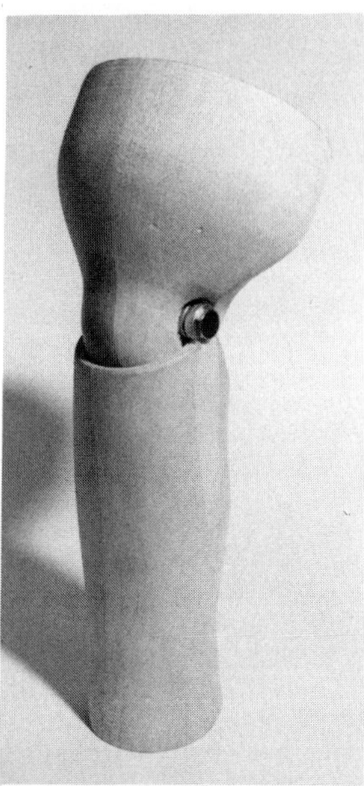

Fig. 25-5. Child-size constant friction knee-shin setup. This is prosthetic knee of preference for children due to its durability and simplicity. (Courtesy U.S. Manufacturing Co., Pasadena, Calif.)

bearing. This feature is called "alignment stability." Prosthetic knees will not function properly if the prosthesis is malaligned. The major differences in prosthetic knees relate to the methods employed to provide stance phase stability and to allow smooth and natural knee flexion during swing phase, especially when patients are walking at different gait cadences.

There are seven different types of prosthetic knee units, varying from the simple fixed-axis hinge type of knee to complicated hydraulic systems. The type of knee to be prescribed will depend on the patient's ability to control the knee, the activity level of the patient, durability and maintenance requirement, and stability requirements necessary to prevent the patient from falling. When there is a choice between two or more separate knee mechanisms the clinic team members and prosthetist should select that unit with which they have the greatest amount of experience. It is important that all members of the amputee team have a clear understanding as to how the knee should function and be able to relate this knowledge to the patient for training and prosthetic use.

Constant friction knee. The constant friction knee is commonly used because of its simplicity. This knee consists of a hinge-type mechanism that swings freely in both flexion and extension.

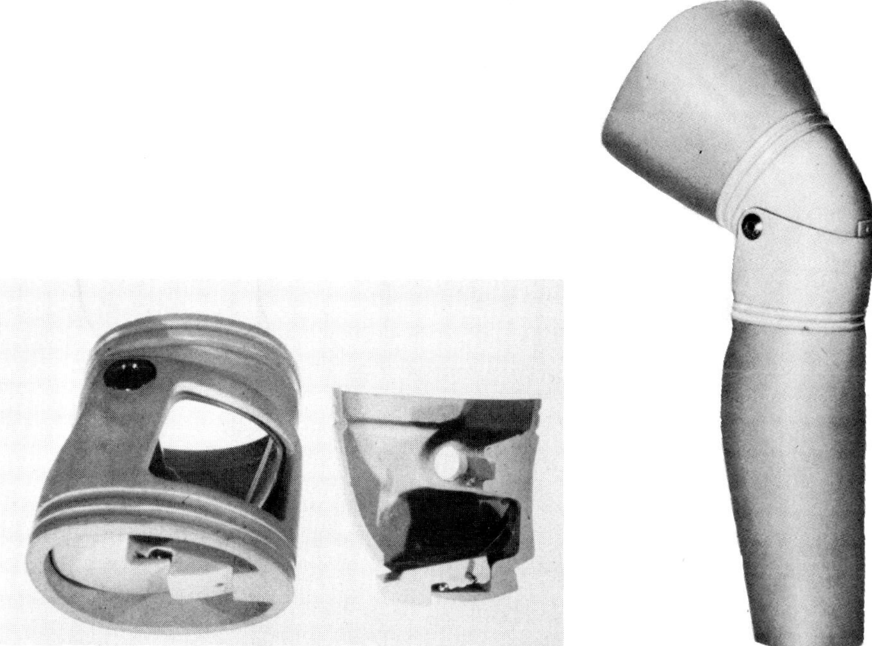

Fig. 25-6. Lightweight, plastic manual lock knee. This unit was designed for geriatric patient who will be marginal walker. It is hollow, yet sturdy enough for geriatric patient. Knee can also function as constant friction unit. (Courtesy Otto Bock Orthopedic Industries, Inc., Minneapolis, Minn.)

Knee swing is dampened by the use of a screw or rubber pad that applies friction to the knee bolt. In this manner, the amount of friction can be adjusted to the patient's normal cadence so that pendulum action of the shank will correspond to the opposite limb.

The constant friction knee is used in most children (Fig. 25-5). The light weight, durability, and small number of mechanical parts present allow it to be easily produced in a number of smaller sizes. The same features are advantageous with adolescent and adult amputees as well. The compact endoskeletal designs allow for good cosmetic shaping around the knee. The major disadvantage of the constant friction knee is that the friction can be set for only one cadence. Should the patient wish to speed up or slow down gait, the prosthetic knee will not flex and extend with the same timing as the natural knee. The constant friction knee obtains its stability during stance phase from prosthetic alignment only. Therefore this knee should not be used on patients who are weak, unstable, have alignment problems because of joint deformities or muscle weakness, or who may have serious problems if they fall. The single-axis constant friction knee continues to be the unit most frequently prescribed. Its simplicity, durability, relatively low cost, and good cosmesis encourage widespread patient acceptance.

Manual locking knee. The manual locking knee consists of a constant friction knee hinge with a positive lock, usually a pin that drops through the knee, locking the knee mechanism in extension. When sitting, the patient can manually release this lock to allow knee flexion. A spring mechanism automatically engages the lock when the patient stands. Manual locking knees generally have the capability of being set in an unlock position if the patient wishes to walk with a free knee. Alignment stability must be incorporated into the prosthesis to allow the patient to walk with a free knee, since it then functions as a constant friction knee when unlocked.

The manual locking knee is generally used for patients who are weak, unstable, and to whom a fall would be serious (Fig. 25-6). It is also commonly used as a temporary prosthesis. The manual locking knee is used by some patients for walking over uneven terrain, as when hiking, hunting, climbing, and carrying heavy objects. Two hydraulic knee units are available with manual lock settings.

Variable friction knee. The variable friction knee differs from the constant friction knee in

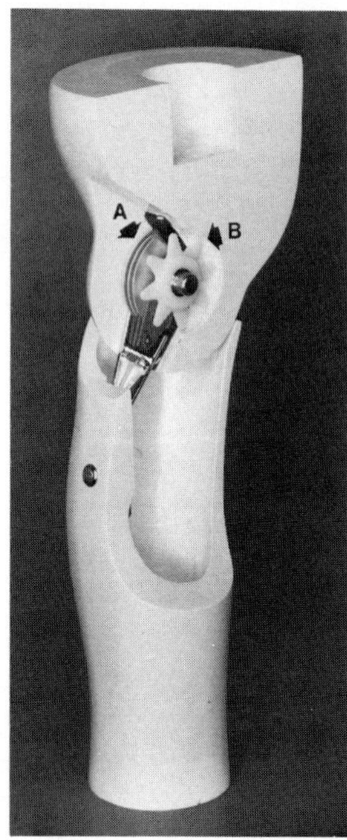

Fig. 25-7. Mechanical cadence control knee unit. This knee unit, designed at Northwestern University, uses three staggered friction bumpers *(A)* to resist knee flexion. Star-shaped adjustment knob *(B)* can be reached by patient. This type of unit generally requires frequent adjustment and is not as smooth as fluid control swing phase units. (Courtesy U.S. Manufacturing Co., Pasadena, Calif.)

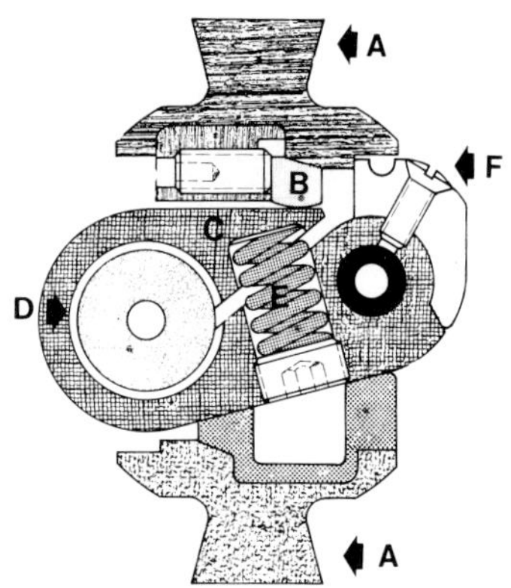

Fig. 25-8. Schematic of endoskeletal weight-activated friction (safety) knee. Pylon tube is attached to upper and lower attachment extensions *(A)*. When weight is applied to top of knee during stance phase, top of joint rotates downward (counterclockwise in this case), forcing pressure block *(B)* against brake lever on lower knee block *(C)*. This narrows diameter of that portion of lower knee block surrounding knee bolt *(D)*, resulting in braking effect. Resistance to knee motion is proportional to weight applied. Amount of weight necessary to initiate braking effect is preset with adjustment screw *(E)*. When weight is released from prosthesis, spring releases friction from knee bolt, and knee functions as constant friction unit during swing phase. Constant friction setting is adjustable by tightening another screw *(F)*. (Courtesy Otto Bock Orthopedic Industries, Inc., Minneapolis, Minn.)

A

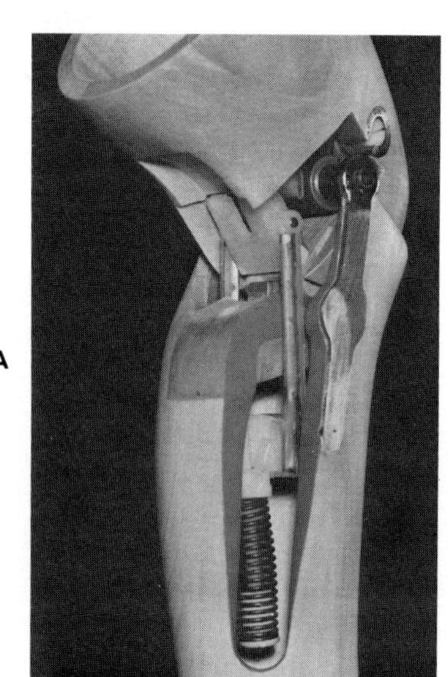

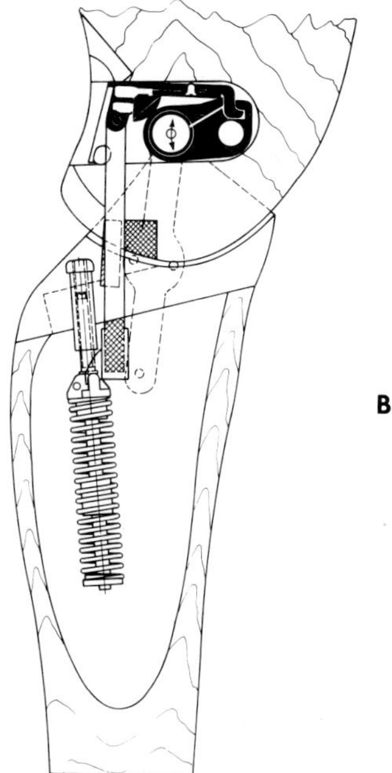

B

Fig. 25-9. A, Weight-activated friction (safety) knee. B, When body weight is applied through knee bolt, friction housing (arrows) engages, preventing knee motion. This knee uses same leverage principle as fingernail clipper. Spring controls knee flexion and extension. Similar knee is available for modular endoskeletal systems (Fig. 25-8). (Courtesy Otto Bock Orthopedic Industries Inc., Minneapolis, Minn.)

that the resistance to knee flexion increases as the knee flexes from the fully extended position (Fig. 25-7). The number of staggered friction pads provides this resistance.

The advantage of the variable friction knee is that it allows "cadence response." Cadence response is the ability to time the knee in swing phase and to allow change when different walking speeds are used, thus matching the timing of the prosthetic knee with the normal knee. Cadence response in the variable friction knee is generally inferior to that provided by fluid control knee mechanisms.

The disadvantage of the variable friction knee is the great number of mechanical parts requiring adjustment for proper function. The components tend to wear quickly and to lose adjustment and become noisy. Considerably more maintenance is required than with the constant friction knee. The variable friction knee is not available in endoskeletal designs, therefore the exoskeletal structure must be used with this knee unit.

Weight-activated friction (safety) knee. The weight-activated friction prosthetic knee is commonly referred to as a safety knee. This unit functions as a constant friction knee during swing phase but when weight is applied through the knee, a housing with a high coefficient of friction presses against the knee mechanism and prevents it from flexing (Figs. 25-8 and 25-9). A number of different designs of mechanical safety knees are available, all of them functioning in an essentially similar manner. The amount of weight required before the knee will "freeze" can be adjusted to meet the patient's requirements, since a 40.5-kg (90-pound) woman will require a different adjustment than a 72-kg (160-pound) man. Safety knees are usually effective from full knee extension to about 20 degrees of knee flexion. Beyond this point the amount of weight passing through the knee decreases, and the bearing surface and breaking action are diminished.

The safety knee is used in most geriatric above-knee amputees. If a geriatric patient falls, fractures can easily occur. The additional margin of safety is important. The safety knee is contraindicated for younger, more active patients, since they usually have the strength and balance to control a more functional constant friction or hydraulic knee. Younger, active patients find the safety knee to be an annoyance because it will lock and not allow them the freedom of movement they desire. Safety knees do not provide cadence response. This poses no problem because patients who use safety knees will usually walk at only one cadence. Safety knees do require minor adjustments, since the friction setting will tend to wear down or change and will make the knee unstable and noisy.

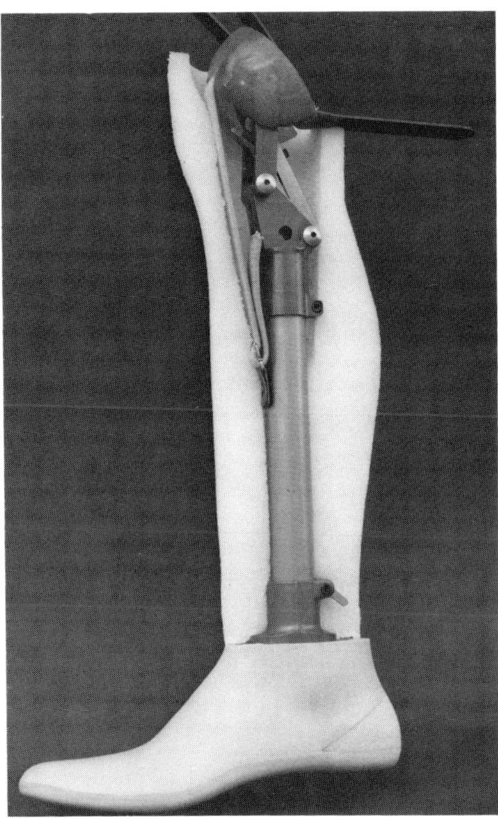

Fig. 25-10. Modular endoskeletal four-bar linkage knee attached to SACH foot. Foam cover provides shape to leg. (Courtesy U.S. Manufacturing Co., Pasadena, Calif.)

Polycentric, or link, knee. The polycentric knee mechanism usually consists of a four-bar linkage that has the ability to change the instantaneous center of rotation between the prosthetic thigh and shank (Fig. 25-10).

A polycentric mechanism is also available that simulates the action of the femoral condyle rotating on the tibial plateau. The advantage of the polycentric mechanism is that the axis of rotation of the knee changes to provide different stability characteristics during the gait cycle. Some polycentric knees also have the advantage of providing an increased range of knee flexion, rotating the shank well underneath the knee during sitting so that the prosthesis does not protrude beyond the level of the normal knee (Figs. 25-11 and 25-12). The polycentric knee helps solve one of the basic anatomical problems in above-knee

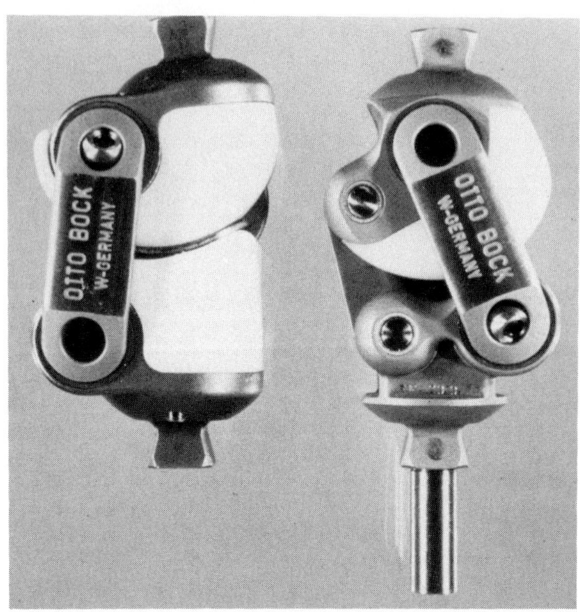

Fig. 25-11. Endoskeletal polycentric knee mechanisms with internal extension assists. (Courtesy Otto Bock Orthopedic Industries, Inc., Minneapolis, Minn.)

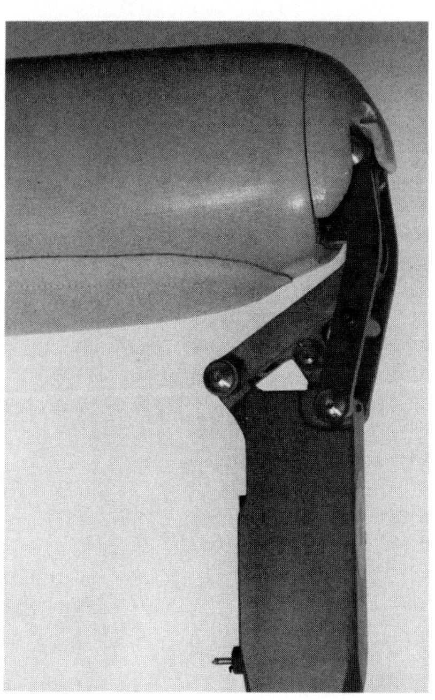

Fig. 25-12. One advantage of polycentric four-bar linkage knee is that it can rotate shank under knee during sitting. This is particularly beneficial to long above-knee and through-knee amputees. (Courtesy U.S. Manufacturing Co., Pasadena, Calif.)

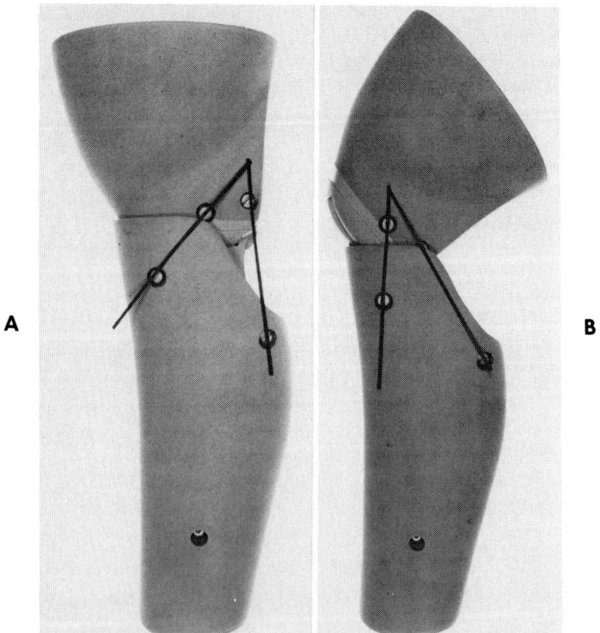

Fig. 25-13. Four-bar linkage (polycentric knee). To determine instantaneous knee center, lines are passed through two vertical linkages. Knee center is wherever these lines intersect. **A,** Knee center moves from posterior to midline during full extension, resulting in knee stability. **B,** Knee center has moved anteriorly with knee flexion, making it easier for knee to be flexed during initiation of swing phase. (Courtesy Hosmer-Dorrance Corp., Campbell, Calif.)

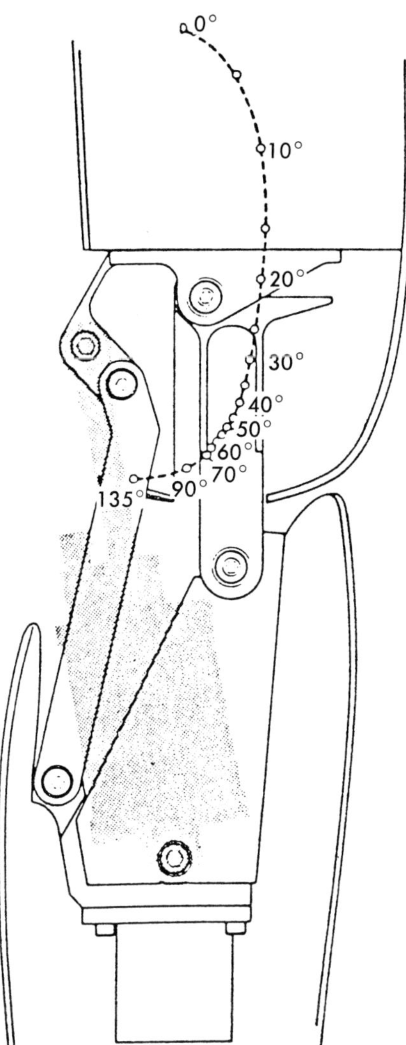

Fig. 25-14. Linkage arrangement and path of instant center for UCBL four-bar linkage polycentric knee. Note that instant center is high and posterior to midline at full extension, affording good control and stability; with slight flexion center moves anteriorly, making it easy to flex knee to initiate swing phase. (From Radcliffe, C. W.: Prosthet. Orthot. Int. 1(3):146-160, Dec., 1977.)

prosthetic design, the location of the center of rotation about the knee. During stance phase knee alignment is very important. From the time the heel strikes the floor until the foot is flat on the floor a flexion moment can occur at the knee, causing it to buckle. The prosthetic knee therefore should be aligned so that the floor reaction resultant force passes through or anterior to the prothetic knee, directing the line of weight bearing posterior to the midline of the limb (Fig. 25-13). At the terminal portion of stance phase, knee flexion is initiated to enable the prosthesis to clear the floor and advance in front of the sound leg during swing phase. If the prosthetic knee center is set too far posterior to the line of neutral weight bearing, it is difficult to initiate knee flexion. Under these circumstances the patient would have a prosthesis that is stable at heel strike but excessively stable when initiating knee flexion. The prosthetist must compromise the location of the single-axis knee to match these contradictory alignment requirements.

The polycentric knee should be designed with the instant center of rotation located posterior to this weight line during heel strike (full knee extension) and anterior to the weight line during heel-off (slight knee flexion) (Fig. 25-14). The polycentric knee also has the advantage of a greater zone of stability than constant friction knees because the instantaneous center of rotation is placed higher on the prosthesis (Fig. 25-15).

Polycentric knees are generally used on three categories of patients. The first is the knee disarticulation patient, in whom the high instant center of rotation is advantageous, so that the polycentric knee will swing under the thigh when the patient sits. Patients with short above-knee amputations (femur length less than 50%) will benefit from this unit because they also can take advantage of the higher instant center of rotation and the increased zone of stability provided by the polycentric unit. The third group of patients benefiting from the polycentric knee mechanism is those individuals with weak hip extensors.

The disadvantage of the polycentric knee is the increased weight and bulk due to the numerous linkage mechanisms. With certain designs, a greater than normal amount of moving parts are needed for proper function. The size and weight usually contraindicate this knee unit for females. The endoskeletal condylar design can be used if a cosmetic polycentric knee is desired.

Hydraulic control knee mechanism. The hydraulic knee is preferred over the constant friction knee because of two major problems inherent in the constant friction mechanism. First, the constant friction unit can be only set for one cadence; when the patient changes pace, the timing of the prosthesis is not the same as the normal limb, and the patient must compensate for his gait or "limp." Also, the energy the patient imparts into constant friction units during the initiation of swing phase is absorbed and given off as heat rather than stored (as a spring mechanism) to help extend the leg during the latter part of swing phase. Both hydraulic and pneumatic con-

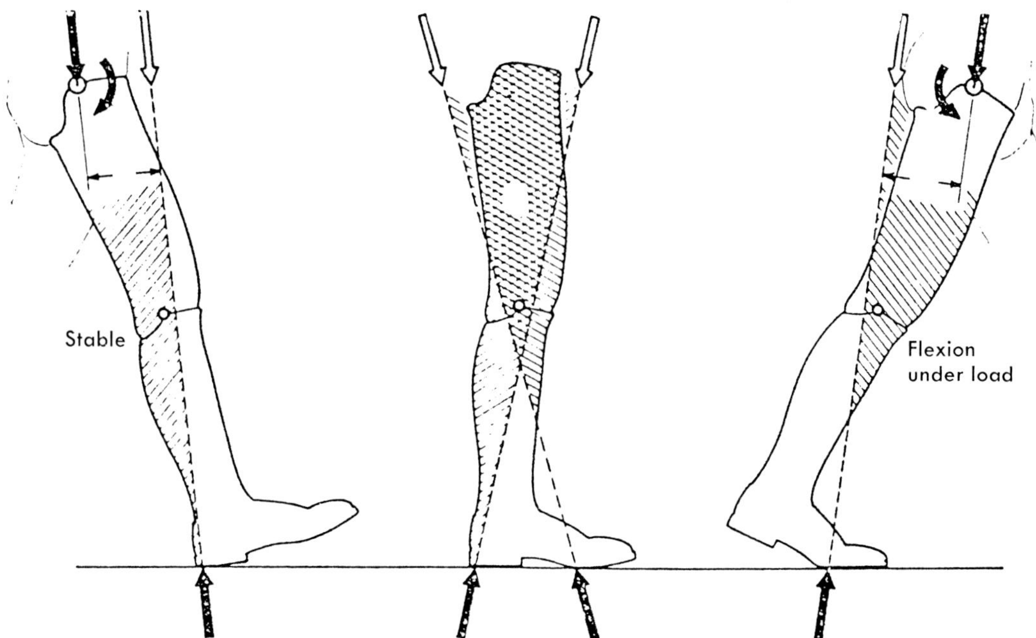

Fig. 25-15. Zone of voluntary stability, as described by Radcliffe,[3] is range of motion in which knee of above-knee prosthesis is stable during stance phase. Factors affecting stability are alignment, inertia, and muscle force. (From Radcliffe, C. W.: Prosthet. Orthot. Int. 1(3):146-160, Dec., 1977.)

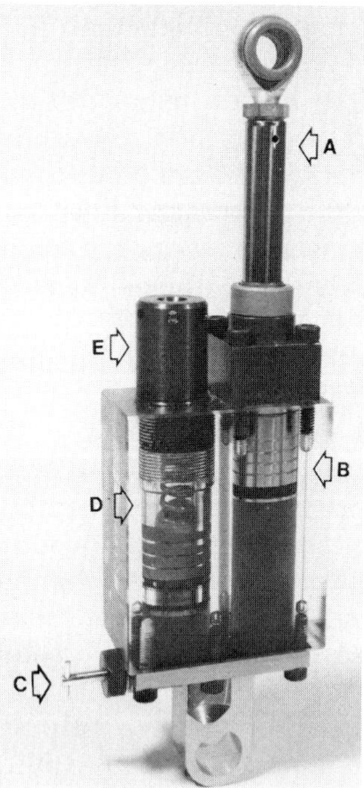

Fig. 25-16. Hydraulic swing phase control. Piston rod *(A)* is attached to thigh section on separate bolt behind knee. As knee flexes, piston *(B)* is forced down cylinder, forcing oil out through bypass channel located at bottom of cylinder. Adjustment screw *(C)* controls rate of oil flow by changing diameter of valve in bypass channel. Spring *(D)* is provided for extension bias control, which can be set by means of adjustment knob *(E)*. (Courtesy U.S. Manufacturing Co. Pasadena, Calif.)

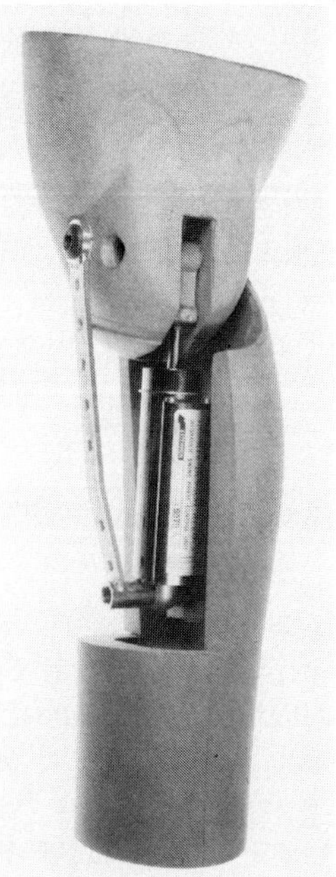

Fig. 25-17. Cutaway of hydraulic swing phase control unit in prosthetic knee-shin setup. Note that attachment of piston on upper (thigh) section is posterior to knee joint. Polyurethane foam is used as structural material for this particular knee unit. (Courtesy Hosmer-Dorrance Corp., Campbell, Calif.)

trol prosthetic knee systems are responsive to the patient's cadence. This cadence response allows the patient to change cadence without having to vault or use other gait compensation techniques. The hydraulic knee will adjust its timing by increasing resistance to knee flexion.

The physical law that liquids are essentially incompressible is employed in hydraulic mechanisms. As the knee flexes a piston is pushed into an oil-filled cylinder, and as the piston moves down the cylinder the oil is forced out through one or more bypass channels (Figs. 25-16 and 25-17). Some knees use a number of bypass channels that are successively covered by the piston as it moves down the cylinder. As these channels are covered the fluid flow rate is decreased, thereby providing greater resistance to knee flexion. Fluid that flows from the cylinder through the bypass channels is forced upward through a check valve and back into the cylinder above the piston. Adjustment screws allow the prosthetist to vary the cross-sectional area of the bypass channel, thus increasing or decreasing resistance to flexion and extension. Heel rise is limited by the effects of gravity, mechanical friction of the hydraulic seals, and the hydraulic resistance itself, which is adjustable. During knee extension the piston rod is pulled up the cylinder and forces the oil back to the check valves at the top of the cylinder, through the bypass channels, and back into the bottom of the cylinder. Full extension of the piston blocks further knee extension.

Present designs of the hydraulic knee mechanism result from years of research to determine the exact size and configuration of the orifices in the cylinder wall, which will provide the optimum resistance to heel rise in flexion and also control extension. Present hydraulic knee mechanisms allow excellent cadence response and are very durable and easily adjusted by the prosthetist (Fig. 25-18).

The hydraulic knee mechanism is indicated for patients who can take advantage of the cadence response function. Adult males are the greatest number of hydraulic knee users. Their activity level requires the cadence response function, and the additional weight and bulk of these units is usually of no consequence. Adult females also use hydraulic units, but to a lesser degree, because it is more difficult to obtain a cosmetically acceptable calf shape when a hydraulic unit is used. Endoskeletal structures are being used with increasing frequency on females, which often contraindicates the hydraulic knee unit, since it is difficult to shape the foam cover around the hydraulic knee and calf.

Pneumatic control knee mechanism. The pneumatic control knee mechanism physically resembles the hydraulic system and also provides cadence response. The difference between these two knees relates to the fact that a hydraulic unit is filled with oil, which is essentially incompressible, and the pneumatic unit is filled with air, a compressible medium that acts like a spring (Fig. 25-19). The pneumatic knee mechanism stores energy that is placed in the system as the piston is pushed down in the cylinder during knee flexion and returns this energy to help extend the knee during the latter part of swing phase. It is not desirable to have the knee extend as quickly as it would if all the energy stored in the fluid control system were released during knee extension. So a certain amount of this energy (which is stored as compressed air) must be leaked off to decrease terminal impact of the knee in full extension.

The pneumatic control knee mechanism consists of a piston rod that is attached to the thigh

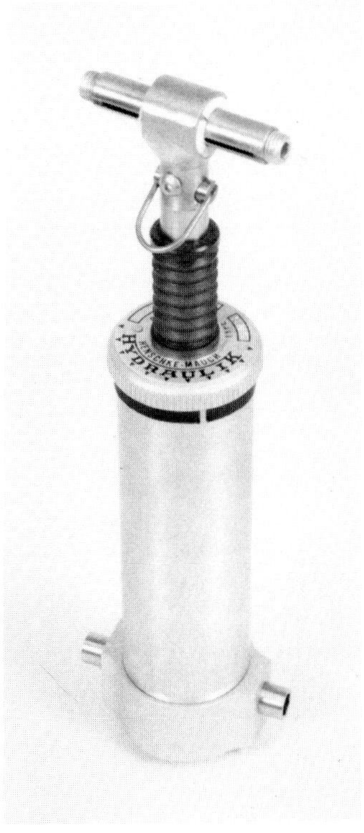

Fig. 25-18. The Henschke-Mauch S'n'S provides both swing phase cadence response and positive stance phase stability. Third feature of this unit is manual lock that can be set by patient. Designer of this unit is presently working on hydraulic foot. (Courtesy Mauch Industries, Inc., Dayton, Ohio.)

section of the prosthesis behind the knee bolt. Knee flexion forces the piston down the cylinder, which in turn forces air through a bypass channel at the bottom of the cylinder. The air travels upward around the side of the cylinder, through a port at the top of the cylinder, and back into the cylinder above the piston. Resistance to knee flexion can be adjusted by a screw that lowers a needle valve into the port at the top of the cylinder. If the needle valve completely blocks this port, knee flexion is blocked. If the needle valve is raised completely, no pneumatic resistance is possible, so the unit functions as a constant friction mechanism. A second adjustment screw regulates the distance the needle valve can float out of the port during knee extension.

The pneumatic swing control unit is generally lighter and smaller than the hydraulic swing unit and easier to maintain. Should it malfunction, the pneumatic swing control unit then works like a constant friction knee, and there is no oil leakage problem. The simplicity of the system makes it easy for the prosthetist to disassemble the system to replace seals, without having to send the unit back to the manufacturer, as is usually necessary with hydraulic units.

The pneumatic swing control unit differs functionally from the hydraulic unit in that it tends to

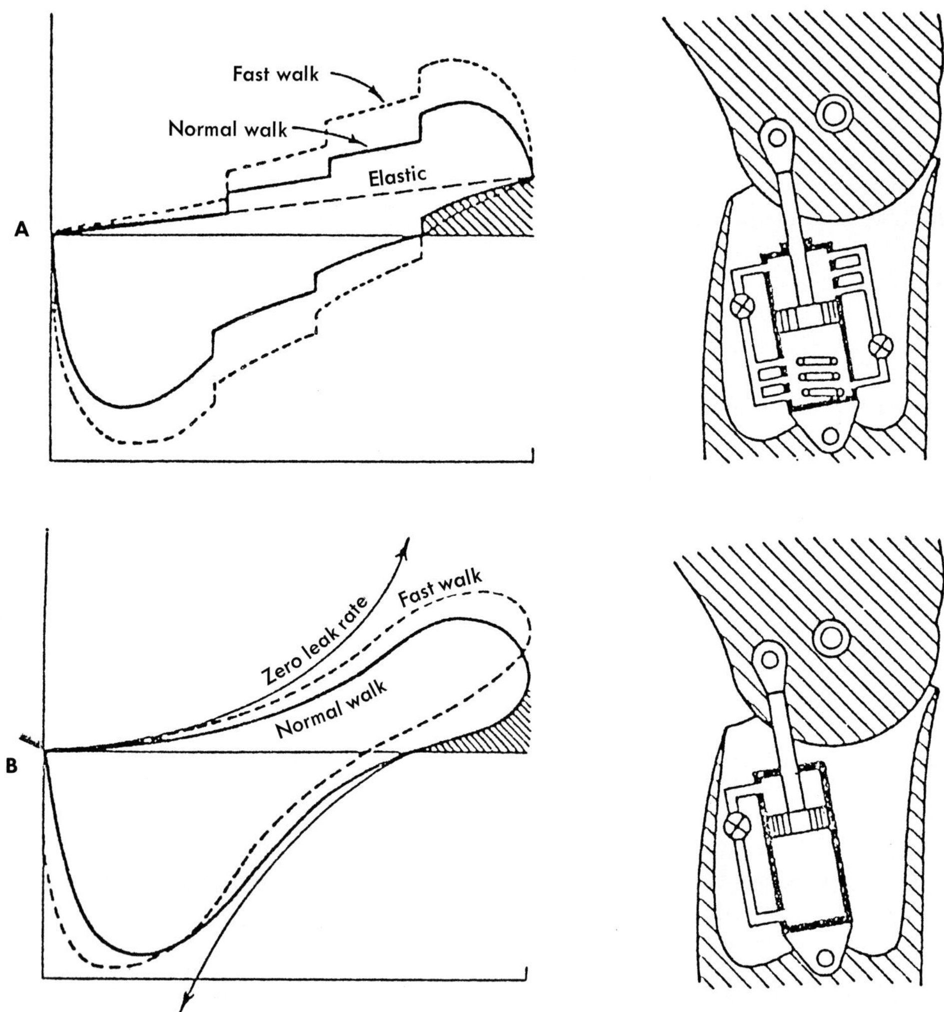

Fig. 25-19. A, Characteristic moment pattern for hydraulic unit. Resistance in unit increases with increased walking speed. **B,** Characteristic moment pattern for pneumatic swing phase control. Increased walking speed allows less time for air to pass through bypass channel, creating resistance. (From Radcliffe, C. W.: Prosthet. Orthot. Int. **1**(3):146-160, 1977.)

have more of a "bounce" or "spring" at the end of heel rise to initiation of extension. Some prosthetists and patients consider the advantages (weight, simplicity) of the pneumatic swing control system to outweigh the functional disadvantage, but most prefer the smoother action of the hydraulic knee unit.

The pneumatic swing control unit is indicated for the same type of patient who could use a hydraulic unit. It is preferred when cadence response is desirable and light weight is also required. Extremely low temperatures may affect the viscosity of the hydraulic unit and the pneumatic unit may be preferred, although pneumatic units are also affected by temperature changes because the seals harden, and the metal may expand and contract to different degrees.

Summary. When determining which knee unit should be used for an above-knee amputee several facts must be considered. First is safety (stability). If the patient has poor coordination, weakness, multiple injuries, or may receive severe injuries if a fall occurs, a manual locking knee is the unit of choice. Other patients who are able to walk around the home or community on a limited basis but are not highly active or have limited strength should use weight-activated friction or safety knees. When durability and ease of maintenance are major factors, as with children and many adult patients, the constant friction knee is the unit of choice.

Fluid control mechanisms (hydraulic, pneumatic) are generally used on active adult males, but can be used on adult females if satisfactory cosmesis can be obtained. Hydraulic knees function smoother than pneumatic knees and are generally preferred for that reason. Knee stability is always the first consideration. Function and cosmesis follow closely. Durability and ease of maintenance of the knee mechanism must also be considered.

Total-contact quadrilateral socket for above-knee amputations

The two basic functions of an above-knee prosthetic socket are support and stability. The

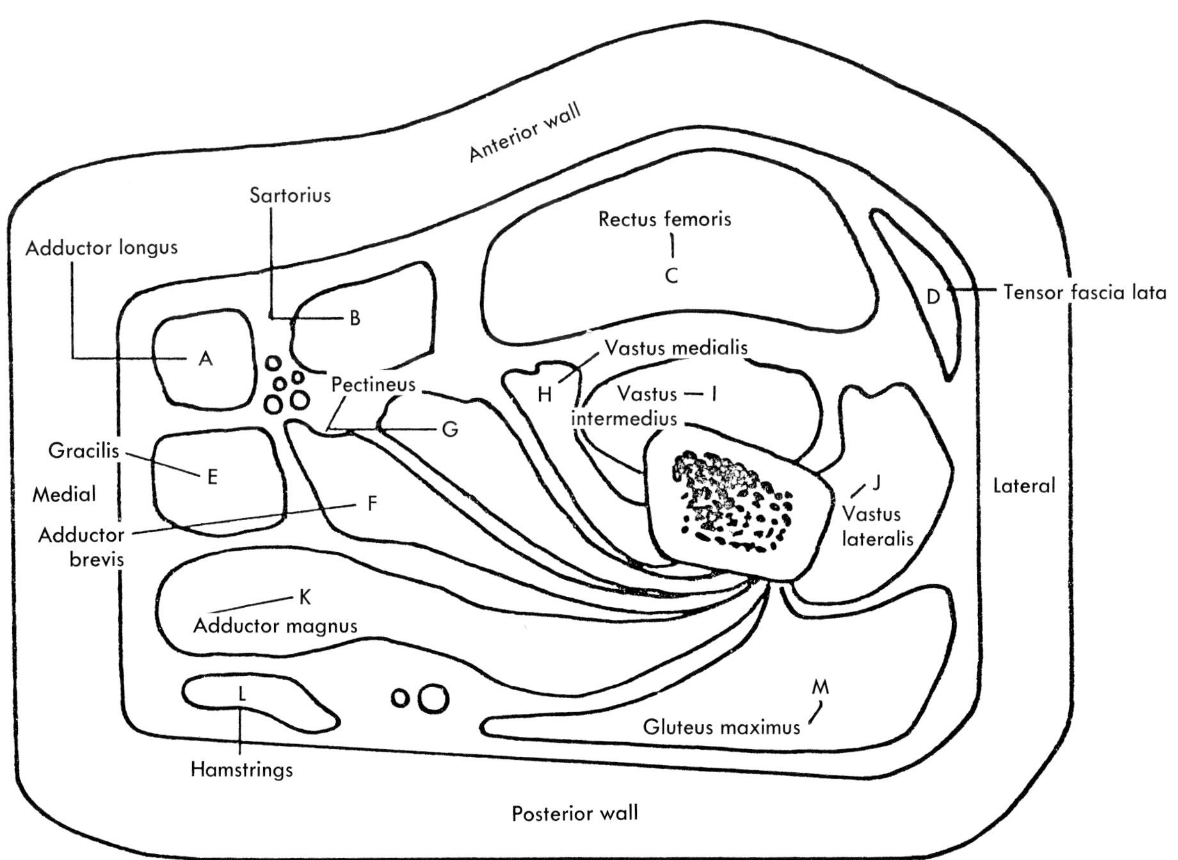

Fig. 25-20. Transverse cross section of quadrilateral socket. (Courtesy Northwestern University, Evanston, Ill.)

socket must be able to comfortably support the body while being subjected to forces greater than body weight during walking and other activities; it must also be designed and aligned to stabilize the femur and the musculature controlling the hip to enable the prosthesis to respond quickly to muscle action.

A number of socket designs are available for the above-knee amputee, but the one that has proven to provide the most support and stability is the quadrilateral design. The term quadrilateral refers to the appearance of the socket when viewed in the transverse plane (Fig. 25-20), since there is a medial wall, posterior wall, lateral wall, and anterior wall. The origin of this socket is attributed to Striede of Austria. This design was brought to the United States by Dr. V. T. Inman and Professor H. D. Eberhart in 1949. They extensively studied the biomechanics of the quadrilateral socket at the University of California Biomechanics Laboratory in Berkeley. The Berkeley studies resulted in an excellent biomechanical rationale for the shape of the socket, and a relationship was made between socket design and the alignment of the knee joint, shank, and foot under the socket.

There are five basic principles of quadrilateral socket design. These principles, as described by Hall[2] are as follows:

1. The socket must be properly contoured and relieved for functioning muscles. Relief must be made in the socket for the muscles that will contract during activity. Although the residual limb may be conical at rest, the shape will change considerably when the muscles are activated. In addition, the normal insertion for the muscles is gone, and the muscles have generally retracted and reattached, resulting in disturbed length relationships that cause the muscles to contract much harder than normal to achieve the same force.

2. Stabilizing pressure should be applied on the skeletal structures as much as possible, avoiding areas where functioning muscles exist. The socket should be in contact with the skin in all areas to prevent swelling and to increase proprioception and control. In certain areas high pressures are intentionally placed to stabilize the femur and maintain the ischial tuberosity in its proper place in the socket. These stabilization forces may be of considerable magnitude because they will frequently have to withstand forces greater than the patient's body weight during ambulation.

3. Functioning muscles, where possible, should be stretched to slightly greater than rest length for maximum power. The hip extensors and hip abductors must be maintained in slight stretch in the socket so they can contract at near maximum strength during stance phase. The socket is therefore slightly adducted to put the hip abductors under stretch and slightly flexed to put the hip extensors under stretch.

4. Properly applied pressure is well tolerated by neurovascular structures. This is an interesting concept for orthopaedic surgeons who are painfully aware of the results of unrelieved plaster of Paris cast pressure over neurovascular tracts. Surprisingly, these vessels and nerves will tolerate firm pressure over extended periods of time, if it is applied properly, yet the same degree of pressure over functioning muscles will prove to be intolerable.

5. Force is tolerated best if it is distributed over the largest available area: pressure = force − area. Therefore to decrease high-pressure areas, which can cause discomfort, choking, or skin breakdown, forces are distributed over the largest area possible. However, it is first necessary to know where these forces will occur and what area can tolerate pressures. Typically the end of the femur is subjected to high pressures because the hip abductors pull it against the lateral wall of the socket during midstance. If these pressures are not accommodated, discomfort will result in a gluteus medius-type limp. Occasionally, a bursa may form over the distolateral femur when these pressures persist. To prevent these problems, the prosthetist must distribute force along the distolateral third of the femoral shaft and provide relief for the cut end of the femur so that the patient will only feel a generalized pressure on the lateral aspect of the residual limb.

Specific socket design characteristics

The ischial tuberosity is the most important bony landmark used in above-knee prosthetics. The total length of the prosthesis is measured on the sound side from the ischial tuberosity to the floor. The ischial tuberosity is also used as a reference for measuring the length of the residual limb and as a starting point for the prosthetist when he modifies the positive plaster mold of the patient when designing a socket. Extending from the posterior wall of the socket is a ledge, or seat, for the ischial tuberosity. This "ischial seat" is generally about 3.1 cm (1½ inches) wide, extending from the medial wall and tapering to a widely flared area at the lateral wall to provide gluteal support.

Since the majority of weight is carried by the ischial tuberosity and gluteal muscles, it is important that this posterior wall be contoured properly. However, the ischial tuberosity and gluteal muscles will not remain in their proper location in the socket unless counterforces are used to hold them in place.

To prevent the ischial tuberosity from moving anteriorly and falling into the socket during weight bearing, the anterior wall is contoured to provide a stabilizing force over the femoral area, or Scarpa's triangle. The dimension from the anterior socket to the posterior wall at the location of the ischial tuberosity is commonly called the anteroposterior dimension. It is measured from the abductor longus tendon to the ischial tuberosity and then decreased by 1.3 cm (1/2 inch) to force the ischial tuberosity firmly on the seat.

Mediolateral migration of the ischial tuberosity and gluteal muscles is prevented by a proper socket width. Should the socket be too wide at the level of the ischial tuberosity, the residual limb will slide laterally, where the anteroposterior dimension is greater, and the ischial tuberosity will then slip into the socket, resulting in poor support and improper pressure distribution. The mediolateral dimension of the socket at the ischial tuberosity level should be slightly less than one third of the patient's limb circumference at that level.

Stabilization of the femur and hip musculature is accomplished in two ways. First the socket is designed so that the lateral wall is adducted 8 to 12 degrees, stretching the gluteus medius muscle (Fig. 25-21). The gluteus medius can then fire rapidly and with adequate strength during midstance to support the body. The lateral wall of the socket is made relatively flat to evenly distribute the high forces resulting from the firing of hip abductors, which prevents these forces from being resolved at the distal end of the femur.

The entire socket is flexed approximately 5 degrees to put the gluteus maximus on stretch and to provide for a greater range of hip extension (Fig. 25-22). Socket flexion allows the patient to take a more normal stride length on the sound side because the hip extension range on the prosthetic side can remain within normal limits.

The total volume of the socket matches that of the patient's residual limb as closely as possible, especially when suction suspension is to be used. The prosthetist uses a number of measurements, including circumference of the patient's limb, and modifies the plaster positive mold until the resulting contours and volume are in accordance with his modification technique. Typically when suction suspension is used, the circumference of the socket is slightly smaller than that of the patient's limb in order to provide some slight compression of the tissue to ensure a snug fit and good

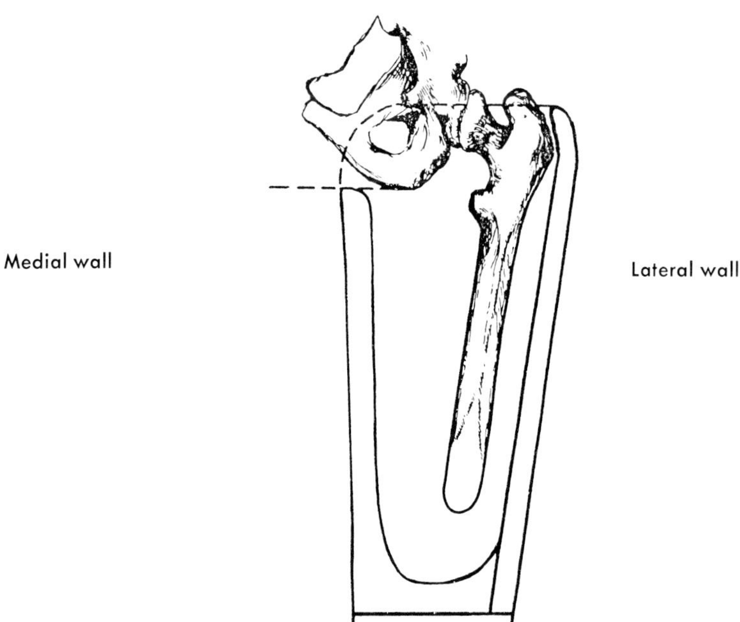

Fig. 25-21. Anteroposterior view of quadrilateral socket. Lateral wall of socket is adducted to put gluteus medius on stretch and is contoured to stabilize femur. (Courtesy Northwestern University, Evanston, Ill.)

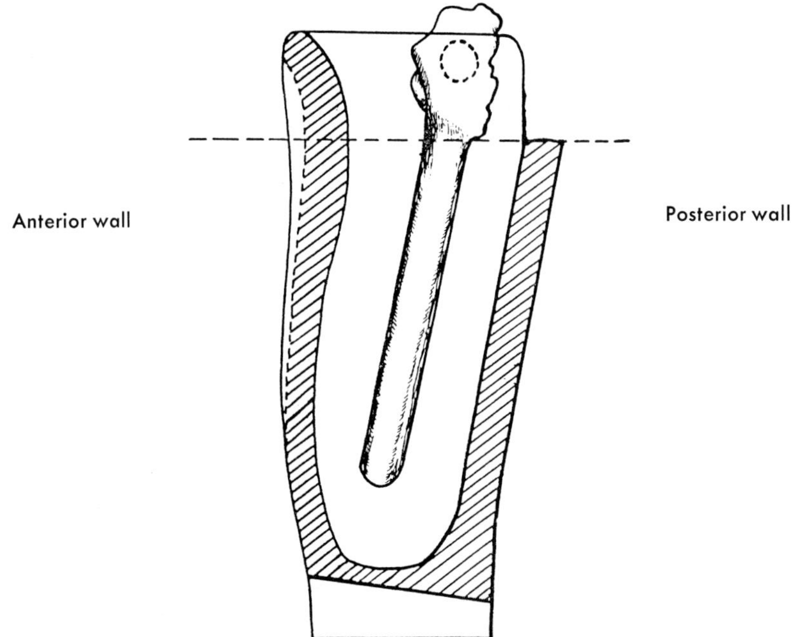

Fig. 25-22. Lateral view of quadrilateral socket. Socket is flexed about 5 degrees to put gluteus medius in tension and to allow greater range of hip extension. (Courtesy Northwestern University, Evanston, Ill.)

seal in the socket. The socket should be in contact with the skin at all points during weight bearing to reduce the incidence of swelling and to increase the patient's proprioception.

In summary, socket shape is influenced by both the anatomy of the residual limb and by biomechanical requirements. The socket must provide support for forces greater than the patient's body weight and must stabilize the femur properly, while at the same time not impinge on muscle contraction or cause discomfort, choking, or swelling. The basic principles of above-knee socket design hold true whether suction, a Silesian belt, or a hip joint and pelvic band are used for suspension.

Suspension

The prostheses must be firmly held in place on the patient's residual limb if the patient is to have adequate control. A prosthesis that tends to move up and down (piston) on the patient's limb will result in unsatisfactory gait deviations. Poor suspension makes it difficult to control the prosthesis, and the prosthesis will feel heavy and skin abrasions may result from piston movement. Three separate types of suspension are used on above-knee prostheses: (1) suction, (2) Silesian belt, and (3) hip joint and pelvic band. Suction suspension can also be combined with the other two methods.

Suction suspension. Suction suspension refers to the technique of maintaining the prosthesis by negative air pressure in the socket during swing phase. This is accomplished by the use of an air expulsion valve at the distal end of the socket and a very well-contoured socket that fits around the patient's leg directly against the skin to form a seal (Fig. 25-23). No prosthetic socks are used with this design because air would tend to leak through the weave of the sock, resulting in a loss of suspension. Suction suspension is relatively sophisticated and is therefore not recommended for all types of patients. To maintain the proper fit of the residual limb in the socket the patient must apply the prosthesis properly. The patient must pull himself into the socket by applying a piece of stockinette around the residual limb, putting the end of the stockinette through the valve hole at the distal end of the socket, and pulling the residual limb down into the socket. After the limb is in the socket the entire piece of stockinette is removed and pulled out of the socket. The valve is then screwed in place, and negative pressure is achieved. This donning procedure requires some skill and exertion.

Suction sockets are indicated for patients with average to long above-knee amputations who have a stable residual limb. The patient must not be experiencing significant volume fluctuations,

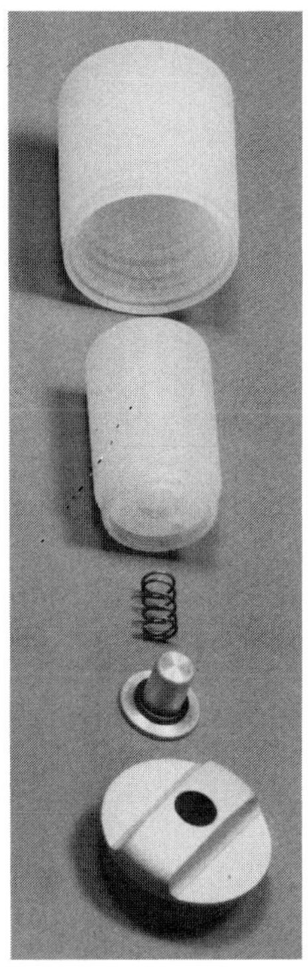

Fig. 25-23. Components of air expulsion valve. This valve allows one-way air passage expulsion to assure constant negative pressure (suction) to suspend above-knee prosthesis. Push button releases suction. From top to bottom: plastic valve housing, shaft, spring, push button, valve head. Spring tension can be changed to adjust amount of negative pressure. Other valves are available that have controlled leak rates to prevent embarrassing noises from fast air expulsion.

balance problems, upper limb disabilities that would make donning the prosthesis difficult, heart disease, or other physical problems that will not allow the exertion required to don the prosthesis. Suction sockets are also contraindicated for certain patients who are extremely active and subject the prosthesis to situations that may cause a loss of suction. Examples of this are children who climb fences and trees or adults who do a great amount of hiking, hunting, or other physical activities. For these patients the Silesian belt may be added to suction as a safety precaution.

A number of valves are available to be used when suction suspension is desired. The most popular type is the one-way air expulsion valve, which allows air to pass freely from the socket when the residual limb presses down into the socket during weight bearing, but does not allow air to enter from the inside. These valves typically have a button that can be pushed or pulled (depending on the design) to allow free passage of air, but still employ the button to allow removal of the prosthesis (Fig. 25-24). Generally, springs inside the valve determine the amount of air that can be expelled from the socket. These springs can be adjusted to allow air to escape easily, therefore increasing the negative pressure. The most common problem with these valves is corrosion, which will cause small leaks in the valves. These leaks generally result in either a loss of suspension or an embarrassing noise.

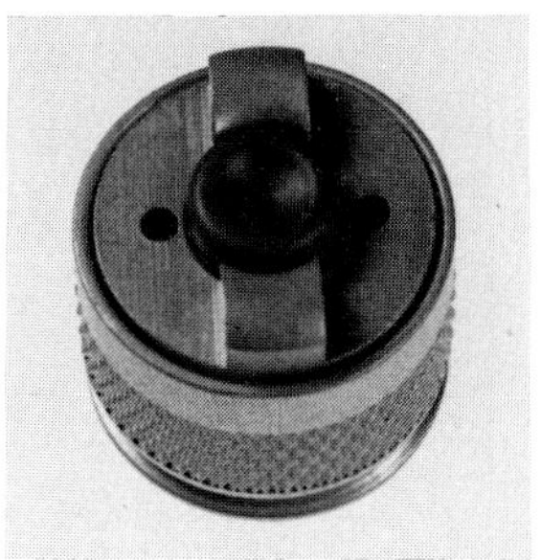

Fig. 25-24. Anodized aluminum valve. Housing is laminated into distal socket at anteromedial aspect, and valve is screwed in. Patient releases suction by pushing button in center of valve or by unscrewing valve.

Although the term "suction" is employed to describe this type of suspension, the intimate socket fit around the musculature of the residual limb is the most important factor in socket design. Patients using suction suspension generally employ their muscles very actively during gait to grasp the socket for suspension. This is best illustrated when a patient wearing a suction socket relaxes his muscles and the prosthesis falls off the leg. Suction therefore is a valuable adjunct to proper socket design but will not suspend a prosthesis properly if the patients muscles are not properly accommodated in the socket.

Silesian belt suspension. The Silesian belt, also called the Silesian bandage, can be used by itself or together with suction suspension. The Silesian belt consists of a flexible belt usually made of cloth or leather. The belt is attached at a pivot point at the lateral aspect of the socket at the approximate location of the trochanter and extends around the back over the iliac crest to the anterior midline where it terminates in a D ring. The Silesian belt is attached to the anterior socket by a strap that extends from 2.5 cm (1 inch) anterior to the ischial level through the D ring on the Silesian belt and down to a buckle, which is attached 2.5 cm (1 inch) distal to the ischial level of the prosthesis on the anterior wall of the socket. The Silesian belt provides a very comfortable, positive suspension of the prosthesis and can also be used to control undesirable rotation of the prosthesis and aid in adducting the prosthesis.

Table 7. General guidelines for above-knee prostheses

Patient type	*Cosmesis*	*Durability*	*Stability*	*Fluid control mechanisms*	*Suspension*	*Ankle-foot rotator unit*	*Adjustability*	*Weight**
Juvenile (1 to 11 years)	Low priority	High priority	By alignment	Not necessary	Pelvic suspension may be used with suction	SACH	Lengthen shank 2.5 to 5 cm (1 to 2 inches)	Average to heavy
Adolescent								
Male	Low to medium priority	High priority	By alignment	Occasionally required	Suction and/or pelvic suspension	SACH light foot	Lengthen shank 2.5 to 5 cm (1 to 2 inches)	Average to heavy
Female	High priority	Medium priority	By alignment	Rarely used	Suction and/or pelvic suspension	SACH light foot	Not required	Light to average
Adult								
Male	Medium priority	Medium priority	By alignment and/or fluid control	Frequently required	Suction and/or pelvic suspension	Any type (rotator may be used here)	Not required	Light to average
Female	High priority	Medium priority	By alignment	Used when cosmesis is not affected	Suction and/or pelvic suspension	SACH (rotator rarely used)	Not required	Average
Very active								
Male	Low priority	High priority	By alignment and/or fluid control	Used only if proven durable	Suction and/or pelvic suspension	Any type	Not required	Average
Female	High priority	High priority	By alignment and/or fluid control	Used when cosmesis is not affected	Suction and/or pelvic suspension	SACH	Not required	Average to heavy
Geriatric†	Medium priority	Low priority	Safety knee, manual lock, polycentric, and alignment	Not necessary	Silesian or flexible pelvic band	SACH or single axis	Adjustable socket volume often preferred	Light
Short amputation (less than 50% of femur)	Refer to age and sex	Refer to age and sex	Polycentric, fluid control, or alignment	Frequently used	Suction and/or pelvic suspension	Single axis or multiaxis	Refer to age	Refer to age and sex
Bilateral above-knee – below-knee or above-knee Syme amputation	Refer to age and sex	High priority	Safety knee or manual lock adjustment	Not necessary	Suction and/or pelvic suspension	Single axis or multiaxis (rotator may be used here)	Not required	Light to average

*Weight definitions: light, 2.03 to 3.2 kg (4½ to 7 pounds) (adult); average, 3.2 to 4.7 kg (7 to 10½ pounds); heavy, 4.7 kg (10½ pounds) and heavier.

†The term "geriatric," as used here, refers to persons over 60 years of age with low activity and amputations, usually resulting from vascular disease.

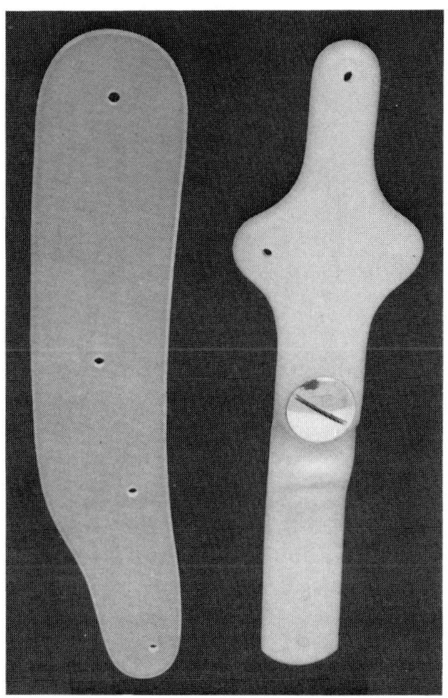

Fig. 25-25. Polypropylene hip joint and pelvic band. (Courtesy U.S. Manufacturing Co., Pasadena, Calif.)

The Silesian belt is primarily indicated for those patients in whom suction is not adequate as the sole means of suspension. Patients using Silesian belts wear prosthetic socks, which must be prescribed whenever this type of suspension is to be employed.

The advantages of Silesian belt suspension are that it is a very positive type of suspension; it is lightweight and comfortable, and it is not affected by weight fluctuations or many of the other factors that will affect suction suspension. It is easy to use because it functions similar to a waist belt. A Silesian belt is not as restrictive as a metal or plastic hip joint with a pelvic band, it is more cosmetic under clothes, and can provide a definite control of rotation adduction of the prosthesis. The disadvantages of the Silesian belt are that (1) it is more cumbersome than the suction suspension, (2) it will restrict the patient's control of the prosthesis to some degree, and (3) it is less cosmetic than suction suspension. The Silesian belt does not provide the same degree of control of flexion, extension, adduction, and abduction as does the hip joint and pelvic band suspension.

Hip joint and pelvic band suspension. The hip joint and pelvic band provides positive suspension and control to an above-knee prosthesis. Hip joints and pelvic bands are typically made of metal, although plastic designs are now available (Fig. 25-25). The hip joint is placed anterior and proximal to the greater trochanter to approximate the location of the anatomical center of hip movement. The metal extension from the proximal hip joint is used for attachment of the pelvic band. The pelvic band should be located between the greater trochanter and the iliac crest and should be contoured to fit snugly on the patient and extend from the anterosuperior iliac spine to approximately the posterosuperior iliac spine. The hip joint should be aligned to allow for a normal plane of motion in flexion and extension and ease of sitting without pinching the flesh between the anterior brim of the socket and the pelvic band. The pelvic band is attached to a wide cloth or leather waist belt that wraps around the patient's waist and buckles anteriorly.

Hip joint and pelvic band suspension is indicated for patients who have poor ability to control their prosthesis and need a very positive suspension. Geriatric patients are the most common users of hip joint and pelvic band suspension. Obese patients frequently require this type of suspension because they have little control over the socket due to the lack of muscle definition, and a Silesian belt will frequently not provide enough control. Hip joint and pelvic band suspension is also very easy to understand for patients with poor cognitive abilities, since it functions the same as a normal waist belt. The hip joint is also indicated for patients with short amputations or with weak hip abductors because the additional lever arm will help absorb lateral forces.

Partial suction suspension. Many patients who are not candidates for suction suspension may benefit from partial suction. Partial suction means that the socket is designed to contour around the muscles of the limb, but enough volume is allowed for the patient to wear a prosthetic sock. An air expulsion valve is placed at the distal end of the socket, and a Silesian belt or hip joint and pelvic band is used as a primary means of suspension. The negative pressure created by the air expulsion valve will improve the suspension slightly during the initiation of swing phase.

REFERENCES

1. Eberhart, H. D., et al.: Summary of European observations, Summer, 1949, Report to Advisory Committee on Artificial Limbs, Washington, D.C., October, 1949, National Research Council.
2. Hall, C. B.: Prosthetic socket shape as related to anatomy in lower extremity amputees, Clin. Orthop. **37**:32-46, 1964.
3. Radcliffe, C. W.: Above-knee prosthetics, Prosthet. Orthot. Int. **1**(3):146-160, Dec., 1977.

CHAPTER 26

Hip disarticulation and hemipelvectomy amputation

ROBERT E. TOOMS
FREDERICK L. HAMPTON

Hip disarticulation is the surgical removal of the entire lower limb by transection through the hip joint. Hemipelvectomy is the surgical removal of the entire lower limb plus all or a major portion of the ilium. Ablative surgery of this magnitude is indicated most often to eradicate a malignant tumor of the bone or soft tissues about the thigh, hip, or pelvic region. Less frequent indications are extensive trauma or uncontrolled infections, especially gas gangrene. On rare occasions, the function and prosthetic fit of a congenital limb anomaly may be improved by surgical conversion to a hip disarticulation.

SURGICAL TECHNIQUES

The basic surgical techniques outlined here may require selective modification because of limb scarring, draining sinus tracts, or the location of a tumor. In most instances, however, the techniques are followed as presented.

Hip disarticulation

The technique of hip disarticulation as described by Boyd[1] is the basic procedure in general use. In developing his technique, Boyd attempted to minimize blood loss by transecting muscles at either their origin or insertion, these areas being relatively avascular. The resultant stump is well padded and provides an excellent weight-bearing surface for prosthetic use.

Placement of the incision may be varied to avoid large areas of scarring or to provide access to the retroperitoneal lymph nodes when excision of this tissue is indicated in certain malignancies.[8] The standard incision is an anterior racquet incision, which begins just inferior to the anterosuperior iliac spine and curves medially about the upper thigh just inferior to the inguinal ligament (Fig. 26-1, *A*). Posteriorly, the incision passes distal to the ischial tuberosity and then curves laterally to pass about 8 cm distal to the base of the greater trochanter. From this point, the incision swings anteriorly and proximally to join the beginning of the incision. After ligation and division of the femoral vessels and transection of the femoral nerve, the superficial muscles about the anteromedial aspect of the hip are transected at their origin on the pelvis. The iliopsoas and the short external rotator muscles are divided at their insertion on the femur. The obturator artery is carefully ligated and divided, and the obturator nerve is transected (Fig. 26-1, *A*). The hip abductors are then divided at their insertion on the greater trochanter and the gluteus maximus is detached from its insertion on the femur. The hamstring muscles are detached from their origin on the ischial tuberosity, and the sciatic nerve is ligated and divided. The hip joint capsule is then circumferentially incised and the ligamentum teres divided to complete the disarticulation (Fig. 26-1, *B*). The wound is closed by suturing the gluteus maximus to the remnants of the adductor

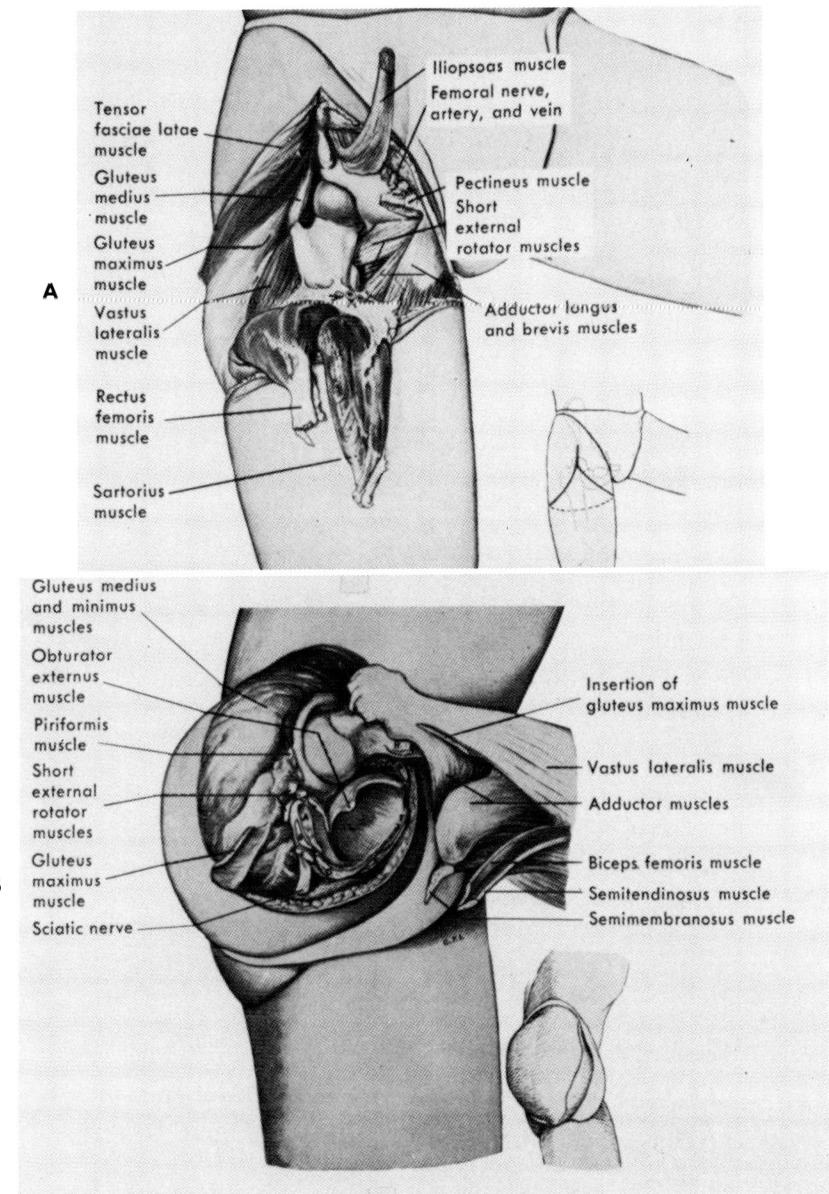

Fig. 26-1. Boyd hip disarticulation. **A,** At this stage femoral vessels and nerve have been ligated, and sartorius, rectus femoris, pectineus, and iliopsoas muscles have been detached. Inset shows line of skin incision. **B,** Glutei are separated from their insertions, sciatic nerve is divided, short rotator muscles are severed, and hamstring muscles are detached from ischial tuberosity. Inset shows final closure of stump. (Modified from Boyd, H. B.: Surg. Gynecol. Obstet. **84**:346, 1947.)

muscles and approximating the skin edges (Fig. 26-1, *B*).

Hemipelvectomy

This formidable procedure is performed almost exclusively for treatment of malignant tumors about the hip and pelvis. Numerous methods for performing a hemipelvectomy have been described,[2,5,8,10] but the operative technique follows the same general pattern in each of the various methods. For purposes of this article, the technique as described by King and Steelquist[3] will be outlined.

The patient is positioned on the operating table in the lateral position with the sound side down. In this position the abdominal contents fall away from the part of the pelvis to be removed, eliminating the need for excessive retraction of the abdominal viscera. The operation is divided into three parts: anterior, perineal, and posterior, performed in that order. The initial incision begins at the pubic tubercle and is extended laterally along the inguinal ligament and then posteriorly along the iliac crest (Fig. 26-2, *A*). The abdominal muscles and the inguinal ligament are detached from the iliac crest, and the fossa between the iliacus muscle and the peritoneum is dissected. The inguinal ligament and rectus abdominis muscle are severed from the pubis and retracted medially along with the spermatic cord and the bladder. This provides exposure of the external iliac artery and vein, which are ligated and divided, and the femoral nerve, which is divided (Fig. 26-2, *B*). The limb is then widely abducted and the skin incision extended from the pubic tubercle along the pubic and ischial rami to the ischial tuberosity. After stripping the perineal muscles from the rami, the ligaments and fibrocartilage of the pubic symphysis are completely divided (Fig. 26-2, *C*). Having completed the anterior and perineal

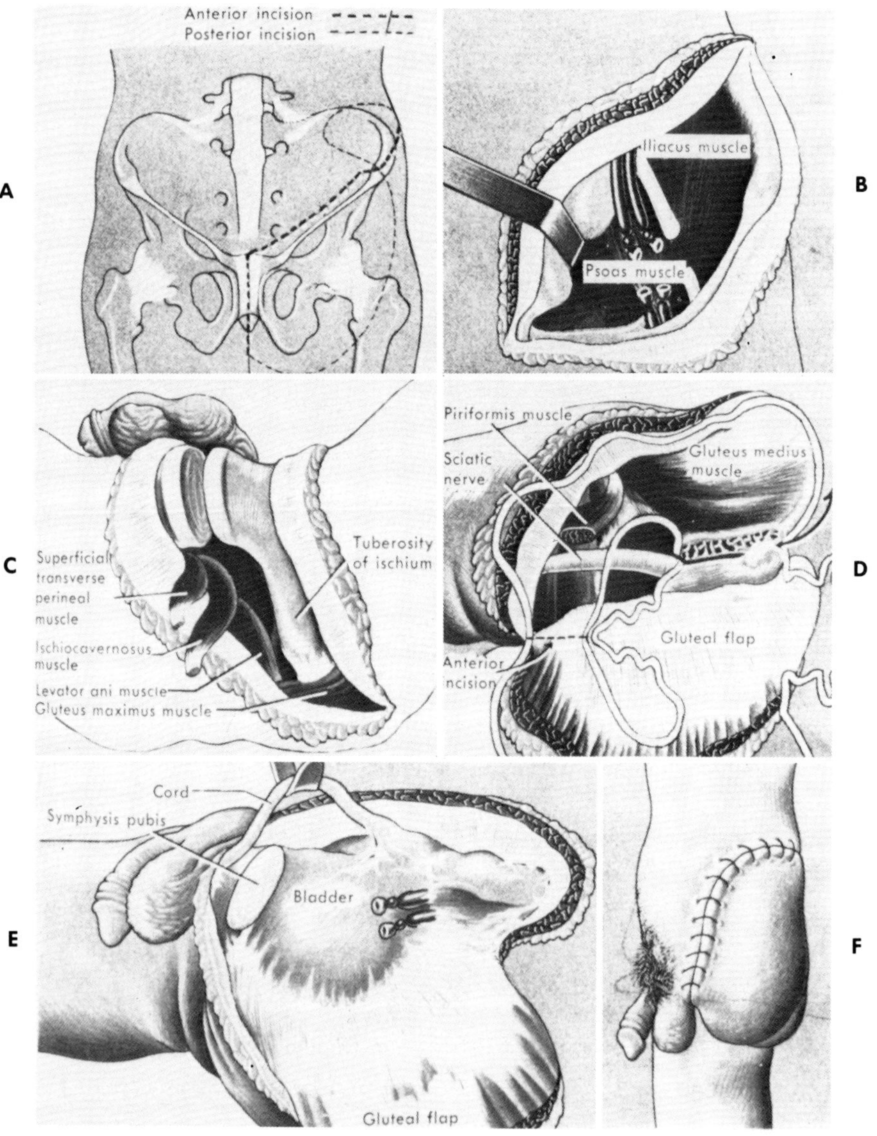

Fig. 26-2. King and Steelquist hindquarter amputation. **A,** incision. **B,** Anterior incision (bladder retracted). Section of femoral vessels and nerve. **C,** Perineal view of division of pubic symphysis and section of perineal muscles. **D,** Posterior view showing section of ilium. White line indicates pelvis. **E,** Lateral view after removal of extremity. **F,** Completed amputation. (Modified from Slocum, D. B.: An atlas of amputations, St. Louis, 1949, The C. V. Mosby Co.)

portions of the procedure, the initial anterior incision is continued posteriorly along the iliac crest to the posterosuperior iliac spine. From this point the incision swings laterally to the greater trochanter and then follows the gluteal crease into the perineum to join the perineal part of the incision. The aponeurosis of the gluteus maximus is divided in line with the skin incision, and this muscle is elevated with the overlying fat and skin as a large flap. The sciatic nerve is then identified, ligated, and divided. The ilium is then divided adjacent to the sacroiliac joint and rotated laterally to expose the intrapelvic structures (Fig. 26-2, *D*). After ligating and dividing the obturator vessels and nerves, the psoas and the levator animuscles are transected, completely freeing the ilium and entire lower limb (Fig. 26-2, *E*). The wound is closed by suturing the gluteal flap to the abdominal muscles and approximating the skin edges (Fig. 26-2, *F*).

Postoperative treatment

After surgery the soft tissues of the amputation site should be firmly supported. This can be accomplished by using a soft compression dressing in the conventional manner or by applying a rigid dressing of plaster of Paris according to the immediate postsurgical prosthetic fitting technique. Resolution of edema from the surgical site is quite rapid after treatment by either of these postoperative management techniques.

After an initial enthusiastic application of immediate postsurgical prosthetic fitting to hip disarticulation and hemipelvectomy amputations, many surgeons discovered that the available prosthetic components of this system do not permit comfortable sitting, nor do they provide a satisfactory gait. Furthermore, suspension of the temporary prosthesis is rather cumbersome. These problems, plus rapid maturation of these amputation stumps when treated in the conventional manner, have led most surgeons to discontinue using the immediate postsurgical prosthetic fitting technique for amputations at the hip disarticulation and hemipelvectomy levels.

When a soft compression dressing is used, the patient is mobilized from bed as soon as comfort allows—usually on the third or fourth postoperative day. In younger individuals, standing in parallel bars can be instituted at this time and rapidly followed by crutch ambulation. Stump wrapping is continued until a definitive prosthesis is fit, often at 6 to 8 weeks after surgery.

PROSTHETIC MANAGEMENT

Hip disarticulation

The hip disarticulation amputation produces a stump with excellent weight-bearing characteristics. However, the lack of a femoral shaft acting as a lever arm on the prosthesis results in poor mediolateral trunk stability and the loss of voluntary control of hip flexion, knee stability, stride length, and alterations in cadence. The design of the hip disarticulation prosthesis must therefore compensate for these missing functions.

Historical review. Early prosthetic designs were basically of three types: a saucer prosthesis, tilting table prosthesis, and single-axis prosthesis. The *saucer prosthesis* (Fig. 26-3) consisted of an above-knee prosthesis with the proximal portion of the socket contoured to the shape of a saucer. The prosthesis was suspended by a sturdy pelvic belt and a shoulder strap. The pelvic belt provided a minimal amount of mediolateral trunk stability during stance phase, but hip and knee locks were usually required to provide adequate stability of the limb during ambulation. Ambula-

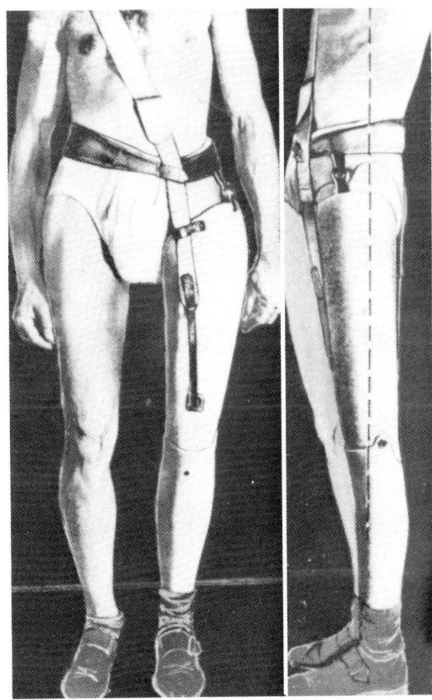

Fig. 26-3. Saucer-type socket for very short (and usually flexed) above-knee stumps approaching hip disarticulation level. It is best suited to rounded contour of stump, which will fit into shallow socket while standing, yet allow socket to slide neatly around stump for sitting. Generally, hip lock is needed, although in some cases patient can use free hip joint. (From Thomas, A., and Haddan, C. C.: Amputation prosthesis, Philadelphia, 1945, J. B. Lippincott Co.)

tion was accomplished by flexion and extension of the pelvis.

The *tilting table prosthesis* (Fig. 26-4) consisted of a reinforced molded leather socket with a wide pelvic band that was attached to the thigh section by a heavy hip joint positioned on the lateral side of the socket. A medial roller or track was positioned between the socket and thigh section to relieve the extreme bending moments on the lateral hip joint during stance phase. A strap under the rollers helped to suspend the prosthesis during swing phase. Mediolateral trunk stability was improved by this prosthetic design, but a hip lock was required for stability during ambulation and, unless alignment stability was quite good, a knee lock was also required. Ambulation was accomplished by flexion and extension of the pelvis.

In the *single-axis prosthesis* (Fig. 26-5) a wide single-axis hip joint was positioned directly beneath the pelvic socket and attached to the thigh section. This design was much simpler and sturdier than the tilting table type, but still required a hip lock for ambulation. A knee lock was also needed unless alignment of the prosthesis provided stability. Mediolateral trunk stability in the stance phase was satisfactory. As with the tilting table design, placement of the hip joint resulted in a poor sitting posture. Ambulation was accomplished by pelvic flexion and extension.

In 1957, McLaurin[7] introduced the Canadian hip disarticulation prosthesis (Fig. 26-6). The unique feature of this design is the use of hip, knee, and ankle joint placement in relation to the weight-bearing line to achieve stance phase stability, while permitting free motion at the hip and knee during the swing phase of gait. This prosthesis continues to be the standard fitting for amputations at the hip disarticulation level. The molded plastic socket encloses the ischial tuberosity for weight bearing, extends over the crest of the ilium to provide suspension during swing phase, and affords excellent mediolateral trunk stability. The hip joint is attached to the socket anteriorly, thus lying anterior to the weight-bearing line and, in conjunction with a stop just posterior to the hip joint, produces excellent stance-phase stability at the hip. The anterior position of the hip joint also permits level sitting. The axis of motion of the knee joint is positioned slightly posterior to the weight-bearing line to produce stance-phase stability at this joint.[9]

Prosthetic prescription. Most young and middle-aged adults will learn to walk quite satisfactorily with a hip disarticulation prosthesis, although some will require at least a cane in the opposite hand for balance. However, older indi-

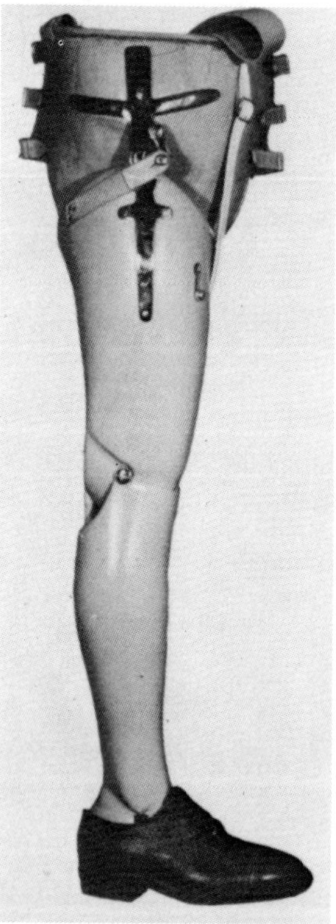

Fig. 26-4. "Tilting-table" prosthesis for very short above-knee stump or true hip disarticulation, with locked hip joint between thigh portion and reinforced molded leather socket with broad pelvic band. Knob in thigh piece engages or releases simple mechanical knee lock.

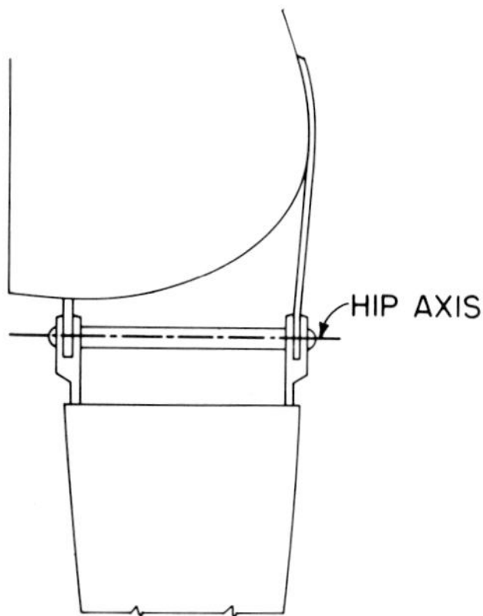

Fig. 26-5. Hip disarticulation prosthesis with axis below socket, allowing broad and sturdy weight bearing but causing clothing wear and shortening of thigh during sitting. (From Human limbs and their substitutes by P. E. Klopsteg, and P. D. Wilson. Copyright © 1954 McGraw-Hill Book Company. Used with the permission of McGraw-Hill Book Company.)

viduals frequently find the amount of energy necessary to ambulate with a prosthesis excessive. These older persons usually elect to use crutches or a walker for indoor activities and a wheelchair for distance mobility. Children rarely have difficulty in mastering ambulation with a hip disarticulation prosthesis, but often find their gait is objectionably slowed by the prosthesis. As a general rule, a prosthesis is prescribed for almost all children and for young and middle-aged adults, but only selectively in older individuals. Medical problems such as heart disease or chronic pulmonary disease are contraindications for prosthetic fitting at the hip disarticulation level because of the energy expenditure required for ambulation. Lambert[4] has clearly documented the fallacy of denying or even delaying prosthetic fitting in individuals undergoing amputation for malignancy, providing there is no evidence of local recurrence or distant metastasis of the tumor.

Components. The standard components of the Canadian hip disarticulation prosthesis are the socket, hip joint, thigh section, constant friction single-axis knee joint, shank section, and single-axis articulated foot. A wide array of alternative components may be selected for various reasons. Swing phase control knee mechanisms of the hydraulic or pneumatic variety may be sufficiently used by younger and more active individuals to justify the extra expense of these items. In contrast, older or weaker amputees may require a knee joint incorporating stance phase stability. In unusual instances, manually locking hip or knee joints may be necessary. A SACH foot may be used whenever the extra knee stability afforded by the articulated foot is not needed. The endoskeletal system for a hip disarticulation prosthesis has many advantages over the conventional exoskeletal system (Fig. 26-7). It is light in weight, cosmetically superior, and permits the incorporation of a variety of knee and foot components to satisfy the requirements of the individual amputee.

Training. During the early postoperative period, the amputee is instructed in stump wrapping, hygiene, and general body strengthening. Ambulation with crutches is instituted as soon as comfort and strength permit. On delivery of the hip disarticulation prosthesis, the amputee is first instructed in proper donning of the prosthesis to ensure correct positioning of the ischial tuberosity in the socket. Prosthetic gait training is initiated by having the amputee transfer his body weight from the sound limb to the prosthetic

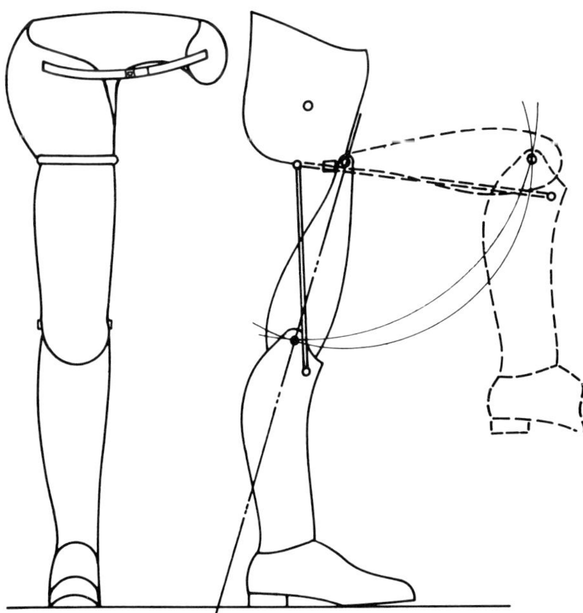

Fig. 26-6. Alignment principle of Canadian hip disarticulation prosthesis.

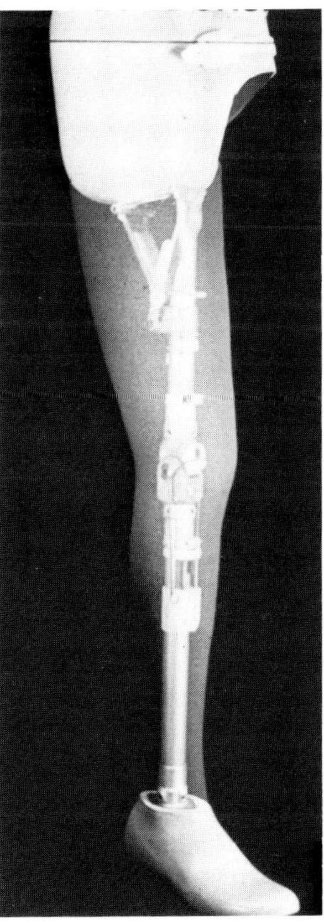

Fig. 26-7. Endoskeletal hip disarticulation prosthesis.

limb. This helps the amputee develop confidence in the stability of the prosthesis. Pelvic flexion exercises are practiced, since ambulation in the hip disarticulation prosthesis is accomplished by flexion and extension of the pelvis. The amputee is instructed to maintain an erect stance and to "walk into" the prosthesis rather than to take a long prosthetic step and wait for reverse heel contact. When attempting to sit, the amputee is instructed to first flex the knee and then flex the hip of the prosthesis.

During the course of gait training various prosthetic gait deviations may become obvious. Some of these can be corrected by further training, but others are due to prosthetic causes and require alterations in the prosthesis for correction. It is appropriate to identify the more common of these gait deviations and their prosthetic causes. Knee instability in the stance phase may be due to improper alignment of the prosthesis so that the weight-bearing line passes posterior to the knee axis of motion, the plantar flexion bumper of the articulated foot or the heel cushion of the SACH foot being too firm, or the hip bumper contacting the socket too soon. In contrast, difficulty in flexing the knee will occur if the knee axis of motion is placed too far posterior to the weight-bearing line. Excessive knee flexion in the swing phase occurs if the extension aid is too weak or the friction in the knee bolt is inadequate. Medial or lateral whip of the shank and foot section during swing phase is due to excessive external or internal rotation of the knee bolt. Circumduction of the prosthesis during swing phase or vaulting on the sound side may be due to excessive length of the prosthesis, inadequate suspension, or excessive knee stability.

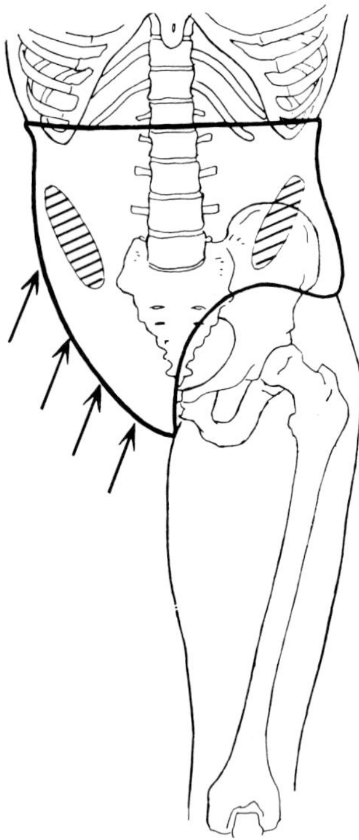

Fig. 26-8. Hemipelvectomy socket. Arrows indicate pressure applied by socket to "stump," upward and medially. Shaded areas indicate bulges produced by use of hip sticks. Bulges aid in suspension of prosthesis, in preventing rotation, and serve as guides for correct alignment while donning prosthesis.

Hemipelvectomy

In addition to all the functional deficits created by hip disarticulation, the hemipelvectomy amputee has also lost the excellent weight-bearing capabilities of the ischial tuberosity and, in a prosthesis, must bear weight on the semisolid abdominal viscera. The socket design for this amputation level must therefore produce weight forces on the abdominal viscera in a manner that is tolerable to the amputee and not injurious to the viscera. Otherwise, the component parts and alignment principles are the same as in the hip disarticulation prosthesis. Lyquist[6] has developed a socket for the hemipelvectomy amputee that produces an upward oblique pressure on the abdominal viscera and yet does not stretch the soft tissues in the perineum (Fig. 26-8).

Many hemipelvectomy amputees reject a prosthesis because of the bulk and weight of the prosthesis and the energy expenditure required for ambulation when wearing it. These individuals often elect to wear a lightweight plastic container socket to support the abdominal viscera and provide a firm comfortable seating surface. Younger patients adjust to the prosthesis and ambulate satisfactorily, although most will require at least a cane for support.

The endoskeletal system is equally applicable to the hemipelvectomy amputee as it is for the hip disarticulation patient. The significant reduction in weight, improved cosmesis, and ability to vary the components of the prosthesis have made this prosthetic design the one of choice for hemipelvectomy and hip disarticulation amputees in many clinics.

REFERENCES

1. Boyd, H. B.: Anatomic disarticulation of the hip, Surg. Gynecol. Obstet. **84:**346-349, 1947.
2. Gordon-Taylor, G., and Munro, R. S.: Technique and management of "hindquarter" amputation, Br. J. Surg. **39:** 536-541, 1952.
3. King, D., and Steelquist, J.: Transiliac amputation, J. Bone Joint Surg. **25:**351-367, 1943.
4. Lambert, C. N.: Limb loss through malignancy. In The child with an acquired amputation, Washington, D.C., 1972, National Academy of Sciences.
5. Lazarri, J. H., and Rack, F. J.: Method of hemipelvectomy with abdominal exploration and temporary ligation of common iliac artery, Ann. Surg. **133:**267-269, 1951.
6. Lyquist, E.: Canadian-type socket for a hemipelvectomy, Artif. Limbs **5:**130, 1958.
7. McLaurin, C. A.: The evolution of the Canadian-type hip disarticulation prosthesis, Artif. Limbs **4:**22-28, 1957.
8. Pack, G. T., and Ehrlich, H. E.: Exarticulation of the lower extremities for malignant tumors; hip joint disarticulation (with and without deep iliac dissection) and sacroiliac disarticulation (hemipelvectomy), Ann. Surg. **123:**965-985, 1946.
9. Radcliffe, C. W.: The biomechanics of the Canadian-type hip disarticulation prosthesis, Artif. Limbs **4:**29-38, 1957.
10. Sarondo, J. P., and Ferré, R. L.: Amputacion interilio-abdominal, Ann. Ortop. Traumatol. **1:**143, 1948.

CHAPTER 27

Physiological variances in lower limb amputees

JACQUELIN PERRY
ROBERT L. WATERS

Walking is such a natural activity for the healthy person it has been assumed to require virtually no effort. Some also claim no work has been done because, during each stride, the body's upward displacement was countered by an equal degree of downward travel. This relates strictly to the physical concept of net mechanical work. If, however, the physiological definition that work is the expenditure of energy is used, the outcome of walking is no longer zero.

Energy is used whenever muscles contract, and during walking there is continuous muscular activity. In the swing phase of gait, flexors must rapidly advance the limb and lift the foot to clear the floor, whereas in stance phase, the extensors actively restrain the influences of momentum and gravity, which threaten weight-bearing stability. Both patterns of muscular activity must combine to create the force needed to propel the body forward. With physical impairment, these patterns of muscle action have to be modified. Amputations require that proximal muscles increase their effort because they substitute for the functions that have been lost. Efficiency of gait is correspondingly decreased.

Artificial legs of older design substituted so poorly for lost limb function that prosthetic improvement became the primary focus of concern at the end of World War II. Significant gains in function accompanied the progress of these modern prosthetic programs. During the initial postwar decades the major patient group consisted of young persons who had suffered limb loss through the events of war, from congenital anomalies, or by various accidents. Their athletic potential made the expenditure of "a little extra energy" secondary to doing what they wanted. This was especially true now that prostheses were available which were comfortable and permitted a more normal gait. Such a response established the model of a well-motivated patient.

These modern prosthetic advantages, even with the added benefit of the very latest designs, are not resulting in the same walking capability in today's patient groups as was formerly experienced. Often the difference is attributed to lower motivation, but in reality it is a matter of age. Amputations in civilian life now largely result from the sequelae of peripheral vascular disease with or without diabetes. The average age of these amputees is 60 years. Physiologically this is a significant contrast to the 20-year-olds of the postwar era or the youngsters with congenital amputations. That "little extra effort" required to walk may impose an overwhelming demand on the dysvascular amputee.

Muscles primarily obtain the energy necessary for contraction force by burning glycogen with the aid of oxygen. For this to occur, an adequate amount of oxygen must be available to the tissues. Therefore a person's energy production capability depends on the combined oxygen delivery

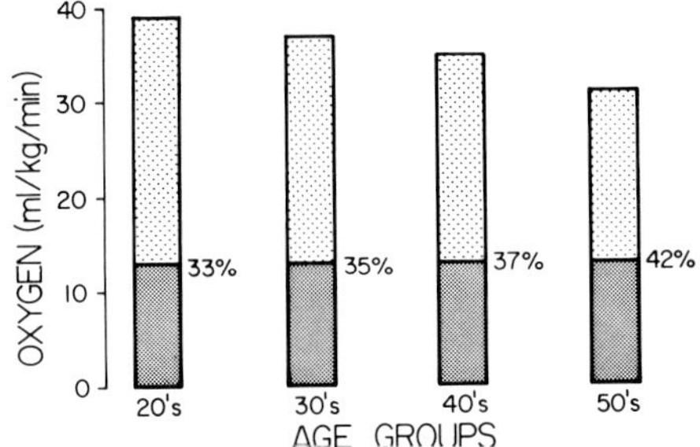

Fig. 27-1. Normal aerobic capacity and percent used in walking. Shaded area identifies percent of total aerobic capacity used for walking.

capacity of the cardiovascular and pulmonary systems (technically called aerobic capacity). These systems gradually became less effective as adults age to the extent that each decade shows a change. As a consequence, the average aerobic capacity of normal adults age 60 years is 21% less than that available to 20-year-olds.[2] The elderly will use a larger percentage of their available energy to walk, since the same limb mechanics are used to travel at the same velocity. A study of the walking habits and energy costs of persons between 20 and 60 years of age demonstrated that during the 5-minute test period the average gait velocity for each age decade was the same, but the energy cost as a percent of their maximum aerobic capacity rose (Fig. 27-1). This average velocity correlated well with that of a large city population, which was unaware of being measured.

The elderly amputee must accommodate to two energy-consuming disabilities: age and limb loss. Actual measurements of energy costs are now available to substitute fact for presumption.

ENERGY COST DETERMINATION

Because muscles use oxygen as they generate their contraction force, a reasonable and technically convenient way of determining the energy cost of an activity is to measure the oxygen consumed. For this purpose the pulmonary air exchanged during a specified period of time is collected in a portable container (plastic bag). This air sample is analyzed for total volume and the content of oxygen and carbon dioxide. Timing of the air sample collection is critical, however.

For a brief time (1 to 2 minutes), the muscles can work without oxygen (anaerobic energy production) by using the high-energy phosphates and supportive substances stored in the muscles.[1] Physiologically this initiates muscle action before adequate oxygen has been delivered to the tissues and maintains an effort level greater than that permitted by the immediate oxygen supply.

To avoid the error of including this unmeasurable (anaerobic) energy source in the determination, the activity must be continued until the person has reached the oxygen-dependent state prior to collecting any air. This generally means a 5-minute test with 3 minutes for stabilization of the energy source and 2 minutes for the measurement. Data from shorter tests will understate the energy cost of an activity. To accommodate to variations in body size, the gas values are generally reported as milliliters per kilogram of body weight (ml/kg). In young children, body surface is substituted for weight. The amount of oxygen used also is related to the duration of the activity, making the basic measurement of energy cost as oxygen use per minute (O_2 ml/kg/min).

By increasing the intensity of a person's activity, the level of energy demand and therefore the physiological response is increased porportionally. This technique has been used to determine the maximum aerobic capacity of normal persons and to estimate that of patients. The pattern of oxygen used at the different levels of effort identified the increase in energy production (O_2 ml/kg/min) with workload. Whereas normal data were determined by having the patient perform to exhaustion, testing was limited to slow, habitual, and fast walking trials. Their maximum capacities were predicted from reference tables relating oxygen usage and heart rate.

AMPUTEE PERFORMANCE

The way amputees accommodate to the dual disabilities of age and limb loss is best demonstrated by citing the results of a series of energy cost studies of healthy persons and five groups of patients with diabetic and traumatic amputations. They were classified by their levels of amputation and the etiology of either vascular (mainly diabetic) or traumatic (also congenital). This information can be used by clinicians to judge the patient's performance potential so that realistic treatment plans can be made.

Physiological stress and gait efficiency must be considered, since both contribute to the person's ability to walk.

Physiological stress

During any activity the cardiovascular and pulmonary systems attempt to provide the oxygen required by the muscles. The amount of stress placed on these systems during the effort is indicated by the ratio between the immediate demand (minute energy cost) and the combined effectiveness (aerobic capacity) of minute oxygen delivery and tissue uptake. Heart rate and respiratory rate are parallel physiological indicators.

Minute energy cost. While walking at a comfortable velocity healthy persons had an average minute energy cost of 12 to 13 ml/kg/min.[2] This also proved true of all the diabetic amputees and those with above-knee amputations from trauma.[3] Only the patients with traumatic below-knee amputations displayed a higher average minute energy cost (15 ml/kg/min).

Since this latter group consisted of young persons with relatively low amputations, their higher minute energy cost first appeared paradoxical. The answer lay in considering two other factors: aerobic capacity and gait velocity.

Aerobic capacity. The traumatic below-knee amputees were in the best physical condition with an aerobic capacity of 45 ml/kg/min. Comparable physical conditioning (aerobic capacity) for their age also was found in diabetics with below-knee and Syme amputations. The age variations (averages of 30 versus 60 years) made a considerable difference in their aerobic capacities, however, with normal values for these ages being 42 and 33 ml/kg/min respectively. Both above-knee amputee groups (traumatic and diabetic) evidenced subnormal physical conditioning. Their aerobic capacities of 35 and 20 ml/kg/min were only 81% and 67% of the normal values for their age groups (Fig. 27-2). This suggests that their disabled limb compromised their ability to exercise at an intensity sufficient to challenge their energy production systems. These involve the heart, blood vessels, lungs, and muscles for adequately delivering and extracting the necessary oxygen.

These differences in available aerobic capacity significantly modify the interpretation of the oxygen consumption measurement recorded during walking. The seemingly high minute energy cost of the traumatic below-knee amputees (16 versus 13 ml/kg/min) was really a normal 35% of their aerobic capacity. A comparable relative energy cost also was displayed by the traumatic above-knee amputees because their absolute aerobic capacities were sufficiently high to accommodate their minute energy cost, even though it was slightly greater than normal for their age group. The relative energy cost of the diabetic below-knee and Syme amputees also was within normal limits, but because of their greater age, a higher percentage of their aerobic capacity was used, 47%. Elderly above-knee amputees far exceeded the normal range with a relative energy cost of 65%. The added physiological stress also is reflected in their abnormally high respiratory quotient of 0.96 compared to a normal ceiling of 0.90 (0.87 ± 0.03). This latter measurement means these patients were obligated to include some anaerobic energy production despite its inefficient nature.

Heart rate. The patterns just described of acceptable and excessive use of aerobic capacity during walking are reflected in this convenient clinical test. Unless there is cardiac disease or medication to prevent it, the heart rate parallels oxygen consumption. Healthy persons average 104 beats/min during free velocity walking. All the amputee groups except the diabetic patients with above-knee amputations approximated the normal rate, with their averages ranging between 105 and 111. The elderly above-knee amputees had an average of 126 beats/min.

Gait efficiency

Patients are obligated to travel specific distances many times during the course of their daily life. Their functional ability to walk these dis-

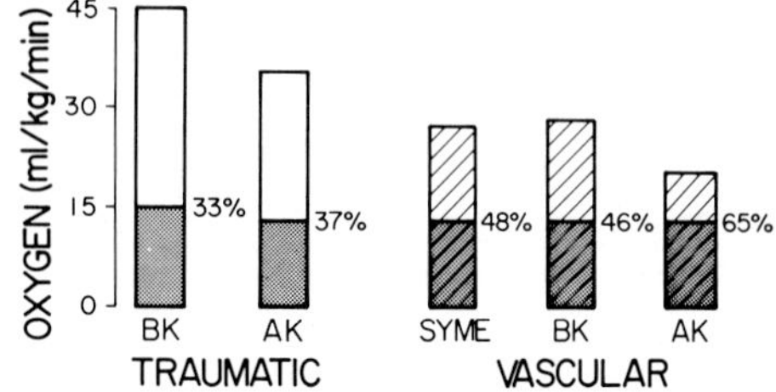

Fig. 27-2. Amputee aerobic capacity and percent used in walking. Shaded area identifies percent of total aerobic capacity used for walking.

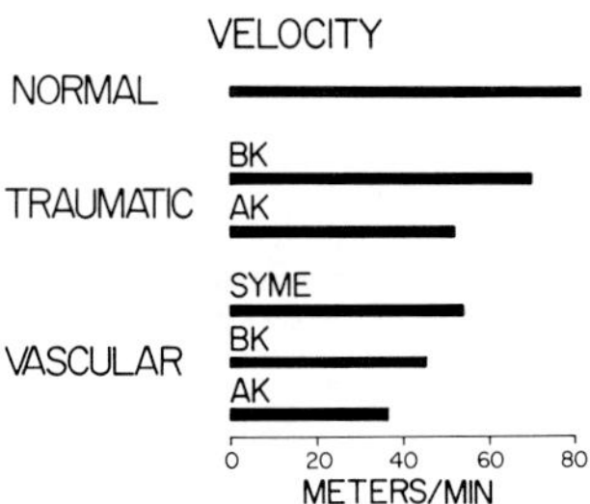

Fig. 27-3. Average gait velocity for healthy persons (normal) and each amputee group.

tances in an acceptable period of time is dictated by their gait efficiency. By correlating the two measurements of gait velocity and minute energy cost gait efficiency is defined.

Gait velocity. Although all the groups averaged the same energy cost per minute (except the traumatic below-knee amputees), the velocity of their gait varied considerably, indicating a corresponding difference in walking efficiency.

The normal average velocity of 82 m/min was not realized by any of the patient groups. Only the traumatic below-knee amputees approached it (71 m/min, or 87% of normal), and they had to use a higher minute energy cost to attain this speed. The others (who maintained normal minute energy costs) walked significantly slower, with gait velocities averaging 47% of normal (Fig. 27-3).

Both age and amputation level proved to be direct influences on gait efficiency. For a given amputation level the elderly patients were 34% slower than their younger equivalents. Each higher level of amputation imposed an additional 20% loss in gait velocity. The combination of these two findings resulted in young traumatic above-knee amputees walking as rapidly as the elderly with Syme amputations (64% and 66% normal). In contrast, the average velocity of elderly above-knee amputees was only two thirds that of the elderly Syme amputation group, or 44% of normal.

Energy cost per meter walked. Correlation of the patient's oxygen consumption with the number of meters traveled during the test period made the significance of amputation level and age immediately evident (Fig 27-4). Elderly (diabetic) above-knee amputees had an energy cost per meter 120% greater than normal requirements (0.35 versus 0.16 O_2 ml/kg/m). This additional demand for energy decreased to 60% in elderly below-knee and young above-knee amputees (0.26 and 0.25 O_2 ml/kg/m). Elderly Syme and young below-knee amputees needed only 30% additional energy per meter (0.21 and 0.20 O_2 ml/kg/m) compared to the normal population. Thus each higher level of limb loss doubled the additional energy requirement per meter. Age doubled this factor for each amputation level as well.

Crutches versus prosthesis. Patients with above-knee amputations frequently choose not to wear a prosthesis and walk with crutches instead. This group includes persons, who by their dress, show concern with their appearance. When skin problems or pain are not difficulties, one reason for using crutches has to be gait efficiency. Energy cost studies have confirmed this assumption.

Both the diabetic and traumatic patient with above-knee amputations walked significantly faster (with one third and one fourth more velocity respectively) while using crutches without a prosthesis. Their minute energy costs, however, were slightly increased, but the resultant energy cost per meter was 11% less for the diabetics and no different for the traumatic amputee compared to walking with the prosthesis.

These findings contrasted significantly with the performance of the other amputee groups. They all displayed a distinct loss in gait efficiency with

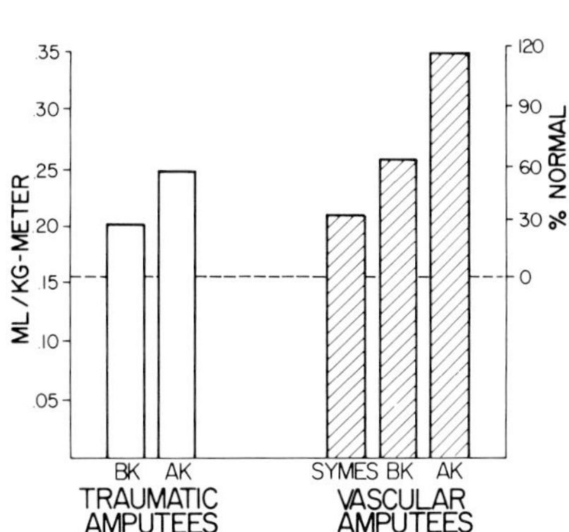

Fig. 27-4. Energy cost per meter of patients with traumatic and vascular amputations. Left scale indicates oxygen in milliliters per kilograms per meter used in walking. Right scale relates these values in amputees to healthy persons. (From Waters, R. et al.: J. Bone Joint Surg. **58A**:42-46, 1976.)

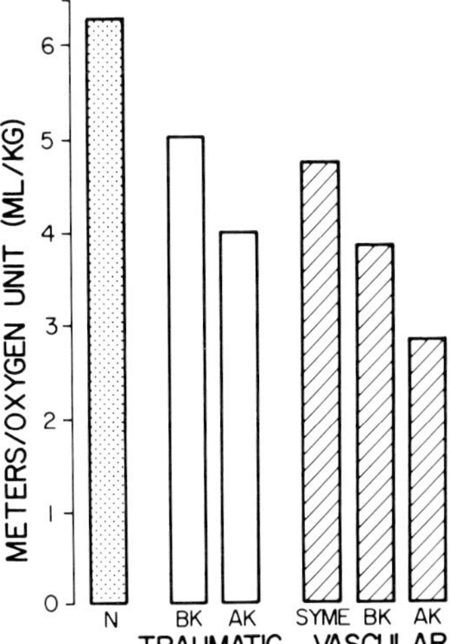

Fig. 27-5. Gait efficiency. Number of meters traveled per oxygen unit (ml/kg) per minute by each amputee group compared to normal gait.

crutches. Among the diabetics the loss in gait velocity and moderate rise in minute energy cost resulted in a 31% loss in gait efficiency. A similar decrease in gait efficiency with crutches was evidenced by traumatic below-knee amputees because of the increased minute energy cost used to maintain the same gait velocity.

Efficiency rating. An analogy may be drawn between the familiar miles per gallon of gas concept of automobile performance to the physiological requirements of walking, in which gait efficiency is measured in meters per unit of oxygen. This is a direct ratio of gait velocity (m/min) and minute energy cost (O_2 ml/kg/min). The normal value of 6.3 O_2 m/ml/kg was not realized by any of the amputee groups. Traumatic below-knee and vascular Syme amputees were comparable, both approaching 78% of normal. Another equality in efficiency was displayed by the traumatic above-knee amputee and the vascular Syme amputee with an average 62% value. Patients with vascular above-knee amputations realized a gait efficiency only 45% of normal (Fig. 27-5).

Correlations of normal maximum output and energy use have identified that as a machine the human body is only 25% efficient. Consideration of this fact makes the penalty of an above-knee amputation in the elderly person even more evident. Comparable interpretation of their data reveals that their machine efficiency is a mere 12%, almost the point of no return for effort expended.

Limb mechanics

Common to all the amputees tested was an anesthetic foot (prosthetic), the insecurity of a soft-tissue interface between the limb's bony lever and the prosthetic socket, and an artificial ankle joint. The latter was either a rigid unit (SACH foot), which must transmit the floor reaction forces of walking proximally, or an insensitive mobile unit with predetermined passive restraints. Above-knee amputees had the added disadvantages of an anesthetic knee joint whose controls were partially dependent on exaggerated body or limb actions and hip musculature rendered subnormal by thigh transection. The two patient populations, classified by traumatic and vascular amputations, differed in age and limb vascularity. Both these factors restricted the strength capability of the vascular group.

The finding, during energy cost measurements, that even healthy, young adults with traumatic amputations walked at a slower than normal velocity demonstrated a functional limitation from the anatomical variants just described. Further confirmation came from the fact that the velocity of the different patient groups reflected the amputation level and etiology. The impact of these factors becomes clearer when the patient's gait measurements are fractioned into the components of velocity. Velocity is defined as distance per unit of time. In gait, the distance factor is stride length. Although cadence refers to timing, both are dually dependent on the swing and stance performance of the limbs.

These values were determined with bilateral insole, contact-closing foot switches as the patients traversed the designated middle 6 m of a 10-m walkway. A built-in forceplate identified the foot-floor reaction forces.

Stride length. Among the amputees studied, two stride-length patterns were displayed. A normal distance was attained by the young, traumatic below-knee group. All others showed a moderate loss. Traumatic above-knee amputees evidenced the advantages of youth with a stride length 86% of normal. All the vascular patient groups had a shorter stride, averaging 74%. Those with Syme amputation averaged 78%. Below-knee patients approximated the average, and the group with above-knee amputations averaged 71%. These differences reflect the influence of the prosthetic limb's stance stability on the amount the contralateral limb can swing forward. Two mechanisms are involved: weight-bearing tolerance and rocker action.

During the period of time one limb is swinging forward the body's full weight has been shifted onto the other foot. Momentum also tends to pull the body forward over the weight-bearing foot. Both events challenge the stability of the stance limb. Limited tolerance of these demands because of prosthetic insecurity, muscular weakness, or sensory impairment has bilateral significance, since inability to bear weight on one limb correspondingly shortens the swing time available to the other limb. A sensitive measure of stance security is the patient's single-limb support time. The absolute time period, however, is not significant because even normal values vary with gait velocity. Thus single limb support is expressed as a percent of normal (for that velocity). This measurement proved to be sensitive to the amputee's pathological condition, both as an independent value and when the two limbs (prosthetic and sound) were compared.

The composite effect of amputation level and

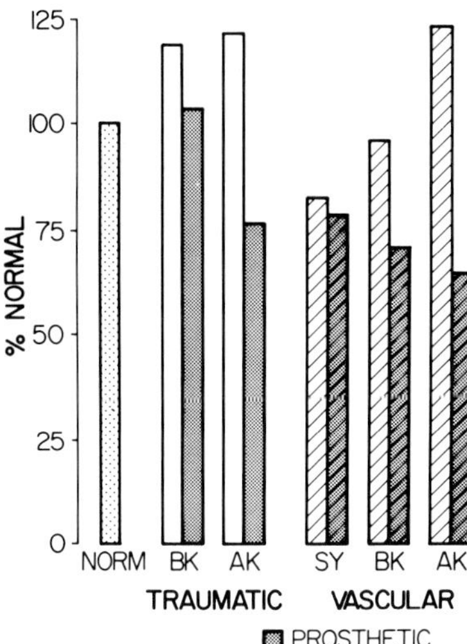

Fig. 27-6. Single-limb support of intact and prosthetic limbs. Note decreasing support capability with each higher level of amputation and corresponding increased dependency on intact limb.

age were reflected in the single-limb support values recorded. In each group, classified as either vascular or traumatic, there was serial shortening of the prosthetic limb's single support period and corresponding lengthening of time spent on the sound side for each higher level of amputation (Fig. 27-6). Youthfulness improved the patient's prosthetic limb single support time far more than it lessened the bilateral disparity. The difference in single support capability of the prosthetic and sound limbs carries two implications. It identifies the amount the patient depends on the sound limb's better functioning capability for the velocity accomplished. This difference also indirectly demonstrates the added penalty the patient would experience with a bilateral amputation of that level. Those with Syme amputations registered only a 2% disparity and therefore would lose little substitutive capability. This supports the common clinical finding that patients with bilateral Syme amputations continue as independent walkers. In contrast, vascular above-knee amputees showed a 48% difference, even with the aid of crutches, and those with traumatic above-knee amputations had a 36% disparity. These data explain why bilateral above-knee amputations carry such a poor functional prognosis.

Between heel strike and toe-off, normal foot and ankle motions create a rocker action that allows the body to travel smoothly forward. The amount of trunk advance normally contributes half the total step length. Stance limb strength proved to be a major determinant of this distance. A comparison of single-limb support ratios and stride lengths suggested that the type of amputation and limb strength exerted a direct influence on the patient's rocker mechanism. Those with Syme and below-knee amputation of vascular origin displayed a disproportionate loss of stride length, indicating that they also suffered some limitation from their prosthetic rocker action (17%). In contrast, the two traumatic amputee groups had proportionally longer stride lengths for their single support periods. These patients had sufficient strength to use the full prosthetic rocker action and exercise additional substitutions by the sound limb as well. Vascular above-knee amputees also had proportionally longer stride lengths for their abbreviated single-limb support periods, but they substituted by relying heavily on bilateral crutches. This dependence was demonstrated by the high heart rate recorded during the energy cost measurements. It equalled that recorded when they walked on crutches without their prosthesis.

Cadence. Quickness of step rather clearly displayed the disability incurred by the mixture of amputation level and age group. None walked at a normal pace (116 steps/min), but those with the least physical impairment (dysvascular Syme and traumatic below-knee amputations) averaged 85% of normal rate. The most disabled patients (those with vascular above-knee amputations) had a cadence averaging only 62% of normal. An intermediate value, 75% of normal cadence, was the average for the others (vascular below-knee and traumatic above-knee amputees).

The rate at which a patient swings the limb forward to take a step determines the impact of loading on that limb at the onset of stance. Therefore patients must not only have the strength to swing the limb rapidly, but must also be able to control its position during loading. Caution in limb loading is indicative of limb instability and is reflected in the percentage of the stance period that is used to reach maximum weight bearing during forceplate recordings. This is the rate of loading. Such measurements are not available for all the patient groups reported here, but a clinically pertinent trend was displayed by data on ten vascular below-knee amputees. These data evidenced a significantly slower loading rate on their prosthetic limb (26%) compared to the normal loading rate of 10%. Among the healthy persons (n = 24), there was no dominance of faster loading rates in right or left limbs. Similar measurements of persons with unilateral degenerated hips confirm the implication of these data because they too displayed slower loading rates on the involved limb.

An indirect measure of loading capability is the patient's double stance period. This increases when patients have difficulty weight bearing in a single stance on an impaired limb. All the vascular amputees had prolonged double stance times (average 13%), yet this was not seen in the traumatic groups. The difference between these two populations is in limb strength. This is a factor which must be considered seriously when estimating walking potential. Muscles cannot be strengthened without the presence of an adequate vascular supply. Disease of the small arteries is one characteristic of diabetic limb pathology. Clinically, physical therapists have found a very limited strengthening capability among the diabetic patients, despite intensive exercise. This has been true even for those in their forties. Therefore age alone is not the determinant.

The very prolonged contralateral single-limb support period recorded by above-knee amputees (traumatic and vascular) implies a second factor retarding cadence. Observation of their gait has revealed difficulty in toe clearance to be common. Persistence of full knee extension throughout stance for weight-bearing security denies these patients the normal amount of preswing knee flexion (passive) that prepares the limb for swing. Loss of this passive arc of knee flexion requires that some substitute action be exerted during initial swing for the toe to safely clear the ground. Most used a deliberate pelvic hiking motion (subtle or obvious). This added effort takes time, thereby slowing the patient's cadence.

SUMMARY

The muscular activity of normal walking employs a significant portion of an individual's energy production capability. As aging decreases oxygen delivery and extraction capability (aerobic capacity), the fraction used in walking rises from 33% for the 20-year-old to 43% for those age 60. In addition, patients with primary vascular disease or diabetic ischemia have restricted muscle oxygenation, which limits their potential for strengthening.

Limb impairment of any type increases the energy cost of walking by the added muscular effort involved in substitution. Decreasing velocity is a natural means of reducing the immediate-energy demand (minute value), although the added time required to travel a desired distance results in a net increase of energy cost (meter value). Therefore gait efficiency is lowered.

Both factors (energy production and limb loss) proved significant to the amputee. Each higher level amputation was characterized by a slower velocity. Age further reduced this value. For all but elderly above-knee amputees velocity reduction maintained the patient's minute energy cost and aerobic capacity fraction within normal limits (physiological comfort), but gait efficiency was proportionally decreased with the additional energy cost per meter being doubled for each amputation level and again doubled by the age differential between 30 and 60 years. The 47% greater demand on aerobic capacity of the elderly diabetic with above-knee amputation appeared related to limb inefficiency, depriving them of adequate physical conditioning. These findings dictate that age and the extent of limb loss, as well as cause of the amputation should be used to predict walking capabilities.

REFERENCES

1. Astrand, P., and Rodahl, K.: Textbook of work physiology, New York, 1970, McGraw-Hill Book Co.
2. Blessey, R., Hislop, H., Waters, R., and Antonelli, D.: Metabolic energy cost of unrestrained walking, J. Am. Phys. Ther. Assoc. **56:**1019-1024, 1976.
3. Waters, R. L., Perry, J., Antonelli, D., and Hislop, H.: Energy cost of amputees: the influence of level of amputation. J. Bone Joint Surg. **58A:**42-46, 1976.

CHAPTER 28

The bilateral lower limb amputee

NEWTON C. McCOLLOUGH, III
ANNE R. HARRIS
FREDERICK L. HAMPTON

The bilateral lower limb amputee presents a special problem in rehabilitation. Although loss of both limbs secondary to trauma may occur, by far the majority of these patients lose their limbs secondary to vascular disease. Silbert[6] studied 294 diabetic amputees and found that 41% lived longer than 5 years after surgery and that 51% of those who survived surgery lost the remaining limb within 5 years. Mazet et al.[4] have reported that a patient who has already lost one lower limb due to ischemia stands a 33% chance of losing the other limb within 5 years. Other authors have established the incidence of bilateral lower limb loss at 21% to 26.5% in various series of amputations done for diabetic ischemia.[1, 2, 7] On the other hand, Whitehouse et al.[9] have emphasized the fact that the majority of diabetic patients who have lost one limb will lose their lives as a result of the disease process before they lose their second leg. In their 12-year study of sixty-seven diabetic amputees, only twenty were alive at the end of the study, and four of these (20%) were bilateral amputees. McCollough et al.[5] in a study of bilateral below-knee amputations, reported that of twenty-seven patients who had been unilateral amputees secondary to vascular disease, twenty lost their second limb within 2 years and seven lost their second limb by 6 years after amputation of the first.

The relatively high frequency of bilateral limb loss in the patient suffering from vascular disease further emphasizes the importance of amputating below the knee whenever possible (Fig. 28-1). Bilateral limb loss below the knee is compatible with functional prosthetic rehabilitation, whereas higher combinations of double amputations routinely carry a much poorer functional prognosis.

In nearly all reported series, loss of both lower limbs appears to be much more common in the diabetic than in patients with arteriosclerosis uncomplicated by diabetes. The lower limb in the diabetic not only is ischemic but frequently exhibits peripheral neuropathy and decreased sensation, predisposing to pressure sores and skin breakdown. Added to this is the predisposition to infection in the diabetic and the difficulty in eradicating such infection once it becomes established. In terms of level of amputation, in our experience, diabetes accounts for 80% to 90% of bilateral below-knee amputations. Arteriosclerosis without diabetes accounts for the majority of bilateral above-knee amputations, frequently in association with a major block to circulation in the distal aorta or iliac arteries.

In the patient with vascular disease who has suffered the loss of one limb, it is most important for the surgeon to instruct the patient in the proper care of the remaining foot. These patients are generally quite receptive to carrying out any program to avert loss of the remaining limb, but they must be impressed with the importance of foot hygiene and proper shoe wear. They must also be advised about the importance of reporting to the

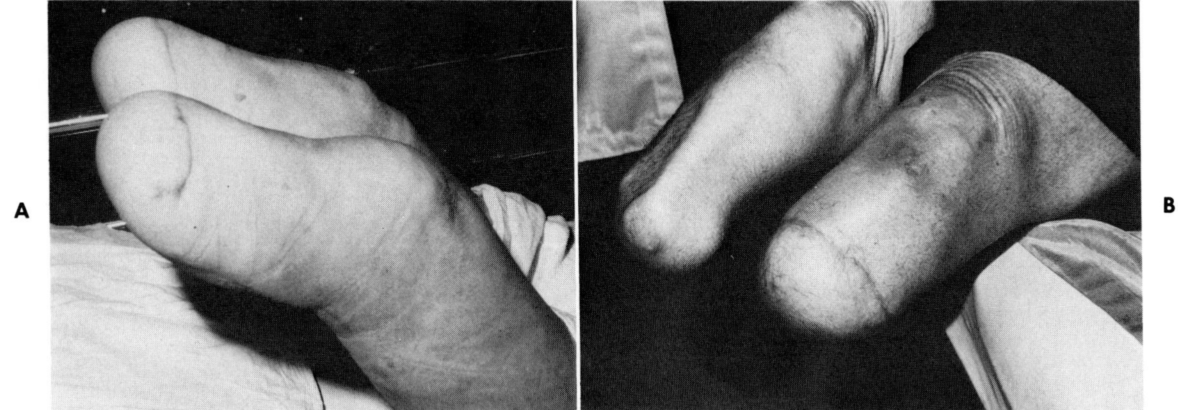

Fig. 28-1. A, Bilateral below-knee dysvascular amputation, long posterior flap technique. **B,** Left, modern muscle-stabilized long posterior flap technique. Right, conventional surgical technique without muscle stabilization.

physician at the earliest sign of infection or skin breakdown and warned against using a hot foot bath, which may contain any number of home remedies. The patient should also be warned against self-administered minor foot surgery, such as trimming calluses or toenails. These instructions are quite simple and straightforward and may seem obvious, but it is this very fact that frequently leads to neglect on the part of the physician to properly inform patients.

SURGICAL CONSIDERATIONS

Every effort must be made to keep the amputation as low as possible, especially in the patient whose second limb is threatened. In some, transmetatarsal amputation may be successful. This procedure, even if it fails, usually does not compromise the below-knee level as a secondary site of election. If at all possible, a transmetatarsal amputation should be performed and the wound left open for secondary closure if infection is present. A Syme amputation can be successfully performed in selected patients with an infection of the forepart of the foot, if the posterior tibial pulse is palpable and the skin of the hindfoot is warm and hyperemic. As a general rule, the longer the residual limb, the better will be the gait and endurance of the bilateral below-knee amputee. Patients with one below-knee and one Syme amputation walk better than those with two below-knee amputations with residual limbs of conventional length. Patients with bilateral Syme amputations have an even more stable and better controlled gait due to the long lever arms of their residual limbs, as well as increased proprioception and end-bearing qualities provided by this amputation level.

In patients who sustain major trauma to both lower limbs, necessitating bilateral amputation, the surgeon should again strive to save all possible length. Such patients, if young and free from vascular disease, do much better when the amputation is through the lower third of the leg, if possible, rather than through the "site of election" 12.5 to 15 cm (5 or 6 inches) below the knee joint.

There has been a mistaken and widespread notion that bilateral amputees do better if their amputations are at the same level. *This is simply not true,* and such thinking should not influence the surgeon in selecting the site of amputation of the second limb. Unfortunately, some have even recommended routine amputation above the knee for patients whose first amputation was above the knee.[3] The absolute rule to follow is to save all length possible when amputating the second leg, regardless of the level of the previous amputation.

PROSTHETIC CONSIDERATIONS

Considerations in fitting

The degree of success in prosthetic fitting of bilateral lower extremity amputations varies according to the patient's age and cardiovascular status and according to the levels of amputation. It should be remembered that many of the patients under consideration have lost their limbs as a result of peripheral vascular disease and are suffering from a systemic disorder. These patients have increased incidence of hypertension, coronary artery disease, and cerebral vascular disease. The prosthetist must give careful consideration to the increased energy cost imposed before attempting to rehabilitate the bilateral amputee.

It is our conviction that these costs are prohibitive for the bilateral above-knee amputee who has lost limbs from vascular disease and that a wheelchair is the best form of locomotion for these individuals. We have not encountered a single bilateral above-knee amputee suffering from arteriosclerosis who has been functionally rehabilitated prosthetically. These observations are at variance with those of Watkins,[8] who reported a 70% success rate in the rehabilitation of 50 bilateral amputees, of whom the majority had bilateral above-knee amputations. In earlier years, we occasionally were successful with ambulation in a small number of such amputees, only to find that they inevitably return to the wheelchair by preference within a few months. We no longer fit or recommend fitting for these individuals.

The younger bilateral above-knee amputee, in whom trauma is usually the reason for the amputation, may indeed be prosthetically rehabilitated, but the increased energy demands for ambulation are enormous, and success in rehabilitation will be directly related to the patient's motivation and physical endurance. Even these patients prefer a wheelchair for traveling other than short distances. In addition, the patient is more likely to stand and walk if the residual limbs are relatively long, so that adequate control over the prosthesis can be obtained. Even under the best of conditions, these patients require external support, and walking is tedious and slow.

A combination above-knee–below-knee amputee can be expected to function at a level superior to that of the bilateral above-knee amputee. Patients who have this combination of amputation level as a result of peripheral vascular disease still carry a relatively limited prognosis for functional ambulation. These individuals also quickly learn that the investment of effort and time required to arise from a sitting position, walk 10 feet, and sit down again, is many times that required to roll a wheelchair the same distance.

Prosthetic rehabilitation is more likely to succeed in patients who already have an above-knee amputation and have learned successfully how to ambulate on an above-knee prosthesis prior to losing the second leg below the knee. The reverse situation, in which a prior below-knee amputee must learn to use an above-knee prosthesis on the opposite side, is more difficult. The most difficult of all tasks from the rehabilitation standpoint is to attempt to train a patient who has lost both limbs at different levels simultaneously. Fitting as a bilateral amputee is recommended with this combination of levels in older patients who have been successful above-knee prosthesis users prior to losing the second limb below the knee and in all young patients regardless of the timing of the amputations.

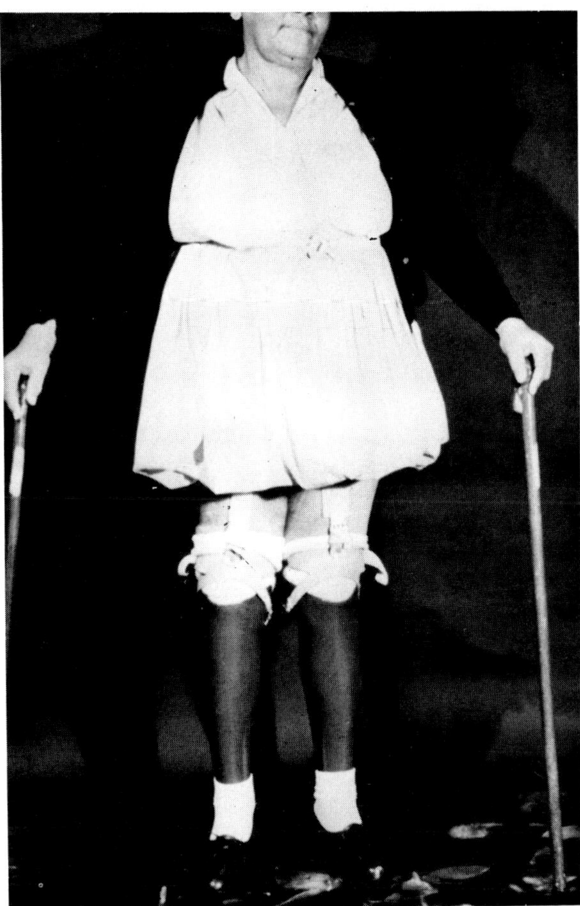

Fig. 28-2. Elderly diabetic bilateral below-knee amputee successfully rehabilitated to ambulatory status using two canes.

The bilateral below-knee amputee can be given a much more favorable prognosis for functional ambulation. Even the elderly patient with bilateral below-knee amputation secondary to peripheral vascular disease has an excellent chance of prosthetic rehabilitation, provided he was ambulatory prior to the second amputation.[2] Elderly patients who lose both limbs below the knee simultaneously carry a more guarded prognosis, but if they were actively ambulatory prior to the onset of their disability, attempted fitting is worthwhile. In a University of Miami study of thirty-one bilateral below-knee amputees over the age of 50, thirty achieved functional prosthetic rehabilitation, and several were independently ambulatory without the use of external support.[2] In others, canes, crutches, or a walker was necessary, but independence of ambulation was still achieved (Fig. 28-2). Young patients with bilateral below-knee amputations should be able to ambulate with a relatively normal gait and without the use of external support. In our experience the older bilateral below-knee amputee has a greater potential for prosthetic rehabilitation than the unilateral above-knee amputee. Fitting is recommended for all bilateral below-knee amputees, unless they were unable to sucessfully ambulate as a unilateral below-knee amputee, or unless their level of activity was relatively limited prior to the simultaneous loss of both limbs.

Prescription considerations

Although immediate postsurgical rigid dressing and early prosthetic fitting is recommended in the bilateral as well as the unilateral amputee, no patient who becomes a bilateral amputee should begin weight bearing on the recently amputated stump until there is good evidence of wound healing as confirmed by visual inspection. The obvious reason for this precaution is that the bilateral amputee is unable to control safely the amount of weight bearing to which the residual limb is subjected. Particularly in the patient who has lost a second limb from vascular disease, the consequences of injudicious early weight bearing may be disastrous, with stump breakdown necessitating reamputation to a higher level. The tilt table is useful in progressively proceeding to upright stance as rehabilitation progresses.

In the bilateral above-knee amputee who suffers loss of both limbs simultaneously, prosthetic rehabilitation is best initiated by the use of "stubbies" (Fig. 28-3). These are nothing more than above-knee quadrilateral sockets to which prosthetic feet have been attached, so that the patient's CG is close to the ground with a broad base of support. This will frequently enable the amputee to gain trunk balance and lends an early sense of security. Some patients may prefer these prostheses as definitive for ambulation within the home environment.

When the patient has become proficient with the use of stubbies he may graduate to bilateral above-knee temporary legs with articulated knees with manual locks. When he becomes independent, ambulates with crutches or other external support, is able to don and doff the prosthesis, and is able to arise from a sitting position independently, he is then ready for definitive prosthetic prescription. Quadrilateral total-contact sockets are recommended, but suction suspension is contraindicated because of the inability of the patient to don the prostheses in the sitting position. Suspension should be accomplished by the hip joint and pelvic band system. The knee joints selected should have stance phase locking features, and a manual lock on one or both knees may be recommended. Prosthetic alignment considerations in the bilateral above-knee amputee include having the feet outset more than usual to provide a somewhat broader base gait and placing the knee bolts sufficiently posterior to provide alignment stability at the knee. Shortening the prostheses to lower the body CG will achieve better stability.

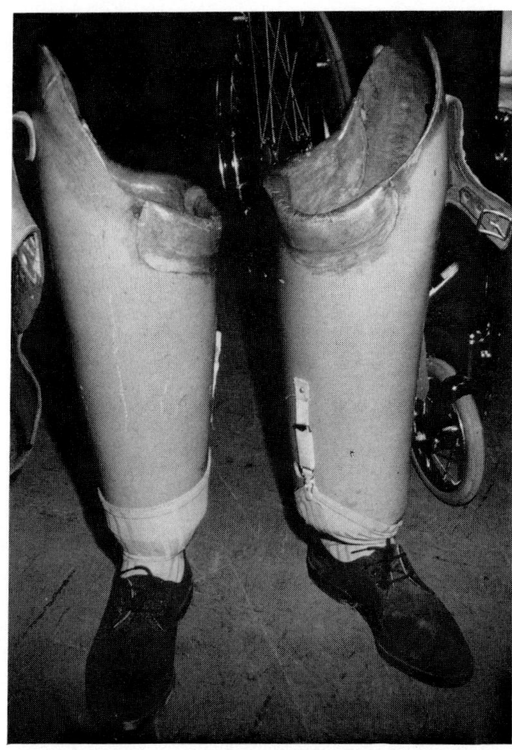

Fig. 28-3. "Stubbies" are used in rehabilitation of above-knee amputee who suffers loss of both limbs simultaneously.

In the case of the patient who has a combination of below-knee and above-knee amputations, the same prescription considerations as just mentioned pertain to the above-knee amputation. With the below-knee amputation, the use of a thigh corset with side joints may improve the patient's stability. Younger patients who have the balance necessary to stand on the below-knee prosthesis while donning the above-knee artificial limb may use a suction socket on the above-knee amputation side.

Prosthetic considerations in the bilateral below-knee amputee include outsetting both feet somewhat more than for the unilateral below-knee amputee so that a stable stance is achieved. In addition, the heels of the prosthetic feet should be quite firm to eliminate the tendency of the amputee to tilt backward. Prosthetic feet should be somewhat longer than the patient's previous foot size to give the amputee additional leverage and balance. It may also be desirable in the bilateral below-knee amputee to fabricate the prosthesis somewhat shorter than the previous limb length for reasons of stability. With regard to socket design for the bilateral below-knee amputee, the supracondylar-suprapatellar design provides improved mediolateral stability over other total-contact designs and is generally preferable. In patients who have short stumps the addition of a thigh corset and outside knee joints is recommended.

Rehabilitation

Rehabilitation of the bilateral amputee to an ambulatory status is contingent on four factors: (1) physiological age and strength of the patient, (2) time between amputations or whether they were performed simultaneously, (3) previous ambulatory ability of the patient, and (4) level of the amputations. As with all amputees, the patient should be evaluated completely and a realistic goal set, whether that goal be ambulation or wheelchair independence. The amputee then begins a program of exercises and functional activities to reach those goals.

The bilateral below-knee amputee who was a good walker as a unilateral amputee with one cane or no external support will in most instances learn to ambulate with one or two canes and will not need to use a wheelchair except for occasional long distances. In this particular instance, extensive gait training is not necessary. Ambulation should begin in the parallel bars and progress rapidly to crutches or two canes. In case of the elderly bilateral amputee, the therapist should not try to change the gait pattern from a three-point to a four-point gait after the loss of the second limb. This often causes confusion and in many instances needless falls.

One precaution to be considered when training the bilateral amputee is to be sure the stumps can tolerate full weight bearing. The bilateral amputee cannot control the amount of weight placed on the stump due to the loss of both limbs. The bilateral amputee should also be discouraged from walking with only one prosthesis. Balancing is difficult, and the forces are too great on the residual limb.

The bilateral below-knee amputee who loses both limbs simultaneously is a more difficult problem. These patients do not have the benefit of time and experience in using one prosthesis. They require more gait training, especially in balancing and becoming accustomed to the pressure of the prostheses. They usually progress more slowly and use more external support for a longer period of time.

The bilateral amputee who has had one amputation below the knee and one above the knee is a more difficult rehabilitation problem than the bilateral below-knee amputee. In this case, the level of independence and expertise developed depends on which leg was lost first. If the above-knee amputation was performed first and the individual was a satisfactory ambulator, he will usually attain that level of ambulation again. If the opposite is true, then ambulation is often very difficult, sometimes requiring the use of a locked, above-knee prosthesis. Long-distance ambulation is not a realistic goal. In many cases the wheelchair is the main mode of transportation. This soon becomes obvious to the patient due to the difficulty in coming to the standing position, and the amount of external support and energy required to walk. Gait training for these individuals is of a longer duration than the bilateral below-knee amputee and usually requires the use of bilateral support.

The bilateral above-knee amputee presents the greatest problem for successful ambulation. Ambulation at this level is usually minimal, even if the individual was a successful walker as a unilateral amputee. In general, the younger the person at the time of loss of the second limb or at the time of simultaneous loss of both limbs, the more successful he will be at using bilateral above-knee prostheses. It is most important, therefore, that the individual gain the highest degree of wheelchair independence possible; considerable time should be spent in this effort. A special wheelchair is essential to prevent the chair from tipping backward, due to the loss of weight normally present at the front on the chair.

If ambulation is to be attempted, it is of utmost importance that the patient have no contractures and is not obese. Time should be spent in balancing activities with the knees locked prior to ambulation. In most instances, it is beneficial to have the prosthesis lowered from the normal height. Stubbies are an excellent tool to use in teaching balance. This type of prosthesis, however, is not always acceptable cosmetically for permanent use.

When ambulation is started in the parallel bars the knees should be kept locked and later unlocked, one at a time. Some individuals elect to always walk with one knee locked for stability. As independence increases, progress should be made to the proper external support. The most difficult activity for these people to master is getting up from the sitting position. Some patients find the use of one locked knee beneficial to this activity.

Most bilateral above-knee amputees eventually discontinue walking as their main mode of locomotion. They find that it is not functional due to the tremendous energy expenditure and the slow gait they must assume. A satisfactory alternative at this stage may be the use of cosmetic prostheses, with a wheelchair as the primary means of locomotion.

REFERENCES

1. Baddeley, R. M., and Fulford, J. C.: A trail of conservative amputations for lesions of the feet in diabetic mellitus, Br. J. Surg. **52:**38, 1965.
2. Cameron, H. C., Lennard-Jones, J. E., and Robinson, K. P.: Amputation in the diabetic: outcome and survival, Lancet **2:**605, 1964.
3. Clark-Williams, M. J.: The elderly double amputee, Geront. Clin. **11:**183-193, 1969.
4. Mazet, R., Schiller, F. J., Dunn, O. J., and Neufeld, A. J.: The influence of prostheses wearing on the health of the geriatric amputee: Project 431, Office of Vocational Rehabilitation, Washington, D.C., March, 1963, Department of Health, Education, and Welfare.
5. McCollough, N. C., Jennings, J. J., and Sarmiento, A.: Bilateral below the knee amputation in patients over fifty years of age, J. Bone Joint Surg. **54A**(6):1217-1223, Sept., 1972.
6. Silbert, S.: Amputation of the lower extremity in diabetes mellitus: follow-up of 294 cases, Diabetes **1:**297-299, 1952.
7. Smith, B. C.: A twenty year follow-up in fifty below knee amputations for gangrene in diabetics, Surg. Gynecol. Obstet. **103:**625, 1966.
8. Watkins, A. L., and Liao, S. J.: Rehabilitation of persons with bilateral amputations of the lower extremities, J.A.M.A. **166:**1585-1586, 1958.
9. Whitehouse, F. W., Jurgensen, C., and Block, M. A.: The later life of the diabetic amputee: another look at the fat of the second leg, Diabetes **17:**520, 1968.

CHAPTER 29

Prostheses and assistive devices for special activities

BERNICE KEGEL

Throughout the world, the attention of professional personnel and the general public is increasingly being drawn to sports as an important aspect of overall treatment and rehabilitation of the disabled. Numerous people with physical disabilities have discovered new and unsuspected levels of achievement through participation in physical recreation.

Progress in development of avocational activities for those physically limited people who are not confined to wheelchairs has been slow. Recently, however, interest has been generated in facilitating activities for ambulatory amputees. Recreational prostheses and adaptive equipment are gradually coming to the forefront.

This chapter presents some special prostheses and adaptive devices currently available and offers an idea of activities in which amputees are able to participate. Many of the adaptations and prostheses described are fairly new and have been used by relatively small numbers of amputees. For this reason, they cannot be considered suitable for every amputee.

SKIING

Skiing is an enormous delight to the amputee because by this means he can again move with speed, grace, and ease. He enters a new world of freedom and competes as an equal with able-bodied devotees of the sport. The average amputee can learn to ski intermediate and expert slopes in one fourth of the time an able-bodied skier needs and with a far greater degree of proficiency.

The concept of amputee skiing originated in Austria and Germany in 1948. The Swiss subsequently introduced "crutch skiing." It was not until the 1960s that genuine interest appeared in the United States. In 1967, the National Amputee Ski Association was formed by a group of Sacramento businessmen. Now amputee skiing is being taught in organized classes in several states.

The unilateral below-knee amputee has essentially two options available. He can ski either with or without a prosthesis. Above-knee prostheses have not yet been refined adequately for use on ski slopes; therefore most above-knee amputees ski on the intact leg only, using the three-track skiing technique (Fig. 29-1). The bilateral below-knee amputee uses the four-track technique, with two prostheses, two skis, and outriggers. Antitip crossing devices on the skis are useful.

The bilateral above-knee amputee could use short prostheses without knee mechanisms or may be happier tobogganing.

The below-knee skiing prosthesis[3]

It is important that the CG of the snow skier be located ahead of the ball of the foot to achieve proficiency while skiing. This position helps to maintain balance, facilitate turning, and compensate for increases in speed. In normal circumstances, the correct location of body weight is accomplished with either ankle dorsiflexion or a forward lean of 23 to 25 degrees. Modern ski boots reflect this forward lean in their design. A conventional prosthesis can be modified by placing a 2.5-cm a (1-inch) wedge under the heel of the boot on the ski to achieve dorsiflexion or by wedging the heel inside the ski boot to obtain forward cant. However, one problem results from these changes. The subsequent increase in socket flexion raises the posterior brim of the socket in relationship to the patellar tendon bar. When the amputee applies weight to the ski on the prosthetic side during a turn, the hip and knee on that side are in considerable flexion, more so than during any part of stance phase in normal gait. The result is an excessive and uncomfortable amount of pressure on the hamstring tendons in the popliteal area of the socket.

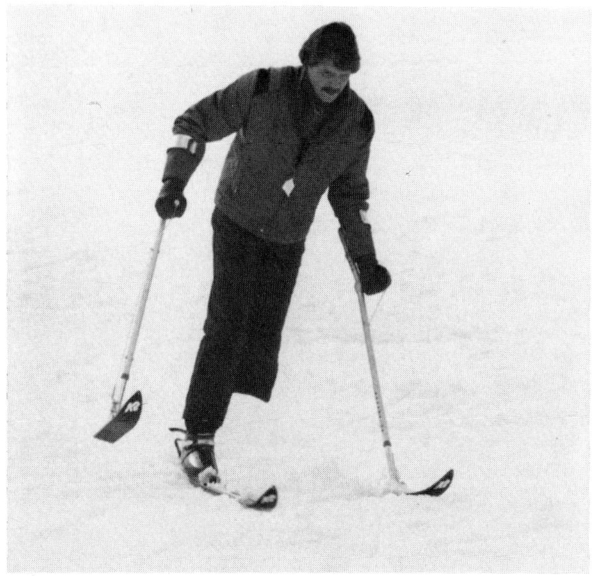

Fig. 29-1. Above-knee amputee doing three-track skiing.

An effective solution to this problem is to move the socket forward of the foot in a linear fashion without significantly increasing socket flexion. Thus with the socket flexed about 12 to 15 degrees and anterior to the foot so that the forward lean or dorsiflexion is approximately 23 degrees, the amputee is able to bear weight comfortably in the prosthesis with his CG ahead of the ball of the foot (Fig. 29-2). The most important biomechanical reason for moving the socket forward linearly without increasing socket flexion is that the skier is more effectively able to raise and lower his CG. With a greater amount of initial socket flexion, any amount of hip flexion will result in a correspondingly greater amount of anatomical knee

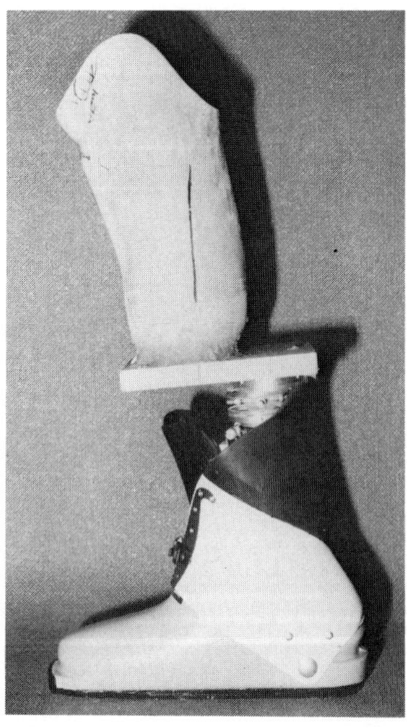

Fig. 29-2. Below-knee skiing prosthesis, showing prosthetic alignment.

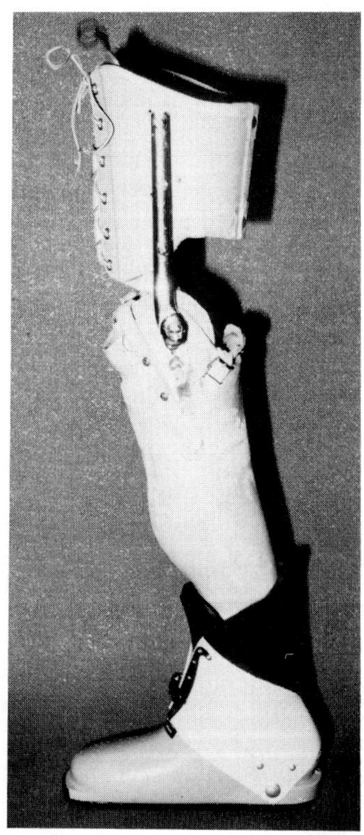

Fig. 29-3. Completed below-knee skiing prosthesis, showing anterior "bulge" caused by moving socket forward.

flexion. The prosthetist simply aligns the limb in a conventional manner. After doing so, the socket is moved forward in a linear fashion so that the anterior brim falls approximately 2.5 cm (1 inch) behind the toe of the foot. Moving the socket forward does decrease cosmesis (Fig. 29-3). Finally, the overall length of the prosthesis is reduced to equal that of the intact lower extremity when that ankle is dorsiflexed 23 to 25 degrees. A SACH foot can be incorporated into the prosthesis because there is usually no need for an ankle joint. For more proficient skiers who desire greater flexibility, a four-way ankle joint could be used to provide the additional forward flexion required on steeper terrain.

Flexion and extension at the knee and hip are basic to the activity of skiing and create a rather unusual residual limb–socket interaction. The interface used should offer as much protection and cushioning as possible. The most effective interface at this time appears to be the silicone gel insert. The insert acts like a protective layer of fatty tissue and distributes pressure evenly.

To eliminate or to minimize the reaction time between leg movement and movement of the prosthesis, there must be little or no "piston" action. The skiing prosthesis, therefore, incorporates a removable medial wedge, supracondylar cuff, and a waist belt with an elastic "pickup" strap. The cuff is particularly useful while the skier rides the chairlift. The wedge not only aids in prosthetic suspension, but enhances mediolateral and rotational stability of the socket.

A step-in binding is most convenient for the amputee who skis without the prosthesis. The newer "rear entry" ski boots facilitate donning. A lightweight ski boot is recommended.

Residual limb protection

It is advisable that amputees skiing without a prosthesis pad their residual limb to protect themselves against injury and cold. For the below-knee amputee, several stump socks are adequate. For the above-knee amputee, a modified socket can be fabricated. The protector is made to match the knee length of the intact limb, thus

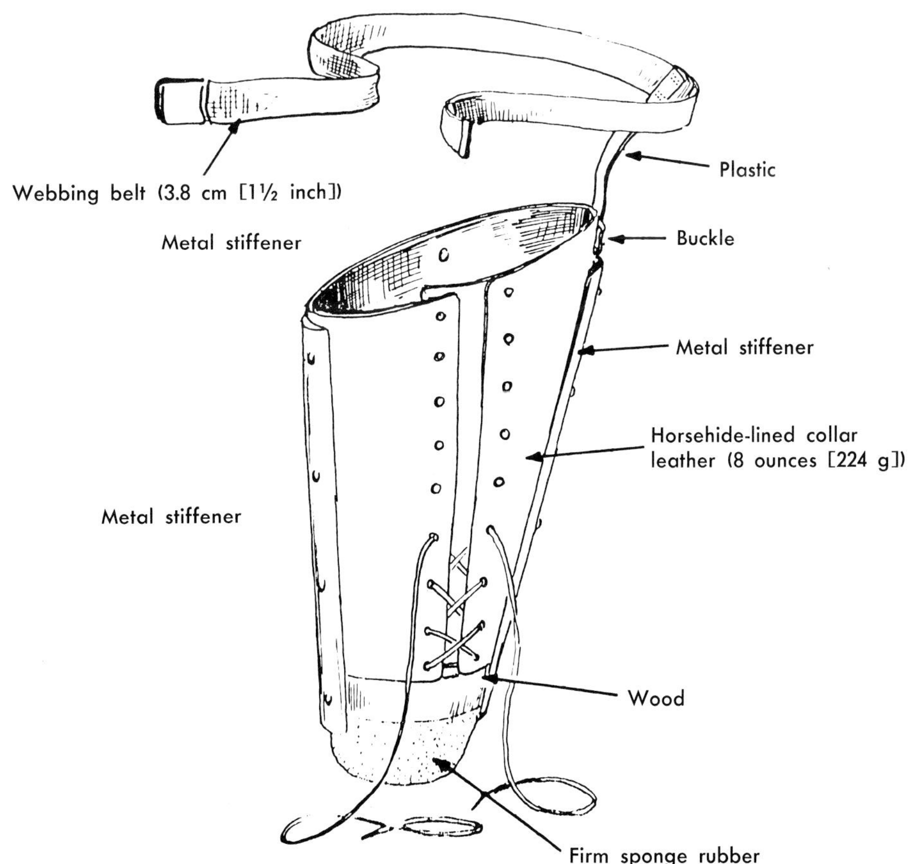

Fig. 29-4. Residual limb protector. (Courtesy Portland Junior Chamber of Commerce, Portland, Ore.)

significantly facilitating resting and getting up from the ground (Fig. 29-4).

The outrigger

Outriggers are specially adapted ski poles that are a cross between a crutch and a miniski, which enable a person to balance and maneuver better than with standard poles (Fig. 29-5). They are made from a pair of Lofstrand crutches attached to 50-cm ski tips, allowing approximately 30 degrees of motion at the junction. The outriggers should be adjusted to a length that allows the skis to hang 2.5 to 5 cm (1 to 2 inches) above the snow surface when the skier is standing erect and holding the outrigger handles. The skier should be wearing a ski boot and ski when making this length test. Two general types of outriggers are available: those which allow the ski tip to flip up for walking (Flipski) and those which do not (Standard). Some standard outriggers are equipped with a plunger device to bring a spike down into the snow when the skier is progressing over flat snow or up a small hill. Unfortunately, obtaining a satisfactory plunger from both operational and cost viewpoints has been difficult. The Flipski changes from a skiing outrigger to a skid-resistant walking crutch (Fig. 29-6). The amputee merely squeezes a cord located at the handgrip, and the ski flips up to lock in a vertical position, producing a walking crutch. Metal claws attached to the tail end of the skis provide additional braking action. The Flipski makes it easy for the amputee to get around when not actually skiing, and in using them, the skier finds he has more energy remaining to ski. Walking with the nonflip-up ski is done by pushing the ski tip edges against the snow. This maneuver takes a significant amount of practice and usually quite a few spills to master.

Several manuals are currently available re-

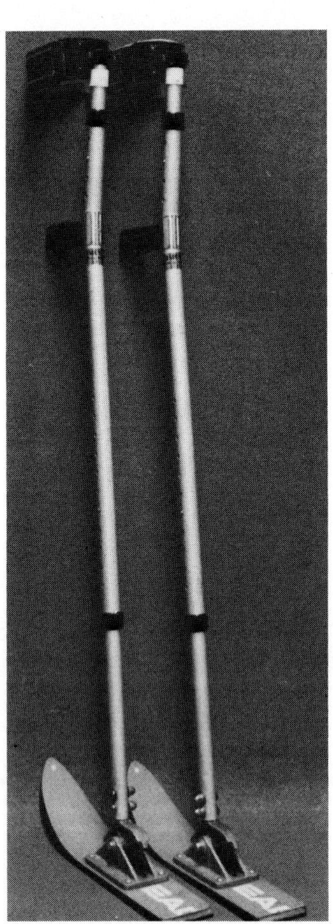

Fig. 29-5. Standard outrigger.

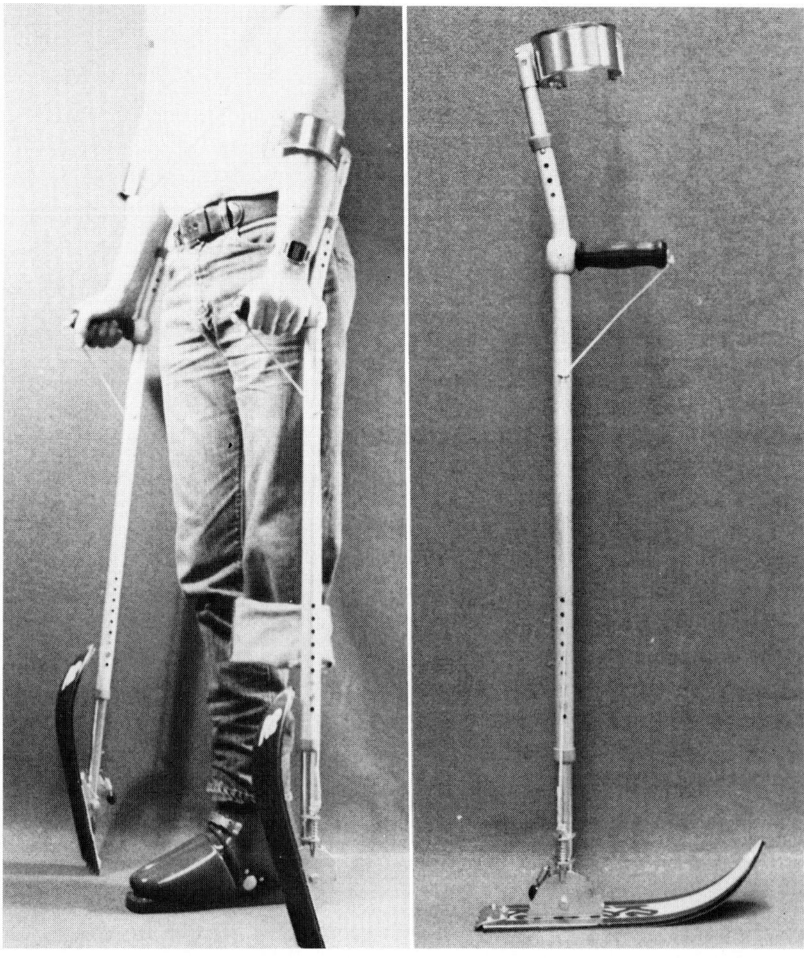

Fig. 29-6. Flipski.

garding actual skiing techniques; this subject therefore will not be dealt with here. (See appendix at the end of the chapter.)[2, 5, 8, 9]

Cross-country skiing

Cross-country skiing can be done by the below-knee amputee, but assistance is usually necessary for the person with an above-knee amputation who may require a strong biped to tow him up gradual slopes. Obviously, selection of proper terrain is most important. Touring routes that require the least amount of climbing are desirable. The only special equipment required is a 6-m (20-foot) length of tow rope. The rope is slung over either one of the skier's shoulders until it is needed, at which time the rope is attached to both skiers at the waist. The amputee again may use outriggers for assistance.

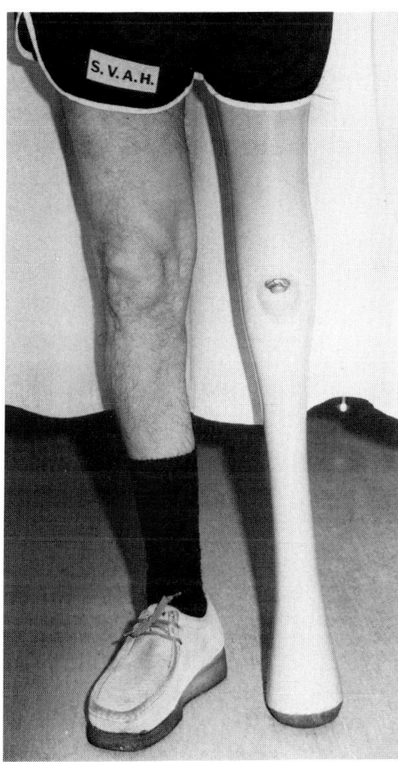

Fig. 29-7. Above-knee waterproof peg leg used for swimming.

WATER ACTIVITIES

Swimming

For many disabled people swimming is one of the few forms of pleasurable exercise available, and it has several intrinsic advantages over other sports. Practically all age groups can swim, either alone or with others; swimming provides freedom to many disabled people who are otherwise immobile; and it may be a welcome challenge to many who lead a relatively sheltered and risk-free life. Facilitites should be readily and cheaply available in most areas. The swimmer may not be very powerful, but this does not matter as long as he or she stays safely afloat, and progress can easily be assessed by participants themselves. Following are several options available to the amputee swimmer:

1. Swimming without a prosthesis
2. Peg legs for use on the beach and possibly for swimming as well (Fig. 29-7)
3. Sockets attached directly to swim fins (Fig. 29-8)
4. The utility, or beach, prosthesis, which is used to get to and from the water, but is not usually used for swimming
5. The swimming leg, which is worn while in the water

Whether or not it is essential to have a swimming leg is a question only the individual amputee can answer. Many lower limb amputees are excellent swimmers and have even performed competitively without a prosthesis. The three intact extremities do most of the work when the

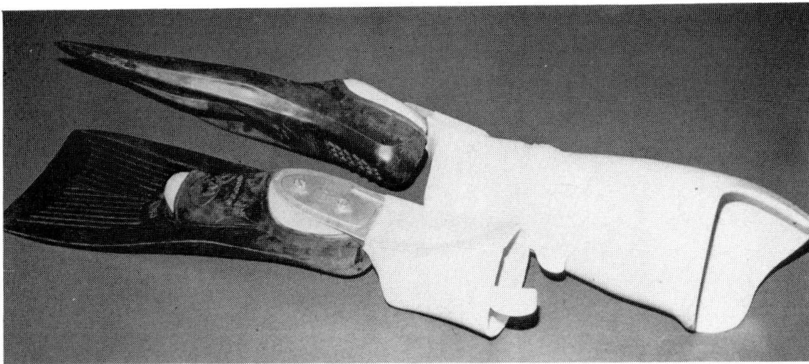

Fig. 29-8. Prosthetic sockets attached to swim fins.

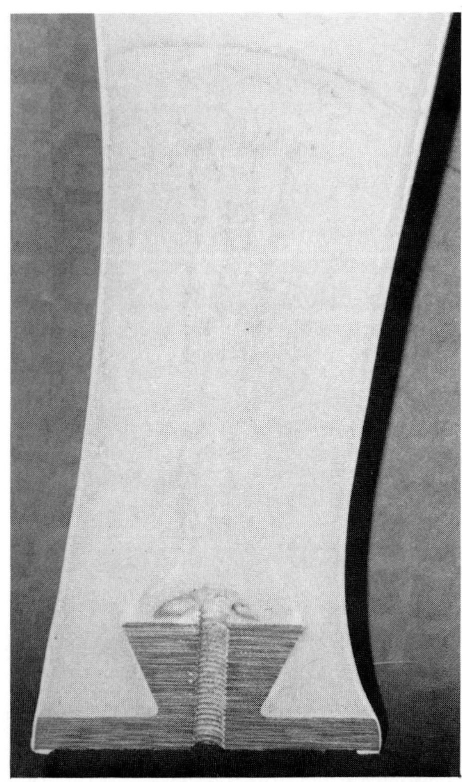

Fig. 29-9. Phenolic ankle block for use in utility prosthesis.

amputee is swimming without a prosthesis. The backstroke is the easiest for the amputee, since he can compensate to a large degree by using his arms and upper body strength. The sidestroke is relatively easy, with the residual limb on the underside. The crawl and breaststroke are very tiring, and the amputee has difficulty maintaining direction of choice. He has a tendency to swim in a circle. One disadvantage to swimming without a prosthesis is that the amputee may have difficulty getting his prosthesis back on after swimming, because the residual limb may become slightly edematous.

There are several distinct advantages in wearing a prosthesis while swimming. Swimming with a prosthesis is an excellent way to exercise the entire body. If the amputee is using some form of "kick" for propulsion in swimming, he is also exercising the residual limb musculature. (This does not necessarily mean that the amputee will swim more proficiently with a prosthesis.) Wearing a swimming leg has other advantages, including the ability to climb out of a swimming pool where there is a ladder, added stability when diving, and some protection against injury to the residual limb.

The beach, or utility, prosthesis. The beach, or utility, prosthesis is used for walking along the beach, standing in a pool to teach children to swim, boating, waterskiing, or wading through streams while fishing. This prosthesis can also be used in the shower, eliminating the need for a stool or grab bars.

The prosthesis can be worn with or without a shoe. It is made waterproof by incorporating an

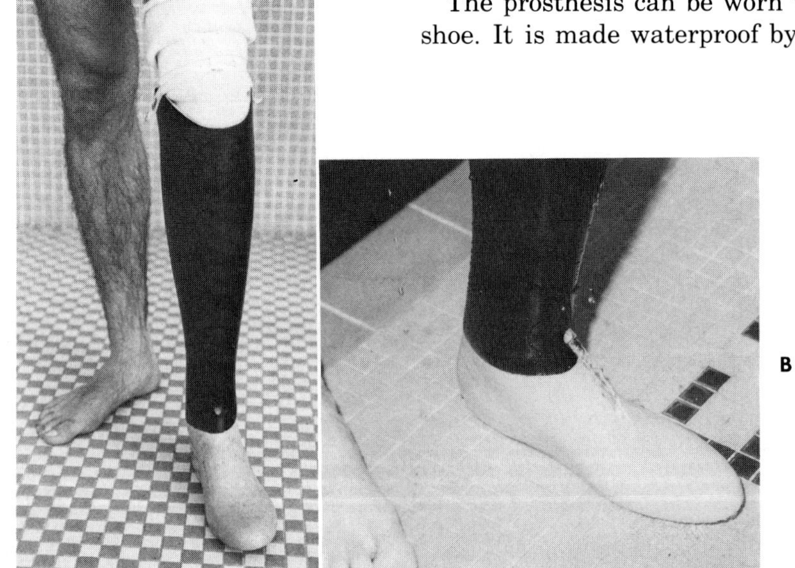

Fig. 29-10. A, Otto Bock swimming leg for below-knee amputee. **B,** Water outflow. (From Kegel, B.: Arch. Phys. Med. Rehab. J., in press.)

undercut, waterproof phenolic ankle block (Fig. 29-9), rather than wood, to join the polyurethane shank to the SACH foot.[7] Since the development of the phenolic block, a foam block has also been manufactured that is lighter and may be preferable. If a soft liner is used, it can be fabricated from Cordo and Plastazote or Pelite. If a SACH foot is used, some adaptations need to be made to the heel to allow the amputee to walk barefoot. Scheinhaus[7] has developed a removable "heel leveler," fabricated of polypropylene molded over the SACH foot. A rubber heel and Velcro closure are then added. The bolt opening should be sealed to prevent water seepage to the wooden keel. An alternative would be to use a flat-heeled postoperative foot (Kingsley), which would allow the amputee to change readily from street shoes to tennis shoes for other activities.

The Otto Bock swimming leg. The Otto Bock swimming leg (Fig. 29-10, *A*) is constructed with an airspace between the two walls of the prosthesis. A hole drilled through the ankle block allows the airspace between the two walls to partially fill with water during swimming and to drain when on land. The draining process is rapid, not causing any cosmetic problem (Fig. 29-10, *B*).

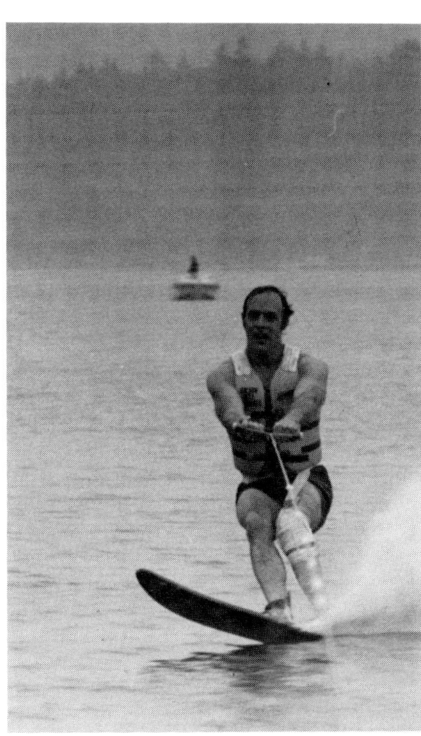

Fig. 29-11. Below-knee amputee skiing on one ski, using prosthesis.

This filling process increases the weight of the prosthesis and therefore reduces the buoyancy enough to permit effective swimming action. Furthermore, the Otto Bock limb is weighted to facilitate proper balancing between the shank and the toe of the prosthesis. Thus when the airspace fills with water, the toe will point at the correct angle to provide an effective swimming "kick." The swimmer may also wear a swim fin with this device. Because of their increased strength characteristics, acrylic resins, rather than polyesters, are used to fabricate the Otto Bock limb. If a supracondylar cuff is used, it should be constructed of a pliable plastic material that is impervious to water.

The Otto Bock above-knee swimming leg incorporates the same double-wall construction. In addition, this prosthesis uses a quick-release knee lock mechanism in conjunction with a waterproof nylon axle. For convenient storage, the amputee may easily disassemble the prosthesis into two parts by removing the axle. The knee mechanism, which is completely functional in water, has a friction lock especially designed for various purposes, such as walking or sitting on the beach. For suspension, a light harness can be made out of waterproof material. Some suction socket wearers manage to keep the limb on with no harness at all.

Waterskiing

Waterskiing on one ski is recommended, with the prosthetic leg placed behind the intact leg (Fig. 29-11). The waterproofed prosthetic leg can be made a little shorter to place weight further back on the ski. Regarding alignment, the prosthetic knee can be outset and externally rotated to allow space for clearance of the knee of the opposite limb.

Many amputees prefer to ski without a prosthesis. Several of them have attached a "bucket" to the ski on which to rest the residual limb. For the bilateral above-knee amputee who does not use prostheses, waterskiing in a "saucer" has also proved successful.

Boating

Skills required in this activity include the amputee transporting himself, equipment, and boat to the launching area, as well as portage and self-rescue. Often he will encounter steep, slippery, or rocky banks that require extreme dexterity to walk on. For these activities, most amputees prefer to wear a prosthesis, since hopping any distance while carrying equipment is exhausting.

For those people getting into a boat from a wheelchair, a hydraulic hoist (Hydro hoist) may prove invaluable. The hoist lifts the boat completely out of the water on large fiberglass pontoons. Lateral motion is prevented by four mechanical arms attached to the side of the slip, and they keep the boat centered in an immovable position. Those who have difficulty boarding boats can now lower the boat so that the gunwale is level with the seat of the wheelchair. The amputee then slides from the wheelchair to the gunwale to the pilot's seat. If the person is using crutches or a walker, he simply backs up to the gunwale, sits down on it, then swings his legs over and into the driver's seat. The amputee should check boat docks in the area to determine which of them are equipped with hydraulic hoists. Hydraulic hoists, of course, were designed for another purpose—to keep the hull of the boat out of the water, so it would remain clean and free from floating oil, algae, and barnacles. Once in the boat, the amputee usually encounters no significant problems.

Those amputees who kayak may fear being trapped during a capsize because of the protrusion of the prosthetic foot. Because of this, some amputees prefer to strap their prosthesis to the boat rather than to their body.[1] Also, for this reason, the amputee may choose to use a peg leg.

It is also important for the amputee to remember that the buoyancy of the prosthesis will counteract the effect of a life preserver and cause the user's head to go underwater if the boat capsizes.

GOLFING

The unilateral amputee has relatively few problems playing golf. Bending over to "tee up" requires a greater than normal sense of balance (Fig. 29-12). The amputee may achieve a little less distance due to the lack of follow-through in his swing and difficulty in rotating on the prosthesis.

The only prosthetic adaptation available to the amputee golfer at this time is a rotator, a device which is also useful for playing baseball and cricket. The rotator, incorporated into the shank of the prosthesis, simulates skeletal rotation by allowing the hips to rotate independently from the position of the foot (Fig. 29-13). The rotator can be incorporated into conventional wood setups or modular systems. Three axial rotation devices are commercially available.[6] Once installed, the rotator provides reduced shear action at the residual limb–socket interface, which in turn, lessens the possibility of skin breakdown and abrasion in this area. The amputee is then able to twist with a greater degree of agility. Daw sheaths may also be used to decrease friction and protect the skin at the residual limb–socket interface. Some amputees prefer not to wear golf shoes with spikes, because this further decreases their ability to rotate on the prosthetic limb. A

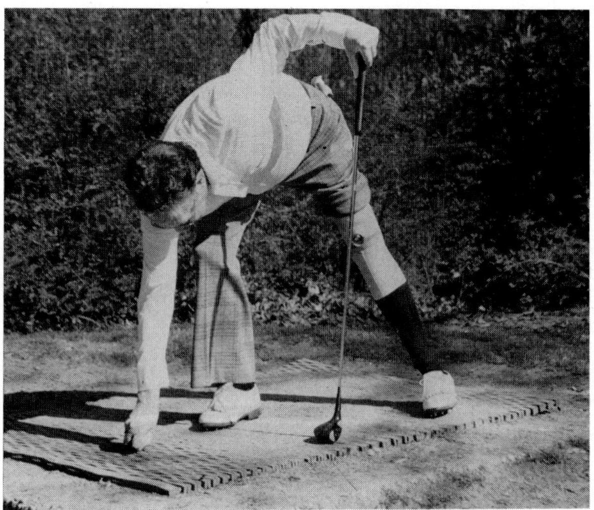

Fig. 29-12. Above-knee amputee "teeing up."

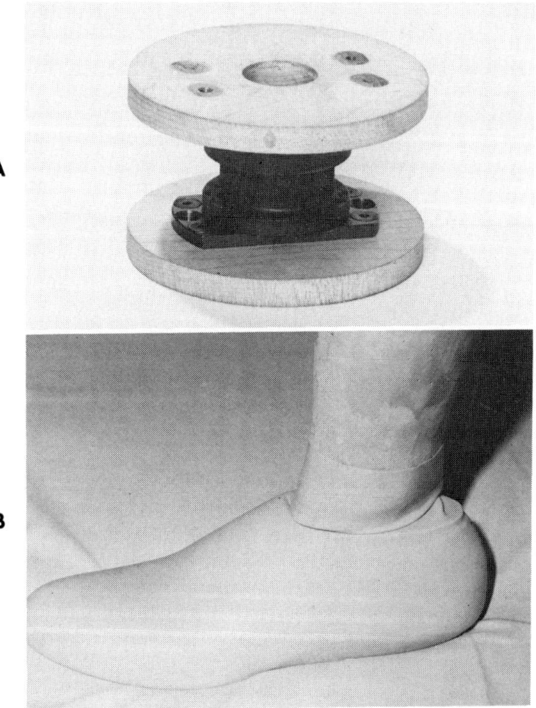

Fig. 29-13. A, STAR (shank torque absorber rotator). **B,** Rotator incorporated into prosthesis.

four-way ankle is preferred by certain amputees, since it allows the foot to remain flat on the ground while teeing off.

The amputee golfer should also give some consideration to the type of terrain on which he plays. Some golf courses have more hills than others. The use of golf or electric carts helps to reduce fatigue.

WHEELCHAIR SPORTS

Prior to World War II, there were no known organized competitive wheelchair sports. Between 1946 and 1948, wheelchair sports were introduced in the United Kingdom and the United States. Since then, wheelchair sports have grown by leaps and bounds, culminating in the initiation of international competition. Wheelchair athletes are those individuals who have a significant permanent physical disability who would be denied athletic competition were it not for wheelchair sports. Because these athletes have such diverse disabilities, competition is regulated by classification to maintain fair competition for all degrees of disability, both in men's and women's divisions. The classification system is as follows: cervical lesions, class I, A, B, and C; thoracic lesions, classes II, III, and IV; lumbar lesions, class V; disability below L4, and scoring 40 points on the rating scale, class VI. Unilateral amputees and bilateral below-knee amputees would compete in class VI, combination above-knee-below-knee amputees in class V, and bilateral above-knee amputees in class IV.

Today, wheelchair basketball, bowling, table tennis, field events, and archery are commonplace for people with multiple amputations. Wheelchair square dancing is also coming into vogue. For the most part, no adaptive equipment is necessary, other than a wheelchair with good wheels and brakes. There are special front wheel brakes, which some amputees prefer to use as an additional safeguard. Specialized wheelchairs, designed specifically to facilitate agility during wheelchair sports, are also becoming popular (Fig. 29-14). Also available are several special bowling devices to aid the more severely handicapped. The ball holder is a "ring" device that clamps to the wheelchair arm so that the bowler can carry the ball from the ball return to the foul line. The snap-handle bowling ball is fitted with a spring-loaded retractable handle. The bowler holds the ball by the handle and swings the ball for delivery. On release, the handle "snaps" back into the ball, which rolls down the lane for a score. The bowling ramp, which is usually made from aluminum tubing, is a device on which the ball is placed. The player then points the ramp in the desired direction and rolls the ball down the ramp and onto the lane. The bowling stick, which can be handcrafted from rigid aluminum tubing, is similar to a shuffle board stick. This device propels the ball up to the foul line where the ball rolls down the lane for a score.

FLYING

Flying is a challenging, stimulating, and exciting experience that does not necessarily require four limbs. The increase of interest in flying by disabled people is becoming more noticeable every year. Portable hand controls for rudder pedals may be installed or removed in a matter of minutes and are easy to use with several models of the popular Piper Cherokee airplane. The control, approved by the Federal Aviation Authority, may be rented for $10 a month (maximum of 3 months) or purchased for approximately $200. There are presently three manufacturers of flying hand controls.

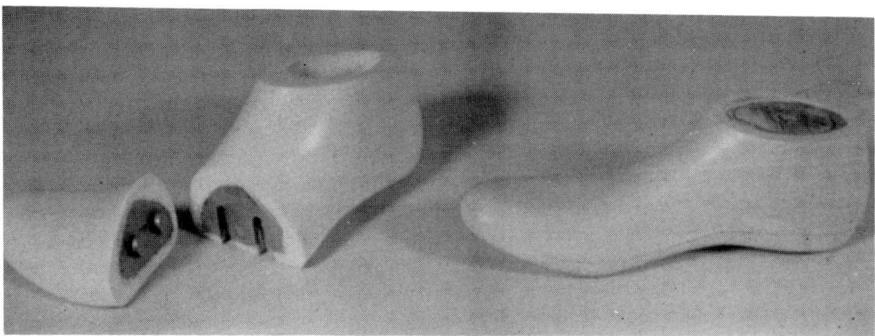

Fig. 29-14. Modified foot from "Hydra-Cadence" unit used by amputee in piloting airplane. (Courtesy Harry N. Hughes, C.P., Gene Helmuth, Navy Prosthetics Research Laboratory, Naval Regional Medical Center, Oakland, Calif.)

For those amputees who choose to pilot airplanes, modification of the conventional prosthetic foot is necessary so that the rudder pedal can be operated without the foot inadvertently hitting the brake pedal. Amputees need to be cautious of the prosthetic foot becoming "hung up" in the cockpit, should bailing out be necessary. Hughes and Helmuth[4] have addressed this problem admirably by designing a two-part SACH foot. The amputee flier can disconnect the toe section when in the cockpit and then reassemble the foot for regular prosthetic use (Fig. 29-14).

HORSEBACK RIDING

For horseback riding, modifications to the saddle and stirrup may be necessary. The individual wearing an above-knee prosthesis may choose to use a four-way hip joint to allow sufficient abduction for comfortable seating on the saddle. Safety straps to keep the prosthesis in the stirrup may be necessary. For the amputee who chooses to ride without a prosthesis, a custom saddle will probably be necessary to maintain balance on the horse. If mounting or dismounting presents a problem, an approach ramp could prove to be invaluable.

BICYCLE RIDING

Bicycling for anyone is exhilarating. To many people it supersedes all other forms of energetic exercise because of its grace, speed, and utility. By bicycling, one can keep in shape, commute, run errands, avoid the need for a second car, "walk the dog," and save money.

The below-knee amputee should encounter no difficulties while riding. The above-knee amputee has to decide whether or not to use the prosthesis. The amputee will usually use a toe strap for the uninvolved leg and ride in a push-pull fashion. There is only one crucial rule for the amputee to remember—he must always keep both hands on the handlebars when exerting leg power. When pushing with only one leg, the whole bicycle is grossly unbalanced, and both arms are used to correct the imbalance. If one hand is taken off the handlebars while pumping uphill, the amputee is likely to fall. When coasting, the hands can be removed from the handlebars without any problem. To keep both hands on the bars, all necessary bike functions must be performed from one posture. The gearshift levers can be arranged so that the amputee can grip the handlebar with his palm and outer two fingers, while the other three fingers work the levers.

Other optional modifications include removing the unused pedal and/or crank, padding the saddle, and turning it slightly away from the good leg. Because one-legged bikers pull hard with their uninvolved leg, they sit down hard on the saddle; therefore extra padding may be very helpful.

SUMMARY

Recreational activities provide enjoyable physical and social outlets for persons with few opportunities and neglected needs for physical movement. Sports often improve physical ability in such areas as overall strength, coordination, and balance. Improvements in the participant's functioning in daily life, physical strength, self-confidence, and other psychological or social aspects are often seen. Sports often improve the handicapped person's attitude toward himself, changing a negative attitude for what his body cannot do to pride in what it can do. They provide an opportunity for the person with a physical handicap to experience enjoyment as a participant, rather than a spectator.

REFERENCES

1. Brandt, M. K.: Kayaking with a prosthesis, Canoe **52:**52-53, March-April, 1976.
2. Clift, S., and Johnston, J.: Instructor's manual for disabled skiers, Banff, Alberta, 1976, Canadian Association for Disabled Skiing.
3. Graves, J. M., and Burgess, E. M.: The extra-ambulatory limb concept as it applies to the below-knee amputee skier, Bull. Prosthet. Res. **10-20:**126-131, 1973.
4. Hughes, H. N., and Helmuth G.: A modified prosthetic foot for pilots, Orthot. Prosthet. **29**(1):33-34, 1975.
5. O'Leary, H.: The Winter Park amputee ski teaching system, ed. 2. Available from P.O. Box 76, Hideaway Park, Colorado, 1974.
6. Racette, W., and Breakey, J. W.: Clinical experience and functional considerations of axial rotators for the amputee, Orthot. Prosthet. **31**(2):29-33, 1977.
7. Scheinhaus, A.: A water resistant patellar-tendon bearing prosthesis. In Amputation, Toronto, Ontario, War Amputations of Canada and the Key Tag Service, pp. 100-101, no date.
8. Schroeder, H., and Perry, L.: Amputee ski techniques. Available from Portland Junior Chamber of Commerce, 824 S.W. 5th Ave., 1965, Portland, Oregon.
9. Winthers, J.: National amputee ski technique. Available from National Amputee Skiers Association, 3738 Walnut Ave., Carmichael, California, 1970.

SUGGESTED READINGS

Adams, R. C.: Bowling for the physically handicapped, Inter-Clin. Info. Bull. **10**(1):9-13, 1970.

Adams, R., Hakala, M. and Oppelt, K.: Ice skating therapy, The Physician and Sportsmedicine, March, 1978, pp. 71-81.

Corrie, B. A.: From "poodle" to "turkey" for an amputee, Am. Correct. Ther. J. **31:**25-28, 1977.

Dean, R. C.: Monoped bicycling, Fragment, **115:**75-76, Summer, 1977.

Ditmer, J.: Fun on one leg and three skis, Denver Post, March 31, 1968.

Hamilton, R. C.: The juvenile amputee in athletics, Inter-Clin. Info. Bull. **6**(1):1-9, Oct., 1966.

Haskin, M. R., Erdman, W. J., Bream, J., and Mac Avoy, C. G.: Therapeutic horseback riding for the handicapped, Arch., Phys. Med. Rehabil. **55**:473-474, 1974.

Johnstone, K.: Wheelchair competitor's classification, swim, track, and field, Sports 'N Spokes **3**(5):16-17, Jan.-Feb., 1978.

Kuhlthau, L.: Equitation for amputees, Inter-Clin. Info. Bull. **10**(5):9-12, 1971.

Lancaster-Gaye, D.: What about leisure? Intr. Rehabil. Rev. **24**(1):6-9, 1973.

Lipton, B. H.: The role of wheelchair sports in rehabilitation, Int. Rehabil. Rev., second quarter, 1970, p. 19.

Lorenzen, H.: Sports for the physically handicapped, Int. Rehabil. Rev., first quarter, 1970, pp. 14-15.

Messner, D. G.: A modified outrigger for "three-track" skiing, Inter-Clin. Info. Bull. **9**(12):9-11, 1970.

Messner, D. G., and Williams, W.: The three-track ski club and the national amputee ski championships, Inter-Clin. Info. Bull. **13**(1):1-4, 1973.

Muller, V. S., Bauer, F., and Stoger, F.: Ein ski-fahrbehelf fur beidseitig oberschenkela, amputierte (A special skiing device for bilateral above-knee amputees), Orthopadie-Technik **12**(77):164-165.

Neishloss, L.: Adapted wheelchair basketball for handicapped children, Inter-Clin. Info. Bull. **13**(1):9, 1973.

O'Morrow, G. S.: Recreation counseling, a challenge to rehabilitation, Rehabil. Lit. **31**(8):226-233, Aug., 1970.

Roberts, G.: Sport for the disabled, Physiotherapy **60**(9):271-274, 1974.

Rullman, L.: A new concept in outriggers for "three-track" skiing, Inter-Clin. Info. Bull. **10**(11):13-17, 1971.

Smith, J. P.: In what sports can patients with amputations and other handicaps successfully and actively participate? Phys. Ther. **50**(1):121-126, 1970.

Stanek, W. F.: Report of the juvenile amputee ski program, Inter-Clin. Info. Bull. **8**(9):1-10, June, 1969.

Stein, J. U.: Recreation and leisure for special populations, Am. Correct. Ther. J. **31**(1):10, 1977.

Stieler, W. E.: Kick the handicap—learn to ski, ed. 2, Marlette, Mich., 1977.

Swimming legs, Fragment, Winter, 1976, pp. 28-36.

Witchel, D. B.: For the handicapped, it's tough, it's fun, it's therapy, Skiing, Dec., 1975, pp. 114-116.

APPENDIX

Organizations involved in recreation for the disabled

Adapted Sports Association, Inc.
Communications Center
6832 Marlette Road
Marlette, Michigan 48453

Adaptive Sports Program
Kinesiotherapy Clinic
University of Toledo
2801 West Bancroft Street
Toledo, Ohio 43606

Aircraft Hand Controls
Ed Stadleman
P.O. Box 207
Sturgis, Kentucky 42459

Alberta Amputee Ski Association
Box 1373
Banff, Alberta, Canada T0L 0C0

American Association for Health, Physical Education, and Recreation Programs for the Handicapped
1201 16th St., N.W.
Washington, D.C. 20036

American Wheelchair Bowling Association
Don Pinault, Executive Director
2424 N. Federal Highway
Suite 109
Boynton Beach, Florida 33435

The Amputee Golfers Association
Lakeview Terrace
Watchung, New Jersey 07060

Amputees in Motion
Irene Jansen
14248 Burbank Boulevard
Van Nuys, California 91401

Canadian Association for Disabled Skiing
Box 2077
Banff, Alberta, Canada, T0L 0C0

Canadian Wheelchair Sports Association
333 River Road
Ottawa, Ontario K1L 8B9

Committee for the Promotion of Camping for the Handicapped
2056 South Bluff Road
Traverse City, Michigan 49684

Disabled Skiers Association of British Columbia
Box 3433
Main Post Office
Vancouver, British Columbia, Canada V6B 3Y4

Dumark Manufacturing Company (archery equipment)
P.O. Box 268
543 Timothy Street
Newmarket, Ontario, Canada L3Y 4X7

Indoor Sports, Inc.
3445 Trumbell
San Diego, California 92106

International Council on Therapeutic Ice Skating
P.O. Box 13
State College, Pennsylvania 16801

International Society for Rehabilitation of the Disabled
(Rehabilitation International)
219 East 44th Street
New York, New York 10017

International Sports Organization for the Disabled and International Stoke Mandeville Games Federation
Stoke-Mandeville Spinal Injury Center,
Aylesbury, England

National Amputation Foundation
Whitestone, New York 11357

National Amputee Golf Foundation
George C. Beckman, Trustee
St. Joseph's Mercy Hospital
11705 Mercy Boulevard
Savannah, Georgia 31606

The National Archery Association
40-24 62nd Street
Woodside, New York 11377 or Ronks, Pennsylvania 17572

National Beep Baseball Association
3212 Tomahawk
Lawrence, Kansas 66044

National Handicapped Sports and Recreation Association
10 Mutual Building
4105 E. Florida
Denver, Colorado 80222

National Inconvenienced Sportsman's Association
3738 Walnut Avenue
Carmichael, California 95608

National Park Guide for the Handicapped
Superintendent of Documents
U.S. Government Printing Office
Washington, D.C. 20402
Stock #2405-0286, $.40

National Therapeutic Recreation Society National Recreation and Park Association
1700 Pennsylvania Avenue, N.W.
Washington, D.C. 20006

National Wheelchair Athletic Association
40-24 62nd Street
Woodside, New York 11377

National Wheelchair Basketball Association
101 Seaton Building
University of Kentucky
Lexington, Kentucky 40506

National Wheelchair Marathon
Bruce Marquis
369 Elliot Street
Newton Upper Falls, Massachusetts 02164

National Wheelchair Softball Association
Box 737
Sioux Falls, South Dakota 57101

North American Recreation Equipment
P.O. Box 758
Bridgeport, Connecticut 07701

North American Riding for the Handicapped Association (NARHA)
Whitepost, Virginia 22663

Portable Aircraft Hand Controls
In-residence pilot training for handicapped people
Union Aviation, Inc.
Sturgis Airport-G
Sturgis, Kentucky 42459

Sport for the Physically Disabled
333 River Road
Ottawa, Canada K1L 8B9

Sports 'N Spokes
6043 North Ninth Avenue
Phoenix, Arizona 85013
(magazine for wheelchair sports and recreation)

Track Three Ski
Box 1260
Station Q
Toronto, Ontario, Canada M4T 2P4

U.S. Ski Association
Central Division
Amputee Skiers Committee
P.O. Box 66014
Chicago, Illinois 60666

Wheelchair Motorcycle Association
101 Torrey Street
Brockton, Massachusetts 02401

Wheelchair Pilots Association
John Green
3953 West Evans Drive
Phoenix, Arizona 85023

Women's Wheelchair Bowling Competition
W. Bennet Avenue
Milwaukee, Wisconsin

CHAPTER 30

Research trends in lower limb prosthetics

GUSTAV RUBIN
A. BENNETT WILSON, JR.

Some of the most important contributions to lower limb prosthetics as a result of the North American research program that began in 1945 are the procedures now universally accepted for fitting and alignment of artificial legs. These procedures, developed primarily at the University of California and at the Department of Veteran Affairs, Canada, were based on sound biomechanical principles and have formed the basis for management of all levels of lower limb amputations. During the past 10 to 15 years progress in lower limb prosthetics has generally been in the form of refinements to already established techniques and devices.

Although a great deal has been learned during the past 30 years about the function of the knee, foot, hip, and spine in normal human locomotion, this knowledge still has not had a great deal of influence on the availability of inexpensive, practical devices for artificial legs, with the possible exception of the SACH foot.

As a result, the present practice of lower limb prosthetics consists basically of the following principles:

1. Surgery to produce the most functional stump that is practical
2. Early or immediate postoperative fitting with temporary prostheses (in any event, a rigid dressing is used immediately postoperatively)
3. Systematic fitting and alignment procedures
4. Simple functional hardware (very little sophisticated equipment is used)

Plastic laminates have largely supplanted wood for sockets and, to some extent, for shanks. Modular prostheses seem to be the system of choice for the patient with hip disarticulation and hemipelvectomy, but high maintenance requirements and inadequate strength of some designs for heavy-duty use, together with their relatively heavy weight have kept them from being used widely for above-knee, knee disarticulation, and below-knee amputees. Following are some of the reasons that use of sophisticated devices is not widespread:

1. Swing phase control knee units available for tests have been designed primarily for the younger, healthy amputee. Some of these have been well-received, but initial costs and maintenance problems have been deterrents to widespread acceptance.
2. The simplicity of the SACH foot in fitting and maintenance, as well as its low cost, has made it quite popular. Many clinicians prefer to prescribe an articulated foot-ankle unit routinely for above-knee prostheses, but this tendency has been decreasing through the years. There are, however, specific indications for the articulated foot, such as the case of the blind amputee who finds the feedback signal provided by foot-slap useful.

3. The strength-weight requirements in sophisticated articulated ankle designs are formidable.

The research efforts begun in the United States and other countries toward the end of World War II were supported almost entirely by agencies concerned with the welfare of war veterans, and thus emphasis was placed initally on young adult amputees. Later, some attention was given to prostheses for children, and, still later, consideration was given to geriatric patients as their relative numbers increased due to arteriosclerosis with and without diabetes. However, relatively little attention has been paid until recently to the special problems of the older amputee.

ULTRA-LIGHTWEIGHT PROSTHESIS

For the older amputee three major problems seem to exist: energy consumption, volumetric changes in the stump, and suspension of the prosthesis. All of these problems, of course, are present in our current concept of leg prostheses, but they are accentuated in the case of elderly patients. Furthermore, these factors to a great degree are interrelated.

Energy consumption depends at least partly on the total weight of the prosthesis. The weight of the prosthesis affects suspension. Stability of the connection of the prosthesis to the patient and suspension of the prosthesis also depend on constancy of the volume of the stump. Therefore improvement in lower limb prosthetics, in general, must be considered from a systems viewpoint.

To simplify suspension and reduce energy requirements the weight of lower limb prostheses must be reduced. Weight reduction of below-knee prostheses does not seem to present a problem with respect to control. Reduction in weight for knee disarticulation, above-knee amputation, and hip disarticulation prostheses must be made judiciously, making sure that adequate control of the shank is provided.

Very little attention has been given in the United States to a reduction in weight of lower limb prostheses. This is probably because during fitting and alignment studies and evaluation of hydraulic knee control units, patients report that the new limb, because of improved function, *felt* lighter than their conventional limb, when actually it was heavier. However recent experience with patients in all age groups has shown that when all other factors are equal, weight reduction is appreciated.

At the Moss Rehabilitation Hospital in Philadelphia and in other centers, pioneering research is being directd to developing ultra-lightweight prostheses. Below-knee limbs, weighing considerably less than 0.9 kg (2 pounds) have been fabricated almost entirely of polypropylene and have been worn successfully by selected patients. Work is proceeding toward the fabrication of clinically useful prostheses for high levels of amputation.

With a similar aim, the Veterans Administration Prosthetics Center* has been developing lightweight prosthetic components such as graphite-epoxy keels for SACH feet, graphite-epoxy rotators, and graphite endoskeletal structures for the Multiplex-type of prosthesis for the above-knee patient. A graphite-nylon material becomes flexible enough to bend when heated to 238° C (460° F), and when cooled the strength is restored. It can be used for such purposes as the fabrication of rigid lightweight external below-knee joints.

To improve on the stability of the connection between the patient and prosthesis more must be known about the effects of pressure on the soft tissues of the stump and the mechanisms of edema. With this kind of information it might be possible to develop sockets that could be adjusted during the day to compensate for stump volume changes. Workers at the Texas Institute for Rehabilitation and Research are currently working on this problem using photogrammetry and other methods.

Early attempts to fabricate adjustable above-knee sockets have not been successful. Currently such centers as that at Rancho Los Amigos Hospital and the Veterans Administration Research Center for Prosthetics are involved in efforts to develop such sockets. Polypropylene socket shells have been used for temporary prostheses, allowing for the shrinkage of the stump by progressive closure of the shell components.

SKELETAL ATTACHMENT OF PROSTHESIS

The ultimate approach to stability short of regenerating limbs is what has popularly been called "skeletal attachment." This is attachment of a rigid structure directly to the stump bone in such a manner that it can in turn be used for attachment of an external prosthesis. Work in this area has been supported at a low but appropriate level throughout the past 20 years, and a good

*As of July 1, 1980, the name Veterans Administration Prosthetics Center was changed to Veterans Administration Rehabilitation Engineering Center (VAREC).

deal of progress has been made even though a practical technique, safely applicable to humans, has yet to be developed.

Hall, of the Southwest Research Institute, has worked extensively with animals to achieve positive results in this field, whereas Mooney at Rancho Los Amigos Hospital has carried out experiments on humans. A major difficulty which has not been overcome, is that presented at the corridor of exit of the fixations device from its internal body milieu to the outside. According to Hall,[1] "no material has yet been found that is ideal, although Dacron and nylon velour fabrics bonded to a solid surface so as to form impervious laminates have offered the most suitable solution thus far." Bone interfacing also has not been satisfactorily accomplished. Various types of porous ceramics, as well as sintered metals, have been used. Sandblasted Vitallium has been employed for the longitudinal extension. Interference with the blood supply led to attempts to use cortical cone-shaped bone attachment devices.

To date, this experimentation has only been done using goats and horses. Extensive further development will be necessary before a practical, safe, and harm-free method can be applied to humans.

FITTING AND ALIGNMENT

The fitting and alignment procedures used in teaching programs are based on biomechanical data collected 20 to 30 years ago and have proven to be extremely useful in daily practice. However, a great deal of skill and judgment are required in arriving at the optimum condition. Better measurement techniques to display the course of the weight line and the amount of pressure exerted on soft tissues will make it possible to refine the present procedures. Techniques to demonstrate the course of the weight line have been developed quite recently and are being used in alignment studies, as well as in clinical situtations.

ENERGY COST MEASUREMENTS

Present methods of energy expenditure evaluation involving oxygen consumption are unwieldly and costly and thus are available only at a few centers. An inexpensive method of measuring the change in energy expenditure is needed. It would be ideal to be able to measure the exact amount of energy used, but for an interim period the ability to measure the change in an energy index would be extremely useful in determining the effectiveness of a treatment program or the application of a device.

KNEE DEVICES

Ideally the above-knee amputee should be able to better control the artificial knee joint. The present designs are more or less preprogrammed. The most sophisticated design available commercially is the Henschke-Mauch S'n'S (swing and stance) hydraulic unit. This unit provides a programmed control sequence of the shank during the swing phase of walking based on the speed assumed by the amputee, and a braking action of the knee is brought about automatically when the patient stumbles during stance phase. Needed, however, is a unit that permits the amputee to control the shank voluntarily at all times. The availability of minicomputers may make this practical. Pattern recognition of myoelectric signals about the hip could conceivably be used as a control source.

The electromyograph (EMG) actuated knee lock being developed at the Veterans Administration Prosthetics Center is another promising approach to the solution of this problem. EMG control of the knee locking function could enable the above-knee amputee to lock the knee reflexively to regain stability should he trip or stumble. Rectified and integrated myoelectric signals from the quadriceps are being used to control the lock in this study.

Radcliffe, at the University of California, Berkeley, has been instrumental in popularizing polycentric knee mechanisms, particularly for the through-knee amputation. Four-bar linkages are universally accepted. Radcliffe is working to develop a six-bar design that presents a better appearance, while allowing a greater range of motion than has been possible with the four-bar designs. The major aim in the development of such units has been to seek ways in which the bulky and noncosmetic steel side joints could be replaced by mechanisms located entirely below the stump, but which provide an effective center-of-rotation passing through the femoral condyles. A second objective has been to improve the swing phase control and to provide function at least equal to knee replacement devices available to the higher level amputee.

FOOT AND ANKLE DEVICES

Mauch Laboratories of Dayton, Ohio, are developing a hydraulic ankle that is ready for clinical testing. Presently, the initial reports from the test wearers have been favorable, but some mechanical difficulties persist, such as noise and wear problems. Solutions to these problems seems to be within reach. Function will be achieved about all three axes. Hydraulic plantar flexion and dorsiflexion control provides toe-slap damping and toe pickup. A variable dorsiflexion stop adapts itself automatically to any change in inclination of the walking surface. Eversion and inversion control optionally yields either in the eversion *and* inversion direction, in the inversion direction only, or in neither direction; and transverse rotation control optionally yields either during forward *and* backward rotation of the pelvis, during forward rotation only, or in neither direction.

MISCELLANEOUS DEVELOPMENTS

A relatively new device that may soon be generally used is the concept of controlled environment treatment, developed at the Biomechanical Research and Development Unit, Queen Mary's Hospital, Roehampton, England, and the Veterans Administration Prosthetics Research Study, Seattle, for the immediate postsurgical amputation period. The stump is inserted into a flexible transparent PVC bag that has a special air seal proximally to avoid any tourniquet effect. Filtered sterile dry air, or other gas mixtures, at controlled pressure and temperature is fed to the dressing bag from a control console at the bedside. Direct observation of the stump is possible.

Physiological suspension of prostheses is being investigated by Burgess at the Veterans Administration Prosthetics Research Study, Seattle. Muscle-stabilized residual limbs are examined by photogrammetric measurement, volume displacement, electromyography, and computerized axial tomography to study contour and interface pressure suspension capability. Biofeedback training techniques are employed. This information can be used to redefine socket design concepts.

A design close to general acceptance is the Veterans Administration Prosthetics Center open-mesh, distal end, soft socket insert, which was developed for the purpose of minimizing the problem of hyperhidrosis for the below-knee amputee. Yet to be developed is a similar solution to that problem for the above-knee suction socket user.

Many other items of research of varying degrees of potential usefulness are under development. Some, such as the polypropylene partial foot prosthesis, border on general acceptance. Rubin's extensive experience with this device has shown that it should not be used for a true Chopart amputation with a fixed equinus contracture, in which instance the plastic-laminated anteroposterior shell prosthesis is usually indicated. However, it is very useful for the Lisfranc to the transmetatarsal levels of amputation, in which active dorsiflexion and plantar flexion are present, but adequate stability and push-off are absent.

At the Veterans Administration Prosthetics Center, a polypropylene vacuum-formed socket fitted into a trefoil polypropylene adaptor with a Staros-Gardner coupling attached has been developed and has undergone testing for more than a year. This design permits fitting a vacuum-formed socket in a system that retains alignment adjustability.

Bennett, of the Veterans Administration Research Center for Prosthetics, has under development a flexible brim for an above-knee suction socket in an attempt to eliminate the frequent skin problems that occur at the junction of the brim and the soft tissues of the stump. It is anticipated that such a socket will redistribute stresses arising within the stump from static and dynamic loading. The investigators believe that shear stresses and stress concentration zones inherent with rigid prosthetic sockets can probably be avoided with an appropriately flexible socket design.

At George Washington University, investigators under Veterans Administration contract are attempting to develop a cosmetic "skin." Presently, a compostion of acrylic latex, color pigment, ammonium hydroxide, and acrysol is applied to a soft polyurethane foam cover.

Also under development are items such as an artificial foot with adjustable heel height, a method of determining easily the load borne by the prosthesis, a friction-stabilized knee unit with potential for incorporation in a lightweight modular device for the geriatric patient, and a below-knee suction socket.

This discussion briefly reviews many of the projects currently under development. It cannot be complete, but it does reflect progress in major areas. New projects will undoubtedly surface prior to and immediately after publication.

It would be a truism to point out that some of the devices categorized as research items at the time of this writing will no longer be considered to be such by the time this book is published. Some will be accepted and others discarded. Nevertheless, based on our present knowledge, this discussion can be summarized into the following broad classifications:

1. Devices still on trial that appear to be close to general acceptance
2. Devices requiring extensive further development
3. Concepts that have not yet reached the laboratory

DEVICES READY FOR GENERAL ACCEPTANCE

1. Lightweight below-knee polypropylene prostheses
2. Weight line measurement techniques
3. Partial foot prostheses
4. Total-contact, open-mesh PTB sockets for hyperhidrosis
5. Vacuum-formed polypropylene below-knee sockets with trefoil adjustable shank attachment adaptor
6. Graphite Multiplex pylon
7. Graphite-epoxy SACH foot

ITEMS REQUIRING EXTENSIVE FURTHER DEVELOPMENT

1. Lightweight above-knee and hip disarticulation prostheses
2. Skeletal attachment for an external prosthesis
3. Flexible-brim above-knee socket
4. Adjustable above-knee socket
5. Mechanical foot with adjustable heel height
6. UCBL six-bar linkage knee
7. EMG knee lock
8. Mauch hydraulic ankle
9. Graphite-nylon below-knee joint
10. Prosthetic skin
11. Below-knee suction socket
12. Prosthetic Research Study Moore load cell
13. Friction-stabilized knee for modular prosthesis

CONCEPTS

1. Voluntary control of the shank of an above-knee amputee with power assist
2. Above-knee hyperhidrosis control
3. An inexpensive method for measuring changes in energy expenditure
4. Power assist controls for hip joint of hip disarticulation amputees
5. Three-dimensional shape sensing using photogrammetry
6. Physiological suspension

SURVEYS

A research area that is crucial to the development of clinical engineering devices is the amputee survey, such as that conducted by the Veterans Administration Prosthetics Center in cooperation with the Disabled American Veterans. The country-wide survey of amputees (1977 to 1978) is designed to determine the prevalence, not only of specific prosthetic problems, but of possible secondary problems that may be attributable directly to the amputation. The investigation will be very thorough, and the results are being awaited with a great deal of interest.

The Prosthetics Research Study, Seattle, has recently concluded a comprehensive series of surveys: "Functional Capabilities of Lower Extremity Amputees," "A Survey of Lower-Limb Amputees: Prostheses, Phantom Sensations, and Psychosocial Aspects," and "Recreational Activities of Lower Extremity Amputees."

REFERENCE

1. Hall, C. W.: Skeletal extension development: Criteria for future designs, Bull. Prosthet. Res. **10-25:**70, Spring, 1976.

PART FOUR

Management of complications in the amputee

CHAPTER 31

Skin problems in amputees

FRED LEVIT

Skin problems affecting amputees may be directly related to the fact of being an amputee, but may be the same problems encountered by nonamputees. In addition to the difficulties that anyone with a skin disease might encounter, the amputee has the special problem of protecting the skin of the stump. A skin disease that would merely be a nuisance otherwise can be a disabling problem if it occurs on the stump and prevents the wearing of a prosthesis. For this reason it is desirable to recognize and treat skin problems in the amputee promptly.

STUMP HYGIENE

Questions often arise concerning routine care of the skin of the stump. Because the amputee's attention is attracted to the stump, there is a great tendency to want to do things to it. Patients have applied to the stump innumerable substances obtained at the drugstore, supermarket, and hardware store, ranging from antiseptics to zinc. All are unnecessary and best avoided.

In general, it is only necessary to keep the stump clean. This is best done by washing it with a cloth, soap, and water. The stump must be thoroughly rinsed after washing and dried well. This should be done at night so that the skin is permitted to become thoroughly dry.

The socket of the prosthesis must also be kept clean. This can be done by nightly cleansing with a cloth dampened with soap and water. The socket is then rinsed well with clean water and dried with a towel. It should be permitted to dry overnight.

If the socket is not cleansed, debris accumulates that can produce dermatitis by mechanical action. Cleansing the stump prevents the accumulation of keratin on the surface of the skin and also removes salt (from sweat), lint, and other materials that may also accumulate and irritate the skin. Permitting the stump and socket to dry overnight helps reduce bacteria on the skin by the process of desiccation.

DERMATOLOGICAL PROBLEMS PECULIAR TO THE AMPUTEE

Reactive hyperemia

Reactive hyperemia, as the name implies, is evidence of an increase in the flow of blood to the skin in reaction to some kind of trauma. In the case of the amputee, the trauma is simply the initial wearing of the prosthesis, which will produce some irritation and consequent reddening and tenderness of the skin. Usually the symptoms are mild enough so that the prosthesis can still be worn. In most cases the symptoms will subside, even though the patient continues to wear the prosthesis. If the symptoms do not subside, a prosthetic cause should be considered.

Verrucous hyperplasia

If the keratin, the surface layer of the skin, is not removed by such natural actions as friction against clothing, washing, or scrubbing, it accumulates and forms a layer that grows thicker and thicker. As keratin thickens, it dries, becomes less flexible, shrinks, and will finally tear. In tearing, it often ruptures the underlying epider-

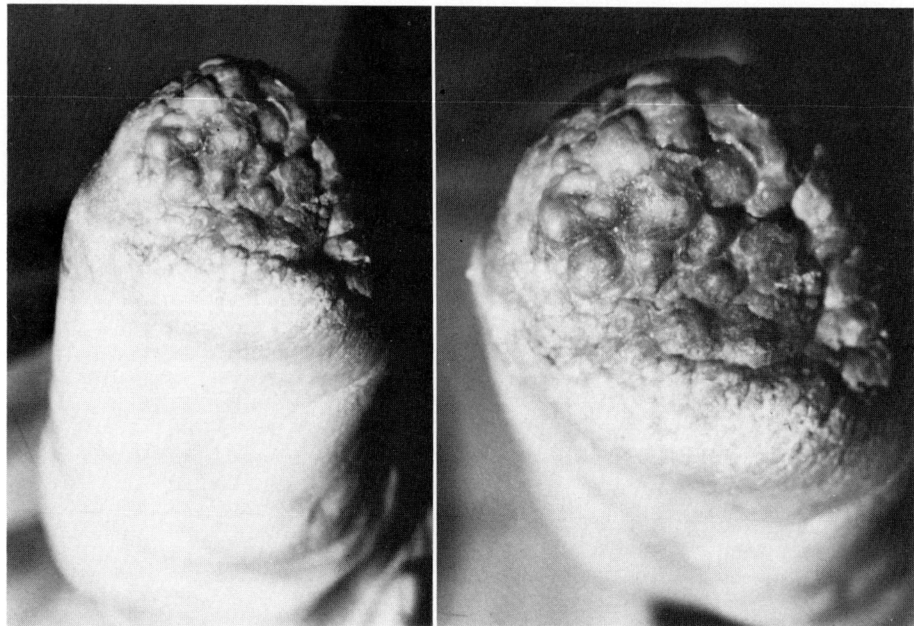

Fig. 31-1. Verrucous hyperplasia.

mis with resultant oozing and bleeding. The mass of keratin looks like a huge wart, hence the designation verrucous. Infection commonly occurs, and the skin surrounding the hyperkeratotic area becomes red, swollen, and painful (Fig. 31-1).

The infection must be treated first. Oral and topical antibiotics, together with intermittent compresses are usually effective. The hyperkeratotic mass can then be softened with a keratolytic agent, such as 12% to 20% salicylic acid in a cream or petrolatum base. The causes, which are failure to scrub the stump and lack of total contact in the prosthesis socket, must also be eliminated.

Epidermoid cysts

Normally the socket brim does not move across the skin very much during walking. If there is too much movement of the socket brim together with excessive pressure, friction is developed along the skin. With this friction keratin can be stripped off the surface of the skin and carried in the direction of the movement of the socket brim. The keratin tends to accumulate at the end of the stroke and is forced down into the skin. When it penetrates to the dermis, it induces a severe foreign body reaction. Dermal tissue is liquefied to form sterile pus with a great deal of inflammation. These sterile abscesses are called "epidermoid cysts."

Epidermoid cysts are better prevented than treated. They are painful and prevent the wearing of a prosthesis. Incision and drainage are helpful, but antibiotics are of little value. These cysts tend to recur, and heal very slowly.

A properly fitted and aligned prosthesis should not cause epidermoid cysts. When they do occur, fit and alignment should be carefully rechecked. If this is adequate, other means of relieving friction should be employed, including silk stump stockings and increased suspension to prevent pistoning.

COMMON DERMATOLOGICAL PROBLEMS ALSO SEEN IN THE AMPUTEE

Contact dermatitis

Contact dermatitis, as the name implies, is a dermatitis caused by something that has come in contact with the skin. Primary irritants are substances that cause dermatitis because of their chemical or physical nature. Strong acids or strong bases, such as nitric acid or sodium hydroxide, and caustics, like silver nitrate, are examples of primary irritants. Less well-known primary irritants include soap, detergents, and formaldehyde.

One may wonder why soap can be considered a primary irritant, since most people wash frequently and few have dermatitis. Soap that is soon rinsed away does not have time to cause irritation. But soap kept in contact with the skin for 12 to 48 hours acts as a fairly effective primary irritant. It is for this reason that the amputee's stump and prosthesis socket must be well rinsed after washing.

The most common kind of dermatitis, both in the amputee and the nonamputee, is allergic contact dermatitis. This occurs when a substance to which the patient is allergic comes in contact with the skin. The person whose skin has become allergic is said to be sensitive, and the substance to which he is allergic is an allergen. No one is born allergic. Allergy is an acquired state and can develop only after a first exposure to the allergen. Following the first contact, the allergen penetrates the epidermis and stimulates lymphocytes to produce antibodies. About a week after the sensitizing exposure, the patient has produced enough antibody to react to a subsequent exposure. Thus the second time the allergen contacts the skin a dermatitis develops.

When a person has been sensitized, the entire skin surface has become allergic. Thus it makes no difference where on the skin the original sensitizing contact was made or where on the skin the subsequent dermatitis-producing contact is made. This explains why a patient may not react for a week or more to a newly applied substance, and why the dermatitis appears only at those places on the skin where subsequent contact is made.

Thousands of chemicals can cause allergic contact dermatitis. It would be difficult to list them all; however, a few that are common causes of contact dermatitis in the amputee are as follows:

1. Chromium
2. Nickel
3. Antioxidants in rubber
4. Unpolymerized epoxy and polyester
5. Accelerating agents used for polymerizing plastics
6. Soap and detergents
7. Formaldehyde

Chromium is found both as a metal and as a salt that is used in tanning leather. It is easily leached out of leather by moisture and sweat. Nickel is used as the surface plate on metal objects and is often found as the layer under chromium plating. The nickel is exposed as the chromium wears off.

Both soap and formaldehyde were discussed as primary irritants. They may also act as sensitizers, and very tiny amounts can cause allergic contact dermatitis.

The hallmark of contact dermatitis is limitation of the dermatitis almost exactly to the area of contact with the offending material. Thus the allergic contact dermatitis frequently takes the shape of the foam rubber pad or the leather strap that causes it. In the case of a metal buckle, which may move around over the skin, the outline may not be as sharp and distinct.

The skin may be merely red and slightly swollen, but severe forms of contact dermatitis have vesicles, blisters, and oozing. Itching is usually severe. The dermatitis is treated with cool compresses and topical steroid creams. Provided that the allergen can be avoided, it will usually heal promptly.

The fact that the entire skin surface becomes allergic provides a method of testing for skin allergy. In the patient who is suspected of being allergic to nickel, for example, a solution of nickel sulfate can be applied to a small patch of gauze and placed on normal-appearing skin for 24 to 48 hours. If the patient is allergic, a miniature dermatitis will appear under the patch. The dermatologist has available a kit of materials containing the common sensitizers with which patch tests can be done on patients suspected of having allergic contact dermatitis.

Infections

Pyogenic infections. Pyogenic infections are those bacterial infections which result in the production of pus. In most cases these are not serious in that they are not life threatening, but if they occur in locations that prevent the use of a prosthesis, they can be extremely troublesome for the amputee.

Folliculitis. When a prosthesis is worn for the first time over a hairy area, a bacterial infection of the hair follicles may be superimposed on the reactive hyperemia that commonly occurs. Folliculitis is characterized by the presence of pustules, each surrounding a hair follicle. The hairs involved become tender, and a stinging pain is felt when they are moved or pressed on. This is usually not severe enough to seriously hamper the patient, and the folliculitis will often subside even without treatment. A topical antibiotic cream may speed healing. Occasionally, the prosthesis will need to be removed for a few days until the condition begins to subside.

Furuncles. When a furuncle, or common boil, occurs on the stump, the patient is usually unable to wear the prosthesis because of the extreme tenderness associated with this condition. Furuncles respond slowly to treatment, although incision and drainage at the appropriate time will relieve the pain and get the patient back into the prosthesis somewhat sooner.

Hidradenitis. "Adenos" is a gland, and "hydros" refers to water or sweat. Thus hidradenitis is an infection of the sweat glands. However, the sweat glands involved are not those producing the temperature-regulating sweat, which are the most familiar. Hidradenitis involves the apocrine sweat glands, which are found almost exclusively in the axilla and groin. These sweat glands produce a secretion that contains a greater variety of substances than is found in eccrine sweat. Apocrine sweat is also produced much more slowly, and the apocrine gland often empties into a hair follicle, a natural habitat for a variety of bacteria. For these reasons, the apocrine sweat gland is more prone to infection. In hidradenitis, the axilla or groin develops tender, pus-exuding swellings. Deep abscesses may form and coalesce. Movement of the arms or legs may become difficult because of the pain.

This infection responds poorly to treatment. Antibiotics are of limited value. Incision and drainage must often be done and are helpful, but new lesions tend to keep forming. Sometimes it is necessary to remove large areas of involved skin and replace them with full-thickness grafts.

Fungus infections

Common dermatophytes. Most fungus infections are caused by a group of organisms called the "dermatophytes" because of their tendency to invade the skin. They live in the keratin layer and usually do not produce symptoms. Occasionally, they become active and will produce redness, scaling, itching, and sometimes blisters or fissures.

In the amputee, fungus infections are most commonly seen in the groin. Here, a gradually enlarging red patch appears, often with an advancing, well-demarcated scaly border. It causes itching, which is made worse by heat and sweating.

Response to treatment is usually good. Oral griseofulvin, an antifungal antibiotic, together with a steroid cream to relieve the itching, will clear up most dermatophyte infections in 2 to 4 weeks. The intermittent use of a topical antifungal agent afterwards can prevent most recurrences.

Candidiasis. Candida albicans, a yeast, produces skin lesions that are somewhat different from those previously described. The skin tends to be moist where Candida organisms grow. The lesions also tend to expand, but the advancing border shows no scale. Pustules will be seen around the lession. These appear on smooth skin and not around hairs like the pustules of folliculitis.

Candidiasis does not respond to oral griseofulvin, and topical agents must be used. A variety of drugs are available, including nystatin in various topical forms. Exposure of the skin to air is also useful. Because candidiasis is more common where skin is pressed against skin, as in the groin and axilla, it is believed that failure to evaporate sweat is one of the predisposing causes. Candidiasis is also more common in diabetics and may be the first clue to that diagnosis.

All of the dermatophytes can be identified by culturing the scales or the content of the pustules. *Candida albicans* will grow in a few days. The other dermatophytes may take 3 weeks or more to be identifiable in culture. Often an earlier diagnosis can be obtained, since scales or pustule contents can be placed on a slide and dissolved in 20% potassium hydroxide solution and examined under a microscope. Characteristic forms of the yeast can often be seen.

BENIGN TUMORS OF THE STUMP

All of the small growths common to skin can occur on the stump. Warts, seborrheic keratoses, hemangiomas, and dermatofibromas commonly occur. They are harmless except when they grow large enough to produce pressure against the prosthesis socket. The resulting pain can interfere with the wearing of the prosthesis, and for this reason such benign growths should be removed.

MALIGNANT TUMORS OF THE STUMP

Malignant tumors of the stump are rarely encountered. If the amputation was done originally for a malignancy, recurrences or metastases may be encountered at any time. Primary malignancies such as basal cell carcinoma or squamous cell carcinoma are uncommon. They are also slow growing and can almost always be identified before they become serious. Both of these begin as nodules of the skin, which gradually enlarge and then ulcerate. Excisional biopsy is most often the procedure used when they are encountered.

Malignant melanoma is uncommon but dangerous. It has often metastasized by the time the primary lesion is identified. The appearance of malignant melanoma may range from a light tan flat lesion to a fungating, ulcerated, black mass. Any lesion that is suspicious to the clinician should undergo a biopsy.

GENERALIZED SKIN DISEASE

Because a patient has had an amputation does not mean that everything which happens thereafter is invariably related to the amputation. An amputee who has had psoriasis before the amputation will most likely have it again. The simple question "Have you ever had this kind of skin trouble before?" may make the diagnosis.

In addition to psoriasis, such diseases as lichen planus, atopic eczema, and seborrheic dermatitis may cover large areas of the body and may be present on or near the stump. These should be readily diagnosed by their clinical appearance on other areas of skin. Treatment can usually be carried out without difficulty in the amputee.

SUGGESTED READING

Levy, S. W. et al.: Skin problems of the leg amputee, Arch. Dermatol. 85:65-81, 1962.

CHAPTER 32

Management of musculoskeletal complications

JOHN H. BOWKER
ROBERT G. THOMPSON

For simplicity, this chapter is divided into two discussions. The first deals with problems that may delay permanent fitting. These may be properly termed "preprosthetic complications." The second, termed "postprosthetic complications," deals with difficulties arising during the time of active use of the prosthesis. In general, preprosthetic and postprosthetic complications seem to appear less often in the practice of the surgeon with a keen interest in the problems of amputation; one who keeps abreast of more recent innovations. Casual or defeatist attitudes toward amputation surgery engender many of the problems to be discussed.

PREPROSTHETIC COMPLICATIONS

Delayed healing

Delayed healing, associated with dehiscence of the amputation wound, may be caused by several factors. Instances of skin necrosis at the wound edge may be related to an excessively tight closure (Fig. 32-1) or to improper selection of level, especially in the dysvascular patient. Removal of skin sutures before the amputation wound has firmly healed may also lead to dehiscence. Sutures should be left in place as many weeks as necessary whenever slow tissue healing is expected, as in dysvascular disease or after chemotherapy or radiotherapy.

If the separation is not significant, it may be allowed to heal by secondary intention, controlling infection by conservative debridement and fine mesh gauze dressings. In patients capable of controlled weight bearing, walking in a temporary plaster of Paris limb will not impede healing if vascularity is adequate.

In cases of significant wound separation, a secondary closure may save considerable time if the wound can be adequately debrided and sufficient skin for a loose closure is present (Fig. 32-2). More commonly, sufficient skin is not available, and a split-thickness skin graft may be required to effect healing. Debridement of separated or locally necrotic wounds in dysvascular patients must be done so as to avoid trauma to skin of marginal viability. This can be accomplished during debridement by leaving a 2- to 3-mm rim of necrotic tissue behind, allowing this to separate spontaneously. Fine mesh gauze dressings, removed daily when thoroughly dry, will assist in preparing a suitable bed for grafting. If the vascular supply is not sufficient to prevent further necrosis or produce granulation tissue, revision to a higher level may be inevitable (Figs. 32-3 and 32-4).

If the dehiscence has been caused by wound infection, it should be treated by appropriate antibiotics, conservative local debridement, and daily dressings. The wound may be allowed to heal by secondary intention, but if clean granulation tissue develops, a secondary closure may accelerate healing.

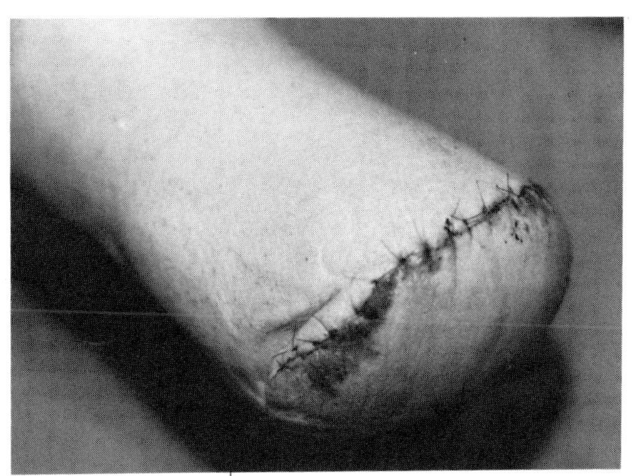

Fig. 32-1. Wound edge necrosis secondary to tight wound closure.

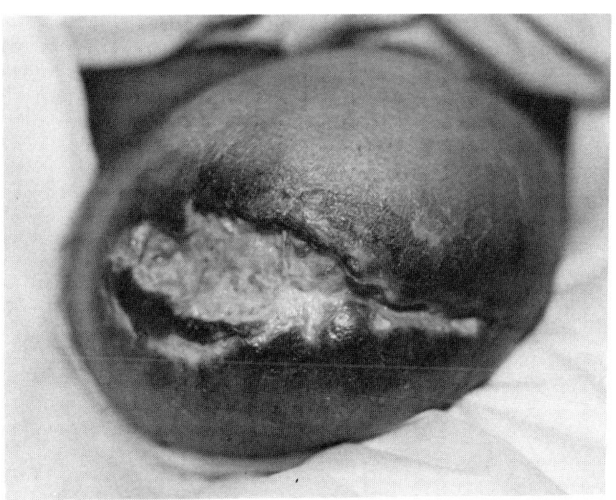

Fig. 32-2. Significant wound necrosis and wound separation. Adequate debridement and secondary closure should lead to healing.

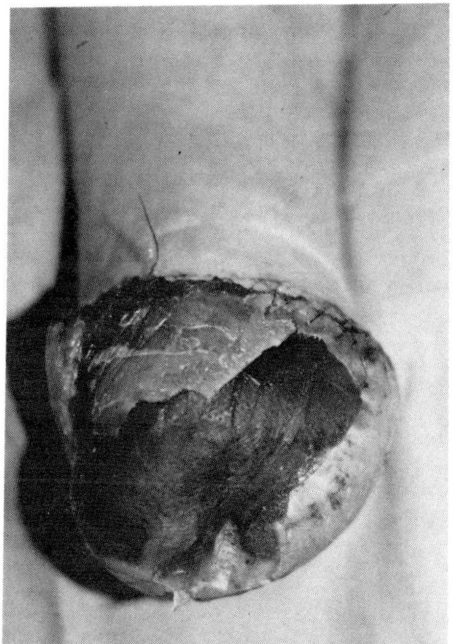

Fig. 32-3. Total necrosis of Syme heel flap necessitating revision to higher level.

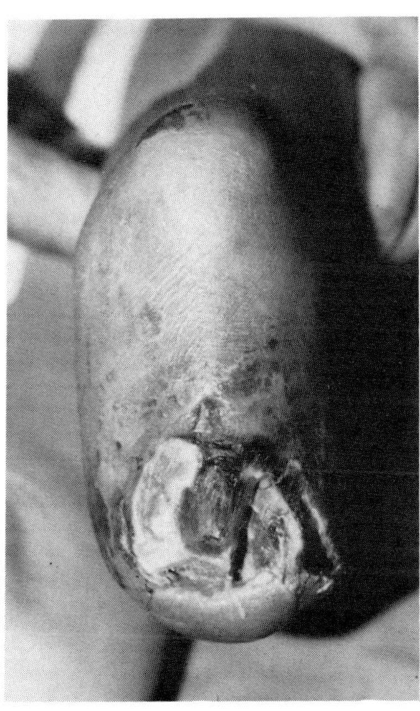

Fig. 32-4. Necrosis of anterior skin flap with infection. Secondary closure required bone shortening but preserved below-knee level.

In cases of infected nonunion, open amputation through the site of nonunion is the usual procedure. The wound may be packed open until healing is well advanced, or alternately, delayed closure over a suction-irrigation system may be employed to better preserve length. Despite these measures, osteomyelitis may recur. In that case, adequate drainage and debridement must be instituted, but it may be possible to leave the skin flaps partially attached to maintain their length and prevent revision to a higher level. This is especially crucial in below-knee amputations. If the bone becomes secondarily infected following protrusion through inadequate soft tissues, it should be shortened to allow closure. A wide dehiscence, caused by a fall directly onto the end of the partially healed residual limb, should be treated as an emergency. Secondary closure should be effected, if the wound is clean, within 6 to 9 hours, as for any other fresh wounds (Fig. 32-5).

Skin adherence to bone of residual limb

If sufficient skin was not available at the time of amputation to cover a stump of functional length, a split-thickness skin graft may have been used to effect a healed, dry wound. These grafts may endure prosthetic use provided they have been laid on adequate soft tissue, such as that provided by myoplasty (Fig. 32-6). Laid directly on bone, they are likely to ulcerate when a prosthesis is used (Fig. 32-7). The patient should be taught to mobilize the adherent graft by gentle fingertip massage, carried out daily over several weeks.

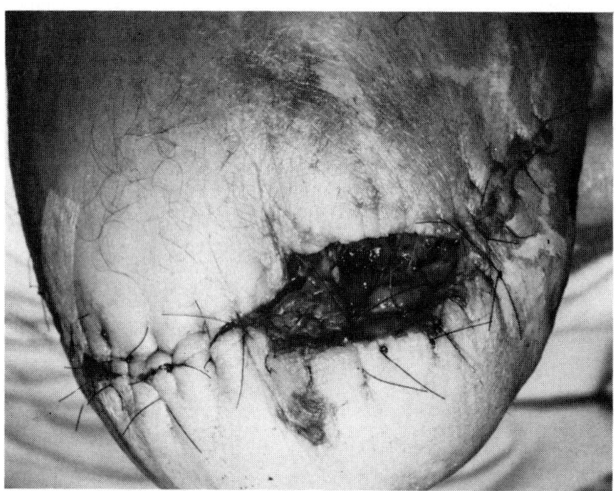

Fig. 32-5. Dehiscence caused by fall onto residual limb, requiring immediate debridement and resuturing.

Problems in stump shaping

A great deal can be done at the time of amputation to produce a residual limb that will rapidly achieve a shape suitable for fitting of a prosthesis. Conversely, many problems that delay the application of a definitive limb are a direct result of poor operative technique.

Wound edge tension on closure of an amputation should be minimal. However, a very loose closure, with redundant skin, may lead to slow shrinkage with persistent distal edema, despite good wrapping technique.

The introduction of myoplasty and myodesis has been a major advance in ensuring permanent stability of stump shape. Myodesis, which means the suturing of surrounding muscle tissue to the bone end, is best applied in nondysvascular cases. In these, the placement of sutures through muscle tissue is not likely to produce necrosis and drainage. Myoplasty, in which sutures are placed only in the fascial portion of the myofascial flap, is more suited to the dysvascular case with marginal muscle viability. The muscle, especially at the midcalf level, should be tapered carefully to avoid excessive bulk.

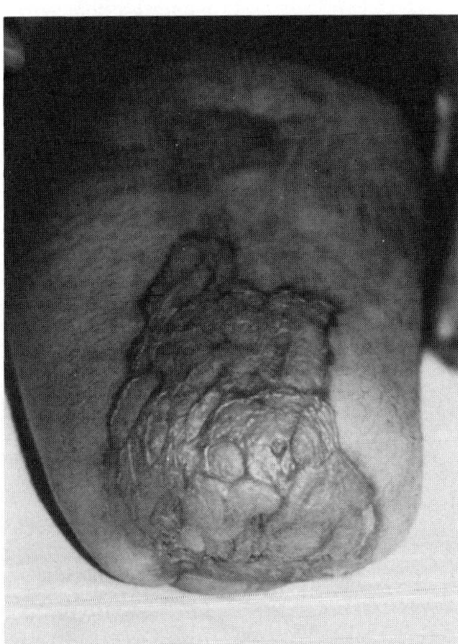

Fig. 32-6. These split-thickness skin grafts, with adequate soft tissue base, have endured 3 years of suction suspension socket usage.

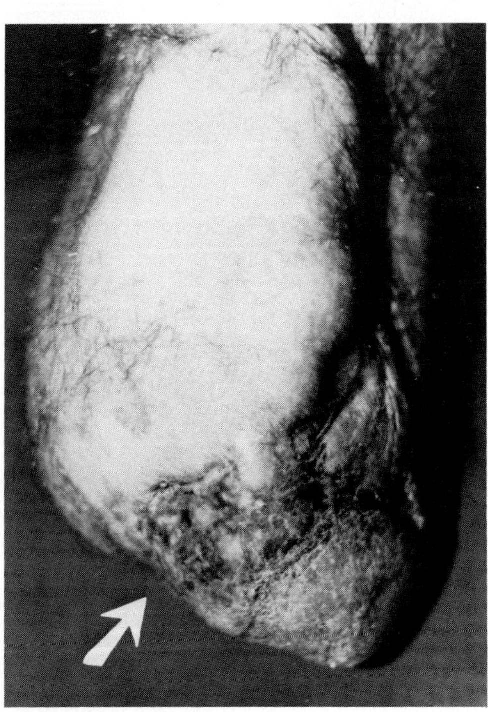

Fig. 32-7. Split-thickness skin graft laid directly onto tibia. Ulceration (arrow) occurred with prosthesis use.

In situations when ablation of a limb for malignancy is to be followed by chemotherapy, it has been recommended that nonabsorbable sutures be used to close the fascia and other deep structures. This is because fascial structures retract secondary to chemotherapy, altering the structure of the residual limb. (See Chapter 33.)

The Syme amputation presents a special case. If the heel pad is well centered, the patient will be able to tolerate a great deal of end bearing. If it has migrated posteriorly or to one side but is passively correctable, it can be held in proper weight-bearing position by a carefully made prosthesis (Fig. 32-8). However, if the heel pad is fixed off center by a deep scar, it should be revised prior to fitting.

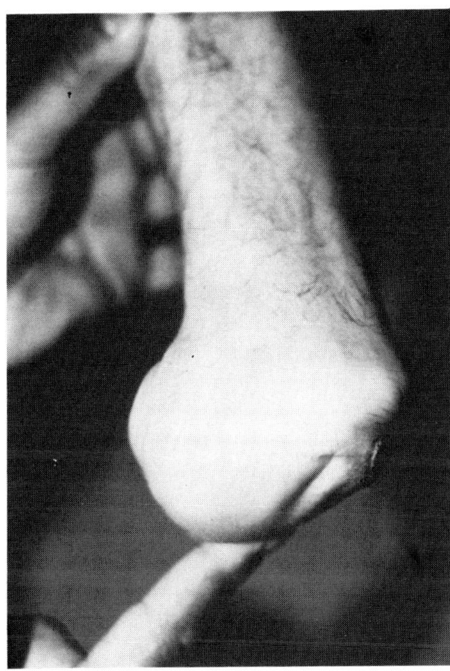

Fig. 32-8. Hypermobile Syme heel pad. Its position may be controlled to some degree by proper fabrication of prosthesis.

Problems in stump shaping related to postoperative factors

The time-honored method of shrinking and shaping a residual limb has been by use of an elastic bandage. Unfortunately, it is easy to produce a poorly shaped stump by less than expert application of this method (Fig. 32-9). The bandage is properly applied on the bias with gradually decreasing pressure as the wrapping proceeds proximally. The layers of bandage tend to shift with movement, requiring frequent rewrapping to avoid circumferential constriction with distal edema formation (Fig. 32-10). Elastic shrinker socks may be used instead, especially when the patient or attendant is unable to learn proper wrapping technique. The sock should be of heavy elastic construction throughout, including the distal end. It must be snug and fitted with a waist belt to keep it in place. In addition, tucks may be sewn in on either side every 7 to 14 days to keep it snug as the stump shrinks. The sock is briefly removed twice daily for skin care.

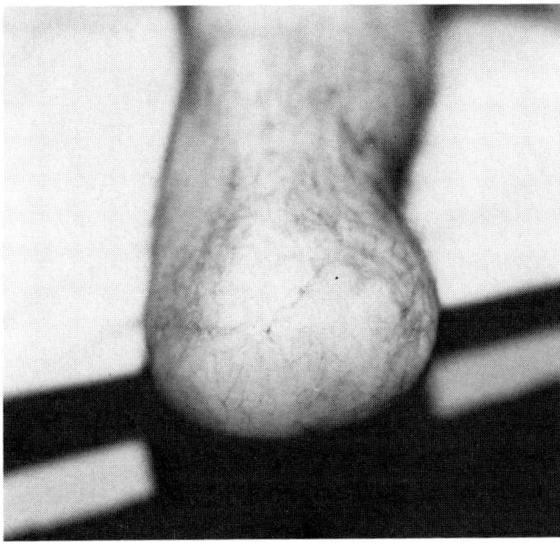

Fig. 32-9. Poorly applied shrinker bandage produced dumbbell-shaped below-knee residual limb.

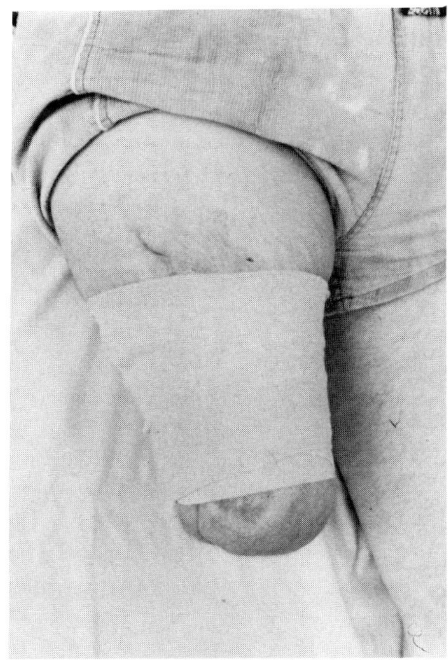

Fig. 32-10. Elastic bandage improperly applied to above-knee residual limb.

Very muscular or fat patients may experience extremely slow shrinkage of their residual limbs by wrapping. Both the bulky triceps surae and the fat thigh shrink most rapidly when fitted with a temporary prosthesis as soon as the wound is soundly healed. Shrinkage may be further enhanced by removing the temporary socket at night and applying a snug elastic shrinker sock. Weekly circumferential measurements of the residual limb should be made, so that a permanent prosthesis may be fitted when a definite plateau in shrinkage has been reached.

Proximal joint problems

Contractures. Contractures tend to develop in the joint immediately proximal to the site of amputation. They often appear in the early postoperative period as a result of the patient placing the joint in the most comfortable position.

The two most common contractures seen in upper limb amputees are an adduction contracture at the shoulder in the short above-elbow amputation and an elbow flexion contracture in the short below-elbow amputation. Either can be prevented by institution of range of motion exercises as soon as postoperative pain has subsided, at 5 to 7 days. Gentle muscle strengthening exercises, begun at 2 to 4 weeks, are also helpful. If contractures are fixed, an extensive physical therapy program may be required. Occasionally, selective releases of contracted muscles are necessary.

In the lower limb amputee, a variety of contractures may occur. The patient with a short above-knee amputation is subject to a hip flexion-abduction contracture, particularly if the wheelchair is used excessively. A flexion contracture up to 25 degrees, at this level, may be accommodated by prosthetic alignment.

As one progresses to the midthigh level, it is difficult to compensate prosthetically for contractures of more than 15 degrees. Even so, the resulting cosmesis of the prosthesis may leave something to be desired. More than 15 degrees of hip flexion contracture will require a compensatory increase in lumbar lordosis, which, even if available, may lead to low back discomfort.

Prevention of contracture is the key. Pillows under the lower limbs are forbidden. Within a few days of surgery, the patient should be taught to lie prone to stretch out any incipient hip flexion contracture and to actively adduct the thighs to prevent abduction contracture. Active extension of the residual above-knee limb, while hugging the opposite limb to the chest, should be taught. Early walking with crutches or a walker, which gets the patient out of the wheelchair, is to be encouraged. Use of a temporary above-knee prosthesis as soon as the wound is healed is excellent preventive treatment.

Below-knee amputees, especially with a short leg segment, are very prone to develop knee flexion contracture, usually in the first or second

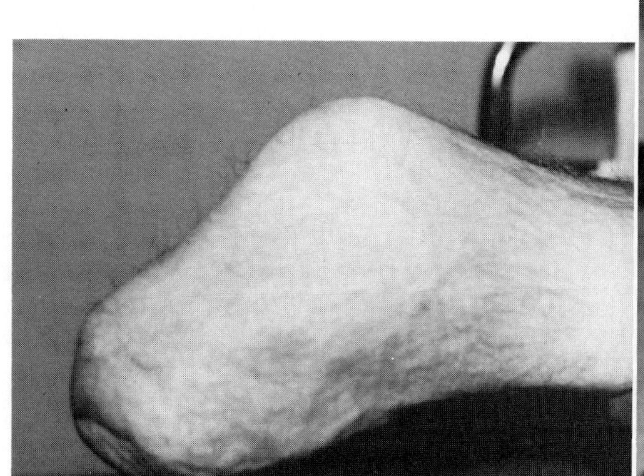

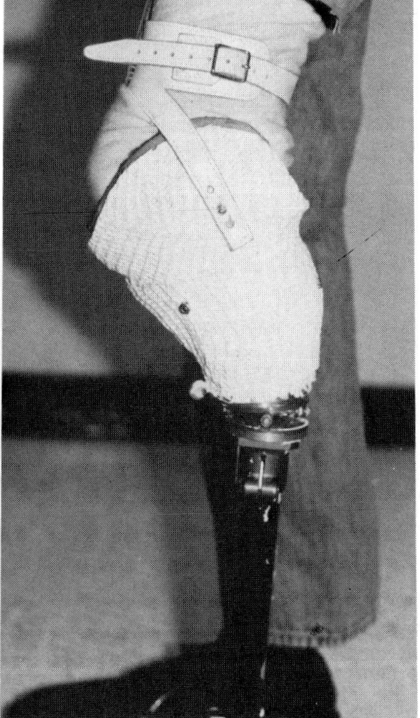

Fig. 32-11. A, Flexion contracture of knee in short below-knee residual limb. **B,** Residual limb with flexion contracture of knee fitted with temporary prosthesis that can be adjusted as ambulation reduces contracture.

week postoperatively. For this reason, the use of a rigid plaster dressing or splint is advised until the wound is healed sufficiently to allow active range of motion exercises. At no time should pillows be placed under either lower limb.

Severe knee flexion contractures are virtually impossible to reduce by exercise (Fig. 32-11, *A*). If the amputation was not done for a vascular problem, hamstring lengthenings and release of the posterior knee joint capsule should be considered. The dysvascular amputee with a short, contracted residual limb usually must be fitted with a bent-knee prosthesis. Occasionally, a contracture in the range of 35 to 40 degrees in a long below-knee stump may be improved by fitting a prosthesis aligned to provide a knee extension moment on foot contact (Fig. 32-11, *B*).

Patients with partial foot amputations, between the transmetatarsal and Syme levels, are likely to develop equinus deformity due to the unopposed action of the triceps surae (Fig. 32-12). This may be partially alleviated during Lisfranc (tarsal-metatarsal) and Chopart (midtarsal) amputations by reattaching the anterior tibial and toe extensor tendons to more proximal bony structures in a balanced fashion and lengthening the Achilles tendon percutaneously. In addition, a plastic ankle-foot orthosis, fitted with an anterior ankle strap, can be used to maintain the residual foot in a plantigrade position. If, despite these precautions, a contracture develops, a second percutaneous Achilles tendon lengthening or revision to the Syme level may be required.

Degenerative arthritis. Presently, approximately 80% of amputations are done for dysvascular disease. Since most of these people are middle-aged or elderly, many have arthritis of the joints proximal to the site of amputation.

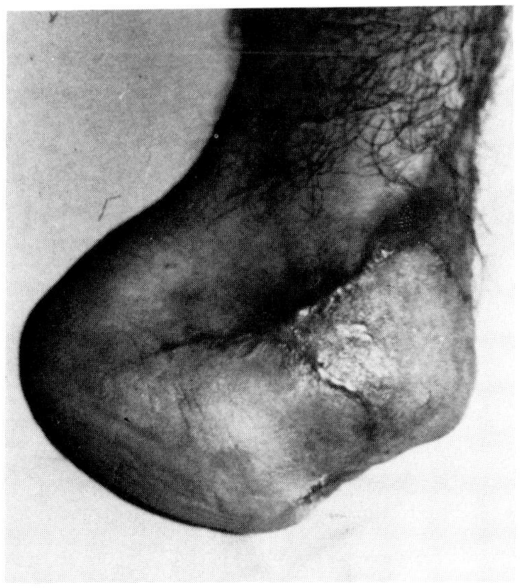

Fig. 32-12. Equinus deformity in Chopart level amputation.

Arthritis of the hip joint in the above-knee amputee may be alleviated to some degree with the standard quadrilateral socket, which uses ischial weight bearing, with a pelvic belt and rigid hip joint. In addition, the lightest possible prosthesis should be fabricated to allow less forceful contraction of the muscles crossing the hip joint, thus reducing joint compression. If pain is unrelieved, a total hip arthroplasty may be considered.

Below-knee amputees with significantly symptomatic hip joint arthritis should not be denied the benefits of total hip arthroplasty if it is otherwise indicated. Weight-bearing pain in the knee, secondary to femorotibial joint arthritis, may be partially relieved by the addition of knee joints and a thigh corset to the standard PTB prosthesis. This will allow sharing of weight bearing between the knee joint and thigh. Patellofemoral arthritis has not proved to be a major concern.

POSTPROSTHETIC COMPLICATIONS

Painful residual limb

In above-knee amputations, if myodesis has not been performed, the femur may drift anterolaterally through the soft tissues to present its distal end subcutaneously. This will produce local tenderness with the use of a prosthesis. Prosthesis modifications may include socket relief over the bony prominence or lateral filling in of the socket just above the prominence. If socket adjustments do not produce relief, a stump revision, including myodesis, may be necessary. Pain-producing bone spurs may develop at the cut end of the femur and require similar socket relief or excision (Fig. 32-13). Adventitious bursae develop over bony prominences and occasionally need treatment other than socket relief.

Above-knee amputees may complain of a burning sensation in the ischial weight-bearing area, particularly in the early phases of using a quadrilateral socket. Examination of the residual limb often reveals areas of local inflammation secondary to pressure.

A common site of discomfort and skin breakdown in below-knee amputations is over the distal anterior tibia. This is usually due to inadequate beveling of the tibia at the time of amputation. This can often be corrected by local socket relief, but may require surgical revision.

Even with adequate beveling, discomfort can

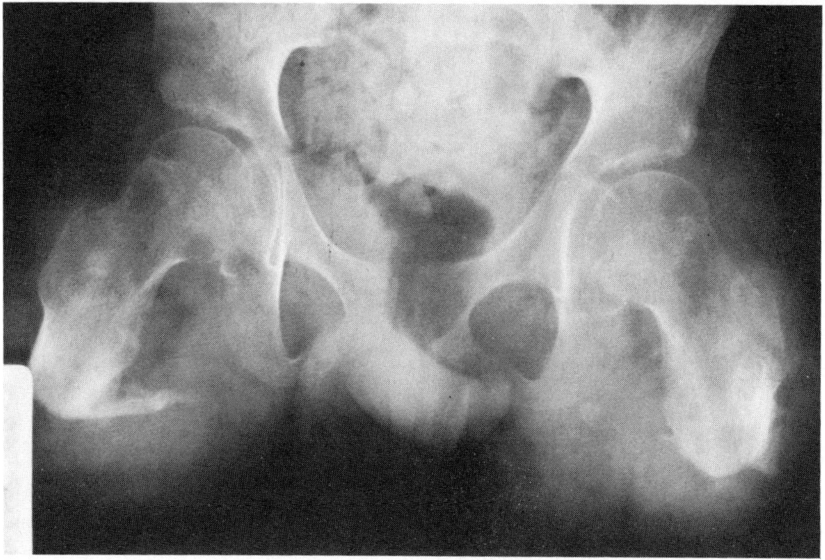

Fig. 32-13. Bone spur on femur; this one did not require resection.

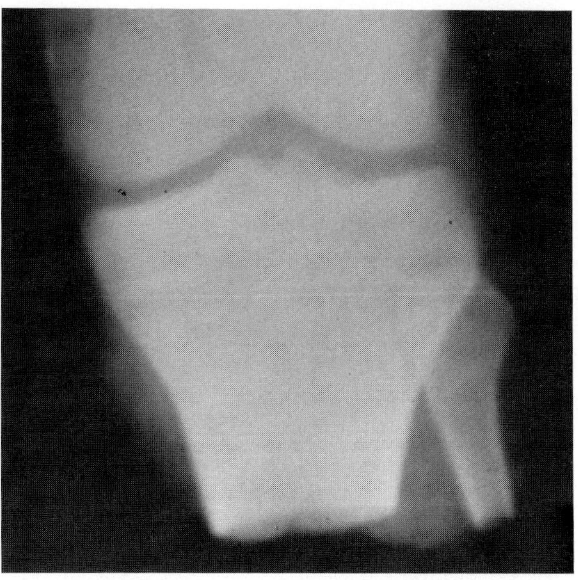

Fig. 32-14. Long fibula that produces pain when patient wears PTB prosthesis.

occur in the same area following circumferential shrinkage. The residual limb may then move in the socket like a clapper in a bell, striking the anterior wall of the socket each time the knee is extended. This may be corrected by filling in the socket.

If the fibular stump is inadvertently left longer than the tibia, the resulting bony prominence may be weight bearing and tender (Fig. 32-14). Socket modifications should be attempted, but surgical revision may be necessary. In very short below-knee stumps, the fibula may be excessively mobile or prominent and may require complete primary or secondary resection (Fig. 32-15).

In the below-knee amputee, torn knee ligaments may result in painful instability while wearing the standard PTB prosthesis. This instability may be controlled by using a prosthesis that better encloses the distal femur. Prostheses that meet this criterion include the supracondylar-

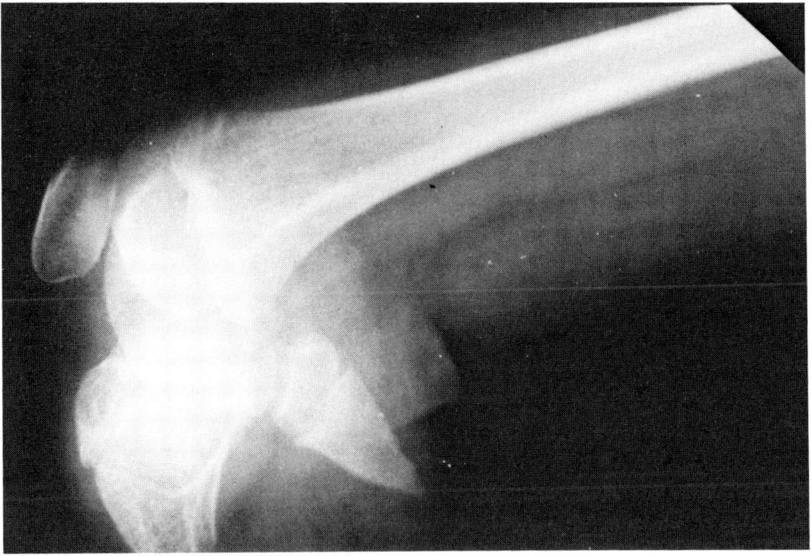

Fig. 32-15. Mobile displaced residual fibula required complete resection.

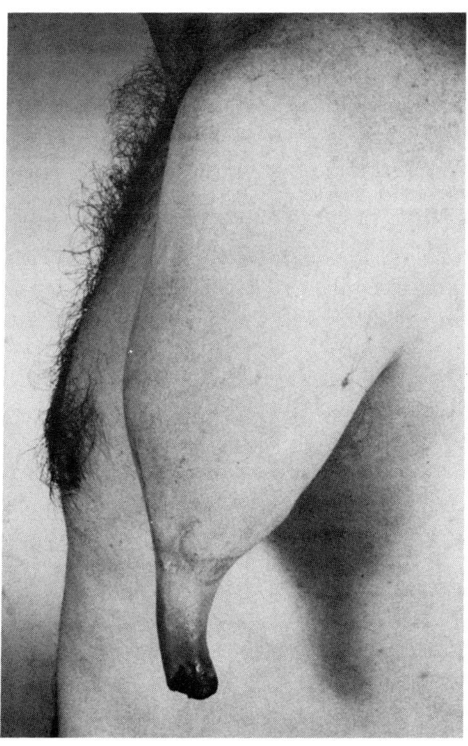

Fig. 32-16. Overgrowth of humerus in adolescent above-elbow amputee.

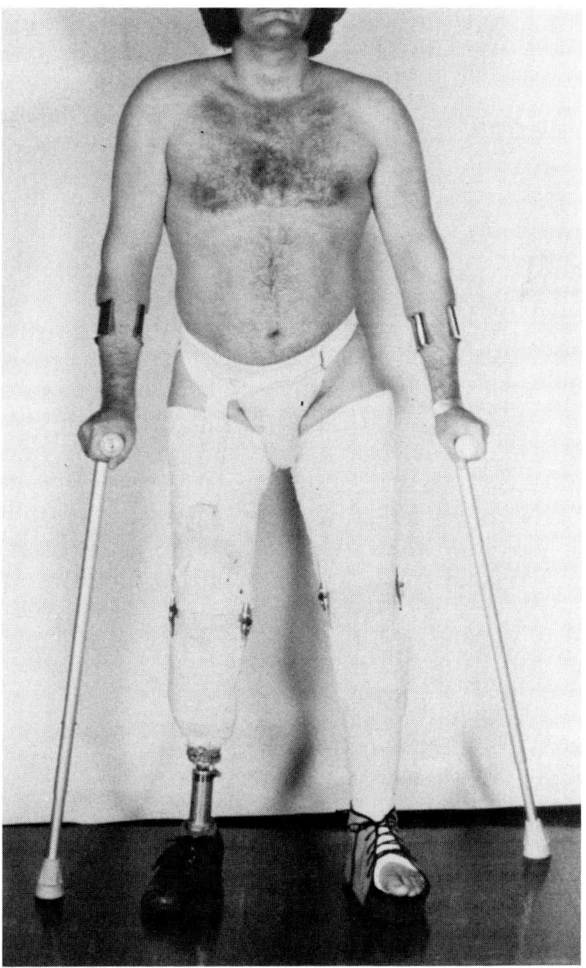

Fig. 32-17. Patient with comminuted, short oblique right supracondylar fracture of residual below-knee limb and left femoral shaft fracture treated by bilateral cast-brace technique for 5 months after 8 weeks of bilateral skeletal traction.

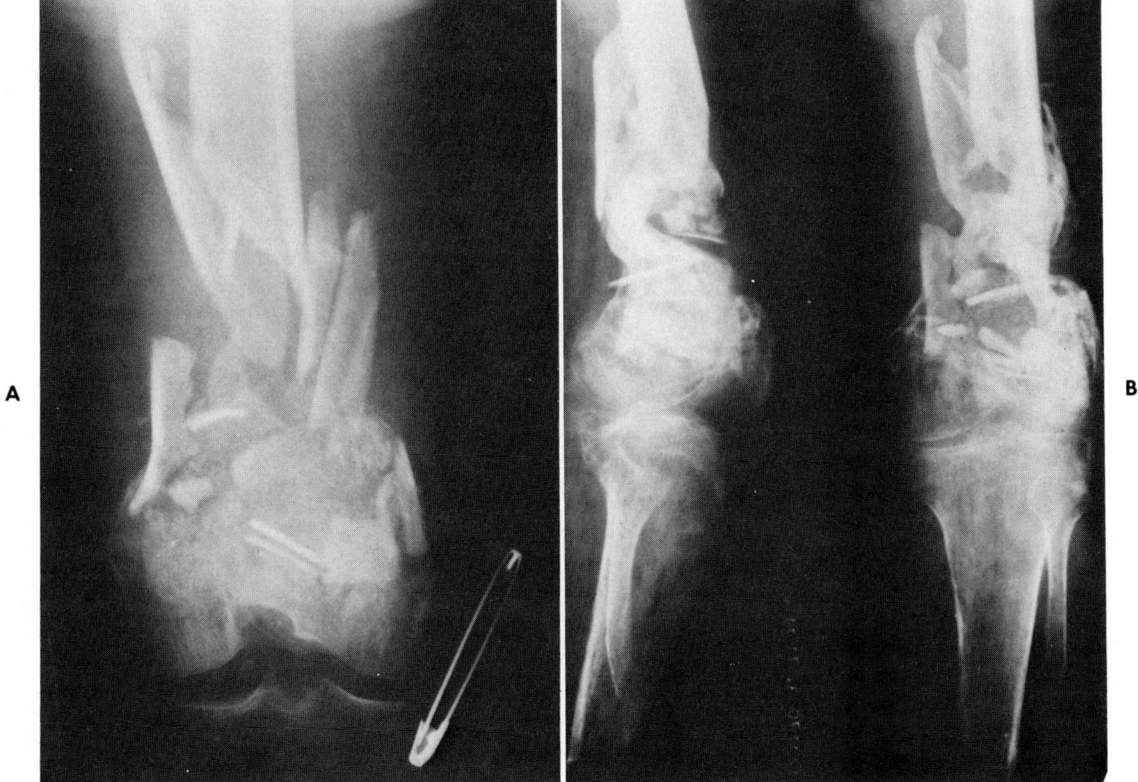

Fig. 32-18. A, Severely comminuted open supracondylar fracture in below-knee residual limb, treated with single spica cast. At 6 months, patient had bone graft to anteromedial defect. **B,** Radiographs of same fracture 9 months later. Patient successfully using PTB prosthesis along with 10- to 40-degree knee range of motion.

suprapatellar, supracondylar, and PTB with thigh corset.

Neuroma formation is the natural consequence of nerve section. If nerves are divided at a level that both prevents their inclusion in the wound scar and avoids weight bearing or other significant pressure from the prosthesis, they will rarely be symptomatic. If a mass is suspected of being a symptomatic neuroma, direct manipulation should produce discomfort in a dermatomal distribution of the missing portions of the limb. Firm, fibrous nodules, which are only locally sensitive, are probably not neuromas. The treatment of neuromas should begin with socket accommodation. If this is unsuccessful after several attempts, resection of the nerve at a higher level may be done.

Whenever a limb is amputated because of tumor, local recurrence is a possibility because tumor may have been left behind. The proper course of action depends on the type of tumor involved and may range from radiation or chemotherapy to amputation at a higher level. Consultation with an oncologist is essential before proceeding (Chapter 33).

Adherence of skin to bone by scar tissue

In any residual limb, but especially in the below-knee amputation, the adherence of skin to bone by scar tissue may rapidly lead to pain and ulceration with prosthesis use. This is because scar without underlying soft tissue has little resistance to shear forces. It may be possible, however, to develop a bursal layer that will allow movement between the scar tissue and bone by gentle persistent massage over an extended period of time. The socket should be modified and a compressible end pad provided to reduce direct and shear forces. Surgical revision should be done only as a last resort.

Insensitive skin

Amputees with diminished sensation in the residual limb are being seen more frequently than in the past. The largest group are diabetics, but a variety of neurological disorders, such as

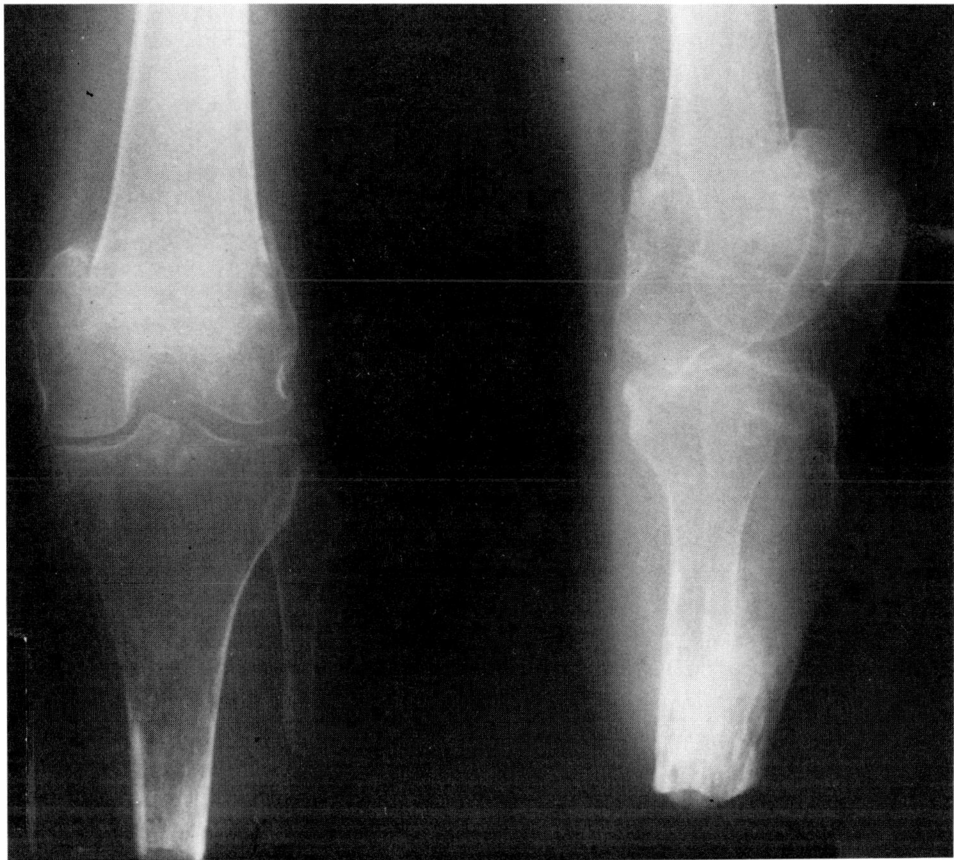

Fig. 32-19. Below-knee amputee with 30-degree flexion contracture sustained impacted supracondylar femoral fracture. This was allowed to heal in full extension with 30-degree posterior angulation in cast and brace. Prosthetic fitting was successful with 0- to 110-degree knee range motion.

myelomeningocele, is also seen. These patients are not deterred by pain from continued walking on an ulcerated stump and must be taught to remove their prosthesis at frequent intervals for skin inspection, especially during the early phases of prosthesis use. Inflamed areas should be shown to the prosthetics team for prompt corrective action. Short periods of ambulation will allow gradual skin adaptation.

If a residual below-knee limb continues to show skin breakdown despite competent socket adjustments, other methods may be helpful. The addition of a rotator unit may decrease shear forces. Partial unloading of the stump by addition of knee joints and a long thigh corset or the use of ischial weight bearing may be necessary to allow continued function.

Poor fit

After a variable period of use, most amputees find that the prosthesis socket can no longer be practically adjusted. It just does not fit any longer, and a new socket is needed if dangerous, costly skin breakdown is to be avoided.

Bony overgrowth in children

The adolescent traumatic amputee may experience rapid growth in length of the residual limb bone, especially of the fibula, humerus, or tibia, to the point where the bone grows through the skin (Fig. 32-16). This is appositional bone growth and has nothing to do with proximal epiphyseal growth, even though bony overgrowth usually ceases when epiphyseal growth ceases. This may occur several times during childhood and adolescence, but usually is easily treated by resecting sufficient bone to allow soft tissue closure. Caps, plugs, chemical cautery, or electrocautery have not proven to be consistently useful in controlling overgrowth. Proximal epiphysiodesis is contraindicated, since this has no influence on distal bony overgrowth.

Fractures

Although not common, fractures in a residual limb do occur sufficiently often to warrant careful design of treatment methods to allow early, effective return to use of a prosthesis.

A survey of the world literature indicated that fractures of residual upper limbs are very rare. It is recommended that humeral shaft fractures be treated by splinting. If delayed union or nonunion ensues, open reduction, internal fixation, and bone grafting should be considered, especially in below-elbow amputees. Fractures about the elbow may be managed by open or closed methods so long as they are designed to maintain elbow range of motion.

Fractures in residual lower limbs have been reported with more frequency. A recent combined American and Canadian study produced ninety cases with sufficient information to give both epidemiological data and some specific recommendations for management.

The average age at injury was 50 years. A fall while wearing the prosthesis was the usual cause of injury. Knee joints and a thigh lacer did not prevent supracondylar fractures in below-knee amputees, nor did a hip joint with pelvic belt prevent fractures about the hip in above-knee amputees.

An important treatment goal in both below-knee and above-knee groups is the restoration of a normal neck-shaft angle in intertrochanteric fractures to restore hip abductor function. Although manipulation and casting often sufficed in a two-part intertrochanteric fracture, those amputees with unstable fractures are best served by open reduction and internal fixation. Displaced femoral neck fractures in both below-knee and above-knee amputees may be managed either by endoprosthetic replacement or reduction and internal fixation. Excision of the femoral head alone will lead to an unstable gait.

Because of the small residual limb mass and length of lever arm in above-knee amputees, most impacted femoral neck or intertrochanteric fractures and shaft fractures can be successfully managed by nonweight bearing alone or by minispica casts after appropriate manipulation of malaligned fractures.

In below-knee amputees, restoration of limb alignment, especially in the more proximal fractures, and preservation of knee motion are paramount. Patients with stable supracondylar femoral fractures can be mobilized rapidly by the use of the cast-brace technique (Fig. 32-17). Unstable supracondylar fractures may be managed by plaster casts with or without preliminary skeletal traction and/or manipulation (Fig. 32-18). Moderate malunion or loss of length at this level is easily compensated by prosthetic adjustment, but an effort should be made to avoid flexion contracture of the knee, which is much less compensable (Fig. 32-19). In the case of displaced intra-articular fractures at the knee, joint congruity should be restored as accurately as possible.

Below-knee amputees were more likely to resume use of their prosthesis than above-knee amputees, due to lesser energy demands. Operative scars did not interfere with the fitting or use of prostheses. Only 25% required a prosthesis modification following fracture. All of these were below-knee amputees. Revision of amputations through the fracture site was not found to be necessary or desirable.

In short, good results in the management of fractured residual lower limbs may be expected if they are treated with the same care accorded fractures occurring in intact limbs.

CHAPTER 33

Special considerations in amputations for malignancies

HUGH G. WATTS

Prior to the advent of chemotherapy, the treatment of osteosarcomas was the purview of the surgeon. Amputation was the usual treatment, and debate was focused on the extent of the limb required for tumor ablation. The introduction of chemotherapy with its many complex regimens led to intimidation of the surgeon, leaving him to play the role of ablative technician. This is not appropriate if the patient is to receive optimum therapy. The biopsy must be done properly, and the surgical options need to be known. The consequences of chemotherapy or radiation on the surgery and postsurgical rehabilitation must be understood.

BIOPSY

The biopsy of potentially malignant bone tumors should be as much a part of the overall planning for the patient as the subsequent surgery. If an amputation is anticipated, the biopsy obviously has to be placed at a site that will not interfere with the amputation flaps.

Recent changes in treatment allow for resection of some osteosarcomas without amputation. In such situations, the location of the biopsy site is critical, since the biopsy site must be removed en bloc with the tumor. If such an operation is anticipated, it is a kindness to all if the biopsy is left to the surgeon who will ultimately perform the resection.

Primary bone malignancies are often histologically heterogeneous. Needle biopsies by and large do not provide satisfactory tissue. The consequences of misdiagnosis are enormous, and needle biopsy is best reserved for areas that are difficult to reach surgically, such as vertebral bodies, or for confirming that a secondary lesion in bone contains tumor where there is a previously diagnosed primary lesion elsewhere.

It is advisable to obtain a frozen section of the biopsy specimen. This is not used for immediate diagnosis, but to establish that the specimen taken is adequate to make a diagnosis when the tissue is finally prepared.

BIOPSY AND RADIATION

Pathological fracture through an irradiated bone is a frequent problem, especially when chemotherapy is superimposed. This should be considered when planning the biopsy if radiation therapy is a potential mode of treatment. If such tumors have extended outside the bone, an adequate biopsy can be obtained without violating the cortex. If the cortex of the bone must be invaded, the cortical hole should not be a "window" but a "porthole." A rectangle with sharp corners creates four areas of stress concentration with an increased possibility of pathological fracture.

If the radiograph suggests that the tumor will be one best treated by radiation, the radiation therapist should be consulted *prior* to the biopsy. The biopsy location may pose problems in planning radiation ports where unradiated skin strips must be left for adequate lymphatic drainage.

If a fracture occurs through an irradiated bone and the patient is receiving chemotherapy, healing of the fracture cannot be expected until chemotherapy is completed—often 2 years. Such fractures require internal fixation. Treatment by traction will impede radiation therapy, as well as lead to further osteoporosis, complicating the ultimate internal fixation. Excessive bleeding is not a feature of these operations and should not deter the surgeon from internal fixation.

AMPUTATION

Despite recent enthusiasm for limb-sparing resections, amputation is still the mainstay for removing the primary malignant tumors of bone, such as osteosarcomas. However, the introduction of massive doses of very toxic chemotherapeutic agents has altered the surgeon's management.

Timing

Current practice in many centers is to amputate an affected limb at the same operation immediately after the biopsy is reported to show malignancy. There are a number of reasons *not* to follow this practice: (1) amputation of an extremity immediately after the biopsy has not led to an increase in patient survival, (2) bone tumor diagnosis by frozen section alone can be disastrous, (3) a limb-sparing procedure may be feasible, and (4) a patient usually does better both in the trip to the operating room and in postoperative care if he has had an adequate mental preparation for an amputation. This is particularly true for children. A short interval between the biopsy and amputation allows several days to prepare the patient by talking over problems, such as phantom limb sensation and range of activities after the amputation. Preamputation crutch walking can be learned, and when possible, the patient can meet with other amputees who are farther along in the treatment.

Level

The choice of the level for amputation in osteosarcoma has always been a point of debate. Should the surgeon remove the entire bone or cut across the bone at some level above the tumor? Since distal femoral lesions account for 60% of osteosarcomas, this debate evolves to the choice of an above-knee amputation with its functional and aesthetic advantages or a hip disarticulation, which eliminates the fear of leaving the tumor behind. Surgeons who recommend whole bone removal cite a "local recurrence" rate as high as 21% with transosseous amputations, implying that primary tumor has been left behind.[6] Those who recommend transosseous amputations report a "local recurrence" rate of less than 5%[1,2,4,5] and blame inappropriate surgical technique for the higher rate cited by others.

Enneking[3] has clearly documented the presence of clinically undetectable intramedullary foci of tumor separate from the primary lesion (so-called skip lesions), whose existence had previously been questioned. The question is no longer, "Are there skip lesions?" The question is, "Do skip lesions make any significant difference?" I have adopted a treatment policy of amputation through the bone and have had no instances of recurrent tumor. Whether this represents a careful selection of the level at which the bone is transected or the efficacy of chemotherapeutic drugs in eliminating "skip lesions" cannot be stated. Presently, there are no data to demonstrate that survival is enhanced by removing the entire bone.

Where should the bone be transected if cross-bone amputation is to be done? Some surgeons will remove the bone as high as the lesser trochanter for a distal femoral lesion. Dahlin and Coventry[2] demonstrated that transosseous amputation 7.5 cm (3 inches) proximal to the tumor as seen on plain radiographs can safely remove the tumor. There have been a number of instances where tumor extended beyond the limits seen by plain radiographs, yet could be detected by bone scan. To avoid the possibility of leaving residual tumor, the bone scan may be used to help in determining the level of bone removal.

At the time of the bone scan, using technetium 99 labeled diphosphonate, a drop of radionuclide is placed at one end of a tube (usually the needle cap of a tuberculin syringe) (Fig. 33-1). The surgeon places this radioactive pointer on the skin of the affected limb. This will show up as a bright dot on the oscilloscope screen. The marker is moved proximally or distally on the extremity until the dot is at the level of the most proximal margin of increased radioactive uptake. A Polaroid photograph of the oscilloscope screen is then taken to confirm the location of the radioactive pointer, and the skin is marked with an indelible pen. At the time of amputation, a threaded Steinmann pin is inserted into the bone, 7 cm proximal to the skin mark. The amputation is carried out with bone transection at the level of the pin. Curettage of the marrow is always done, but using the technique just described, tumor has never been found.

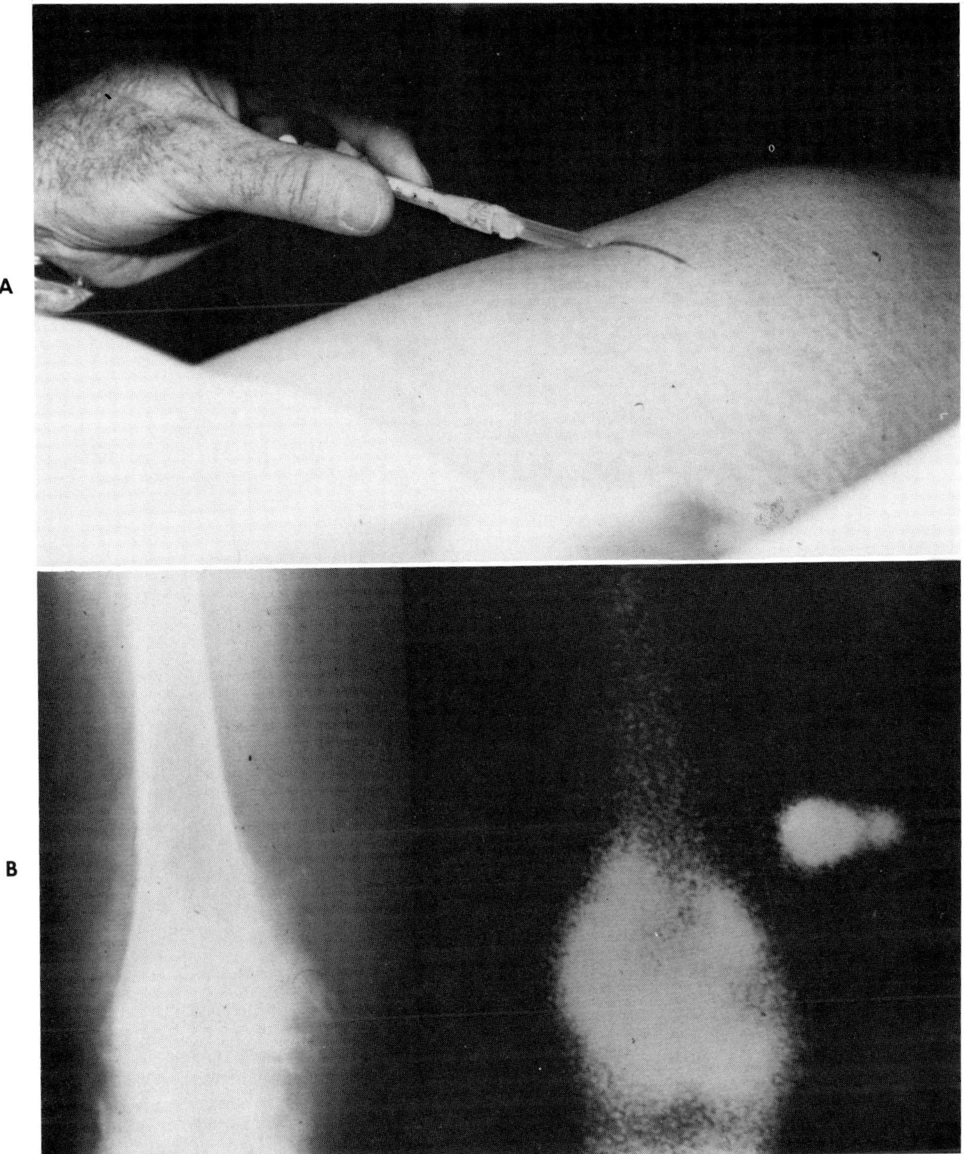

Fig. 33-1. Selecting amputation level with aid of bone scanning. **A,** Syringe cap containing drop of isotope at its tip is moved along thigh while oscilloscope is being observed. **B,** Plain film on left with corresponding scan on right showing "hot spot" of radioactive marker.

Systematizing my selection of amputation level by this technique has resulted in longer stumps than when the level was chosen by guesswork, since surgeons tended to remove extra bone "to be on the safe side." There have been no local recurrences.

Technique

The standard techniques of amputation must be altered for patients who will receive postoperative chemotherapy. High-dose methotrexate produces some inhibition of healing of the skin, considerable inhibition of healing of the fascia and soft tissues, and significant inhibition of healing of bone. Laboratory examination of the collagen extracted from the skin, fascia, and bone of patients who have had high-dose methotrexate, demonstrated marked alteration in the cross-links.

Almost invariably after amputation, when methotrexate has been used, there has been significant soft tissue retraction. This can be sufficient to cause protrusion of the underlying bone through muscle and fascia to the subcutaneous layer. This is not due to bony overgrowth, a phenomenon that is common in childhood amputees. This soft tissue retraction is decreased if *nonabsorbable* sutures are used to attach the muscles to each other or to bone, as well as for the subcutaneous tissues. Skin sutures are best left in place at least 3 weeks.

TIMING OF CHEMOTHERAPY

When chemotherapy was initiated in the recovery room, two patients had generalized seizures. In addition, more episodes of drug toxicity were experienced. A possible explanation for these phenomena is that methotrexate is a low-molecular weight substance that is readily able to enter into the edema space, whereas citrovorum is not. Following the "rescue" and cessation

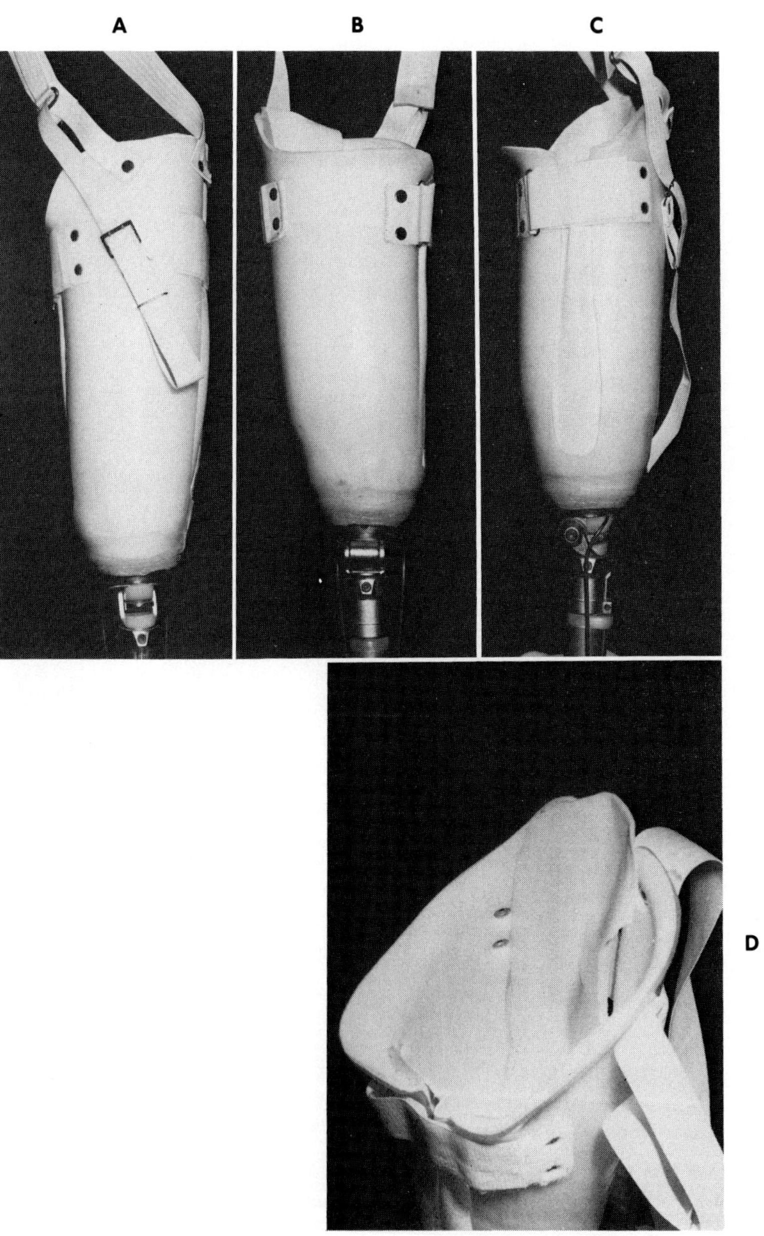

Fig. 33-2. "Intermediate prosthesis" adjusts to accommodate changes in stump size resulting from chemotherapy. **A,** Anterior view. **B,** Posterior view. **C,** Medial view with cutout and Velcro closure. Lateral cutout is identical. **D,** Internal view showing closed-cell foam lining to reduce skin problems from chemotherapy.

of citrovorum factor, the methotrexate can leak back from the edema space into the general circulation and produce a rebound toxic episode. Consequently, I arbitrarily start chemotherapy 2 weeks after amputation.

POSTOPERATIVE MANAGEMENT

All of the patients are treated with an immediate postsurgical prosthetic fitting. Generally, the patients are able to walk in 2 to 4 days and are discharged within 7 to 10 days, so they have several days at home before commencing chemotherapy.

The use of high-dose methotrexate may alter the stump volume with an increase in size during each course of chemotherapy. This must be taken into consideration in prosthetic fitting. The use of suction as the only suspension is unwise. It is preferable to use an auxiliary Silesian belt, which may be discontinued at the end of the use of chemotherapy. Most recently, a polypropylene "intermediate prosthesis" has been used, which is split medially and laterally to allow an adjustable socket fit (Fig. 33-2). This "intermediate" socket is attached to the final endoskeletal limb and worn until several months after the completion of chemotherapy. At that time the socket is changed to the final one. This adjustability also aids in maintaining prosthetic fit in patients who have significant weight loss during an episode of drug toxicity.

Any irritation of the skin from the prosthesis can be accentuated by the use of chemotherapeutic agents, and extra care should be taken to avoid injury by the prosthesis. The "intermediate prostheses" are made with a closed-cell polyethylene foam liner to reduce skin irritation.

Postoperative infection in stumps occurred in two patients following amputation. They were given chemotherapy on schedule starting at 2 weeks after amputation, while the infections were treated by open debridement and closures of the stump over irrigation tubes. Both amputation stumps healed satisfactorily despite continued administration of chemotherapy.

As a result of chemotherapy, the number of patients surviving malignant bone tumors has increased enormously. This has necessitated a change in the philosophy with regard to postoperative care. No longer can these patients be denied a prosthesis because of a diagnosis of malignancy, nor relegated to a "wait and see" category concerning rehabilitation. They deserve exactly the same treatment as any other person who has undergone an amputation.

REFERENCES

1. Coventry, M., and Dahlin, D.: Osteogenic sarcoma: a critical analysis of 430 cases, J. Bone Joint Surg. **39A:**741-758, 1957.
2. Dahlin, D., and Coventry, M.: Osteogenic sarcoma: a study of 600 cases, J. Bone Joint Surg. **49A:**101-110, 1967.
3. Enneking, W. F., and Kagan, A.: "Skip" metastases in osteosarcoma, Cancer **36:**2192-2205, 1975.
4. Lee, E. S., and MacKenzie, D.: Osteosarcoma: a study of the value of preoperative megavoltage radiotherapy, Br. J. Surg. **51:**252-274, 1964.
5. Moore, G., Gertner, R., and Brugarolus, A.: Osteogenic sarcoma, Surg. Gynecol. Obstet. **136:**359-366, 1973.
6. Sweetnam, R.: Osteosarcoma, Ann. R. Coll. Surg. **44:**38-58, 1969.

CHAPTER 34

Management of pain in the amputee

MAURICE D. SCHNELL
WILTON H. BUNCH

For those individuals who have sustained the loss of a limb, the possibility of developing various painful conditions is all too common. These frustrating problems may arise from either intrinsic causes, that is, from the amputation and its underlying disease, or extrinsic causes, from the prosthesis and its complications. The etiology of some of these pain problems is relatively easy to identify, whereas others are formidable in their effect on the amputee and the obscurity of their origins. Often the pain may profoundly impede the functional readjustment and life-style of the prosthesis wearer.

With amputation the patient is not only deprived of a segment of the normal limb, but is faced with alterations in functional capabilities secondary to impairment of weight bearing, prehension, sensory feedback, proprioception, and muscle power. Due to unavoidable structural changes of the involved limb, it is not unrealistic to expect obstacles in functional readjustment. The major challenge to the clinician is analyzing the various physiological and psychological factors that inhibit the rehabilitation of the patient. The most apparent abnormalities, such as changes in peripheral nerves, vascular structures, muscle, and bone, represent a convenient focal point for specific treatment to eliminate these pain factors. Unfortunately, an unrelenting search for the pathomechanical cause of pain in the amputee may overlook less obvious dysfunction of the central nervous system. Treatment directed toward only organic causes of pain often falls short of complete resolution of the pain problem.

In view of the morbidity incumbent among amputees with significant pain problems, a skilled amputee manager must be prepared to investigate the wide scope of extrinsic and intrinsic causes of pain. To achieve this he must have an adequate understanding of the basic mechanisms involved in both central and peripheral pain.

INTRINSIC CAUSES OF PAIN

Pain mechanisms

Pain is a phenomenon that consists of complex circuits of cellular communication and integration elicited by stimulation of peripheral tissues, such as skin, joints, tendon, ligaments, and viscera.[23,36] It is a personal experience, differing somewhat from one individual to another as influenced by cultural experiences, personal attention, the importance of a specific situation, and other cognitive activities.[24] Although there is no evidence of control mechanisms affecting the sensitivity of peripheral nerve receptors, pain is not simply a transmission of a neural message, but rather a reaction that involved interpretative processes within the central nervous system.

Several types of peripheral nervous receptors have been identified: mechanoreceptors, thermoreceptors, and nociceptors, or pain receptors.[3,14,15] Mechanoreceptors and thermoreceptors consist of either free nerve endings or specialized capsulated receptors (Pacini and Ruffini endings, Merkel spots, and Iggo corpuscles). Impulses from these low-intensity receptors are carried by large myelinated fibers. The thermoreceptors and mechanoreceptors are characterized by low threshold for certain stimuli. For example, thermoreceptors have distinctive sensitivity to high and low skin temperatures, but can be excited by firm pressure. On the other hand, nociceptors have a high threshold to an appropriate stimulus and a relatively small field of reception.[3,14,15] The two subclasses of nociceptors are thermal nociceptors and mechanical nociceptors. These receptors are terminal endings of small myelinated and nonmyelinated fibers and are activated by intense mechanical stimulation and low (less than 15° C) or high (above 50° C) temperatures.

There is considerable controversy regarding the existence of specific chemoreceptors.[3,14,15,16,17] Although past studies have failed to substantiate unique chemoreceptors, there is abundant evidence from experimental work that extracellular chemical substances (such as bradykinin, histamine, and prostaglandins) released into extracellular fluid following tissue damage secondary to injury or disease act in some way to produce pain.[3]

Once depolarization is initiated, the generated action potential flows along sensory nerve fibers to superficial and deep cutaneous complexes and ultimately to the dorsal root ganglion, where cell bodies of the afferent neurons are located. The axions of the ganglion cells enter the apex of the dorsal horn of the spinal cord and terminate in a complex array of synaptic arrangements (Fig. 34-1). The dorsal horn has been divided into six laminae on an anatomical and functional basis.[31] Sensory input from the periphery is roughly distributed according to fiber size. The large myelinated fibers give off a collateral, which enters the dorsal horn and forms synaptic connections with cells and various laminae, especially laminae II and III. The small myelinated sensory afferent fibers proceed into the Lissauer tract, where they divide into ascending and descending divisions extending over one and two segments and establish synapses with marginal neurons and gelatinosa cells (Fig. 34-2).[16]

The long ascending afferent pathways are formed by axions of neurons from laminae I, IV, V, and VI.[3,6,16,26,37] The majority of these axions ascend in the contralateral spinothalamic tract. Some fibers arising from lamina V cells enter the dorsolateral and ventrolateral white matter both ipsilaterally and contralaterally to join the spinothalamic tract (Fig. 34-3).

The spinothalamic system is composed of two

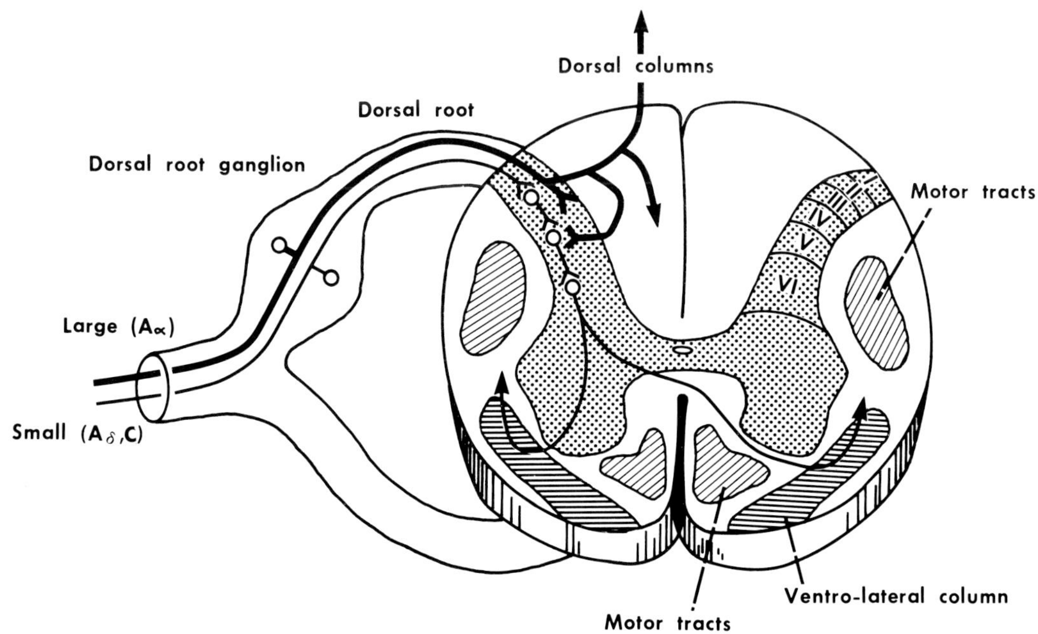

Fig. 34-1. Cross section of spinal cord showing connections of small type (A delta and C) and large type (A alpha) of peripheral afferents (right) and six laminae of dorsal horn (left). (From Bonica, J. J.: Arch. Surg. **112:**750-761, June, 1977.)

divisions: the neospinothalamic tract and the paleospinothalamic tract.[3,16,39] The neothalamic system is characterized by long fibers that make direct connections to the ventrolateral and posterior thalamus. The third relay of fibers at the thalamic level is relayed to the postcentral gyrus, which represents the primary somatosensory cortex of the brain. This system provides rapid transmission of somatosensory information regarding the location of peripheral stimulation in space, time, and intensity. Although it has only three neurons involved in its transmission, the system sends numerous collaterals to the paleospinothalamic system, which ascends medially to it.

The paleospinothalamic system is associated wih short fibers that project to the reticular formation, the pons, and the midbrain. It then connects with the medial intralaminar thalamic nuclei and from there to the limbic forebrain, hypothalamus, and other diffuse areas of the brain. This older system has frequent synapses and slow transmission. Functionally, it provokes a nondiscrete, deep unpleasant sensation that motivates the individual into action. Also, it is involved with suprasegmental reflex responses that play a role in respiratory, circulatory, and endocrine functions of the organism.[3]

Another important projection system for transmission of pain is the lemniscal system.[3,37,38] It consists of large alpha fibers that enter the dorsal root and pass cephalad through the dorsal columns to synapse with the nucleus gracilis and cuneatus in the medulla. Second-order neurons cross the medulla and ascend in the medial lemniscus to the ventral and medial thalamus.[6] Finally, third-relay neurons project through the internal capsule and corona radiata to the sensory cortex. The large, fast-conducting fibers of this system carry information concerning touch, pressure, vibration, and proprioception. Moreover, the lemniscal sysem assists in central analysis, assessment, and localization of sensory messages and then modulates through corticofugal impulses the sensory input before the action system is activated.[3]

More recently other ascending pathways have been recognized as being important in the study of pain. The spinoreticular multisynaptic ascend-

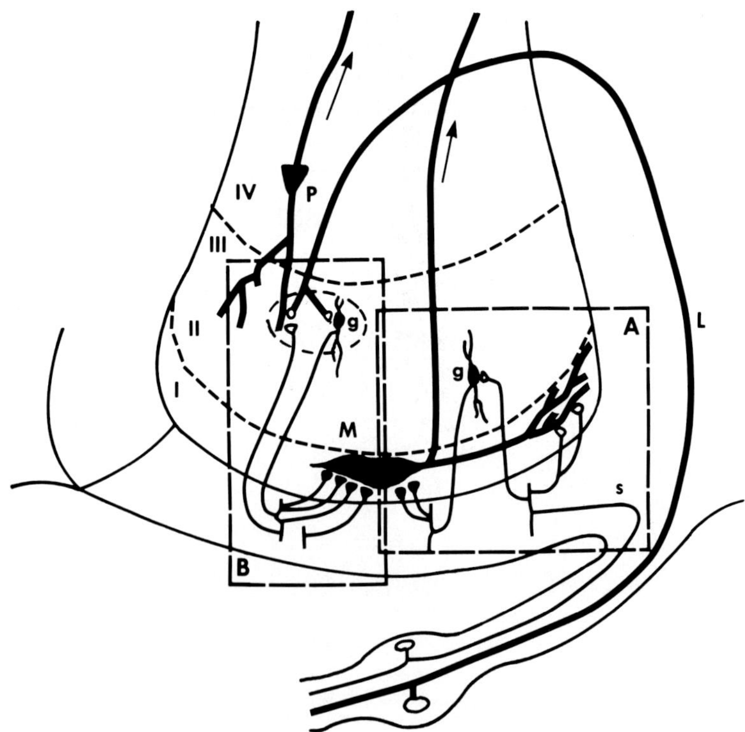

Fig. 34-2. Central relationships between primarily nociceptive input from small fiber *(s)* to circuit *A* and from large *(L)* predominantly nonnociceptive fibers to circuit *BM* marginal neuron projecting to spinothalamic system. *P*, projection neuron of lamina *IV*; *g*, gelatinosa neurons. (From Kerr, F. W. L.: Segmental circuitry and spinal cord nociceptive mechanisms. In Bonica, J. J. and Albe-Fessard, D.: Advances in pain research and therapy, vol. 1, New York, 1976, Raven Press.)

ing system, spinocervicothalamic system (SCT), the dorsal intracornu tract, and other propriospinal systems may play a role in transmission of nonciceptive impulses.[3] Information regarding these alternate systems is sketchy, and their precise function in pain has not been described.

During the past 20 years investigators have attempted to unravel the complexities of the poorly understood, although extremely imporant, inhibitory and facilitory mechanisms of pain, acting at all levels of the central nervous system. Dorsal horn cells are modulated by peripheral sensory input. Lamina I cells are inhibited by stimulation of the sensitive mechanoreceptors and high threshold afferents near the excitatory receptive field, but are strongly excited by high-intensity thermal and mechanical stimuli.[36] In contrast, lamina V cells have a wide range of inputs from skin, subcutaneous tissue, muscle, viscera, and other deep structures and are quite responsive to noxious stimuli in their respective field.[22] Inhibition of lamina V cells is produced by stimulation of low-threshold afferents at the periphery of the receptive field.

In addition to local and segmental factors that participate in modulation of sensory information

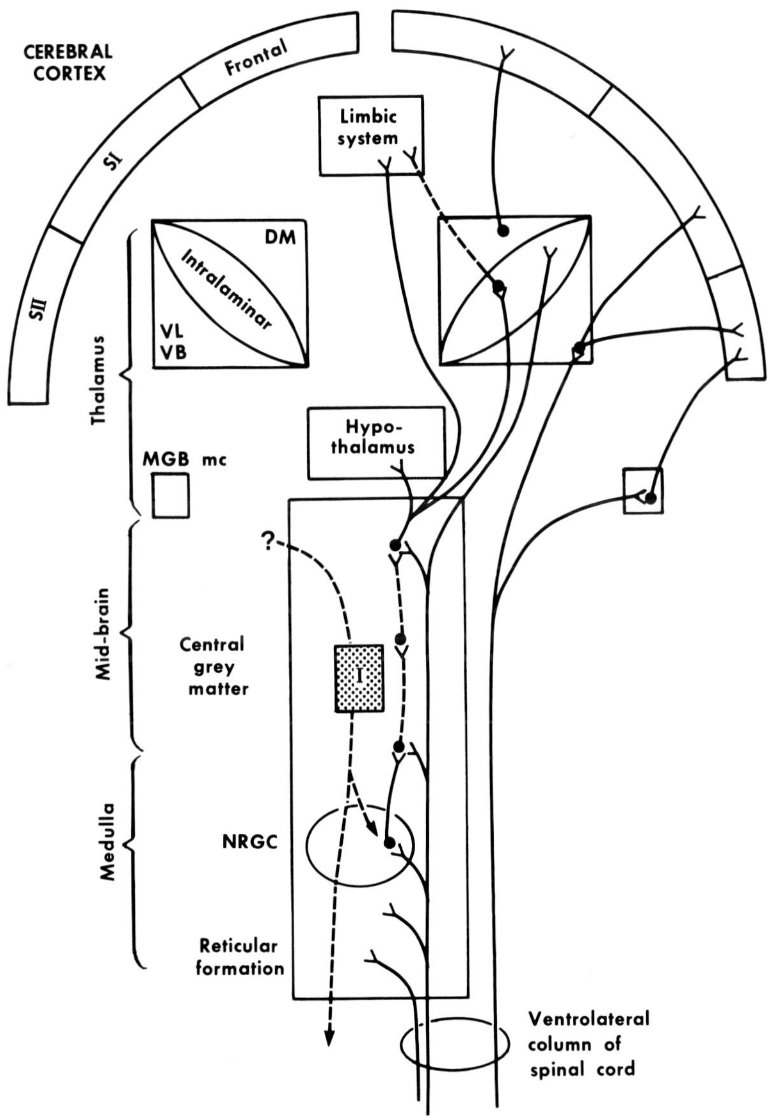

Fig. 34-3. Principal projections of ventrolateral volumn of spinal cord. For clarity, crossed pathways are not shown. *DM*, dorsomedial nucleus; *VL*, ventrolateral nucleus; *VB*, ventrobasal nucleus; *I*, midbrain inhibitory area; *MGB mc*, medial geniculate body – magnocellular portion; *NRGC*, nucleus reticularis gigantocellularis. There is considerable uncertainty about details of dashed pathways. (From Wilson, M. E.: Anaesthesia **29**:407-421, July, 1974.)

from the periphery to the brain, supraspinal descending neural systems strongly influence the synaptic transmission in the dorsal horn and along the course of the ascending somatosensory tracts.[3] The pyramidal tract, rubrospinal tract, and reticulospinal tract have been shown to inhibit firing of the cells in the dorsal horn and other parts of the spinal cord. The descending fibers from the cortex of the brain affect transmission in the thalamus, reticular formation, and dorsal column relay station. Other fibers from each of these structures descend to lower relay stations and influence their transmission.

Psychological factors play an important role in the total pain experience.[11,22] Scientific data suggest that various emotional, motivational, cognitive, and affective factors can stimulate areas of the brain which have the ability to inhibit transmission of painful impulses at the spinal cord and various other levels of the neuraxis. Paradoxically, psychological factors can enhance the transmission of noxious impulses to the brain under certain conditions and consequently increase the severity of the pain problem.

To summarize, impluses from afferent fibers are not simply transmitted to the brain by a group of spinal cord cells that are specific for each type of afferent receptor. Rather, the situation is one of convergence, interaction, and control. The gate control theory, proposed by Melzack and Wall in 1965[24] (Fig. 34-4), is one of the basic pain theories used to explain the complex anatomical and physiological mechanisms that perform this integration process. This concept of pain suggests that the substantia gelatinosa in the dorsal horn of the spinal cord functions as a gate control mechanism which increases or decreases the transmission of neural impulses from peripheral fibers to the central nervous system. The somatic input is modulated by the gate mechanism before it promotes pain perception and response. The degree of modulation by the gate is determined by the relative activity in the large (A beta) and small (A delta and C) fibers and the descending influences from the brain. The neural areas that are responsible for pain perception and responses are only activated when the flow of neural impulses through the gate exceeds a critical level.[22]

Phantom sensation

In 1551, Ambroise Paré first described the phenomenon of phantom limb sensation.[8] After the Civil War (1871), Silas Weir Mitchell[25] wrote a classic essay on his experience with phantom sensation. His observations resulted from management of ninety amputees from the 15,000 individuals who were estimated to have lost limbs during the conflict. His work pointed out that phantom sensation, with its remarkably constant subjective pattern, is almost universally a sequel of a major amputation.

The term "phantom sensation" is usually reserved for those individuals who have an awareness of the missing portion of their limb in which the only subjective sensation is mild tingling. It is rarely unpleasant; in fact, the majority of am-

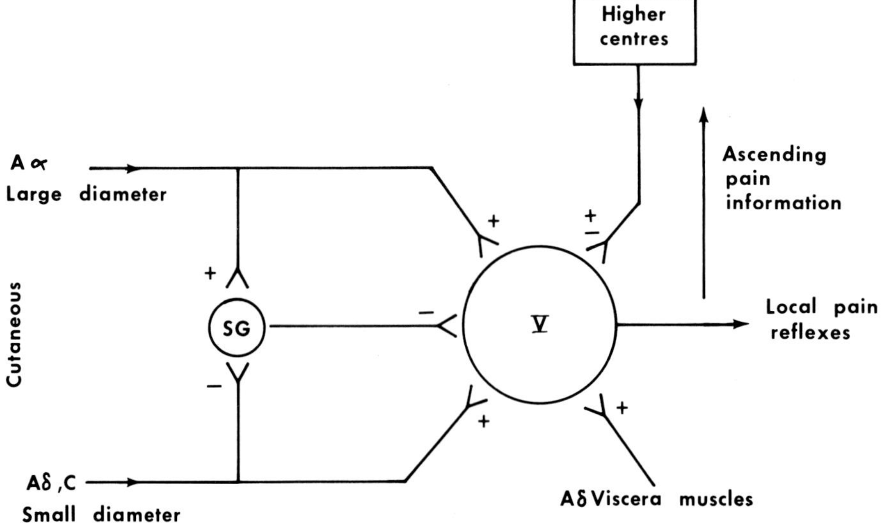

Fig. 34-4. Gate theory of pain. *SG,* substantia gelatinosa cell; *V,* central trigger cell of lamina V; +, excitatory effects; −, inhibitory effects. (From Wilson, M. E.: Anaesthesia **29**:407-421, July, 1974. Based on data from Melzack, R., and Wall, P. D.: Science **150**:971-979, 1965.)

putees describe their phantom sensations as painless. The presence of this phenomenon is usually described in terms of numbness, pressure, position, temperature, or needles and pins. These sensations seem to vary in intensity in individual patients, and the type of sensation described differs with each.

Since the phantom sensation is a painless image, no treatment is necessary. However, consultation with the patient both in advance of amputation and postoperatively is imperative for acceptance of phantom limb sensation as an expected sequel to this type of surgery. The phantom limb may change in its position and character in response to an external stimulus, such as wrapping the stump, use of a postoperative rigid dressing, or wearing a prosthetic device. Amputees should be warned that in instances of altered consciousness after the use of certain medications or arousal from a deep sleep there may be a momentary tendency to use the phantom limb for weight bearing or external support with the possibility of an associated injurious fall. Most amputees are aware of the phantom limb immediately after surgery. The pattern of the phantom sensation is usually the most distal portion of the limb, namely the hand or foot. The extent to which the more proximal segments of the ablated limb are present varies widely among individual amputees. In some patients the limb progressively shortens with telescoping of the segments proximal to the hand or foot. The duration of the sensation is a matter of years with only rare instances of complete disappearance of the phantom limb.

Phantom pain

In contrast to phantom limb sensation, the patient with phantom pain tends to fall into certain broad categories.[8,13] The three most commonly described painful sensations are (1) postural type of cramping or squeezing sensation, (2) burning pain, and (3) sharp, shooting type of pain. Many patients may complain of a mixed type of pain, but often the major sensation falls into one of these categories.

Variation in the degree of discomfrot of the phantom sensation led Feinstein[8] to suggest "that the painful state may be an accentuation or exaggeration of the type of feeling orrdinarily experienced in the painless phantom. Thus tingling or pins and needles may become a stabbing type of pain; temperature variations, a burning pain; postural or positional abnormalities, a cramping pain."[21,22,23]

Melzack has listed four major characteristics of phantom limb pain: (1) the pain endures long after healing of the injured tissues and may last for years; (2) trigger zones may spread to healthy areas, and stimulation of these zones will produce pain; (3) phantom limb pain is more likely in patients who have suffered pain in the limb for sometime; (4) phantom pain may be abolished by changes in somatic input.

The causal mechanism of phantom pain remains controversial.[32] Peripheral nerve irritation, abnormal sympathetic function, and psychological factors all contribute to the pain in some manner,[22] yet none of these mechanisms satisfactorily explains the phenomenon of phantom limb pain. Recently it has been proposed that a central biasing mechanism in which the reticular formation exerts a tonic inhibitory influence (bias) on transmission at all synaptic levels of the somatic projection system.[21,22,23] When amputation surgery destroys a large number of sensory fibers to the reticular formation, the inhibitory influence is diminished. This results in self-sustaining neural activity at all levels that can be initiated by the remaining fibers. If the self-sustaining activity reaches a critical level, pain results.

In 5% to 10% of amputees, painful sensations may occur in the phantom limb from immediately after surgery to years later. They may be episodic or continuous and are variously described as shooting, burning, cramping, or crushing. The pain is usually localized to anatomical regions of the foot or hand because of their greater cortical representation. Exacerbations of phantom pain may be triggered by seemingly innocuous stimuli such as cooling, local heat, or dependent positioning of the stump. Yawning, micturition, defecation, or coughing may suddenly precipitate more severe pain. Emotional disturbances such as anxiety, depression, sleeplessness, and emotional stress can elicit painful attacks, but are not the primary cause. In some patients pain can be stimulated by touch or pressing over sensitive areas of the stump called "trigger points." If phantom pain persists for long periods of time, the trigger zones may spread to other unrelated healthy areas of the body.

The psychological status of the amputee has a heavy impact on the course of the painful phantom.[11,28] Several studies indicate that patients with phantom pain are often individuals exhibiting psychological aberrations. Typically, this type of individual may be withdrawn, easily depressed, introspective, has a compulsive, professionistic personality, and is obviously anxious about the inability to adjust to the limb loss (Chapter 35).

Although the management of phantom pain is exceedingly frustrating, the task can be less onerous by a systematic approach to evaluation and subsequent treatment. Initially, a thorough examination of the stump is mandatory to eliminate other causes of stump pain, such as adherent scars, neuromas, bursitis, tendinitis, joint contractures, vascular insufficiency, vasomotor and sudomotor disturbances, soft tissue infection, tumors, or pathological conditions of underlying bone. A detailed workup should include selected vascular studies and appropriate radiological studies. The value of a careful psychiatric assessment cannot be overemphasized.

Simple treatment measures that create increased peripheral central input may provide at least temporary partial relief of the phantom pain. Certainly one of the more effective adjuncts to the treatment program is extensive use of the prosthesis. Other treatment modalities include gentle manipulation of the stump by massage or a vibrator, stump wrapping, baths, and application of heat with hot packs, microwaves, or ultrasound. Most of these noninvasive techniques are easily learned and can be carried out as a home treatment program without expensive equipment.

No singular drug is proven effective in long-term control of phantom pain. The use of other than mild analgetic drugs may lead to a serious drug addiction.

Specific "trigger points" on or near the stump may be injected with local anesthetic agents in combination with aqueous steroid preparations. Occasionally, prolonged relief of phantom pain is obtained. However, all too frequently pain recurs at a later date, but repeat injections of the trigger point can be performed at will with little risk or morbidity to the patient.

Amputees with generalized tender areas in the distal portion of the stump that aggravate phantom pain sometimes obtain excellent and prolonged relief with repeated injections of local anesthetic and steroid preparations.[1]

Although the sympathetic nerve system seems to contribute to phantom pain in some way, the success of sympathetic blockade in relief of agonizing phantom pain is unpredictable. At times, abnormal sympathetic manifestations such as excessive seating, vasoconstriction, decreased skin temperature, or hypersensitivity to light touch may be relieved for prolonged periods by anesthetic block of the sympathetic ganglia. Unfortunately, the phantom pain may not be affected. The greatest success with sympathetic blockade seems to occur when this type of therapy is instituted soon after the onset of pain. Since sympathetic activity is not a major cause of phantom limb pain, surgical removal of a segment of the sympathetic ganglia rarely produces lasting relief of this frustrating pain.[22]

Transcutaneous nerve stimulation has been reported as being successful in reducing phantom limb pain on a temporary basis.[1,7,19,20] Even if this technique is only partially successful, it may reduce the patient's requirement for more potent analgetic drugs. This safe and simple technique of neuromodulation is designed to diminish chronic pain through low-level stimulation of large myelinated afferent fibers. Since the equipment is portable, patients are able to treat themselves at home. The intensity of stimulation and the length of each treatment session are individualized. The combined use of transcutaneous nerve stimulation and appropriate psychotherapy may represent one of the most realistic approaches to the management of phantom pain.

Further exploitation of the inhibitory action of large myelinated afferent fibers in peripheral nerves and the dorsal columns of the spinal cord have been attempted by implantable peripheral nerve stimulators and dorsal column stimulators respectively.[9,27,35] Although both of these techniques have proven partially effective in the relief of chronic pain, they appear to be no more effective than transcutaneous nerve stimulation without the attendant potential surgical hazards.

Interruption of the anatomical pathways of somatosensory input has lead to a wide range of ineffective surgical intervention at all neuroanatomical levels.[9,18] Surgical procedures for sensory interference range from neurectomies at the periphery, rhizotomies, cordotomies, tractotomies to thalamotomies, cortical ablation, and lobotomies. In general, the long-term results of these surgical procedures have been disappointing, particularly in view of the associated complaints and risks. Surgical innervation should be approached with extreme caution, and any hasty surgical decisions should be avoided at all costs.

Phantom pain may be controlled or abolished by distraction conditioning, hypnosis, and other forms of psychotherapy. *The Minnesota Multiphasic Personality Inventory* is a useful means of evaluating the presence of depression, hypochondriasis, and other personality disorders that may be influencing the degree of phantom limb pain.

When considering the multiple treatment modalities suggested for control of phantom pain, it is quite apparent that none of these methods is highly efficacious. Therefore the treatment of every amputee afflicted with this difficult problem must be approached on an individual basis. The ultimate treatment program should consist of carefully selected treatment techniques combined with ongoing psychotherapy and counseling.

Neuromas

The development of a neuroma is a natural repair phenomenon that occurs in any transection of a peripheral nerve. During the repair phase of the nerve the axons lose their architectural parallelism and tend to turn back on themselves and combine with the fibrous repair tissue to form a small enlargement at the distal end of the nerve.

Surgeons have varied in their recommendations regarding the handling of peripheral nerves during the performance of an amputation. Some adhere strictly to gentle traction on the nerve, followed by its division with a sharp scalpel, allowing the nerve to retract several inches above the distal end of the stump. Other surgeons add a single ligature, placed slightly proximal to the transection of the nerve, to control bleeding from the nutrient vessels. They believe that the ligature per se adds little to the degree of neuroma formation. Virtually no one now advocates injection of a nerve with noxious substances such as alcohol, phenol, or radioactive isotopes.

The importance of neuroma formation is its size and location. If the neuroma is located well above the distal end of the stump and buried in adequate soft tissue, pressure and traction will not be sufficient to produce any local symptoms. Moreover, large neuromas located superficially may not be symptomatic when covered by a carefully fitted prosthetic socket. The pressure of the socket wall can be so well distributed over a large surface area of the stump that no symptoms are elicited at the neuroma site. If the prosthesis does trigger discomfort by stimulation of the neuroma, relief of the socket will generally alleviate the pain.

Injection of the neuroma site with local analgesics and steroids may alleviate the pain. Since pain relief may be only temporary, several injections may be necessary before a lasting remission is obtained.

Large neuromata buried in scar or located in an exposed position may be so symptomatic that the amputee is severely impaired. Although surgical excision is the treatment of choice, resection of neuromata has failed to yield uniform results. Commonly, relief of pain is quite transient due to the eventual development of a new neuroma. Some of these neuromas may be more easily handled by a proxomal neurectomy rather than an extensive exploration of the stump.

Encasement of the nerve stump in a microporous filter sheath (H. A. Millipore) occluded by a Silastic rod has been recommended. Not only has this technique been effective in some cases of preventing recurrent symptomatic neuromata, but has also decreased phantom limb pain in some patients as well. Similar results have been achieved producing slow atrophy of the intact nerve above the level of transection. Prolonged nerve compression is obtained by turning a Silastic rod around the nerve trunk twenty to forty times.

Reflex sympathetic dystrophy

Amputations as a result of trauma, particularly partial hand and foot amputations, may be followed by severe unremitting pain that is entirely out of proportion to the injury or the apparent state of the limb. This burning pain, originally called causalgia,[2] and its variants may be considered together as reflex sympathetic dystrophy.

The cause is thought to be an abnormal prolongation of the normal sympathetic response to injury.[2] This produces vasospasm, hyperhidrosis, and erythema. The pain impulses to the cortex are amplified, causing intense discomfort.

In the early stages the remaining dorsal portion of the limb is swollen, warm, and erythematous. There is hyperesthesia, particularly to light touch and extreme sensitivity to cold. These symptoms make wrapping and wound care extremely difficult.

After about 3 months, the swelling in the remaining digits becomes fusiform. Palmar nodules and fasciitis become evident. Fixed contractures are present because of the lack of active motion.

By 6 to 9 months after the injury, the skin is pale, cool, and dry. The joints are fixed. If pain is still a predominant feaure, it is quite likely it will be persistent indefinitely. Hopefully, this stage of the process is prevented by prior treatment.

Radiographs of the distal bones will show patchy osteopenia, particularly in periarticular areas. There is loss of bone substance, with up to one third of the inner aspect of the cortex being resorbed. If a technetium 99m Etidronate sodium (EHDP) scan is performed, it will be positive before the bone resorption is visible on plane films.

The early treatment is interruption of the abnormal sympathetic reflex. This is done by sympathetic blocks, such as a stellate ganglion block for the upper limb.[2,5] These may be repeated daily until the pain subsides.

Transcutaneous nerve stimulation has afforded pain relief for patients who have not responded to nerve block. Stilz and Carron[34] have shown an increase in cutaneous blood flow with a 1.5° to 2.5° C rise in skin temperature with this technique. Nerve stimulation should be strongly considered for those patients whose pain persists after stellate ganglion block.

Bursitis and tendinitis

Although uncommon as sources of pain in the amputee, bursitis and tendinitis must be considered in the differential diagnosis of aggravating limb pain. Localized tenderness, slight swelling with mild erythema of the overlying skin, increased localized skin temperature, and occasional soft tissue crepitation are signs of possible bursitis or tendinitis. Passive stretching of the suspected involved tendon should increase the pain significantly if tendinitis is present. Radiographs of the affected limb segment may demonstrate a calcific deposit in some cases of tendinitis.

Treatment may consist of any combination of several of the following modalities: (1) elimination of any activity that has produced overstress to the involved tendons or localized trauma to affected bursae, (2) rest through reduced use of the involved limb, (3) temporary discontinuance of the prosthesis, (4) possible rigid dressing immobilization for 14 to 21 days, (5) compression of swollen bursae by elastic wraps, (6) application of heat modalities to involved structures, (7) injection of bursae or tendon sheaths with local anesthetic agents combined with steroid preparations, (8) appropriate analgesic drugs, (9) and modification of the prosthetic socket to alleviate local pressure to the stump.

Pain not associated with an amputation

The prosthesis draws the amputee's attention to the involved limb. Thus any pain in the limb may be immediately associated in the patient's mind with the amputation and the prosthesis. This is not always the case. A large number of upper limb referred pain syndromes are entirely independent of the amputation or the prosthesis. These need to be remembered and eliminated as the cause.

Referred pain from the neck may masquerade as limb pain. This may be due to cervical disc disease or osteoarthritis and foramenal narrowing. Similarly, lumbar disc disease may produce referred pain to an amputated lower limb. The various vascular and nerve compression syndromes in the neck and axilla are occasionally the cause of pain in an amputee. Cardiac pain may be referred to the limb after an amputation as well as before.

Finally, not all pain has an organic basis. Pain on the basis of a neurotic syndrome or unresolved anxiety may persist long after the wound is healed and the physician has assumed that the patient has completed the acceptance of amputation.

EXTRINSIC CAUSES OF PAIN

Lower limbs

Syme amputation. Two common problems that arise in the management of the Syme amputee are (1) hamstring pressure when the patient is seated and (2) pain with or without associated skin breakdown over the anteriodistal portion of the stump.

The stump of some Syme amputees cannot tolerate full end bearing in the prosthesis. In such cases the proximal portion of the socket can be modified similar to a PTB socket with resultant distribution of partial weight bear proximally.[33] With faulty socket design patients may complain of soreness and pressure over the posterior aspect of the knee. Usually the patient is relatively comfortable in the upright position, but has significant discomfort when sitting with the prosthetic foot resting squarely on the floor.

Pressure on the biceps femoris and semitendinosus produce hyperemia of the skin in the area of the distal portion of these tendons. The involved skin and tendons are tender to palpation. If the pressure gradient increases, superficial skin ulceration may occur.

Lowering the posterior brim of the socket to a point just distal to the center of the patellar bar and increasing the flare of the brim are ordinarily ample to alleviate the hamstring pressure.[12]

High floor reaction forces are generated between heel-off and toe-off, and these forces must be dispersed over a large enough area of the anterior portion of the stump to prevent pain and possible skin breakdown. The anterior trim line of the socket must be placed at the level of the inferior pole of the patella to provide an adequate area of interface between the anterior stump and the front of the prosthesis.

Below-knee amputation. Common causes of prosthetic pain in the below-knee amputee are (1) excessive end bearing, (2) uneven skin pressure, (3) frictional skin loss, (4) loss of total contact, (5) hammocking phenomenon, and (6) inlet impingement. Evaluating the complaint of pain is simply a systematic process of ruling out each of these causes and then applying the appropriate solution for its correction.

Excessive end bearing. If end bearing is a source of limb discomfort, commonly specific physical signs are present on examination of the stump. Often a callus is located over the distal end of the tibia and/or fibula. Also, there may be palpable bursae over the distal end of the tibia or fibula as further evidence of end bearing.

When the prosthesis is applied, the stump descends too deeply into the socket. The addition of an appropriate number of stump socks to raise the stump from the distal portion of the socket should provide prompt symptomatic relief.

If a physical examination is inconclusive and the possibility of end bearing warrants further evaluation, other techniques will aid in the diagnosis. The simplest method is to put a small ball of clay in the bottom of the socket and ask the patient to walk. Clay that is severely compressed, is a crude indicator of excessive load bearing at the distal end of the stump.

A more informative test is the use of a Brand microcapsular stocking.[4] This system is composed of cotton fabric with a polyurethane lining into which encapsulated blue dye has been sprinkled. A stump sock is constructed from the basic material and then placed carefully over the stump. Next, the prosthesis is applied, and the patient is asked to walk. With increasing gradients of pressure, the microcapsules of dye are ruptured, and there is a color change from light yellow to various hues of green to deep blue. The use of this stocking locates any area of pressure quite precisely, but the amount of pressure is only grossly quantified.

Other careful tests include radiographs of the stump through the socket, with or without dye contrast medium injected around the stump; thermography; thermistor studies; and the use of a polycarbonate check socket. Although radiographs provide information solely in a static loading condition, they are helpful in determining the adequacy of total contact of the socket. This is particularly true if a contrast medium is injected between the interface of the stump and the socket wall.

The use of a polycarbonate check socket gives similar information but under conditions of both static and dynamic loading. A polycarbonate socket can be made from a plaster positive mold of the existing socket, and then the degree of end bearing can be analyzed by direct visualization and probing the stump surface through multiple holes drilled in the socket distally. If evidence exists of excessive loading of the distal end of the stump, a new cast should be taken of the stump from which a new below-knee prosthesis is fabricated. This can be preceded by the use of a second polycarbonate check socket to confirm total contact in the new socket.

Positive thermograms will demonstrate an increased skin temperature in the area of end bearing. Repeat thermograms after appropriate prosthetic adjustment should show a reversal of the temperature gradient toward normal at the end of the stump. Such evidence corroborates the resolution of excessive end bearing as a source of stump pain.

The most frequent reason for end bearing is a reduction in stump volume. Although this problem may be temporarily alleviated by adding more socks, there is a limit to which this solution may be used. A large number of stump socks will cause increased pressure on the stump at the inlet of the socket and may further complicate the existing problem by producing choking of the stump or skin pressure problems of the proximal stump. If the patient is using a socket liner, exterior pads may be added at various locations on the liner to compensate for the stump volume loss. Again, the benefit in regaining improved socket fit through this technique may be offset by problems produced by increased skin pressure at the level of the adjustment pads. Unless the problem is easily resolved, in the long run, it is preferable to fit the patient with a new socket.

Uneven skin pressure. A common problem produced by an ill-fitting socket is uneven distribution of skin pressure over bony prominences. Frequently, involved areas are the head of the fibula, tibial tuberosity, distal pole of the patella, and distal end of the fibula and tibia. Occasionally, the condyles of the tibia may show evidence of increased soft tissue pressure.

Fluctuating stump volume is a major cause of unequal skin pressure distribution. With reduction of stump size secondary to the loss of edema, muscle atrophy, or excessive weight loss, the intimate contact between the surface of the stump and the socket is altered. Thus the stump may shift slightly distal in the socket. Even minor distal displacement may produce forces of a higher magnitude being applied over various surface contours.

Other causes of uneven skin pressure include excessive use of stump socks, increased stump growth, and increased stump volume due to muscle hypertrophy, weight gain, or edema. On physical examination there is significant erythema of the skin overlying involved bony prominences. Although this skin has good capillary refill, the redness will persist for several minutes to several hours after removal of the socket. Even with minimal skin changes, the patient is usually very specific about areas of tenderness and can point directly to the involved area. With higher pressure gradients, the skin may have a deep violaceous color and is tender to palpation. With the use of multiple stump socks, ridges or indentations in the skin from the weave of the stump sock material may be present in areas of high pressure. In amputees who persist in walking, despite considerable discomfort, superficial skin ulceration or blistering may occur. If the skin has resisted breakdown, the area of involvement may respond by formation of a callus or corn. The distal portion of the stump may have chronic lymphedema with associated generalized rubor, both of which are secondary to choking because of the tight fit at the inlet of the socket.

When the patient dons the prosthesis, the stump may be in the socket to the proper depth, but the anteroposterior or mediolateral diameters may be very snug. Frequently, an extensive number of stump socks is being worn. The stump socks will elevate the stump from the socket with resultant loss of distal stump contact and alteration in the interface between the contours of the socket and stump surface.

The first step in evaluating this problem is checking the relative lower extremity lengths by comparing the level of the iliac crests in the standing position. If the patient is long on the prosthetic side, this may indicate that the stump is not in the socket to the proper depth. Removing a few of the stump socks might correct this misfit and substantially relieve the patient's discomfort during standing and walking.

If the patient's socket is too tight as a result of increased stump volume or limb growth, skin redness, localized tenderness, and vivid stocking marks will be present. The use of a microapsular stocking will dramatically outline the areas of increased pressure. Radiographic studies are seldom necessary in this situation, unless the examiner is concerned about the adequacy of total contact at the distal end of the stump. More precise information regarding areas of specific skin loading can be determined by use of a polycarbonate check socket.

An easy therapeutic, as well as diagnostic tool, is reduction of the thickness of the socket wall in areas of skin discoloration and pain. If the patient is comfortable in standing and walking after adjustment of the socket, the problem is both identified and resolved. If all conservative measures of socket readjustment fail, fabrication of a new total-contact socket may be the only solution.

Frictional skin loss. Superficial frictional blisters are a deterrent to prosthetic comfort and effective gait training. This phenomenon is predominantly seen in new amputees. Possible underlying pathomechanics include (1) highly localized shear forces to skin over bony prominences, (2) immature epithelium in areas of secondary healing of the surgical incision, (3) venous and lymphatic outflow is obstructed with vertical positioning of the limb, causing localized edema blebs in regions of secondary healing, or (4) presence of an extension contracture of the knee.

Physical examination reveals a superficial blister or shallow ulcer with surrounding erythema. The skin appears thin, shiny, and immature. The lesion may be surprisingly devoid of significant tenderness. However, if the condition is not recognized and treated, the lesion will increase in size and be accompanied by progressive discomfort.

Slight alteration of socket fit due to increased stump volume is a common cause of this type of skin breakdown. Among new amputees variability in stump volume from day to day is a constant hazard. Despite extensive efforts toward excellent stump compression and judicious inspection of the limb during gait training, development of a skin blister or small ulcer is likely to occur even under the supervision of an experienced prosthetic team. The transient change in socket fit is subtle, and it is sometimes difficult to detect. Consequently, the combination of increased skin compression over localized areas of the stump surface with alteration of socket fit and possible greater shear stress secondary to piston action of the socket, resulting from inadequate suspension, will produce a friction blister or ulcer.

Improper socket fabrication can create skin

breakdown. If the anteroposterior diameter of the socket is too large, during sitting the anterior wall of the socket will displace forward from the anterior surface of the stump, generating increased compression and shear forces over the anterodistal portion of the stump. This error can be compounded by inaccurate placement of the pivotal axis for the suspension straps on the mediolateral aspect of the socket. If the posterior trim line is too high, or there is an extension contracture of the knee, the stump will be levered upward from the distal end of the socket, and, again, the forces against the anterodistal stump surface are significantly increased. Provided stump volume control is not a problem, ulceration over the anterodistal surface of the stump should direct the clinician's attention to careful scrutiny of the anteroposterior diameter of the socket in the standing and sitting positions. While the patient is seated, the anterior wall of the socket can be forced backward against the front of the stump. By placing the hand inside the posterior wall of the inlet, one can determine the tightness of the anteroposterior diameter. At the same time the location of the pivot point of the suspension system should also be checked.

In the early stages of gait training recent amputees have difficulty controlling the forces against the stump by proper coordination of knee and body action.[10] If a prosthetic foot with a firm heel wedge is used, the end of the stump may be thrust forward against the anterior socket wall as the patient attempts to control the prosthesis at heel strike with active knee extension. The resultant discomfort and potentially hazardous skin pressures can be corrected by switching to a softer heel wedge, increasing plantar flexion of the foot (or extension of the socket), or moving the foot forward.[10]

The occurrence of a blister or ulcer should signal the discontinuance of the prosthesis until the lesion is healed. During this time proper stump wrapping must be done continuously. Range of motion and muscle strengthening exercises should be carried out at the knee and hip. Any design discrepancies of the socket should be corrected before the patient returns to walking. With closure of the lesion and gaining control of the stump volume, prosthetic training can be initiated with skin inspection at frequent intervals and graduated periods of stump loading until skin tolerance is achieved.

Loss of total contact. Satisfactory total contact over the distal portion of a stump is difficult to maintain when stump shrinkage or loss of weight occurs. The use of multiple stump socks to maintain a proper fit at the inlet of the socket is insufficient to regain total contact over the lower portion of the stump. The patient may complain of excessive tightness about the knee while still feeling loose in the distal portion of the socket. Subsequently, choking of the stump may occur with gradual development of lymphedema in the lower portion of the stump. Chronic edema encourages the development of stasis pigmentation and hemorrhagic papules and nodules of the distal portion of the stump. In some instances, the skin takes on a characteristic hypertrophic fissuring called verrucous hyperplasia. In individuals with vascular insufficiency, particularly those with diabetes mellitus, progressive lymphatic and venous outflow obstruction may produce a stasis ulcer at the distal end of the stump. Failure to recognize this condition and to take appropriate corrective steps will only lead to gradual worsening of the soft tissue ulceration.

The first step in the remedy of this condition is removal of the ill-fitting socket and application of appropriate topical treatment combined with continuous stump wrapping. With reestablishment of proper limb volume and healing of the stasis ulcer, a new total-contact below-knee socket should be prescribed.

Hammocking phenomenon. A somewhat uncommon, but frustrating problem, is the development of localized skin abrasion or ulceration produced by the hammocking effect of a stump sock. This peculiar problem is the result of two major factors. First, there is a lack of total contact over the distoposterior aspect of the stump. Second, because of snug anteroposterior and mediolateral diameters at the midportion of the socket, the stump sock is suspended at this level as the prosthesis is donned. Consequently, the posterior side of the stump sock is drawn tightly against the distal posterior aspect of the stump. Edema gradually develops in the lower portion of the stump with use of the prosthesis. The combined effect of the tight sock and stump edema is significantly increased compression and shear forces over the posterior flap that may produce a skin ulcer. The unusual location of this ulcer should be a clue to its possible cause. More definite proof of the cause can be obtained by radiographs through the socket and the use of a polycarbonate socket taken from the existing prosthetic socket.

A temporary solution to the problem may be obtained by altering the anteroposterior and mediolateral diameters of the socket, the use of a Daw nylon sheath, and Silastic foaming of the distal aspect of the socket. The definitive solution is refitting the amputee with a new total-contact socket with proper dimensions.

Inlet impingement. If the posterior trim line of a below-knee socket is too high posteriorly or the channels for the biceps femoris and semitendinosus tendons are inadequate, discomfort may result from pressure being applied against the hamstring tendons or the skin of the popliteal area with increased flexion of the knee. The amputee complains of tenderness and chafing of the skin behind the knee and in the region of the biceps femoris or semitendinosis tendons. The discomfort is made worse by sitting or excessive bending of the knee.

Physical examination reveals redness and chafing of the skin along the course of the involved tendon with associated point tenderness. The skin may have a superficial ulceration where the pressure is maximal. The diagnosis is self-evident by inspection of the relationship of the posterior aspect of the socket with the back of the knee and hamstring tendons as the knee is flexed. Elimination of the source of the problem can be achieved by lowering the posterior trim line or deepening the channels for the hamstring tendons.[30]

Above-knee amputations. Prosthetic causes of pain in the above-knee amputee include (1) exsessive pressure on the ischial tuberosity, (2) adductor roll, (3) choking, (4) malalignment, (5) inlet impingement, (6) excessive end bearing, (7) pressure from a high anterior wall, and (8) high medial wall. As in the below-knee amputee, one must systematically eliminate each of these problems as the cause of the patient's complaint.

Excessive pressure on the ischial tuberosity. Improper design of the ischial seat may result in significant discomfort with either standing or walking.[29] Any decrease in stump volume that allows greater distal displacement of the stump results in increased compression and shear forces over the ischial tuberosity. The patient often finds that he can obtain transient relief of his discomfort by sitting or lying down. Although if the ischial seat is too wide, even sitting may produce ischial symptoms.

Localized tenderness and skin changes ranging from hyperemia to frank skin breakdown are the hallmark of ischial seat pressure. If the increase in pressure is gradual, the involved skin will respond by forming a typical callus.

Checkout of the socket fit reveals no obvious problems except firm contact of the ischial tuberosity against the ischial seat. When the patient is asked to stand will full weight bearing on the contralateral limb and then to shift the weight gradually onto the prosthetic side, the degree of compression against an examining finger between the tuberosity and the ischial seat is obviously high. Further corroboration of ischial seat pressure can be demonstrated with the use of microcapsular stocking or thermography.

When the pressure over the tuberosity is marginal, the addition of more stump socks will elevate the stump slightly and distribute some of the load bearing to the surrounding gluteal musculature. In the case of a suction socket the prosthetist may apply a liner pad along the interior of the posterior wall that will tighten the anteroposterior diameter and accomplish the same purpose. Lowering the ischial seat or increasing its radius may produce effective results for some patients. If these simpler measures fail, a new total-contact above-knee suction should be prescribed.

Adductor roll. With improper stump wrapping, increased stump volume or unsatisfactory socket fit, a horizontal bulge of soft tissue or adductor roll may develop high on the medial aspect of an above-knee stump. The size of this roll may eventually prevent the amputee from donning the prosthesis properly. If the roll is excessive, the patient may complain of pain and tenderness along the inferior border of the roll due to impingement against the upper edge of the medial wall of the socket.

An adductor roll causes a relative lengthening of the prosthetic limb, producing a variety of gait deviations. When standing, the iliac crest on the involved side is higher than on the contralateral side. The patient may be forced to circumduct the prosthesis or vault on the opposite lower limb to clear the foot during swing phase. Or the patient may walk with the limb in abduction to reduce the medial wall pressure against the adductor roll. Palpation confirms the position of the ischial tuberosity well above the ischial seat. The adductor roll is easily felt on the inside of the stump above the brim of the medial wall.

Examination following removal of the prosthesis reveals a somewhat firm, tender roll of soft tissue with a horizontal orientation in the adductor region of the thigh. Inspection of the inferior margin of the roll may reveal considerable erythema but rarely any evidence of superficial ulceration. Often there is associated brawny edema of the distal end of the stump, with early stasis changes of the skin because of the loss of total contact distally.

A combination of correct stump wrapping with modification of the prosthetic socket is quite likely to resolve the adductor roll problem. If the roll is small, drilling a hole in the distomedial aspect of the socket and using a pull-through sock to advance the proximal stump tissues into the socket will compress the roll against the medial wall. Subsequent atrophy of the roll provides an improved socket fit. When adductor roll is extensive, it is preferable to fit the amputee with a new total-contact quadrilateral socket, anticipating the fabrication of a second socket at a later date as the proximal stump changes shape.

Choking. Constriction of the proximal portion of an above-knee stump impedes venous and lymphatic outflow from the remainder of the stump. Excessive use of stump socks, weight gain, musculoskeletal growth, and limb swelling are some of the causes of stump choking. Resultant stump abnormalities include absence of stump sock markings over the distal part of the stump, with associated palpable edema, generalized skin redness, and a possible adductor roll. If severe, the skin may show typical stasis changes that eventually lead to verrucous hyperplasia. Stasis ulceration may be a late-stage sequela, but it is rather uncommon.

Usually careful assessment of the amputee while wearing the prosthesis will suffice in elucidating the nature of the problem. Almost inevitably the stump is riding partially out of the socket. Therefore the ischial tuberosity is well above the ischial seat; the ipsilateral iliac crest is elevated, creating pelvic obliquity; and the patient walks with some type of gait deviation such as abduction of the hip, circumduction of the prosthesis, or vaulting on the intact extremity.

If confirmation of the loss of total contact is necessary, a clay ball compression test, roentgenograms through the socket, or a microcapsular stocking are helpful techniques. Seldom is a polycarbonate check socket necessary.

The resolution of choking should be approached initially by improving the socket fit by removal of unnecessary stump socks, use of a pull-through sock, improved stump wrapping, socket relief, and foaming the lower end of the socket to regain total contact. If these measures are only partially effective, the definitive solution is fabrication of a new socket.

Malalignment. In the short above-knee amputee, the degree of adduction of the lateral wall should be as much as conditions permit.[29] Also, the lateral wall must be precisely contoured to evenly distribute the socket pressures over the largest possible surface area during midstance. Despite careful socket design, the patient may complain of progressive pain and soreness over the distolateral aspect of the stump. To alleviate the concentration of forces in this area during walking, he must incline the trunk lateralward over the prosthesis to shift the weight line closer to the support line. His base of support may be widened by abduction of the hip as well.

Examination of the stump reveals no striking features except for varying degrees of skin erythema and localized tenderness in the area of increased pressure. The socket fit is nearly always satisfactory. Use of a microcapsular stocking or thermography are the most practical means to verify the increased local pressure to the stump.

Alignment adjustment through reducing the adduction of the socket and out-setting the prosthetic foot usually eliminates this problem.

Inlet impingement. An occasional source of pain in the anteromedial aspect of the above-knee stump is irritation of the upper portion of the adductor longus and gracilis muscles. This occurs when the adductors are impinged by a narrow adductor channel of the socket. Physical examination rarely demonstrates any evidence of change in the stump except for point tenderness over the adductor longus and gracilis. This finding should suggest the cause of the patient's complaints. A diagnostic, as well as treatment, method consists of routing the adductor channel to increase its size. With this relief modification the patient is frequently relieved of his pain.

Excessive end bearing. As in the below-knee amputee, the reduction of stump volume or a significant drop in body weight will change the socket fit dramatically. The stump is able to descend deeper into the socket, since all total contact with the socket surfaces has been lost. The rate and magnitude of stump volume loss determine the degree of pain and associated soft tissue changes in the distal stump. The physical findings are comparable to those of a below-knee stump, namely hyperemia of the skin with possible bursitis over the distal femur, localized soft tissue tenderness, callus formation, and occasional superficial ulceration.

Positive physical findings include (1) relative shortening of the prosthetic limb, (2) displacement of the ischial tuberosity forward and distal to the seat, and (3) gait abnormalities, consisting of a rapid swing phase with reduced stride length of the uninvolved limb and a shortened stance phase on the prosthetic side. Patients with minimal end bearing may be more accurately diagnosed by a trial of additional stump socks, a clay ball compression test, microcapsular stockings, socket radiographs, or a polycarbonate check socket. In suction sockets or sockets with openings for pull-through socks, the stump may be evaluated both visually and manually.

The addition of more stump socks may be the only treatment required in amputees with mild end bearing. Relief of the distal end of the socket and lining the socket to decrease the anteroposterior and mediolateral diameters may suffice in moderate cases. In more advanced circumstances the best remedy is fabrication of a new total-contact quadrilateral socket.

Any associated skin ulceration can be treated with appropriate topical care and stump wrapping. The underlying bursitis often responds to the relief of socket pressure and stump wrapping. Aspiration combined with injection of a local anesthetic agent and a corticosteroid preparation administered under sterile technique will often eradicate a more persistent bursitis that has failed to respond to noninvasive treatment. In the small number of amputees who are greatly disabled by chronic bursitis, surgical excision may be necessary.

Pressure from a high anterior wall. The purpose of the anterior brim of the socket is to maintain the ischium in proper relationship to the ischial seat to prevent discomfort with ischial weight bearing. This is accomplished by building the anterior brim 5 to 6.5 cm (2 to 2½ inches) higher than the ischial seat, flaring the margin of the brim generously and bulging the inner wall of the brim in the area of Scarpa's triangle. Ordinarily, the high front does not interfere with sitting or bending over, provided there is no contact with bony prominences of the pelvis, and a channel is provided for the rectus femoris muscle. However, an obese above-knee amputee with a protuberant abdomen or massive panniculus may experience pinching of lower abdominal soft tissues with sitting or bending over. It is rare to have any difficulty with standing or walking.

Customarily, the socket fits well otherwise. When the patient sits or leans forward, palpation demonstrates high compression against the lower abdominal tissues. With the prosthesis removed, the only localizing signs are erythema of the skin, varying degrees of tenderness in the areas of pressure, and occasional small hemorrhagic lesions secondary to contusion of the skin. Judicious lowering of the anterior wall and increasing the flare of the brim usually provide prompt relief.

High medial wall. In a properly fitted quadrilateral socket essentially no weight should be borne by the medial wall. The upper third of the medial wall should be flattened and the superior brim flared to prevent skin irritation. Although the medial wall should be as high as tolerated, it is usually 0.3 to 0.6 cm (⅛ to ¼ inch) lower than the ischial seat. With pelvic tilt, excessive adduction of the socket or too much length of the medial wall, the amputee will develop pain and tenderness in the region of the origin of the adductor muscles as well as along the pubic ramus. The patient compensates for these changes while walking by maintaining a wide base of support by abduction of the hip during both stance and swing phase. Relief is provided by lowering the medial wall and flaring the superior brim.

Summary

The major prosthetic causes of pain in the lower limb are volumetric changes, malalignment, and inlet impingement. Comparison and contrast are best summarized in Table 8.

Upper limbs

Partial hand devices. Strict adherence to the surgical dogma of preserving all possible segments of an injured hand may result in chronic pain compounded by significant functional problems. For example, digits afflicted with posttraumatic vasomotor changes secondary to altered sympathetic innervation can be detrimental to

Table 8. Major Causes of pain in lower limb levels

	Presenting signs	
Problem	*Above-knee*	*Below-knee*
Volume (increased)	Adductor roll	Skin blistering or superficial ulceration
	Choking	Loss of distal total contact
Volume (decreased)	Ischial seat pressure End bearing	End bearing
Malalignment	Skin pressures of distolateral stump	Skin pressures of anterior stump
Inlet impingement	Adductor muscle tenderness	Biceps femoris or semitendinosis compression

patients because of episodic pain associated with increased cold sensitivity. Should reflex sympathetic dystrophy or causalgia develop, the recovery of hand usefulness is obstructed, and the difficulty of fitting the patient with an appropriate orthotic or prosthetic device is definitely magnified. Massive damage to joints and their related tendons may virtually assure extensive permanent functional loss and pain, when associated vascular and neurological recovery of the hand is marginal at best. Unfortunately, insufficient venous and lymphatic drainage creates chronic swelling of the hand, adding another factor that enhances hand impairment. Worse yet, poor skin coverage and diminished epicritical sensation further complicate functional retraining of an injured hand with or without a special device.

To maximize the rehabilitation process of an injured hand, critical decisions regarding the preservation of those segments of the hand which have a reasonable likelihood of regaining nonpainful, useful function must be made by the attending surgeon during initial treatment. If the patient fails to make satisfactory progress during the rehabilitative period, consideration should be given to secondary reconstructive surgery that would convert the patient to a higher functional amputation. Removal of part or all of a painful, functionless hand with subsequent replacement by a well-designed prosthesis is welcomed by most patients.

In general, partial hand prostheses have neither satisfied the cosmetic or functional needs of the hand amputee. Faulty design, poor material properties (weight, thermal conductivity, surface friction characteristics, strength, durability, etc.), inadequate device suspension, reduction of sensory feedback, and possible restriction of proximal joint motion are only a few of the reasons for prosthetic failure.

If, after prosthetic fitting, the patient with a hand amputation complains of discomfort, every effort should be directed toward evaluation and elimination of all potential pain sources. Assessment of the adequacy of skin coverage is simple but absolutely essential. Tethered, noncompliant scar is unyielding to shear forces that produce definite skin tenderness and discomfort with possible associated skin breakdown. Careful inspection and palpation of the involved hand provide sufficient information to estimate the probable skin tolerance to compression and shear stress from a proposed prosthetic device. If it is questionable whether the skin can tolerate such forces directly, the device should be lined with Plastazote, Pelite, polyurethrane, or comparable materials that will protect the damaged skin surfaces.

The painful hand with increased cold sensitivity often manifests coolness, cyanosis, edema, and excessive sweating. These vasomotor and sudomotor disturbances are similar to those of sympathetic reflex dystrophy. Characteristic signs of Raynaud's phenomenon may be elicited by exposure of the hand to a cold environment. These amputees should be instructed to avoid any exposure of the hand to environmental temperatures below 10° C without an insulated glove. Furthermore, all partial hand devices used in a cold environment should be constructed of material with poor thermal conductivity and lined with a synthetic substance with excellent insulation properties.

Wrist disarticulation. Almost without exception the major reason for pain in individuals wearing a wrist disarticulation prosthesis is irritation of the soft tissue over the ulnar and radial styloid processes. With any reduction of total contact in the region of the distal radioulnar joint, the distal end of the stump tends to rotate independently of the prosthetic wall during pronation and supination of the forearm. The torsion of the prosthesis creates a high shear force across the skin in the region of the radial and ulnar styloid processes. In addition to localized pain, repetition of these forces across the involved skin produces reactive hyperemia, localized soft tissue tenderness, and possible skin ulceration.

Detection of the source of pain and irritation is often a simple matter of careful inspection of the distal end of the amputation stump. If localizing signs are scant, the use of a microcapsular stocking may demonstrate increased localized pressure in the resgion of the ulnar and radial styloids. Seldom is it necessary to resort to radiographs through the socket, polycarbonate check socket, or thermogram.

Foaming of the distal end of the socket with Silastic to regain satisfactory total contact is usually adequate in relieving this problem. If the volumetric loss of stump is high, it is preferable to fabricate a new wrist disarticulation socket. When the problem may be the result of increased soft tissue edema or a tight distal socket, relief in the area of skin pressure provides an easy solution.

In those few patients with chronic skin problems despite frequent adjustments and redesigning of the wrist disarticulation socket, surgical revision of the stump may be necessary. In the presence of adequate skin flaps, resection of prominent ulnar or radial styloids can be accomplished without the loss of important radioulnar joint motion, which is critical to the preservation of forearm pronation and supination.

Below-elbow amputation. Three frequent causes of pain in the below-elbow prosthetic wearer are (1) pressure over the anterodistal end of the stump, (2) choking of the stump, and (3) inlet impingement.

Amputees with acquired short below-elbow stumps are vulnerable to high compression and shear forces across the anterodistal aspect of the stump when lifing heavy loads with the elbow in a flexed position. Conditions are only made worse by (1) poor total contact of the socket distally as a result of stump shrinkage, (2) inadequate soft tissue coverage over the distal end of the radius and ulna, and (3) osteophyte formation or appositional bone growth of the forearm bones.

Whatever the cause, the symptoms and signs are similar—localized stump pain, tenderness of the distal stump, reactive hyperemia of the skin, possible presence of an underlying bursa, and occasionally a skin ulcer. A lack of total contact may result in edema and induration of the distal portion of the stump as well.

Careful inspection of the stump localizes the area of increased skin pressure. With the artificial limb applied, strong resistance during elbow flexion will usually produce discomfort at the distal end of the stump. Seldom is it necessary to use a microcapsular stocking, socket radiographs, or thermography to determine the nature of the patient's complaints. Roentgenograms of the stump are valuable, however, in the detection of offending osteophytes or excessive appositional bone growth in the juvenile amputee.

Treatment should be directed initially toward healing the skin ulceration and reduction of stump edema if present. Next, socket relief distally or foaming the end of the socket with Silastic may eliminate skin pressure. In certain patients, a new total-contact socket is required.

The juvenile amputee is faced with periodic loss of socket fit as a result of musculoskeletal growth. With increased circumference and length of the stump, the socket is too small to accept the entire stump. As a result, increased forces over the distal end of the stump create painful pressure symptoms that reduce the functional efficiency of the amputee. Recognition of an improper socket necessitates replacement with a properly fitted one.

Below-elbow amputees with stump soreness will often increase the number of stump socks to relieve pressure against the end of the stump. This leads to elevation of the distal portion of the stump from the end of the socket and obstructs venous and lymphatic outflow from the stump because of constriction of the proximal portion of the stump. The resultant choking of the stump is painful and may produce skin changes of the distal end of the stump.

Inspection of the stump reveals an absence of sock markings over the distal portion of the stump. The lower portion of the stump is swollen and tender. There may be generalized reactive hyperemia of the skin of the stump. The proximal portion of the stump may have stump sock indentations, indicating increased skin pressures. With the prosthesis donned the olecranon lies above the trim line of the posterior aspect of the socket, indicating a loss of socket fit.

Removal of some of the stump socks will often achieve an improved fit of the socket. If edema prevents continued use of the socket, it may be necessary to resort to continuous wrapping for a few days. With elimination of the edema of the stump, satisfactory total contact and stump protection can be obtained by foaming the socket with Silastic. If a tight inlet is responsible for choking the stump, routing the socket walls will aid in opening the inlet.

A Muenster socket may produce impingement of the humeral condyles or the olecranon during the application of a vertical traction force with the elbow flexed to 90 degrees or with the elbow in maximum extension. Since this type of socket must be designed with restriction of complete extension of the elbow to maintain adequate suspension, excessive traction in the extended position would be expected to produce some discomfort over the humeral condyles or olecranon with high axial loads. However, some amputees find that with active flexion of their elbow they feel pressure over these bony prominences. This leads to localized pain and skin changes that usually can be corrected by socket relief or alteration of trim lines without sacrificing good socket suspension. Failure to diminish elbow impingement by means of socket adjustments dictates fabrication of a new socket in greater extension.

Above-elbow amputation. As in the below-elbow prosthesis wearer, the magnitude of forces applied to the anterodistal aspect of the above-elbow stump is significantly increased with progressive loading of the prosthesis. If the stump is quite short, total contact is poor, or soft tissue coverage of the stump is less than optimal, the symptoms and physical findings of the involved stump are identical with high soft tissue forces over any bony prominence. Careful physical examination is usually adequate to identify the cause of the problem. If necessary, confirmatory tests with a microcapsular stocking, thermography, or radiographic studies can be performed. Prosthetic solutions include relief of the distal portion of the socket, foaming of the distal end of the socket to regain total contact, or fabrication of a new socket. Stump revision may be required in the presence of poor skin coverage, bony overgrowth of the humerus, or extreme soft tissue redundancy.

In the short above-elbow amputation, the anteroposterior walls of the socket must be extended medially over a large portion of the shoulder joint to provide rotational stability. Excessive tightness of the anteroposterior diameter of the medial portion of the inlet will produce pressure against the skin along the edges of the socket brim. Altering the trim lines, heating and rolling the brim edges, or increasing the anterposterior diameter of the inlet will eliminate the pressure problem.

Children with acquired above-elbow amputations are plagued by troublesome appositional bone growth of the humerus. The gradual lengthening of the humerus compresses the skin over the distal end of the bone against the bottom of the socket. Associated pain when wearing the prosthesis interferes with its optimal use. Soon skin changes appear and may be accompanied by a swollen bursa over the end of the bone. As discomfort increases, the child periodically removes the prosthesis or refuses to wear it at all.

Early in the evolution of the problem, removal of an existing socket liner and/or deepening of the end of the socket will provide temporary help. However, with further bony overgrowth, the amount of stump change exceeds the improvement obtained with socket adjustments. Now the treatment of choice is surgical revision of the stump, which includes excision of the bony overgrowth and removal of any bursa. Since appositional bone growth is unrelated to epiphyseal growth, epiphysiodesis is absolutely contraindicated. This condition tends to recur periodically so that the child is likely to have several surgical procedures until reaching skeletal maturity when general bone growth ceases. A Silastic bone plug has been recommended to prevent recurrence of appositional bone growth. However, its use has not been widespread.

Shoulder disarticulation. Achievement of proper prosthetic suspension and total-contact fit of the socket is difficult in the shoulder disarticulation amputee. The weight of the prosthesis tends to create a downward displacement and rotation over the acromion. Combined high compression and shear forces generated over the tip of the acromion cause localized pain and concomitant skin changes. Lining the involved portion of the socket wall with Plastazote, Pelite, or similar synthetic materials distributes the forces over a larger skin surface area, thus making the soft tissue pressure tolerable. Adjustment or redesigning the suspension system will also reduce the rotary action of the socket.

Meticulous socket design usually minimizes soft tissue pressure problems over the anteroposterior aspect of the shoulder girdle. Subsequent alterations of tissue forces as a result of soft tissue shrinkage, edema, or musculoskeletal growth can be managed by socket relief, socket lining, or increased socket dimensions by routing the socket wall.

Forequarter amputation. Most of the discomfort associated with fitting a forequarter prosthesis is caused by uneven distribution of soft tissue pressure. Suspension problems with this type of prosthesis are immense, and contouring the socket wall to accommodate uneven bony prominences and bulky soft tissues is most difficult. The use of the lightest possible prosthetic components minimizes the downward displacement of the device. Lining the socket wall with compliant synthetic materials improves soft tissue pressure distribution. Usually adjustments of the trim lines, periodic checking of socket contact with the thoracic wall, base of the neck, and opposite shoulder region, and alteration of the suspension system will prevent considerable prosthetic discomfort.

REFERENCES

1. Blankenbaker, W. L.: The care of patients with phantom limb pain in a pain clinic, Anesth. Analg. **56**(6):842-846, Nov.-Dec., 1977.
2. Bonica, J. J.: Causalgia and other reflex sympathetic dystrophies. Postgrad. Med. J. **53**:143-148, May, 1976.
3. Bonica, J. J.: Neurophysiologic and pathologic aspect of acute and chronic pain, Arch. Surg. **112**(6):750-761, June, 1977.

4. Brand, P. W., and Ebner, J. D.: Pressure sensitive devices for denervated hands and feet, J. Bone Joint Surg. **51A**(1): 109-116, Jan., 1969.
5. Carron, H., and Weller, R. M.: Treatment of post traumatic sympathetic dystrophy. In Bonica, J. J., editor: Advances in neurology, vol. 4, Pain, New York, 1974, Raven Press.
6. Casey, K. L.: Pain: a current view of neural mechanisms, Am. Sci. **61**:194-200, March-April, 1973.
7. Ersek, R. A.: Transcutaneous electrical neurostimulation: a new clinical modality for controlling pain, Clin. Orthop. **128**:314-324, Oct., 1977.
8. Feinstein, B., Luce, J. C., and Langton, J. N. K.: The influence of phantom limbs. In Klopsteg, P. E., and Wilson, P. D., editors: Human limbs and their substitutes, New York, 1954, McGraw-Hill, Inc., pp. 79-138.
9. Ferguson, J. P. et al.: Neurosurgical management of intractable pain, N. C. Med. J. **34**:707-710, Sept., 1973.
10. Foort, J.: The patellar-tendon-bearing prosthesis for below knee amputees: a Review of technique and criteria, Artif. Limbs **9**:4-13, 1965.
11. Frazier, S. H. et al.: Psychiatric aspects of pain and the phantom limb. Orthop. Clin. North Am. **1**:481-495, Nov., 1970.
12. Hampton, F. L.: Prosthetic principles in the lower extremity amputee, Orthop. Clin. North Am. **3**:339-347, July, 1972.
13. Henderson, W. R., and Smyth, G. E.: Phantom limbs, J. Neurol. Neurosurg. Psychiatry **11**:88-112, May, 1948.
14. Iggo, A.: The case for "pain" receptors. In Tanzen, R., Keide, W. D., Herz, A., Steichele, C., Payne, J. P., and Burt, R. A. D., editors: Pain, Baltimore, 1972, The Williams & Willkins Co., pp. 60-61.
15. Iggo, A.: Pain receptors. In Bonica, J. J., Procacci, P., and Pugni, C. A., editors: Recent advances on pain: pathophysiology and clinical aspects, Springfield, Ill., 1972. Charles C Thomas, Publisher.
16. Kerr, F. W. L.: Segmental circuitry and spinal cord nociceptive mechanisms. In Bonica, J. J., and Albe-Fessard, D., editors: Advances in Pain Research and Therapy, vol. 1, New York, 1976, Raven Press, pp. 75-89.
17. Lim, R. K. S.: Neuropharmacology of pain and analgesia. In Lim, R. K. S., Armstrong, D., and Pardo, E. G., editors: Pharmacology of pain, vol. 9, New York, 1968, Pergamon Press, Inc., pp. 169-217.
18. Loeser, J. D.: Neurosurgical relief of chronic pain, Postgrad. Med. J. **53**:115-119, May, 1973.
19. Loeser, J. D. et al.: Relief of pain by transcutaneous stimulation, J. Neurosurg. **43**(3):308-314, March, 1975.
20. Long, D. M.: External electrical stimulation, Minn. Med. **57**:195-198, March, 1974.
21. Melzack, R.: Phantom limb pain: implications for treatment of pathologic pain, Anesthesiology **35**:409-419, Oct., 1971.
22. Melzack, R.: The puzzle of pain, New York, 1973, Basic Books, Inc., Publishers.
23. Melzack, R.: Central neural mechanisms in phantom limb pain. In Bonica, J. J., editor: Advances in neurology, vol. 4, Pain, New York, 1974, Raven Press, pp. 319-326.
24. Melzack, R., and Wall, P. D.: Pain mechanism: a new theory, Science **150**:971-979, Nov., 1965.
25. Mitchell, S. W.: Phantom limbs, Lippincott's Mag. **8**:563, 1871.
26. Nathan, P. W.: Pain, Br. Med. Bull. **33**(2):149-155, May, 1977.
27. Nielson, K. D. et al.: Pahntom limb pain. Treatment with dorsal column stimulation, J. Neurosurg. **43**(3):301-307, March, 1975.
28. Parkes, C. M.: Factors determining the persistence of phantom pain in the amputee, J. Pschosom. Res. **17**:97-108, March, 1973.
29. Radcliffe, C. W.: Functional considerations in the fitting of above knee prostheses, Artif. Limbs **2**:35-60, 1955.
30. Radcliffe, C. W., and Foort, J.: The patellar-tendon below knee prosthesis manual, Berkley, Calif., 1961, University of Califnroia, Biomechanics Laboratory, Department of Engineering.
31. Rexed, B.: The cytoarchitecture organization of the spinal cord of the cat, J. Comp. Neurol. **96**:415-496, 1952.
32. Riding, J.: Phantom limb: some theories, Anesthesia **31**(1):102-106, Jan.-Feb., 1976.
33. Sinclair, W. F.: Below the knee and Syme's amputation prostheses, Orthop. Clin. North Am. **3**:349-357, July, 1972.
34. Stilz, R. J., Carron, H., and Sanders, D. B.: Reflex sympathetic dystrophy in a 6-year-old: successful treatment by transcutaneous nerve stimulation, Anesth. Analg. **56**(3): 438-443, May-June, 1977.
35. Sweet, W. H. et al.: Stimulation of the posterior columns of the spinal cord for pain control: indications, techniques and results, Clin. Neurosurg. **21**(0):278-310, 1974.
36. Wall, P. D.: Physiological mechanisms involved in the production and relief of pain. In Bonica, J. J. Procacci, P., and Pagni, C. A., editors: Recent acvances on pain: pathophysiology and clinical aspects, Springfield, Ill., 1974, Charles C Thomas, Publisher, pp. 36-63.
37. Webster, K. E.: Somesthetic pathways, Br. Med. Bull. **33**: 113-120, May, 1977.
38. Whidden, A., and Fiddler, M. R.: Pathophysiology of pain, In Jacox, A. K., editor: Pain: a source book for nurses and other health professions, Boston, 1977, Little, Brown, & Co., pp. 27-56.
39. Wilson, M. E.: The neurological mechanisms of pain. A review, Anaesthesia **29**:407-421, July, 1974.

CHAPTER 35

Management of psychological problems

CHARLES A. HOFMANN
WILTON H. BUNCH
JOANNE SIMON KESTNBAUM

Every amputee clinic has its unhappy patient. Nothing is right in his eyes. The physician is brusque and never explains anything, the prosthesis is unsightly and hurts, and the prosthetist is a money-grubbing entrepreneur. The physical therapist is not helpful, the clinic nurse is rude, and the social worker asks questions that are none of her business. One wonders how this individual can identify so many errors when the rest of the patients are satisfied or even grateful.

It requires little insight or imagination to realize that the problem is not with the clinic team but with the individual. However, it requires a great deal of patience to deal with this person and help him accept his loss and proceed with living.

The purpose of this chapter is to discuss the psychological reactions that accompany the loss of a limb and the resultant disturbance of self-image. If the personnel of the clinic team appreciate the psychological loss, as well as physical loss, they can offer additional support to the patient and positively influence the treatment plan.

PREOPERATIVE PERIOD

In any consideration of managing psychological problems of the amputee it is important to remember that the process of adjustment to loss begins before the operation. The time immediately prior to the operation, the postoperative period, and subsequent life are three major areas of uncertainty and stress for the patient. Adequate preparation by medical attendants before surgery can, to some extent, avert some of the fear and uncertainty.

The surgeon, anesthetist, and medical staff can do much to ensure that the patient understands why surgery is necessary and what the operation entails. Medical personnel must, however, keep in mind that patients vary greatly in their ability to understand such matters, and indeed, some seem to prefer not to be told too much about the technical aspects of their case. Psychologically, the wish to be kept in ignorance is sometimes a defense against overwhelming fears of the fantasied situation.

That communication between medical personnel and the patient can be effective, a good empathic relationship with the patient is necessary. Such relationships can be established only if the medical personnel is willing to spend some time getting to know the patient before the operation.

Egbert et al.[3] and Lazarus and Hagens[13] have clearly demonstrated the positive value of preoperative preparation in promoting postoperative recovery. Preoperative preparation should include the following:

1. An adequate explanation of why the operation was necessary.

2. An explanation, in simple terms, of what the operation entails.
3. A prediction of how the patient can expect to feel after the operation; this should include a description of phantom reactions and stump pain.
4. Instruction about pain. In addition to being instructed to tell the nurse when he is in pain, the patient may be able to be taught to help himself by means of relaxation exercises. Aside from whatever their effect might be on the local lesion, the relaxation exercise will give the patient the feeling that he is contributing to his own recovery.
5. Reassurance that the pain will pass.
6. An introduction to and explanation of prosthetic services.
7. Realistic information regarding the probable effect of the operation on working life and other functions.

Parkes and Napier[20] state that there is some evidence to suggest that efficient prevention of pain before and after surgery may minimize the risk of persisting postoperative pain in the phantom limb. They note that in this, as in other situations, it is easier to prevent pain by the proper use of analgesic drugs in small, regular dosages, than to relieve pains that have become established.

It is also important during the preoperative period for members of the medical team to get to know the principal family members of the patient, so that their needs might become known and their potentialities as allies in the rehabilitation process might be used.

POSTOPERATIVE PERIOD

Personal grief – acquired amputation

Grief is the universal reaction precipitated by the loss of a limb.[20] Various authors choose differing words but all support this position. Wittkower[24] states that "Mourning is the normal reaction." Fisher[5] writes that "The reaction to loss of a limb, and for that matter the loss of function of a vital part, is grief and depression." According to Dembo,[2] "A person may mourn his loss because the personal satisfaction which the object of loss gave him in the past is denied him!" Kessler[11] suggests that "The emotional investment persons feel when told that they must lose a limb can be compared with the emotion of grief at the death of a loved one."

Grief can be considered to take a definite, predictable course. The events may be divided into those of the acute immediate impact, the recall, and finally the reconstruction or psychological rehabilitation. It is the immediate impact or acute grief that is the most obvious.

Lindemann,[14] in his classic paper on the symptoms and management of acute grief, noted that acute grief is a definite syndrome which has both somatic and psychological components. He described three classes of symptoms that he thought were pathognomonic for the acute grief reaction. These are somatic reactions, emotional reactions, and behavioral reactions. Somatic distress includes anxiety, tension, increased awareness, weight loss, and sleep disturbances. Emotional reactions include fear, guilt, anger, and withdrawal, as well as a tendency to preoccupation with themselves and thus emotional distancing from others. Changes in behavior that are pathognomonic for the grief reaction are mental and motor retardation or excitation, an unwillingness to initiate activity, lack of motivation, and/or dependency on others.

It must be understood that all grief reactions are not the same, and each individual reaction is conditioned by the basic personality type. A stoic individual may show little. A person who has a basically hysterical personality will continue to have this personality throughout and after the grief reaction.

Parkes[18,19,20] studied the similarities between the grief reactions in amputees and the grief reactions in the recently widowed. For both groups the grief process is one of accepting the loss and giving up hope of retrieving the lost object. Just as a wife may initially experience shock, numbness, and disbelief when she loses her husband, the amputee will experience similar reactions on loss of a limb. The amputee commonly denies the significance of the handicap or illness. Prior to surgery, he may even deny amputation as a possibility. Following amputation, the patient may refuse to look at the stump, and many amputees report an initial feeling of numbness and persistence of the lost limb.

Somatic complaints and anxiety are not unusual in both the bereaved person and the amputee. Both experience a sense of helplessness, the amputee because of the physical disability, the widow due to the loss of her husband. Each may have a sense of vulnerability and fear of loss of physical and financial support. Both may be faced with learning new vocational skills and with assuming new or different responsibilities.

Both the bereaved individual and the amputee may react with anger and/or guilt in their grieving process. Frequently the anger is directed at the caretaker or anyone who attempts to make the individual accept his loss. It is this individual who is described in the opening paragraph of the chapter. Guilt is frequently present at the death of a loved one; it may also be present in amputees. The amputee, like the bereaved person, must deal with the feeling of internal loss. The sense of loss varies depending on the amputated part and its psychological significance. The amputee may be forced to change professions; he may become dependent or infantilized; he may see himself as less competent.

Changes in behavior and depression are common in the loss of a loved person, as well as loss of a limb.[20] The amputee tends to feel sorry for himself and jealous of others who have not suffered the way he has. He also often blames himself for acts of omission that might have contributed to the loss or for his reaction to it. The psychotherapeutic task during the acute grief phase is realization and acceptance of the loss. Only after these have been accomplished will the amputee be able to reorder his life, regain self-esteem, and return to an active life. As with the widow, only if grieving is prolonged or distorted should the patient's response be considered pathological.

After acute grief has subsided there is a period of putting the past life into memory. In the phase of recall it is acceptable to talk about the loss and even joke about it but only in terms of the past. Parkes[19] notes that both widows and amputees may be preoccupied with an image of the lost object or with an urge to search for a new way of coping with the loss.

In general, all people try to give meaning to every event in their lives. In loss of a spouse or limb the search is for the meaning of the loss. "Why did this happen to me?" As in the acute phase, this may produce many variations and widely differing answers. Newton[16] reported on three widows whose husbands were simultaneously killed in a small plane crash. Despite their closeness before the loss and their obvious identical involvement in the loss, their searching took vastly different courses. Similarly, the amputees will approach the question in widely differing ways.

Finally, both the widow and the amputee reconstruct the shattered life. Lindemann[14] suggests that the sequence of "grief work" is that process by which the bereaved individual frees himself "from the bondage of the deceased." The usual course of a grief reaction is one of a gradual adjusting to the reality in which the deceased is missing. The final state consists in the formation of new relationships and patterns of interaction that are satisfying and rewarding. The amputee still has much work remaining. He will have to make adjustments, at times radical, in his lifestyle so as to cope with various problems engendered by amputation. The problems are, indeed, multiple: psychological, physical, social, vocational, and recreational.

With regard to treatment, Pasnau and Pfefferbaum[21] maintain that in both the ubiquitous acute response and the occasional chronic pathological response, the nursing staff may be very helpful. They suggest that mental health professionals should be consulted to provide psychological support and education to the nursing and medical personnel directly involved with the patient. Only with more resistant pathological responses should mental health professionals be called on to provide direct support and/or treatment for the patients and their families. They expect that nursing and medical staff can deal with the majority of grief responses to amputation provided they have ready access to mental health professionals for support when needed.

Friedmann[7] agrees and thinks that deep psychic intervention is rarely needed, provided there is a well-trained staff willing and able to give proper guidance to the patient. He notes that there are indeed patients who need active psychiatric care by someone experienced in the care of amputees and the reactions to amputation. These patients are usually older, withdrawn individuals, frequently from the lower socioeconomic and educational strata. They usually become more depressed, irritable, and aggressive; they sometimes drown in a sea of self-pity.

To summarize, a grief reaction to the loss of a limb is to be expected. It may take any number of forms. It may be extreme, apparently absent, or distorted. The response might be expected to be more prolonged in the amputee than in the widow. The widow buries her loss and frequently remarries. The amputee, however, after the acute crisis is resolved, must learn to live with a daily reminder of the assault to his emotional and physical well-being.

Parental grief – congenital limb-deficient child

To effectively understand the parents of a defective child, a brief consideration of two processes is imperative[8]: (1) the psychological preparation that one goes through prior to giving birth, and (2) the concept of narcissism.

Assume that the woman wants to be pregnant. The long wait, labor, and finally delivery give the mother time for psychological "sorting out" of adolescent ambivalences and adjustment to the adult acceptance and nurturing of a new individual. During this time she composes an image of the expected child and builds a composite picture that includes herself and significant love objects (mother, father, husband, and siblings). In this phase she mentally constructs the child in the image her mother conveyed to her, thus allowing for the emergence of old issues, conflicts,and fears that she had with her own mother. This recalling and review is a normal part of pregnancy. The adjustment to motherhood starts with this process, continues after birth, and can be seen through the interactions between mother and child. The mother anticipates much during her 9-month wait. She wishes for a perfect child. She fears a defective child.

> It is very likely that there is always some discrepancy between the mother's wishes and the actual child; to work out this discrepancy becomes one of the developmental tasks of motherhood that is involved in the establishment of a healthy mother-child relationship. However, when the discrepancy is too great, as in the birth of a defective child or where the mother's wishes are too unrealistic, a trauma may occur.[23]

This trauma is best characterized by the mother's feelings of incredible disappointment, helplessness, and sense of failure at bearing a blighted child. The feelings are evoked because the mother has suffered what is termed a "narcissistic injury."

In this context narcissism simply means the concentration of psychic energy on the self. A narcissistic injury, then, is a blow to one's sense of omnipotence and self-esteem. Because of this, the mother's previously developing ability to accept and nurture this totally dependent being may be diminished or halted.[5]

One extreme reaction is increasing dedication to the welfare of the infant to the detriment and often neglect of the rest of the family. This will be explored further. Another reaction is abhorrence and the urge to deny the relationship to the child. This relates directly to the blow to both parent's self-esteem. The narcissistic injury is intolerable.

The two reactions just described are the extremes. The majority of parents suffer from universal reactions of grief and anger, but inevitably through a series of successive adjustment phases, they learn to accept. Parents must (1) experience a period of grief, (2) acknowledge and learn to manage their anger, (3) deal with the anxieties stirred up by the impact of the child's handicap on their ordinary adaptive patterns, and (4) make certain adjustments in their manner of living that will affect the handicapped child and the family as a whole.[1]

Let us explore these four stages of acceptance. A radical change from what has been expected or the occurrence of what has previously never been considered usually elicits shock. Parents who have hoped for and expected a normal infant, and suddenly do not have one, experience shock. This moves into a period of grief in their search for the "why" of the occurrence. Guilt creeps in as the mother blames herself for inadequate prenatal care. Both parents seek to rid themselves of this misfortune through this mental search. Just as in the process of death and dying in which they mourn the total loss of a loved one, parents seek to deny the misfortune.

If parents are not aided or if parents have suffered much in the way of narcissistic injury throughout their childhoods, then fixation at this first stage is highly possible. During this phase parents do much shopping around for second opinions and seemingly do not "hear" the diagnosis that has perhaps been repeated many times. This is the norm. The normal initial reaction to grief is denial. The best stance for the medical personnel to take is one of patience and understanding; they should answer questions, reiterate the nature of the child's handicap, and discuss how it can be cared for best. At this time social workers and psychologists should do little but allow this process to run its course. Time is often the best healer. Often in their zeal to be helpful and to move the parents on to more active paths for dealing with the child, mental health personnel misconstrue this early grief period as the parent's resistance to accepting the handicap.

Olshansky,[17] in his article "Chronic Sorrow: A Response to Having a Mentally Defective Child," intimates that although acceptance does eventuate, such parents, in response to a tragic event, always feel somewhat sad. This is a normal rather than neurotic reaction. Through recognition and acceptance of this response, mental health professionals are able to step back and allow the parents time to absorb the shock. At this time placement in a group with others who have had to make similar adjustments can be quite effective in aiding the parent's process of working through their grief.

Learning to handle anger is the second adjustment phase of parents moving toward acceptance. Since anger is one of the responses for which society holds negative views, parents are often hard pressed to express it. They may not realize that they are angry. They feel cheated and identified at the same moment. Cheated, in that their incredible investment of time, love, and psychic energy in this new being has been essentially squandered; identified, in that they are isolated, chosen by fate to bear this dastardly blow. These facets of anger can be incapacitating. It often moves parents into a cave from which they exit only when carefully composed and only when necessary. They fear rebuff for their hostilities. They feel sorrowful and move around licking their wounds for prolonged periods of time. This self-pity is another form of anger. Lack of empathy on the part of the rest of the world often heightens parent's angry feelings and responses. Such a narcissistic injury requires calm understanding, patience but not pity. Pity seems only to serve to increase the anger. At this time the caregiver's role is to allow the anger to be vented. This frequently is better managed by mental health professionals than by surgeons and nurses. Anger is a plea for help, gushing forth from a well of "how could this have happened to us?"

Parents' anxieties about the cause and repercussions of bearing a handicapped child are as troublesome as grief and anger. Old, subconscious wishes of ill rear their heads in need of punishment; the punishment being the addition of this "bad self," the handicapped child. The parents' inability to successfully separate from their parents also elicits dissonance within themselves and their system. If previous dissatisfactions with their mate were dealt with head-on, the parents will not use the child as the dumping ground for their frustrations with one another. In the guise of "discussions" about Jimmy's care, the child becomes the repository of the parents' unmet marital needs. Wives feeling depreciated become "super moms"; husbands feeling neglected may stray from family life; other sibs losing out in this process seek attention by feigning somatic distress. The mental health professional's role at this time should move from being the sounding board comforter to one who helps in sorting out and reality focusing to set the family train back on the tracks through each member regaining his/her own inner balance.

Living with a handicapped child may be difficult. "How will I care for this child?" "What kind of a financial burden are we talking about?" "What will this mean in terms of deprivation for other family members?" "What will be this child's future?" These questions haunt parents and fuel the chronic sorrow that in all likelihood they will feel the rest of their lives. However, these questions and the sorrow are workable. With the aid of the medical team the task of implementing therapy programs, coordinating clinic visits, and maintaining a smooth household can move from overwhelming to manageable.

All of this arranging, planning, and scheduling can produce anger. Anger in these parents should not be construed as direct rejection of the child. It is a normal reaction to a constant hassle. In availing themselves to such families, the medical team must keep in mind that parents feel their anger is related to their investment in the betterment of the child.[22]

All is not bleak. Many families unite and form strong bonds between each other because of their concern for the handicapped child. These families are most often the ones who initiate education programs and general understanding about the handicapped in their communities.

> Because they are compelled by circumstances to understand themselves and their own need, the parents of a handicapped child often become more sensitive to the needs of others. In many instances these parents have sought professional help in resolving their own personal problems. As they have matured through this therapeutic experience, they have begun to think about what they have to offer others rather than what they can get from others. A wife who has been afraid to turn to her husband for help or to reveal her dependency on him begins to look for support after they have worked together on planning for the care of their handicapped child. The very narcissistic person begins to grow up after he has worked through some of his feelings of grief and bewilderment. As the parents' understanding of the needs of the handicapped child increase, they may become better parents to all of their children.[23]

This discussion has considered the general case of the birth of a handicapped child. Specifically, a child born with a congenital amputation induces all of these reactions in parents, siblings, and the world at large. However, the child who is a congenital amputee or who loses a limb soon after birth fares somewhat better psychologically than does a child who suffers such a loss later in life. The congenitally blind individual adapts to the vicissitudes of life without sight with greater facility than those who have seen the world and traumatically are thrust into darkness; this is also true for congenital amputees. For those who have never experienced running freely on a beach or making a great catch in the outfield, there is less to miss. Working through a loss (i.e., the grieving process) within such a child is almost nonexistent. It is the blow the parents suffer, the chronic sorrow that they carry with them and naturally transmit to the child, which can isolate the child and eventually make them feel inadequate and grieve the loss.

Body image

Not only has the amputee sustained a loss in ability and function, he has sustained a loss to his psychological being. This internal concept of the body is referred to as "body image." Its mutilation may be more disruptive to the overall rehabilitation than the actual physical loss of the limb.

We consider the body image to be our view of ourselves. It is our view of how we look, how we move in space, and the extent of our physical abilities. It is the result of lifelong proprioceptive, optic, and tactile sensations that become cortical perceptions. The meaning of these perceptions can be modulated by interpersonal and environmental values placed on bodily parts as well as bodily changes that occur with time.

However, the concept of body image is overly broad and may not be completely useful in a therapeutic sense. Kolb[12] has suggested that the term can be better understood if it is broken down into four components: body percept, body concept, body ego, and body ideal.

Body percept is the accumulated sensory experiences of the body that establish the preconscious body schema postural model. This is the phenomenon studied by neurologists and from it emerges the body phantom sensation that occurs after loss of parts.

Body concept includes those thoughts, feelings, attitudes, and memories that have evolved over time as the individual views and experiences his body with others. Comparisons of athletic powers would be included in body concept.

Body ego is the perceiving or viewing of the personality as it concerns body image. Thus a person with a generally positive outlook will tend to view his body image positively.

Body ideal is the idealized image of the body that each person projects. Against this ideal he measures the body percepts and body concepts.

There may be great disparities between the expectations of the body ideal and the experiences of the body concept, which may lead to the arousal of either painful or pleasurable feelings. The ego functions to alleviate the pain or to integrate to pleasant affective response. The result of this ego function is the body image.

The concept of disturbances in body image evolves from observations of an individual's failure to perceive his body and its parts and adapt to them as they actually exist. The outstanding examples of acute disturbances of body image occur as a result of traumatic or surgical dismemberment. In such disturbances the basic body image persists despite the visible or apparent loss of a body part. Where the consequences of disturbance of body image do not follow the general expectation of the recognized healthy adaptation, the influence of neurotic or psychotic personality development or social factors will be found operative.

Phantom phenomena. Following an amputation, the individual normally feels as if the nonexistent limb were still present. Ewalt and his coworkers,[4] studying over 2000 soldiers undergoing amputation of a limb in the army during World War II, reported that phantom limb sensation was almost universal. Insofar as the phantom limb is such a common experience after an amputation, it can be considered to be the expected healthy response following sudden loss of a limb.

The sensory phenomena of the phantom limbs have been characterized as consisting of three general types.[9] The first is a mild, tingling sensation, the basic phantom phenomenon. The second experience is a stronger, momentary pins and needles sensation such as that felt in the phantom limb when the neuromata in the stump are touched. The third type consists of certain superadded disagreeable or painful sensations that are described as "twisting," "burning," "pulling," "itching," or various other complaints of a similar nature. Most phantom sensations, regardless of type, are intermittent and more annoying than agonizing.

Frazier and Kolb[6] have presented an excellent summary of various aspects of the phantom phenomenon. They note that the life of the phantom has been variously reported but is generally considered to be a normal sensation that persists from 6 months to 20 years. As the phantom sensation disappears, it frequently undergoes a perception change known as telescoping, in which the hand or foot feels as if it were directly attached to the stump area; the last parts of the phantom phenomenon to disappear are those that are best represented in the cortex, such as the thumb, index finger, and great toe. The amputee normally experiences the phantom phenomena immediately after the operation and may be even more aware of the phantom than the contralateral normal limb. The phantom may feel as the original limb did in every respect as to shape, size, consistency, position, sensation, and ability to move. Rings, watches, and the like, which were formerly worn on the amputated limb, may be incorporated into the phantom. Upper limb phantoms are stronger and longer lasting than those of the lower limb. If the limb had been deformed a long time prior to amputation, the phantom may be perceived as being deformed.

It is also reported that burning and tingling sensations may occur in phantom legs with urination, defecation, sexual intercourse, and even smoking; upper limb phantom limbs are usually unaffected by such acts. Phantom arms are more easily moved than legs, and there is greatest movement in the thumb, index finger, and great toe. The amputee perceives the phantom as passing through objects instead of bending or moving around them.

The phantom is the expected healthy response after sudden loss of a limb. The account of this phenomena just presented is meant to be an aid in distinguishing the healthy psychophysiological response to amputation from the psychologically and emotionally maladpative response.

Painful phantom. An entirely different dimension of the phantom phenomenon is the painful phantom. Although the nonpainful phantom is considered to be a normal condition following amputation, the painful phantom is a pathological circumstance. Phantom pain is described as a burning, twisting, cramping, sharp, shooting, cyclic pain perceived in the vicinity of the absent body part. Those patients who experience hand or forearm amputations usually describe the pain as a clenched fist with fingers bent over the palm, so that the entire hand is painful and fatigued. If the pain becomes chronic, other responses of the body may become trigger zones or areas so sensitized that mere touch may evoke spasms of severe pain in the phantom limb. Emotional upsets, even arguments, may provoke the attacks as well.

It is important to distinguish between phantom phenomenon, phantom pain, and stump pain. Phantom phenomenon can and usually does occur at once after amputation, and the patient may refuse to believe that the limb has been removed. Phantom pain is also referred to the lost extremity. It can be stimulated emotionally, often by anger or by discussion of the patient's plight as it affects the family or occupational status. It can disappear when attention is distracted by a discussion of pleasant, unrelated subjects. Phantom pain is intense after orgasm in the male and during orgasm in the female. Stump pain takes time to develop. It is usually associated with point tenderness and can be excited directly by tactile stimulation of the stump.

Melzack[15] reports that up to 35% of amputees feel some occasional phantom pain, and approximately 5% to 10% of all amputees experience severe phantom pain that may become worse over the years. This is in significant contrast to Ewalt's[4] report that only eight of 2284 amputees experience phantom pain. When this group studied the few patients who experienced phantom pain, they found that there were individuals with significant preexisting psychopathological conditions and that they tended to interpret their phantom sensations as painful. They also reported that the pain would come and go along with other symptoms of emotional disorder without a clear relationship to external treatment. Surgeons have tended to assume a peripheral cause for phantom pain, and this explanation is developed in detail in Chapter 34. However, the same peripheral sensory deprivation exists for all amputees, yet only a few develop phantom pain.

Frazier and Kolb[6] believe that the painful phantom is generally indicative of psychopathological conditions. The temporary phantom sensations of the distal portion of a severed limb are experienced normally, but the sensations gradually disappear as the patient learns to accept the loss of part of himself and to modify his body image accordingly. People whose phantom sensation becomes chronic, painful, and disabling are expressing their inability to accept the loss and are turning on themselves the resentment and hate connected with their misfortune.[10]

Whether the origin is peripheral or central, there will always be a psychological factor present to influence these patients. This may be in the personality that predisposes the individual to be more prone to pain or less able to cope with loss. It may be in the psychology of an amputation per se and related to the fantasy of the illness and the attendant anxiety. Finally, it may reside with maladaptive use of the pain for secondary gain, as with a so-called pain personality.[21]

Treatment consists of vigorous attempts to aid in the establishment of a healthy, reorganized self-image. These embrace all those therapeutic procedures which allow for increased facility in use of the body musculature, as in athletic games, dance, and posture, as well as correction of bodily defects through surgery, and cosmetic and rehabilitation efforts. The various means that are used to strengthen the body image and thereby to enhance ego functioning and self-esteem are seen as positive techniques.

Medical personnel may aid considerably in the prevention of serious disturbances through proper use of the knowledge at hand when a patient is confronted with an elective surgical procedure known to produce deformity. In the case of amputation, the patient should be made aware of the occurrence of the phantom. Considerate inquiry into the patient's fears and anxieties is desirable. If a limb is to be amputated, the patient's desire as to its disposal and possible burial should be ascertained.[12] Some initial discussion of the disability, its meaning to the patient, and compensation for it are advisable.

The family and other persons who are significant to the patient should be advised as to the expected posttreatment psychological and emotional phenomena. In this way their aid may be immediately enlisted in the rehabilitation process and especially in ascertaining the possibility of severe emotional reaction to the operation.

When disruption of the body structure leads to personality disorder, treatment should be instituted as quickly as possible. Failure to do so can result in fixation of chronic psychopathic reactions. Treatment depends on the particular reaction and is beyond the scope of this book.

REFERENCES

1. Cohen, P. C.: The impact of the handicapped child in the family, Social Casework, vol. **43,** March, 1962.
2. Dembo, T., Ladieu-Leviton, G., and Wright, B. A.: Acceptance of loss—amputations. In Garrett, I. F., editor: Psychological aspects of physical disability, ser. no. 210. Washington D.C., 1952, Federal Security Agency, Office of Vocational Rehabilitation.
3. Egbert, L. D., et al.: Reduction of postoperative pain by encouragement and instruction of patients. A study of doctor patient rapport, N. Engl. J. Med. **270:**825-827, April, 1964.
4. Ewalt, J. R., Randall, G. C., and Morris, H.: The phantom limb, Psychosomat. Med. **9:**118, 1947.
5. Fisher, S. H.: Psychiatric considerations of hand disability, Arch. Phys. Med. Rehabil. **41:**62-70, 1960.
6. Frazier, S. H., and Kolb, L. C.: Psychiatric aspects of pain and the phantom limb, Orthop. Clin. North Am. **1:**481, 1970.
7. Friedmann, L. W.: The psychological rehabilitation of the amputee, Springfield, Ill., 1978, Charles C Thomas, Publisher.
8. Heinz, R.: The psychoanalytic study of the child. Monograph 4: The analysis of the self, New York, 1974, National University Press.
9. Henderson, W. R., and Smyth, G. E.: Phantom limbs, J. Neurol. Neurosurg. Psychiatry **11:**88, May, 1948.
10. Kapp, F. T.: Psychogenic pain. In Freedman, A. M., Kaplan, H. I., and Sadock, B. J., editors: Comprehensive textbook of psychiatry—II, vol. 2, Baltimore, 1975, The Williams and Wilkins Co.
11. Kessler, H. H.: Psychological preparation of the amputee, Industrial Med. **20** (2):107-108, Feb., 1951.
12. Kolb, L.: Disturbances of the body-image. In Arieti, S., editor: American handbook of psychiatry, vol. 4, New York, 1975, Basic Books, Inc., Publishers.
13. Lazarus, H. R., and Hagens, J. H.: Prevention of psychosis following open-heart surgery, Am. J. Psychiatry **124:** 1190-1195, March, 1968.
14. Lindemann, E.: Symptomatology and management of acute grief, Am. J. Psychiatry **101:**141, 1944.
15. Melzack, R.: The puzzle of pain, New York, 1973, Basic Books, Inc., Publishers.
16. Newton, J. H.: First year of bereavement: a clinical study bulletin. Special Edition on Pastoral Care, vol. XLII, no. 2., 1978, American Hospital Association.
17. Olshansky, S.: Chronic sorrow: a response to having a mentally defective child, Social Casework, vol. 43, April, 1962.
18. Parkes, C. M.: Bereavement studies of grief in adult life, New York, 1972, International Universities Press, Inc.
19. Parkes, C. M.: Components of the reaction of loss of a limb, spouse or home, Psychosomat. Res. **16:**343-349, Aug., 1972.
20. Parkes, C. M., and Napier, M. M.: Psychiatric sequelae of amputation, Br. J. Psychiatry **9:**440, 1975.
21. Pasnau, R., and Pfefferbaum, B.: Psychologic aspects of post-amputation pain, Nurs. Clin. North Am. **11**(4): 679-685, 1976.
22. Plank, E. N., and Horwood, C.: Leg amputation in a 4-year-old: reactions of the child, her family and the staff, Social Casework **43:**405-422, April, 1962.
23. Solnei, A. J., and Starle, M. H.: Mourning and the birth of a defective child. Psychological study of the child, vol. 16, New York, 1961, International Universities Press, Inc.
24. Wittkower, E.: Rehabilitation of limbless; joint surgical and psychological study, Occup. Med. **3:**20-44, Jan., 1947.

PART FIVE

The juvenile amputee

CHAPTER 36

Introduction to the child amputee

GEORGE T. AITKEN
RAYMOND J. PELLICORE

The identification and departmentalization of the treatment of the juvenile amputee is a relatively recent development. Immediately following World War II there was a renaissance in the area of prosthetic fabrication, fitting and alignment techniques, and training modalities. The large volume of postwar amputees stimulated a renewed interest in amputee rehabilitation. During World War II the army and navy had established amputee centers. The success of these multidisciplinary centers was a great stimulus to all interested in the care of the amputee. In this postwar period the Veterans Administration continued this philosophy with the establishment of amputee centers for those discharged amputees. In parallel manner, civilian amputee centers were created. Finally, an educational program was developed to disseminate the knowledge so gained to a broad spectrum of physicians, therapists, and prosthetists, thereby making available to the endemic amputee population the advantages in medicine, prosthetics, and training that had been acquired from the treatment of the postwar epidemic of amputees.

Some observers of this phenomenon believed that many of these advantages could be applied to children with amputations.[6] Several astute directors of crippled children's programs, impressed by the success of "centers" for adults, considered this concept for their juvenile wards, since past experience in the habilitation of the child amputee had been generally discouraging. Industry was importuned to scale down to child size commercially available components. Improved fabrication and alignment techniques were found to be as applicable to children as to adults. Early success seemed to justify further investigation of the juvenile amputee and his problems.

Historically, the treatment of the juvenile amputee was carried out in, or in close proximity to, a general crippled children's clinic. In the light of this new interest in prosthetics, congenital limb deficiency problems suddenly were viewed in a new perspective. As these limb deficiency problems were reviewed, it became evident that an adequate descriptive classification did not exist. Efforts were generated to develop a suitable classification, and these efforts continue (Chapter 37).[8,10,11]

Skeletal limb deficiency problems should be classified anatomically as a matter of good record keeping and also to enable all disciplines involved to communicate with each other in an intelligent manner. The transverse deficiencies are homologues of acquired amputations and as such are amenable to immediate application of the improved techniques developed for acquired limb losses. Proper classification, however, does not lead to accurate prescription writing, and this is particularly true in patients with longitudinal deficiencies. In such patients, the deformity must be analyzed carefully to locate the "key joint." This is the most distal stable joint beyond which there is sufficient tissue to function as a stump. When this has been identified (usually by clinical and x-ray evaluation), then one can determine the amputation type of which the deformity is a homologue. With this as a basis, a prescription for a nonstandard prosthesis of the appropriate type may be formulated, and eventual surgery planned. Analysis of this bizarre group of upper and lower limb anomalies led to an elucidation of the following biomechanical losses:

Lower limb biomechanical losses

1. Inequality of leg lengths
2. Malrotation
3. Inadequacy of proximal musculature
4. Instability of proximal joints

Upper limb biomechanical losses

1. Varying losses of prehension
2. Inequality of arm lengths
3. Malrotation
4. Inadequacy of proximal and distal musculature
5. Instability of proximal joints

In the severe total limb anomaly, some degrees of all types of the listed biomechanical losses were evident; however, not all losses were present in each case. Inequality in length seemed to be the most common loss. Theoretically, prosthetic application should be assistive to this group. A prosthesis could easily equalize leg length discrepancy, and malrotation would be improved, if not eradicated, by prosthetic alignment techniques. Instability of the proximal joints could be improved, at least partially, by special techniques of fabrication, fit, and alignment. In upper limb deficiencies, although body-powered prostheses could offer only marginal gain in the area of proximal musculature inadequacy, special harnessing techniques could be valuable in this area. Absence of prehension could be replaced by those prehension devices already available, especially since a full range of sizes from infancy to maturity had now become available.

If one accepts these theoretical hypotheses, then prosthetic application in this complicated group of anomalies is feasible. With the knowledge that in many such cases traditional orthopedic surgical and nonsurgical treatment offered only marginal to inadequate functional gain, several clinics proceeded with prosthetic care for this group of patients.

It is important at this time to recognize the involvement of a complete clinic team in the discussion of the prosthetic prescription because of the complexities of fabrication, alignment, stability, and harnessing that are implicit in the fitting around these often bizarrely shaped limbs, as compared with standard amputation stumps.

PHYSIOLOGICAL DIFFERENCES BETWEEN THE CHILD AND THE ADULT

There is justification for the segregation of the juvenile amputee group from the adult population. Physiologically the child is a growing dynamic organism as opposed to the aging, decelerating adult. The child has the potential of longitudinal growth, and his patterns of circumferential growth are not directly related to diet. The adult has no potential for longitudinal growth, and his circumferential variations are primarily diet related. The most dependable indicator of immaturity is the presence of open epiphyses. If open epiphyses are present, the patient is skeletally immature. By correlating the chronological age and ascertained bone age, it is possible to determine quite accurately the degree of immaturity. Thus one may define the child amputee as a skeletally immature individual with either an amputation or a congenital deficiency of one or more limbs. Tissues in children are quite different from those of adults. Blood supply, healing potential, and general tissue metabolism usually are maximal in children. The presence of these favorable factors has many surgical implications as discussed elsewhere in this chapter. This is yet another manifestation that the child is not a small adult. Tissue tolerance in children is superior to that in most adults. Circulation is abundant, and the wounds can be expected to heal more readily. Split-thickness skin grafts can be used to preserve length in amputation surgery for children. Experience demonstrates that such grafting techniques will stand up under socket-stump interface stresses. For cases in which trauma is the cause, the use of grafts will often preserve skeletal length in the presence of extensive skin loss.

When a physician performs amputation surgery on an adult, he can plan in most instances so that a stump of adequate length, proper contour, and comfort is achieved. This is because the underlying skeletal and soft tissue structures are mature and not undergoing longitudinal growth. Contrarily, amputation surgery in juveniles is carried out on a growing organism.[12] Longitudinal growth is to be expected, and its duration and extent can be assessed accurately by chronological and bone age studies. The desired goal of good juvenile amputation surgery is to fashion a stump that is not only satisfactory now, but will either continue to be satisfactory during the course of proportionate longitudinal growth or else, when required, may be refashioned at the time of com-

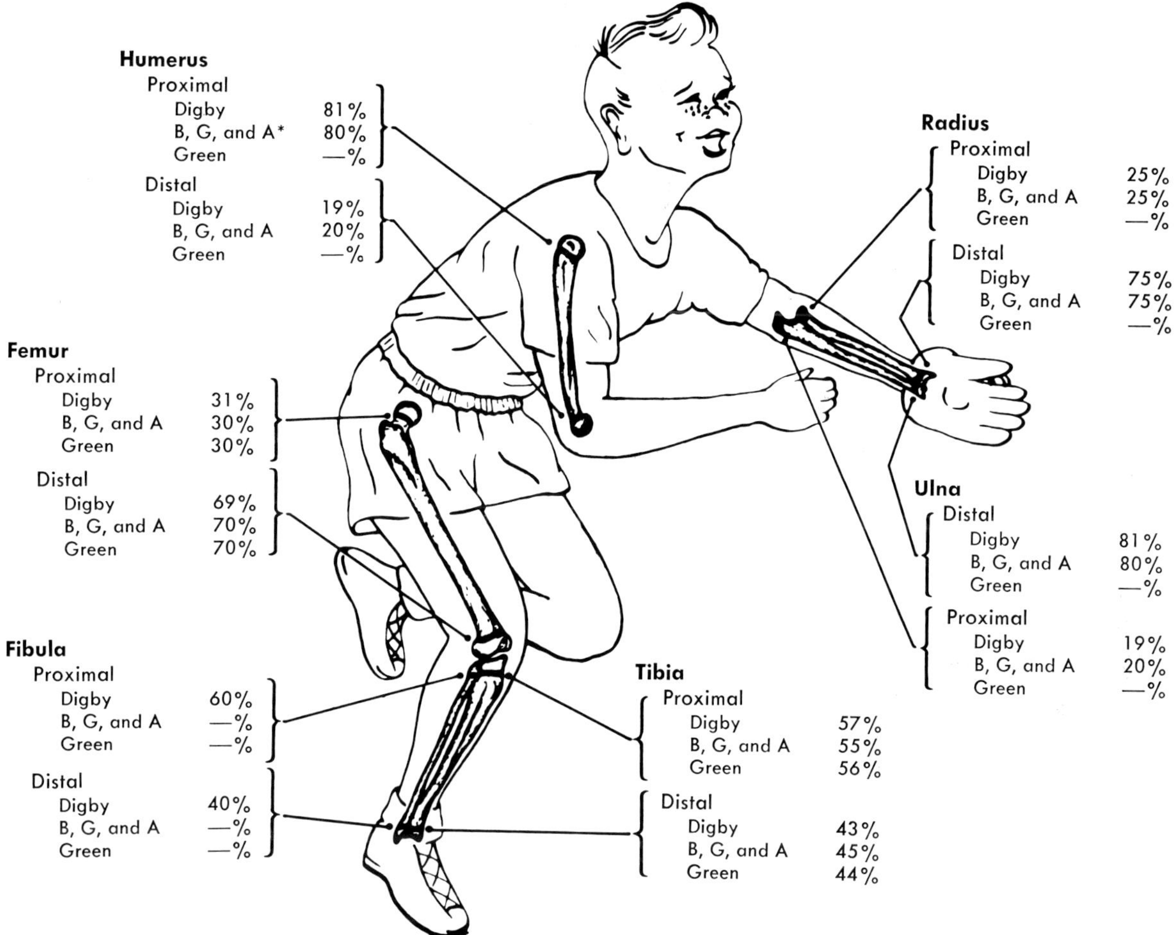

Fig. 36-1. Epiphyseal contributions to longitudinal bone growth. Percentages represent contribution of each epiphysis to total growth of each bone. *B, G,* and *A,* Bisgard, Gill, and Abbott. (From Aitken, G. T.: Inter.-Clin. Info. Bull. **7**(8):6, 1968.)

pletion of bone growth. In adults there may be sites of election. In children there are no ideal levels of amputation. The basic surgical dictum is to save all length possible. Each epiphysis that can be preserved contributes to a more satisfactory length of stump at maturity and prevents the most common complication in children's amputation surgery, bony overgrowth (Fig. 36-1). If the choice is between a supraepiphyseal amputation or a disarticulation, do the disarticulation. This is not to imply that a knee disarticulation is better than a below-knee amputation, but means that a knee disarticulation is better in children than is the classical above-knee amputation. Sacrifice of the distal femoral epiphysis reduces the retained potential of growth of the femur by 70%. Retention of that epiphysis maintains the growth potential of the entire bone.

The major complication of amputation surgery in children is bony overgrowth (Fig. 36-2).[2] The cause of this phenomenon is obscure. It is not a complication of disarticulation surgery, but only follows metaphyseal or diaphyseal transection. Histologically, this is appositional bone growth from the end of the skeletal stump. Implantation of a metal marker at the time of amputation and serial followup by x-ray examination have conclusively shown that this is an additive phenomenon, not the vis-a-tergo of the next proximal epiphysis. Usually there is a bursa formation between the bone and the soft tissue of the stump. As the overgrowth progresses, the soft tissue cushion is invaded, and the bursa becomes subcutaneous and increasingly painful. In neglected cases, the skin may erode, and a low-grade superficial infection develops.

Surgical management of the transected bone or manipulation of the periosteal sleeve do not seem to have any favorable effect. The use of Silastic caps or plugs has been tried,[14,15] but the results

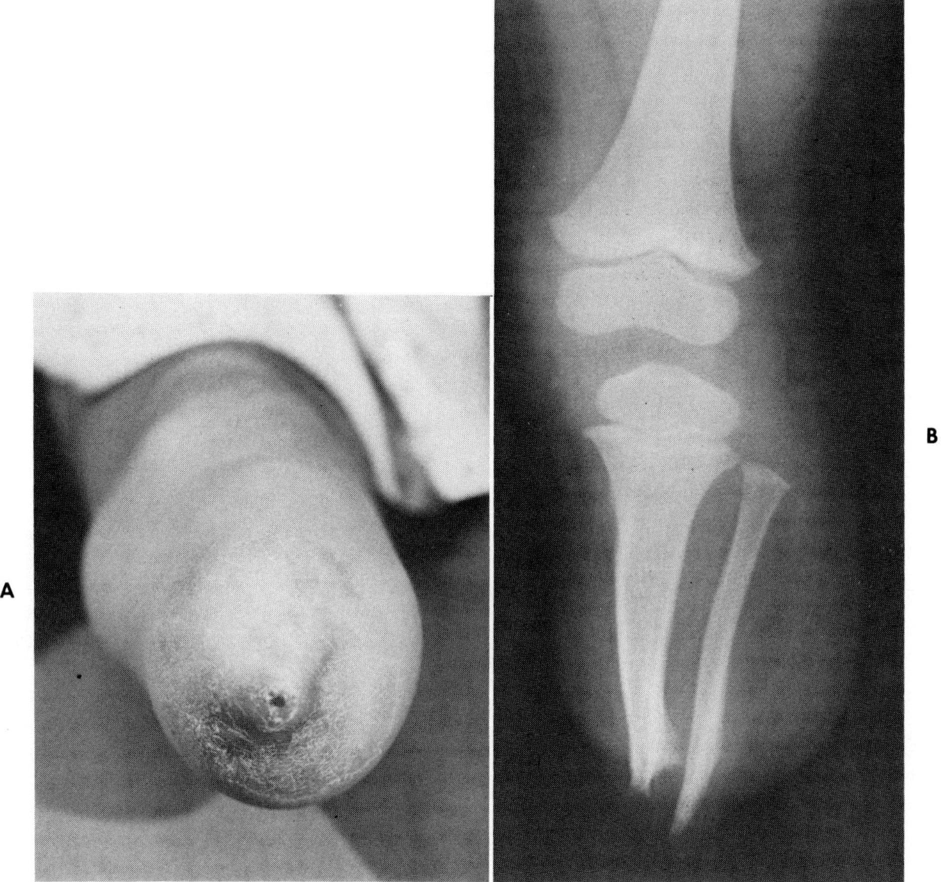

Fig. 36-2. A, Clinical appearance of bony overgrowth in below-knee amputation. Note sinus tract, indicating perforation of skin by bony overgrowth. **B,** Roentgenogram of stump shown in **A.** It is evident that perforation of soft tissue covering is from excessive overgrowth of fibula.

have been disappointing. There is some animal experimentation that would indicate that the denervation of the stump may control bony overgrowth.[7] A rabbit model experiment seems to show that transplantation of a metatarsal epiphysis to the transected long bone will prevent overgrowth.[16] The present state of the art is such that in the human there is no certain way of preventing this complication (pp. 601-608).

Treatment is revision of the stump, removal of the bursa and overgrown bone, and then prosthetic reapplication when healing is secure. The incidence of this complication is variously reported in ranges of 10% to 30%, with 15% being a reasonable incidence figure. Actual appositional bone growth may be present on x-ray examination in a stump that is asymptomatic. Contrarily, a symptomatic painful stump can be present before unequivocal x-ray evidence is developed. Limited bone scans may be valuable for cases in which there is some question concerning the relationship of the patient's symptoms and the plain x-ray evidence of equivocal bony overgrowth. Early, limited use of this technique has seemed to indicate that unless there is definitely increased uptake of the radioactive material, the stump skeleton is not *actively* overgrowing, regardless of the appearance of the plain x-ray film. The threat of this complication should not be a contraindication to the indicated elective or emergency amputation surgery in children.

As experience was obtained and documented, it became evident that in some of the longitudinal deficiencies, it was necessary to convert the presenting anomaly to a suitable stump.[1-6,9] It was evident that such conversions were more frequently necessary in the lower limb group than in the upper limb group. A recent analysis of 1605 patients with congenital limb deficiencies indicates that approximately 50% of the lower limb group and only 8% of the upper limb group required conversion.

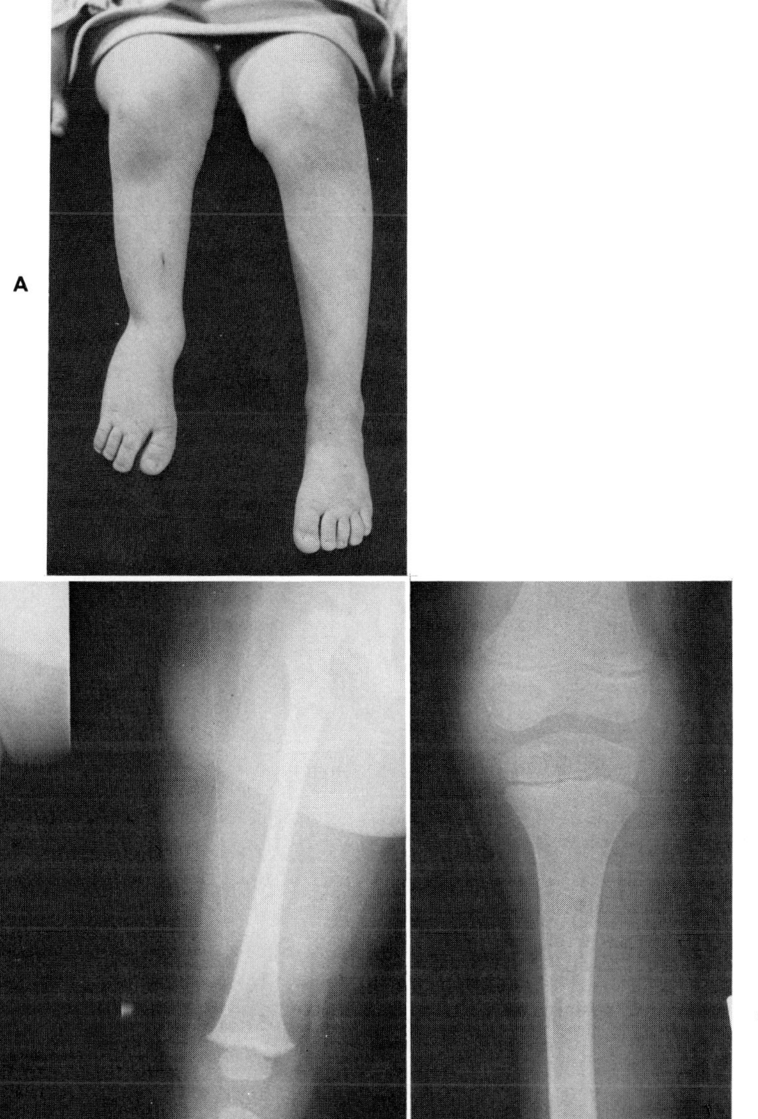

Continued.

Fig. 36-3. A, Clinical appearance of terminal longitudinal fibular deficiency. Note shortening of shank as compared to opposite side, four-rayed foot, and skin dimple over anterior bow of tibia. **B,** Roentgenogram of limb shown in **A**: complete absence of fibula, shortening of tibia, anterior bow at juncture of middle and distal thirds of tibia, and anomalies of bony hindfoot, **C,** X-ray film of patient shown in **A** after ankle disarticulation with Syme-type closure. No surgical manipulation of retained epiphyseal plate or medial malleolus has been accomplished.

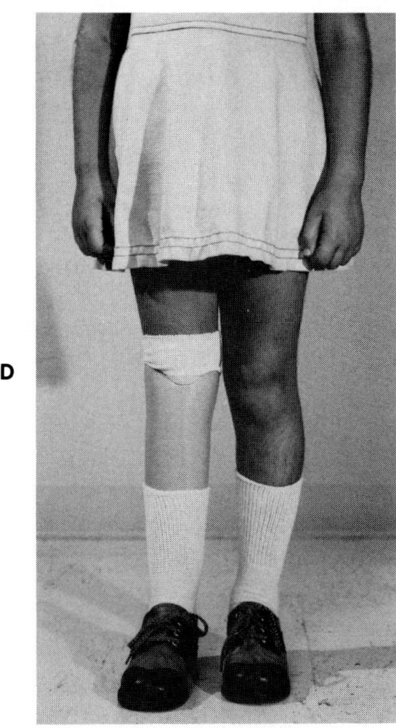

Fig. 36-3, cont'd. D, Prosthetic fitting of patient shown in **A.** PTB prosthesis with Syme end-bearing characteristics has been applied. PTB-type top enhances rotary stability.

Conversion may be primary or delayed. Primary conversion is reserved for those anomalies in which the life history is so well known that at whatever age the patient is seen, one can accurately predict what the anomaly will be like at maturity. When experience has demonstrated that conversion eventually will be indicated and necessary, then the conversion surgery may be done as a primary procedure (Fig. 36-3). Secondary conversion is reserved for those cases in which experience has indicated that functional gain can be obtained in a reasonable number of cases without refashioning the limb. In such cases, the patient is fitted around the anomaly and trained to use a prosthesis. If, after adequate fitting, training, and wearing, it is evident that function and comfort will be enhanced by conversion, then the indicated surgery can be done. It is our current opinion that there are no indications for primary conversion in upper limb deficiencies.

PSYCHOLOGICAL DIFFERENCES BETWEEN THE CHILD AND THE ADULT

From a psychological aspect, the child is quite different from the adult.[5] The mental and emotional maturity of children, of course, varies with age but in general is less than expected from an adult. The manifestations of immaturity have many influences on prescription writing, training modalities, rehabilitation goals, and educational and vocational recommendations. The child in many areas is dependent, the adult independent. The child as opposed to the adult is untrained in life's disciplines. He is an individual who can accept responsibility only in a limited manner, whereas the adult supposedly is capable of being independently responsible, at least in the economic and social areas. The child is malleable physically, socially, emotionally, and vocationally, whereas the adult is at least less malleable and, in some instances, is rigid or fixed in his patterns.

When one attempts to establish the rehabilitation goals for a juvenile patient, they must be realistically related to the age of the child. Since the child is a growing organism, these goals rightly may be expected to increase with the patient's growth. The primary aim is to develop prosthetic acceptance and functional gain that is realistically related to his or her specific age and development. With growth and development, prosthetic equipment and training may be altered and augmented to provide an orderly progression in functional skills that mimic the orderly development of the intact juvenile.

The child's most important influence emanates from the family. It is essential in juvenile amputee management that the family becomes convinced of the desirability of prosthetic application. If they become so convinced, then by their authoritarian role they will insist on wear and practice until functional gain is acquired. Unless such cooperation can be obtained, prosthetic habilitation will be less than ideal. This is particularly true of patients with upper limb loss.

CLINIC TEAM APPROACH

The "team approach" concept of amputee management is as applicable to the juvenile as it is to the adult. There should be a physician director who is interested and skilled in the care of the child with an acquired amputation or a congenital limb deficiency. The other members of the basic team should include representatives of physical and occupational therapy, nursing, and prosthetists and orthotists. It is presumed there is an adequate social services department and a full spectrum of medical and surgical consultative services. Such consultative services generally are episodic in their needs, and regular clinic attendance of such disciplines frequently is unnecessary.

The additional service of a biomedical engineer on an ongoing basis is very desirable. A keen engineer is an attribute to any prosthetic clinic. His analysis of the man-machine combination, that is, an amputee with his prosthesis, is very helpful. Often it is the machine and not the man that needs the treatment, and the engineer often may spot the fault and have suggestions for correction before the medical and allied health team members have defined the problem. A serendipitous gain is either a new gadget approach to an old problem or a basic innovative new device development.

Adjunctive services such as psychological testing and counseling, electromyographic studies, speech therapy, recreational therapy, drivers training, and schooling are all very desirable and should be an integral part of the juvenile amputee management program.

It would seem desirable to have all new patients processed through an orderly, systematic routine that would include the basic intake data of name, age, address, etc. The patterned social service interview would include an assessment of the family/patient needs and the potentials for solution. At such times, some often evident (but nearly equally often repressed) anxieties of patients and families will surface, and they can be enumerated and dealt with in the interview. Laboratory studies and indicated x-ray examination with routine intake photographs and appropriate release forms may also be obtained. If this routine is followed and all available medical histories are obtained before the clinic visit, valuable patient and clinic time is preserved. A treatment regimen is developed and its timing and organization ordered. Prefitting surgery can be planned and scheduled, as can any physical or occupational therapy. If prosthetic fitting is decided on as the initial treatment, then the prosthetic prescription is formulated, with all representative disciplines entering into the decision. The patient subsequently wears the prosthesis for a full clinic team evaluation and checkout.

At the time of the checkout, recommendations are made concerning the training routine to be employed and whether it should take place on an outpatient or inpatient basis.

Regularly scheduled return visits are an essential part of the program. Since children grow longitudinally and circumferentially, they must be seen frequently enough to make the necessary corrections of prosthetic fit, alignment, and length to accommodate growth. At such regular followup visits, functional evaluations can be made, and remedial therapy may be indicated for correction of faulty functional patterns. New skills may be introduced if the motor kinetic development of the patient so indicates. The clinic team must be on guard at all times against overprescribing both components and training. No child should be fitted with a complexity of components that exceeds his mental and physical development. This is particularly true in upper limb prosthetics,[13] in which there is a tendency to overgadget those children more gifted neuromuscularly. Similarly, training modalities and goals should not exceed the functional patterns of the norms at a similar mental and physical developmental age. It is important to evaluate the total patient as well as the presenting deformity. Elements such as alertness, attention, and nature of the total family response to the problem are integral parts of the evaluation. The recognition of the brevity of the attention span of the young child is important to the therapist who designs a training program and sets training goals for that child. Similarly, the supportive role of the family must never be underestimated. It is somewhat axiomatic to point out that it is easier to habilitate a lower limb—deficient child than the child with the severe upper limb deficiency.

REFERENCES

1. Aitken, G. T.: Amputation as a treatment for certain lower-extremity congenital abnormalities, J. Bone Joint Surg. **41A**(7):1267-1285, Oct., 1959.
2. Aitken, G. T.: Osseous overgrowth in amputations in children, In Swinyard, C. W., editor: Limb development and deformity: problems of evaluation and rehabilitation, Springfield, Ill., 1969, Charles C Thomas, Publisher.
3. Aitken, G. T.: Proximal femoral focal deficiency, In Swinyard, C. W., editor: Limb development and deformity: problems of evaluation and rehabilitation, Springfield, Ill., 1969, Charles C Thomas, Publisher.
4. Aitken, G. T.: Tibial hemimelia. In Aitken, G. T., editor: Selected lower limb anomalies: surgical and prosthetic management, Washington, D.C., 1971, National Academy of Sciences.
5. Aitken, G. T.: The child amputee: an overview, Orthop. Clin. North Am. **3**(2):447-472, July, 1972.
6. Aitken, G. T., and Frantz, C. H.: The juvenile amputee, J. Bone Joint Surg. **35A:**659-664, 1953.
7. Bunch, W. H., Deck, J. D., and Romer, J.: The effect of denervation of bony overgrowth after below knee amputation in rats, Clin. Orthop. **122:**333-339, 1977.
8. Burtch, R. L.: Nomenclature for congenital skeletal limb deficiencies: a revision of the Frantz and O'Rahilly classification, Artif. Limbs **10:**24-35, 1966.
9. Frantz, C. H., and Aitken, G. T.: Complete absence of the lumbar spine and sacrum, J. Bone Joint Surg. **49A**(8): 1531-1540, Dec., 1967.
10. Frantz, C. H., and O'Rahilly, R.: Congenital skeletal limb deficiencies, J. Bone Joint Surg. **43A:**1202-1224, 1961.
11. Hall, C. B., Brooks, M., and Dennis, J.: Congenital skeletal deficiencies of the extremities: classification and fundamentals of treatment, J.A.M.A. **181:**590-599, 1962.
12. Lambert, C.: Amputation surgery in the child, Orthop. Clin. North Am. **3**(2):473-482, July, 1972.
13. MacDonell, J. A.: Age of fitting upper extremity prostheses in children, J. Bone Joint Surg. **40A:**655-662, 1958.
14. Meyer, L. C., and Sauer, B. W.: The use of porous, high-density polyethylene caps in the prevention of appositional bone growth in the juvenile amputee: a preliminary report, Inter-Clin. Info. Bull. **14**(9-10):1-4, Oct., 1975.
15. Swanson, A. B.: Bony overgrowth in the juvenile amputee and its control by the use of silicone rubber implants, Inter-Clin. Info. Bull. **8**(5):9-18, Feb., 1969.
16. Wang, G. W., Baugher, W. H., and Stamp, W. G.: Epiphyseal transplants in amputations, Clin. Orthop. **130:**285-288, 1978.

CHAPTER 37

International terminology for the classification of congenital limb deficiencies

LEON M. KRUGER

When, in 1961, Frantz and O'Rahilly presented their paper on the classification of skeletal limb deficiencies at the American Academy of Orthopaedic Surgeons, many thought that the ultimate need for such a classification or system of nomenclature had now been developed. Throughout the United States the terminology became fairly widely accepted. Increasingly, it was used in the orthopaedic literature by many American authors. In Europe, however, it was poorly accepted by those involved in the treatment of limb deficiencies, and numerous other systems of terminology were in use there. In 1966, a special group of consultants to the subcommittee on Childrens Prosthetic Problems of the Committee on Prosthetic Research and Development offered a revision of the Frantz and O'Rahilly classification. This received some interest, but never replaced the original Frantz and O'Rahilly classification, which continued to be used to a large extent in this country.

During this period, one who was very interested in classification of limb deficiencies was Hector Kay, the assistant executive director of the Committee on Prosthetic Research and Development. At many meetings, Kay would discuss the possibility of developing an internationally acceptable classification. In 1968, he hosted a small luncheon meeting that included guests from Germany. At that time, the major discussion was around the possibility of developing such a classification. No progress was made, and it was apparent that there was little commonality of thought. It seemed that sufficient interest could not be stimulated to proceed with any work. Persistent individual that he was, Kay did not give up, and, in June of 1973, under the auspices of the Research and Development Committee of the International Society for Prosthetics and Orthotics, a workshop was convened in Dundee, Scotland, charged to study the problem and make a recommendation. Kay chaired that workshop. A terminology was developed that was descriptive in nature and easily translated into any language. Following the 1973 workshop, the terminology was tested on an international basis and found to be acceptable. In the meantime, under the leadership of Dr. Frank H. Stelling, of the Shriners Hospital for Crippled Children, Greenville, South Carolina, the Shriners Hospitals were developing a parallel classification, which, in fact, was almost identical with this so-called new international terminology.

To write a chapter on terminology would only be to paraphrase the original report published by Hector Kay. That report is therefore reprinted here with permission of the publishers.

A Proposed International Terminology for the Classification of Congenital Limb Deficiencies

The Recommendations of a Working Group of the International Society for Prosthetics and Orthotics

Hector W. Kay, *Chairman* (U.S.A.);
H. J. B. Day (England);H.-L. Henkel (West Germany);
Leon M. Kruger, *Rapporteur* (U.S.A.); Douglas W. Lamb (Scotland);
Ernst Marquardt (West Germany); Ross Mitchell (Scotland);
Alfred B. Swanson (U.S.A.); H.-G. Willert (West Germany)

Prepared for the Group by
HECTOR W. KAY

Assistant Executive Director
Committee on Prosthetics Research and Development
National Academy of Sciences—National Research Council
Washington, D.C.

During the past twenty years the treatment of children with limb deficiencies has emerged as a recognizable subspecialty in both medicine and prosthetics. These children can be divided into two broad categories—those whose amputations are acquired as the result of trauma or disease, and those who are born with a limb defect or anomaly.

With the first group, classification of the presenting condition usually poses little difficulty either nationally or internationally as the terms used are common throughout the world. For example, a partial limb loss described as a short below-elbow stump in English would be reported as a kurzer Unterarmstumpf in German, and the translation is straightforward. However, in the case of congenital deficits or anomalies, the situation has been quite the reverse in that different systems of nomenclature are used in different parts of the world. In some cases there are even different systems in use within the same country.

TWO PRIME SYSTEMS OF TERMINOLOGY

The two mainstreams of nomenclature for congenital limb deficiencies are those developed and in vogue in the United States of America, and those which originated in Germany and are used extensively in European countries.

U.S. terminology

In the U.S.A. the classic work of Frantz and O'Rahilly,[2] published in 1961, provided a clear, concise, and comprehensive system of nomenclature which was rapidly adopted by clinicians in that country. However, although this system offered many advantages, it did contain a number of terms, chief among them hemimelia, which were unacceptable to European orthopedists. Fig. 37-1 shows the elbow-disarticulation and knee-disarticulation types of what might be called true forms of *terminal transverse* hemimelia, or half a limb. Fig. 37-2 shows the above-elbow and above-knee forms of the same defect. Fig. 37-3 illustrates the deficiency classified as terminal transverse *partial* hemimelia. The terminal longitudinal defects identified as complete *paraxial* hemimelia are shown in Fig. 37-4, and the incomplete forms of these deficiencies are shown in Fig. 37-5. The complete and incomplete forms of the *intercalary longitudinal* type of paraxial hemimelia are indicated in Fig. 37-6. Hemimelia literally means

☐ From Kay, H.: Inter-Clin. Info. Bull. 13(7), April, 1974.

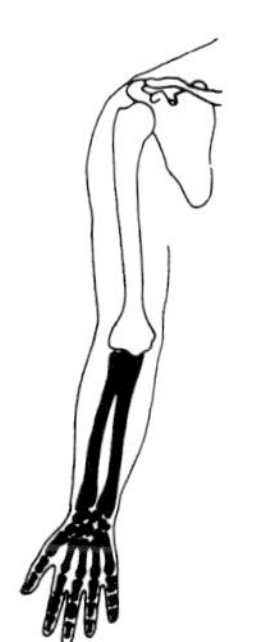
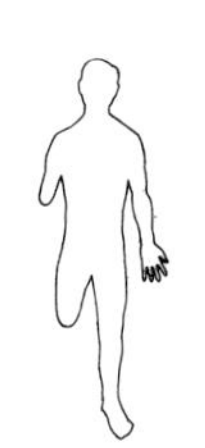
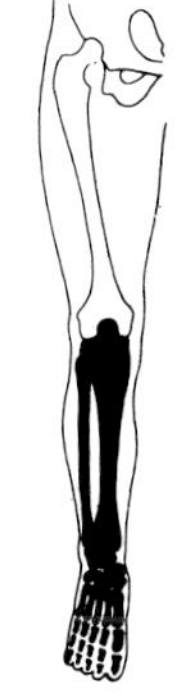

	NOMENCLATURE	
Hemimelia (T-) (E-D type) right	Original Frantz-O'Rahilly	Hemimelia (T-) (K-D type) right
Peromelia, at level of right elbow	European	Peromelia, at level of right knee
Meromelia (T-) radioulnar right	Revised Frantz-O'Rahilly	Meromelia (T-) tibiofibular, right

Fig. 37-1. Absence of forearm and hand or leg and foot.

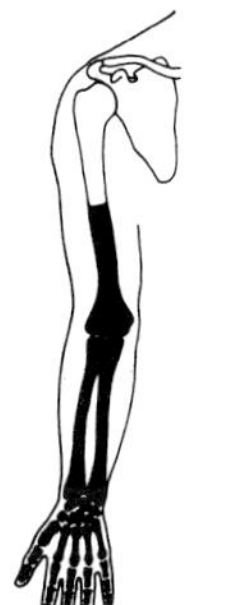
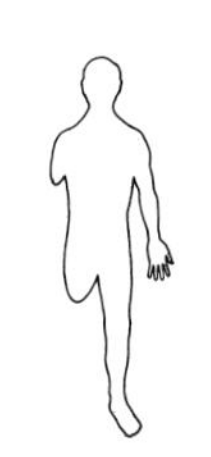
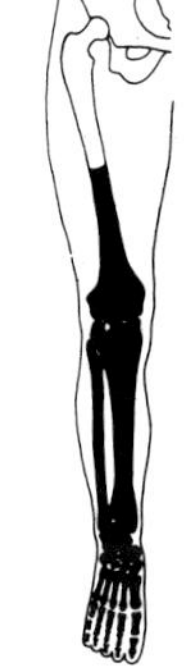
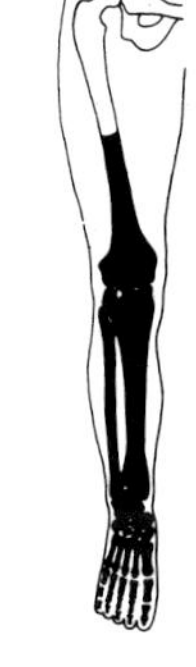

	NOMENCLATURE	
Hemimelia (T-) (A/E type) right	Original Frantz-O'Rahilly	Hemimelia (T-) (A/K type) right
Peromelia, upper right, midhumeral level (short, above-elbow stump)	European	Peromelia, lower right, midfemoral level (short, above-knee stump)
Meromelia (T-) humerus M, right	Revised Frantz-O'Rahilly	Meromelia (T-) femur M, right

Fig. 37-2. Absence of part of arm and all of forearm and hand or part of thigh and all of leg and foot.

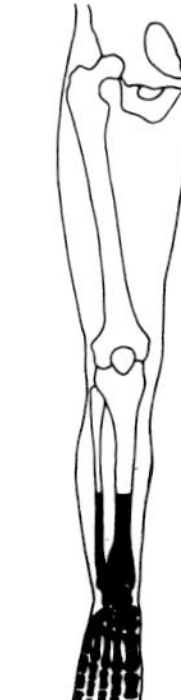
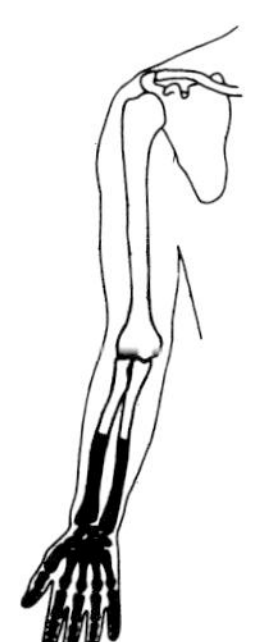
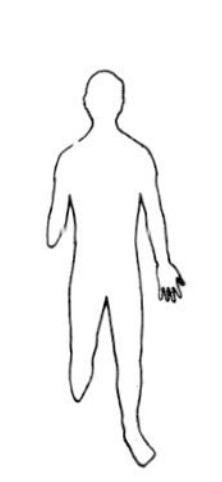
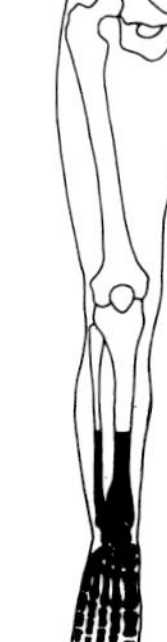

	NOMENCLATURE	
Partial hemimelia (T-) right	Original Frantz-O'Rahilly	Partial hemimelia (T-) right
Peromelia at midradioulnar level; partial aplasia of radius and ulna, right	European	Peromelia at midtibiofibular level; partial aplasia of right tibia and fibula
Meromelia (T-) radius M, ulna M, right	Revised Frantz-O'Rahilly	Meromelia (T-) tibia M, fibula M, right

Fig. 37-3. Absence of part of forearm and hand or part of leg and foot.

Fig. 37-4. Absence of radius and corresponding skeletal elements of wrist and hand or absence of tibia and corresponding skeletal elements of ankle and foot.

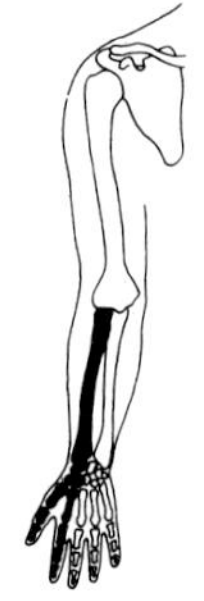
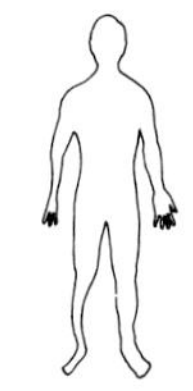
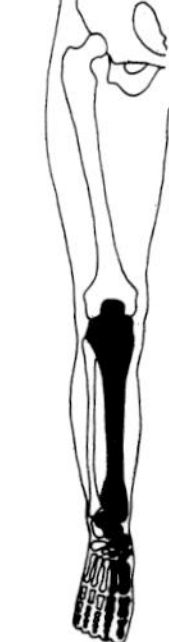

	NOMENCLATURE	
Complete paraxial hemimelia, radial (T/) upper right	Original Frantz-O'Rahilly	Complete paraxial hemimelia, tibial (T/) lower right
Ectromelia with axial aplasia; radial, carpal, metacarpal, and phalangeal; right	European	Ectromelia with axial aplasia; tibial, tarsal, metatarsal, and phalangeal, right
Meromelia (T/) radial	Revised Frantz-O'Rahilly	Meromelia (T/) tibial

Fig. 37-5. Absence of part of radius and corresponding skeletal elements of wrist and hand or part of tibia and corresponding skeletal elements of ankle and foot.

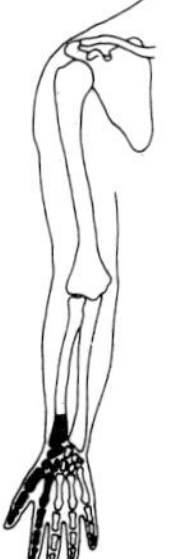
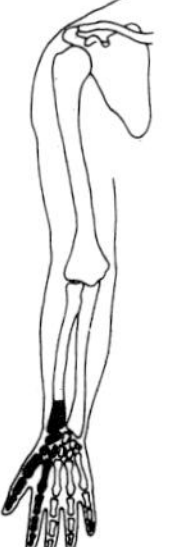
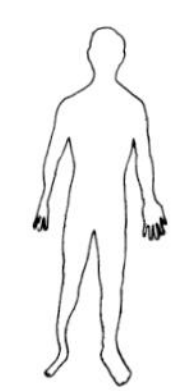
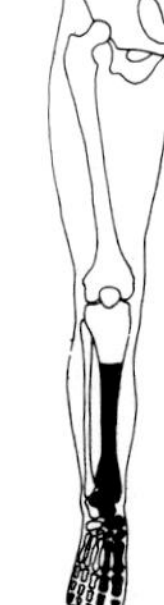

	NOMENCLATURE	
Incomplete paraxial hemimelia, radial (T/) upper right	Original Frantz-O'Rahilly	Incomplete paraxial hemimelia tibial (T/), lower right
Ectromelia with partial aplasia of radius and complete aplasia of the carpals, metacarpals, and phalanges, right	European	Ectromelia with partial aplasia of the tibia and complete aplasia of tarsals, metatarsals, and phalanges, right
Meromelia (T/) radial D, right	Revised Frantz-O'Rahilly	Meromelia (T/) tibial M, D, right

Fig. 37-6. Left, absence of one of skeletal elements of forearm (or leg, not shown). Right, partial absence of one of skeletal elements of leg (or forearm, not shown).

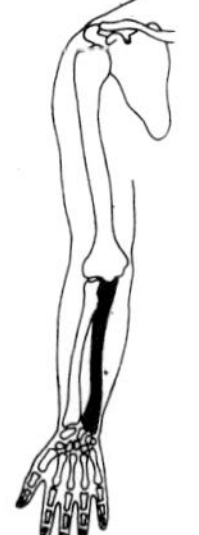
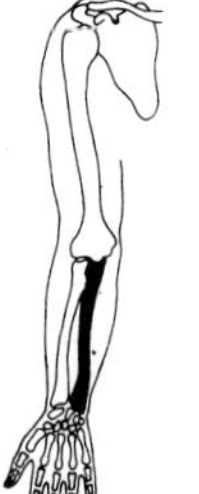
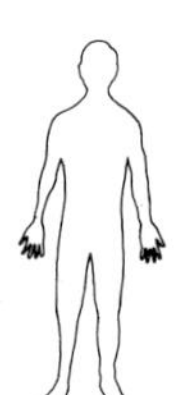
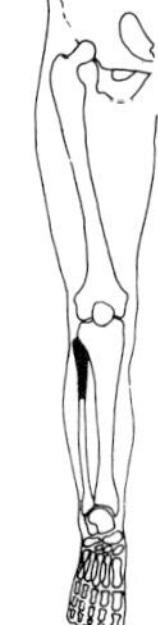

	NOMENCLATURE	
Complete paraxial hemimelia. (L/) upper right	Original Frantz-O'Rahilly	Incomplete paraxial-hemimelia fibular (L/) lower right
Ectromelia with complete axial aplasia, ulnar, right	European	Ectromelia with partial axial aplasia, proximal third of the fibula, right
Meromelia (L/) ulnar, right	Revised Frantz-O'Rahilly	Meromelia (L/) fibular P, right

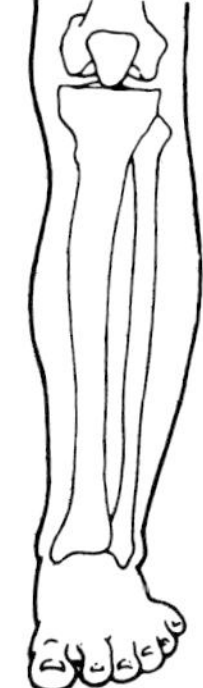

Fig. 37-7. Duplications of foot.

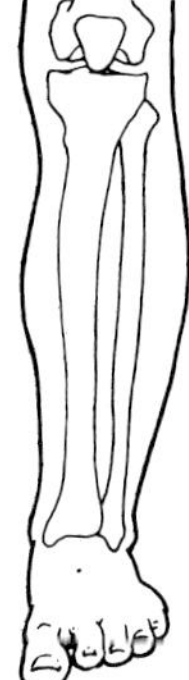

Fig. 37-8. Overgrowth of foot.

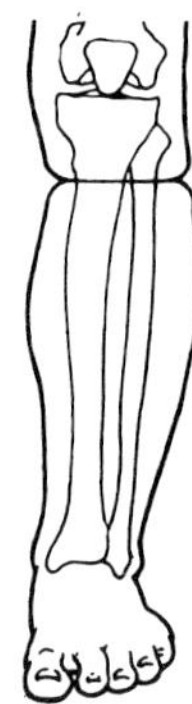

Fig. 37-9. Congenital circular constriction band syndrome of leg.

half a limb, which may be variously interpreted as being present, absent, or affected. Hence these terms admittedly could be somewhat confusing to the uninitiated.

In an effort to eliminate features of the Frantz-O'Rahilly system that were objectionable to overseas clinicians and to provide a means for classifying conditions not classifiable by the earlier work, a proposed revision of the Frantz-O'Rahilly scheme was published in 1966.[1] This revision eliminated the term hemimelia by calling all partial-limb absences meromelias, but it did retain the four major Frantz-O'Rahilly categories (terminal transverse, terminal longitudinal, intercalary transverse, and intercalary longitudinal), as shown in the previously cited illustrations (Figs. 37-1 to 37-6). However, instead of serving to replace the original Frantz-O'Rahilly classification system in the U.S.A., the proposed revision came into use as an additional classification method, i.e., it has been adopted by some practitioners while others have continued to use the original Frantz-O'Rahilly terminology.

The third component in the U.S.A. picture is the classification procedure first proposed by Swanson in 1964[6] and amplified in 1966.[7] This system covers soft tissue as well as skeletal considerations, and such anomalies as duplications (Fig. 37-7), overgrowth (Fig. 37-8), and the congenital constriction band syndrome (Fig. 37-9) which are not included in the other (skeletal deficiency) classifications.

German terms

In Germany nomenclature for the classification of limb deficiencies followed a different course and by the early 1960s such terms as peromelia, ectromelia, and dysmelia, which are not used at all in the U.S.A., were common in the German literature.[3,4,5] The only terms in fact on which there has been some degree of general agreement in Europe and America have been amelia and phocomelia (Figs. 37-10 through 37-12). It remained for Willert and Henkel, in 1969,[8,9] to attempt a systemization of the German nomenclature based on a pattern of orderly

Fig. 37-10. Absence of entire limb.

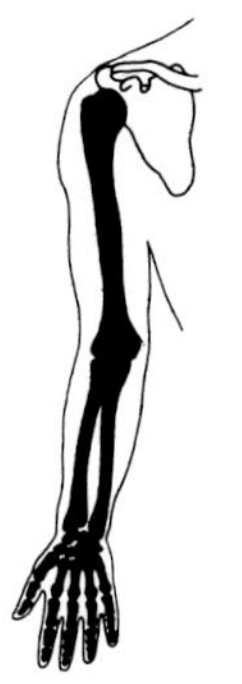
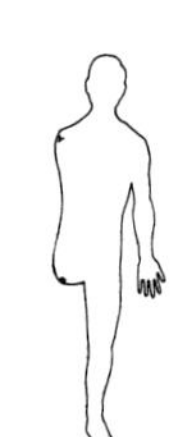
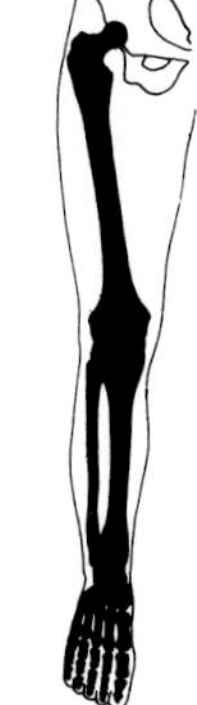

	NOMENCLATURE	
Amelia (T-) upper right	Original Frantz-O'Rahilly	Amelia (T-) lower right
Amelia, upper right (shoulder-disarticulation)	European	Amelia, lower right (hip-disarticulation)
Amelia (T-) upper right	Revised Frantz-O'Rahilly	Amelia (T-) upper right

Fig. 37-11. Absence of skeletal elements of arm and forearm with hand attached to trunk or absence of elements of thigh and leg with foot attached to trunk.

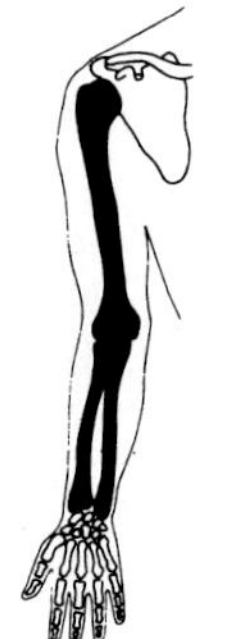
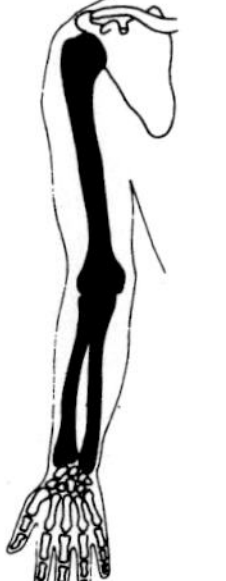
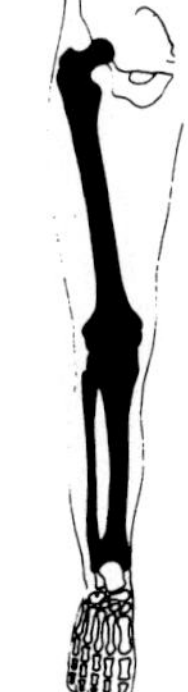

	NOMENCLATURE	
Complete phocomelia (L/) right	Original Frantz-O'Rahilly	Complete phocomelia (L/) right
Phocomelia, upper right	European	Phocomelia, lower right
Meromelia (L/) humeral, radioulnar, right	Revised Frantz-O'Rahilly	Meromelia (L/) femoral, tibiofibular right

Fig. 37-12. Left, absence of arm elements with forearm attached directly to trunk, or absence of thigh elements with leg attached to trunk. Right, absence of leg elements with foot attached directly to thigh, or absence of forearm elements with hand attached to arm (not shown).

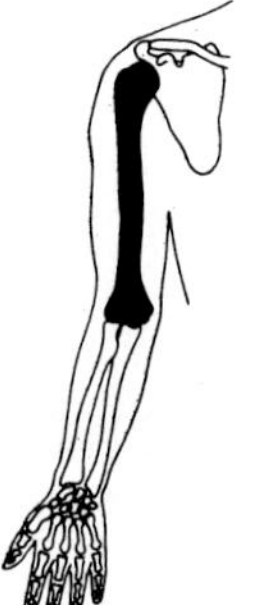
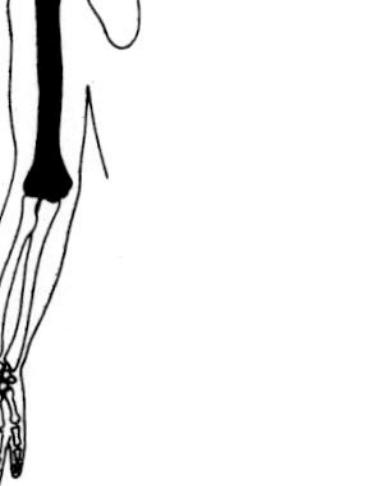
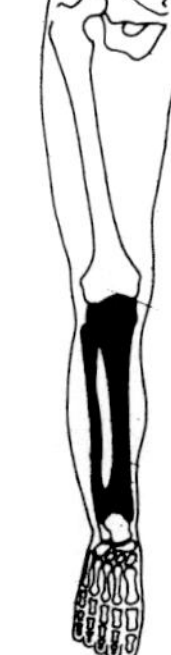

	NOMENCLATURE	
Incomplete (distal) Phocomelia (L/) right	Original Frantz-O'Rahilly	Incomplete (proximal) Phocomelia (L/) right
Ectromelia, proximal type	European	Ectromelia, distal type
Meromelia (L/) humeral, right	Revised Frantz-O'Rahilly	Meromelia (L/) tibiofibular, right

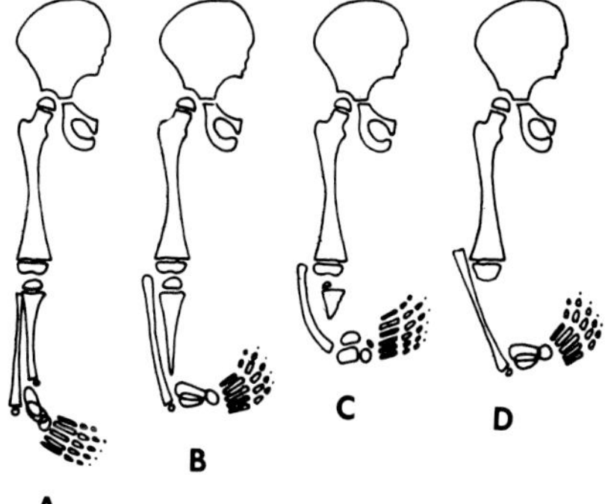

Fig. 37-13. Distal form of ectromelia. **A,** Tibia hypoplasia. **B,** Partial tibia aplasia. **C,** Subtotal tibia aplasia. **D,** Total tibia aplasia.

"Reduktion" or progression in the severity of a defect, and characterized by such terms as hypoplasia, partial aplasia, and total aplasia (Fig. 37-13).

THE DUNDEE WORKSHOP

It was against this background then that a working group met in Dundee, Scotland, under the auspices of the International Society for Prosthetics and Orthotics, charged with the responsibility of proposing a terminology which might be acceptable internationally.

The proceedings opened with brief presentations by members of the working group concerning terminology systems in current use, plus some preliminary thoughts as to procedures for the development of some unanimity of opinion on nomenclature.

In the discussion which followed it was readily agreed that, while the use of words derived from Greek and Latin roots was common in medicine and was theoretically attractive for a classification nomenclature, the implementation of this practice in the past had led to considerable confusion. People had tended to invent Greek- or Latin-derived words and attach their own special meanings to them. Moreover many languages in the world were not related to the classical languages and translations were sometimes difficult. Hence it was decided to eliminate such terms as peromelia, ectromelia, hemimelia, and meromelia, and attempt to describe deficiencies in the simplest yet most precise language which would be understandable by all the English-speaking world and be easily translatable into other languages.

Subcategories

Attention was directed to a consideration of the four basic categories of limb deficiencies proposed in the original Frantz-O'Rahilly work. These categories were:

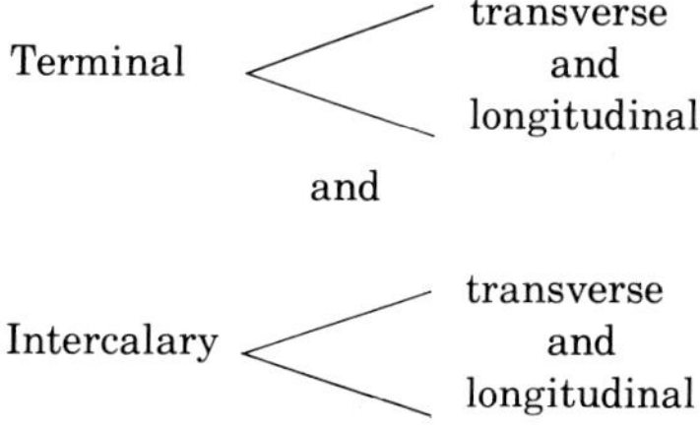

Unanimity of opinion was reached immediately concerning terminal transverse conditions, i.e., those presenting a congenital amputation-type stump. However, the existence of true intercalary deformities was questioned.

After considerable discussion and review of prior presentations involving both x-rays and diagrammatic representations of limb deficiencies, general agreement was reached that true intercalary deficiencies rarely if ever existed. It was postulated that all "phocomelias" or "intercalary deficiencies" had some terminal manifestation—be it a tarsal or carpal aberration, a defect of a finger or toe, or a deficiency of muscle, tendon, skin, or nail. From this evolved an approach to classification which suggested that these intercalary defects were in reality variable degrees of longitudinal deficiencies. It was concluded that with the single exception of the previously mentioned transverse deficiencies all others were a manifestation of some longitudinal aberration in the formation of parts—thus even that condition described as "hypoplasia" of a limb or skeletal element in reality had a longitudinal (in the sense of the long axis of each bone) failure. Similarly, although "phocomelia" had a major manifestation of failure of formation in the long bones, there was also a lesser and perhaps minimal failure in the peripheral elements which, although present, were never truly normal. This concept of progressive longitudinal reduction can be carried to a point where only a single digital remnant of a limb of a limb remains and ultimately to the situation in which even this vestigial peripheral element failed to form—the true amelia. This, therefore, might be considered a maximum longitudinal deficiency although presenting as a transverse-type defect. For simplicity of designation, however, amelia might best be categorized as a transverse deficiency. It was recognized that in clinical practice the use of such well-established terms as amelia, phocomelia, and proximal femoral focal deficiency (PFFD) would likely continue.

Based on this line of reasoning, a decision was reached to consolidate all limb deficiencies into two groups:

1. Transverse
2. Longitudinal

The transverse defects would encompass all so-called congenital amputation-type conditions and include what heretofore were referred to as terminal transverse deficiencies. The second major category would then become the longitudinal deficiencies which would encompass in effect all deficiencies which were not in the transverse category. It was agreed that the longitudinal category would require subdivision into (1) proximal longitudinal, (2) distal longitudinal, and (3) combined longitudinal deficiencies.

In further discussion of subdivisions under these two major categories, it was generally agreed that transverse deficiencies could be described and characterized by the level at which the limb terminated, but that in the longitudinal deficiencies such a description was unnecessary and that each deficiency could be described by naming the bone(s) affected and indicating whether they were completely or partially absent. It was recognized that conditions referred to as hypoplasia or underdevelopment in any one or all of the bones of the limb did exist, and could be described in the proximal, distal, or the combined form, again by naming the bone(s) affected and indicating the presence of hypoplasia.

OVERALL CLASSIFICATIONS OF MALFORMATIONS

At the request of Dr. Swanson the overall classification for congenital malformations, which had been accepted previously by the American Hand Society, was considered. This system encompassed seven categories:

I. Failure of formation of parts
II. Failure of differentiation (separation) of parts
III. Duplication
IV. Overgrowth (gigantism)
V. Undergrowth
VI. Congenital constriction band syndrome
VII. Generalized skeletal abnormalities

While there was tacit acceptance of the rationality of these categories, it was unanimously agreed that the prime and virtually sole concern of the workshop was with nomenclature and classification in congenital *skeletal limb deficiencies*. In terms of the classification categories listed above these conditions would generally fall into the grouping designated as "failure of formation of parts," although some conditions might also involve failure of differentiation of parts, e.g., synostosis, or even occasionally undergrowth, e.g., a radius which was complete but hypoplastic.

PROPOSED INTERNATIONAL NOMENCLATURE FOR CLASSIFICATION OF DEFICIENCIES

The workshop members then proceeded to the development of a schema which was unanimously proposed for international adoption as follows:

Failure of formation of parts

1. Transverse limb deficiencies (congenital amputations)

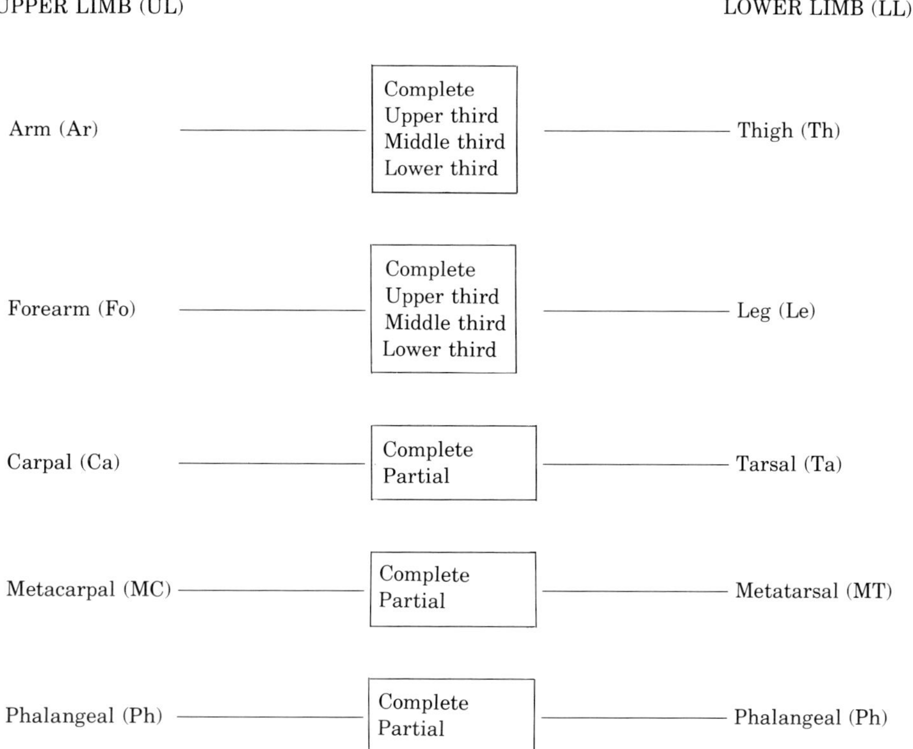

Discussion

A few illustrations are presented to clarify the application of this classification procedure. It should be noted that in each case *the designation indicates the level of absence,* it being understood that all skeletal elements distal to that level are also absent. Each classification would, of course, include right (R), left (L), or bilateral (Bil).

1. Complete absence of an upper or lower limb (Figs. 37-14 and 37-15) would then be a transverse deficiency – arm (Ar), or thigh (Th), complete. The term amelia (Fig. 37-10) would probably continue in clinical use to characterize this condition.

2. A transverse deficiency, Ar, upper, would indicate a short above-elbow amputation-like limb which terminated in the upper third of the humerus (Fig. 37-16); a transverse deficiency, Th, lower, would be the term applied to a long above-knee amputation-like stump which terminated in the distal third of the femur (Fig. 37-17).

3. An elbow-disarticulation-type deficit (Fig. 37-18) would be classified as a transverse deficiency, forearm (Fo), complete; while below-elbow-type stumps would be designated Fo, upper, middle, or lower, depending on the third of the forearm in which the limb terminated (Figs. 37-19 to 37-21).

4. For transverse deficiencies which terminate in the carpal, tarsal, metacarpal, metatarsal, and phalangeal areas, only the designations complete and partial are used to denote the level of loss in that particular area. For example, carpal (or Ca), complete, would indicate a wrist-disarticulation-type stump (F-O'R's acheiria); MC, complete, a F-O'R adactylia, and Ph, com-

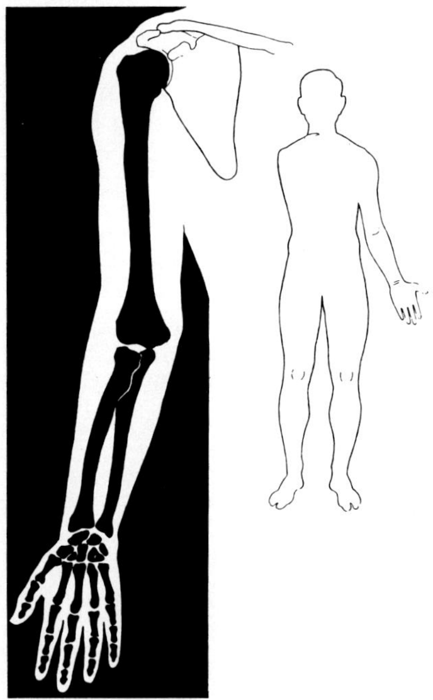

Fig. 37-14. Transverse deficiency: right arm (AR), complete.

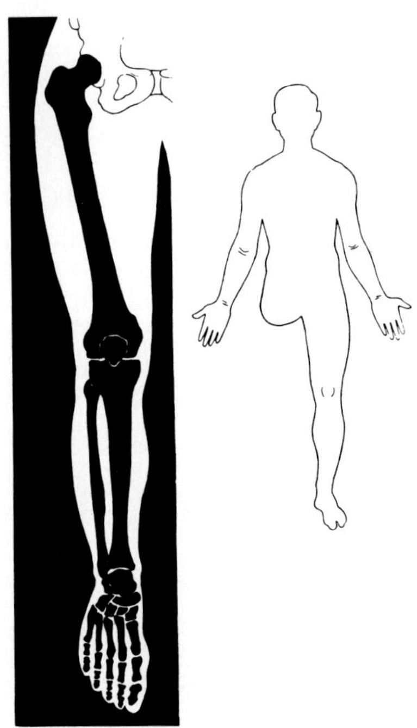

Fig. 37-15. Transverse deficiency: right thigh (Th), complete.

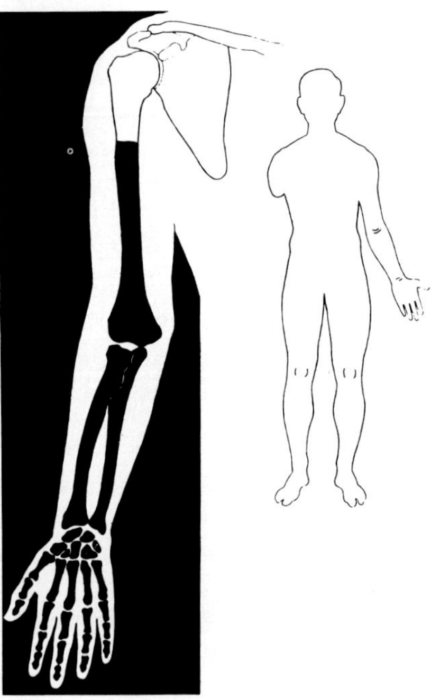

Fig. 37-16. Transverse deficiency: right arm (Ar), upper.

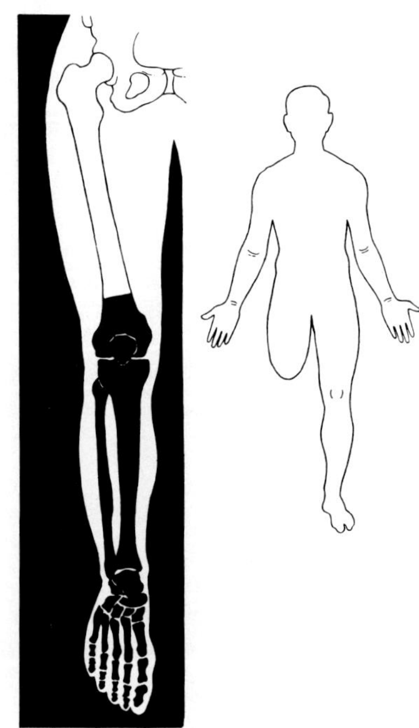

Fig. 37-17. Transverse deficiency: right thigh (Th), lower.

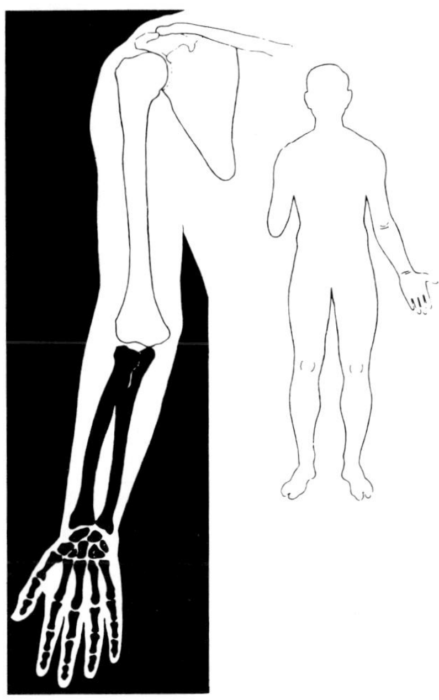

Fig. 37-18. Transverse deficiency: right forearm (Fo), complete.

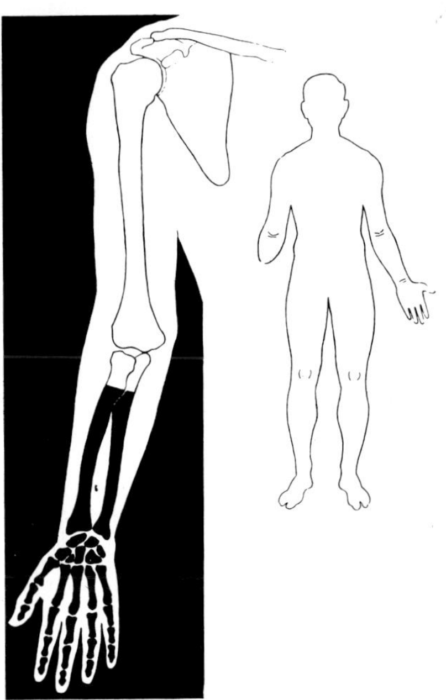

Fig. 37-19. Transverse deficiency: right forearm (Fo), upper.

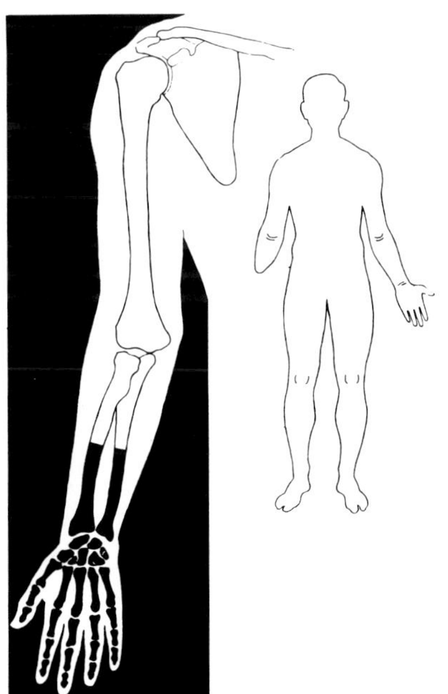

Fig. 37-20. Transverse deficiency: right forearm (Fo), middle.

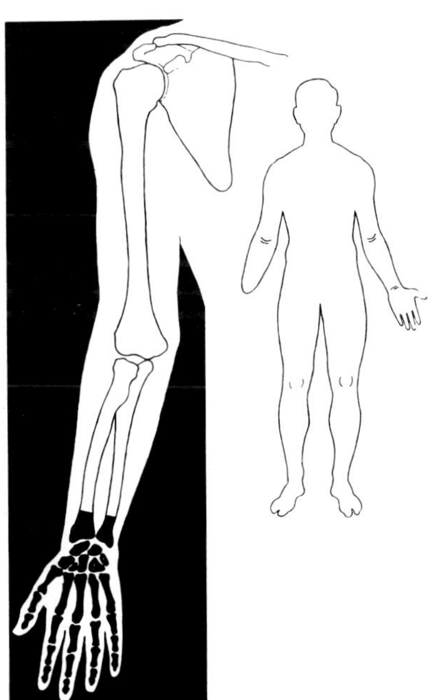

Fig. 37-21. Transverse deficiency: right forearm (Fo), lower.

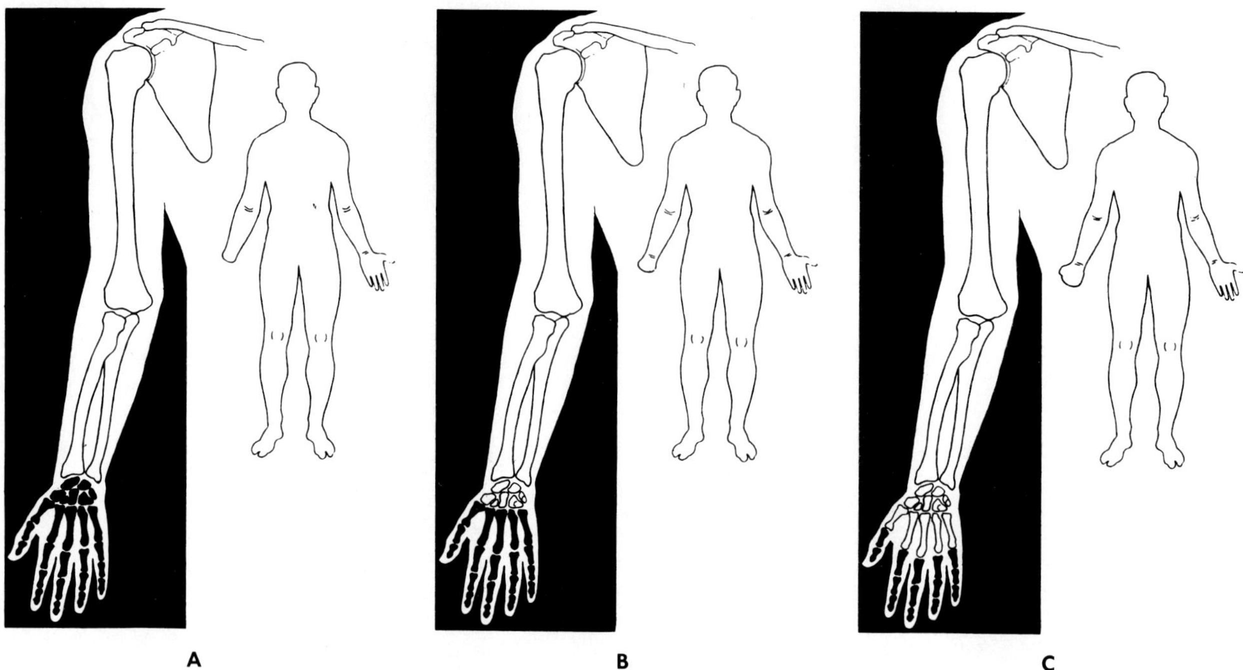

Fig. 37-22. A, Transverse deficiency: right carpal (Ca), complete. **B,** Transverse deficiency: right metacarpal (MC), complete. **C,** Transverse deficiency: right phalangeal (Ph), complete.

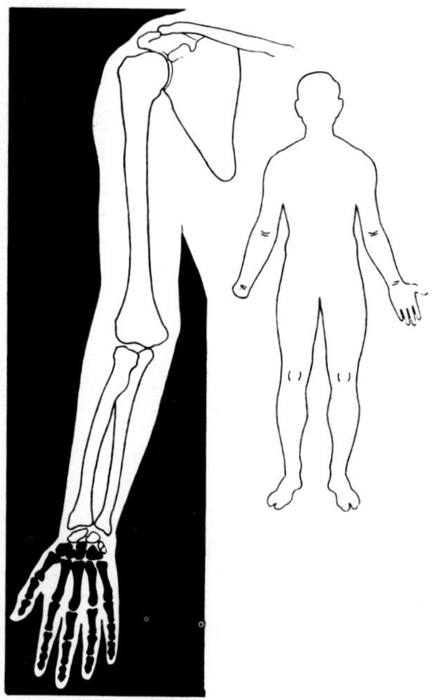

Fig. 37-23. Transverse deficiency: right carpal (Ca), partial.

plete, a F-O'R aphalangia (Fig. 37-22). If for example one row of carpals still remained, the term used would be Ca, partial (Fig. 37-23).

It is obvious that although all limb deficiencies will fall into the broad categories of upper- or lower-limb deficits it is unnecessary to spell out this identification in classifying them, since the information will be self-evident from the bone(s) named.

In developing the examples presented the author found it tedious to write out the general category each time. He suggests, therefore, that the abbreviation (T-) from earlier classification systems be used. Fully abbreviated then the deficit shown in Fig. 37-18 would be written: (T-), R, Ar, upper.

2. Longitudinal deficiencies

Naturally the application of the proposed schema for longitudinal deficiencies is considerably more complex than that involving the transverse variety, since the longitudinal category now includes deficits which, in earlier American systems, had been divided into three groups—terminal longitudinal, intercalary transverse, and intercalary longitudinal.

However, if we proceed from the simplest situation to the more complicated and relate new terms to old, a pattern is readily discernible. It should be noted that the principle followed in earlier systems, that of naming bones that were absent rather than those that were present, is also followed here. It is also worthy of note that while the term intercalary has been eliminated from the proposed international terminology, this condition, both in its transverse and longitudinal forms, is readily describable in the new system.

The classification system applicable to longitudinal deficiencies is presented in the following chart:

2. Longitudinal deficiencies—all bones named to be designated as partially or completely absent

UPPER LIMB (UL)

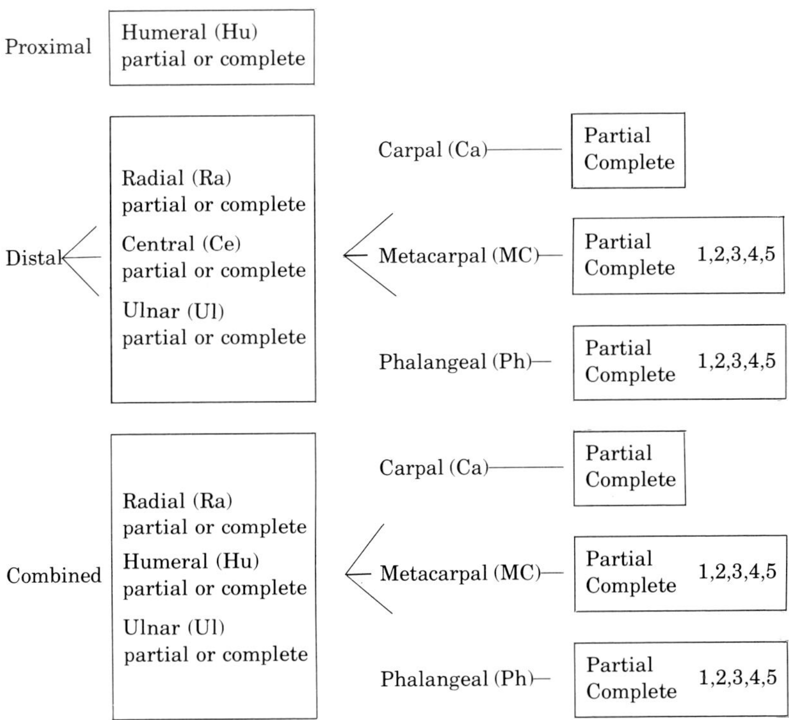

LOWER LIMB (LL)

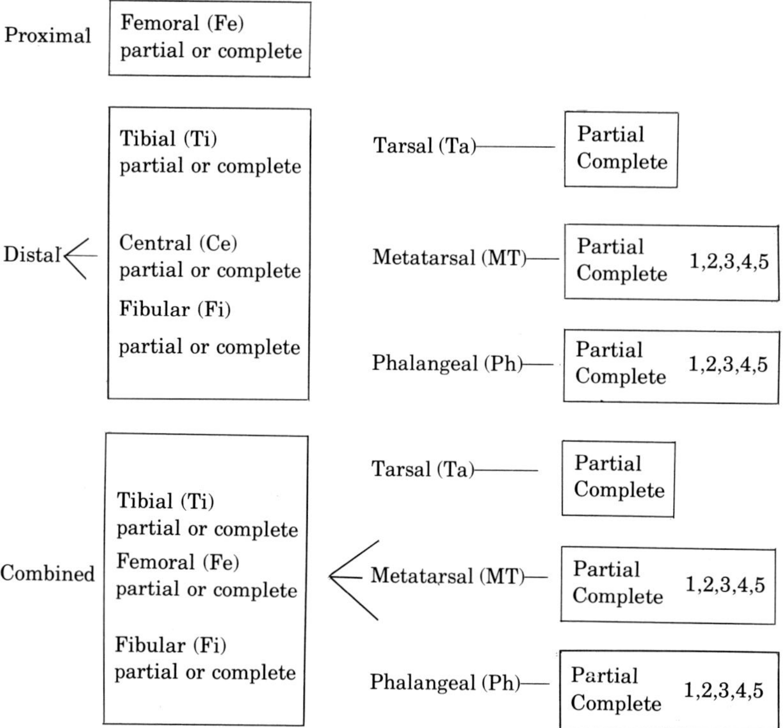

Examples

Application of the classification scheme for longitudinal deficiencies is illustrated in the examples which follow:

1. A longitudinal deficiency (proximal), Hu or Fe, complete, would correspond to the intercalary transverse defect – proximal phocomelia – of Frantz-O'Rahilly (Fig. 37-24). Similarly

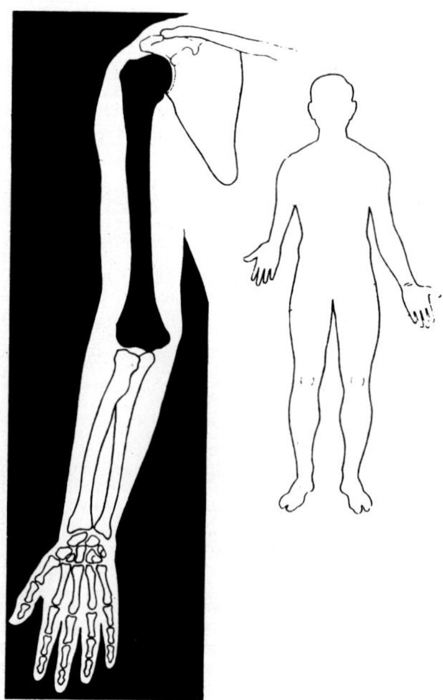

Fig. 37-24. Longitudinal deficiency: right humeral (Hu), complete.

the distal forms radial-ulnar (Ra-Ul) or tibial-fibular (Ti-Fi), complete, would correspond to Frantz-O'Rahilly's distal phocomelia (Figs. 37-25 and 37-26).

2. In other distal forms, radial (Ra), ulnar (Ul), tibial (Ti), or fibular (Fi), complete, would be the new terms for the old Frantz-O'Rahilly intercalary longitudinal defects—complete paraxial hemimelia radial, ulnar, tibial, or fibular (Fig. 37-27). Ra, Ul, Ti, or Fi, incomplete, would, of course, be the incomplete forms of these same conditions (Fig. 37-28).

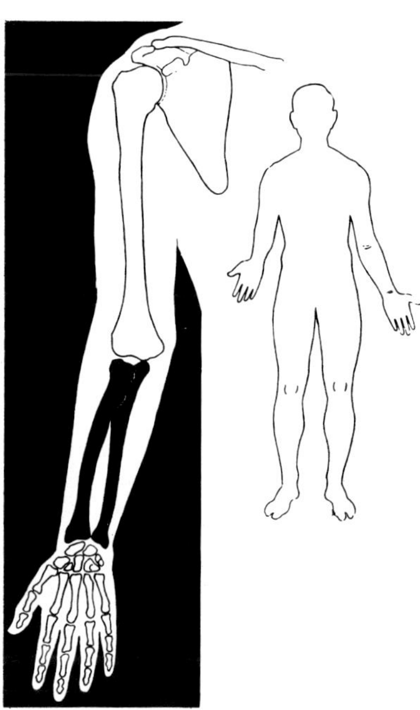

Fig. 37-25. Longitudinal deficiency: right radial-ulnar (Ra-Ul), complete.

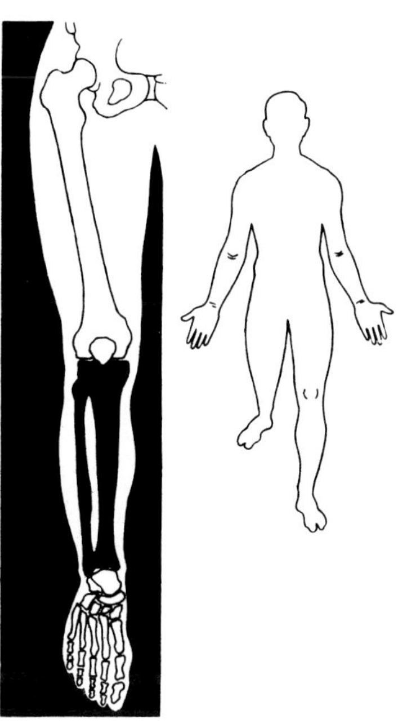

Fig. 37-26. Longitudinal deficiency: right tibial-fibular (Ti-Fi), complete.

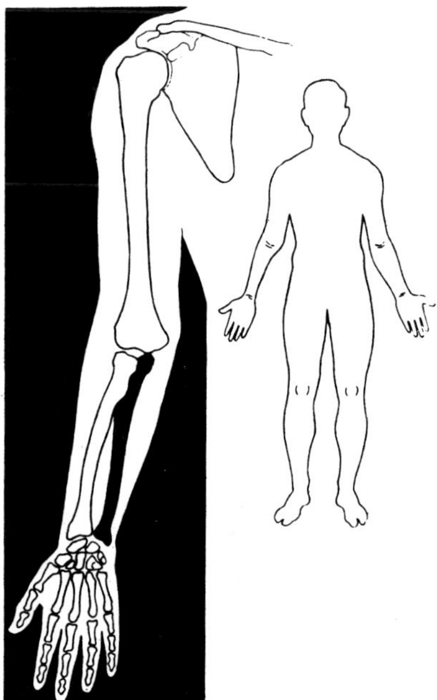

Fig. 37-27. Longitudinal deficiency: right ulnar (Ul), complete.

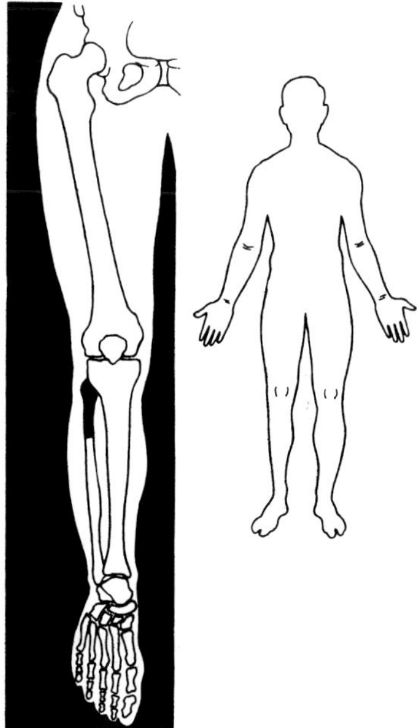

Fig. 37-28. Longitudinal deficiency: right fibular (Fi), partial.

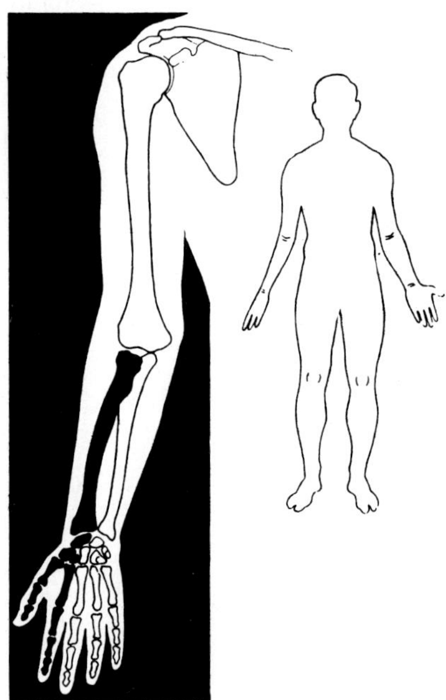

Fig. 37-29. Longitudinal deficiency: right radial (Ra), complete; carpal (Ca), partial; metacarpal (MC) 1.2, complete; phalangeal (Ph) 1.2, complete.

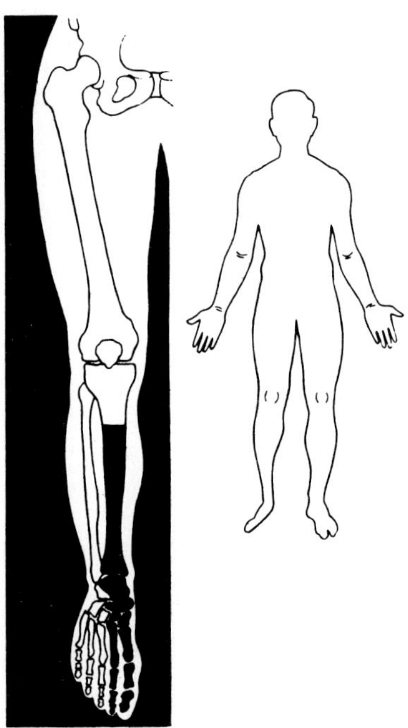

Fig. 37-30. Longitudinal deficiency: right tibial (Ti), partial; tarsal (Ta), partial; metatarsal (MT) 1.2, complete; phalangeal (Ph) 1.2, complete.

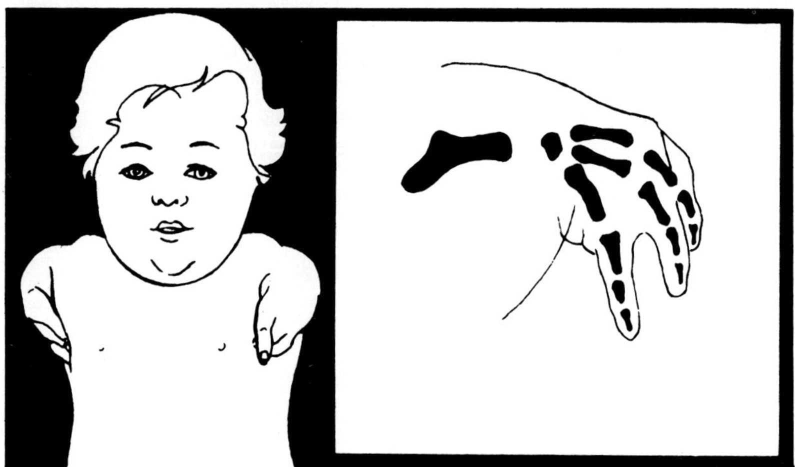

Fig. 37-31. Longitudinal deficiency: left humeral (Hu), complete; radial-ulnar (Ra-Ul), partial, with synostosis; carpal (Ca), partial; metacarpal (MC) 1.2, complete; and phalangeal (Ph) 1.2, complete.

3. Samples of distal forms which also involve hand or foot elements would be (a) Ra, complete; Ca, partial; MC 1.2, complete; Ph 1.2, complete, to describe what had been known heretofore as the terminal longitudinal deficiency—complete paraxial hemimelia, radial, of Frantz-O'Rahilly (Fig. 37-29); or (b) Ti, partial; Ta, partial; MT 1.2, complete; Ph 1.2, complete, to describe the defect shown earlier as incomplete paraxial hemimelia, tibial, in the Frantz-O'Rahilly terminology (Fig. 37-30).

4. Combined types of longitudinal deficiencies would essentially be those erstwhile phocomelias in which elements were defective or absent at all levels of a limb. An example is shown in

Fig. 37-31 from Willert and Henkel. Described by these authors as an "Axiale Form der Ektromelie" (kurzer Achsentyp mit radioulnärer Synostose), its full description in the proposed international terminology would be a longitudinal deficiency; Hu, complete; Ra and Ul, partial with synostosis; Ca, partial; MC 1.2, complete; and Ph 1.2, complete. Clinically the condition would doubtless still be called a phocomelia, or perhaps a proximal phocomelia.

It should be emphasized that in the longitudinal deficiencies only the absent bone (or bones) is cited no assumptions being made that more distal elements are also absent.

Again it is evident that, while the categories of UL and LL, and proximal, distal, or combined would be useful in organizing statistical or census data, these terms are not essential for classification. As in the transverse deficiencies this information is self-evident from the bone(s) named.

In preparing the examples for this paper the author again found it tedious to have to write out "a longitudinal deficiency" each time. Use of an abbreviation L slash in parentheses (L/)—to avoid confusion with L for left—is proposed.

It should also be emphasized that the examples presented in this section are for illustrative purposes only. Some of the deficiencies classified may not exist clinically in as "pure" a form as depicted here.

FURTHER RECOMMENDATIONS

Following the development of the proposed international nomenclature as described, members of the working group tried out the new system by reclassifying a number of the deficiencies presented in slides earlier in the workshop. No difficulties were experienced. However, it was recognized that more extensive trials were desirable. Members of the workshop agreed to continue trying out the new system themselves but also recommended that field trials be carried out internationally under the auspices of the International Society for Prosthetics and Orthotics. These trials could be conducted in the U.S.A. through the medium of the Subcommittee on Child Prosthetics Problems of the Committee on Prosthetics Research and Development, and elsewhere in the world through selected child amputee clinics. Plans are now being made to implement these recommendations.

It was further recommended that the proposed international terminology for the classification of congenital limb deficiencies, as described in this paper, be brought to the attention of the World Health Organization for possible inclusion in the revision of standard nomenclature now being undertaken by that body. This recommendation has since been followed.

LITERATURE CITED

1. Burtch, Robert L., Nomenclature for congenital skeletal limb deficiencies, a revision of the Frantz and O'Rahilly classification. Artif. Limbs, **10:**1:24-35, Spring 1966.
2. Frantz, C. H., and R. O'Rahilly, Congenital skeletal limb deficiencies. J. Bone and Joint Surg., **43-A:**8:1202-1224, December 1961.
3. Hepp, Oscar, Frequency of the congenital defect—Anomalies of the extremities in the Federal Republic of Germany. Inter-Clin. Inform. Bull., **1:**10:3-12, July-August 1962.
4. Jentschura, G., E. Marquardt, and E.-M. Rudel, Behandlung und Versorgung bei Fehlbildungen und Amputationen der oberen Extremität. Georg Thieme Verlag, Stuttgart, Germany, 1963.
5. Jentschura, G., E. Marquardt, and E.-M. Rudel, Malformations and Amputations of the Upper Extremity: Treatment and Prosthetic Replacement. Grune & Stratton, New York, 1967.
6. Swanson, A. B., A classification for congenital malformations of the hand. New Jersey Bull., Academy of Medicine, **10:**166-169, September 1964.
7. Swanson, A. B., Classification of limb malformations on the basis of embryological failures: A preliminary report. Inter-Clin. Inform. Bull., **6:**3:1-15, December 1966.
8. Willert, H.-G., and H.-L. Henkel, Klinik und Pathologie der Dysmelie: Die Fehlbildungen an den oberen Extremitäten bei der Thalidomid-Embryopathie. Springer-Verlag, Heidelberg, New York, 1969.
9. Henkel, H.-L., and H.-G. Willert, Dysmelia, a classification and a pattern of malformation of congenital limb deficiencies. J. Bone and Joint Surg., **51-B:**3:399-414, August 1969.

SUGGESTED READING

Henkel, H. L. et al.: An international terminology for the classification of congenital limb deficiencies, Arch. Orthop. Traumat. Surg. **93:**1-19, 1978.

CHAPTER 38

Congenital limb deficiencies

Section I

Upper limb deficiencies

RAYMOND J. PELLICORE
CLAUDE N. LAMBERT

A congenital limb deficiency is often erroneously categorized as a congenital amputation. This latter is a rare phenomenon in which one or more limbs are delivered separately from the fetus.

Restoration and rehabilitation of the limb-deficient child should strive to accomplish normal development and function equal to that of a fully formed child of the same age. Congenitally limb-deficient children present a complex group of problems, all of which are different, but interrelated and cannot be separated or dealt with individually. Satisfactory rehabilitation requires all facets to be coordinated. Most children with a congenital abnormality of a limb other than terminal transverse deficiencies also have other abnormalities. At birth, recognition of the emotional impact on the parents takes precedence over immediate treatment of the limb-deficient child, yet these two entities cannot be dealt with separately. The child's physical appearance is of primary importance to the parents at birth, whereas later, self-image[10,15] of the child is preeminent in the treatment program. The clinic team[8] concept offers the best approach in evaluating and treating the total needs of the limb-deficient child and his family. The resources of a well-structured clinic are the primary tools for problem solving. The emotional impact of a limb-deficient child on the parent can be greatly alleviated by another parent[19] who has encountered the same traumatic experience. In addition to clinic team members such as a physician, nurse, therapist, prosthetist and others, the parent and child must be considered as important members. It is their interaction with other parents and patients that is so invaluable in developing the treatment program. Questions and doubts can be discussed frankly, with care and concern, and should be carefully orchestrated by the clinic chief. This dialogue offers parents and the patient more awareness of the problems and information for the solutions.

Every child depends on the parents' response to his needs, but this is especially true for the limb-deficient child. The nucleus of self-concept begins with the parents' understanding and ability to accept this "special" child as an individual with the need for complete fulfillment. The prosthesis aids in achieving this fulfillment. Ideally, this device will be integrated into the patient's normal activities and eventually become part of his body and body image. A child's achievement usually indicates the parents' acceptance of the deficiency and the relationship existing between the child and parent. Prosthetic acceptance and use can be directly related to the reinforcement and care given by the parents. Sorby[17] of Sweden indicated that with early fitting of a prosthesis, the child can achieve almost normal natural use of the limb. Although his patients have been few, his early results appear impressive.

It is essential that the child be fitted with the most current prosthetic devices available for the specific level of amputation. The goals of prosthetic restoration include optimum function, comfort, and cosmesis. Having achieved these goals, appropriate training must follow, remembering that this is a prosthetic substitution and not a replacement of a normal limb. It is important to reiterate that we should strive for function and restoration compatible with a nonlimb-deficient child of the same age. At times, in our enthusiasm, we lose sight of our rehabilitation goals and have a tendency to "overgadget" these children, with less than desirable results. With certain limb deficiencies, a prosthesis actually interferes with or diminishes available function in the residual limb. Specifically, tactile sensation or grasping function of remaining digits should not be interfered with or covered by a prosthetic device. This is especially true of the most distal levels of upper limb deficiencies. The most difficult prosthetic restorations to achieve are those with the most proximal and most distal deficits. Until external power becomes more sophisticated, functional, and durable, we will have the ongoing problem of restoring adequate function for high-level deficiencies. The age[23] for fitting upper limb-deficient children has undergone an interesting evolution. In past years it was taught that upper limb–deficient children should be fitted 6 months to 1 year prior to admission to an educational system (school). At this age the child is capable of developing a pattern of purposeful grasp and release and has an adequate attention span to effect satisfactory prosthetic training. Early fitting (less than 1 year of age) is now advocated by the majority of clinics. Prosthetic tolerance and prehension patterns at normal arm's length from the body are two of the desirable goals to be achieved with early fitting. Substitution patterns are avoided, and sensory function of the stump at the interface with the prosthesis will stimulate visual clues. Some centers teach that upper limb–deficient children may be fitted when good sitting balance is established, but a 3-month-old infant can execute useful gross grasp in a supine position. The fitting of a 3-month-old with a passive mitten prosthesis has been a successful and an accepted early fitting prescription.

The duration of attention span and patterns of prehension and release have been well documented[9] for various ages. Therefore the age of training and functional goals are for the most part standardized and accepted. At age 18 months the child fitted with a single-control below-elbow prosthesis should be ready for training by a competent therapist. The child with an above-elbow deficiency fitted with a prosthesis with dual control, including an elbow locking mechanism should be at least 36 months old if training is to be successful. As a generalization, a unilateral or bilateral upper limb amputee can be fitted with a prosthetic appliance to furnish gross grasp as soon as adequate development for such function is present.

SURGERY

Most experienced surgeons believe there are few indications for primary conversion in congenital upper limb deficiencies. Surgical procedures should be undertaken only by a surgeon who has had ongoing experience in dealing with the congenital limb-deficient child and is aware of the natural history of the deficiency. Although approximately 50% of lower limb longitudinal deficiencies require some form of conversion, only 8% of similar upper limb deficiencies require any type of surgical conversion.[1] The majority of these surgical procedures are performed at the hand and wrist. Vestigial tags that are long and pedunculated and cause difficulty because of torsion may have to be removed. Other procedures include deepening of webs or clefts to enhance grasp, separating of fingers in syndactylism, centralizing procedures for radial deficiencies, osteotomies, and, rarely, amputations. The objective of reconstructive surgery is to develop a terminal motor and sensory end organ to achieve maximum function.

TRANSVERSE DEFICIENCIES

Deficiencies of digits and metacarpals

Transverse deficiencies of digits, single or multiple, rarely require any replacement prosthesis. On occasion, associated syndactyly requires surgical intervention. With deficiency of all digits or of the distal two digits, clefting between the metacarpals may be indicated.[12] This is particularly indicated to obtain prehension when the digits of the thumb are missing. With transverse deficiency of all digits or partial transverse deficiency of metacarpals, although no surgery may be indicated, prosthetic assistance in the form of an opposition post is indicated.

Complete carpal deficiency

Only rarely is any surgical intervention indicated for complete carpal deficiency. As discussed in Chapter 41, with the multilimb-deficient child, there may be an indication to consider the Krukenberg procedure.[20] Children with this deficiency do quite well with prosthetic restoration (Chapter 40).

Forearm deficiency

Partial. The partial forearm transverse deficiency is the most common upper limb deficiency and is said to represent 30% of all congenital deficiencies.[3] These deficiencies are more common in females than males by a ratio of 3:2. The left side is more frequently absent than the right by a ratio of 2:1. Bilateral deficiencies are extremely rare. At birth, the child has not only the deficiency, but very frequently has an invaginated area of skin over the tip. Subluxation of the proximal radioulnar joint or proximal dislocation of the radial head is quite frequent, resulting from the unopposed pull of the biceps tendon.[7] The elbow flexes to a full 135 degrees, and hyperextension of the elbow joint is almost always present. Rarely is any surgical intervention indicated.

Complete. Anatomically, the complete forearm transverse deficiency is an elbow disarticulation with the distal epiphyseal plate present and a flared bulbous contour of the condyles. These deficiencies may, in rare instances, maintain normal contour and growth, but more often the condyles become attenuated, and shortening occurs. The distal stump may be dimpled, smooth, or have a small lobule of fat. Normal musculature of the shoulder arm complex is present, with completely normal motion and strength. Surgical intervention is seldom, if ever, indicated in the very young child.

Arm deficiency

Partial. The partial arm transverse deficiency may have a residual limb from 5 cm (2 inches) to virtual full length. Bony overgrowth of the humerus[11] has been reported in patients with this deficiency. Surgical correction is identical to that recommended for bony overgrowth which occurs after transmetaphyseal amputations. In selected cases with longer residual limbs, Marquardt's osteotomy may be beneficial (Chapter 41).

The function of very short residual limbs, whose motion cannot be captured to activate a prosthesis can be enhanced with surgery. Deepening of the axillary web can, in a few instances, allow sufficient socket interface to capture the residual stump motion. A more extensive procedure entails a skin, fascia, and muscle tube to elongate the stump, followed with a bone transplant.[5] A free bone graft implanted into the tube will usually be absorbed, with only a very small portion of the graft remaining. With the use of microsurgical techniques, a pedicle bone graft should remain viable and preclude reabsorption.

Complete (amelia). When the upper limb is completely absent (amelia), no surgical procedure has been devised to improve function. Prosthetic use is less than ideal (Chapter 11).

LONGITUDINAL DEFICIENCIES

Syndactyly

Syndactyly[4] is the second most frequent congenital anomaly of the hand (polydactyly being the most common). Bilateral involvement, often symmetrical, occurs in approximately 50% of the cases. The male to female ratio is about 3:1. The simplest form of syndactylism is an incomplete skin web between two fingers without bone, joint, or other associated deformity. More complicated cases may occur, varying from partial synostosis to complete failure of segmentation, extending the entire length of the phalanges. The age at which surgical intervention is indicated is determined by the severity of involvement. Correction of webbing, without bone or nail involvement, can be delayed until the child is 3 to 5 years old. However, synostoses that inhibit normal growth or interphalangeal function should have earlier surgical intervention. Middle and ring fingers are the most commonly involved digits. Rarely is the thumb affected.

When three or more adjacent fingers are syndactylized, only two fingers should be separated during one surgical procedure. The major functioning fingers should be separated in the primary surgery. As stated in Chapter 10, these are, in order of importance, the index, middle, ring, and small fingers. Longitudinal incisions for developing flaps should be avoided, since scar contracture will occur when the finger grows, and distortion of the finger will result. Suture lines should be curved or zigzagged[16] to prevent cicatricial contractures. The cleft flaps should be outlined to obtain adequate depth. Dorsal and volar flaps of adjacent fingers should be developed with the objective of covering the volar finger surfaces with tactile skin flaps.[16] Remaining denuded surfaces should be covered by free split-thickness grafts or by full-thickness grafts from the groin. When a double nail is separated, a strip of the cut border should be removed, including the matrix, and the skin reshaped around the nail edge by swinging a flap from the side of the pulp around the angle of the nail.

Clubhand (complete or partial longitudinal deficiency of the radius)

Clubhand is a longitudinal deficiency with complete or partial absence of the radius. The incidence of bilateral involvement in patients with a complete radial deficiency is about 50%.[3]

The deformity is cosmetically unattractive, with a short forearm, radially deviated hand, unstable wrist, and weakness of digital power. As in most longitudinal deficiencies, there exists a total limb involvement with varying associated anomalies. The ulna is short, thickened, and curved, with the convexity directed posteriorly. With absence of the thumb, the scaphoid and trapezium usually are missing. Other deformities include shortening of the humerus with hypoplasia of the shoulder girdle. Humeroulna synostosis may be present. The biceps, brachioradialis, flexor carpi radialis, and extensor carpi radialis muscles may be absent or anomalous. Other forearm muscles may be absent or coalesced into one muscle mass. The radial artery and nerve are frequently absent, but the interosseous arteries are usually well developed. The radial nerve frequently ends at the elbow, but the median and ulna nerves extend to the distal portion of the hand. Sensation to the radial side of the ulna is supplied by the median nerve.

In the unilateral club hand, some type of corrective surgical procedure may be indicated if elbow function is present. Early, it is necessary to correct the radial deviation by stretching or surgically elongating the contractures on the radial side. Splinting alone is seldom successful, and surgical release is necessary to centralize the carpus over the distal portion of the ulna. When a mobile wrist is the desired goal, skin Z-plasties and tendon lengthening should be performed; however, if a fusion is planned, then tenotomies and capsulotomies may be done. Ulnocarpal fusion should only be considered as a late procedure.

Several surgical procedures have been devised for correction of the deformity, improvement of hand function, and cosmesis. One technique is to create an articulation between the distal ulna and carpus, attempting to establish a degree of stability and still allow some mobility.[2] Steindler[18] performed a double osteotomy of the distal ulna, removed the segment in between, and accomplished a Y articulation with the wrist. Others grafted a portion of the fibula to the distal ulna to accomplish the same Y articulation. Riordan[13] grafted the proximal epiphyseal portion of the fibula to the ulna, and in a few cases the fibular epiphysis continued to grow. Sayre,[14] in 1893, was the first to recommend centralization of the ulna. He accomplished this by resecting the lunate and capitate bones and inserting the distal ulna into the gap created.

In bilateral clubhand cases, controversy exists as to whether any surgical procedures should be performed, since radial deviation of the wrist is essential for hand-mouth function. Surgery should be considered only if normal shoulder and elbow function are present.[6]

Phocomelia

Phocomelia is a longitudinal deficiency in which part or all of the forearm and arm are absent with the hand articulating with the residual limb or at the shoulder. In phocomelia, the hand[22] has prehension and sensation, but it cannot be positioned for normal function.

Complete (longitudinal deficiency of the humerus, radius, and ulna). In complete phocomelia, the hand is attached at the shoulder level. In unilateral complete phocomelia, unequal lengths of limbs require awkward torso gyrations for bimanual activity. In this deficiency, sensation of the hand is intact. Finger and wrist function are present, although restricted. These are total limb deficiencies with considerably less than normal musculature of the hand, wrist, and shoulder girdle. Flexion of the fingers can develop pinch forces of 0.45 to 9 kg (1 to 2 pounds). Extension force is much less.

Rehabilitation of patients with unilateral deficits may include prosthetic prescription to permit limbs of equal length. Successful prosthetic restoration is unusual. Surgery is seldom indicated.

Bilateral (longitudinal deficiency of the humerus, radius, and ulna). Patients with bilateral phocomelia usually have associated lower limb deformities that preclude good foot function for activities of daily living. It is axiomatic that if normal lower limbs are present, foot function should not be inhibited.[21]

Early prosthetic fitting is not advocated in either the unilateral or bilateral phocomelic patient. When growth of the head and neck away from the torso makes hand to face and mouth contact difficult, prosthetic aid should be considered for eating and toilet care. Indications for surgery are rare.

Proximal (longitudinal deficiency of the humerus). This is a deficiency in which the forearm articulates with the scapula. This deficiency is rare, constituting about 1%[3] of all congenital anomalies, with bilateral involvement in 40% of patients. Finger motion and power parallel those for other phocomelic deficiencies. Shoulder motion also lacks normal range and power.

Prosthetic restoration should be considered in the bilateral case when hand to mouth contact cannot be made with either limb and when aid is needed for toilet care. Surgery is of little value other than to enhance hand function.

Distal (longitudinal deficiency of the radius and ulna). In this deficiency the hand articulates with the humerus, the distal end of which appears to be forked. This deficit represents about 4%[17] of all anomalies, with 25% of these cases having bilateral involvement. The hand usually lacks one or more rays and lacks normal muscle power. The philosophy of fitting and prosthetic indications are the same as for proximal phocomelia. Surgical considerations are of little value.

Section II

Lower limb deficiencies

LEON M. KRUGER

BASIC PRINCIPLES

The physiological differences between children and adults have already been discussed, as have general surgical considerations and planning for the care of the juvenile amputee. Emphasis should be placed on early prosthetic fitting and habilitation whenever possible. In general, it can be stated that the unilateral lower limb–deficient child can and should be fitted when he shows any tendency to stand. One should anticipate that the child will become ambulatory promptly, whether it is a distal or proximal transverse deficiency. By the same token, in unilateral longitudinal limb deficiency, in which it is likely that surgical revision will be necessary, a treatment plan should be developed so that, if possible, all surgical procedures can be carried out in one stage. The child should be brought to independent ambulation as early as possible, with surgical intervention and resultant scarring kept to a minimum and with the best physiological restoration available.

Surgical intervention on the limb-deficient child, particularly on those with longitudinal deficiencies, should be undertaken only by the experienced orthopaedic surgeon, and preferably in those centers which are accustomed to dealing with these children. By their very nature, and fortuitously, these deformities occur infrequently and therefore are not likely to be seen on any recurring basis in the office practice or general hospital.

Certain basic principles must be understood and applied with regard to surgical intervention on these children: (1) early communication and explanation of treatment concepts to the parents as well as to the pediatrician, (2) maintenance of muscular development in the residual limb, (3) prevention of progressive deformity, especially in joints proximal to the deficiency, and (4) retention of all long bone growth plates.

Early communication with parents and pediatricians

Those clinics caring for limb-deficient children should attempt to establish rapport with pediatricians and obstetricians so that on the birth of such a child the clinic chief will have the opportunity to examine the child in the newborn nursery. Subsequent to this examination he will have an opportunity to discuss with the parents the positive approach to the treatment program, which he may outline for the child's care. Recognition of the shock, grief, and guilt experienced by the new parent of a child with one or more deficient limbs dictates the physician's responsibility to assuage these feelings by presenting to the parent not just the diagnosis or anatomical description of the deficiency, but a positive approach to the child's immediate status and future capabilities. For a positive approach, the physician should emphasize the remaining normal limbs, absence of brain damage, and expectations of the child's physical development. The new parent should be assured of the child's potential for ambulation, independence of daily living, and normal mental development. Assistance in these discussions may be sought from the social worker and pediatrician. If there is a problem with the parent, psychological or psychiatric consultations may be indicated.

It is particularly important to stress to the family that most limb deficiencies occur sporadically and are not genetically transmitted. In those rare instances, such as deficiency of the tibia associated with absence of the first metacarpal ray, in which there is a known heritable defect, genetic consultation is indicated.

Once out of the hospital, and particularly if surgical conversion of the limb deficiency is anticipated, the parents should be invited to the "clinic." There they should be encouraged to observe older children with the same or similar deficiencies and particularly to discuss the child's physical and social development with the parents of these older children. They should be encouraged to ask questions with regards to the child's participation, not only in family activity at home, but also social, play, and school activities. Concerns about social acceptance of the deficiency and, particularly, of indicated prosthetic restoration may subconsciously prejudice a parent against any recommended treatment program. Airing their concerns, through conversations with parents of other children with these problems, eases new parents through this difficult transition period and assimilates them into the clinic team as integral members in the planning and execution of the program to habilitate their child. Such "group therapy" enables the parent to comprehend the need for and accept the recommendation to proceed with ablative surgery when it is indicated. In effect, then, these parents participate in the ultimate treatment decisions. Without this open communication between parent and clinic team the more complicated problems of the limb-deficient child may be insoluble.

Maintenance of muscular development in the residual limb

A congenital limb deficiency may not be simply the absence of a long bone or the peripheral joint distal to the deficiency, but may also include inadequacy of the proximal musculature and deficits in the skin, nail, and nerve. Recognizing the deficits in the proximal musculature at the initial evaluation is important if progressive deformity is to be prevented. To this end a program must be developed to include not only institutional physical therapy but also education of the parents in the techniques of development and maintenance of muscle strength. The parents should be brought into the physical therapy department for instruction by the therapist for a home program.

Prevention of progressive deformity

Prevention of deformity in the child with a lesser deficiency may pose no problem. In fact, even with a major deficiency such as an amelia, there is no concern with progressive deformity. However, in the more complicated limb deficiency, such as proximal femoral focal deficiency (PFFD) and longitudinal deficiency of the tibia and fibula, an exercise program for strengthening or stretching of remaining musculature may be inadequate to prevent deformity of the remaining joints. Orthotic management for the control of foot, ankle, and knee deformities can be pursued until the child is ready for definitive surgical conversion.

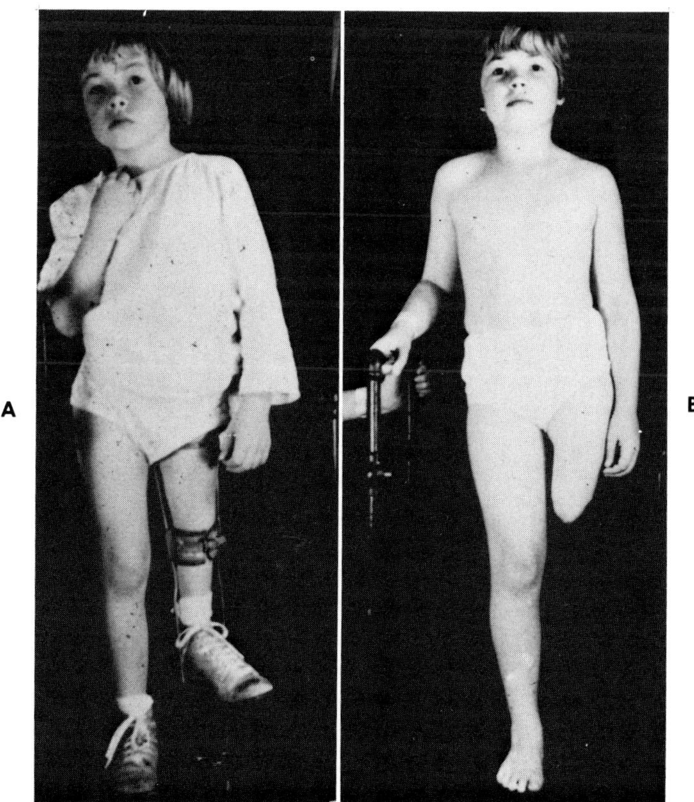

Fig. 38-1. A, Young patient with caliper orthosis for ambulation until definitive surgical intervention. **B,** After amputation.

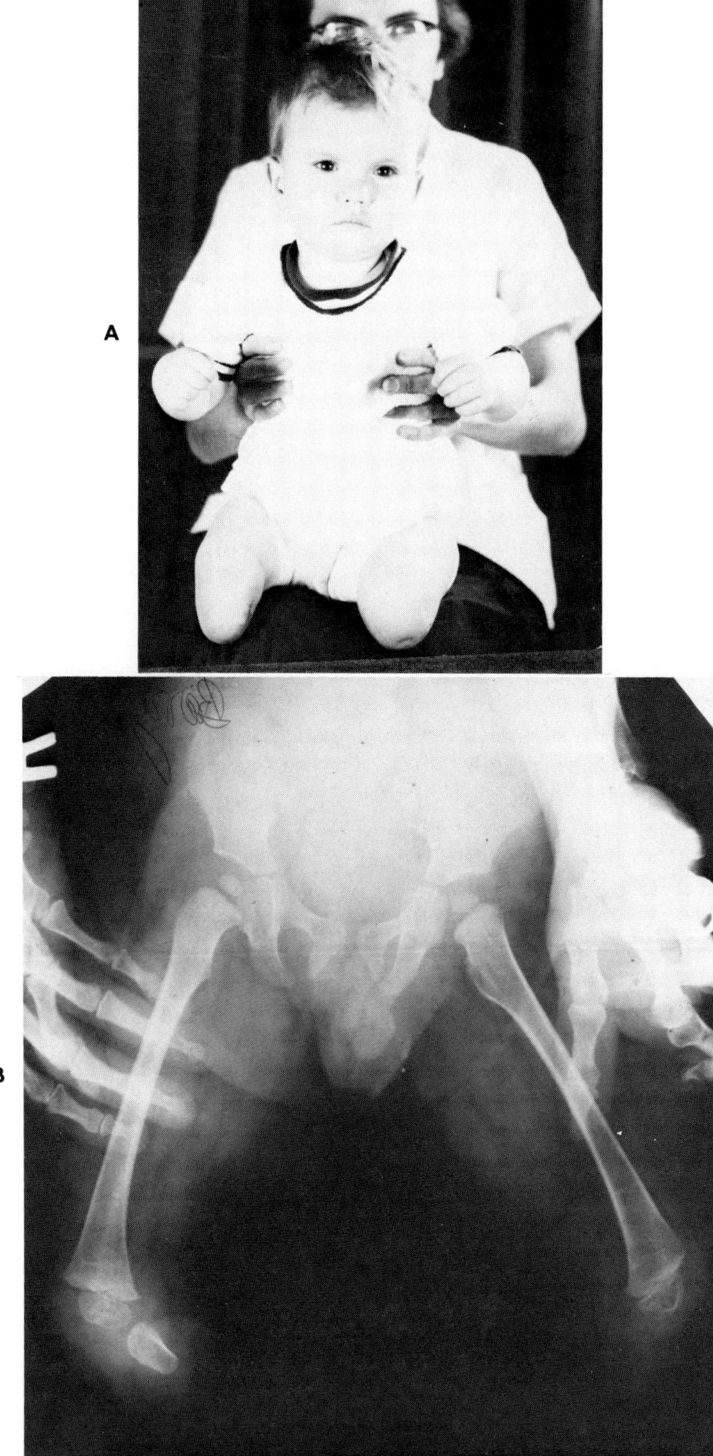

Fig. 38-2. A, At age 18 months, diagnosis of left leg is transverse deficiency, leg, complete; right, right leg transverse deficiency, leg, proximal one fourth, with 50-degree flexion deformity. **B,** Roentgenogram shows short tibial segment, which measures less than 5 cm (2 inches). **C,** At age 11 years, 6 months, there has been continued longitudinal growth of tibial segment with evidence of ossification of small segment of fibula. **D,** At age 19, patient still has good left knee disarticulation stump. Right below-knee stump now measures 10 cm (4 inch) in length, preserving excellent knee function for below-knee prosthesis. **E,** At age 19, patient is employed as welder and enjoys riding motorcycle.

In many patients, particularly those with PFFD, orthotic management without revision may be indicated until the optimal time for surgical intervention is reached (Fig. 38-1).

Prevention of progressive deformity is an important ingredient of the long-range planning for these patients. When surgical intervention is considered, plans should be laid out in such a manner as to anticipate the result in terms of the adult patient. To this end we must consider many facets of surgical intervention, including rentention of all long bone epiphyses, preservation of functional proximal joints, stabilization of proximal joints where necessary, and the judicious use of skin grafting when necessary.

Retention of all long bone growth plates. The percentage contributions to longitudinal growth of the distal femoral, proximal tibial, and distal tibial growth plates are shown on p. 495. Unnecessary sacrifice of any of these three longitudinal growth centers in the infant or very young child may result in major prosthetic problems in adult life. In some instances, the sacrifice of such an epiphysis in the very young child can be catastrophic. As an example, the patient with a longitudinal deficiency of the tibia should be

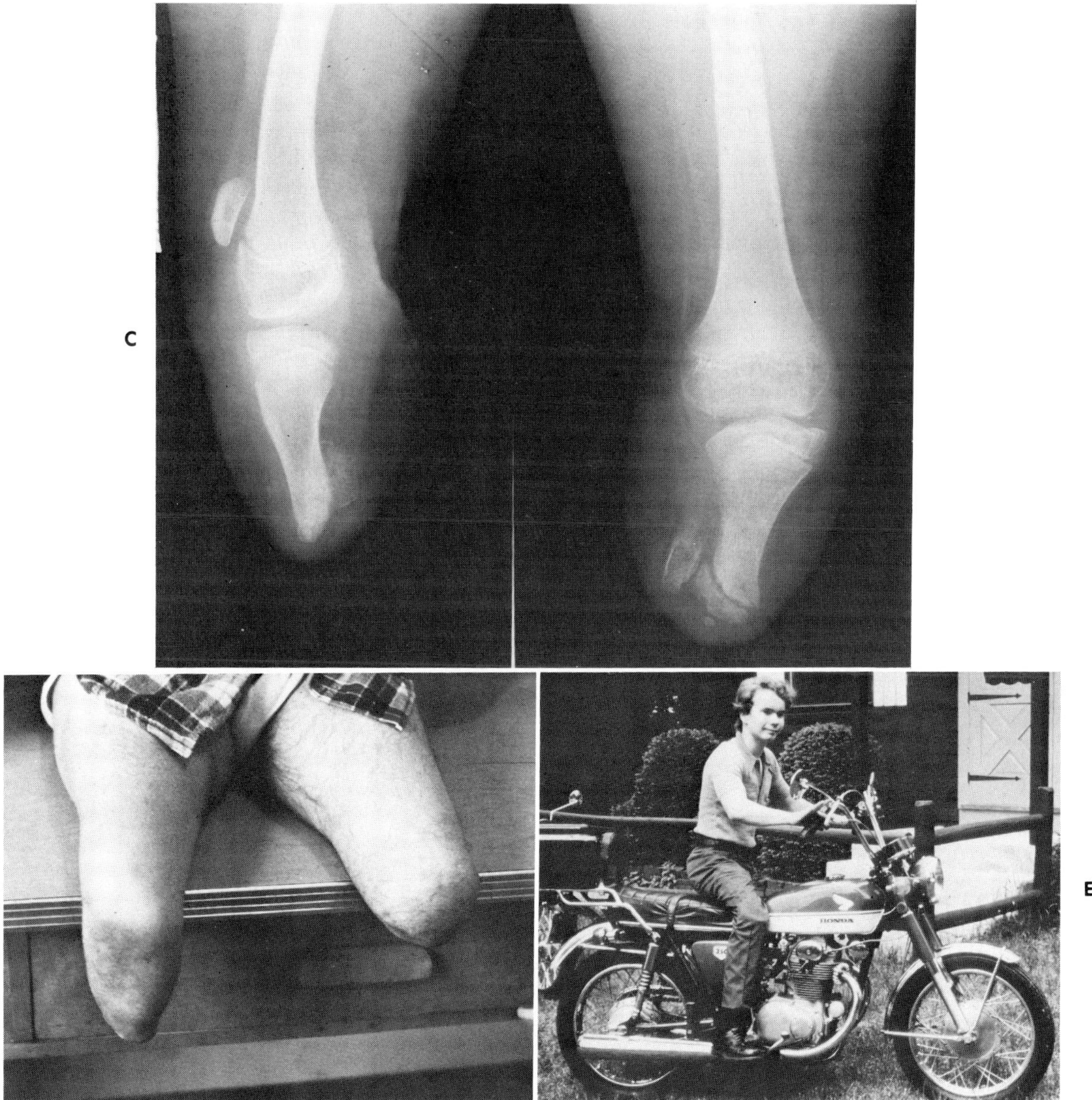

Fig. 38-2, cont'd. For legend, see opposite page.

treated by disarticulation at the knee level, leaving the distal femoral epiphysis intact. Assuming normal growth in the distal proximal femoral growth plates, in adult life, the patient would have a knee disarticulation or a very long above-knee stump, either of which is ideal for prosthetic fitting. Should the surgeon elect to carry out an above-knee amputation with sacrifice of the distal femoral growth plate, this would deprive the child of 70% of the eventual length of the femur, and in adult life the patient would have a very short above-knee residual limb. Disarticulation assures a long residual limb with all of its advantages in adult life.

Preservation of proximal joints. Particularly in transverse deficiencies of the leg, in its upper quarter or higher, preservation of the knee joint is important. Functional restoration of the below-knee patient is far superior to that which can be expected of the above-knee amputee. The sacrifice of a knee joint in the small child may severely limit his ability to climb stairs, manage ramps, and take part in many physical and sport activities. By the same token, efforts to preserve such a very short below-knee tibial segment (Fig. 38-2) may be rewarded in adult life with a competent functional knee joint and a good sturdy sufficiently long below-knee stump.

Patients with classes A and B PFFD are recognized to have a hip joint at birth.[2] It is not possible at this time to be sure of the integrity of that joint or of the stability. Although Lloyd-Roberts[27] had recommended early exploration of all of these joints, he later conceded that it may not be necessary and that early exploration may indeed damage the joint.[15]

Stabilization of proximal joints where necessary. Stabilization of proximal joints is particularly applicable to patients with PFFD. When the hip instability is severe, osteosynthesis in Aitken class A and B deficiencies may produce a near normal hip joint. In very short Aitken class B, C, and D deficiencies, knee fusion becomes important to have a single lever remaining bone in the limb for a good above-knee fitting. These procedures will be described in subsequent discussions.

Bilateral limb deficiencies

With regard to the bilateral limb-deficient child, these decisions will be somewhat altered, but in general the effort should be made to fit prostheses as early as possible based on the team evaluation of the child. Emphasis must be placed on the therapist's evaluation of the child's muscular coordination and ability to manage prosthetic

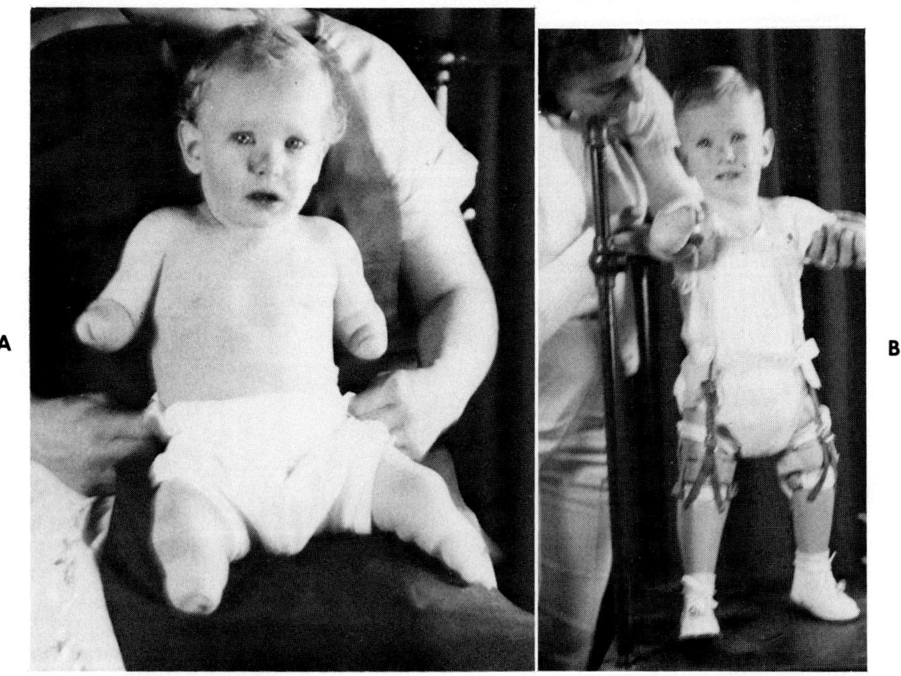

Fig. 38-3. Bilateral partial transverse deficiency of forearm and bilateral partial transverse deficiency of leg (below-elbow and below-knee amputations). **A,** At age 1, child is prepared for first fitting with prostheses. **B,** At age 2, child is independently ambulatory.

devices. Prosthetic fitting may have to be staged or delayed until surgical intervention can reasonably be accomplished. The physiological and, particularly, psychological differences between the child with bilateral limb deficiencies and the adult with a bilateral amputation must be recognized when contemplating the bilateral fitting. When bilateral surgical conversion or a revision procedure is planned, rehabilitation goals for the infant or juvenile should take these differences into consideration. The child who requires bilateral ankle disarticulation should be expected to ambulate independently without crutches or canes (Fig. 40-42). He should be expected to take part in all normal activities, including athletics, and should be able to doff and don the prostheses

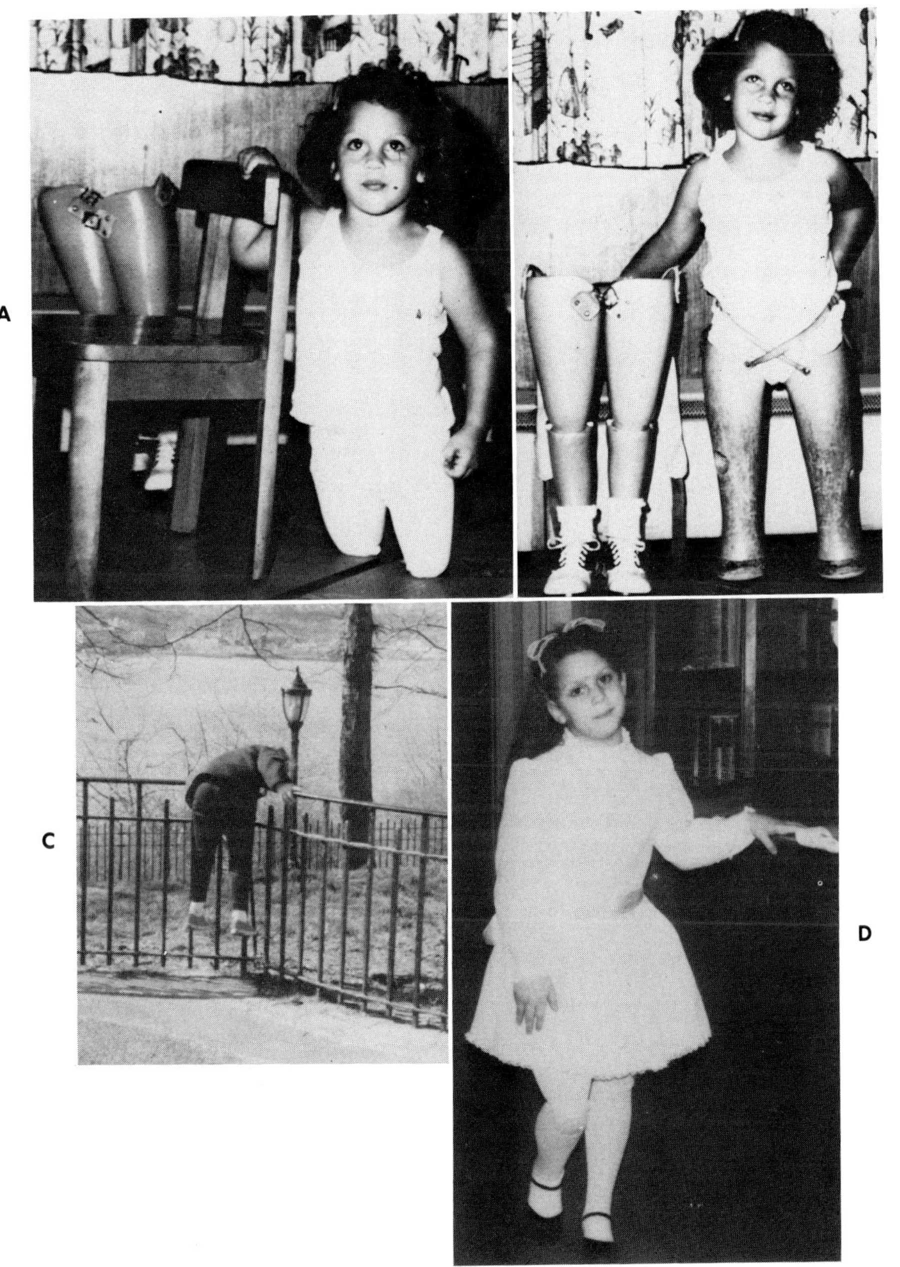

Fig. 38-4. Bilateral complete transverse deficiency of leg (bilateral knee disarticulations). **A,** Patient standing on stumps. **B,** Patient in stubbies and standing by articulated limbs. **C,** Patient playing in articulated limbs. **D,** Patient at age of 9 years, fully independent using public transportation and attending school. At age 19, patient is in her second year of college, drives her own car, and leads an independent life.

independently early in life. Similarly, the child with a bilateral below-knee fitting should have very high rehabilitation goals (Fig. 38-3). Even as the levels of amputation go higher, one should anticipate that as long as the child has functional upper limbs with which to improve balance, he should be independently ambulatory. It is generally appreciated that the adult bilateral above-knee amputee, if he is to walk, will require crutches or canes. The child, on the other hand, can be expected to ambulate independently when properly trained. Early fitting and appropriate training can be a very rewarding experience in such a patient. In the very young child, as in the very old patient with bilateral above-knee amputations, initial fitting with stubbies is used.[23] Stubbies are modified quadrilateral sockets with either a rocker or rubber-soled bottom. The use of stubbies permits the patient to develop balance in the erect position. When ambulation with the stubbies has been accomplished, they may be lengthened. This increases the child's height and increases his confidence in the erect position. The final prescription is for articulated limbs (Fig. 38-4). Ambulation without crutches or other external aids can be anticipated.

The parents of the bilateral lower limb–deficient child must be made aware of the importance of weight control. Instruction and dietary regulation should be available to the family and their responsibility at home stressed (Fig. 40-61).

Although the problem of the bilateral PFFD patient will be dealt with later in this chapter, it cannot be repeated often enough that this is the one situation in which any consideration of amputation of the feet should be deferred (Chapter 5).

Skin grafting

Skin grafting in the child is very well tolerated. Split-thickness skin grafts will mature promptly in children and withstand the shearing or frictional forces of socket contact. Denuding of a short below-knee residual limb is no indication to proceed with higher amputation in a child. Skin grafting should be carried out. The resurfaced limb should then be toughened up in anticipation of prosthetic application.

The surgeon should keep this philosophy in mind when dealing with the limb-deficient child. If preservation of a knee joint requires a posterior release and skin is a problem, split-thickness grafting may be carried out. The surgeon should

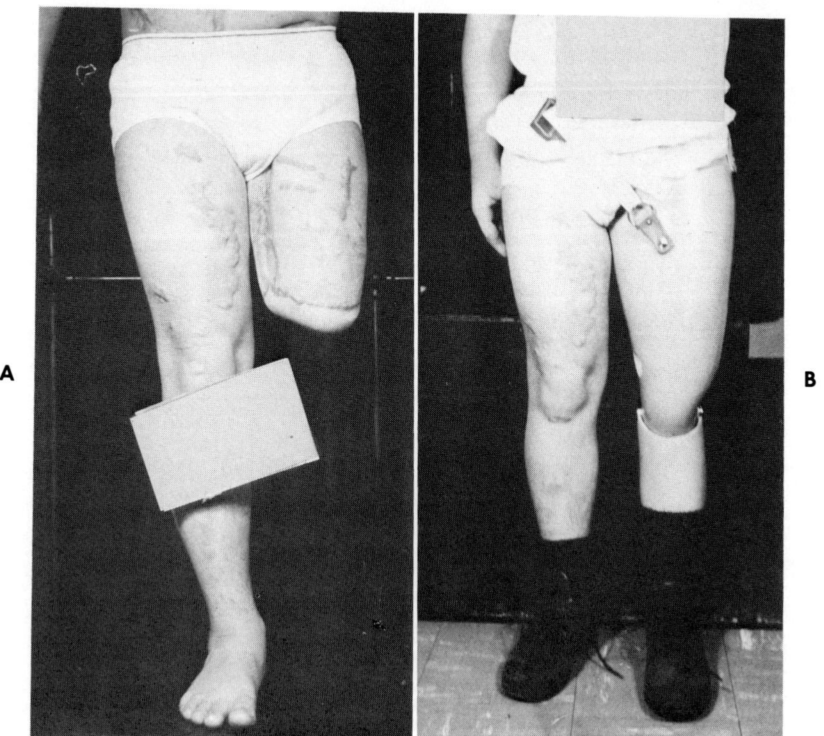

Fig. 38-5. A, Above-knee amputation with entire adductor surface covered with skin graft. **B,** Above-knee prosthetic fitting. Patient required later revision of grafts.

not hesitate to use a skin graft to preserve an epiphysis where there is a deficiency of skin. Split-thickness grafting in weight-bearing areas may ultimately require revision and/or a pedicle graft (Fig. 38-5), but most split-thickness grafts mature rapidly and tolerate prosthetic wear well. Newer improved materials for sockets have been developed to reduce shear forces at the stump-socket interface and lessen the possibility of breakdown of grafted surfaces.

Selection of a donor site for skin graft in the lower limb amputee should not be casually undertaken. Consideration must be given to the ultimate amputation level and the type of prosthesis that the patient will ultimately wear. No area should be chosen as a donor site if there is the possibility that it may later interfere with prosthetic wear. As an example, the thigh should not be chosen as a donor site for skin grafting for a below-knee stump if there be subsequent need for a thigh corset. Similarly, in an above-knee amputation the pelvic brim area should not be chosen, since there may be a need to wear a Silesian bandage.

When there is a need for a pedicle or flap graft, the operating surgeon should take into consideration the patient's ultimate amputation level. These procedures should be planned so that there will be no scarring in areas of weight bearing or in areas where a strap or stump socket interface may occur.

TRANSVERSE DEFICIENCIES

Phalangeal deficiencies

Transverse deficiencies of the phalanges, whether partial or complete, do not usually require revision surgery. If associated with congenital constriction bands, surgical intervention should be directed at the constriction bands, and occasionally proximal amputation of the toes will be necessary.

Partial or complete metatarsal deficiencies

As in transverse deficiencies of the phalanges, revision surgery is not usually necessary for metatarsal deficiencies. Occasionally, it is necessary to remove vestigial phalanges that have either no bony component or insufficient bony component for functional value. These may present not only cosmetic and hygienic problems, but they may also present a serious problem in shoe insert fitting. The vestigial phalanges may become irritated and even ulcerate. With such problems, excision is recommended.

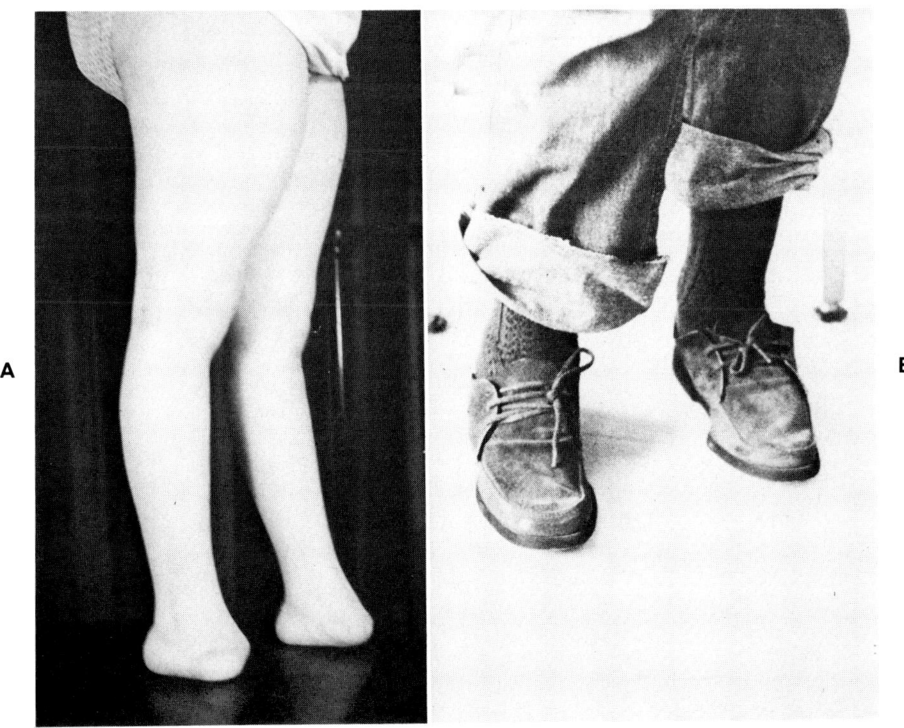

Fig. 38-6. A, Partial transverse tarsal deficiency. **B,** Chopart-type partial foot prosthesis with posterior closure. With shoes on, cosmesis is less than ideal.

When the residual metatarsal elements are extremely small, whether short or atrophied, shoe fitting problems are the major concern. If there is insufficient residual foot on which to fit a shoe with an insert, consideration must be given to other prosthetic restoration. Those patients with very short remaining metatarsal elements and those with complete transverse metatarsal deficiencies must be treated as a tarsal deficiency.

Complete or partial tarsal deficiencies

For the patient with a complete tarsal deficiency (apodia or congenital ankle disarticulation), the deficit may be managed by prosthetic restoration. No surgical intervention is necessary.

Partial tarsal deficiencies with a normal distal tibial epiphysis and no length discrepancy may require conversion surgery. In the very early years, these children may ambulate with a high-top lace shoe. Prosthetic devices are available, but function and cosmesis are less than ideal (Fig. 38-6). Proximal revision for functional as well as cosmetic reasons will be considered (Fig. 38-7). Ankle disarticulation is the procedure of choice. This is frequently referred to as a modified Syme's amputation.[29,40] The articular cartilage is left intact. The Boyd amputation may be considered as an alternative to disarticulation.[21,22,25] In the very small child, up to age 3, the malleoli may be left intact and will present no problem in prosthetic fit or restoration. In the older child, the malleoli may be transversely sectioned at the level of the tibial articular surface to provide a broad, flat end-bearing stump. Care must be taken not to damage the distal tibial epiphysis in this procedure. In the older child, in whom the epiphyses have fused, one may have to model the stump or shave the malleoli to achieve acceptable cosmesis

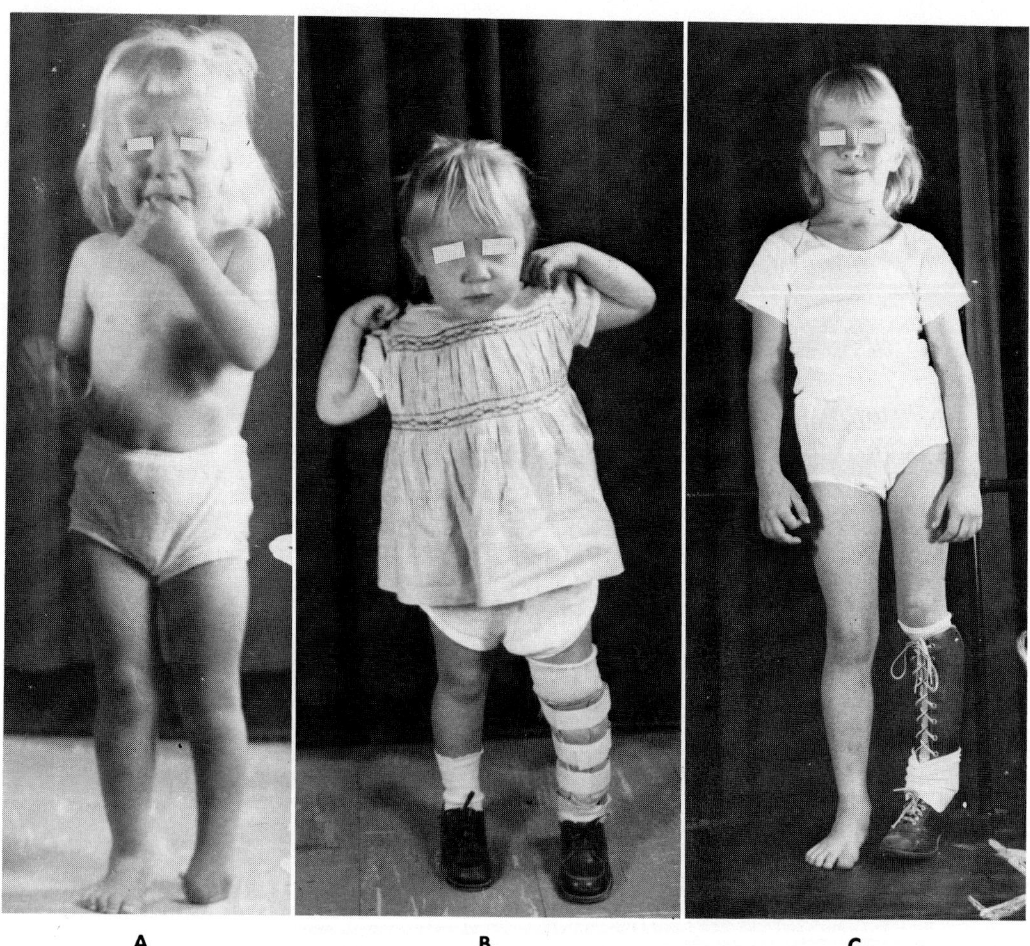

Fig. 38-7. A, Child age 2½, with partial transverse tarsal deficiency. **B,** Syme prosthesis fitted at age 2½ years. **C,** Child at age 6, Syme-type prosthesis restoration is no longer cosmetically acceptable.

in a Syme-type prosthesis. Patients so treated are left with an end-bearing stump that is the best functional stump. The patient may walk without the prosthesis. There is no concern for the phenomenon of bony overgrowth so frequently observed when transtibial amputation is performed.

Procedure for ankle disarticulation

The procedure for ankle disarticulation should be carried out with tourniquet control. The incision starts anteriorly at the tip of the medial malleolus and is carried directly across the ankle joint to the lateral side. The second half of the incision is then carried from these two points to the plantar surface of the foot, describing a slight arc to carry the incision just distal to the calcaneocuboid level (Fig. 38-8). The anterior part of the incision is carried down through the subcutaneous tissue, clamping and ligating the superficial vessels. The anterior tibial tendon and toe extensors are divided and held with a clamp or suture for later attachment. The dissection is carried medially and the posterior tibial vessel identified and traced distalward to preserve the circulation of

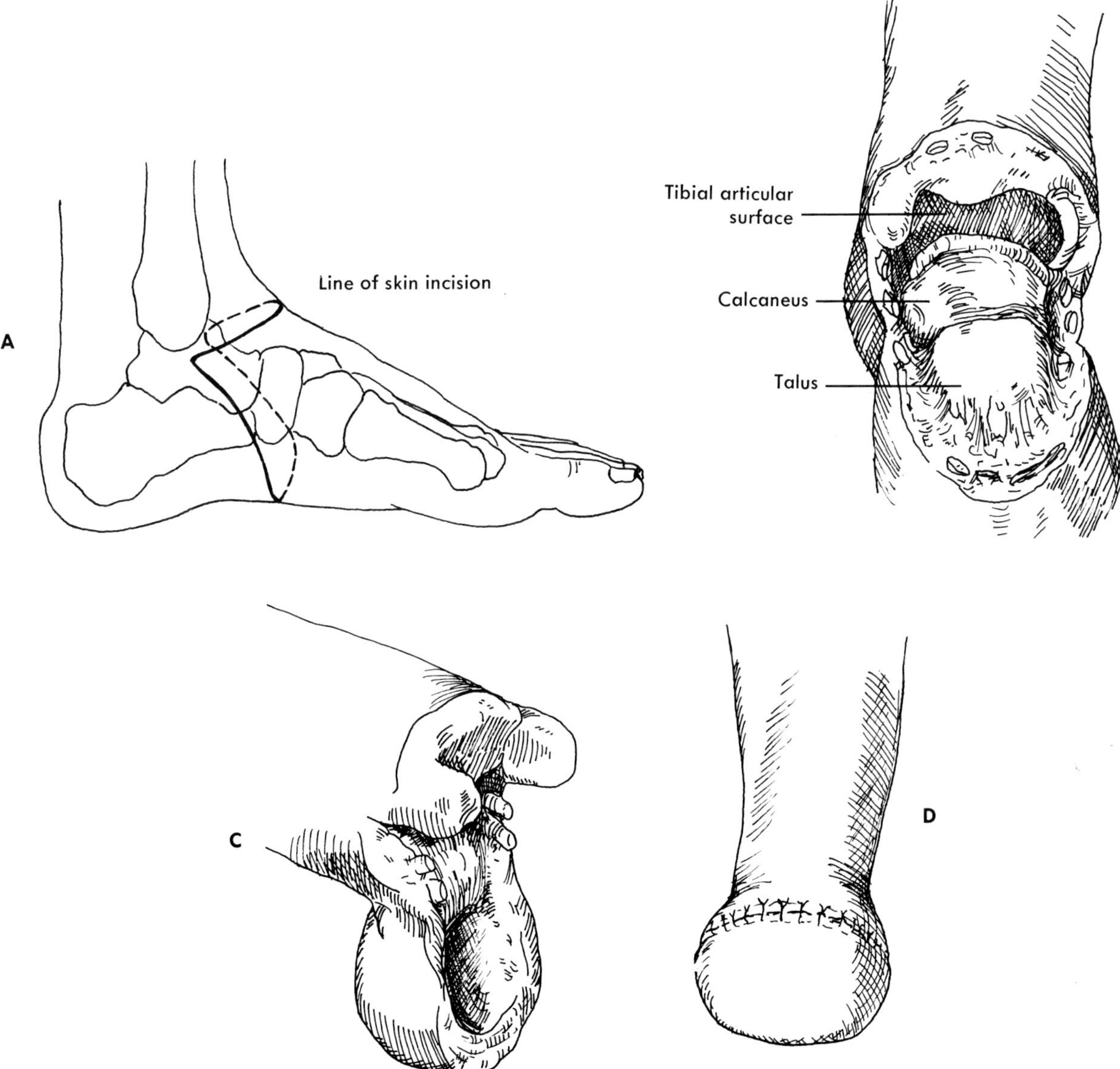

Fig. 38-8. Ankle disarticulation. **A,** Incision starts anteriorly at tip of medial malleolus and is carried directly across ankle joint to lateral side. Second half of incision is then carried from these two points to plantar surface of foot, describing slight arc. **B,** With foot pulled forward posterior capsule is divided and heel cord dissected off superior aspect of os calcis. **C,** Dissection is completed, care being taken not to puncture skin posteriorly. **D,** Wound is closed.

the plantar flap. The anterior capsule is opened, and the medial and lateral ligaments are divided. The plantar portion of the incision is carried directly down to the bone and the plantar flap dissected off the inferior aspect of the os calcis by sharp and blunt dissection. With the foot pulled forward, the posterior capsule is divided and the heel cord dissected off the superior aspect of the os calcis. The dissection is completed by removing the os calcis, taking care not to puncture the skin posteriorly. All major bleeders are ligated, the tourniquet released, and bleeding controlled. The heel cord is now sutured to the posterior capsule. The anterotibial tendon is sutured to the anterior capsule, and the plantar flap is brought forward and also sutured to the anterior capsule. Drainage may be accomplished with a soft tissue drain or suction drainage if desired. The heel pad is now stabilized with a Kirschner wire through the heel pad, the articular surface, and across the epiphysis. The skin is closed with loose interrupted sutures. The rigid dressing technique may be employed or, if desired, dressing may be with dry compression dressing. Drainage is discontinued at 48 hours.

Leg deficiency

Upper third. The transverse leg deficiency (congenital below-knee amputation, partial transverse hemimelia) may occur as a true deficiency or in association with Streeter's dysplasia – the congenital constriction band syndrome. When it is associated with Streeter's dysplasia, surgical attention to other constriction bands may be necessary, either above the level of amputation or on other limbs. In those true deficiencies, vestigial structures may be appended, and these may require surgical removal. Such appendages may range from one metacarpal ray to five vestigial digits.

The deficiency is apparent at the time of birth, and attention should be directed to the maintenance of range of motion in the proximal joints, particularly the knee joint. If the child is born with a flexion contracture of the knee joint, it may be necessary to surgically relieve this prior to considering prosthetic restoration. If the knee joint extends completely at the time of birth, implementation of a range of motion program should maintain this until the child is ready for the prosthesis.

Until recently, it was thought that these congenital amputations were not subject to the phenomenon of bony overgrowth. Pellicore et al.[33] have now reported the observation of bony overgrowth in the remaining tibia of these children and have observed them through the period of symptomatic overgrowth until surgical revision was required.

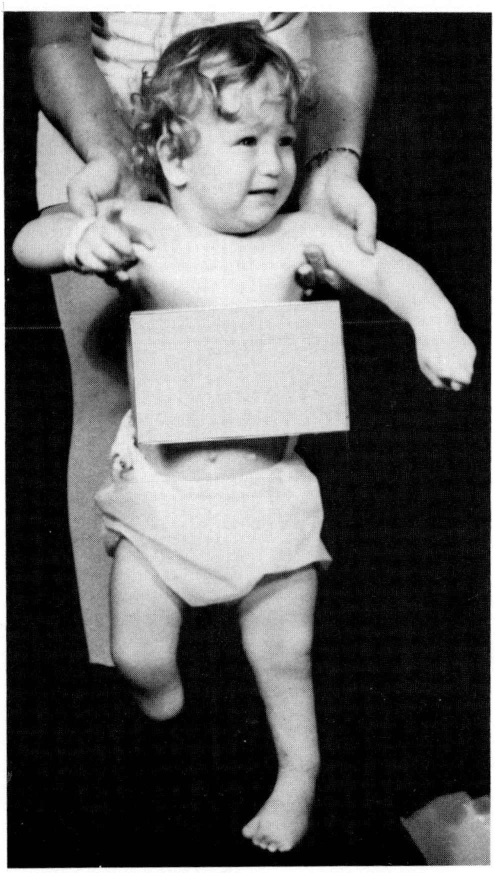

Fig. 38-9. Child at age 19 months, diagnosis of transverse deficiency of leg, proximal third.

Children with transverse deficiencies of the leg in the proximal portion will demonstrate good standing balance on their sound limb somewhere between 9 and 15 months of age, and they are ready for prosthetic restoration at this time (Fig. 38-9).

Complete and lower third of thigh. Above-knee deficiencies occur less frequently in children than do below-knee deficiencies. Surgical intervention is seldom, if ever, indicated. Management is prosthetic restoration (Fig. 38-4).

Complete thigh (amelia). Children with complete transverse deficiency of the thigh (amelia) (Fig. 38-10), should be fitted with their first prosthesis as soon as they are standing independently on the normal opposite side. As with other deficiencies, they may have a vestigial digit attached. This usually is not a problem, since it

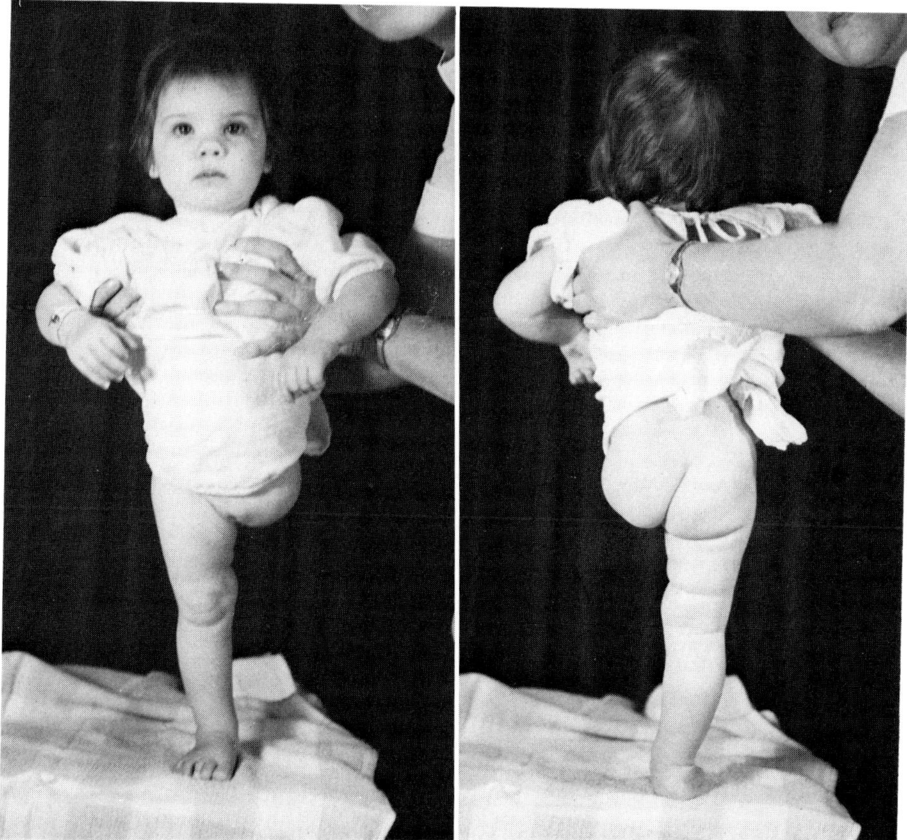

Fig. 38-10. Child at age 1, diagnosis of complete transverse deficiency of thigh (amelia).

has no rigidity and hence can be incorporated into the socket without difficulty. Surgical intervention is seldom indicated.

The infant with bilateral amelia will require a plastic "bucket-type" socket fitted to a firm base to achieve sitting or "standing" balance. As he grows older, he may progress to the swivel walker developed at Ontario Crippled Childrens Center. If the child has normal upper limbs, bilateral articulated hip disarticulation prostheses may be prescribed at about age 4 or 5.

LONGITUDINAL DEFICIENCIES

Deficiency of the fibula

Because of the frequency of its occurrence, longitudinal deficiency of the fibula has received a great deal of attention in the literature.* The titles are varied—congenital absence of the fibula, fibular deficiency, paraxial fibular hemimelia, dysgenesis, etc. In 1951, O'Rahilly[31] reported on 296 cases of this deficiency he had reviewed in the literature prior to 1935. Since that time several hundred cases have been reported. In 1952, Coventry and Johnson[12] reported twenty-nine cases of congenital absence of the fibula and mentioned amputation as a form of treatment but stressed the reconstructive approach. Since Aitken's report of 1959,[1] most authors[22,25,29,40] have emphasized amputation and prosthetic restoration. Although O'Rahilly was only able to find 296 cases in the literature prior to 1935, by 1977 there were over 1100 cases in the Shriners Hospitals in North America alone.

Clinical picture. As with other longitudinal limb deficiencies, one is impressed with the fact that it is a true limb deficiency, not simply the absence of a single bone (fibula). The tibia, in addition to being bowed, usually has an abnormality of the distal epiphysis. There may be a minimal shortening of the femur or coexistent PFFD. A congenitally short femur may be present. Deficiency also exists in the muscles, tendons, nerves, and even in the skin as evidenced by dimpling frequently present over the deformed tibia. The classical clinical picture is a foreshortened limb with equinovalgus foot, with or without

*1, 5, 11, 12, 14, 22, 25-27, 34, 40.

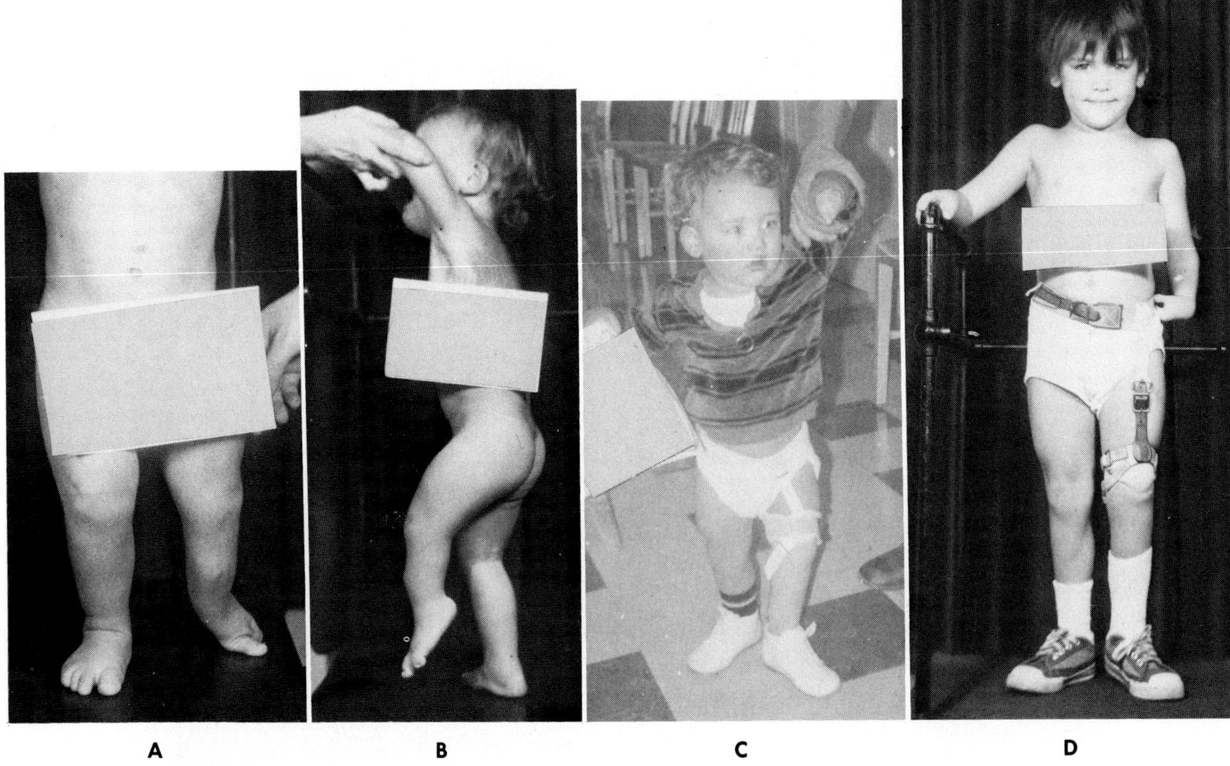

Fig. 38-11. A, Classical unilateral longitudinal deficiency: fibula, complete; tarsal, partial; metatarsal-phalangeal fourth and fifth complete. Note anterior bowed tibia, which is short and has dimple in skin over bow. Note also valgus at ankle and absent fourth and fifth rays. **B,** Side view of same patient. **C,** At age 2, after disarticulation, he is fitted with PTB prosthesis with toddler harness. **D,** At age 5½, he is asymptomatic and fully active at level of peers.

absence of metatarsal rays and tarsal anomalies (Fig. 38-11). For the patient with unilateral deficiency, progressive length discrepancy is the major clinical problem. In the patient with bilateral fibular deficiency, this is translated to failure to attain normal height.

Definitive treatment of patients with this limb deficiency will depend on two major considerations: (1) is it associated with PFFD and (2) is it unilateral or bilateral?

Patients with longitudinal deficiency of the fibula with associated PFFD must be treated primarily as a PFFD, with the fibular deficiency as a secondary consideration. The patient with unilateral fibular deficiency with PFFD on the contralateral side is an exception to this.

Treatment of unilateral fibula deficiencies

Leg length discrepancy is the major problem in the patient with unilateral longitudinal deficiency of the fibula. Experience has shown that this is a progressive discrepancy[25] and that the progress of this discrepancy can be predicted on growth charts. Efforts at equalizing the discrepancy by tibial lengthening have generally been unsatisfactory. Efforts at equalizing discrepancies in excess of 7.5 cm (3 inches) are contraindicated because this amount of loss in overall height of the patient is too great a price to pay. Only rarely can leg length equalization by epiphyseal arrest be accomplished in these patients. In those with lesser length discrepancies, it is likely that there will be a severely deformed foot which will preclude normal shoe wear. Except in the unusual patient in whom the discrepancy is minimal and not progressive and in whom foot development is normal, ankle disarticulation and prosthetic restoration is the treatment of choice. It is therefore recommended that early conversion be carried out (Fig. 38-12) between 9 and 12 months of age or as soon as the child is able to

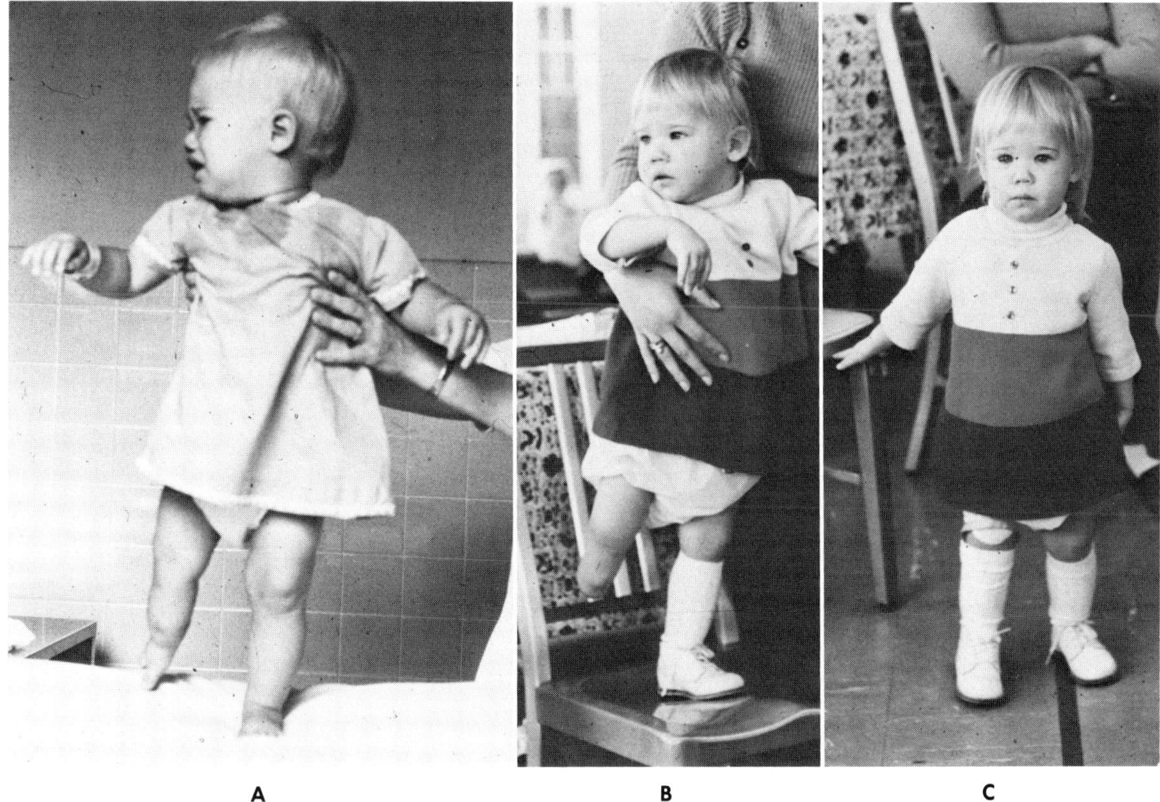

Fig. 38-12. A, Preoperative diagnosis. Unilateral longitudinal deficiency: fibula, complete; tarsal, partial; metatarsal-phalangeal, fourth and fifth complete. **B,** After ankle disarticulation. **C,** Child fitted with first prosthesis—PTB with cuff suspension. Immediate independent ambulation.

stand, indicating a readiness to commence ambulation.

Indications for early conversion and prosthetic restoration may then be summed up as (1) length discrepancy in excess of 5 cm (2 inches) and progressing and (2) foot deformity.

It is mandatory that the procedure be a disarticulation at the ankle joint or Boyd amputation, never transtibial amputation. Transtibial amputation is contraindicated for two major reasons: (1) loss of longitudinal growth at the distal tibial growth plate and (2) bony overgrowth at the amputation site.

The distal tibial epiphysis contributes 20% of growth of the limb as a whole and 45% of growth of the tibia itself. Recognizing that the distal tibial epiphysis may not be normal, it is still important to appreciate that if this epiphysis is sacrificed at age 1 year, the child will be left with a short below-knee residual limb when he attains full growth. On the other hand, if the growth plate is retained, one may anticipate that there will be at worst a long below-knee stump or at

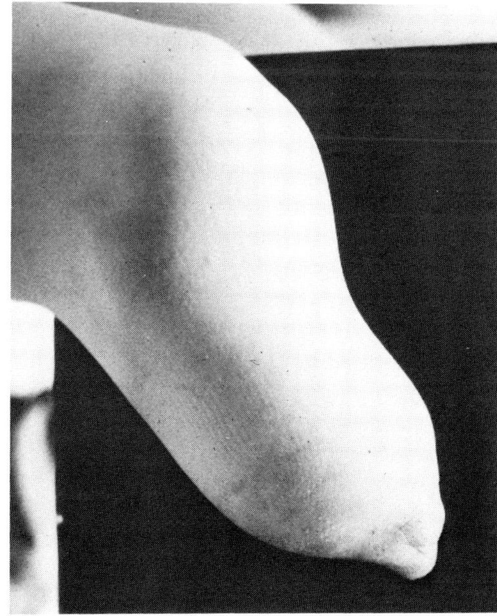

Fig. 38-13. Bony overgrowth at site of transtibial amputation.

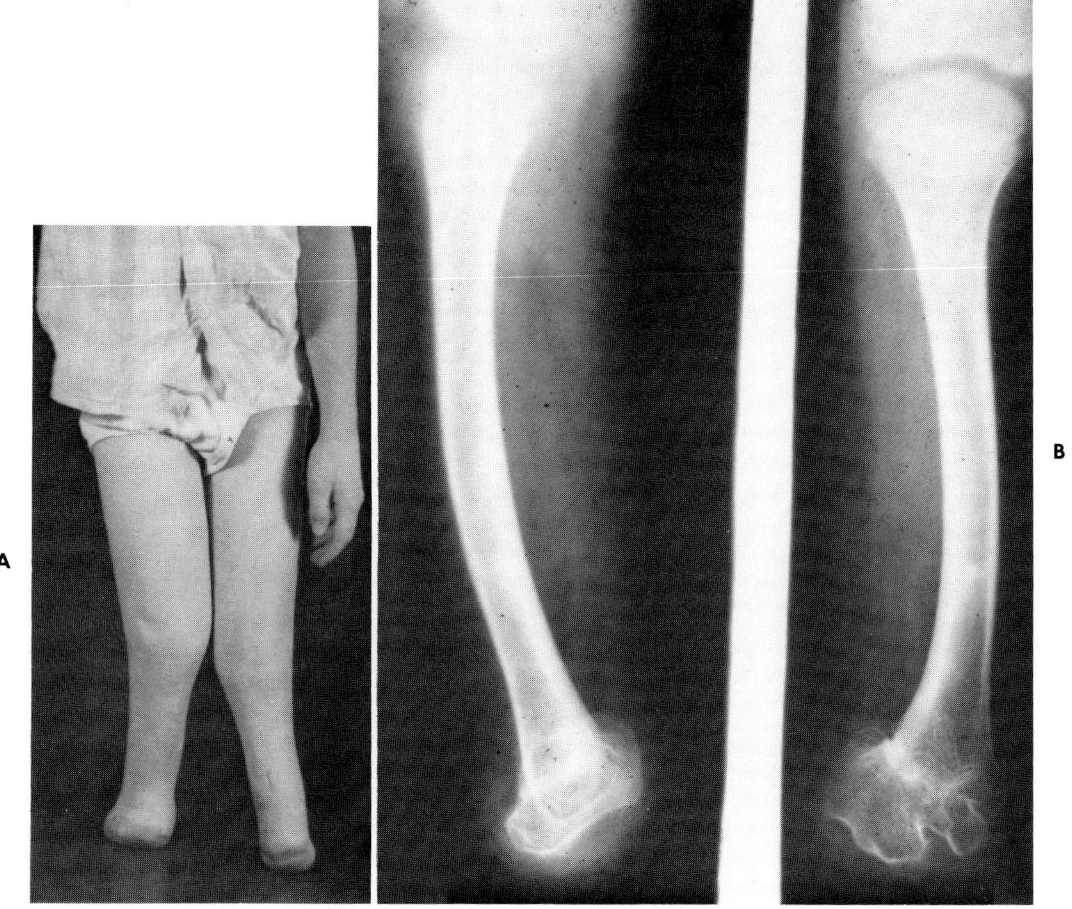

Fig. 38-14. A, Boyd amputation stumps. **B,** Roentgenogram appearance.

best a good Syme-type ankle disarticulation stump. The disarticulation procedure also provides an end-bearing stump on which the child may walk without the prosthesis.

Prior to 8 years of age, transtibial amputation is accompanied by a high incidence of bony overgrowth at the amputation site (Fig. 38-13). Much has been written about bony overgrowth,[33] its prevention, and treatment. It is sufficiently frequent to avoid transtibial amputation if at all possible. When symptomatic, revision of the amputation is necessary. In summary, most children with unilateral fibular deficiency require ankle disarticulation and prosthetic restoration. In the operation the articular cartilage should be left on the distal tibia and the heel pad fixed to it.

Procedure for ankle disarticulation

In the older child, consideration should be given to modification of the disarticulation procedure (p. 531). Many of these children have already had triple arthrodesis or other surgical procedures in an attempt to restore a functional foot. Length discrepancy is progressive and is the indication for amputation. In these patients fusion of the ankle joint and amputation through the midtarsal level or a modified Boyd procedure retains the extra length and normal attachment of the heel pad to the os calcis. The broad stump contour does require a more bulky prosthetic socket and is cosmetically less desirable. The procedure is therefore usually reserved for boys, in whom cosmesis is not so important (Fig. 38-14). Ankle disarticulation is the procedure of choice for girls. In the older girl, there may be sufficient cosmetic justification to consider below-knee amputation.

Bilateral fibula deficiency

There are two major considerations for patients with bilateral longitudinal deficiency of the fibula

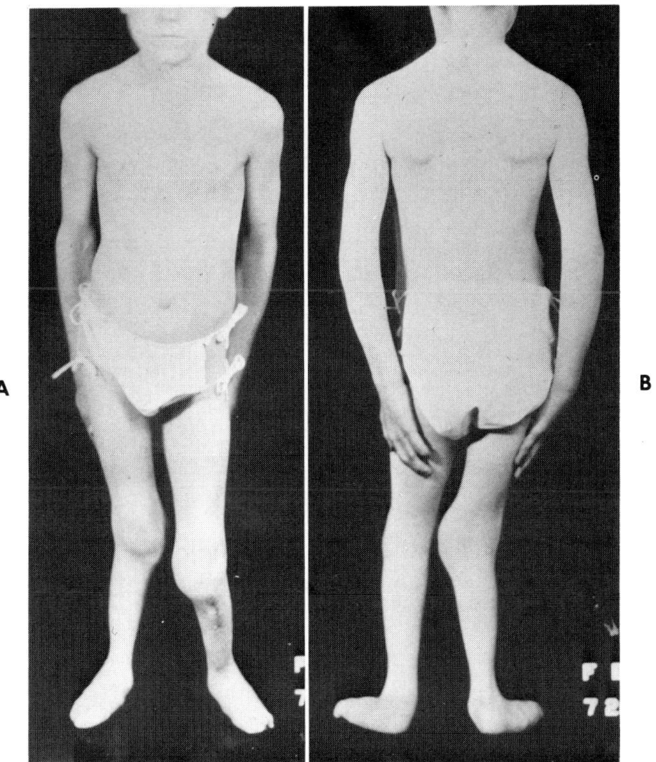

Fig. 38-15. Complete bilateral fibula longitudinal deficiency. **A,** At age 6 years, 7 months, there is disproportionate shortening of tibiae. **B,** Posterior view confirms shortening and reveals residual valgus of feet and ankles. This patient should have been treated by disarticulation and prosthetic restoration.

with a normal femur: (1) the condition of the feet and (2) the anticipated overall height of the patient.

Patients with five-rayed feet, which are reasonably aligned beneath the tibia, will have no problem in shoe wear. On the other hand, those patients with a three- or four-rayed foot with associated severe equinus and valgus may require considerable surgery to align the foot plantigrade. Even after repeated surgical procedures, normal shoe wear may be precluded by the shape and deformity of the foot. Severe foot deformity may then be an indication for amputation and prosthetic restoration.

With fibular deficiency there may be a deficiency of the distal tibia and its growth plate. When the tibiae at birth are disproportionately short as compared with the femur, one can anticipate that this will be a progressive discrepancy. In these patients early ankle disarticulation at age 1 year to 18 months is indicated.

In a small series of unamputated patients studied retrospectively at the Shriners Hospital for Crippled Children in Springfield, Massachusetts, it was believed that 50% should have had amputation (Fig. 38-15) and prosthetic restoration to provide normal stature.[22] When length discrepancy between the tibia and femur is sufficiently great to make this decision at an early age, it is desirable to introduce parents to the clinic scene, where they may see similar children with prosthetic restoration and discuss this with the parents of these children rather than to rely completely on the recommendation of the clinic chief.

If the discrepancy in proportional length of the tibia and femur is small and there is a good foot, consideration of amputation should be deferred, but growth charts should be maintained for the patient. If the discrepancy is a progressive one, and it is apparent that the patient is going to be unduly short in adult life, bilateral ankle disarticulation and prosthetic restoration may be recommended prior to school age (Fig. 38-16). As the child grows older and particularly if he has been permitted to enter his early teens without surgical intervention, the child himself should

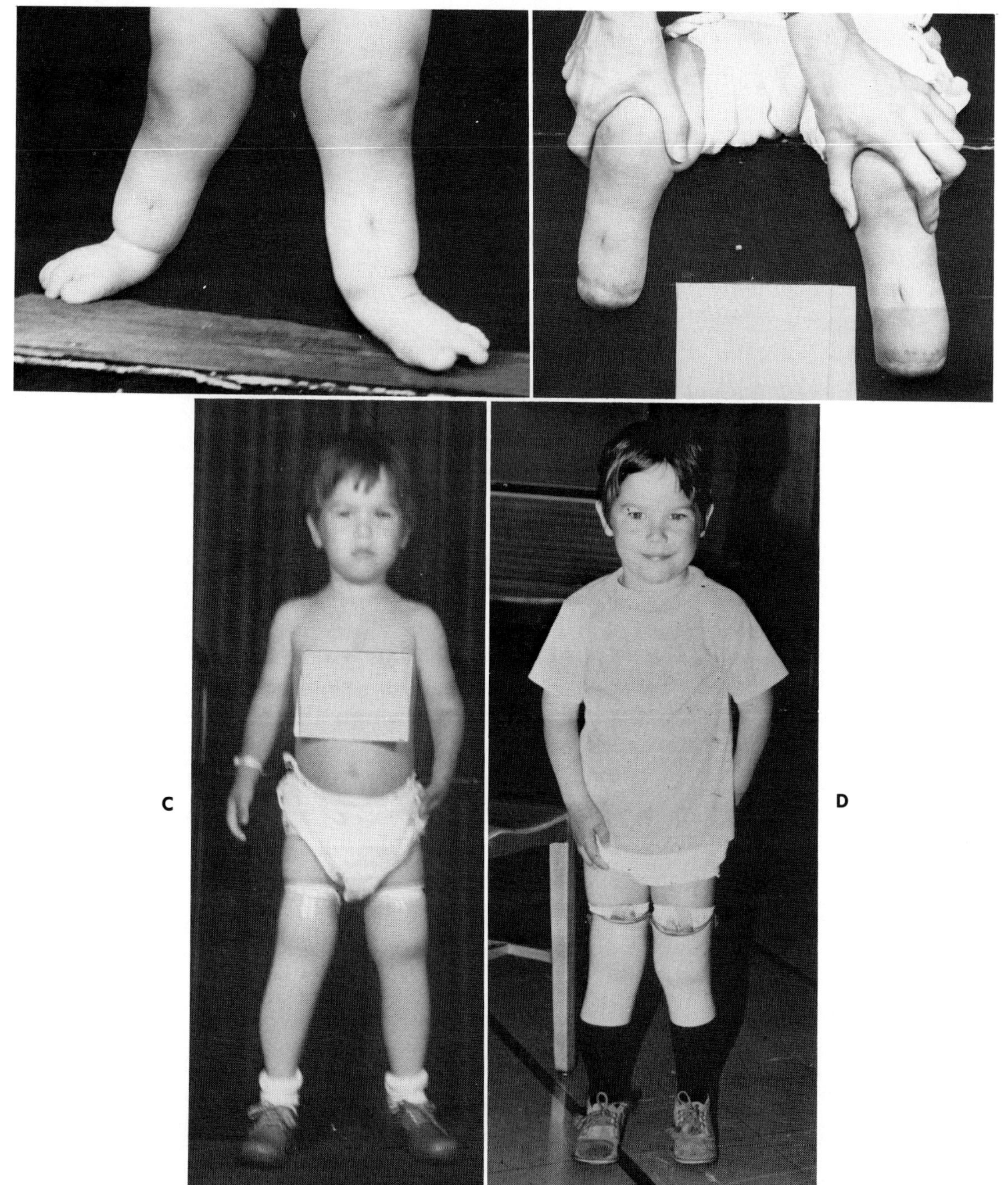

Fig. 38-16. A, Bilateral longitudinal deficiency: fibula, complete; tarsal, partial; metatarsal-phalangeal, fourth and fifth complete. **B,** Child after bilateral ankle disarticulations at age 1 year, 1 month. **C,** Child is fully ambulatory with bilateral PTS prostheses at age 1 year, 2 months. **D,** At age 4, he is completely independent in PTS prostheses.

enter into the decision making to consider such ablative surgery and prosthetic restoration.

Deficiency of the tibia

Longitiduinal deficiency of the tibia may occur either unilaterally or bilaterally. It may be partial or complete. Its occurrence is much less frequent than fibula deficiency. There have been several reports of the association of longitudinal deficiency of the tibia with deficiency of the first metacarpal ray (absent thumb), as well as with polydactyly.* Although Eaton and McKusick,[13] in reporting their four cases, stated that "no familial cases have been recorded," Clark[10] has cited thirteen case reports of familial occurrence of tibial deficiency that she found in literature and added to it her report of a patient with nine affected descendants in three generations.

*10, 13, 31, 32, 41.

The characteristic clinical picture of tibial deficiency[3] can usually be recognized at birth (Fig. 38-17). Gross instability of the knee, with or without flexion contracture and lateral displacement of the fibula, is evident. Severe varus of the foot is present, with the sole of the foot facing toward the opposite leg or even toward the knee or perineum. The knee joint is so unstable that the foot can almost be brought up against the medial thigh. Length discrepancy is the most obvious part of this deficiency. Several patients have an exostosis or osteochondroma of the femur (Fig. 38-18). The deficiency may be complete or partial, but at birth it is difficult to be sure of this differential diagnosis.

Partial. Since the presence or absence of a proximal segment of the tibia is crucial in the

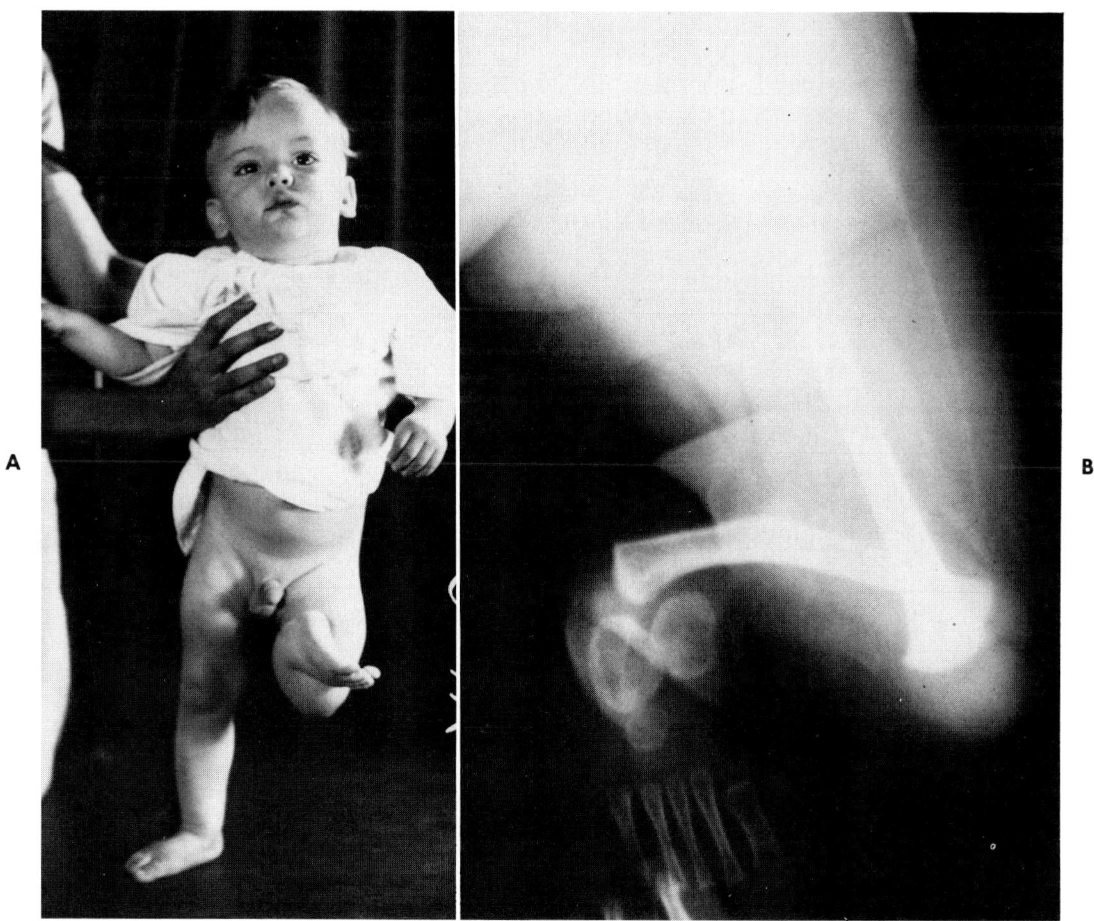

Fig. 38-17. A, Complete longitudinal deficiency of tibia. Foot faces toward groin. There is severe length discrepancy and no stability at knee or ankle. Foot is in varus. **B,** Roentgenogram shows fibula lateral to femoral condyles and foot medial to fibula. Tibia is completely absent.

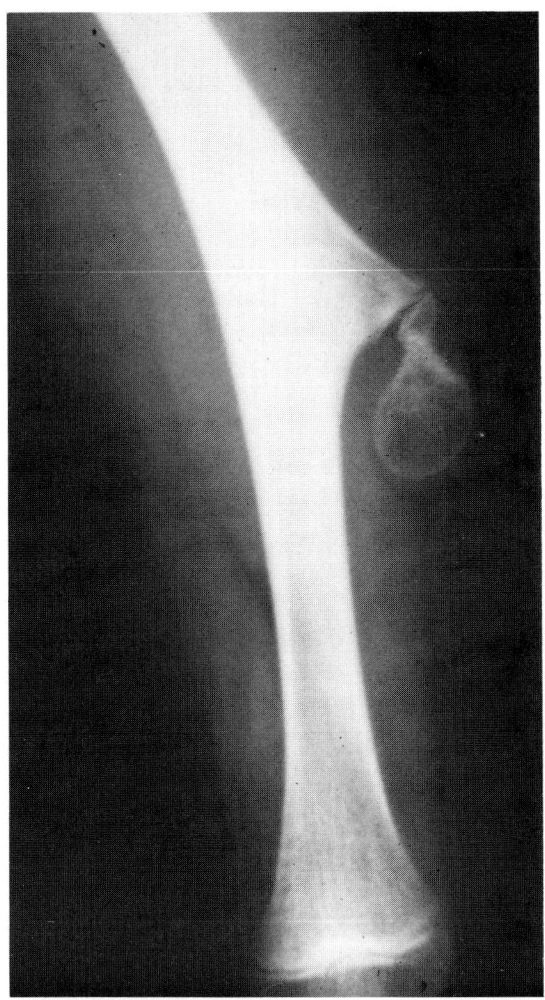

Fig. 38-18. Roentgenogram of femur in patient with deficiency of tibia and large exostosis from shaft. Base of exostosis has fractured.

treatment decision, it is important to establish this knowledge early in life (Fig. 38-19). If there is a suggestion that a proximal tibial segment is present, even though it is not visualized on a roentgenogram, it is important to rely on the clinical examination. Ossification of a proximal tibial segment may not occur for months and even up to 2 years of age. In such patients, arthrography may be of assistance in making a diagnosis. Partial deficiency of the tibia should be treated orthotically until one is certain of the ossification of the remaining fragment and of the presence or absence of the knee joint. Having established the presence of a proximal fragment and knee joint, the size of this tibial fragment is the next concern. If the tibial segment is short, less than one third the length of the normal tibia, the procedure of choice is synostosis of the fibula to the tibia and disarticulation of the foot (Fig. 38-20). This produces a long below-knee stump.

Complete. With complete longitudinal deficiency of the tibia, the clinical picture is the same as just described. The treatment of choice is disarticulation at the knee (Fig. 38-21). In those patients with unilateral deficiency, this procedure may be considered as soon as the individual is standing on the normal limb. Prosthetic restoration and good functional rehabilitation should be anticipated.

In 1965, Brown[8] first reported on his experience with construction of a knee joint in patients with complete longitudinal deficiency of the tibia. His experience dated back to 1957, when he first implanted the fibula beneath the femur and disarticulated the foot. The residual limb was fitted into a below-knee socket with outside hinges. A limb deficiency that had always been considered for above-knee amputation was converted into a below-knee prosthetic restoration (Fig. 38-22). Since that time, many of these procedures have been accomplished.[9] However, at a long-term review in 1975,* the high incidence of recurrent deformity and need for repeated operative intervention with ultimate failure and higher level conversion was such that only a few centers continue to perform this procedure.

Procedure for tibiofibular synostosis

The proximal tibial segment is exposed through an elliptical incision between it and the fibula. The distal portion of this tibial segment is dissected subperiosteally and completely exposed. The fibula is now exposed subperiosteally at the level opposite to the remaining tibia. Using a sharp gouge the medial surface of the fibula is turned proximalward, and the lateral aspect of the tibia is turned distalward. Bone graft is then packed into the defect between the two. The fascia is not sutured. The subcutaneous tissue and skin are closed in layers. Disarticulation at the ankle is then accomplished in the usual fashion. Marquardt[28] has described implantation of the fibula into the os calcis to create an end-bearing stump. This procedure may be employed instead of simple disarticulation. The limb is immobilized in a long leg plaster with the knee in full extension for 8 weeks, or until there is evidence of firm cross union between the tibia and fibula.

If the proximal segment of the tibia is suffi-

*Cooperative Clinic Chief's Meeting, Seattle, Washington, 1975.

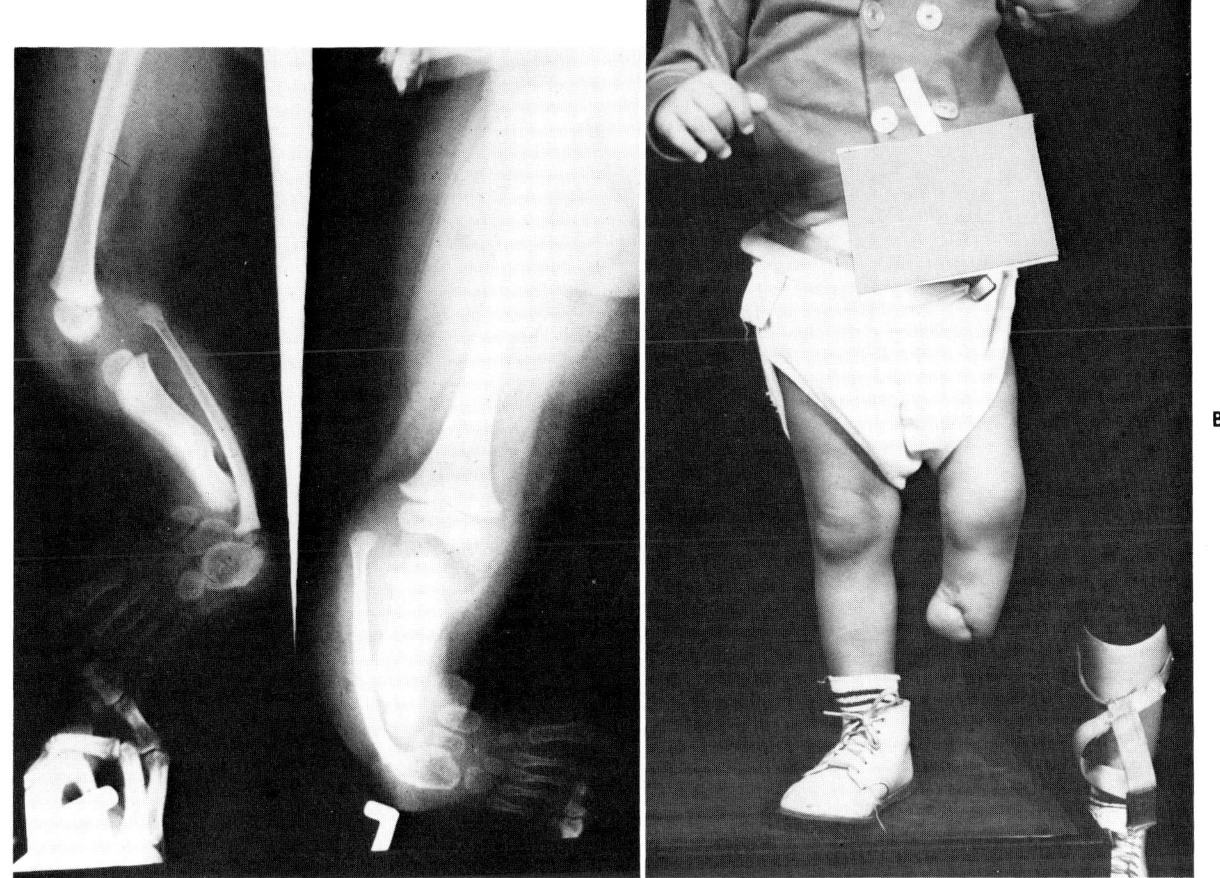

Fig. 38-19. A, Roentgenogram of partial longitudinal deficiency of tibia. Note fibula subluxated proximalward and varus of foot and distal fibula. **B,** Child at age 23 months, after disarticulation at ankle.

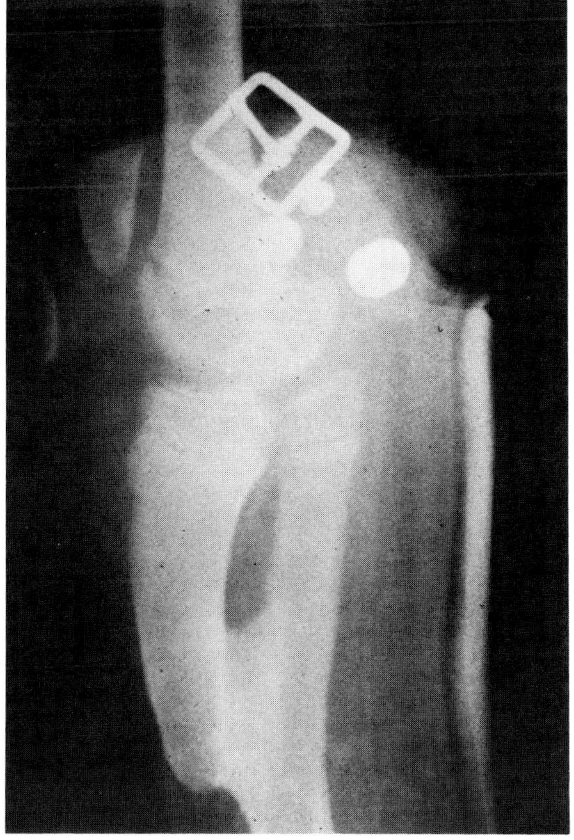

Fig. 38-20. Partial deficiency of tibia with synostosis to fibula.

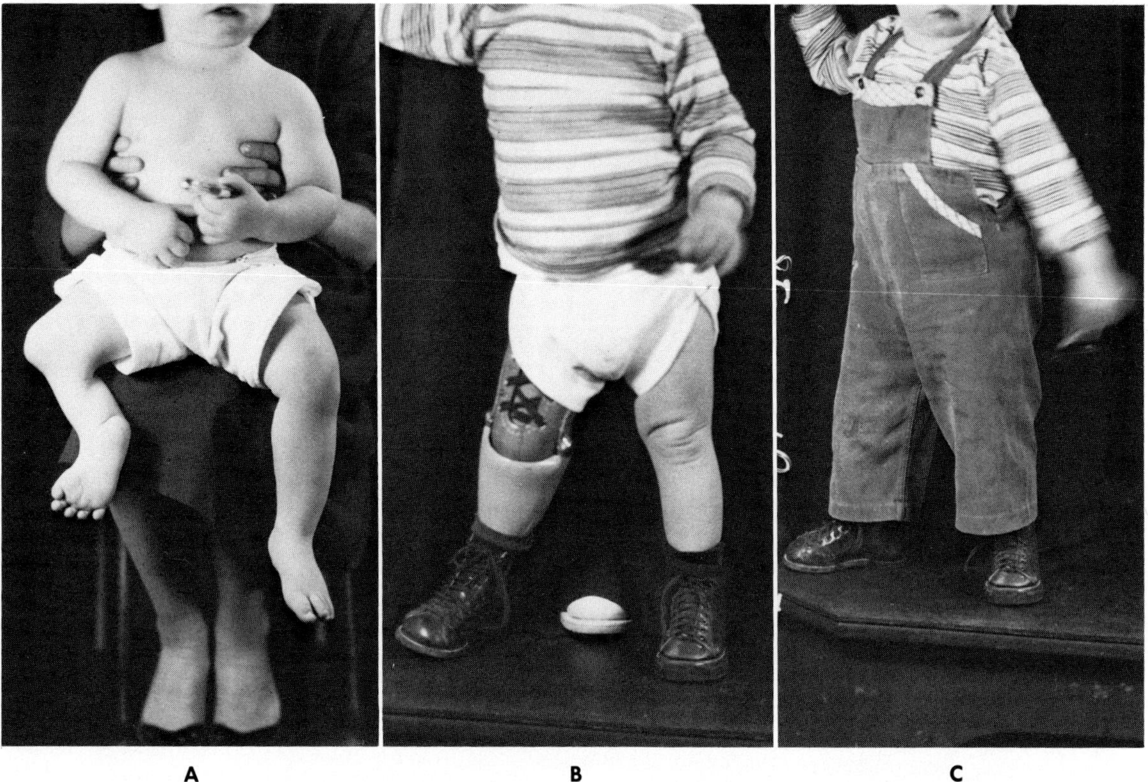

A B C

Fig. 38-21. A, Complete longitudinal deficiency of tibia. Note length discrepancy, varus foot, and subluxated knee. **B,** Child at age 1 year, 4 months, after knee disarticulation and fitting with leather socket knee disarticulation prosthesis with outside knee joint (1955). **C,** Clothed, child appears entirely normal.

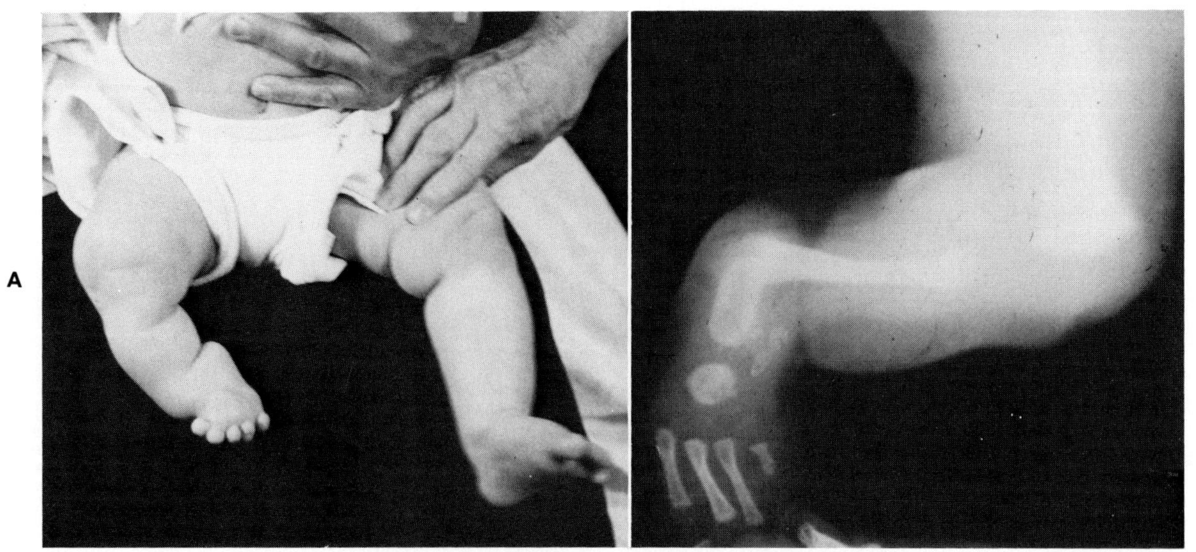

A B

Fig. 38-22. A, Child at age 6 months, complete longitudinal deficiency of tibia. **B,** X-ray film shows good location of proximal fibula, relative to femur, for Brown reconstruction.

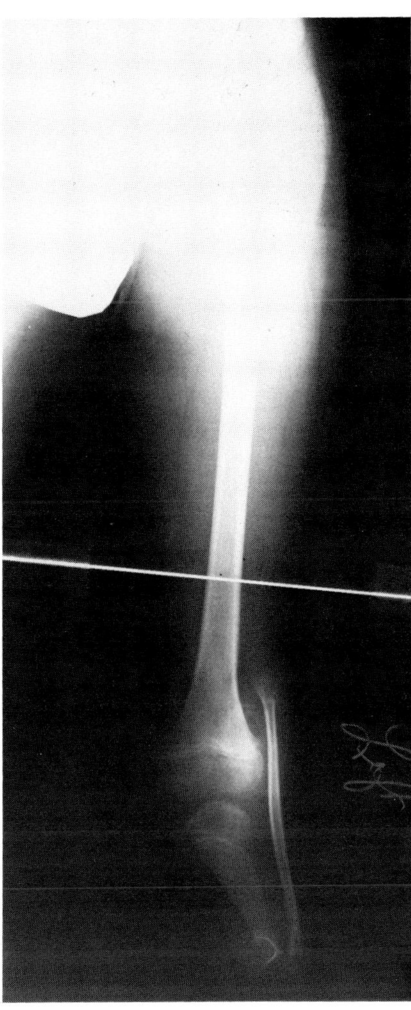

Fig. 38-23. Proximal migration of fibula in patient with partial longitudinal deficiency of tibia.

ciently long, tibiofibular synostosis is not necessary. Disarticulation at the ankle and fitting with a below-knee prosthesis may be carried out early in life. Proximal migration of the fibula may occur. This is appreciated clinically as the fibula rides proximally to the joint level. As a rule, it is asymptomatic. By x-ray examination it appears grossly anomalous, and one would expect that resection is necessary. In our experience, this has not been the case. A resection of this proximal portion of the fibula may create instability at the knee joint (Fig. 38-23). Relief of socket pressure in this area is preferable to surgical intervention.

Procedure for knee disarticulation

In the procedure for knee disarticulation (Chapter 24), a skin incision is marked out with a long anterior flap, which is also wide at its distal portion, and carried to well below the level of the femoral condyles. The posterior portion of the incision should be marked out at or just below the popliteal crease. The anterior incision is made and carried down through the subcutaneous tissues. The anterior capsular structures are divided, entering the knee joint. There may not be a patellar tendon. Posteriorly, the incision is made and deepened, and the hamstring tendons, if identifiable, are divided somewhat long and tagged for later suture. The great vessels are clamped and doubly ligated and the nerves treated in the usual manner. The gastrocnemius origin (if discernible) is severed from the femoral condyles. The capsule and ligaments are divided and the limb removed. At this point, the tourniquet is released and all bleeding controlled. The hamstring tendons are sutured to the capsule or ligamentous structure as available. If a patella and its tendon are present, the patella is left in place, and the tendon is sutured to the stump of the cruciate ligament. The capsule is closed over the cartilage of the femoral condyles. Drainage with either a soft tissue drain or suction is placed, and the closure is completed. It should be noted that the long anterior flap provides good coverage of the femoral condyles and good weight-bearing skin for subsequent prosthetic wear. The postoperative care may be with rigid dressing or soft dressing according to the surgeon's preference.

As the patient grows older, a length discrepancy of the remaining femur may occur that will permit use of a knee joint other than the outside hinge. If this does not occur, distal femoral epiphysiodesis may be considered when the child is 10 to 12 years of age. If the child is seen when it is considered too late for epiphysiodesis, then revision may be carried out as discussed in Chapter 24. Newer design of joints for the knee disarticulation prosthesis may render this option unnecessary.

PFFD longitudinal deficiency of the proximal portion of the femur

Aitken[2] recognized "the existence of a group of partial deficiencies of the proximal femur involving the iliofemoral joint" and, since no appropriate terminology existed, used the designation "proximal femoral focal deficiency." Amstutz[4] has defined PFFD as the "absence of some quality or characteristic of completeness of the proximal femur, including stunting or shortening of the entire femur." Aitken described four classes (Fig.

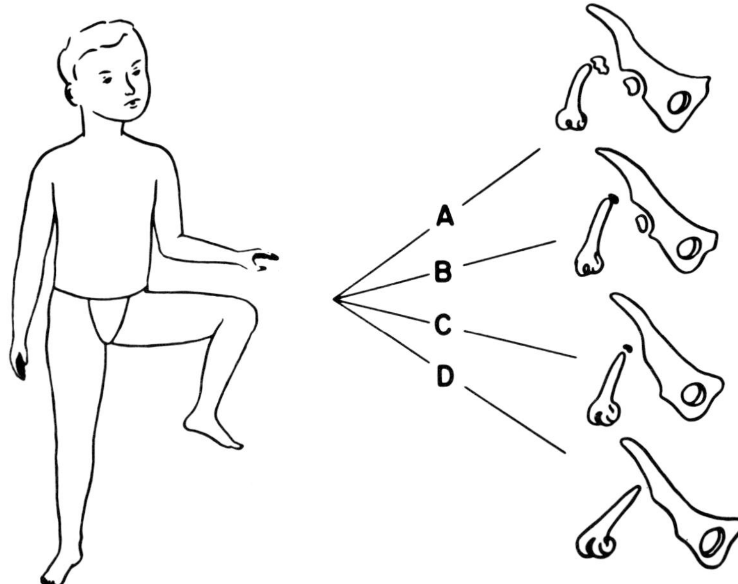

Fig. 38-24. Four radiographic subclasses of proximal femoral focal deficiency (PFFD). (Courtesy National Academy of Sciences, Washington, D.C.)

38-24). In class A there is an acetabulum. The head of the femur is within the acetabulum, and there is a subtrochanteric deficit. In class B there is an acetabulum and a capital fragment within the acetabulum. There is a short shaft fragment with no bony connection between the two. In class C there is no acetabulum. There is a short femoral fragment with a tuft. In Class D there is no acetabulum. A very short triangular femoral segment is present. Amstutz further expounded this classification and developed five types. His type 1 included those patients with what has been described by Aitken as a congenital short femur or coxa vara with bowing. His other four types approximate the Aitken classes A, B, C, and D. These morphological classifications offer assistance in treatment decisions primarily with regard to the hip.

Most reports of PFFD have included only small numbers of cases.* Prior to January 1, 1968, the Area Child Amputee Center in Grand Rapids, Michigan, had only thirty-five cases. In his report, King was able to review over 100 cases of PFFD collected from various juvenile amputee clinics throughout the United States. In 1968, Westin and Gunderson[39] were only able to gather 165 cases collectively recorded from Shriners Hospitals.

Westin and Gunderson reported a 65% incidence of other defects, with 50% of the patients having deficiency of the fibula in the same limb. Amstutz and Aitken noted a high incidence of fibular deficiencies in the same limb as well as other skeletal deficiencies. Kruger and Rossi[24] reported thirty-one of thirty-eight patients to have other limb abnormalities, with fibular deficiency in 50% of their patients.

In his early description of the biomechanical losses of lower limb skeletal deficiency, Aitken has stressed four points[1,2]: (1) inequality of leg length, (2) malrotation, (3) inadequacy of proximal musculature, and (4) instability of proximal joints. PFFD has all four of these elements of biomechanical loss. Although malrotation, inadequacy of proximal musculature, and instability of proximal joints all contribute to the poor gait and complexity of treatment, it is the length discrepancy that is the ultimate indication for definitive surgery – amputation and prosthetic restoration.

Amstutz and Wilson[4] recognized this progressive discrepancy in length of limbs so affected and developed a concept of proportionate inhibition of growth in all patients over the age of 5. Amstutz believed that precise prognostication of the expected discrepancy in limb length was possible and that definitive treatment could be planned on these children as early as 2 years of age. The theory of proportionate growth has been further expanded by Mosley[30] in his technique of charting the proportionate discrepancy as opposed to the growth of the normal limb. Although in most patients with PFFD the discrepancy early in life is

*2, 4, 6, 15, 17, 21, 24, 26, 27, 35, 39

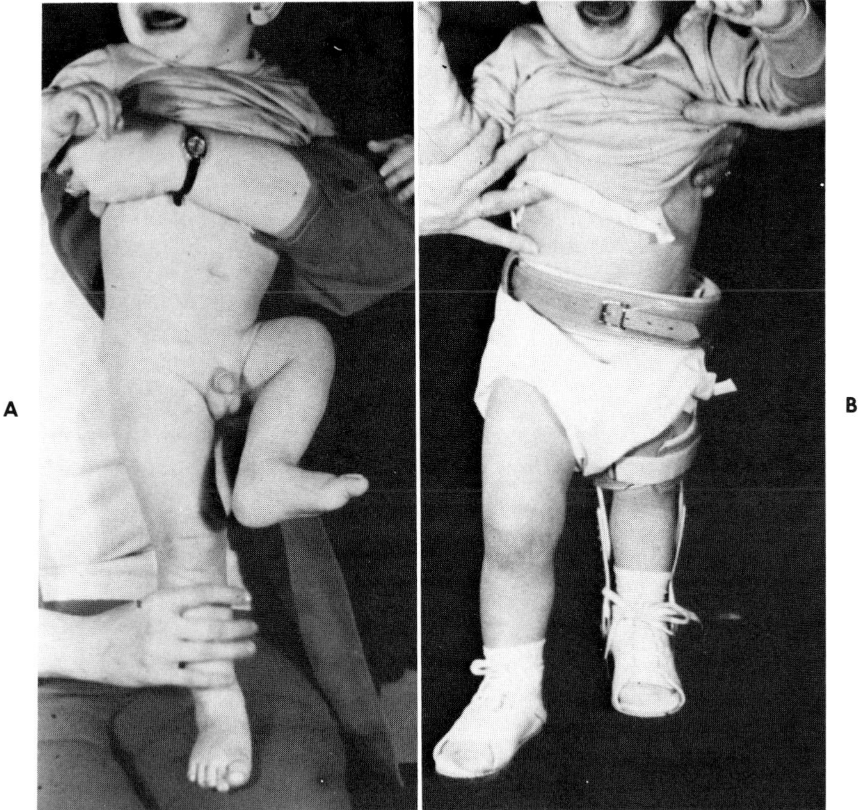

Fig. 38-25. A, PFFD, femur is short. Hip is flexed, abducted, and externally rotated. Knee is flexed. **B,** Orthotic management to prevent fixed deformity until surgical intervention.

sufficient to suggest that eventual amputation will be indicated, growth charts can be of assistance in decisions as to the total treatment plan.

The clinical picture of PFFD (Fig. 38-25) is that of a short femoral segment, which is positioned in flexion and external rotation. If ignored, this may become a fixed deformity with secondary knee flexion deformity. When associated with fibular deficiency, the length discrepancy will be much greater, and foot deformity will be present. If the tibia and fibula are essentially normal, then foot and ankle function willl be normal. It is important to institute an early stretching program to prevent knee and hip deformity.

The hip joint

As described by Aitken, classes A and B PFFD have an acetabulum present by x-ray examination at birth, and this indicates the presence of a femoral head within the acetabulum. Types C and D have no acetabulum present by x-ray examination at birth, suggesting that no femoral head will develop. It is usually impossible to distinguish between type A and B at birth. As ossification of the capital epiphysis, femoral neck, and trochanteric portion occur, the distinction can be made.

Class A PFFD can be recognized by x-ray examination when the cartilaginous anlage of the head and neck have ossified. The head and neck will be noted to be connected to the shaft fragment with subtrochanteric varus deformity that may be progressive. This subtrochanteric varus may be associated with subtrochanteric pseudoarthrosis. Correction of the deformity by subtrochanteric valgus osteotomy may be carried out, and, if a pseudoarthrosis is present, resection and bone grafting are indicated. If correction is deferred, the subtrochanteric valgus may be of such magnitude that it is impossible to correct it completely at a single stage, and the two-stage procedure may be necessary. A part of the deformity is corrected, and then after 1 or 2 years the operation may be repeated to complete the correction. The goals should be the creation of a neck shaft angle of between 120 and 135 degrees.

The Aitken class B PFFD is characterized by

the presence of a head and neck fragment that has no continuity with the shaft fragment which rides proximal to it. Lloyd-Roberts[27] and Lange et al.[26] have indicated that they have found connection either by fibrous tissue or cartilage between the two fragments. In either case, osteosynthesis is indicated to create a stable hip (Fig. 38-26). This should be accomplished some time between the ages of 3 and 6. Efforts at osteosynthesis should be delayed until there is adequate evidence of bone in the neck fragment so that with grafting, firm union between the shaft and neck fragment can be attained. If osteosynthesis is delayed too long, there is a possibility that the capital fragment may fuse to the acetabulum, in which case osteosynthesis should not be carried out, preferring an unstable mobile hip to a rigid hip.

Procedure for osteosynthesis

A lateral incision is made over the proximal shaft of the femur with extension proximally to the anterior spine of the pelvis, as with the Watson-Jones approach. The femoral shaft is exposed subperiosteally and osteotomized at the level of the head-neck fragment. Muscle insertions, especially if abductors are attached to the proximal fragment, are left intact. The neck is now exposed, and the capsule is opened to inspect the hip joint. The lateral portion of the neck is usually covered with fibrous tissue and/or a cartilaginous cap. This lateral aspect of the neck is nibbled away with a small rongeur, exposing a raw bony base in the center of the cartilage. If the patient is very young, only a small area of bone is available. The shaft fragment is now brought into opposition with the exposed neck by wide abduction and fixed to the neck fragment with Kirschner wires. In the case of the older child in whom advanced ossification of the neck fragment is present, a Coventry screw or small Smith-Petersen nail and plate may be used. Bone graft is desirable in an effort to obtain union. The proximal fragment of the femoral shaft is now allowed to fall back into place and may be fixed with wire to the shaft at a more distal point. The wound closure is routine. Immobilization should be in a hip spica with wide abduction for a minimum of 8 to 12 weeks or until good bony union is verified by x-ray examination.

Unilateral PFFD

Since length discrepancy is the major factor in patients with unilateral PFFD, they may be divided into three groups: (1) femoral segment less than 20% of the normal side, (2) femoral segment 20% to 70% of the normal side, and (3) femoral segment greater than 70% of the normal side.

A

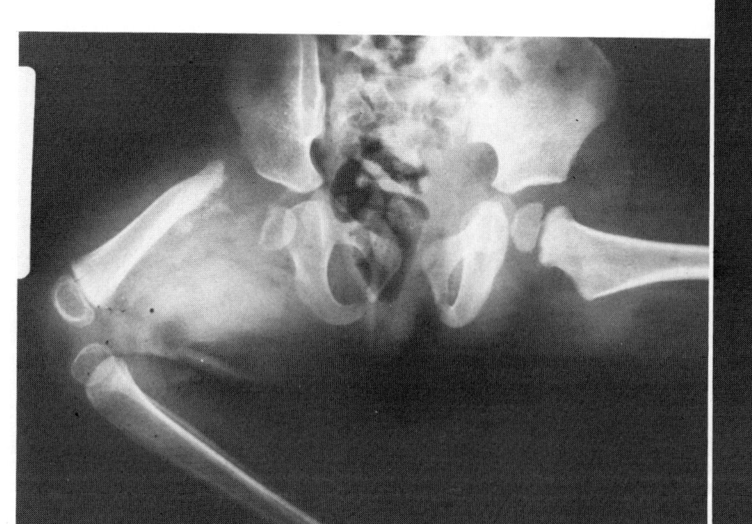

B

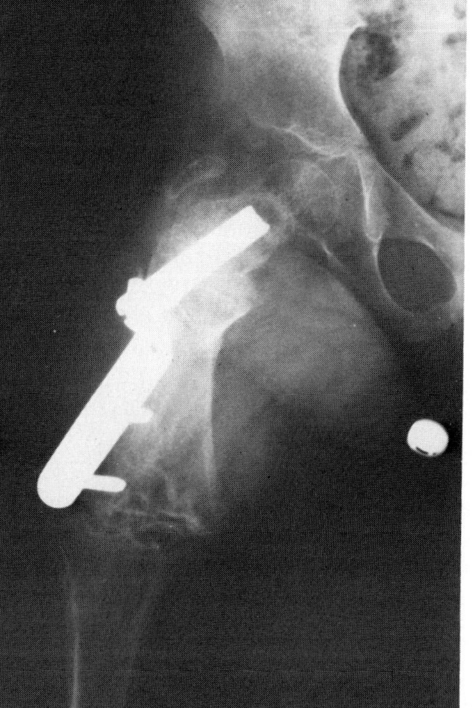

Fig. 38-26. A, Aitken class B PFFD. Head and neck are ossifying. There is no connection between shaft and head neck fragment. **B,** After osteosynthesis and knee fusion. Note that proximal tibial and distal femoral epiphyses have been destroyed to control longitudinal growth.

Short femoral segments. Patients with PFFD whose femoral segment is less than 20% of the length of the normal side are usually either in the Aitken class C or class D. No hip joint is present, and even though the discrepancy may be moderate at birth, it will be a progressive discrepancy with growth. Definitive treatment in these patients will be disarticulation at the ankle level and prosthetic restoration (Fig. 38-27). As with other limb deficiencies, if the parents have been prepared, and especially if they have attended a clinic and had the opportunity to observe other children with similar problems, acceptance of this recommendation can be expected. If the parents are reluctant to accept ablation, then as an alternative, an articulated extension prosthesis can be prescribed. This may be either a temporary measure or permanent if the parents so desire. As a further option, the Van Nes rotation plasty[19, 20] may be considered (p. 549).

Medium length femoral segments. There are many options available in the treatment of patients with PFFD with the femoral segment measuring 20% to 70% of the length of the normal femur. A treatment plan should be developed. Early management should emphasize prevention of deformity at the hip and the knee. Orthoses may be prescribed, as well as a stretching and exercise program. If the parents are resistant to surgical intervention or if surgical intervention is to be deferred beyond the time of expected ambulation, the child may be fitted with a platform orthosis or an extension prosthesis without amputation (Figs. 38-28, *A*, and 40-40).

When the femoral segment approaches 70% of the length of the femur on the normal side and full knee extension and quadriceps power have been maintained, disarticulation at the ankle and prosthetic restoration with a Syme-type prosthesis are indicated (Fig. 40-62). Although knee levels are unequal and therefore stride length is unequal, these patients manage very well.

Children with shorter femoral segments may have developed a flexion external rotation deformity of the hip and associated knee flexion deformity. The weight-bearing line is therefore anterior and lateral to the weight-bearing line of the body, and they do not do well. Knee fusion in full extension will establish a single skeletal lever. King and his associates have pointed out that with knee fusion, the flexion abduction external rotation deformity at the hip will spontaneously

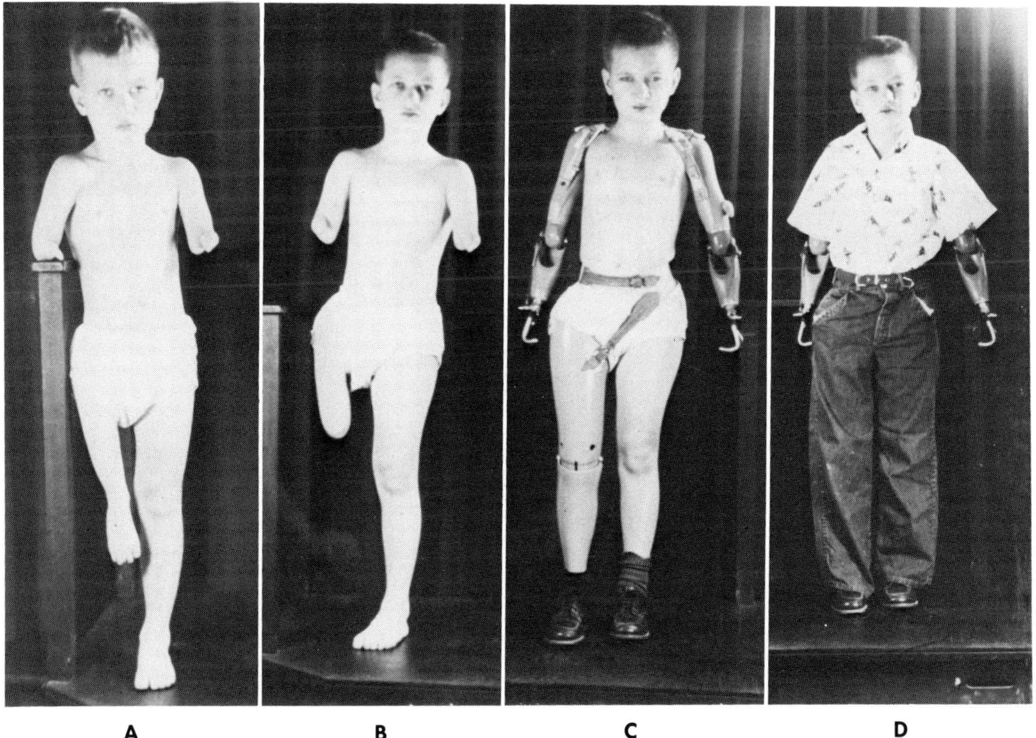

Fig. 38-27. PFFD (20% femoral segment). **A,** Child age 6, before amputation. **B,** Postamputation. **C,** With prosthesis. **D,** Fully clothed.

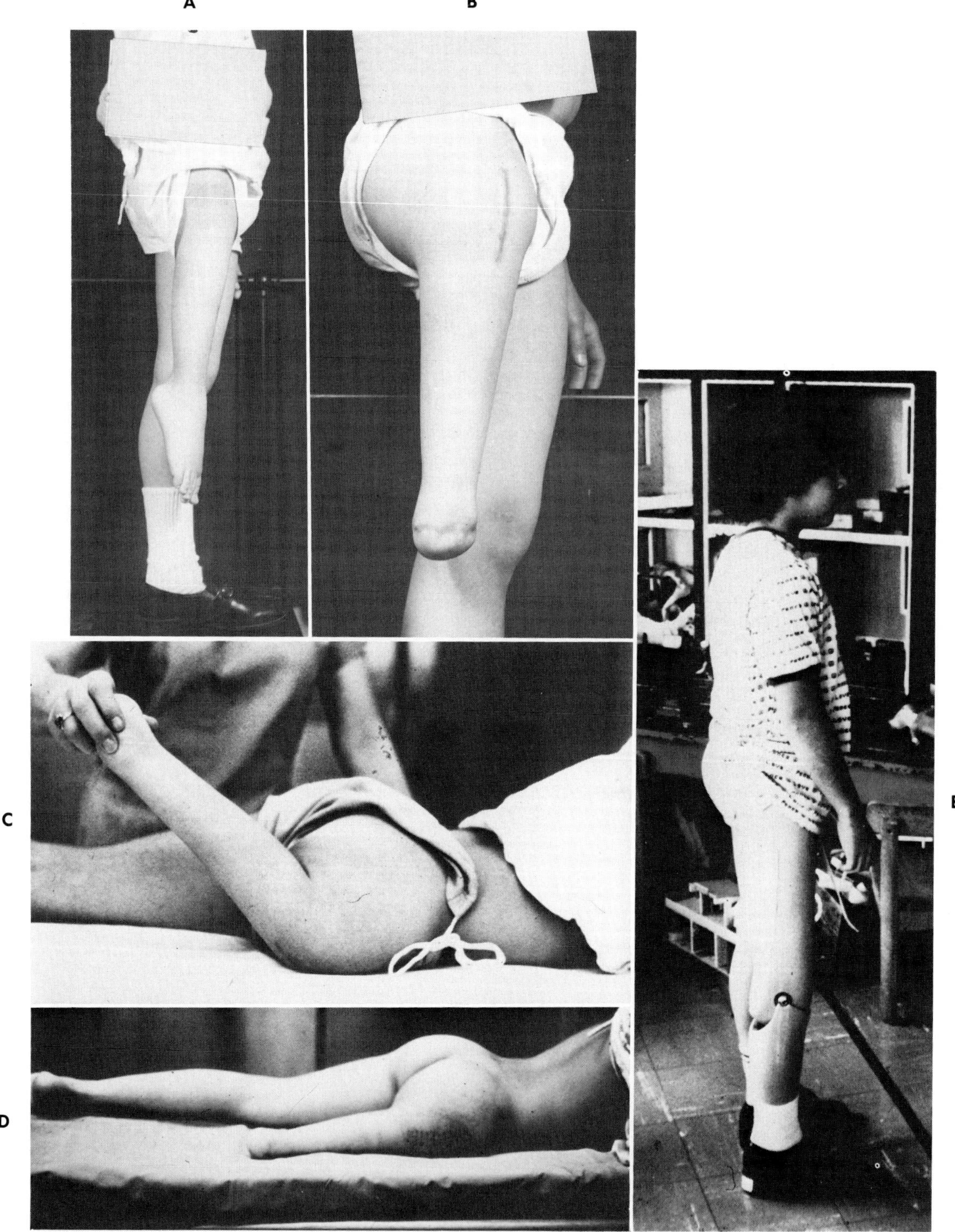

Fig. 38-28. A, Proximal longitudinal deficiency of femur (PFFD). Definitive treatment has been delayed. **B,** After knee fusion and ankle disarticulation, there has been increasing flexion deformity at knee. **C,** Flexion deformity demonstrated with patient lying prone. **D,** After correction, with patient prone, full correction is demonstrated. **E,** Patient with single-axis knee and good ischial bearing. Two years after surgery, correction is maintained.

correct without surgical intervention.[16] The single skeletal lever then comes into the weight-bearing line, and not only does the gait improve but also the strength of the muscles about the hip. The knee fusion should be carried out in full extension. Recurrent flexion may occur through the epiphyses. King and Marks[18] have attributed this to the Hueter-Volkmann law. Recurrent flexion deformity through the knee fusion should be corrected by osteotomy (Fig. 38-28, *B* to *D*).

Options in definitive treatment are disarticulation at the ankle and above-knee prosthetic restoration or Van Nes rotation plasty. Disarticulation at the ankle may leave the prosthetic knee center below that of the normal side. In this case, distal femoral epiphyseal arrest or shortening at the time of knee fusion may be desirable.

The Van Nes rotation plasty may be considered in conjunction with knee fusion.[7,38] The Van Nes procedure requires resection of a segment of the tibia and fibula sufficient to permit rotation of the distal portion of the leg 180 degrees so that the foot then faces backward. Following solid healing, the ankle joint can then be expected to function as a knee joint with dorsiflexion of the ankle providing "knee flexion" and plantar flexion of the ankle providing "knee extension." Prior to making the decision for Van Nes rotation plasty there must be a reasonable expectation that at the completion of growth the ankle joint will be approximately at knee level of the sound side. Use of the Van Nes rotation plasty provides the patient with a "knee joint" and a below-knee prosthesis (Fig. 46-25). The nonconventional prosthesis will have a socket modified to accept the foot as the shank portion, with weight bearing primarily on the heel and longitudinal arch of the foot. Placement of the knee axis must be precise and the thigh corset constructed and padded to prevent pressure over the pretibial region.

Procedure for Van Nes rotation plasty. Tourniquet control is optional in the Van Nes rotation plasty, but preferred. After the usual preparation and draping, an incision is made from the anteromedial proximal tibia slightly obliquely to the anterolateral aspect of the ankle level. The diaphysis of the tibia and fibula (when present) are exposed. Short segments of Kirschner wire may now be inserted into proximal and distal tibia to use as a reference point for rotation, or, if desired, the tibia can be marked prior to resection for this purpose. According to the prior plan, depending on the age of the patient and the amount of shortening desired, 5 to 7½ cm of tibia are resected, and approximately 2½ cm more of the fibula. The fibula may be reserved to use as a central bone graft for added stability. The tourniquet is released and bleeding controlled. If adequate bone has been resected, rotation of the distal segment 180 degrees poses no circulatory problem, and fixation of the tibial fragments may be accomplished with a compression plate and screws. If there is any question of circulatory impairment, either additional tibia may be resected or parallel Kirschner wires may be used above and below the osteotomy resection site for control of the fragments, using the reserved fibula as a central bone graft to prevent displacement. The skin wound is closed, making no effort to close the deep structures. Again circulation of the foot is observed, and, if satisfactory, the limb is immobilized in plaster.

Long femoral segment. Patients with femoral segments greater than 70% of the length of the normal side usually have a variation of coxa vara with bowing, or what Aitken terms, a congenitally short femur. He does not include either of these in the PFFD category, even though they are a manifestation of a deficiency in the proximal end of the femur. These patients must be observed and growth charts maintained, and as a rule they may be treated as a length discrepancy problem. Options to be considered include (1) lengthening of the short femur, (2) growth arrest at the normal knee epiphyses, (3) shortening of the normal femur, or (4) a combination of lengthening and growth arrest. If there is no reasonable hope for equalization of leg lengths, disarticulation at the ankle and a Syme prosthesis are considered as a method of leg length equalization, rather than resorting to excessive shortening of the patient's overall height. Although patients with coxa vara with bowing of the femur or a congenitally short femur appear to benefit from subtrochanteric valgus osteotomy, development of the acetabulum must be carefully observed. If acetabular dysplasia is present, valgus osteotomy is contraindicated.

Bilateral PFFD

Patients with bilateral PFFD may be divided into two groups[24]; the symmetrical, in which the length of the limbs is approximately equal, and the asymmetrical, in which there is a discrepancy in length between the two limbs so that to stand on the feet the patient is required to excessively flex one hip and knee while the other is extended.

Asymmetry may result from a difference in length of the remaining femoral segment or from a concomitant fibula or tibial deficiency on the short side.

Symmetrical. Patients with bilateral PFFD with approximately equal length limbs ambulate despite the severity of their limb anomalies, provided they have functional upper limbs. When seen in infancy, they can begin a physical therapy program to maintain their musculature and prevent fixed deformity. Trunk strengthening exercises should be instituted early in life, and the parents should be encouraged to permit the child maximum activity. When bilateral PFFD is associated with other lower limb deficiencies such as fibular deficiency it may be necessary to consider surgical intervention and/or orthotic management to control the deformity. Although those with severe upper limb deficiencies may be deferred in walking as late as 7 or 8 years of age (Fig. 38-29), most of these patients with functional arms assume independent ambulation sometime between 2 and 3 years of age. It is interesting that these children spontaneously become hand walkers. When the child reaches 5 or 6 years of age an effort should be made to allow him to use "stilts." It is at the time of entering school that a child's deficiency in stature becomes important to him. Prosthetic restoration is directed toward cosmetic, rather than functional, improvement. With development of good balance, the child can ultimately be fitted with articulated limbs *without amputation,* providing adequate height. It must be recognized that the energy consumption required for ambulation is great. Weight control here is very important, and since the child's activity level is usually reduced, weight is gained easily. The parents must recognize this and institute dietary control at home (Fig. 40-61).

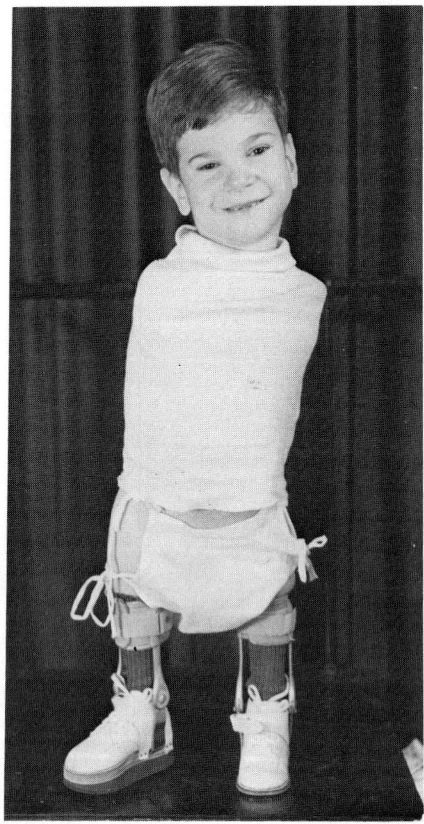

Fig. 38-29. Child with bilateral symmetrical PFFD with bilateral upper amelia is first able to stand and walk at age 7.

This group of patients should not be considered for amputation. The feet and ankles should be preserved so that the patient remains independent without prostheses. We have observed patients continuously using their prostheses up to age 35, but what their ability will be at age 55 or 65 we cannot say. It is therefore important to preserve the feet. It is wise to use a helmet for head protection for children on stilt prostheses, particularly those with upper limb deficiencies. Children with bilateral upper limb amelia and PFFD in the lower limbs prefer to have their feet free so that they may use the feet for prehensile activities. This should be encouraged and is of sufficient importance to contraindicate prescription for prostheses.

Asymmetrical. Patients with asymmetrical PFFD, one leg significantly longer than the other, walk independently despite the severe deformity of both legs. When seen in infancy, the major effort should be directed toward preservation of joint function and prevention of deformity. Orthotic management will be necessary to maintain knee extension, and lifts should be prescribed as necessary to equalize leg lengths. When the discrepancy is great, as occurs when the short side has an associated fibular deficiency, disarticulation at the ankle joint on the short side is indicated. Provision of a Syme-type prosthesis will equalize length and give reasonable stature (Fig. 40-64, *A* and *B*). Restoration of stature by bilateral prosthetic restoration has been attempted in these children. The short side is fitted with an articulated limb, whereas the long side is fitted with an extension prosthesis (Fig. 40-64, *C*). Since the combinations of deficiency may be varied, the treatment plan for each patient must be individualized.

SUMMARY

Amputation or disarticulation and prosthetic restoration offer a method of limb length equalization in children with unilateral limb deficiencies. Since the child with bilateral transverse lower limb deficiencies is already a bilateral amputee, prosthetic restoration is a natural treatment.

A recognition of the natural history of longitudinal limb deficiencies suggests that the child with bilateral fibular deficiency, tibial deficiency, and PFFD will in adult life be a disproportionate dwarf. Restoration of normal height by prosthetic replacement with or without amputation offers a solution to this problem. The psychological implications of the severe limb deficiency should be appreciated at the child's birth and every effort made to educate the parent so that appropriate surgical intervention and prosthetic restoration will be acceptable.

REFERENCES

Upper limb deficiencies

1. Aitken, G. T., and Frantz, C. H.: Management of the child amputee, In American Academy of Orthopaedic Surgeons: Instructional course lectures, Ann Arbor, Mich., 1960, J. W. Edwards.
2. Albee, F. H.: Formation of radius congenitally absent; condition 7 years after implantation of bone graft, Ann. Surg. **87:**105-110, 1928.
3. Birch-Jensen, A: Congenital deformities of the upper extremity, Copenhagen, 1949, Munksgaard.
4. Boyes, J.: Bunnell's surgery of the hand, Philadelphia, J. B. Lippincott Co.
5. Freeman, B. S.: Results of epiphyseal transplants by flap and by free graft, Plast. Reconstr. Surg. **36:**227-230, 1965.
6. Goldberg, M., and Meyn, M.: The radial clubhand, Orthop. Clin. North Am., April, 1976.
7. Kruger, L., and Breyan, N.: A study of radial head dislocation in children with partial hemimelia, Inter-Clin. Info. Bull. **10**(1):1, 1970.
8. Lyttle, T., Spencer, D., and Perry, R.: Satisfaction and self esteem in patients attending a juvenile amputee clinic, Inter-Clin. Info. Bull. **15**(3-4):1, 1976.
9. Northwestern University Prosthetics Manual: Management of the juvenile amputee, Evanston, Ill., 1975.
10. Novotony, M., and LaFleur, J.: A study of human figure drawings by amputee children and verbalization of their general adjustments (unpublished masters thesis), 1979.
11. Pellicore, R., and Sciora, J. et al.: Incidence of bone overgrowth in the juvenile amputee population, Inter-Clin. Info. Bull. **13**(15):10, 1974.
12. Rank, B. K.: Long-term results in epiphyseal transplants in congenital deformities of the hand, Plast. Reconstr. Surg. **61**(3):321-329, 1978.
13. Riordan, D. C.: Congenital absence of the radius, J. Bone Joint Surg. **37A:**1129-1140, 1955.
14. Sayre, R. H.: A contribution to the study of club hand, N.Y. Med. J. **58:**529-532, 1893.
15. Schilder, P.: The image and appearance of the human body, New York, 1950, International Universities Press, Inc.
16. Skoog, T.: Syndactyly: a clinical report on repair, Acta Chir. Scand. **130:**537-549, 1965.
17. Sorby, R.: Clinic chiefs meeting, Grand Rapids, Mich. April, 1978.
18. Steindler, A.: Orthopaedic operations, Springfield, Ill., 1947, Charles C Thomas, Publisher.
19. Sullivan, R., and Celikyol, F.: An ongoing seminar for parents of amputee children, Inter-Clin. Info. Bull. **15**(5-6): 9-14, 1976.
20. Swanson, A.: The Krukenberg procedure in the juvenile amputee, J. Bone Joint Surg. **46A:**1540-1549, 1964.
21. Swanson, A. B.: Les malformations congitales du membre superieur. A propos de leur classification et de leur trailement, Ann. Chirurgie **29**(5):433-462, 1975.
22. Swanson, A.: Phocomelia and congenital limb malformation: reconstruction and prosthetic replacement, Am. J. Surg. **109:**294-299, 1965.
23. Sypniewski, B.: Age of initial fitting, Inter-Clin. Info. Bull. March, 1972.

Lower limb deficiencies

1. Aitken, G. T.: Amputation as a treatment for certain lower extremity congenital abnormalities, J. Bone Joint Surg. **41A:**1267-1285, Oct., 1959.
2. Aitken, G. T.: Proximal femoral focal deficiency—definition, classification, and management. In Proxomal femoral focal deficiency: a congenital anomaly, Publication No. 1734, Washington, D.C., 1969, National Academy of Sciences.
3. Aitken, G. T.: Tibial hemimelia. In Aitken, G. T., editor: Selected lower limb anomalies, Washington, D.C., 1971, National Academy of Sciences.
4. Amstutuz, H. C., and Wilson, P. D., Jr.: Dysgnenesis of the proximal femur (coxa vara) and its surgical management, J. Bone Joint Surg. **44A:**1-24, Jan., 1962.
5. Badgley, C. E., O'Connor, S. J., and Kudner, D. F.: Congenital kyphoscoliotic tibia, J. Bone Joint Surg. **34A:**349-371, April, 1952.
6. Bevan-Thomas, W. H., and Millar, E. A.: A review of the proximal femoral focal deficiencies, J. Bone Joint Surg. **49A:**1376-1388, Oct., 1967.
7. Borggreve, J.: Kniegelenksersatz durch das in der Beinlangsachse um 180° gedrehte Fussgelenk, Arch. Orthop. Chir. **28:**175-178, 1930.
8. Brown, F. W.: Construction of a knee joint in congenital total absence of the tibia (paraxial hemimelia, tibia): a preliminary report, J. Bone Joint Surg. **47A**(4):695-704, June, 1965.
9. Brown, F. W.: The Brown operation for total hemimelia tibia. In Aitken, G. T., editor: Selected lower limb anomalies, Washington, D.C., 1971, National Academy of Sciences.
10. Clark, M. W.: Autosomal dominant inheritance of tibial meromelia, J. Bone Joint Surg. **57A**(2):262-264, March, 1975.
11. Corner, E. M.: The clinical picture of congenital abscence of the fibula, Br. J. Surg. **1:**203-206, 1913.
12. Coventry, M. B., and Johnson, E. W., Jr.: Congenital absence of the fibula, J. Bone Joint Surg. **34A:**941-955, Oct., 1952.
13. Eaton, G. O., and McKusick, V. A.: A seemingly unique polydactyly-syndactyly syndrome in four persons in three generations. In The National Foundation–March of Dimes: Birth defects, **5**(3):221-225, 1969.

14. Farmer, A. W., and Laruin, C. A.: Congenital absence of the fibula, J. Bone Joint Surg. **42A:**1-12, Jan., 1960.
15. Fixsen, J. A., and Lloyd-Roberts, G. C.: The natural history and early treatment of proximal femoral dysplasia, J. Bone Joint Surg. **56B**(1):86-95, Feb., 1974.
16. King, R. E.: Providing a single skeletal lever in proximal femoral focal deficiency. A preliminary case report, Inter-Clin. Info. Bull. **6**(2):23-28, Nov., 1966.
17. King, R. E.: Some concepts of proximal femoral focal deficiency. In Proximal femoral focal deficiency: a congenital anomaly, Publication No. 1734, Washington, D.C., 1969, National Academy of Sciences.
18. King, R. E., and Marks, T. W.: Follow-up findings on the skeletal lever in the surgical management of proximal femoral focal deficiency, Inter-Clin. Info. Bull. **11**(3):1-4, 1971.
19. Kostiuk, J. P., Gillespie, R., Hall, J. E., and Hubbard, S.: Van Nes rotational osteotomy for treatment of proximal femoral focal deficiency and congenital short femur, J. Bone Joint Surg. **57A:**1039-1046, Dec., 1975.
20. Kritter, A. E.: Tibial rotation plasty for proximal femoral focal deficiency, J. Bone Joint Surg. **59A**(7):927-934, Oct., 1977.
21. Kruger, L. M.: Classification and prosthetic management of limb-deficient children, Inter-Clin. Info. Bull. **7**(12):1-25, Sept., 1968.
22. Kruger, L. M.: Fibular hemimelia: a symposium. Selected lower-limb anomalies, Washington, D.C., 1971, National Academy of Science, p. 49.
23. Kruger, L. M.: The use of stubbies for the child with bilateral lower-limb deficiencies, Inter-Clin. Info. Bull. **12**(12): 7-15, Sept., 1973.
24. Kruger, L. M., and Rossi, T. V.: Proximal femoral focal deficiency and its treatment, J. Orthot. Prosthet. **29**(2):37-57, June, 1975.
25. Kruger, L. M., and Talbott, R. D.: Amputation and prosthesis as definitive treatment in congenital absence of the fibula, J. Bone Joint Surg. **43A:**625-642, July, 1961.
26. Lange, D. R., Schoenecker, P. L., and Baker, C. L.: Proximal femoral focal deficiency, Clin. Orthop. **135:**15-25, Sept., 1978.
27. Lloyd-Roberts, G. C., and Stone, K.. H.: Congenital hypoplasia of the upper femur, J. Bone Joint Surg. **45B:**557-560, 1963.
28. Marquardt, E.: Personal Communication, 1979.
29. Mazet, R., Jr.: Syme's amputation. A follow-up study of fifty-one adults and thirty-two children, J. Bone Joint Surg. **50A:**1549-1563, Dec., 1968.
30. Mosley, C. F.: A straight-line graft for leg length discrepancies. J. Bone Joint Surg. **59A**(2):174-179, March, 1977.
31. O'Rahilly, R.: Morphological patterns in limb deficiencies and duplications, Am. J. Anat. **89:**135-193, 1951.
32. Pashayan, H., Fraser, F. C., McIntyre, J. M., and Dunbar, J. S.: Bilateral aplasia of the tibia, polydactyly and absent thumb in father and daughter, J. Bone Joint Surg. **53B:** 495-599, Aug., 1971.
33. Pellicore, R. J., Sciora, J., Lambert, C. N., and Hamilton, R.: Incidence of bone overgrowth in the juvenile amputee population, Inter-Clin. Info. Bull. **13**(15):1-8, 1974.
34. Putti, B.: The treatment of congenital absence of the tibia and fibula, Int. Surg. **50:**42, 1930. (Abstract from Chir. Organi. Mov. **7:**513, 1929.)
35. Scheer, G. B.: Treatment of proximal femoral focal deficiences, Clin. Orthop. **85:**292, 1972.
36. Serafin, J. A.: New operation for congenital absence of the fibula, J. Bone Joint Surg. **49B:**59-65, Feb., 1967.
37. Thompson, T. C., Straub, L. R., and Arnold, W. D.: Congenital absence of the fibula, J. Bone Joint Surg. **39A:** 1229-1237, Dec., 1957.
38. Van Nes, C. P.: Rotation-plasty for congenital defects of the femur, J. Bone Joint Surg. **32B**(1):12-16, Feb., 1950.
39. Westin, G. W., and Gunderson, F. O.: Proximal femoral focal deficiency—a review of treatment experiences. Symposium on Proximal Femoral Focal Deficiency—A Congenital Anomaly, Washington, D.C., 1969, National Academy of Sciences, pp. 100-105.
40. Wood, W. L., Zlotsky, N., and Westin, G. W.: Congenital absence of the fibula: treatment by Syme amputation: indications and technique, J. Bone Joint Surg. **47A:**1159-1169, Sept., 1965.
41. Yelton, C. L.: Certain congenital limb deficiencies occurring in twins and half-siblings, Inter-Clin. Inter. Bull. **1:**1-7, Feb., 1962.

CHAPTER 39

Acquired amputations in children

ROBERT E. TOOMS

Annual surveys of specialized child amputee clinics in the United States have repeatedly shown that approximately 60% of childhood amputations are congenital in origin, and 40% are acquired.[12] In contrast, a survey of prosthetic facilities has revealed that significantly more children with acquired amputations receive prosthetic services than those with congenital limb deficiencies.[8] This discrepancy suggests that children with the more complex congenital limb deficiencies are referred to specialized child amputee clinics, whereas most acquired childhood amputations are managed in less specialized settings. In either case, the number of children with acquired amputations is relatively small, but represents a significant segment of the pediatric population with major orthopaedic problems.

Acquired amputations are secondary to either trauma or disease, with trauma causing roughly twice as many limb losses as disease.[3, 15] Although there are obviously many traumatic incidents that may result in childhood amputations, power tools and machinery are the worse offenders, followed closely by vehicular accidents, gunshot wounds and explosions, and railroad accidents. In the older child, vehicular accidents, gunshot wounds, and power tool injuries are the most frequent causes of limb loss. In the 1- to 4-year-old group, power tools, such as lawn mowers, and household accidents account for most amputations (Fig. 39-1).

Of the disease processes necessitating amputation in children, malignant tumors are responsible for more than half, the highest incidence occurring in the 12- to 21-year-old group. Vascular malformations, neurogenic disorders, and a wide variety of miscellaneous disorders are responsible for the remainder of amputations due to disease (Fig. 39-2).

In over 90% of acquired amputations a single limb is involved, and it is a lower limb that is involved in 60% of the cases. Males outnumber females in incidence of acquired limb loss in a ratio of 3:2, most probably because males tend to engage in more hazardous activities.

SURGICAL PRINCIPLES

The well-established surgical principles for amputation surgery in the adult are just as applicable to amputations performed in children.[2,5,9,14] The cardinal dictum in children is to conserve all limb length possible, consistent with appropriate treatment for the condition that requires the amputation. Trauma is the proximate cause of most acquired amputations in children. In attempting to conserve length in the severely traumatized limb, adequate tissue vascularity of the growing child may allow the surgeon to use surgical techniques that are not successful in the adult. Skin grafts, firm traction, and wound closure under tension may be *judiciously* used in the child to conserve limb length without compromising wound healing or subsequent prosthetic use.[2,7,9,11] Split-thickness skin grafts, even over large areas of the stump, may tolerate prosthetic use quite well in the child. The increased elasticity of the child's skin, coupled with an excellent blood supply, allows the surgeon to apply somewhat heavier skin traction to open amputations in the child than would be safely tolerated in the adult. For the same reasons, open wounds may successfully be closed under slightly more tension in the child than would be permissible in similar adult patients. In each instance, however, good surgical judgment must be used, since even the tissue tolerance of the child has its limitations.

A second surgical dictum is, whenever possible, to perform a disarticulation rather than a transdiaphyseal amputation in a growing child. Disarticulation preserves the epiphyseal growth plate and thereby ensures longitudinal growth of the bone.[2,14] Loss of stump length due to epiphyseal loss is most readily apparent in above-knee amputations in young children. In amputations at this level, the distal femoral epiphysis, which accounts for approximately 70% of the longitudinal growth of the femur, is sacrificed. When a midthigh amputation is performed in a young child, the resultant above-knee stump present at age 16 will be quite short and will be a considerably less than optimal skeletal lever for prosthetic use (Fig. 39-3). Disarticulation also precludes the development of terminal or appositional overgrowth of new bone at the transected end of a long bone — the most common complication of amputation surgery in the growing child. The prominent condyles or malleoli, resulting from disarticulation, usually undergo atrophy with further growth of the child, thereby eliminating the cosmetic objection to this type of surgery when it is performed in the adult.[2,5,9,14]

COMPLICATIONS

Terminal overgrowth is the most common complication of amputation surgery in the skeletally immature individual. This is an appositional overgrowth of new bone at the transected end of a long bone. It is in no way related to epiphyseal plate growth, and previous attempts to prevent this problem by epiphysiodesis have not been successful.[22] Terminal overgrowth occurs most often in the humerus, fibula, tibia, and femur, in that

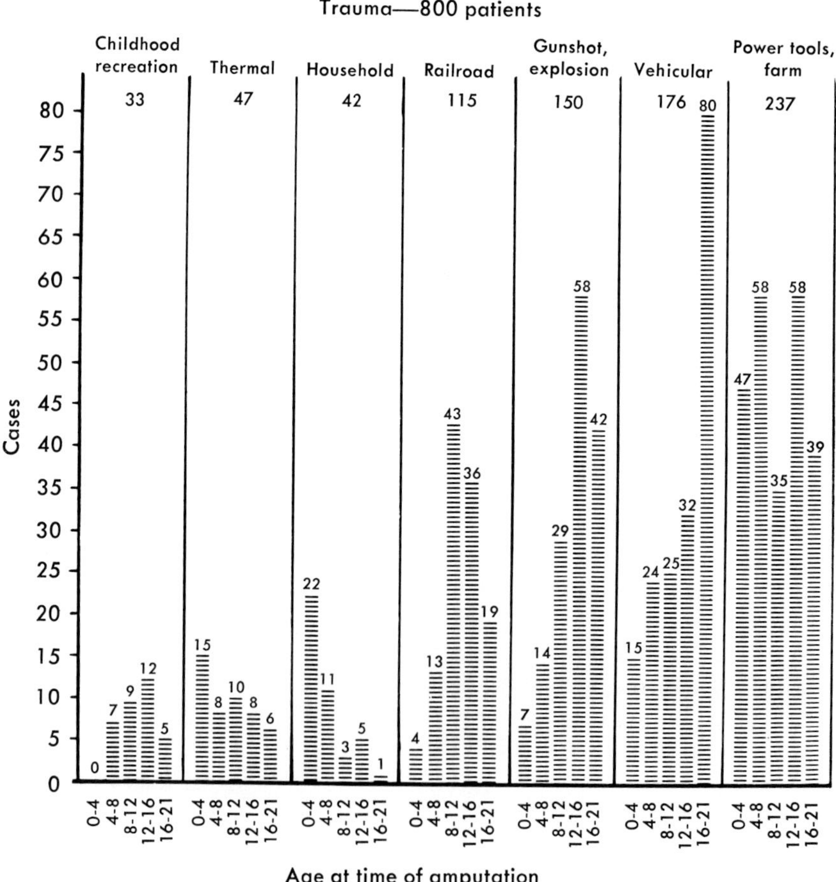

Fig. 39-1. Etiology of acquired amputations due to trauma. (From Northwestern University Medical School Prosthetic-Orthotic Program, Juvenile Amputee Course Manual, Evanston, Ill.)

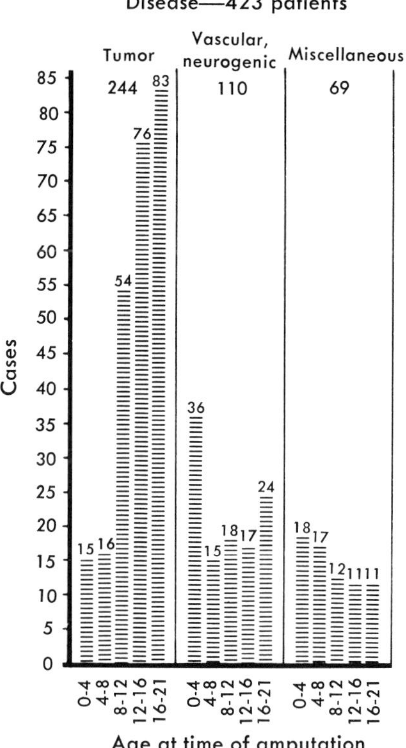

Fig. 39-2. Etiology of acquired amputations due to disease. (From Northwestern University Medical School Prosthetic-Orthotic Program, Juvenile Amputee Course Manual, Evanston, Ill.)

order.[2] In this condition, the appositional growth of new bone may exceed the growth of the overlying soft tissues to such an extent that the bone end actually penetrates the skin (Fig. 39-4). Many surgical techniques have been devised to prevent terminal overgrowth from developing. These include using intramedullary implants of silicone rubber[20,21] or porous polyethylene[16] to cap the resected bone end and prevent terminal overgrowth. This approach may eventually prove to be effective. However, the best treatment method remains stump revision with appropriate resection of the bony overgrowth.[1,14] This has been necessary in 8% to 12% of several reported large series of acquired amputations in children.[1-5,17] Once surgery becomes necessary to correct the problem, recurrences are common and may necessitate repeated stump revision at 2- to 3-year intervals until skeletal maturity (Chapter 41).

Adventitious bursae frequently develop in the soft tissues overlying an area of terminal overgrowth. Conservative treatment of such symptomatic bursae by aspiration, corticosteroid injection, and stump wrapping is seldom more than temporarily effective. Bursae that form over bony prominences subjected to recurrent pressure from a prosthetic socket are effectively managed by appropriate socket modifications. Permanent relief from those symptomatic bursae overlying an

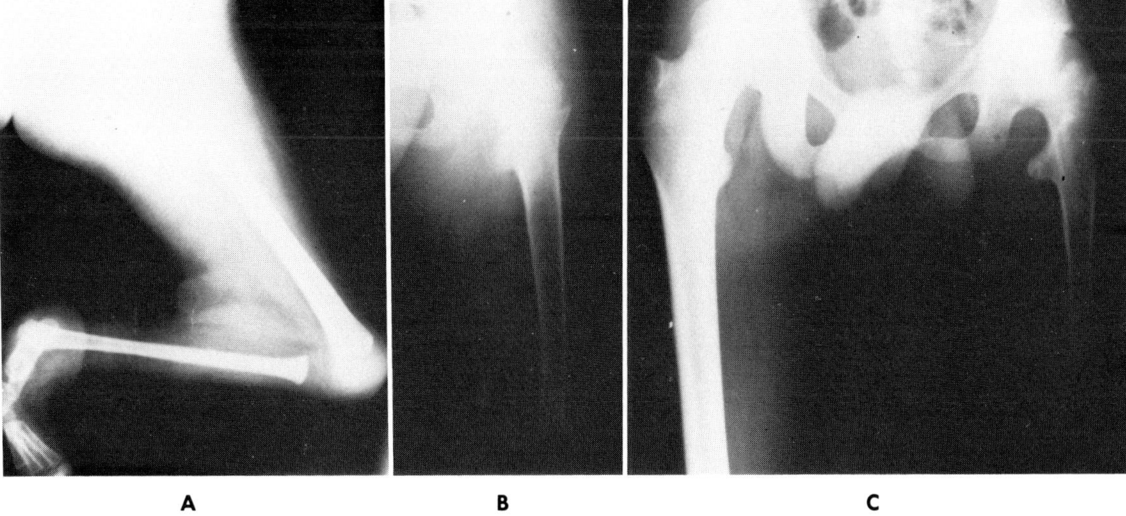

Fig. 39-3. A, Roentgenogram of left lower limb, illustrating tibial deficiency with severe soft tissue webbing in popliteal area. **B,** This limb deficiency was treated by amputation through distal third of femur. **C,** At skeletal maturity there is significant shortening of femur on amputated side due to loss of distal femoral epiphysis, with resultant very short amputation stump. (From Tooms, R. E.: The amputee. In Lovell, W. W., and Winter, R. B.: Pediatric orthopedics, vol. 2, Philadelphia, 1978, J. B. Lippincott Co., pp. 999-1054.)

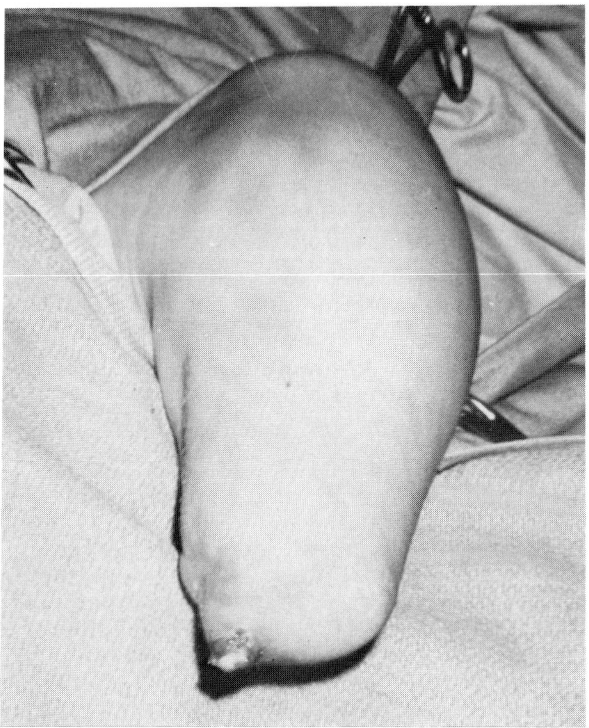

Fig. 39-4. Terminal overgrowth of humerus in posttraumatic above-elbow amputation. Bony overgrowth has actually penetrated soft tissues at end of amputation stump. (From Tooms, R. E.: The amputee. In Lovell, W. W., and Winter, R. B.: Pediatric orthopedics, vol. 2, Philadelphia, 1978, J. B. Lippincott Co., pp. 999-1054.)

area of terminal overgrowth usually requires surgical excision of the bursae combined with appropriate resection of the underlying bone (Fig. 39-5).[3-5]

Bone spurs often form at the periphery of transected bone ends as a response to periosteal stimulation at the time of surgery. Such bone spurs rarely necessitate stump revision and should be easily distinguished from terminal overgrowth.[3]

Extensive stump scarring from trauma, previous surgery, or skin grafting is usually well tolerated by the child amputee. Stump revision is seldom necessitated by scarring alone, but may require prosthetic modification to disperse weight-bearing forces and dminish shear stress at the stump-socket interface.[10] Minor modifications in the prosthetic socket will usually relieve symptomatic pressure that is concentrated over small areas of scarring in relatively nonweight-bearing areas of the amputation stump. Wearing a nylon sheath next to the skin and beneath the stump sock or wearing multiple stump socks may prevent tissue breakdown from stump-socket interface friction over small areas of scarring. More extensive prosthetic modifications may be necessary when the scarred area is larger or is over weight-bearing areas of the stumps. Check sock-

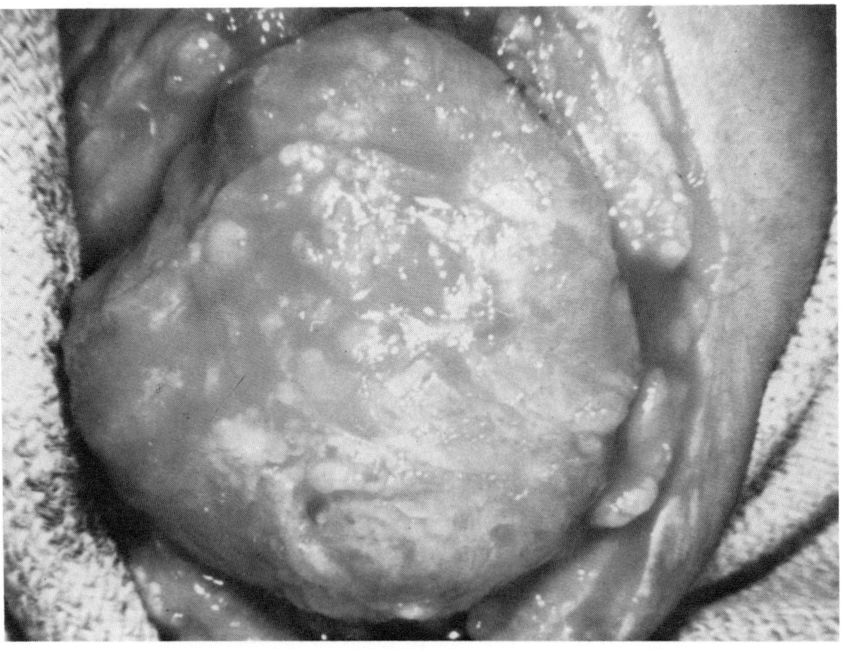

Fig. 39-5. Large bursa developed over end of humerus in acquired above-elbow amputation. Surgical excision of bursa, as well as underlying bony overgrowth, is necessary to eradicate problem. (From Tooms, R. E.: The amputee. In Lovell, W. W., and Winter, R. B.: Pediatric orthopedics, vol. 2, Philadelphia, 1978, J. B. Lippincott Co., pp. 999-1054.)

ets made of transparent polycarbonate plastic[18] and stump socks of pressure-sensitive fabric[6] allow precise identification of pressure-producing areas in the socket at both the below-knee and the above-knee amputation levels. For the severely scarred below-knee stump, the most commonly used method of relieving excessive pressure and shear forces is attaching outside knee joints and a weight-bearing thigh corset to a total-contact socket. Other successful techniques include the use of an air cushion socket[23] or a Silastic gel socket insert with a rubber sleeve for suspension.[13] I have been most successful in eliminating skin breakdown in the extensively scarred below-knee stump by using a meticulously fitted hard-socket PTB prosthesis worn over two or three five-ply stump socks. Suspension is by means of a supracondylar strap or, if necessary, with outside knee joints and a thigh corset.

When upper limb amputations are complicated by extensive trunk scarring, harnessing techniques alternative to the figure-of-eight harness may be necessary. The shoulder saddle with chest strap is an excellent solution in such cases (Fig. 39-6).

Neuroma formation in amputation stumps of children is seldom symptomatic enough to warrant surgical treatment. In reviewing a large series of acquired childhood amputations, Aitken[3] found that only 4% required surgical treatment for neuromata, most being satisfactorily managed by socket adjustment.

Phantom limb phenomenon always occurs in children following acquired amputations. If the amputation is performed under the age of 10 years, the phantom sensation is rapidly lost.[14] *Painful phantom limb sensation* does not occur in growing children, but has been reported in the teenager.

SURGICAL TECHNIQUES

Keeping in mind the previously discussed surgical principles of limb length conservation and the need for performing disarticulations in

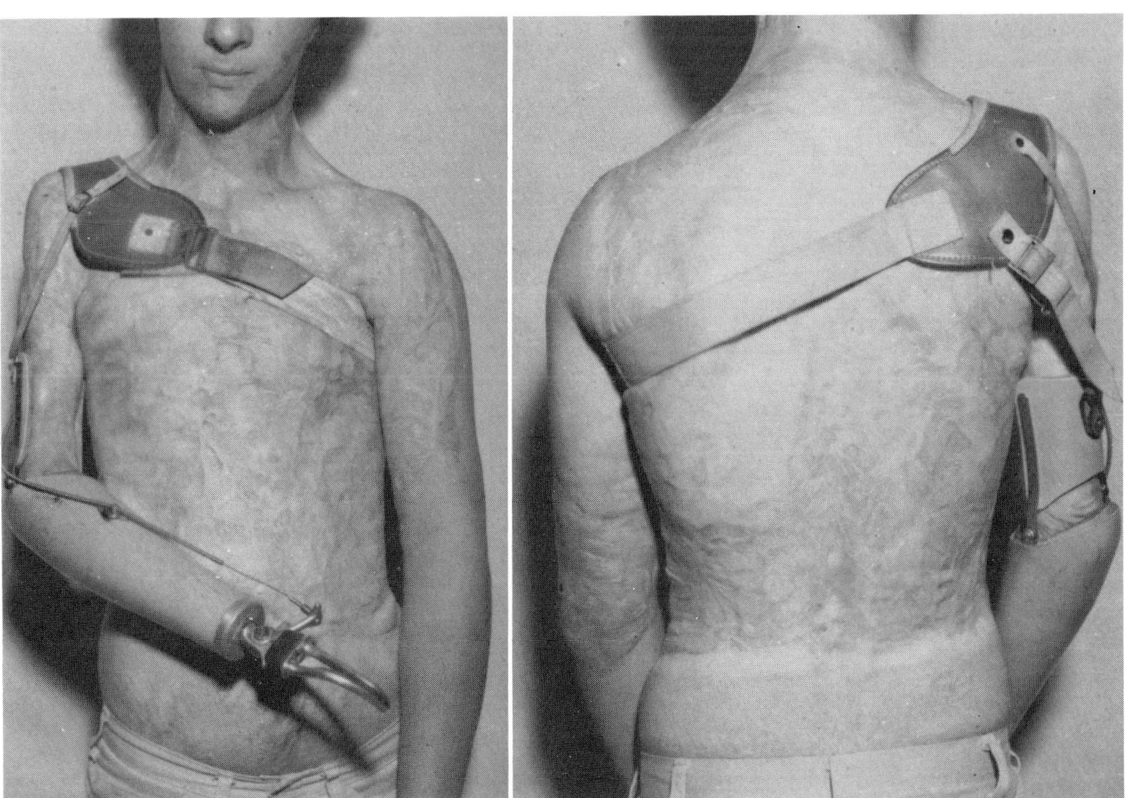

Fig. 39-6. Shoulder saddle with chest strap harness has been used to disperse pressure and shear forces over extensively scarred soft tissues of this child with below-elbow amputation due to severe thermal burns. (From Tooms, R. E.: The amputee. In Lovell, W. W., and Winter, R. B.: Pediatric orthopedics, vol. 2, Philadelphia, 1978, J. B. Lippincott Co., pp. 999-1054.)

preference to transdiaphyseal amputations, surgical techniques in the child do not differ significantly from those used for the adult. Therefore specific surgical procedures will not be outlined for any of the major levels of amputation in the upper or lower limb. However, several specialized surgical procedures do deserve mention.

Biceps kineplasty, which is rarely indicated in the adult below-elbow amputee, is never indicated in the growing child.[14] The skin tunnel rarely remains intact as the child grows, and children are seldom able to maintain the degree of cleanliness so essential in kineplasty tunnels. Furthermore, the limited excursion of the biceps muscle in a small child reduces the function of the kineplasty to a very marginal level. (See also Chapter 15.)

The Krukenberg, or "lobster-claw," operation, on the other hand, may well deserve consideration in the child with a long below-elbow amputation.[19] The Krukenberg procedure provides a crude pinching mechanism with preserved sensation by splitting a long below-elbow stump into radial and ulnar rays that are widely separated and covered with skin possessing normal sensation. The forearm muscles that attach to the two rays provide voluntary opening and closing of these rays. Children who have the operation performed early in life learn to use the pincer and are not often emotionally disturbed by the unsightly appearance of the stump. The procedure has its greatest application in bilateral upper limb amputees, especially in the blind. (See also Chapters 15 and 41.)

Ankle disarticulation is a frequently indicated level of amputation in the growing child. It should be stressed that this procedure should be performed as a true disarticulation with a Syme-type soft tissue closure and not as a supramalleolar amputation as is done in the conventional Syme amputation in the adult. (See also Chapter 22.)

Lawn mower injuries and *severe burns* that result in partial limb loss occur in sufficiently large numbers to justify specific comments on the surgical management of these problems. As in other traumatic incidents, preservation of limb length is of major concern in both of these injuries. The physiological tolerance of growing children fortunately allows the surgeon to preserve limb length by using skin grafts, traction, and soft tissue – shifting plastic procedures.

Most lawn mower injuries sustained by children result in partial foot amputations. Some of these injuries involve only the digits or the distal metatarsal area and present no great treatment problems. Others are quite extensive, involving most of the foot with multiple deep and extensively contaminated wounds. In these latter instances, proper surgical judgment is necessary to determine which injury can reasonably be expected to provide a serviceable partial foot amputation by using skin grafts and soft tissue – shifting plastic procedures and which injury would require revision to a higher level. This decision is seldom obvious, and when doubt exists it is better to err on the side of conservatism. The initial debridement of such injuries should be limited to excision of only that tissue which is absolutely nonviable, preserving any tissue of questionable viability. Initial bone resection should be minimized until sufficient time has elapsed to be certain how much viable soft tissue will ultimately be available for wound closure. Following thorough irrigation and debridement, the wound is lightly packed open.

Five to seven days later the wound is examined with the patient under anesthesia. After further debridement of any nonviable tissue, a decision may be made to revise the amputation to a higher level or to continue with a more conservative approach. For example, an amputation at the midtarsal joint level that requires extensive skin grafting over the plantar surface of the heel and results in loss of the foot dorsiflexors will be less functional and require more subsequent treatment than revision to a higher level. If revision to a higher level (ankle disarticulation or below-knee amputation) is indicated at the time of the first wound dressing, an open amputation is preferable, followed by skin traction until secondary closure is performed 5 to 7 days later. If continued conservatism seems appropriate, it may be possible to partially close the wound at this time with minimal additional bone resection. If extensive skin grafting or tissue-shifting plastic procedures such as a Z-plasty are needed, these are more safely done at the time of a second wound dressing 5 to 7 days later, when granulation tissue begins to cover open areas and the danger of infection is less.

Thermal or electrical burns may cause such widespread tissue destruction that amputation of a major portion of the limb may become necessary. In such circumstances, conservative treatment should be pursued until there is adequate demarcation of nonviable tissue to allow open amputation at the lowest possible level. During this time, appropriate splinting of proximal joints is essential to minimize the development of joint contractures in nonfunctional positions. Despite splinting, late soft tissue releases may be needed to improve joint motion. Extensive skin grafting is usually necessary in children with severe burns, and the resultant scarred stumps may present very difficult problems in prosthetic fitting. The use of pressure dressings over scarred and grafted areas helps to decrease scar hypertrophy. When healing has occurred, gentle massage is often beneficial in mobilizing scar tissue that is adherent to bone. Successful prosthetic use usually necessitates modification of prosthetic sockets and suspension systems as noted previously.

REFERENCES

1. Aitken, G. T.: Overgrowth of the amputation stump, Inter-Clin. Info. Bull. **1**(11): 1-8, Sept., 1962.
2. Aitken, G. T.: Surgical amputation in children, J. Bone Joint Surg. **45A:**1735-1741, 1963.
3. Aitken, G. T.: The child with an acquired amputation, Inter-Clin. Info. Bull. **7**(8):1-15, May, 1968.
4. Aitken, G. T., and Frantz, C. H.: The juvenile amputee, J. Bone Joint Surg. **25A:**659-664, 1953.
5. Aitken, G. T., and Frantz, C. H.: Management of the child amputee. American Academy of Orthopedic Surgeons: Instructional course lectures, vol. 17, Ann Arbor, Mich., 1960, J. W. Edwards, pp. 246-298.
6. Brand, P. W., and Ebner, J. D.: Pressure sensitive devices for denervated hands and feet, J. Bone Joint Surg. **51A:** 109-116, 1969.
7. Cary, J. M.: Traumatic amputation in childhood – primary management, Inter-Clin. Info. Bull. **14**(6):1-10, 1975.
8. Davies, E. J., Friz, B. R., and Clippinger, F. W., Jr.: Children with amputations, Inter-Clin. Info. Bull. **9**(3):6-19, Dec., 1969.
9. Frantz, C. H., and Aitken, G. T.: Management of the juvenile amputee, Clin. Orthop. **9:**30-47, 1959.
10. Hall, C. B., Rosenfelder, R., and Tabloda, C.: The juvenile amputee with a scarred stump. In Aitken, G., editor: The child with an acquired amputation, Washington, D.C., 1972, National Academy of Sciences.
11. Herndon, J. H., and LaNone, A. M.: Salvage of a short below-elbow amputation with pedicle flap coverage, Inter-Clin. Info. Bull. **12**(7):5-9, 1973.
12. Kay, H. W., and Fishman, S.: 1018 children with skeletal limb deficiencies, New York, March, 1967, New York University Post-Graduate Medical School, Prosthetic and Orthotics.
13. Koepke, G. H., Giacinto, J. P., and McUmber, R. A.: Silicone gel below-knee amputation prostheses, U. Mich. Med. Center J. **36:**188-189, 1970.
14. Lambert, C. N.: Amputation surgery in the child, Surg. Clin. North Am. **3**(2):473-482, 1972.
15. Lambert, C. N.: Etiology. In Aitken, G., editor: The child with an acquired amputation, Washington, D.C., 1972, National Academy of Sciences.
16. Meyer, L. C., and Sauer, B. W.: The use of porous high-density polyethelyne caps in the prevention of appositional bone growth in the juvenile amputee: a preliminary report, Inter-Clin. Info. Bull. **14**(9-10):1-4, Sept.-Oct., 1975.
17. Romano, R. L., and Burgess, E. M.: Extremity growth and overgrowth following amputation in children, Inter-Clin. Info. Bull. **5**(4):11-12, Jan., 1966.
18. Snelson, R.: Use of transparent sockets in limb prosthetics, Orthot. Prosthet. **27:**3, Sept., 1973.
19. Swanson, A. B.: The Krukenberg procedure in the juvenile amputee, J. Bone Joint Surg. **46A:**1540-1548, 1962.
20. Swanson, A. B.: Bone overgrowth in the juvenile amputee and its control by the use of silicone rubber implants, Inter-Clin. Info. Bull. **8**(5):9-16, Feb., 1969.
21. Swanson, A. B.: Silicone-rubber implants to control the overgrowth phenomenon in the juvenile amputee, Inter-Clin. Info. Bull. **11**(9):5-8, June, 1972.
22. Von Soal, G.: Epiphysiodesis combined with amputation, J. Bone Joint Surg. **21:**442-443, 1939.
23. Wilson, L. A., Lyquist, E., and Radcliffe, C. W.: Air-cushion socket for patellar-tendon-bearing below-knee prostheses, Bull. Prosthet. Res. **10:**5-34, Fall, 1968.

CHAPTER 40

Prosthetic management

Section I

Upper limb prosthetic management

RAYMOND J. PELLICORE
ROBERT E. TOOMS

In formulating a prescription for prostheses for the child amputee, whether the amputation is congenital or acquired, function is of primary importance but cannot be completely separated from cosmesis. Family acceptance is essential to successful prosthetic wear and function. This is not to say that a prosthesis with a functional hand should be prescribed for a child too young to use it, just to satisfy the psychological needs of the parents. However, thorough explanation and constant reinforcement is necessary to obtain the full cooperation of the parents and thus attain success in fitting young children with prostheses.

Early fitting[7] of the congenital upper limb-deficient child has now become the accepted norm. Some centers adhere to the theory of waiting for adequate and independent sitting balance before fitting. They theorize that useful function is difficult to obtain in other than a sitting posture. However, a 3-month-old child can execute useful gross grasp in a supine position. In addition, an upper limb prosthesis helps to equalize limb lengths, provide aid in crawling, and assist these young children to a sitting position. Therefore fitting at approximately 3 months of age with a passive prosthesis has gained wide acceptance.

Many advantages have accrued from this philosophy of early fitting.[1] The child develops (1) prosthetic tolerance, (2) equalization of limb lengths, (3) a two-handed pattern of activity (bimanual), and (4) more acceptance of the prosthesis as an integral part of the body (self-image).

The proximal and distal limb deficiencies are the most difficult amputation levels to restore to adequate function with present day prostheses. In partial hand deficiencies, up to and including wrist disarticulation, the trade-off of a sensate gross grasp end organ for an insensate prehension device may result in rejection of the prosthesis. With the more proximal levels of amputation, the prostheses are cumbersome and heavy and provide little function because of limited and inadequate motor sources.

Following are six basic prosthetic systems required for the management of the upper limb amputee with congenital or acquired amputations; in addition to these, there are many congenital anomalies that require custom-made nonstandard prostheses:

1. Partial hand restoration
   A. Opposition post
   B. Cosmetic hand
2. Wrist disarticulation prosthesis
3. Below-elbow prosthesis
4. Elbow disarticulation prosthesis
5. Above-elbow prosthesis
6. Shoulder disarticulation prosthesis

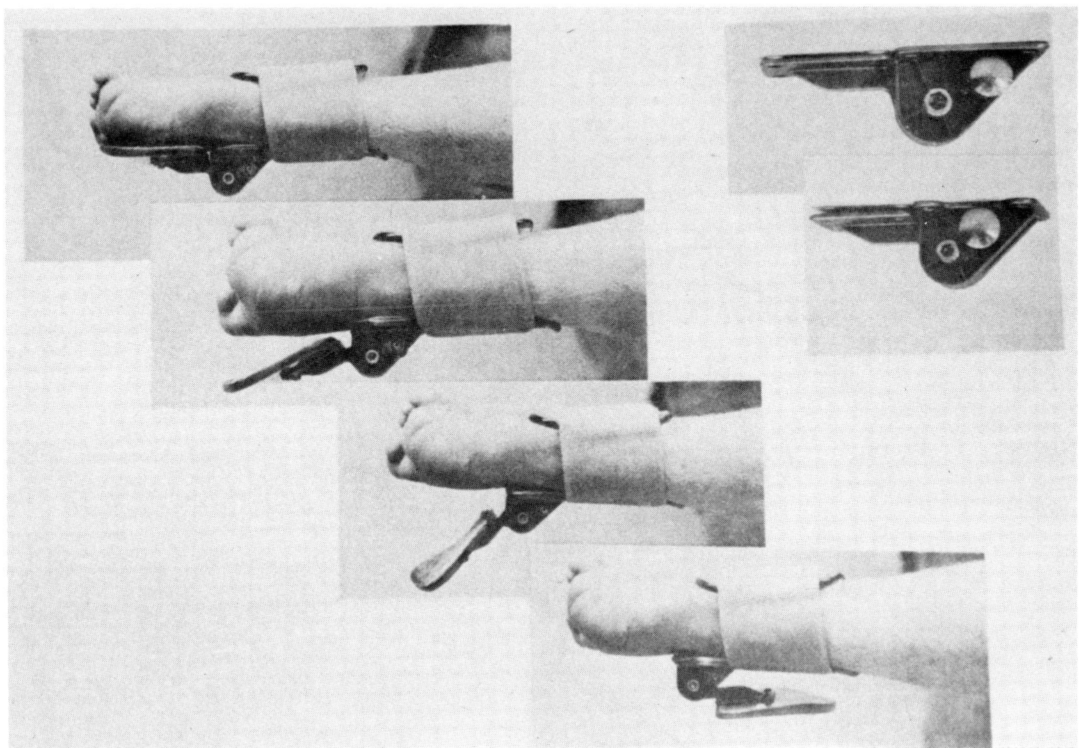

Fig. 40-1. CAPP opposition post, from fully closed, *top*, to folded away, *bottom*.

TERMINAL DEVICES

1. *Opposition post*[3] (Fig. 40-1). The CAPP multiposition opposition post consists of a plastic cuff and projecting post that are hinged at the wrist. The post can be manually locked in any of three positions in relation to the palm to hold different sized objects. It can also be folded against the forearm to permit free use of the exposed stump.

2. *Plastic mitten* (Fig. 40-2). The plastic mitten is used in infants as a passive terminal device for gross grasp and as an aid in turning over and crawling. It can withstand the rigors of this treatment. A plastic passive hand with separate fingers has been developed. This poses the danger of being chewed off and swallowed or having the child choke on a broken finger.

3. *Plastisol-covered hook* (Fig. 40-3). The plastisol-covered hook provides protection from the bare metal and allows the prehension of a voluntary opening hook. As the child grows, this terminal device may be replaced with appropriate sized neoprene-lined hooks.

4. *CAPP terminal device*[5] (Fig. 40-4). An alternative to the 10P or 10X hook that cosmetically seems to be an improvement has been developed at CAPP. It is a voluntary opening device that opens to 6.6 cm (2⅝ inches), with a spring for passive closing. The springs range from size 0 to 4 and provide a pinch force of 0.23 to 0.9 kg (½ to 2 pounds) respectively. These terminal devices can usually be used up to 6 years of age.

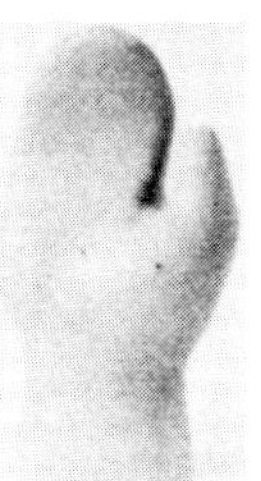

Fig. 40-2. Plastic mitten, 5.6 cm (2¼ inch) long, 56 g (2 ounces), for child 6 to 12 months.

5. *Functional hands* (Fig. 40-5). These hands were available in sizes small enough to be used by toddlers of 2 to 3 years of age and should be made available again. The weight 224 to 280 g (8 to 10 ounces) was excessive for these small children to manage. Prehension with these hands was less than ideal. The gloves were fragile, easily stained, expensive, and therefore impractical.

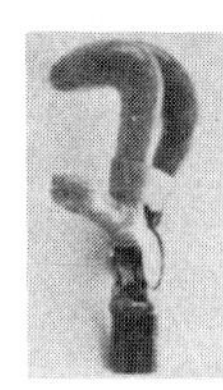

12P
Plastisol-covered fingers
7 cm (2¾ inches) long
56 g (2 ounces), steel
1-4 years

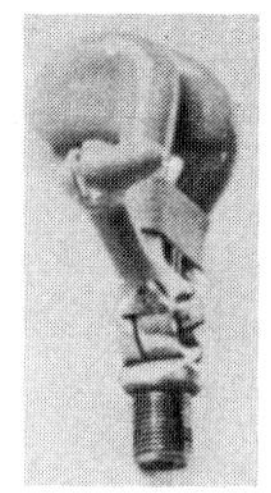

10AW
Plastisol wafer
8.6 cm (3½ inches) long
112 g (4 ounces), aluminum
2-4 years

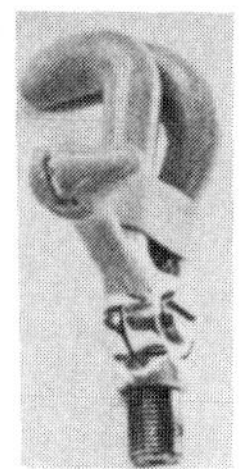

10P
Plastisol-covered fingers
8.6 cm (3½ inches) long
84 g (3 ounces), aluminum
3-6 years

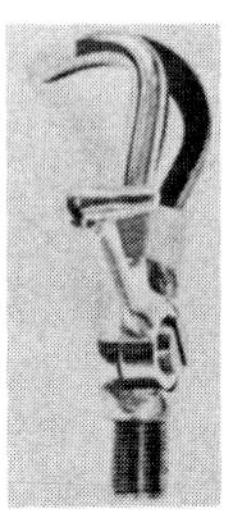

10X
Neoprene-lined fingers
8.4 cm (3⅜ inches) long
56 g (2 ounces), aluminum
3-6 years

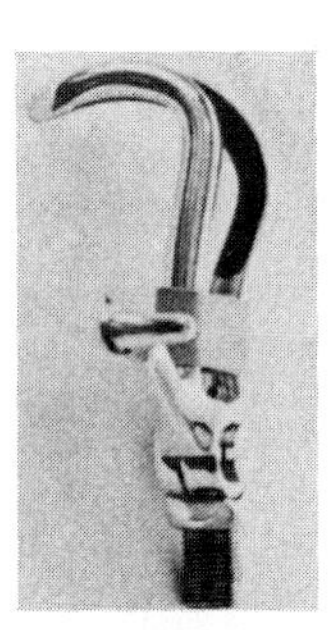

99X
Neoprene-lined fingers
10 cm (4 inches) long
65.3 g (2⅓ ounces), aluminum
6-10 years

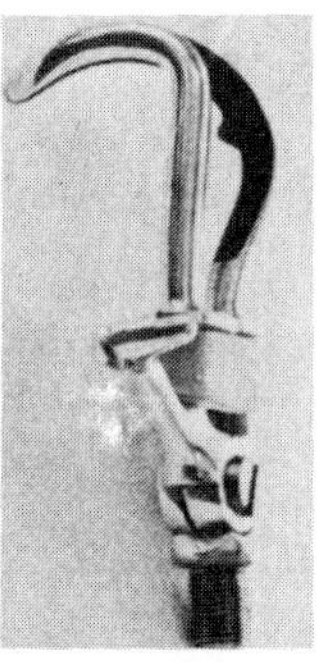

88X
Neoprene-lined fingers
10.9 cm (4⅜ inches) long
84 g (3 ounces), aluminum
10-14 years

Fig. 40-3. Available terminal devices in children's sizes.

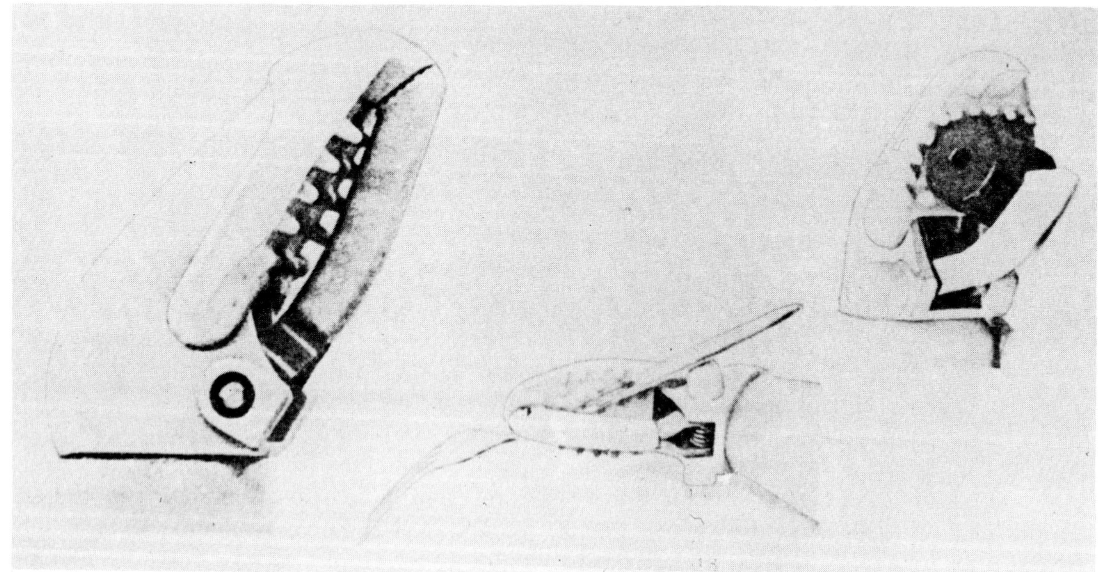

Range of thumb opening, 6.6 cm (2⅝ inches)
Height (not including stud), 7.3 cm (2$\frac{15}{16}$ inches)

Fig. 40-4. CAPP terminal device.

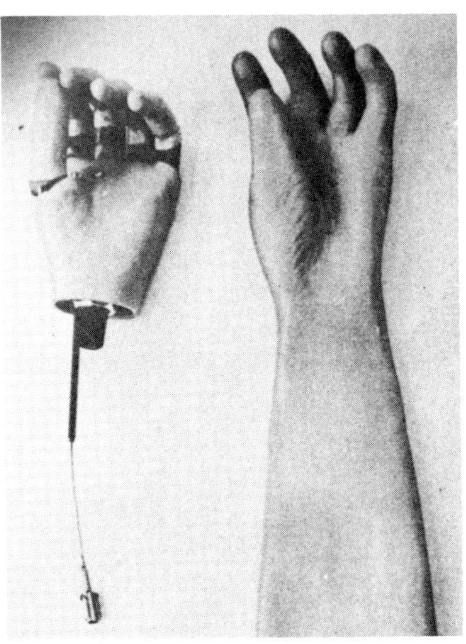

Robin-aids mechanical hand
7.8 cm (4⅛ inches) long
Hand, 226.8 g (8.1 ounces)
Glove, 56 g (2 ounces)
Size 6 and up

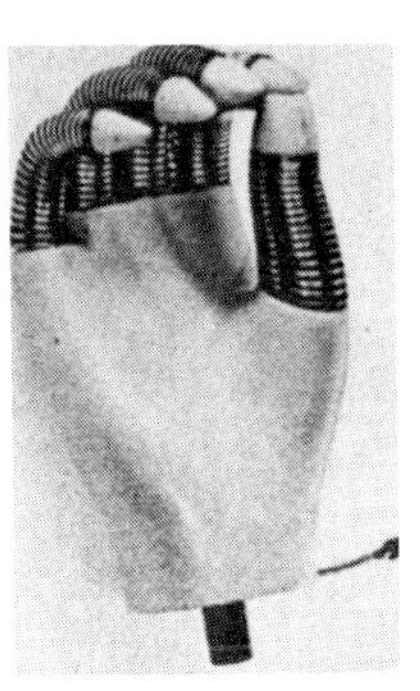

Becker mechanical hand
13 cm (5¼ inches) long
322 g (11½ ounces)
Size 6½ and up

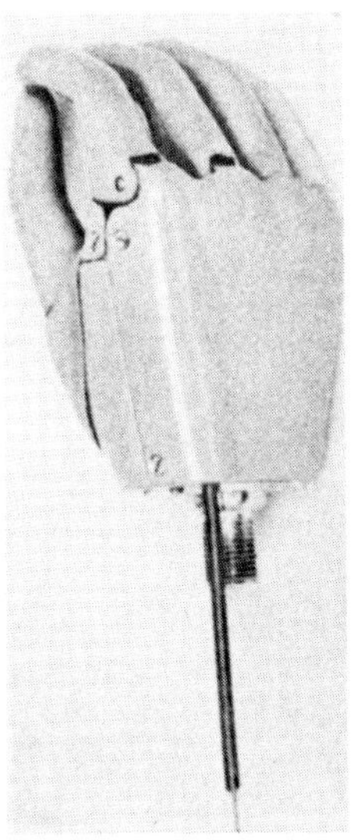

Dorrance hand
Model 1 (size 6½), 10 cm (4 inches) long with fairing; 196 g (7 ounces)
Model 2 (size 7), 10 cm (4 inches) long; 224 g (8 ounces)
Model 3 (size 7), 11.25 cm (4½ inches) long; 336 g (12 ounces)
Glove, 56 g (2 ounces)

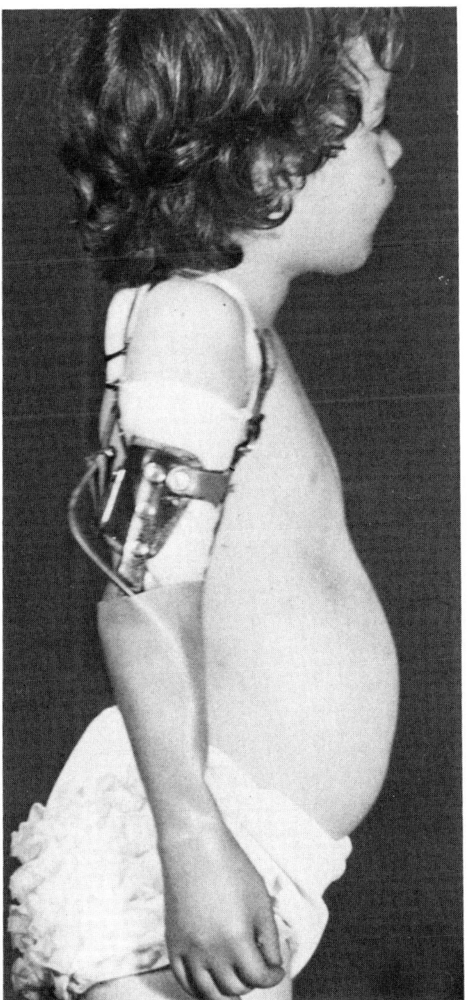

Fig. 40-5. Functional hands.

A

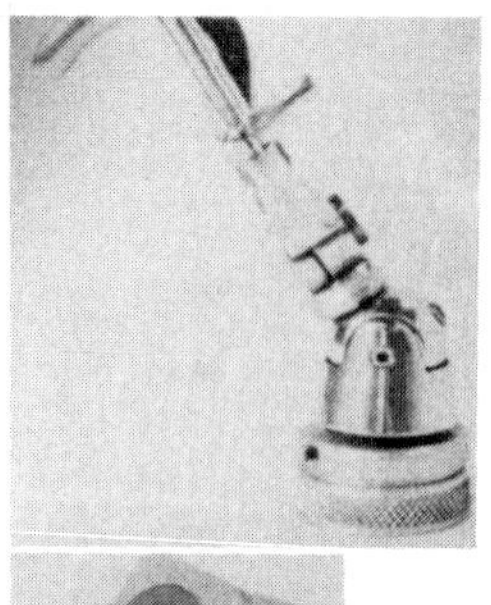

Wrist flexion unit
Makes arm 2.8 cm ($1\frac{1}{8}$ inch) longer
39.2 g (1.4 ounces)
Two positions: straight and 35 degrees

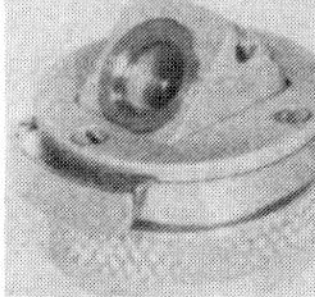

Wrist flexion unit
Child size, 3.7 cm ($1\frac{1}{2}$ inch) outside diameter
Medium size, 4.3 cm ($1\frac{3}{4}$ inch) outside diameter

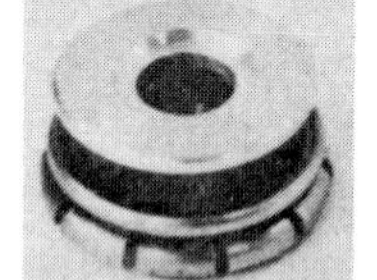

Constant friction wrist for long stumps of
steel, 3.4 cm ($1\frac{3}{8}$ inch) outside diameter

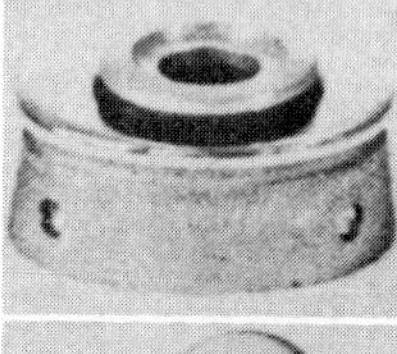

Oval constant friction wrist of aluminum,
4.7 × 4.3 cm ($1\frac{7}{8} \times 1\frac{3}{8}$ inches)

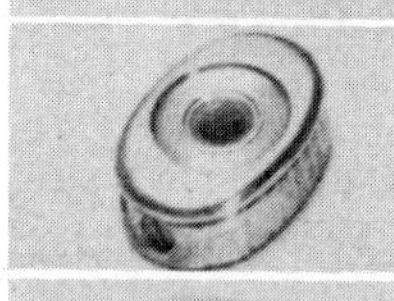

Oval constant friction wrist with nylon threads of
4.7 × 3.8-cm ($1\frac{7}{8} \times 1\frac{1}{2}$-inch) aluminum

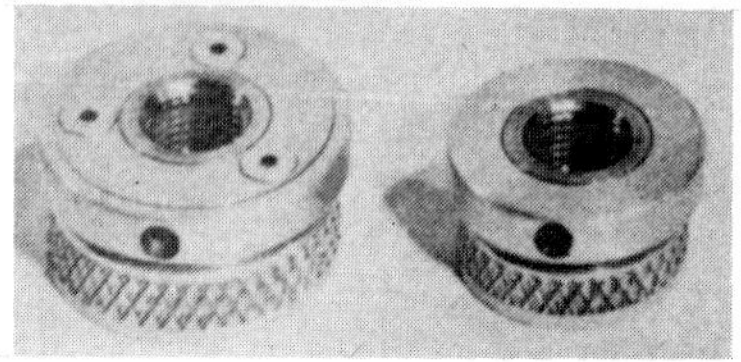

Round constant friction wrist with
Super-Oilite threaded metal insert
Child size, 1.2 cm ($1\frac{3}{16}$ inch) outside diameter
Medium size, 1.4 cm ($1\frac{3}{8}$ inch) outside diameter

B

Fig. 40-6. A, Wrist units. **B,** CAPP terminal device provides wrist flexion by built-in adduction.

WRIST UNITS

A variety of wrist units are shown in Fig. 40-6. Constant friction wrist units are the only types used for children. These are available in round or oval contours. A wrist flexion unit, to adduct the terminal device 30 degrees, is useful for the bilateral amputee. The CAPP terminal device provides wrist flexion through a built-in adduction of 30 degrees.

ELBOW UNITS

1. *Flexible elbow joints* (Fig. 40-7). A flexible metal unit is available, but leather or Dacron tape as hinges are more commonly used. These materials are flexible, wear well, and are easily replaced when worn out. The degree of stability can be varied by the points of attachment to the socket (and triceps pad).

2. *Rigid elbow units* (Fig. 40-8). Rigid elbow units are used in shorter below-elbow stumps, mainly for older boys who participate in extremely strenuous activity.

3. *Polycentric elbow units* (Fig. 40-9). Theoretically, the polycentric elbow joint is advantageous in short, fat, below-elbow stumps because it "circumvents" the piling up of fat in flexion. Practically, it is rarely used for children.

4. *Step-up hinges* (Fig. 40-10). In those rare instances when adequate flexion cannot be accomplished by socket design, and it is necessary for the terminal device to reach mouth level, the

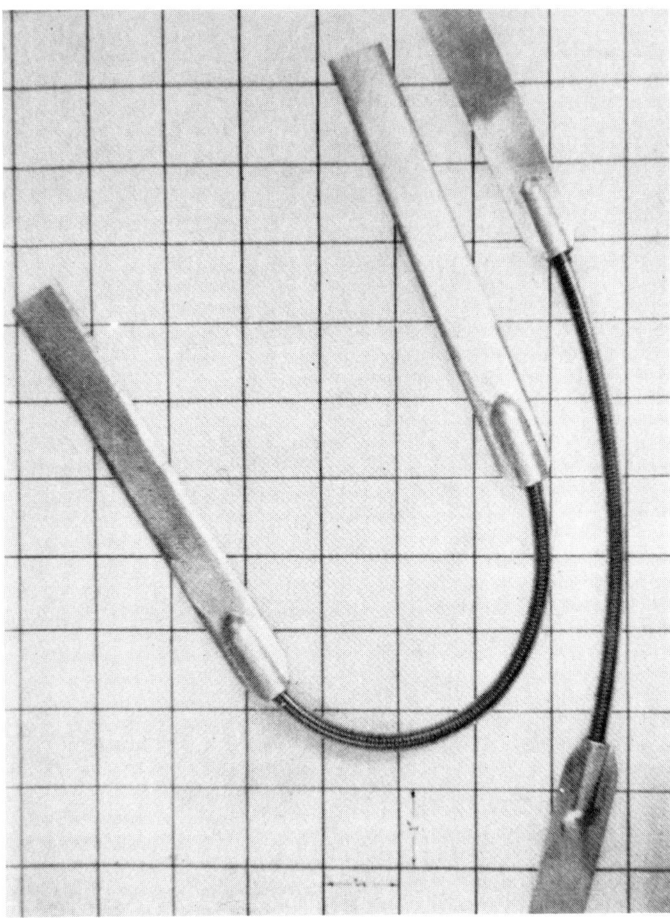

Fig. 40-7. Flexible elbow joints.

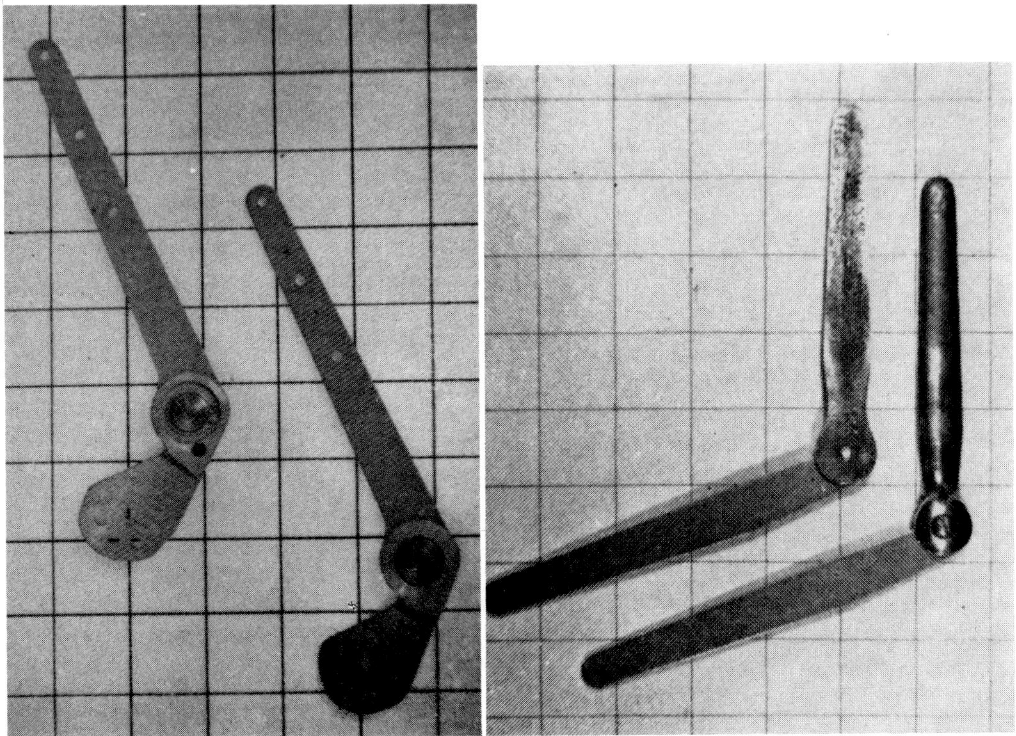

Fig. 40-8. Rigid elbow units.

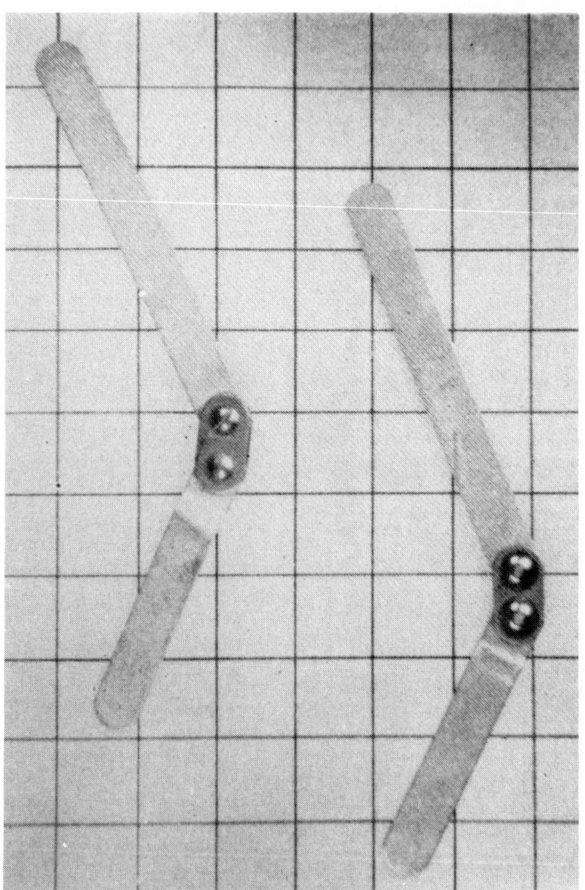

Fig. 40-9. Polycentric elbow units.

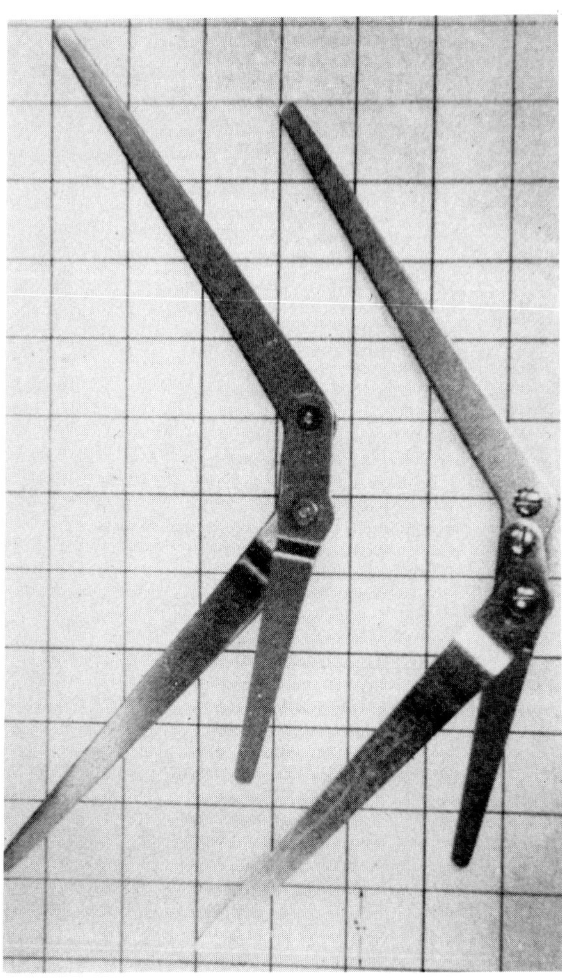

Fig. 40-10. Step-up hinges.

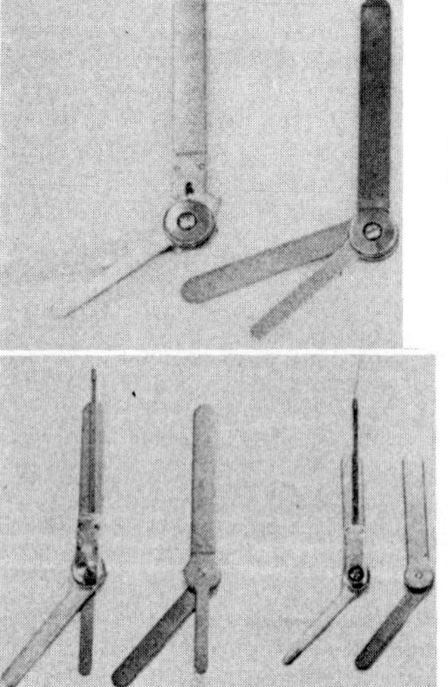

Stump-activated below elbow locking hinge of steel and aluminum
Medium size, head 1.9 cm (3/4 inch) thick, 1.1 cm (1 1/16 inch) diameter

Outside locking hinge, elbow disarticulation of steel and aluminum
Small-locking side, 1.1 cm (7/16 inch) with five positions
Medium-locking side, 1.3 cm (1 1/2 inch) with seven positions

Fig. 40-11. Stump-activated locking hinge, outside locking elbow.

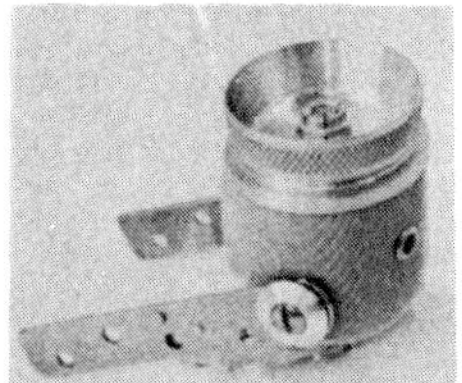

Friction lock elbow with friction turntable, 5 cm (2 inch) outside diameter

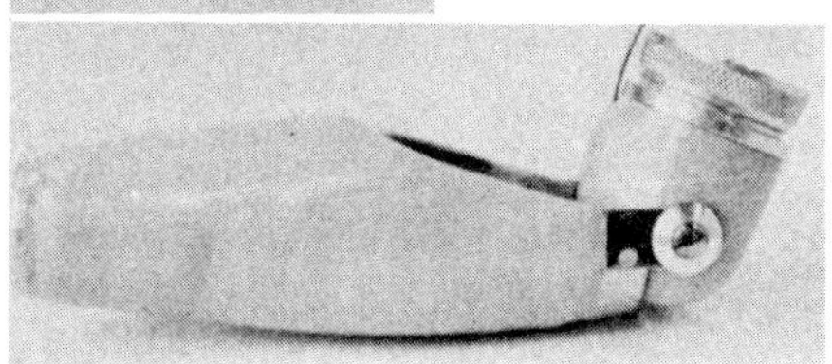

Above elbow setup with turntable

Fig. 40-11, cont'd. Positive locking elbow with turntable.

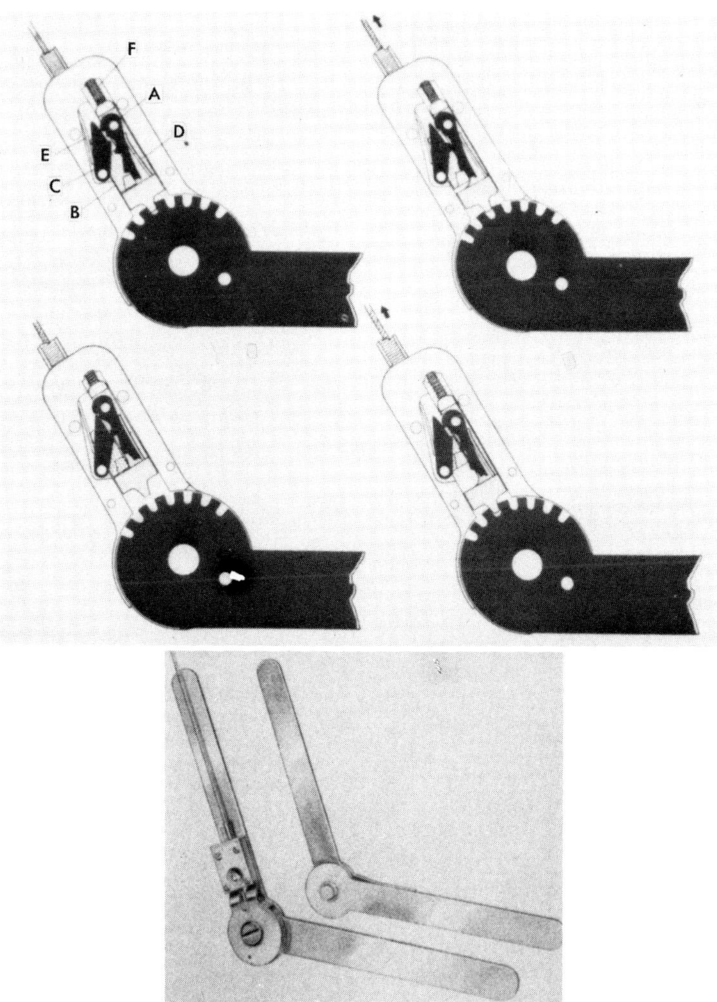

Fig. 40-12. Outside locking elbow. *A* to *F*, locking mechanism for seven-slot gear. (From Manual of upper extremity prosthetics, ed. 2, Los Angeles, 1956, University of California Department of Engineering.)

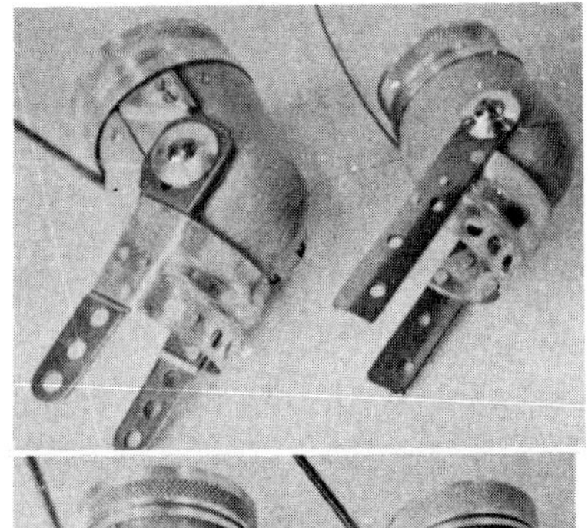

Hosmer positive locking elbows
Child size, 5 cm (2 inch) outside diameter
Medium size, 5.9 cm (2⅜ inch) outside diameter
Eleven locking positions

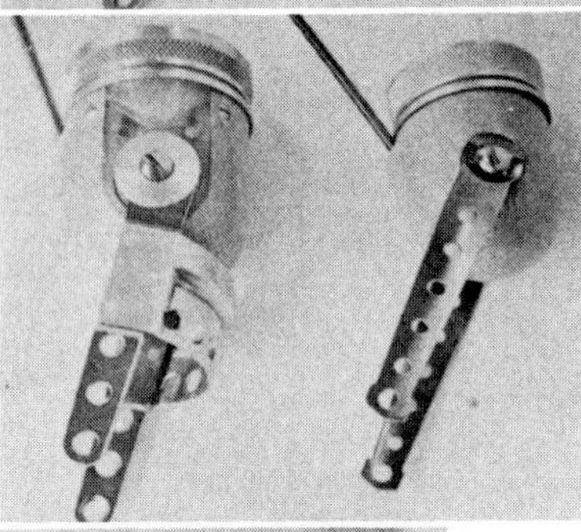

Sierra positive locking elbows
Child size, 5 cm (2 inch) outside diameter
Medium size, 5.9 cm (2⅜ inch) outside diameter
Eleven locking positions

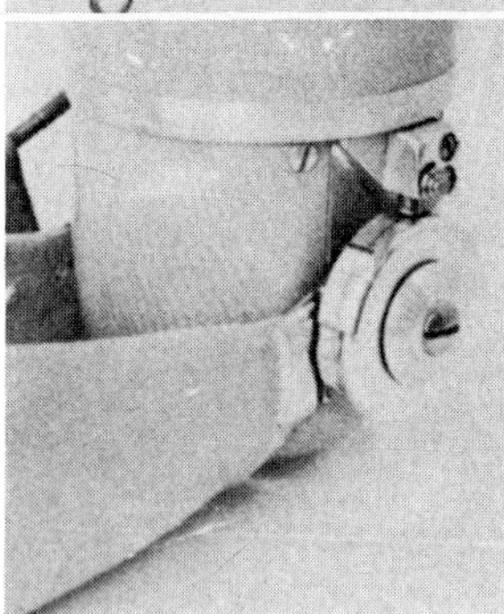

Spring lift assist for medium size
or adult elbows only

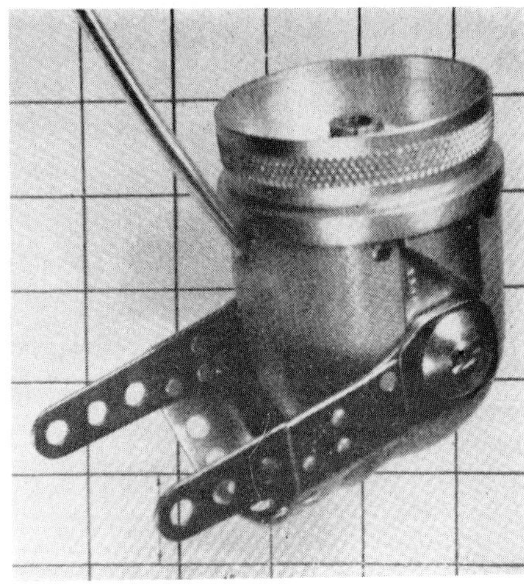

Fig. 40-13. Positive locking elbow with turntable.

step-up hinge may supply the range of motion needed. It does this at the expense of lift strength.

5. *Stump-activated locking hinge* (Fig. 40-11). The stump-activated locking hinge is useful in extremely short below-elbow stumps that cannot effectively be fitted as a below-elbow amputation level. This extremely short stump is used to activate the elbow lock.

6. *Outside locking elbow* (Fig. 40-12). The outside locking elbow is used for long above-elbow and elbow disarticulation prostheses to prevent excessive socket length. It has seven locking positions.

7. *Positive locking elbow with turntable* (Fig. 40-13). Positive locking elbows with a turntable are commonly used in shorter above-elbow levels. Eleven locking positions are available.

SHOULDER JOINTS

1. *Friction abduction unit* (Fig. 40-14). The friction abduction unit is seldom used, since only abduction of the prosthesis is possible.

2. *Shoulder abduction and humeral flexion joint.* This unit is used mainly in small children with their first shoulder prosthesis.

3. *Universal joints.* Up to six different motions are available on some universal joints—flexion, extension, abduction, adduction, and external

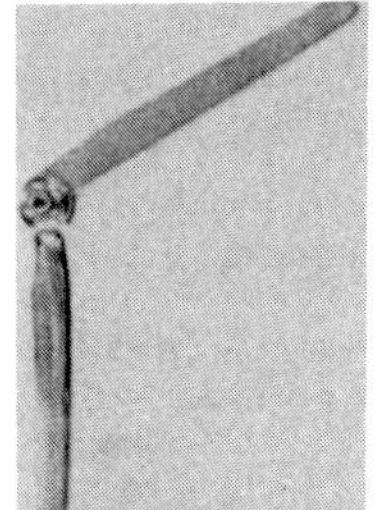

Shoulder abduction joint, head 1.9 cm (3/4 inch) diameter, 0.9 cm (3/8 inch) thick

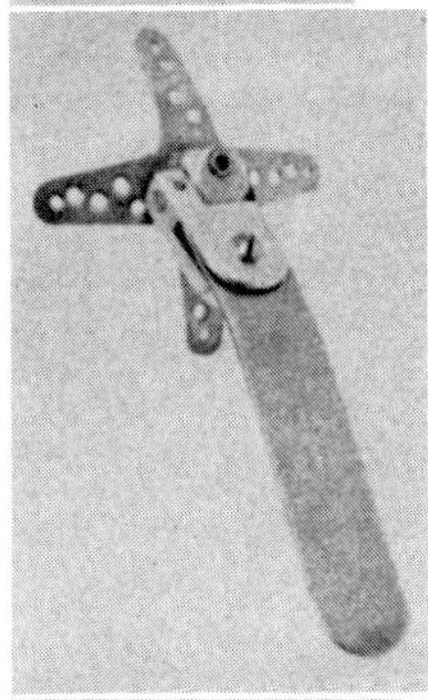

Shoulder abduction and humeral flexion joint

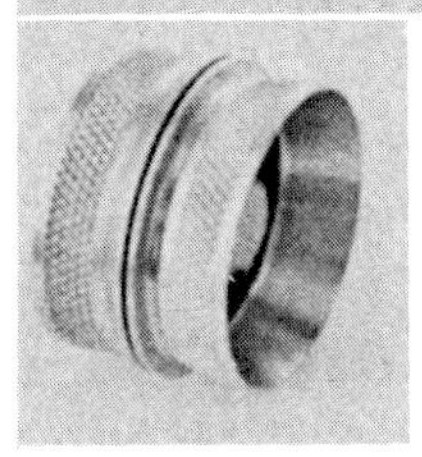

Hosmer shoulder bulkheads
Small, 5 cm (2 inch) outside diameter, 3.1 cm (1 1/4 inch) thick
Medium, 5.9 cm (2 3/8 inch) outside diameter, 4.1 cm (1 5/8 inch) thick

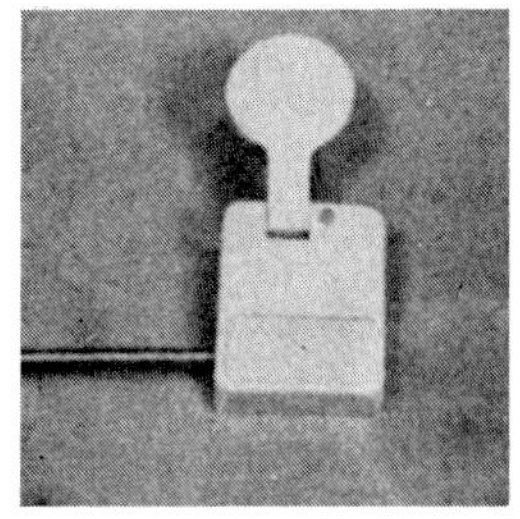

Nudge control

Fig. 40-14. Shoulder units and nudge control for elbow lock.

and internal rotation. This is the most desirable unit available and should be prescribed whenever the size of the child permits its usage.

4. *CAPP two-way shoulder joints* (Fig. 40-15). This gives the patient a narrow, cosmetic shoulder line along with reliable friction control; it is fitted here with Ontario Crippled Childrens Center (OCCC) electric elbows and conventional shoulder disarticulation sockets.

SOCKETS

Sockets in children, with few exceptions, are fabricated from plastic laminate. There is some use of other material such as polypropylene. The advantages of plastic laminate over formerly used materials include a high strength to weight ratio, low raw material cost, and ease in cleaning.

PARTIAL HAND RESTORATION

Opposition post

Children with a single digit or a portion of a hand, without ability for grasping, can be aided with an opposition post (Fig. 40-16). This may be

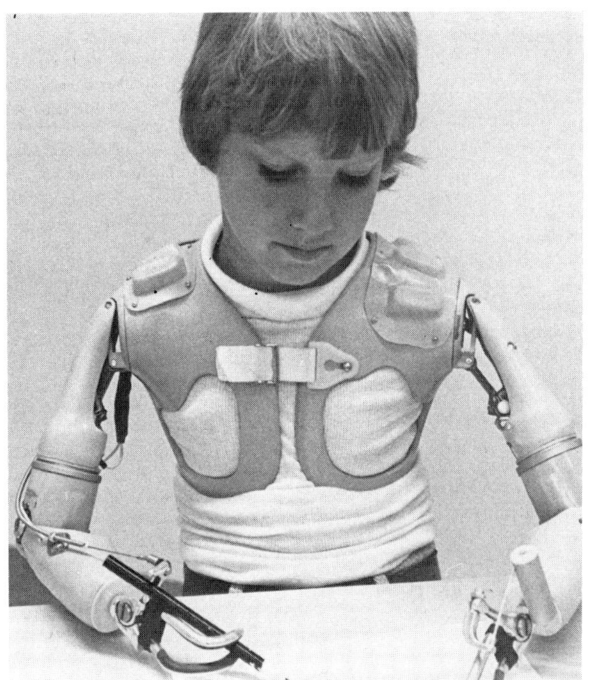

Fig. 40-15. CAPP two-way shoulder joint.

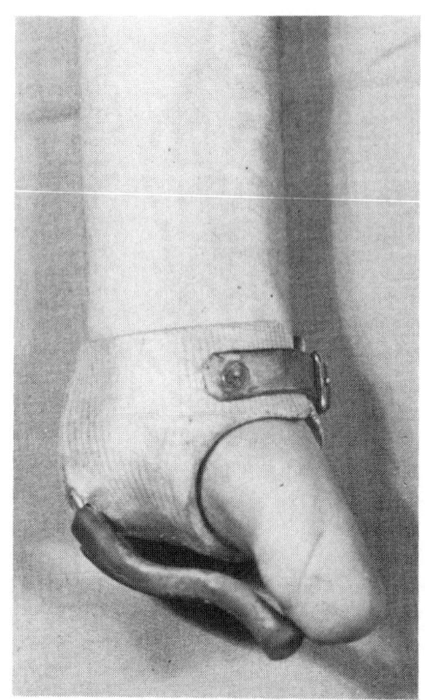

Fig. 40-16. Opposition post.

fabricated from thermoplastic material or metal and attached by a forearm cuff. A highly sophisticated prefabricated variable opening opposition post was developed by CAPP and is available commercially. These devices are of limited use in the very young child. They are usually prescribed for older children, as a gross grasping device for the nondominant side. Other adaptive devices for activities of daily living may be fabricated on an individual basis.

Cosmetic hand

In the older child (at or after puberty) with a hand deficiency, when social awareness takes precedence over the asexual activities of early age, a demand for a cosmetic prosthesis (Fig. 40-17) is frequently made. Although cosmetic hands are heavy, they are aesthetically desirable and sometimes necessary for these children. Experience has shown that cosmetic hands are worn with a degree of regularity for the first month, then with decreasing frequency for the next 3 to 4 months. We have found them worthwhile, for no matter how short a time, to help these children

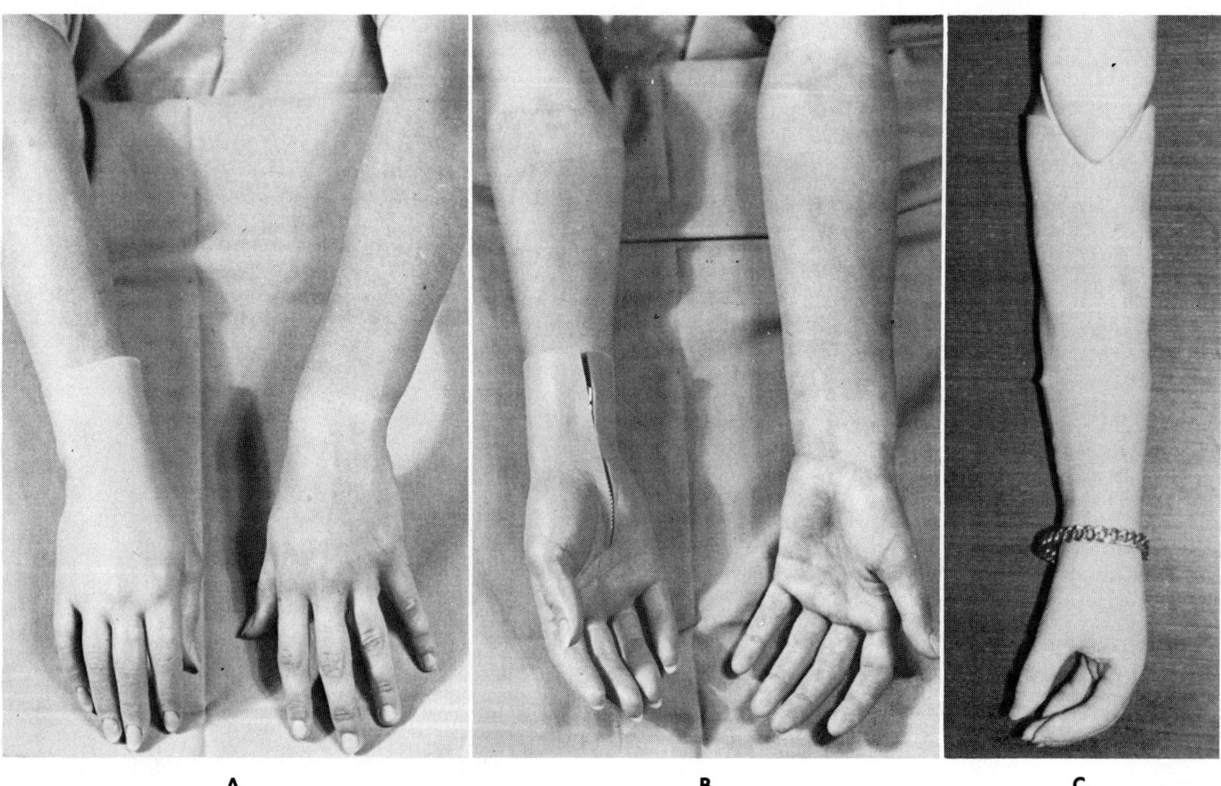

Fig. 40-17. Cosmetic prostheses. **A** and **B**, Cosmetic (nonfunctional) hands. **C**, Myoelectric below-elbow prosthesis with functional hand.

during this important and often traumatic period of growth and development.

WRIST DISARTICULATION PROSTHESIS

Shortly after birth it is extremely difficult to absolutely distinguish between a complete acheiria and a deficiency in which two or more carpal bones are present. Since these carpal bones do not calcify before 6 to 8 months of age, early x-ray examinations are of little value. This is of small importance in the 3-month-old child, but becomes more important later. The child with carpal bones seldom develops shortening of the limb, and if shortening does occur, it is minimal. Atrophy and shortening invariably occur in the wrist disarticulation deficiency (complete transverse carpal deficiency).

Both may be fitted with a below-elbow prosthesis. The prescription should include a plastic laminate socket with a passive mitten terminal device (Fig. 40-18), with or without a wrist unit, flexible elbow hinges, and a triceps pad. The prosthesis is suspended with an inverted Y strap and figure-of-eight harness. For infants, it is preferable to sew the cross of the harness (Fig. 40-19) rather than use a Northwestern University ring. The flexible hinges should be attached distally on the forearm to allow a maximum amount of flexibility, since stability is not a problem in these long residual limbs.

Unlike the screwdriver-shaped adult forearm, the child has a round and flabby contour, so little of the rotation is transmitted to the prosthesis. To prolong the life of the prosthesis, the original fitting should be made with one or two heavy nylon socks. Removal, or use of thinner socks, will then accommodate for the child's growth. Preflexion of the socket is unnecessary, since full elbow motion is present and can be retained when the socket is properly fabricated with low anterior trim lines.

When the child reaches 12 to 14 months of age the passive mitten is replaced with a functional terminal device, either a 10P or 12P (plastisol covered) hook (Fig. 40-20) or a CAPP terminal device (Fig. 40-21). Activation of the terminal device[8] is optional at this stage. If the terminal device is activated at this time, training may be

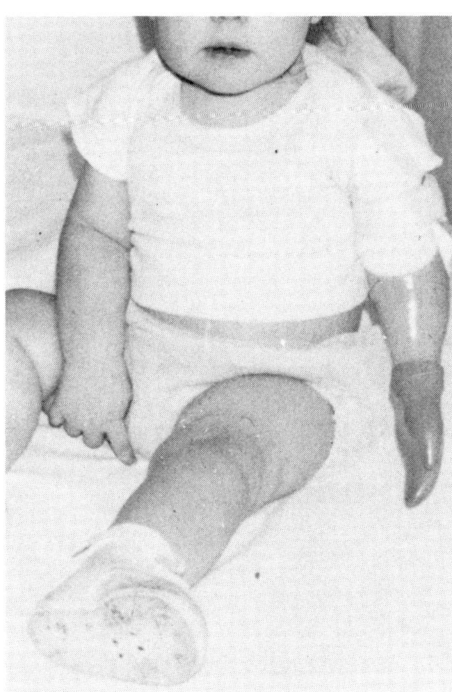

Fig. 40-18. Below-elbow prosthesis passive plastic mitten terminal device.

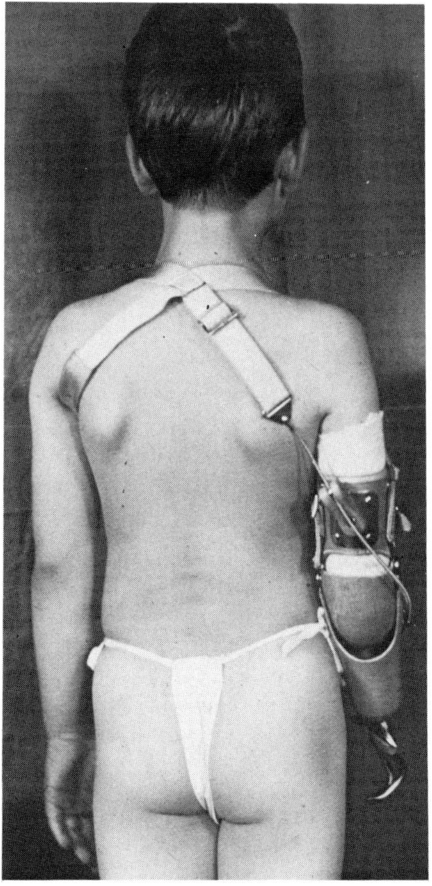

Fig. 40-19. Cross harness sewn. Buckle permits adjustment of cable tension.

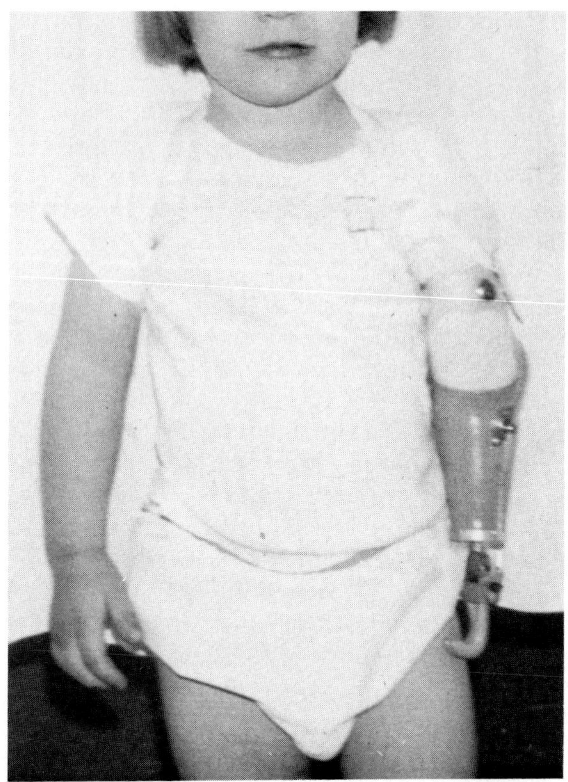

Fig. 40-20. Below-elbow prosthesis. Note anterior strap to retain harness and plastisol-covered terminal device.

postponed until the child is about 18 months of age. The attention span and the physiological capabilities of the child are not adequate for training until this age. Some children may acquire functional use by trial and error.

The CAPP terminal device is useful only to about 6 years of age. At about this age, the prescription should be for a hook or hand. As the child grows, the terminal device prescription is changed for appropriate size.

When carpal bones are present and the child is 3 years or more, an open-end German-type socket (Fig. 40-22) may be used. With the open-end socket, the child has the use of a hook for prehension and yet retains the sensation of the distal stump protruding through the open end of the socket. Experience has shown that most children gain very little by this extra freedom, mobility, and sensation. The noncosmetic appearance of the socket and the confusion to the child resulting from the two use options may be contraindications to this prescription.

The majority of young children with wrist disarticulations, with or without carpal bones, are excellent wearers. However, by puberty many boys may reject their protheses. These children are extremely adaptable and can perform many delicate functions with their residual limbs. The rejection rate by girls at the same age is much

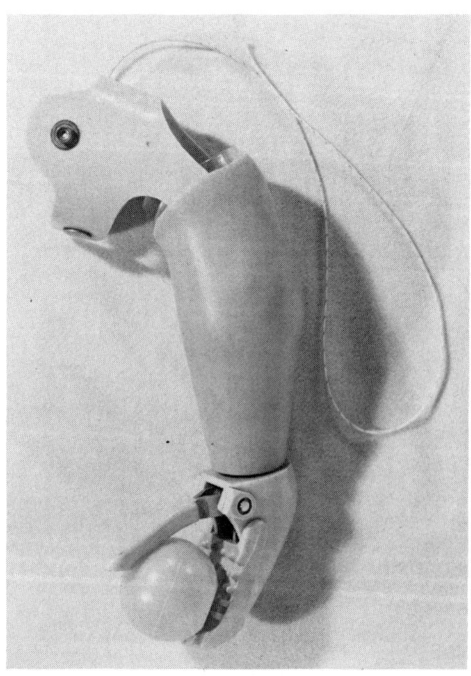

Fig. 40-21. CAPP terminal device on below-elbow prosthesis.

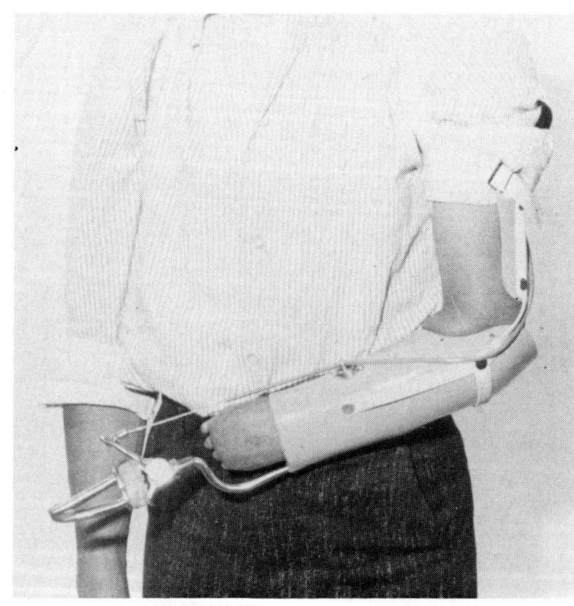

Fig. 40-22. Open-end German-type socket used as prosthesis for patient with functional wrist joint. This preserves tactile sensation.

less, and they usually return as wearers several years after rejecting their prostheses. This phenomenon of rejection, with later acceptance, also holds true for children with below-elbow levels of amputation.

BELOW-ELBOW PROSTHESIS

The prescription for the child with a below-elbow amputation or deficiency should consist of a plastic laminate socket, friction wrist, and appropriate terminal device. Suspension may be attained through elbow hinges and a triceps pad, plus a Y strap off a figure-of-eight harness. Socket prescriptions are of three major types:

1. Standard, or preflexed, socket
2. Split socket
3. Muenster (Hepp-Kuhn) socket

STANDARD, OR PREFLEXED, SOCKET

The standard, or preflexed, socket is a double-wall plastic laminate socket that is fabricated with sufficient preflexion to accommodate for the limited excursion in short, fat bulbous stumps. To obtain better socket interface for good suspension and function in these rounded stumps, the socket has to be fabricated with more proximal trim lines.

SPLIT SOCKET

The split socket (Fig. 40-23) used in the rare bilateral amputee in whom it is necessary for one terminal device to reach the mouth level, and in whom this cannot be accomplished with the standard preflexed fabrication. This prosthesis has the disadvantage of poor cosmesis and loss of lift strength. It is not necessary for the unilateral patient to have the forearm reach mouth level, since the prosthetic side is the assistive limb and not the dominant one. With recent improvement in fabrication techniques and materials it is seldom necessary to prescribe a split socket, since even a 3.8-cm (1½-inch) stump can be satisfactorily fitted with a preflexed socket and still allow an adequate range of elbow flexion.

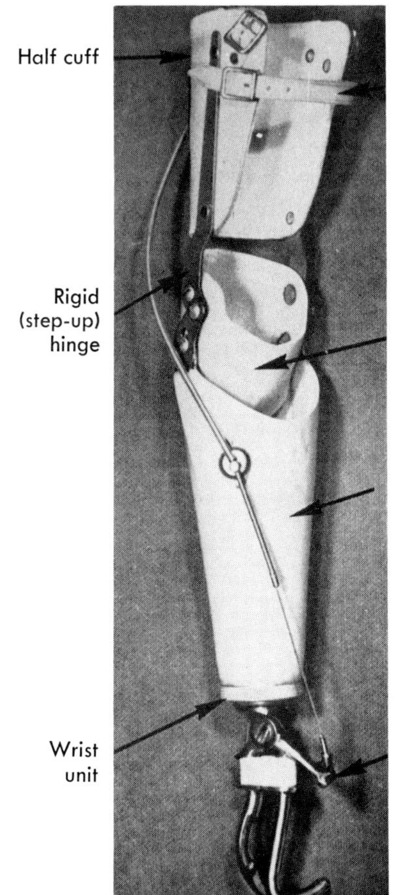

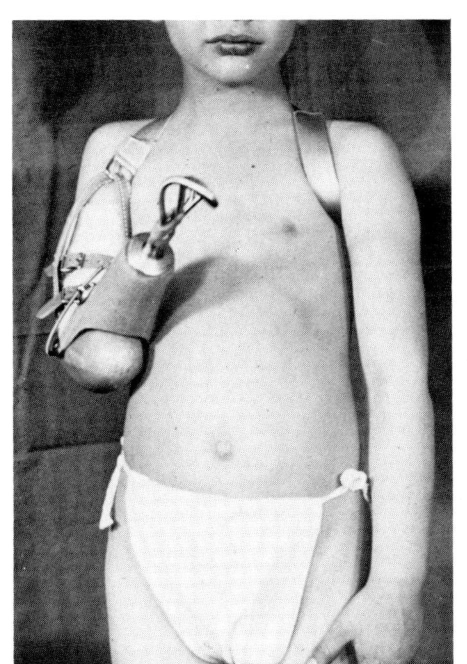

Fig. 40-23. A, Split-socket construction shows in socket and forearm shell connected to upper arm triceps half cuff by step-up hinge. **B,** As stump in socket is flexed, step-up hinge causes forearm to flex at ratio of 2:1. (From Manual of upper extremity prosthetics, ed. 2, Los Angeles, 1956, University of California Department of Engineering.)

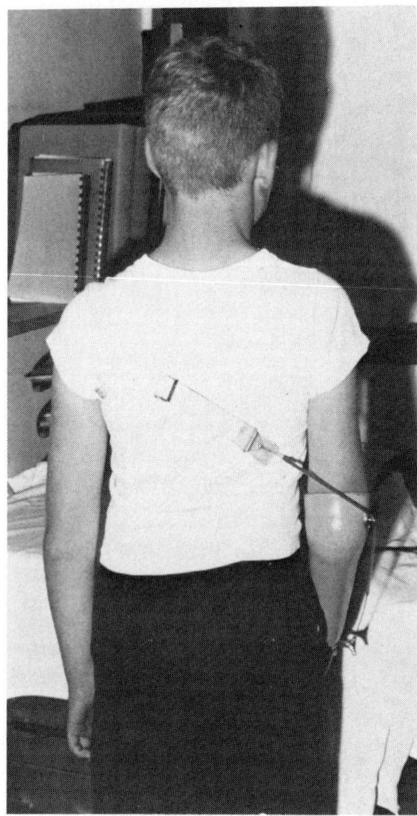

Fig. 40-24. Muenster (Hepp-Kuhn) socket. Note cable is attached to figure-of-nine type harness, since socket is self-suspending.

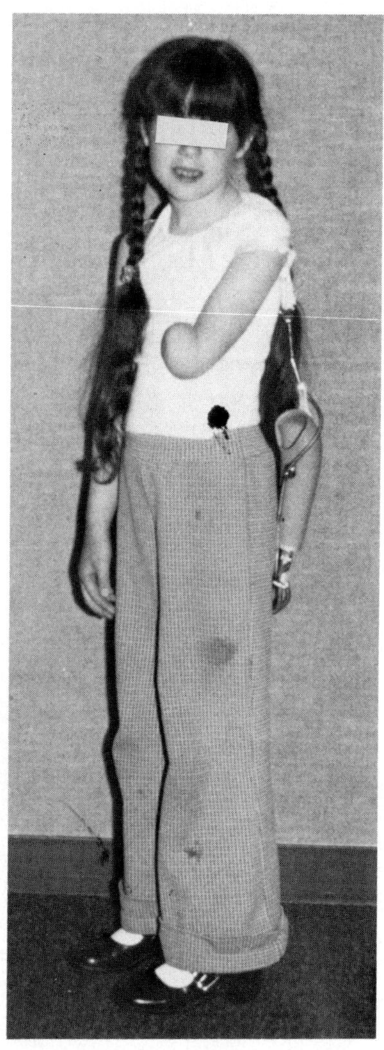

Fig. 40-25. Muenster socket without additional suspension may be used for very short below-elbow stump.

MUENSTER (HEPP-KUHN) SOCKET

The Muenster (Hepp-Kuhn) socket (Fig. 40-24) is fabricated to fit snugly around the olecranon and the epicondyles of the humerus, with counterpressure in the antecubital fossa on the biceps tendon. This becomes a self-suspending socket (Fig. 40-25) and eliminates the need for additional harnessing.

The Muenster socket is contraindicated in very young children for two major reasons: (1) the bulbous stumps of these children deter adequate contouring of the socket and (2) the attention span of the child is so short that it is almost impossible for the prosthetist to accomplish the critical fit needed in this type of socket. Even in the older child the following disadvantages to the Muenster fabrication exist:

1. The range of motion is limited.
2. The intimate fit of the plastic socket becomes uncomfortably hot and moist in warm weather.
3. The critical fit requires expert fabrication and frequent replacement of sockets. This last objection can be partially eliminated by the use of triple lamination. As the child grows, one of the inner laminations can be removed, thus prolonging the life of the prosthesis.
4. Boys who like to carry heavy loads with their prosthesis create an extension force against the olecranon process that may cause a great deal of discomfort.
5. The combination of limited motion and discomfort results in a high incidence of rejection. This is especially true if the child has been a good wearer of a standard preflexed socket.

Billock and Childress[2] of Northwestern University increased the range of elbow motion without sacrificing suspension or stability. This is

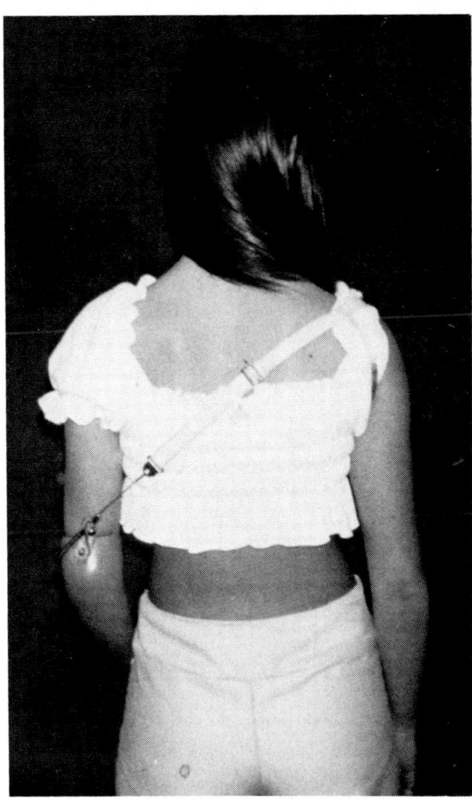

Fig. 40-26. Low take-off of figure-of-nine harness used with Muenster socket.

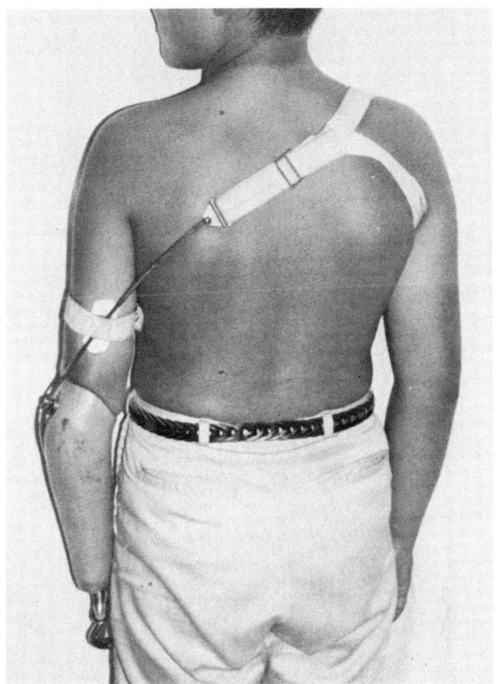

Fig. 40-27. Suspensor about arm to redirect low take-off of cable used with Muenster socket.

accomplished by designing the socket to fit more intimately over the epicondyles and extending the socket more proximally. These higher lateral forces prevent stump withdrawal and permit lower anterior trim lines, eliminating the restriction to elbow flexion.

Since the socket is self-suspending, harnessing for suspension is not necessary. Activation of the terminal device can be accomplished through a single figure-of-nine harness. The single axillary loop from the opposite shoulder results in a low take-off point (Fig. 40-26), which impinges on boy's shirts, but does not affect the loose fitting blouses and sweaters worn by girls. If this becomes a problem, a suspensor can be arranged around the shoulder or arm (Fig. 40-27) of the amputated limb to redirect the activating cable.[9]

ELBOW DISARTICULATION PROSTHESIS

The unilateral elbow disarticulation can be fitted at 3 months of age with a unit arm (Fig. 40-28). The socket is nonarticulated with sufficient preflexion so as to allow two-handed grasp. A figure-of-eight harness with an anterior strap

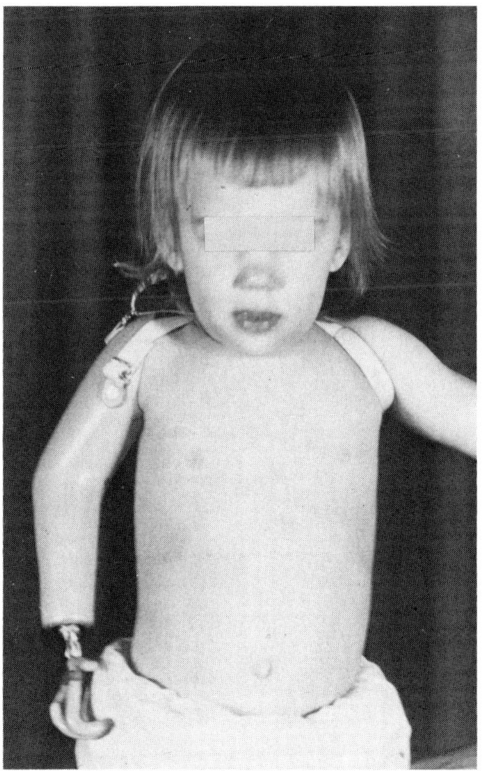

Fig. 40-28. Since this unit arm has no elbow joint, it is used only for infants.

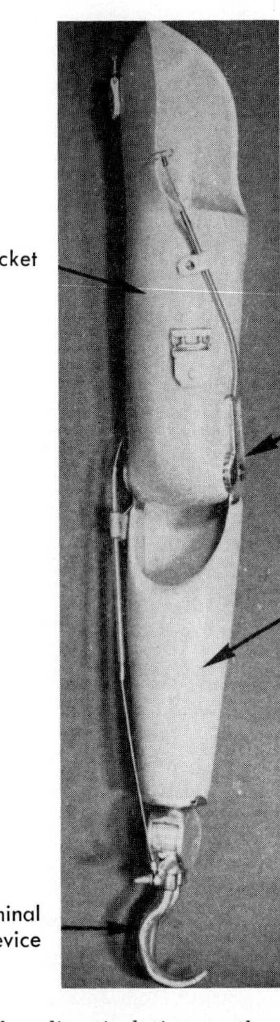

Fig. 40-29. Elbow disarticulation prosthesis. (From Manual of upper extremity prosthetics, ed. 2, Los Angeles, 1956, University of California Department of Engineering.)

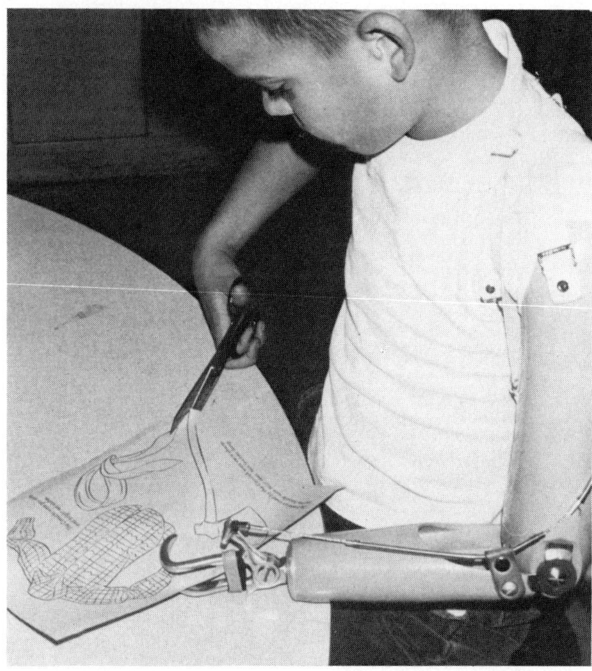

Fig. 40-30. Elbow disarticulation prosthesis with outside locking elbow hinge on medial aspect.

suspends the prosthesis. A plastic mitten passive terminal device completes the unit.

At 14 to 18 months of age, an articulated prosthesis with a passive friction elbow, standard forearm, and 12P hook suspended by a figure-of-eight harness is the prescription of choice. The terminal device may or may not be activated, but training for single-control use is deferred until 18 months of age.

The child, as a general rule, lacks the attention span and neuromuscular development to use a dual control prosthesis until about 36 months of age. At that time a standard elbow disarticulation (Figs. 40-29 and 40-30) prosthesis with dual control is prescribed. The socket is contoured about the condyles for control of rotation and added suspension. This permits low trim lines at the shoulder (Fig. 40-31) and thus allows a greater range of shoulder motion. Suspension is accomplished with a figure-of-eight harness, and the elbow lock is activated with an anterior humeral strap. A friction wrist unit with an appropriate terminal device completes the prosthesis.

Bilateral elbow disarticulation levels can be fitted at an early age in the same sequence as unilateral levels. However, at 3 years of age, only the dominant limb should be fitted with an articulated prosthesis with dual control. As the child becomes proficient in using this prosthesis, the unrelenting desires of the therapists to fit the child bilaterally should be rejected in an unswerving manner. If fitted bilaterally (Fig. 40-32), the child will function admirably, using both prostheses until about 6 years of age. At that time, the new experiences of school and new friends apparently detract from the attention needed for good neuromuscular coordination. Loss of fine coordinated movements and the inability to separate controls, leading to clumsy and frustrating usage may result in a rejection of both prostheses. We would urge all efforts to encourage foot usage and the use of one prosthesis until the child is old enough to demand more.

ABOVE-ELBOW PROSTHESIS

Above-elbow congenital deficiencies with residual limb lengths of greater than 7.5 cm (3 inches)

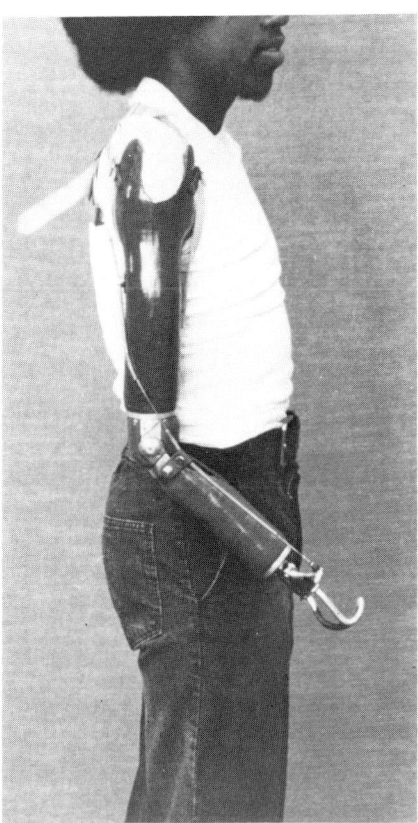

Fig. 40-31. Low trim lines on lateral aspect of socket permit greater abduction of shoulder.

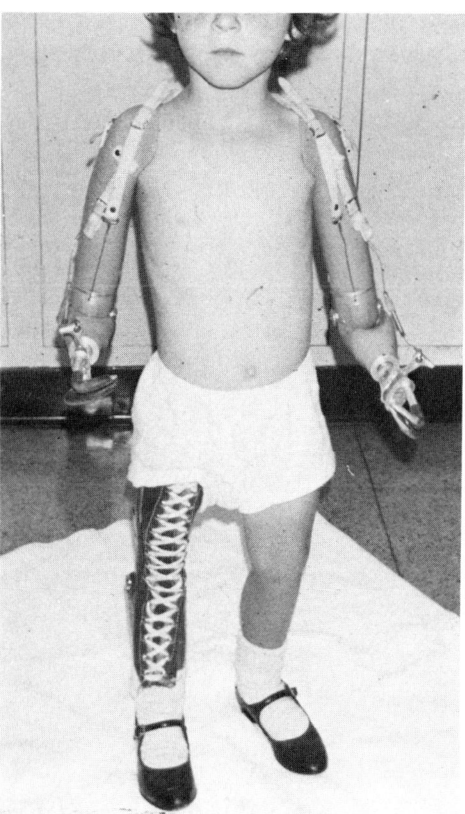

Fig. 40-32. Overgadgeting. Bilateral above-elbow fitting for small child may be effective early, but frustration may lead to later rejection.

distal to the tuberosity can be fitted at 3 months of age. a unit arm with a plastic mitten is used until 14 to 18 months of age, when a prosthesis with a friction elbow and a terminal device with single control can be prescribed.

When the child is 3 years of age, an inside locking elbow (with eleven stops) with a turntable is applied. Because of the loss of rotary stability provided by the condyles in an elbow disarticulation, it is necessary to extend the proximal socket anteriorly and posteriorly to attain this stability. The lateral wall may be cut down considerably for unrestrained abduction movement. Harnessing, suspension, elbow locking, and terminal device function are the same as in elbow disarticulation prostheses.

An electric elbow is available for older children. Present models have several negative aspects. Among these are the high noise level at operation and the slow function they provide for these active children. Breakdown and maintenance are problems when these elbows are used for vigorous activities.

Patients with bilateral above-elbow congenital deficiencies (more common than elbow disarticulation) should follow the program of prosthetic prescription and training as that outlined for the bilateral elbow disarticulation.

When available, foot usage should be encouraged. The child should be fitted with shoes that can be slipped on and off to make the feet available. Socks should not be worn so toes are free. When the dual-control, definitive prosthesis is prescribed at 3 years of age, *only* unilateral fitting of the dominant side should be ordered. The pattern of use and rejection with bilateral fitting has already been described.

SHOULDER DISARTICULATION PROSTHESIS

Total arm deficiency (amelia) (Fig. 40-33) or the equivalent (less than 30% of the humerus) is a most disabling and difficult deficit. Restoration of function and rehabilitation of these patients are equally difficult. At this proximal level, fewer power sources are available for useful, adequate, prosthetic function.

To the child with unilateral amelia, the prosthesis is cumbersome, bulky, heavy, at times uncomfortable, and is of little use as an assistive device. In addition, when the opposite shoulder is harnessed for better function, function of the normal limb is compromised. Presently, no practical externally powered prosthesis has been fabricated for the unilateral amelic child. Therefore, in unilateral total arm deficiencies, early prosthetic fitting is neither practical nor desirable and invariably is unsuccessful.

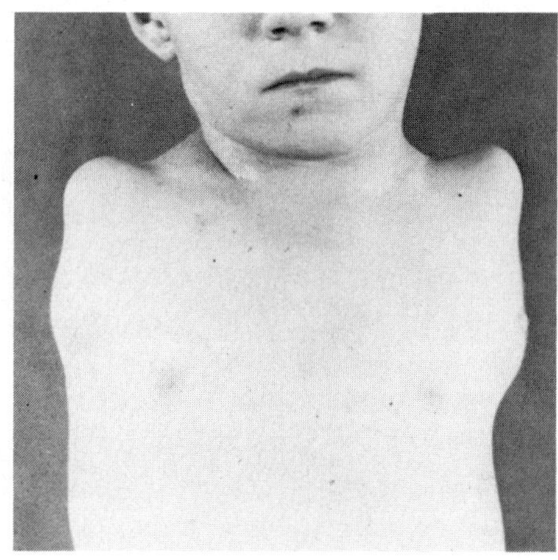

Fig. 40-33. Bilateral amelia.

Frequently, at puberty or earlier, the desire for symmetry and cosmesis will precipitate a request for a prosthesis. A modular, lightweight, soft-covered, passive prosthesis with a cosmetic hand should be prescribed.

Bilateral upper limb amelia levels are the most intractable problems to manage in the child amputee population. The total loss of upper limb prehension mandates that free foot function for prehension not only be permitted but encouraged. Fortunately, no specific training is necessary because these children develop a high degree of skill in foot usage, unless thwarted.

If they are to be freed of complete dependence on foot prehension, a prosthesis that can function as a leading device must be made available. Our goals should be realistic and related to the needs of the child.

Early fitting is advocated to develop prosthetic tolerance and visual clues, but fitting should be delayed until the child has good sitting balance. Bilateral shoulder caps are fitted to impart prosthetic feel and tolerance. When a decision to

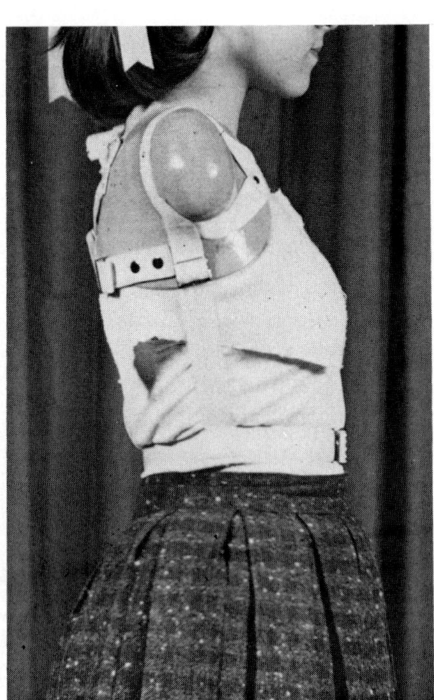

Fig. 40-34. Shoulder cap. In patient with bilateral amelia, one prosthetic arm is fitted, and opposite shoulder cap is used for suspension and fixation point for cable control.

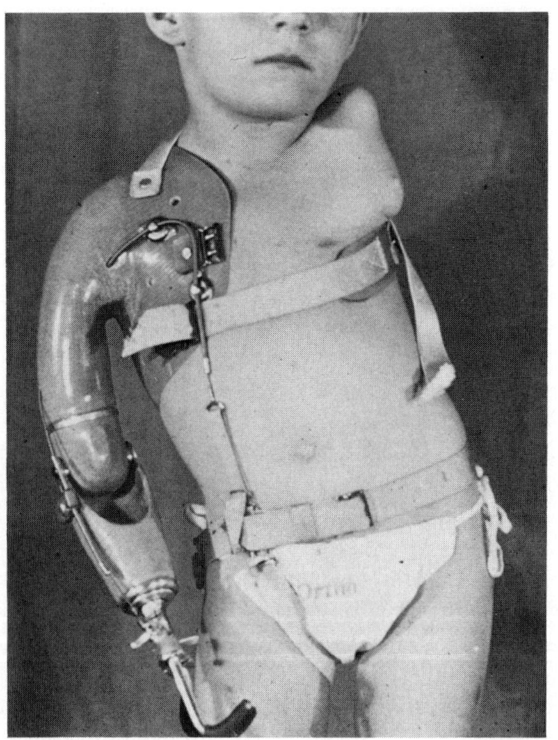

Fig. 40-35. Amelic prosthesis (no shoulder joint) using waist belt for elbow locking.

prescribe a prosthesis is made, about age 2, it is advisable to fit the side corresponding to the lead foot. However, the child will adapt and learn regardless of the side fitted. The contralateral cap will be used later for suspension and work source.

Purposeful terminal device activity with single control can be taught at age 2 if no other mechanical demands are made by excessive gadgeting. Therefore the prescription should specify a friction shoulder and elbow, capable of passive prepositioning, and a 12P hook with friction wrist unit. The socket should be of the frame type or with numerous perforations if made of solid plastic. With the absence of two limbs there is considerable loss of body area for heat dissipation. It is essential that as little of the torso as possible be covered with plastic. This is one of the many reasons why bilateral fitting is not advocated. The opposite shoulder cap plus chest strap (Fig. 40-34) is used for suspension and terminal device activation. The terminal device is powered by bilateral scapular abduction. Primitive marginal feeding patterns can be taught, but are usually accomplished only with contortions of the torso, head, and neck.

At about 4 years of age, a dual-control harness and elbow locking device can be prescribed. Although with growth the torso area has increased,

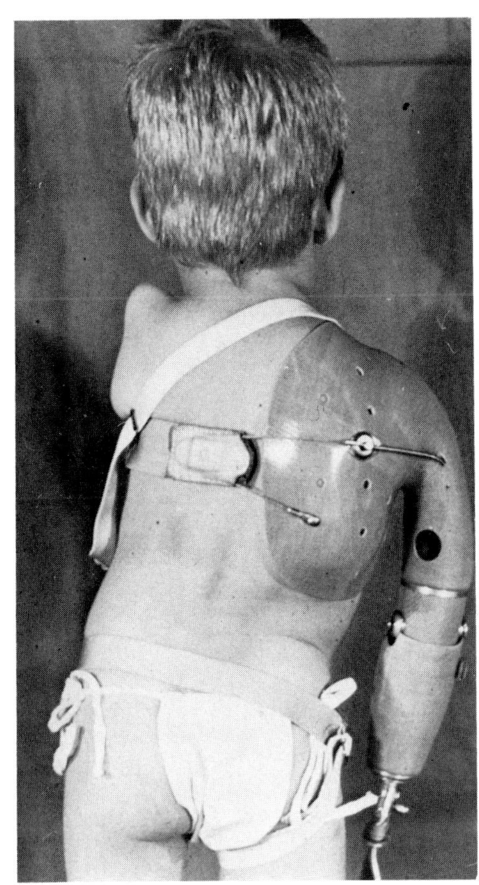

Fig. 40-36. Excursion amplifier.

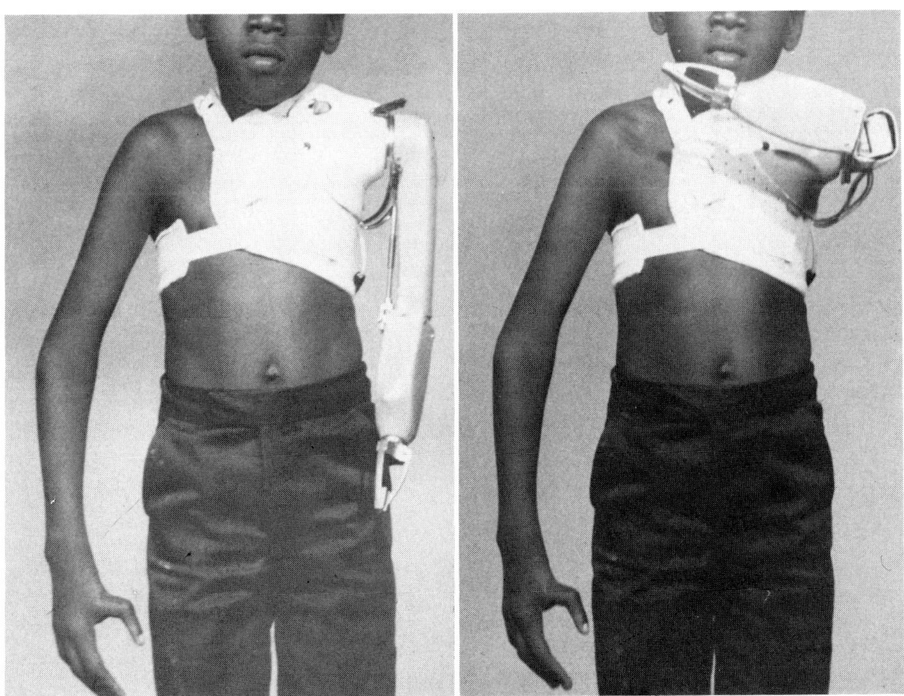

Fig. 40-37. OCCC coordinated arm.

the proportion of heat dissipation from this area remains rather constant, and the same precautions with the socket prevail throughout growth. The prosthetic prescription should include a passive shoulder joint to abduct and flex the arm for dressing and for placing the arm on the table or desk. An inside locking elbow with a turntable, standard forearm, friction wrist, and appropriate size aluminum hook completes the prosthesis.

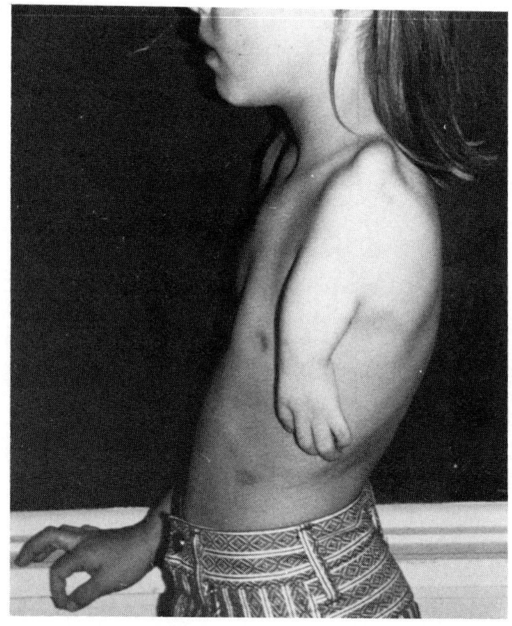

Fig. 40-38. Proximal phocomelia.

Harnessing for suspension, forearm flexion, and terminal device opening is much the same. The shoulder cap and chest strap are used for suspension. Chest expansion at this age can be used for elbow locking and unlocking if a wide Dacron strap is applied. If chest expansion is not adequate, a waist belt, attached to an elbow locking cable (Fig. 40-35) is another alternative. A third method for elbow locking function is to use a nudge control.

Forearm flexion and terminal device activation is accomplished with bilateral scapula abduction. If inadequate, this can be augmented by chest expansion. In case sufficient excursion cannot be obtained to open the terminal device with the elbow flexed, an excursion amplifier may be added (Fig. 40-36).

When female patients approach puberty there is a true test of a prosthetist s ingenuity. Chest straps above and below the breasts may be necessary for adequate suspension, function, and comfort. The bra may be used for attachment of the elbow locking cable, thereby harnessing shoulder elevation to activate the lock.

Several electric arms have been fabricated specifically for patients with bilateral amelia. The Michigan feeding arm and the OCCC coordinated arm (Fig. 40-37) were designed for feeding and not for multipurpose use. There is hope that a satisfactory externally powered prosthetic system will be made available soon.

For older children, an electric elbow is available, operated by switch control, which eliminates the need for an additional work source to activate elbow lock. Present models can with-

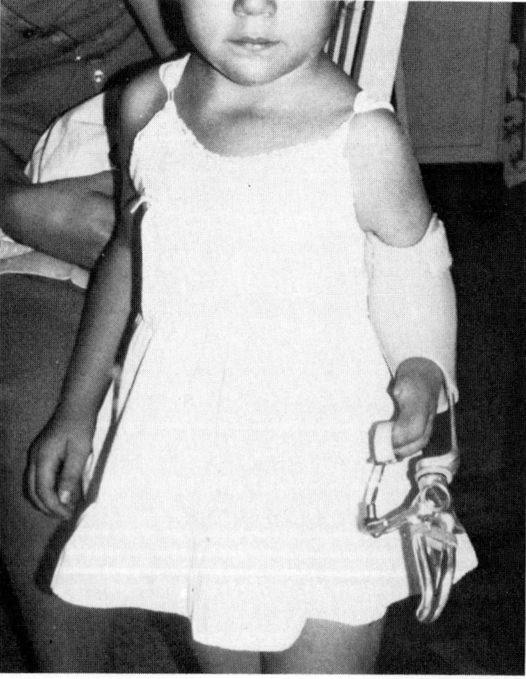

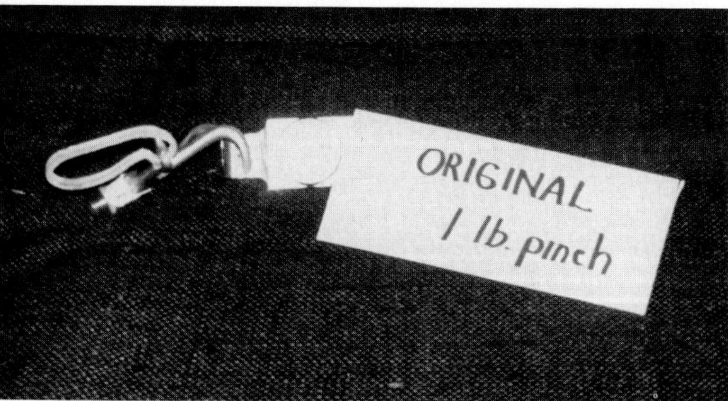

Fig. 40-39. Using phocomelic fingers for opening terminal device, but only 0.45 kg (1 pound) of pinch force can be generated.

stand vigorous function without breakdown, but the noise level and slow operation are two detracting features.

As with the bilateral above-elbow amputee, foot usage should constantly be encouraged. It has been shown that good prosthetic function can be correlated with good foot usage. For these patients, a unilateral fitting of a functional prosthesis is preferred. However, as a young adult, a cosmetic prosthesis may be prescribed if requested. Some patients may request bilateral functional prostheses.

PHOCOMELIA

In fitting phocomelic patients several modifications are necessary. The socket should have a cutout to accommodate the phocomelic hand and allow free finger motion. These fingers can activate the elbow locking device. Theoretically, these fingers could be used for terminal device activation (Fig. 40-38), but insufficient pinch force (Fig. 40-39) makes this impractical.

A shoulder cap with shoulder hinges, inside locking elbow, standard forearm, friction wrist, and appropriate size hook completes the prosthesis. Harnessing for suspension and dual-control activation can be easily accomplished with a chest strap and excursion amplifier. If this proves to be an inadequate motor, a figure-of-eight harness with biscapular abduction may be used alone or with a chest strap. Elbow lock function is by direct pull on the cable by one or more fingers.[6]

In the older child, use of various electrical components, connected to switches can be activated by the phocomelic fingers. Of greatest use at present is the electric elbow. The imperfections are outweighed by transforming a dual-control harness into a single active terminal device control.

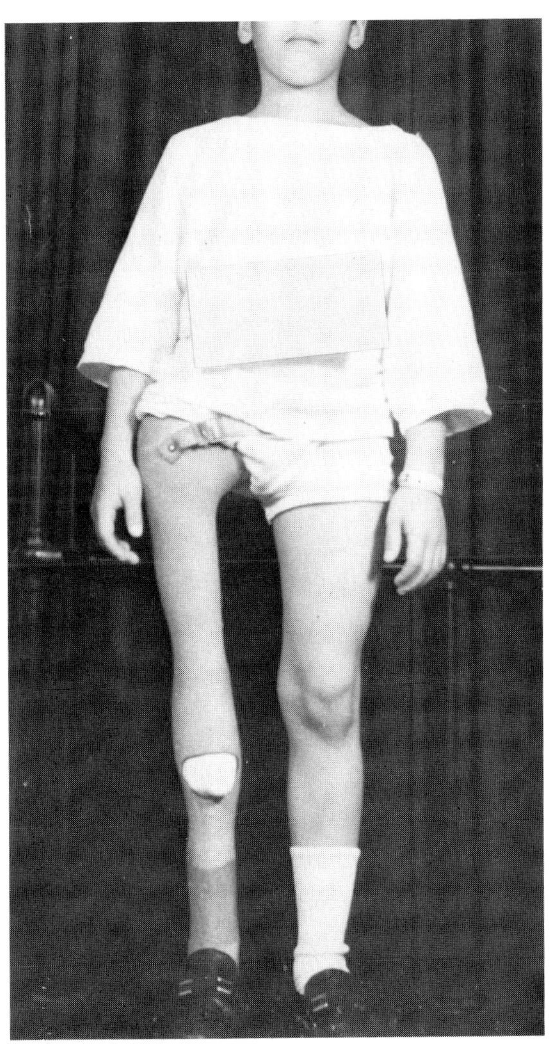

Fig. 40-40. Patient with PFFD right leg is fitted with a customized prosthesis with so-called ship's ventilator-type socket and foot intact.

Section II

Lower limb prosthetic management

LEON M. KRUGER
ROBERT HAYES

PROSTHETIC RESTORATIONS

Five basic prosthetic restorations are required for the management of a lower limb juvenile amputee:

1. Partial foot restorations
2. Syme-type prosthesis
3. Below-knee prosthesis
4. Above-knee prosthesis, including knee disarticulation types
5. Hip disarticulation prosthesis

To this list must be added prostheses that are constructed on a custom basis for limb deficiencies that are fitted without revision. Since each of these must be customized for the individual patient it is not possible to describe any single technique that is applicable. Some of these are modified below-knee prostheses made with the foot fitted into the shank portion above the prosthetic foot, using the patient's normal knee joint (Fig. 40-64, *C*). In others the foot is fitted into the thigh section, with a prosthetic knee and ankle joint below (Fig. 40-61, *B*). Still others are customized ship's ventilator-type prostheses for the PFFD patient (Fig. 40-40). The prosthetic prescription options available are found in Table 9 at the end of the chapter.

In formulating a prescription for the juvenile amputee, either a congenital limb deficiency or a surgically converted amputation, one should be primarily interested in functional restoration, with cosmesis being of secondary importance. The activity levels of the child must be considered, as well as the type of activity. As an example, one would not prescribe an endoskeletal limb with foam cover for a 13-year-old boy who would be playing football or working in a shop with oil and grease soaking through his clothing. Recognizing that fewer moving parts mean less maintenance, the SACH foot or heel wedge is preferred to a more complex foot assembly when prescribing for the juvenile.

Material selection for the socket is not likely to be a problem today. In the past wood, aluminum, steel, and leather sockets were in common usage. Today fabrication with plastic laminate over a plaster cast mold of the stump is considered standard. This provides excellent prosthetic fit as well as a durable socket. Newer materials on the scene include polypropylene, vitrathene, and polycarbonate. The increasing use of vacuum-forming techniques with these thermoplastic type materials may lead to their more frequent use. As of this writing plastic laminate remains the standard material used in the prosthetic sockets.

Partial foot restoration

For those children with transverse deficiencies of phalanges and/or metatarsals, as well as those with surgical amputations at this level, a shoe insert is the standard prescription. The insert is fabricated either from an impression or a cast of the residual foot and constructed to the shape of the patient's shoe. The more distal deficiencies are easily fitted with such inserts. As the deficiency or amputation level occurs more proximally, the deficit is such that there is insufficient residual foot to suspend the shoe on the limb. A supramalleolar suspension technique can be used. This "shoe within a shoe" for partial foot restoration becomes standard when the amputation level is through the tarsal joints or proximal. The Chopart "shoe within a shoe" prosthesis is fabricated with molding leather stretched over a mold of the patient's stump. The toe extension is applied to fill the shoe. The prosthesis may have a toe break, which is adjustable for resistance. A flexible foam plastic or rubber toe may be used (Fig. 40-41).

As an alternative to this, an ankle-foot orthosis

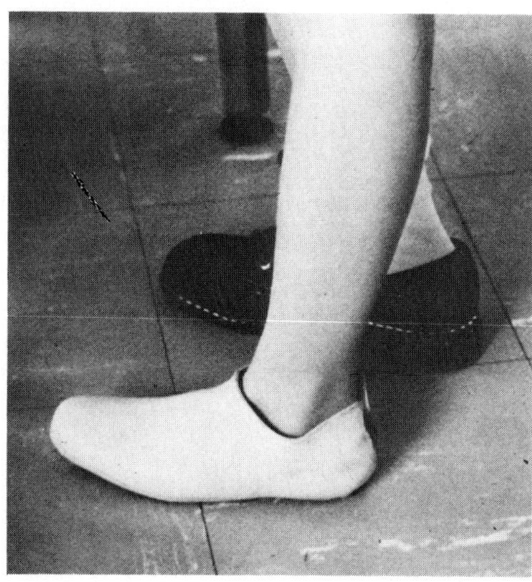

Fig. 40-41. Chopart-type "shoe within a shoe prosthesis" is fabricated over cast of foot and has posterior opening so that residual limb may be slipped into prosthesis, which is in turn fitted into shoe.

with foam toe extension affords good stability at toe-off. Force from the footplate is transferred through the plastic to the padded anterior strap at the proximal tibia. The patient with a sensitive or scarred anterior stump thus has complete relief of the anterior surface of the stump. For those patients in whom scarring is excessive posteriorly, the ankle-foot orthosis may be constructed with a posterior opening and an anterior wall to provide support. This type of prosthesis is also used for the more proximal level partial foot amputation. Either provides better toe-off than does the Chopart insert.

At the time of prescription, it is important for the clinic team to recognize the cosmetic problems that may be created, especially for a girl. The options must be carefully explained to the patient and to the parent so that they enter into the final prescription decision. For many patients the cosmetic loss from supramalleolar suspension is such that they would prefer proximal revision, so that a more cosmetically acceptable prosthesis may be used.

Syme-type prosthesis

Patients with a complete transverse deficiency of the foot or partial tarsal deficiency, as well as those who have had an ankle disarticulation, Syme-, or Boyd-type amputation, will require the use of a Syme prosthesis or a modification of a Syme prosthesis (Figs. 40-42 and 40-43). For the individual who has a length discrepancy of the

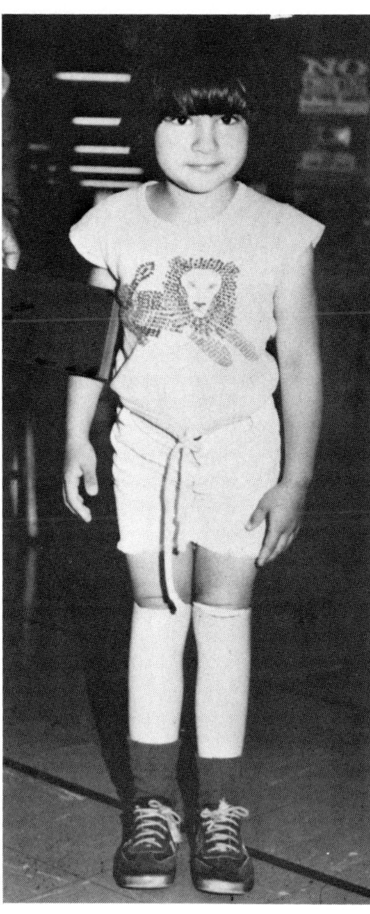

Fig. 40-42. Patient with bilateral longitudinal deficiency of fibula treated by disarticulation at ankle is fitted with bilateral Syme prosthesis of plastic laminate socket with partial soft insert for suspension.

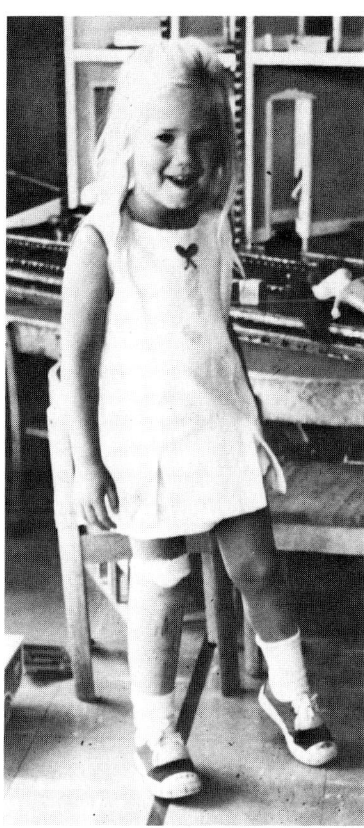

Fig. 40-43. Child with longitudinal deficiency of fibula who has been treated by disarticulation is fitted with Syme-type prosthesis, with partial insert for suspension. Cosmesis may be poor when child is small but improves with growth.

limb, as with congenital deficiency, there is sufficient room for a heel wedge or SACH foot to be incorporated on the prosthesis, and the major concern will be the shape of the residual limb and the resultant problems of socket construction. The circumferential measurement of the distal stump is greater than the midtibial level. This feature is used for socket suspension. If the measurement differential is small, one has the option of using a closed socket with a partial insert or an expandable socket. Where the discrepancy between circumferential measurement of the distal stump and midtibial level is greater, it may be necessary to proceed to the Canadian-type Syme socket with posterior opening or with medial panel opening (Fig. 40-44). Additional suspension is not necessary with these fittings. For those individuals in whom no length discrepancy exists, as with the traumatic amputation or congenital deficiency with the talus and os calcis retained, a

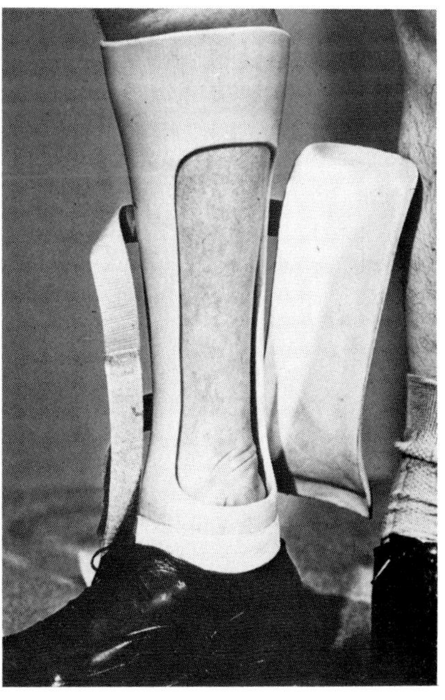

Fig. 40-44. VAPC-type medial opening Syme end-bearing prosthesis with SACH foot.

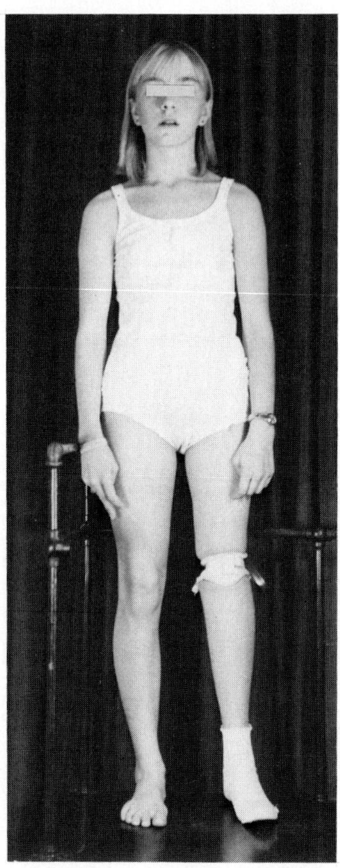

Fig. 40-45. This girl with transtibial amputation has been fitted with PTB socket, soft insert and cuff suspension, and SACH foot, which is conventional fitting for below-knee amputees.

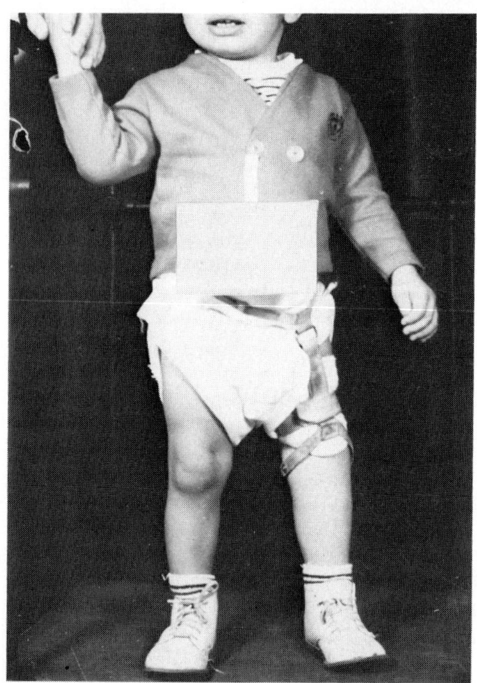

Fig. 40-46. Very small child fitted with PTB socket and cuff suspension will require toddler harness as additional suspension.

length problem exists in the attempted use of the Syme-type prosthesis. In the very young patient a small lift on the shoe of the normal side may offset this problem. In the older child one will have to make a decision between the use of the ankle-foot orthosis with foam extension as previously described or revision of the amputation level proximally.

Below-knee prosthesis

The basic prosthesis for the below-knee juvenile amputee is a total-contact PTB plastic laminate socket with insert, SACH foot, and cuff suspension (Fig. 40-45). The very small child will require a toddler harness or a waistband with an inverted Y as auxiliary suspension (Fig. 40-46).

Some clinic chiefs and prosthetists believe that the very small child requires additional stability and prefer that the initial prosthesis be a modified PTB socket with a thigh corset and side bars as well as a toddler harness (Fig. 40-47). This provides additional knee stability, more flexibili-

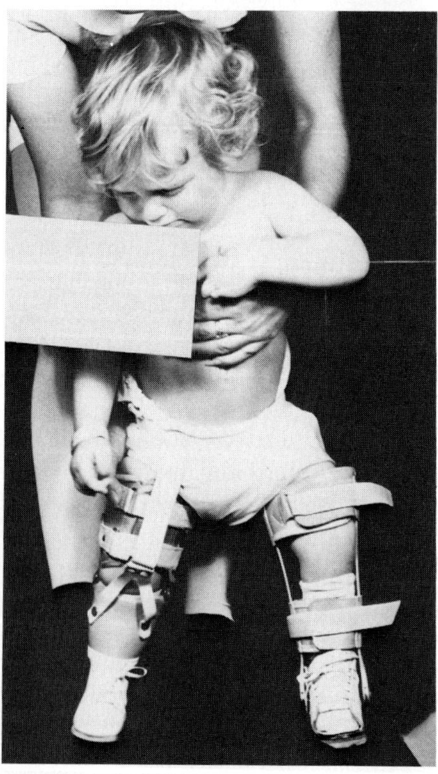

Fig. 40-47. For young child PTB socket may be modified so that thigh corset and side bars may be used, as well as toddler harness for additional suspension. Thigh corset and side bars provide additional knee stability and more flexibility in socket fit.

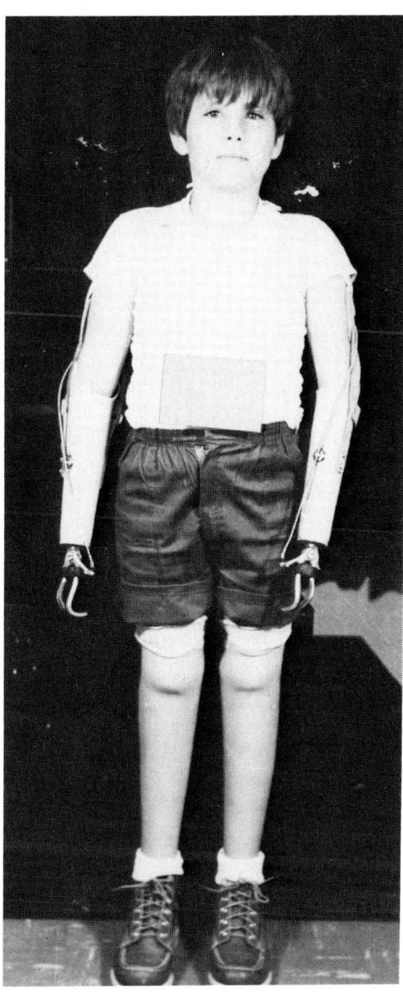

Fig. 40-48. Below-knee prostheses with patellar tendon supracondylar (PTS) suspension provide for ease of donning and diminished maintenance and can be lightweight in construction. Note suprapatellar trim lines for additional stability for this bilateral amputee.

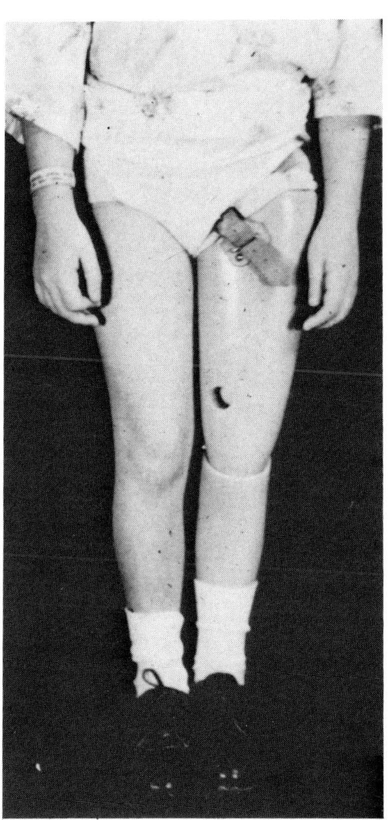

Fig. 40-49. For long above-knee stump, in this case with poor hip joint as result of PFFD, conventional above-knee prosthesis is prescribed. This consists of quadrilateral suction socket with auxiliary Silesian band suspension, single-axis knee, and SACH foot.

ty in socket fit, and partial weight bearing on the thigh corset. At age 3 or 4, the prescription should be changed to a conventional PTB socket with cuff suspension or, better yet, patella tendon supracondylar (PTS) trim lines or supracondylar suspension. The PTS socket provides for knee stability and at the same time diminishes maintenance, since it has no straps or moving parts (Fig. 40-48). If properly constructed, the child can slip in and out of the socket with ease.

Above-knee prosthesis

The basic prosthesis for a child with a knee disarticulation will be a plastic laminate total-contact socket with outside knee hinges, SACH foot, and Silesian suspension. Most children manage a knee joint well. If there is a problem in extension

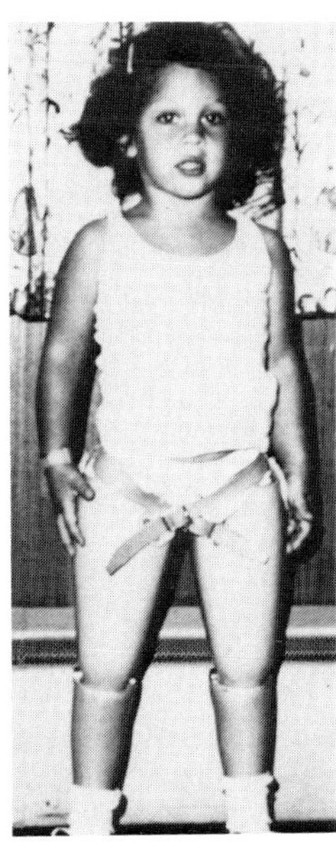

Fig. 40-50. Bilateral above-knee amputee is fitted with conventional quadrilateral sockets with crossed Silesian suspension, single-axis knee, and SACH foot. At an older age this patient's prosthesis will be converted to suction suspension.

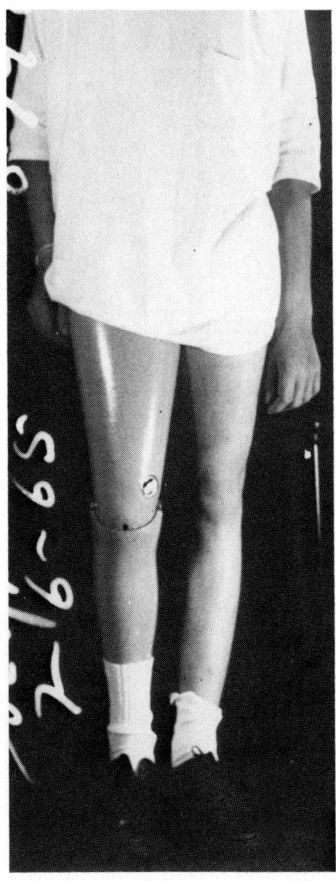

Fig. 40-51. This child's prosthesis, originally fitted with quadrilateral socket with Silesian suspension, has been converted to suction suspension and requires no additional belt.

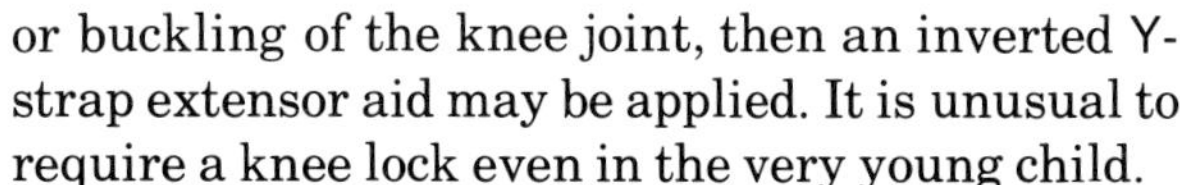

or buckling of the knee joint, then an inverted Y-strap extensor aid may be applied. It is unusual to require a knee lock even in the very young child.

For children with long above-knee stumps, the prosthesis most commonly used is the plastic laminate socket with a single-axis knee joint, SACH foot, and Silesian bandage suspension (Figs. 40-49 and 40-50).

Perhaps the most frequent problem in socket construction for the small child is failure to provide adequate preflexion of the socket, which in turn causes the child to walk with an exaggerated lumbar lordosis. Attention to this detail in socket construction and alignment is important. Suspension modifications are much more frequent. For the child with a very short stump it may be necessary to provide a pelvic belt with hip joint to provide stability and security. The very small child may likewise benefit from additional suspension

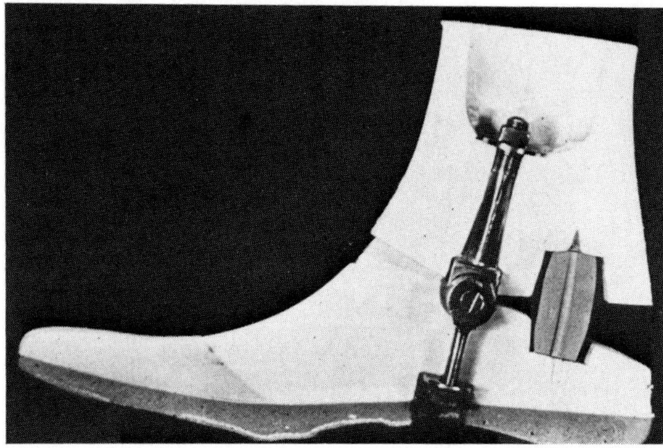

Fig. 40-52. Single-axis ankle joint with molded toepiece and anterior bumper. Single-axis ankle joint and posterior bumper are shown in cut section.

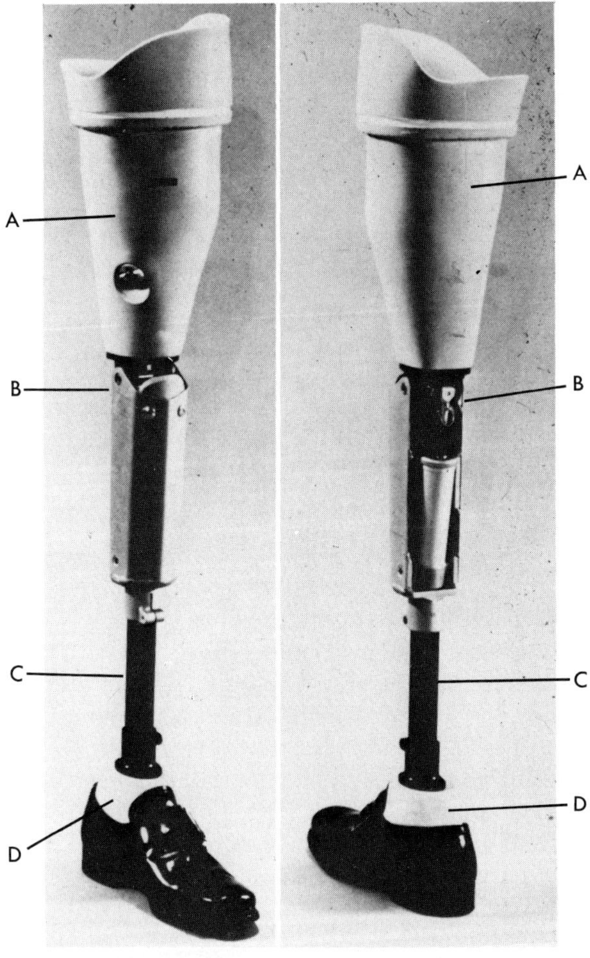

Fig. 40-53. Multiplex endoskeletal above-knee unit. Knee joint depicted here is Mauch unit, but this can accommodate any type of hydraulic knee unit. *A,* Socket. *B,* Knee unit. *C,* Pylon tubing. *D,* SACH foot.

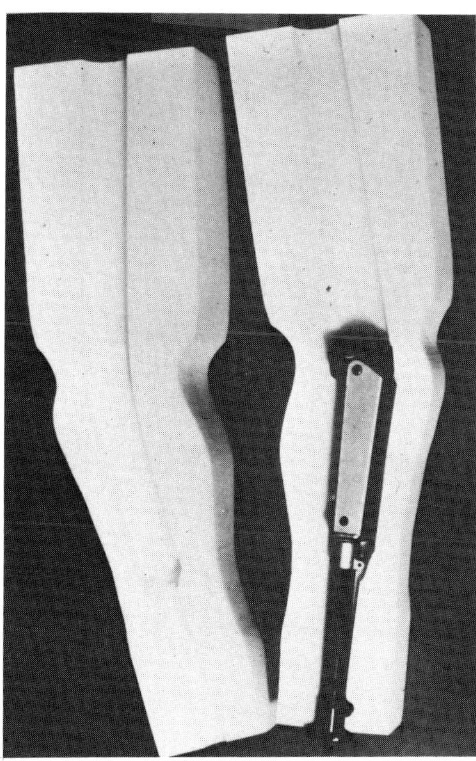

Fig. 40-54. Multiplex unit with unshaped foam cover split in half to demonstrate unit fit into foam.

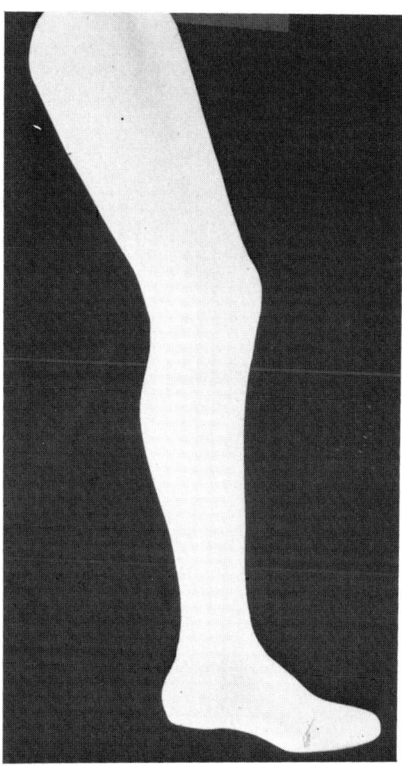

Fig. 40-55. Cosmetically carved foam cover for endoskeletal limb provides excellent cosmesis. "Feel" of this cover is desirable, especially for female patient.

in the form of a shoulder strap or toddler harness.

As the child grows older (at age 6 or 7), conversion, provided the stump is adequate, to suction suspension may be considered (Fig. 40-51). The addition of suction suspension prior to this age is difficult in that the child is usually unable to pull the stump into the socket by himself. This means that accidental loss of suction and loss of the limb may provide a crisis situation for the child. Since socket fit with suction suspension is much more critical, frequent socket replacement will be necessary.

Most children handle the prosthetic knee joint well when the prosthesis is properly aligned. If the knee instability is great, a knee lock may be added. Safety knees are not available for the very small child, but for the older child a variety of hydraulic and pneumatic knee units are available. The addition of such a unit may improve the overall gait of the above-knee amputee in the adolescent years. The weight of the prosthesis is slightly increased when using these units, but most patients believe the advantages of improved gait and knee stability make this worthwhile.

Although the standard prescription for the above-knee adolescent amputee is a SACH foot, consideration should be given to the prescription of other foot-ankle units. The SACH foot simulates anteroposterior and minimal mediolateral motion at the ankle. The single-axis foot-ankle unit provides only motion in the anteroposterior plane (Fig. 40-52). The Greissinger foot will give motion in all planes and is proven to be a help on uneven surfaces and in sports requiring lateral movement. As an alternative, the SACH foot can be used with an ankle rotator unit, the SACH foot providing anteroposterior motion as well as minimal mediolateral motion. The rotator unit reduces shear stress on the stump-socket interface where pivot occurs.

As the child grows older, consideration should be given to the use of an endoskeletal prosthesis, especially in the female patient for whom cosmesis is important (Figs. 40-53 to 40-55). The endoskeletal prosthesis is constructed of a structural support of lightweight aluminum tubing with a very lightweight covering of foamed plastic. The endoskeletal prosthesis is considerably lighter than a conventional limb. The solid foam cover is particularly attractive to girls, not only for its

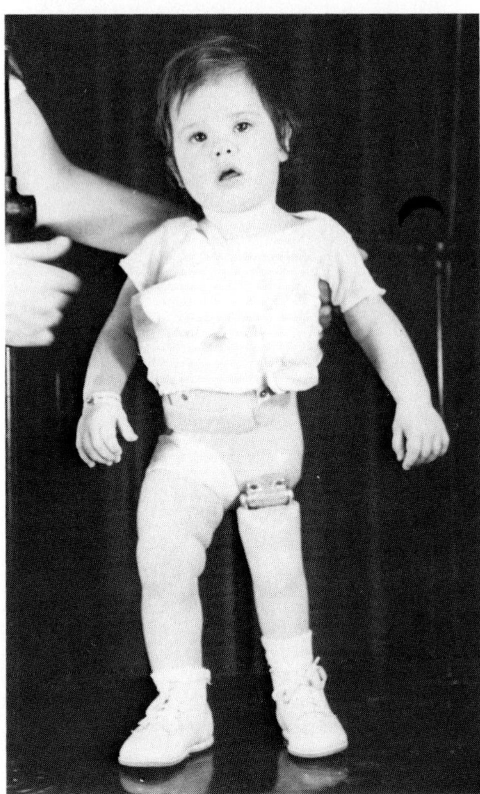

Fig. 40-56. For very young patient with hip disarticulation, prosthetic prescription calls for plastic laminate socket with Canadian hip joint, no knee joint, and SACH foot. Auxiliary shoulder strap suspension is usually necessary.

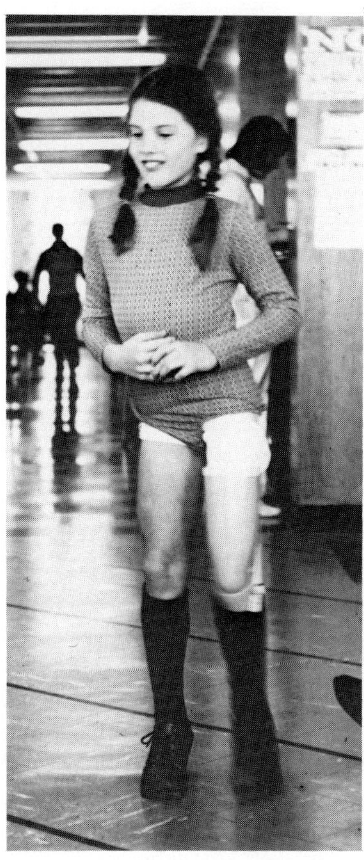

Fig. 40-57. As patient with hip disarticulation grows older, there is adequate room to provide knee joint as well, and shoulder strap suspension may be eliminated.

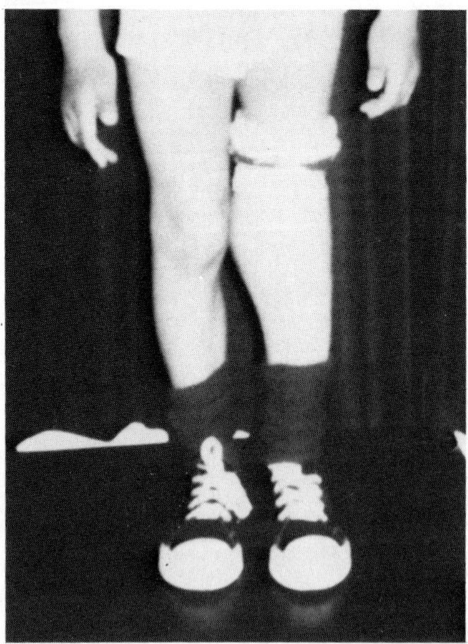

Fig. 40-58. Patient with longitudinal deficiency of tibia, partial, has been converted to below-knee amputation and fitted with PTS suspension prosthesis, despite proximal subluxation of proximal end of fibula.

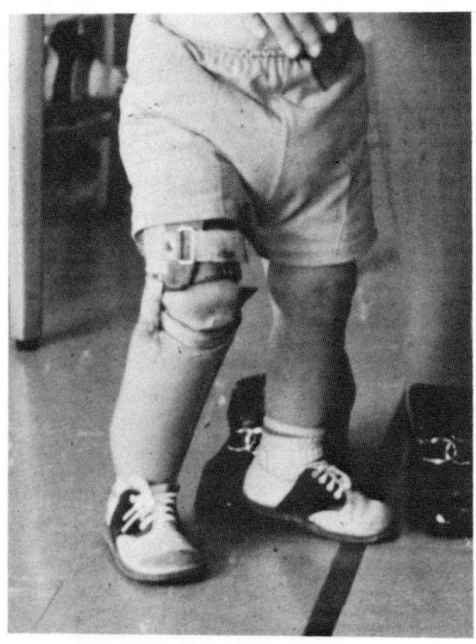

Fig. 40-59. Following Brown procedure child is fitted with plastic laminate socket with side bars and thigh corset. Note knee flexion deformity that has developed here.

cosmetic appearance, but also for "the feel" of the leg (Fig. 40-55). It is much easier on clothing than the rigid structure of a conventional limb. As with the conventional prosthesis, there is a choice of knee joint and foot-ankle assembly. The major benefits of the endoskeletal prosthesis for the child are improved cosmesis and lighter weight. The trade-off is the considerable increase in maintenance.

Hip disarticulation prosthesis

In the very young child, age 1 to 2 years, prescription will include a plastic laminate socket with a hip joint, no knee joint, and a SACH foot (Fig. 40-56). A requirement for auxiliary shoulder strap suspension is frequent because the small pelvis of the child and the critical nature of socket fit may be inadequate to provide suspension. The distance from socket to floor is such that there is inadequate room to accommodate hip, knee, and ankle joints, and the easiest joint to eliminate is the knee joint.

As the child grows and his height increases, the prosthesis should include a single-axis knee joint (Fig. 40-57). Stability of the knee joint is obtained by alignment techniques, as well as the elastic straps that are a part of the hip disarticulation assembly.

As the child approaches the adolescent years, an endoskeletal hip disarticulation prosthesis should be considered. As with other endoskeletal prostheses, a reduction in weight is the important consideration. This is usually accompanied by an improvement in gait pattern. It is also a cosmetically much more desirable limb for girls. Maintenance is increased, and the foam covers do not wear well. They will not withstand the rough usage of an active teenage boy. The advantages of reduced weight of prosthesis and improved cosmesis must be weighed against the disadvantages of increased maintenance and more frequent replacement.

SPECIAL CONSIDERATIONS IN LIMB DEFICIENCIES

Longitudinal deficiency of the fibula

Almost all patients with this limb deficiency are converted to ankle disarticulation or a Boyd amputation and have a more or less bulbous end-bearing stump. There may be valgus and/or anterior bowing of the remaining tibia. The knee joint usually has good stability but may have valgus instability. The usual prescription will be for a Syme-type prosthesis with SACH foot (Figs. 40-42 and 40-43). Sufficient relief must be provided in the socket to prevent skin irriation over the anterior tibial bow. When knee valgus is present, medial displacement of the foot on the socket will accommodate this deformity. The socket bulkiness may be sufficiently objectionable to warrant recommendation for surgical intervention to correct the deformity.

When the valgus is of such a degree as to cause instability of the knee joint, proximal and medial thrust on the knee may require that additional stability be built into the prosthesis.

Longitudinal deficiency of the tibia

Since complete longitudinal deficiency of the tibia is usually treated by disarticulation at the knee level, the prosthesis would be the same as for knee disarticulation for any other purpose.

For those patients with a partial deficiency of the tibia the prosthesis is a below-knee prosthesis, with modification of the socket to accept the abnormal shape of the residual limb. Particular attention is made to a prominent proximal fibula, which may sublux proximalward or across the knee joint. Although the younger child usually requires side bars and a thigh corset, when the child is older, fitting with PTS suspension is more desirable (Figs. 40-46 and 40-58).

For those patients who have had a Brown procedure as treatment for tibial deficiency, the prosthesis will require a plastic laminate socket, side bars and thigh corset, and a SACH foot (Figs. 40-59 and 40-60). Particular attention must be

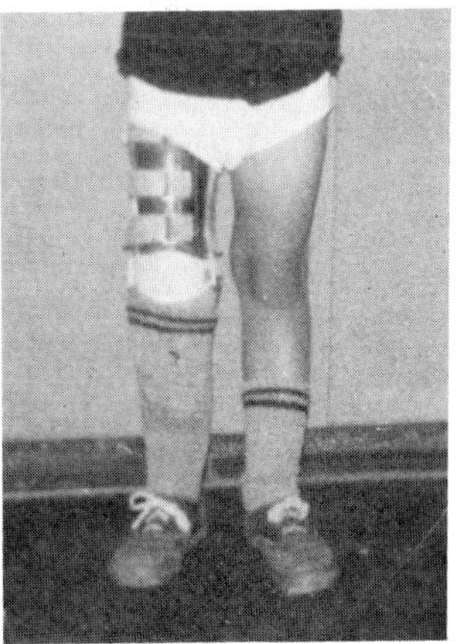

Fig. 40-60. Following correction of recurrent knee flexion deformity after Brown procedure, child is fitted with new below-knee prosthesis with plastic laminate socket, side bars, and thigh corset. On occasion, extensor aid may be used.

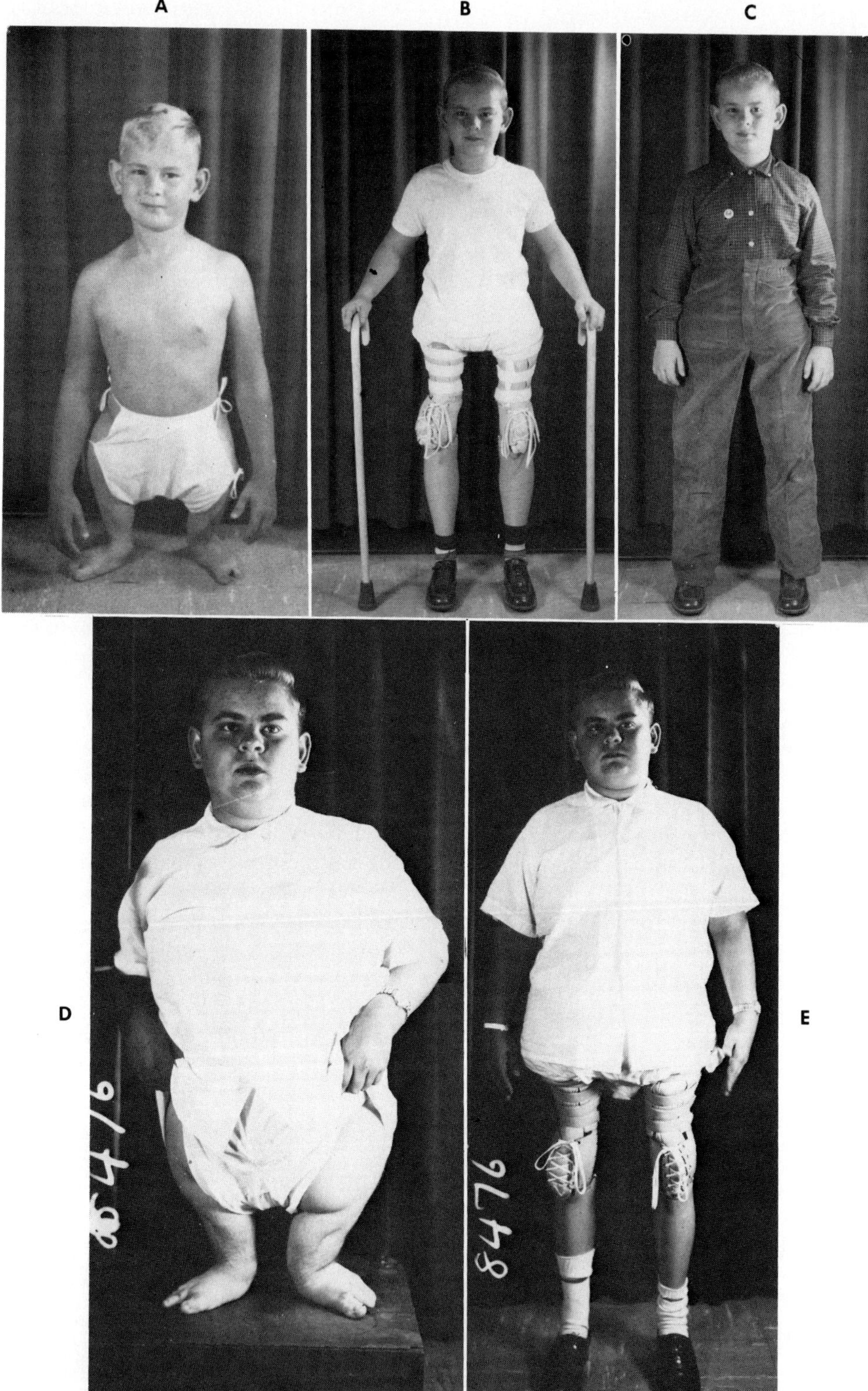

Fig. 40-61. A, Patient with bilateral PFFD has been fitted with prostheses without amputation or revision surgery. **B,** Thigh segment of prosthesis is carved willow wood with lacers over feet and Velcro closure over shank portion. Single-axis knee and SACH foot complete prosthesis. **C,** Clothed patient has normal appearance, even though gait demonstrates severe waddle. **D,** At age 15, he has become obese, a major problem for such a patient. **E,** Despite obesity, he remains fully ambulatory. At age 29, he continues to wear this type limb and is employed full time in responsible position. Overall body habitus must be considered in deciding exactly where knee level will be placed when fitting bilateral PFFD patient without amputation or revision. There is temptation to make patient too tall in which case he may become top heavy and lose stability.

paid to socket fit and to location of the knee joints. If the extensor mechanism is weak, an extensor assist in the form of an inverted Y strap is indicated.

Partial longitudinal deficiency of the thigh (PFFD)

Prior to the definitive surgical intervention in patients with PFFD, the prosthesis must be individualized (Fig. 40-40). Each patient requires not only a custom-built prosthesis, but also a well thought out plan for its fabrication. Casting of the limb is a complicated procedure. The cast must be taken with the foot in the appropriate degree of equinus, since the foot will be used as a weight-bearing end organ. The technique of enclosing the shank portion must be individualized and the decision made by the prosthetist whether this is best accomplished with a solid shell, split and closed with straps, or with a tongue and lacer apparatus. The overall body habitus must be considered in arriving at the decision on placement of a prosthetic knee joint below the patient's foot (Fig. 40-61). Alignment and a final decision on the length of the limb will depend on that position in which the patient is most comfortable with regard to knee and hip extension.

When the limb deficiency has been converted by amputation, many of these difficulties remain. Thus the PFFD patient with a residual femoral segment of 50%, who has had an ankle disarticulation, has a prescription for a Syme-type prosthesis. The basic socket fitting will follow that discussed elsewhere, but the decision on length and alignment will be greatly affected by the position of maximal stability of the patient's remaining knee and hip on the affected side (Fig. 40-62).

The patient with a very short femoral segment and flexed and externally rotated position of the hip and knee will require that these be incorporated into the ship's ventilator-type prosthesis, which incorporates the flexed knee and short femoral segment and is so trimmed as to provide stability as well as partial ischial weight bearing.

After the PFFD patient has had a knee fusion and conversion to an above-knee amputation stump, the prosthesis becomes more conventional—a modified quadrilateral socket with a

A

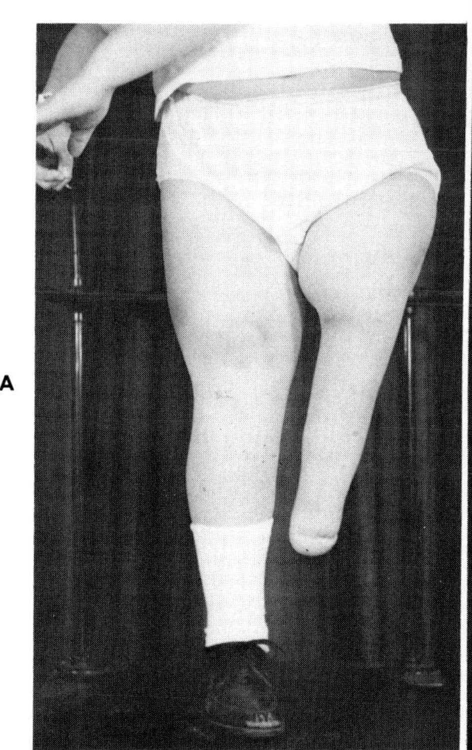

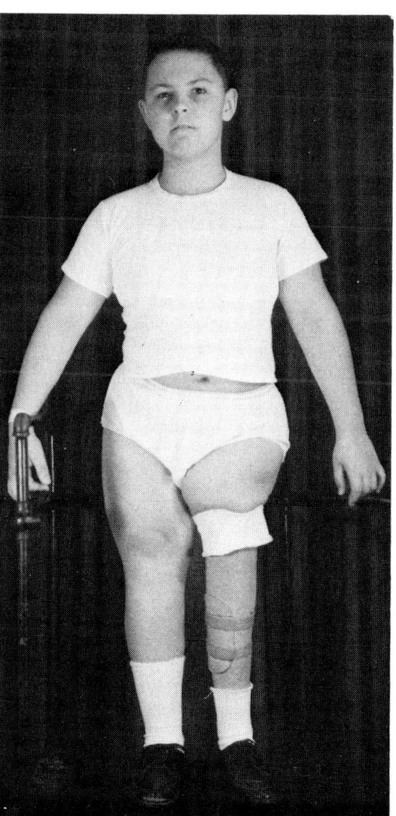

B

Fig. 40-62. A, Following amputation for length equalization prosthesis in patient with PFFD, knee levels are unequal, and there may be residual hip flexion and knee flexion deformity. **B,** Prosthetic length will be determined by that length which provides patient with maximum knee and hip stability, rather than effort at exact equalization of leg lengths.

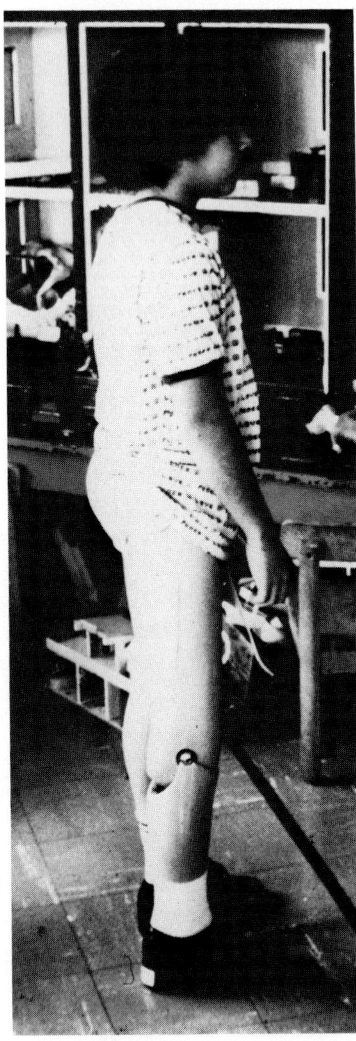

Fig. 40-63. PFFD patient with very short femoral segment has been subjected to knee fusion in full extension followed by amputation. He is fitted with conventional quadrilateral socket with ischial-bearing single-axis knee and SACH foot. Note that alignment is excellent, when knee has been fused in full extension.

single-axis knee, SACH foot, and Silesian suspension (Fig. 40-63). If the thigh segment is quite short and there is a notable bulbous contour of the proximal thigh, the modification of the socket may be extreme. When the knee fusion has not been carried out at a full 180 degrees, the socket will again take on the configuration of a ships ventilator. When the knee has been fused in complete extension at 180 degrees, the socket fabrication is much less difficult. Improved ischial weight bearing and alignment are possible. With excessive hip instability it may be necessary to consider pelvic band and hip joint rather than Silesian suspension.

In the younger child the single-axis knee joint is the standard. As the child approaches the teenage years prescription for the hydraulic or pneumatic knee should be considered to improve the gait pattern and knee stability. The SACH foot is the standard prescription, although in older children a single-axis ankle may have some benefits.

Bilateral PFFD

The child with bilateral PFFD, whose limbs are of approximately the same length, is usually independently ambulatory, and the major concern is for overall height. Prosthetic prescription therefore is not as for other amputees and limb-deficient children, primarily for functional improvement, but in this specific instance is for cosmetic reasons. Since these patients are independently ambulatory, the feet have not been amputated. It is therefore necessary for the prostheses to be fitted about the feet and legs. The variations in socket construction will depend on the length of the femur, the presence or absence of flexion deformities of the hip and knee, and the flexibility of the foot and ankle. It may be difficult to achieve reasonable cosmesis in clothes because the foot and ankle are incorporated into the socket. Below this socket a single-axis knee, wooden shank, and single-axis foot-ankle assembly complete the prosthesis. Alignment should be carried out so that there is good stability at the knee. Although these prostheses provide for cosmetic improvement by increasing stature, they also have a functional capacity and the individual should be made independently ambulatory with the use of a cane (Fig. 40-61).

If discrepancy in leg length exists in the bilateral PFFD patient, disarticulation at the ankle on the short side and prosthetic restoration may be the solution for this limb length discrepancy (Fig. 40-64, *B*). The prosthesis is no different from any other ankle disarticulation prosthesis. Since individuals with PFFD are still disproportionate dwarfs, they may also be interested in stilt prostheses for cosmetic restoration. The longer limb should be fitted without amputation, and the shorter limb then fitted with an above-knee prosthesis (Fig. 40-64, *C*). This then permits the patient the option of cosmetic restoration with the bilateral lower limb prosthetic fittings or the use of the single prosthesis and his normal foot for increased stability and ease of ambulation. Many patients will reject the bilateral fitting because of the increased energy expenditure in ambulation. It is for this reason that the feet should not be removed in the symmetrical patient, and only

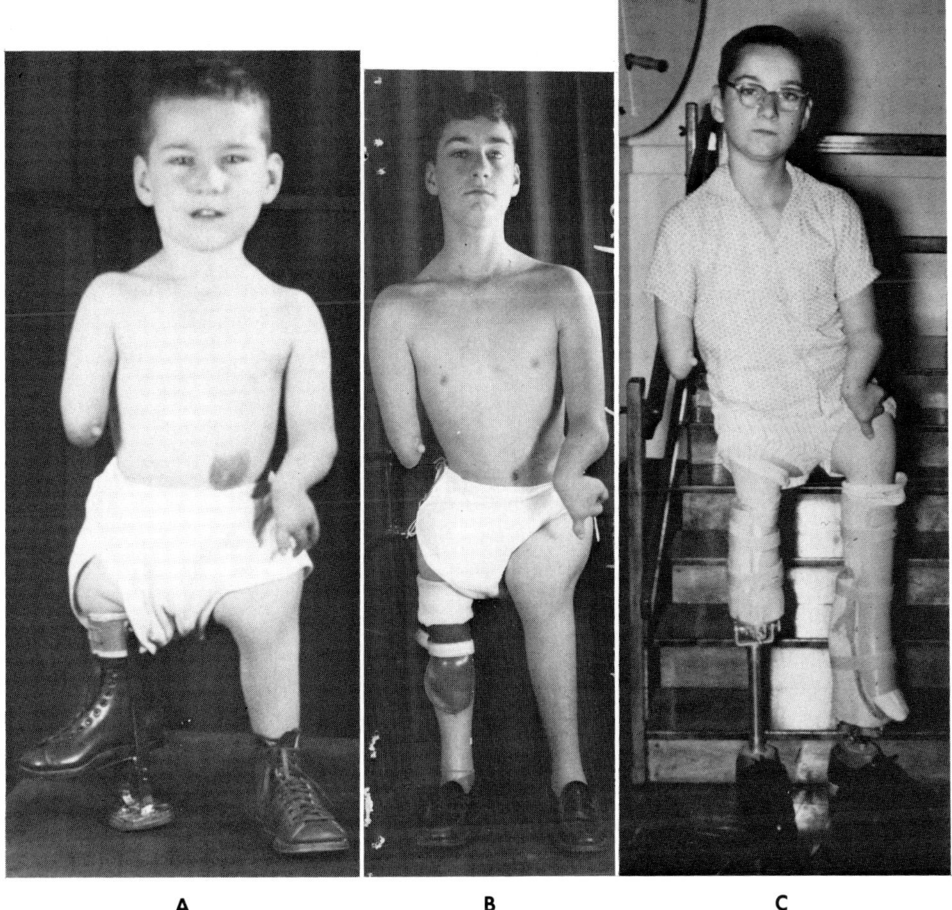

Fig. 40-64. A, Patient with multiple limb deficiencies including bilateral asymmetrical PFFD. **B,** Disarticulation at ankle on right side is followed by fitting with Syme-type prosthesis for length equalization. **C,** For cosmetic purposes, to increase height, patient may be fitted with right above-knee prosthesis, and left leg and foot are fitted into molded plastic socket with patient using his own knee above this prosthesis.

Table 9. Prosthetic prescription options

Level	*Socket*	*Foot-ankle unit*	*Knee joint*	*Hip joint*	*Suspension*
Ankle disarticulation (Syme)	Plastic laminate Molded polypropylene	SACH	–	–	Partial insert Expandable liner Medial panel
Below-knee amputation	Total-contact PTB, PTS Plastic laminate Molded polypropylene (with or without insert)	SACH	–	–	PTB cuff suspension PTS Thigh corset with side bars Toddler harness
Knee disarticulation	Quadrilateral Plastic laminate	SACH rotator unit (older)	Outside hinge Four-bar	–	Insert Silesian bandage
Above-knee amputation	Quadrilateral Plastic laminate	SACH single-axis rotator unit (older)	Single-axis Safety knee Hydraulic (older)	–	Silesian bandage Pelvic belt with hinge Suction Toddler harness
Hip disarticulation	Total contact (Canadian or Northwestern type) Plastic laminate	SACH Single-axis	Single-axis	Canadian	Socket Shoulder strap

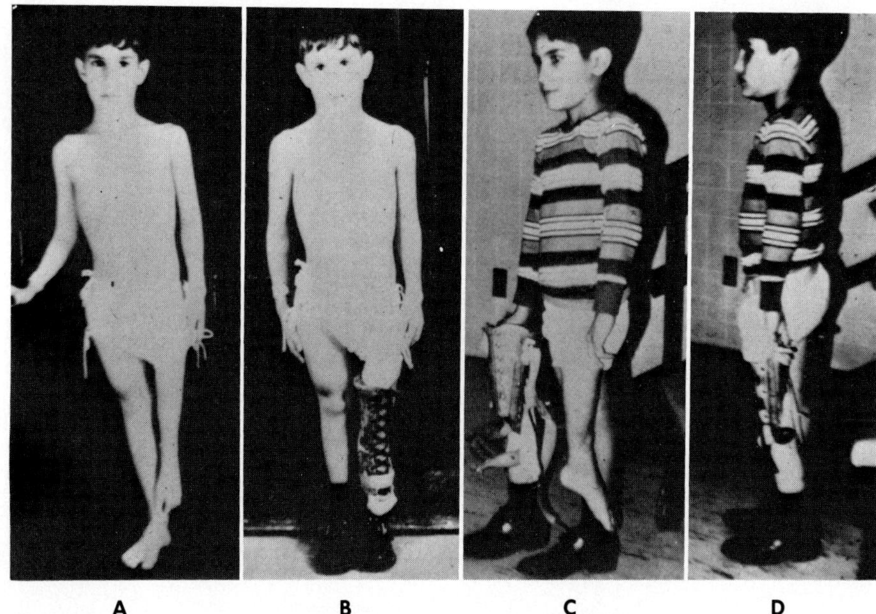

Fig. 40-65. A, Left leg, PFFD, Aitken class C. **B,** Early prosthetic fitting around deformity and without surgery. **C,** After definitive treatment: knee fusion and Van Nes rotation plasty. Foot and ankle are turned 180 degrees. **D,** Below-knee prosthesis with outside knee hinge. With foot in equinus, prosthetic knee is fully extended. When foot dorsiflexes, prosthetic knee will flex 90 degrees. (From Rossi, T. V., and Kruger, L. M.: Orthot. Prosthet. **29**(2):37-57, 1975.)

the short side should be ablated in the asymmetrical PFFD patient.

Van Nes turnplasty

Another special prosthesis is the below-knee modification used for the Van Nes turnplasty. Here the child has been treated by an osteotomy of the tibia (leg) with rotation of the distal portion 180 degrees, so that the ankle, now at knee level, will substitute for the knee joint, and the foot will be used as the shank portion to power the knee. When the foot dorsiflexes it will simulate knee flexion, and when the foot plantarflexes, it will act as an extensor of the shank portion of the prosthesis. This requires construction of a below-knee prosthesis with a thigh corset and side bars and a SACH foot (Fig. 40-65). The socket must be constructed to accept the foot as the shank with weight bearing on the plantar aspect of the foot, in particular the heel and longitudinal arch. Relief must be provided for the toes and for the dorsum of the foot, which is in the posterior part of the socket. Preflexion of the socket is necessary to accommodate for the restricted range of motion of the ankle joint, which is now acting as the knee joint. The thigh corset must conform to the anatomy of the leg with adequate padding over the pretibial area. Since the axis of rotation of a normal knee joint is different from the axis of rotation of this converted ankle joint, alignment of the knee hinges may be difficult. Suitable socket fit and knee joint alignment provide the individual with a below-knee prosthesis that is of great benefit in climbing stairs and ramps or running.

REFERENCES

1. Aitken, G. T., and Frantz, C. H.: Management of the child amputee. In American Academy of Orthopaedic Surgeons: Instructional course lectures, vol. 18, Ann Arbor, Mich., 1960, J. W. Edwards, Publisher.
2. Billock, J., and Childress, D. S.: Supracondylar suspension technique for below elbow amputation, Orthot. Prosthet., Dec., 1972.
3. Kuhn, G.: Treatment of the child with severe limb deficiencies, Inter-Clin. Info. Bull. **10:**1-26, 1970.
4. Setogucci, Y., Sumida, C., and Shaperman, J.: The CAPP two way shoulder, Inter-Clin. Info. Bull., Feb., 1977.
5. Shaperman, J.: The CAPP terminal device, Inter-Clin. Info. Bull. **14**(2):1-12, 1975.
6. Sullivan, R. J., and Celihyal, F.: The functional use of phocomelia and digital appendages, Inter-Clin. Info. Bull., **15:**1-8, 1976.
7. Sypniewski, B.: Age of initial fitting, Inter-Clin. Info. Bull. **9:**11-14, 1972.
8. Trefler, E.: T.D. activation for infant amputees, Inter-Clin. Info. Bull., June, 1970.
9. Vanderwerkan, E., and Paul, S.: Modification of the Hepp-Kuhn arm, Inter-Clin. Info. Bull. **10**(9):15-16, 1971.

CHAPTER 41

The multiple limb – deficient child

ERNST MARQUARDT

Prior to the 1950s adult prosthetics in Germany ranged from good to excellent in both the quality of the prosthesis and medical care. However, for children, each prosthetist had to build on his own personal experiences. There was no systematic treatment of the limb-deficient child; nor were there organized limb-deficiency clinics or child amputee clinics. There was no special education or organized interchange of ideas, practices, and experiences among workers with child amputees. No center was able to claim the presence of a complete clinic team, such as that started in Grand Rapids, Michigan, or other similar teams in the United States of America. There were no special devices or equipment for children's prosthetics. Patients with congenital limb deficiencies were treated on an individual basis in the regular orthopaedic hospitals. In some of these hospitals, such as in Berlin, Hannover, Heidelberg, Muenster, and Volmarstein, experience in certain limb deficiencies existed in the orthopaedic and prosthetic services. However, they did not work together as a full team, and each center developed its own ideas without exchange of ideas with others in the same field.

The philosophy of upper limb devices centered on the development of technical aids for limb-deficient persons. Soft leather sockets for below-elbow amputees had adaptors so that spoons, forks, pencils, or other items could be attached directly to the prosthesis.[40,41] In 1917, Biesalski[2] demonstrated a 9-year-old boy with new bilateral terminal devices. On one side, the boy had the "Finger-Klaue" and on the other side the "Spann-Klaue," both developed by Fischer[5] in Berlin. This boy was able to demonstrate that both of these were as practical as the hook; however, these terminal devices were not widely used and were soon forgotten.

It was widely assumed that children with transverse deficiencies of the upper limbs or children with traumatic amputations should be fitted with prostheses only after they had completed their growth. Because of this philosophy, it is understandable that the Krukenberg procedure[1,12,43] had greater acceptance in Germany than in the United States. With this procedure, the bilateral amputee was able to achieve independence in many of the activities of daily living. For the very high upper limb amputee, the Heidelberg pneumatic prosthesis gave additional independence for some individuals, but did not have a wide sphere of influence.*

Lower limb prostheses for children were even more provincial and personalized. They were generally fitted with the most simple walking devices that could be constructed. Many of these were stirrups fixed by splints or leather sockets that functioned as extensions.

THE BEGINNING OF MODERN PROSTHETICS

The 1950s proved to be an exciting and revolutionary time for children's prosthetics in Germany. Three factors were central to the changes that occurred in the field. The first of these was

*6, 17-20, 22-25, 30, 31, 45.

the visit of the German Study Group to the United States in 1952 and the outpouring of new ideas resulting from this stimulation. The second was the international cooperation that developed with Kessler of New Jersey, providing advice and stimulation to his German colleagues in the development of comprehensive clinic programs. The third event was the thalidomide catastrophe.*

In 1952, the German orthopaedic surgeon, Hepp, and a group of experts in prosthetics came to the United States to review the progress and problems encountered in the prosthetic centers in that country. In the following years, Hepp[7] and his co-worker Kuhn[13] developed special casting techiniques for the upper limb and the fabrication of a new plastic socket. This is now well known as the Muenster socket (Fig. 41-1). They introduced the active hook, which proved to be the most universal and most functional of all terminal devices. Their work in research and development was made easier by the German Federal Government providing money for prosthetic centers, first in Kiel, and later in Muenster. However, despite these advances, there were still no special units for children in all of Germany.

The second of these major factors was my visit to the Kessler Institute for Rehabilitation in New Jersey and the development of a close friendship with Kessler. I also made contact with numerous other prosthetic clinic teams in the United States and a generous exchange of information resulted. While observing Kessler's patients with kineplasty and body-powered, as well as pneumatic, prostheses, I learned of enormous possibilities inherent in the body's own compensatory functions and of the limited value of artificial limbs for congenitally armless persons. By watching the children with and without their prostheses, my colleagues and I realized the need to improve all of the body's own compensatory functions as the child develops activities of daily living.[17-20] Following these experiences, we developed the Pat-A-Cake prosthesis for armless babies, which allowed us to give them simple grasp at an early age. When these were fitted early, combined with prosthetic training that emphasized motivation and play, better results than had previously been thought possible were obtained.

During the years 1958 to 1962, there was an enormous increase in newborn children with multiple, symmetrical, longitudinal limb deficiencies.* In the upper limbs, there was a predominant reduction on the radial side of the hand and forearm, in combination with lower limb deficiencies in either the tibia, femur, or both† These

*14-16, 32, 33, 36, 44.

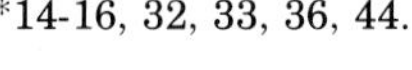

*8, 14, 20, 25, 32, 33, 36, 44.

†5294 upper limbs of 2647 thalidomide victims were reviewed in November, 1978, and registered by the "*Stiftung Hilfswerk für behinderte Kinder*" *Bonn-Bad Godesberg.*

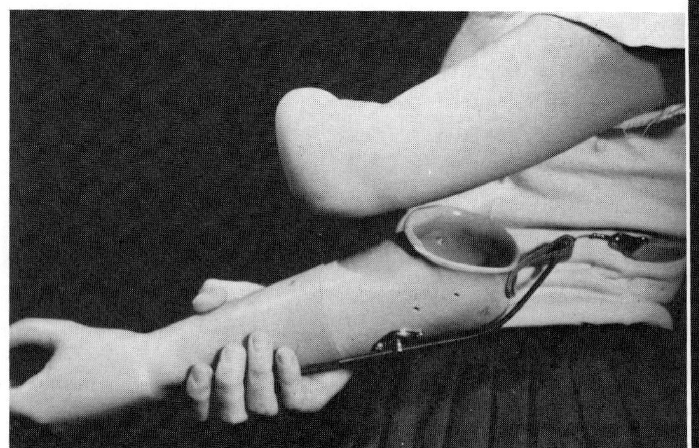

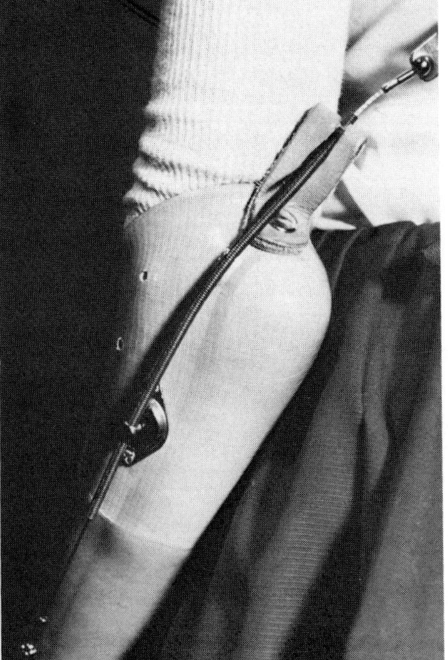

Fig. 41-1. Münster socket for very short below-elbow amputee. **A,** Very short stump flexed at 90 degrees with prosthesis held alongside. **B,** Prosthesis on stump. Note that with elbow extended, fit over proximal end of ulna and distal humerus prevents full extension of elbow.

limb deficiencies were often combined with abnormalities of the spine and potentially with every other body system. These abnormalities were later shown to be associated with maternal ingestion of thalidomide early in pregnancy.

These types of longitudinal deficiencies were not new and had been reported since antiquity. What was new was the enormous number that seemed to be almost an epidemic of multiple limb – deficient children. Prior to the thalidomide episode, between 1953 and 1958, thirty-seven children were seen in the orthopaedic hospital at the University of Heidelberg. However, from 1959 through 1962, 216 children had multiple limb deficiencies. In the following 2 years, after the withdrawal of thalidomide from the market, only ten children were seen with this type of limb deficiency. Faced with these numbers it is understandable that a major investment in time, research, and ingenuity was directed to the multiple limb – deficient child.

PHILOSOPHY OF TREATMENT – 1960s

The simple fitting of a prosthesis or multiple prostheses for these children is not adequate. As we struggled to make them as independent as possible, a whole philosophy of care developed in our center.

The treatment of a limb-deficient child is centered in the family, not in the hospital.[18-25] The mother is the child's best therapist under the supervision of the clinic team – physician, occupational therapist, and physical therapist (Fig. 41-2). All instruction should be channeled through her, or the father, or both. Whenever possible, the training, whether the child uses the prosthesis or not, should be conducted in the home.

It is important that all possible sensory contact with the feet be stimulated. The infant should be permitted to see his feet uncovered and encouraged to play with them (Fig. 41-3). If there are small digits or hands off the shoulder they should be trained to appreciate touch and grasp. Even if they seem functionless, eventually they may have important prosthesis control functions, which will need the most acute sensory input. If there is hip dysplasia, the Pavlik harness or similar treatment is recommended, since the feet will be allowed full freedom. If there are no arms, the head must be protected from bruising as the child starts to walk. A helmet or a ring of sponge rubber or other material can provide such protection until stability of walking has been achieved (Fig. 41-4).

If the child can eat and play, even deformed hands are better than a prosthesis. However, if one side is functionally behind the other and cannot be used in bimanual activity, a prosthesis is necessary. The infant at 6 to 8 months of age can be successfully fitted with a passive prosthesis allowing gross grasp. At this age, it is expected the infant will include the prosthesis into its body

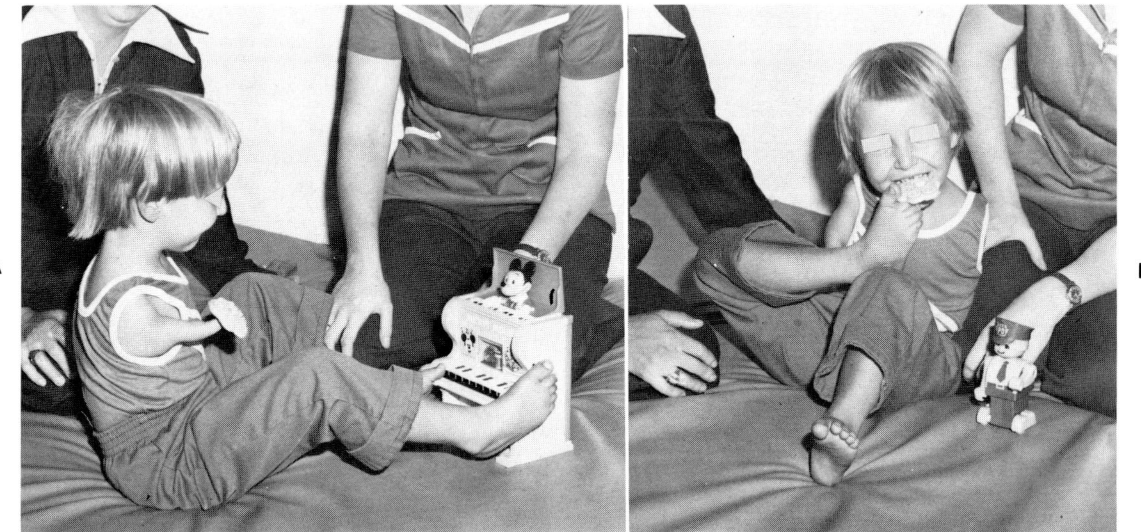

Fig. 41-2. Training in use of foot should include mother as integral part of program. **A,** Therapist instructs child in using toes as hand for play function. **B,** Child is encouraged to use foot to feed himself. Mother is always part of this instruction so that program continues at home, as well as in hospital.

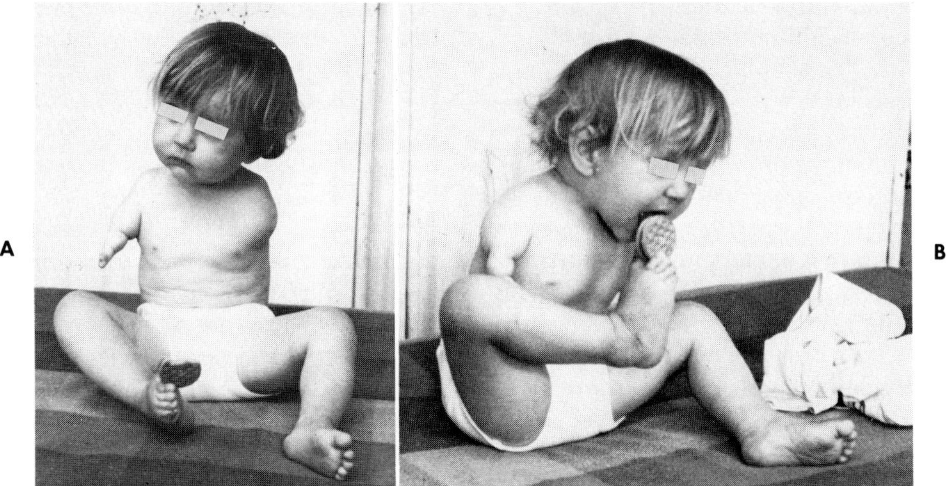

Fig. 41-3. Child with severe upper limb deficiencies is encouraged to learn to use feet as hands. **A,** This child with left upper amelia, upper right severe phocomelia with only one digit. Note use of great toe for prehensile function grasping cookie between it and second toe. **B,** Mobility of ankle, knee, and hip as well as spine is required for child to feed himself.

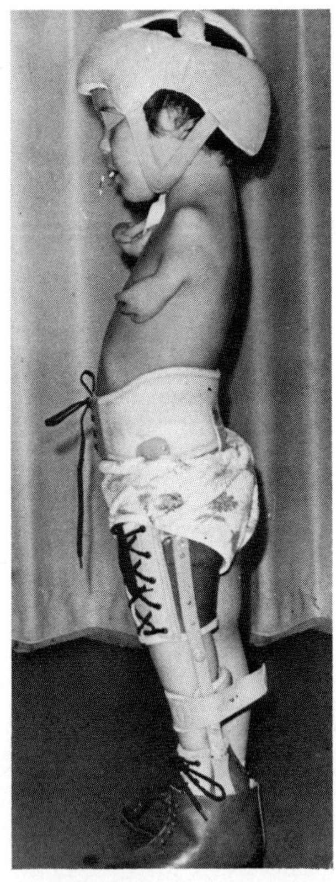

Fig. 41-4. For multiple limb–deficient children, particularly with severe upper limb deficiencies, balance is problem. Helmet or headgear protect against head injury when child falls.

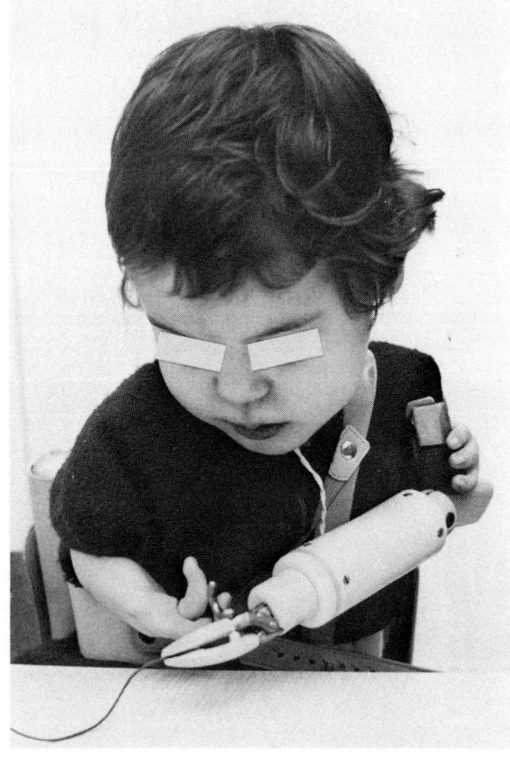

Fig. 41-5. Phocomelic child with specially designed pneumatic prosthesis.

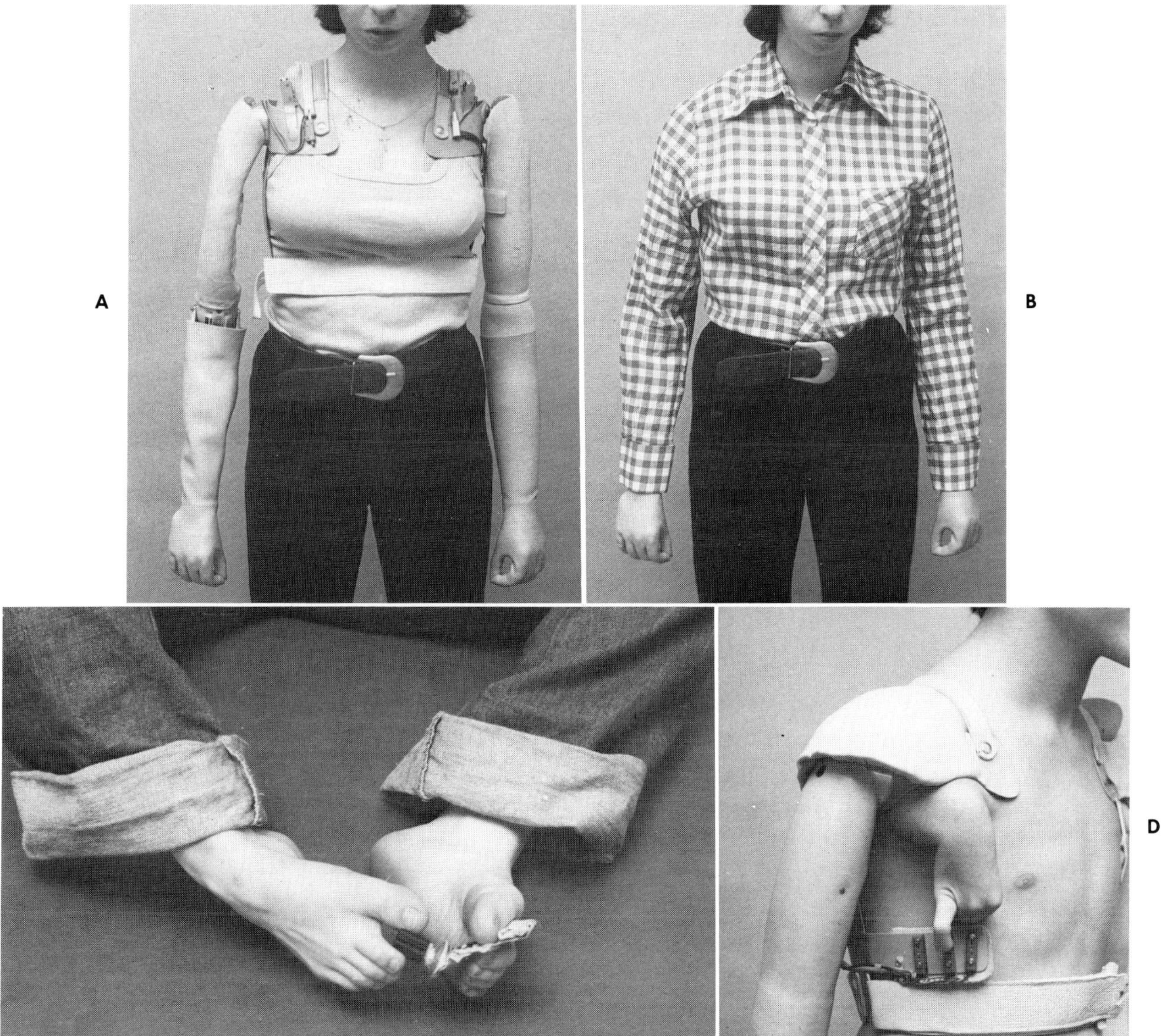

Fig. 41-6. A, Heidelberg hybrid prosthetic system for armless children has been fitted to patient with bilateral upper amelia (note Simpson frame socket). Active function is on right side only. Microswitches in both shoulders are necessary to provide (1) elbow flexion and extension, (2) pronation-supination, (3) shoulder positioning, and (4) opening and closing of hand. **B,** When patient is fully clothed, cosmetic restoration is good. **C,** Even though this girl uses prostheses well, she still preferred to use her feet "as hands" for all fine work, including hygiene and self-care. **D,** Eighteen-year-old boy with phocomelic hands demonstrates use of microswitches activated by phocomelic fingers, replacing switches on shoulder cap used on amelic patients.

image. If it allows for increased function and activity, the prosthesis should be accepted without difficulty.

The provision of an actively powered prosthesis starts about the beginning of the second year of life.[17-20,22,25] Shoulder movements, or if present, small digits emanating directly from the shoulders, can be used to control carbon-dioxide pneumatic-powered prostheses (Fig. 41-5). The active prosthesis for children over the age of 4 has an active grasping function with active wrist rotation and an active elbow joint with automatic lock. Training of the child with the prosthesis is adapted for the stage of development present at that time. The actual technical provision of the prostheses and exercise within a therapy setting are insufficient. If these prostheses are to become functional, they must be supplemented cleverly by individual pedagogical and psychological guidance of the children *and their parents,* which is provided by the prosthetic team. Nevertheless, the success of bilateral arm amputees fitted with pneumatic prostheses cannot be reached by amelic and phocomelic children.[30]

Between 1957 and 1977, in Heidelberg, sixty-seven amelic and phocomelic children were fitted with pneumatic-powered arm prostheses, from ages 2 to 5. During this same interval, 317 children with transverse upper limb deficiencies, mostly unilateral transverse forearm deficiencies, were fitted with body-powered prostheses. It is a significant observation that 80% of this latter group continued to be successful prosthetic wearers. On the other hand, sixty-one of sixty-seven children fitted with different types of pneumatic-powered prostheses have ultimately rejected them, some after years of wearing and with excellent prosthetic accomplishment. Only six of these sixty-seven continued to wear externally powered arm prostheses in their latest version, which is an electropneumatic hybrid system (Fig. 41-6).[31] All sixty-seven are well trained in the use of the feet. Significantly, those prosthetic wearers have been noted to be more interested in the aesthetics of the prosthesis as related to their social life than in the functional value. However, this changes with age as increasing problems of hip stiffness appear. In Heidelberg, we have therefore come to the conclusion that training the infant in the use of his feet is most important and that fitting of externally powered prostheses may be delayed, unless it is recognized early that hip problems will eventually cause stiffness or lack of function. These consequences will prevent the child's foot from reaching the mouth. In this latter instance externally powered prostheses should be fitted earlier.

The Heidelberg philosophy may then be summarized as follows:

1. For the upper limb amelic child, the feet and not the arm prostheses will provide maximum function. For the phocomelic child, all digits, both upper and lower, should be used to compensate for loss of normal function.

2. In general, conventional body-powered prostheses for amelic and phocomelic children provide so little function that they are likely to be rejected, particularly in those who are able to use the feet as hands. By the same token, externally powered prostheses are too heavy and complicated. They provide too little effective function for the patient's need and this, coupled with high cost and discomfort of wearing, causes rejection.

3. Prostheses for amelic and phocomelic children are still in the experimental state. The major problem is in positioning the terminal device in space and not so much the terminal device itself. Simpson[38,39] has developed a brilliant technical solution to this problem, but weight and complexity of the mechanism have precluded its general acceptance.

4. When amelic or phocomelic individuals request an arm prosthesis at or after the age of puberty, this request is considered and discussed with the patient, along with a discussion of all pros and cons. When a decision is made to prescribe prostheses for these individuals, it is our policy to prescribe one functional prosthesis—an electropneumatic hybrid system—for the dominant side and a cosmetic arm with the power pack in it for the nondominant side. Both are fixed on a Simpson frame. This is at best a compromise, providing the best possible appearance, the lightest weight, and some function (Fig. 41-6).[31,35] Practically all of these individuals continue to use the feet as hands.

Of major importance is the recognition of the fact that the prosthesis should never impede the child's function. When it is recognized that wearing a prosthetic device diminishes important functions, the prosthesis should be removed in favor of such function as was present without it.

In 1962 and 1963, the Federal Republic of Germany opened special units for "Dysmeliekinder" in eight other centers, in addition to those clinics which already existed in Muenster and Heidelberg. Programs for research and development of prosthetic devices as well as the testing of prostheses and technical aides for limb-deficient children were developed. Annual workshops and meetings were organized, and, in 1964, I made my first statement about the development of compensatory functions of the clubhand by the patient and warned against early operative intervention. In addition to developing new body-powered and externally powered prostheses for the upper limbs, a new electric driven vehicle was developed in Muenster by Kuhn. My Horowitz lecture in 1968, "The Total Treatment of the Limb Deficient Child"[25] and the publication in 1974 of "10 Jahre Entwicklung und Erprobung von Hilfen und Hilfsmitteln für behinderte Kinder" spelled out concisely the development of prosthetics and technical aids and training for limb-deficient children, which I believe should be integrated into the total philosophy of care. In the years following the thalidomide episode, in which some 2500 children were victimized in the Federal Republic of Germany, such a philosophy was developed at Heidelberg and in the other centers. This was espoused and financed by the goverment and especially by the Social Security System for the benefit of these victims. On the basis of evaluation of 2000 of these 2500 children, my conclusions on the treatment and rehabilitation program have continued to develop and, in instances, to change. The care of these patients continues.

SPECIAL SURGICAL PROCEDURES FOR THE MULTIPLE LIMB–DEFICIENT CHILD

A number of surgical procedures have been used to advantage in children with multimembral deficiencies, which might have application only occasionally in selected cases of single-limb deficiency. Because of the degree of functional disability in patients with multiple deficiencies, procedures that are designed to provide even limited improvement in function are more frequently indicated. Several procedures that have been used to treat bony overgrowth, enhance function of above-elbow prosthetic use, provide surgically assisted prehension in a forearm stump, as well as considerations in the positioning of residual prehensile members are reviewed in some detail.

Stump capping

Contrary to a generally held opinion of a few years ago, bony overgrowth has, in fact, been observed in transverse diaphyseal deficiencies. This overgrowth and its concomitant stump attenuation is particularly troublesome when it occurs in a weight-bearing segment, such as the tibia, and is, of course, most disabling when the opposite limb is also the site of a deficiency. Bony overgrowth of a transhumeral deficiency may be equally disabling. It can eventuate in catastrophe should it occur in a bilateral short above-elbow stump, necessitating revision to a higher level such that the prosthesis would be of the shoulder disarticulation type rather than the above-elbow type.

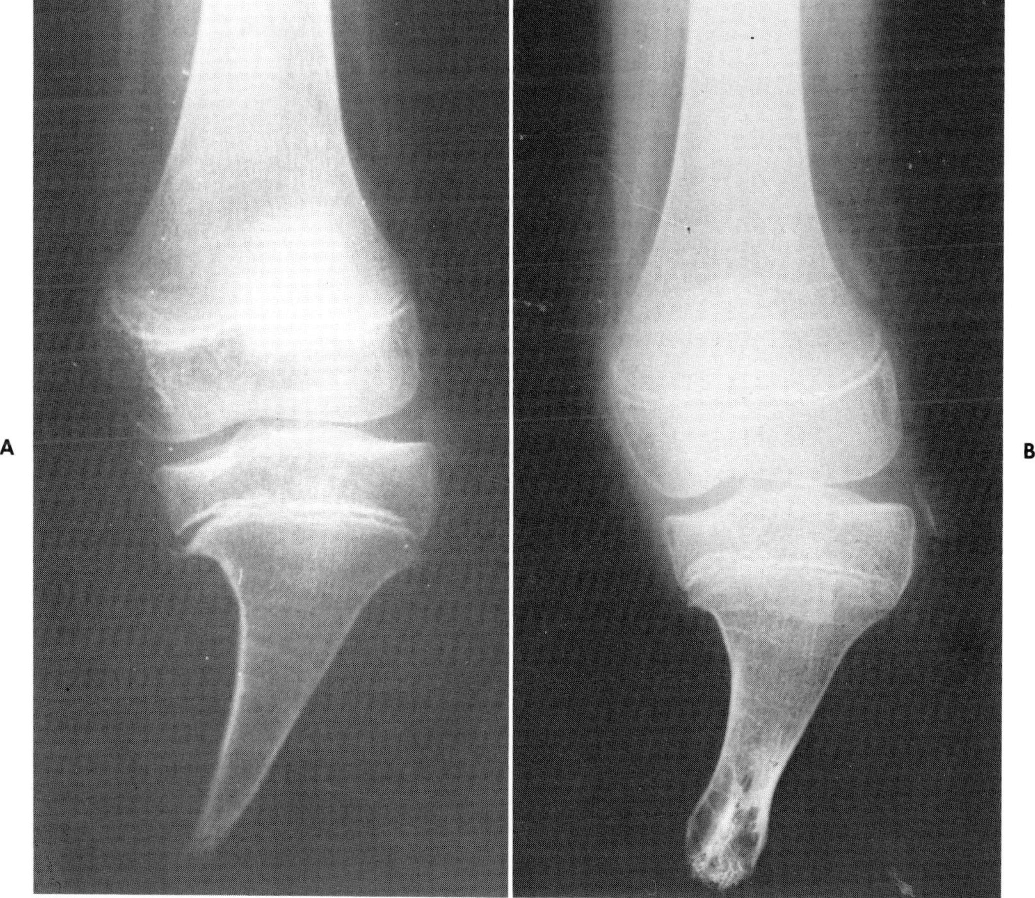

Fig. 41-7. A, Preoperative osseous overgrowth of the tibia–"spiking." **B,** Postoperative stump capping. "Spike" has been converted to "disarticulation stump."

The conventional practice in treating bony overgrowth has, in the past, taken the form of either resection of the overlying bursa and shortening of the bony stump or, in some cases, a formal reamputation at a higher level. In 1972, Swanson[42] reported the development of a silicone rubber implant for capping a transtibial amputation stump. He also used this silicone cap for revising amputation stumps in which bony overgrowth had occurred. Buchtiarow[28] attempted stump capping using a bone and cartilage transplant for transdiaphyseal femoral stumps. Stimulated by these experiences, I have developed a technique for capping stumps with osseous overgrowth using autogenous cartilage–bone transplants.[27,28,35] The goal is conversion of a transhumeral or transtibial amputation into a stump resembling that seen in a disarticulation (Fig. 41-7).

A transplant source is not usually available in cases of single-limb deficiency, but in the quadrimembral-deficient child various reconstructive procedures on other parts may make a transplant source readily available. When a PFFD, for instance, is present, the cartilaginous and bony cap from the femur may be used. In the same condition, when knee arthrodesis is planned, the articular surface of the distal femur may be salvaged for transplant.

The operation may be used in cases of overgrowth in congenital deficiencies of the humerus or in treatment of the condition in a transdiaphyseal femoral or transtibial amputation. In the humerus it seems preferable to use a cartilage-bone transplant without a growth plate, unless there is good quality soft tissue overlying the end of the stump, or the patient has bilateral *short* above-elbow stumps.

In the weight-bearing bones, on the other hand, it is desirable to procure a transplant with an epiphyseal plate to obtain additional length. In those cases where amputation is carried out for trauma, an epiphysis from the amputated limb may be used. When the procedure is done for overgrowth of the humerus an effort is also made to attain optimal growth. In most instances weight-bearing training will stimulate continued growth in the proximal humeral growth plate. If the condition of distal skin permits, transplantation of a growth plate here may be carried out.

Surgical procedure. The incision is planned to avoid scarring in the skin of the end-bearing area. A medial or lateral longitudinal incision is made, starting a few centimeters proximal to the

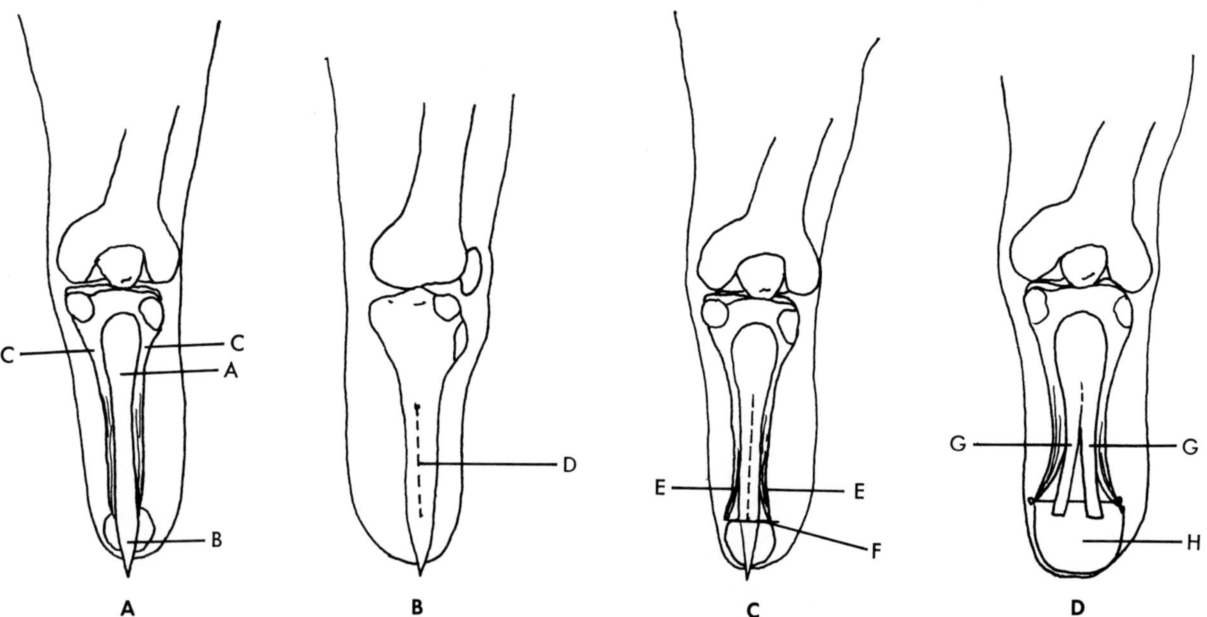

Fig. 41-8. Stump capping surgical procedure. **A,** Tibia is represented by *A* and *C*. Spike is *B*. **B,** From lateral diagram, incision, *D,* should be made in such position that it will not cause prosthetic problems later. It should neither rise to flare of tibia nor extend down over end of stump. **C,** After elevation of musculoperiosteal flaps, *E,* spike is transected at *F* and removed. Tibia is then split longitudinally in proximal direction. **D,** Two pillars of tibia, *G,* are now gently separated and previously prepared stump cap, *H,* is applied over pillars. Stump cap may not be bigger than bursa, which should be closed over cartilage of stump cap. It may be fixed with screw or Kirschner wire.

end of the stump (Fig. 41-8, *B*). The bursal sac is opened, and the bony overgrowth is transected at its entry into the bursa and removed. Two or three periosteal and muscular flaps are then developed on the sides of the diaphysis and are reflected proximally. The diaphysis of the bone is then split longitudinally for a distance of at least 3 to 4 cm proximally from its tip (Fig. 41-8, *C*). The split ends are gently spread apart, with care taken to prevent fracturing. The cartilage and bone transplant is prepared with two grooves fashioned on either side of the bony portion to accept each of the arms of the split long bone (Fig. 41-8, *D*). Fixation of the transplant may be accomplished with two crossed Kirschner wires or with a centrally placed long intramedullary screw. The defect between the split ends of the long bone is packed with additional autogenous cancellous bone (Fig. 41-9). The periosteal-muscular flaps are then reattached to the transplant with sutures passed through small drill holes in the graft. The wound is repaired, avoiding skin tension, and, in lower limb stumps, a rigid plaster dressing is used. In above-elbow stumps a soft compression dressing is preferred.

Postoperative care. It is important to recog-

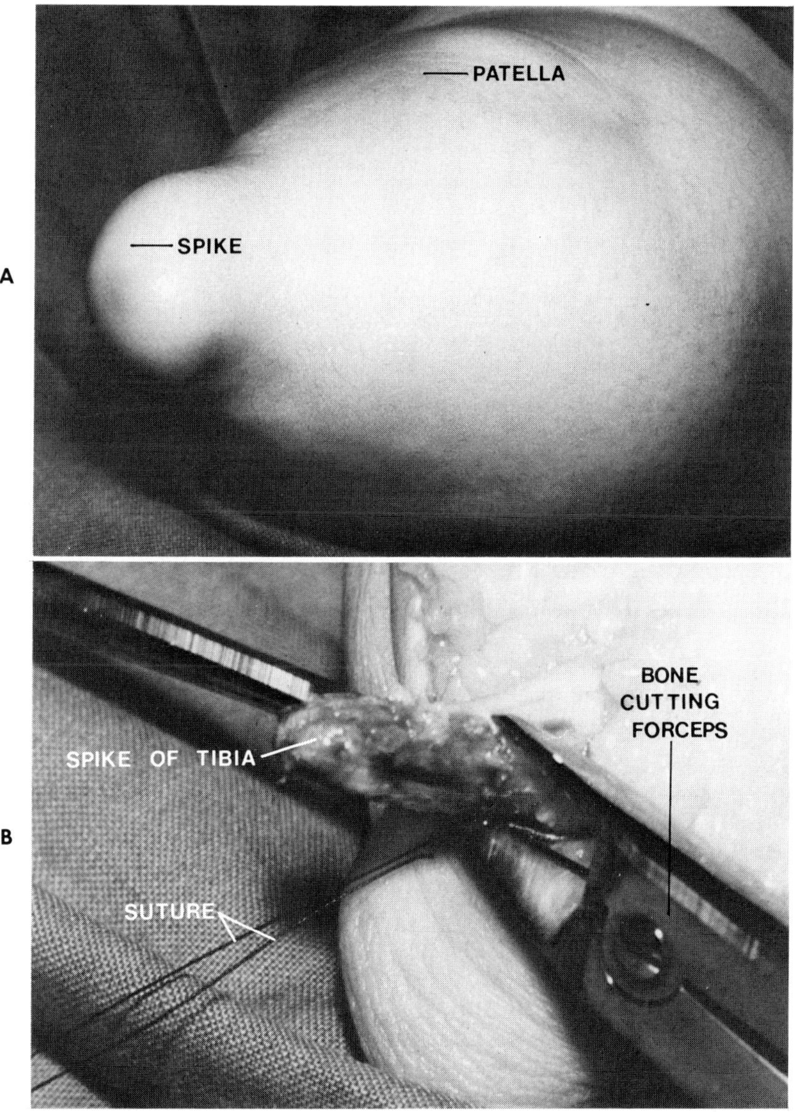

Fig. 41-9. Stump capping surgical procedure. **A,** Tibial stump with spike to left. Patella is at top. **B,** Spike has been exposed, and bone cutting forceps are about to cut off spiked portion of tibia. Note suture in musculoperiosteal flap that has been elevated.

Continued.

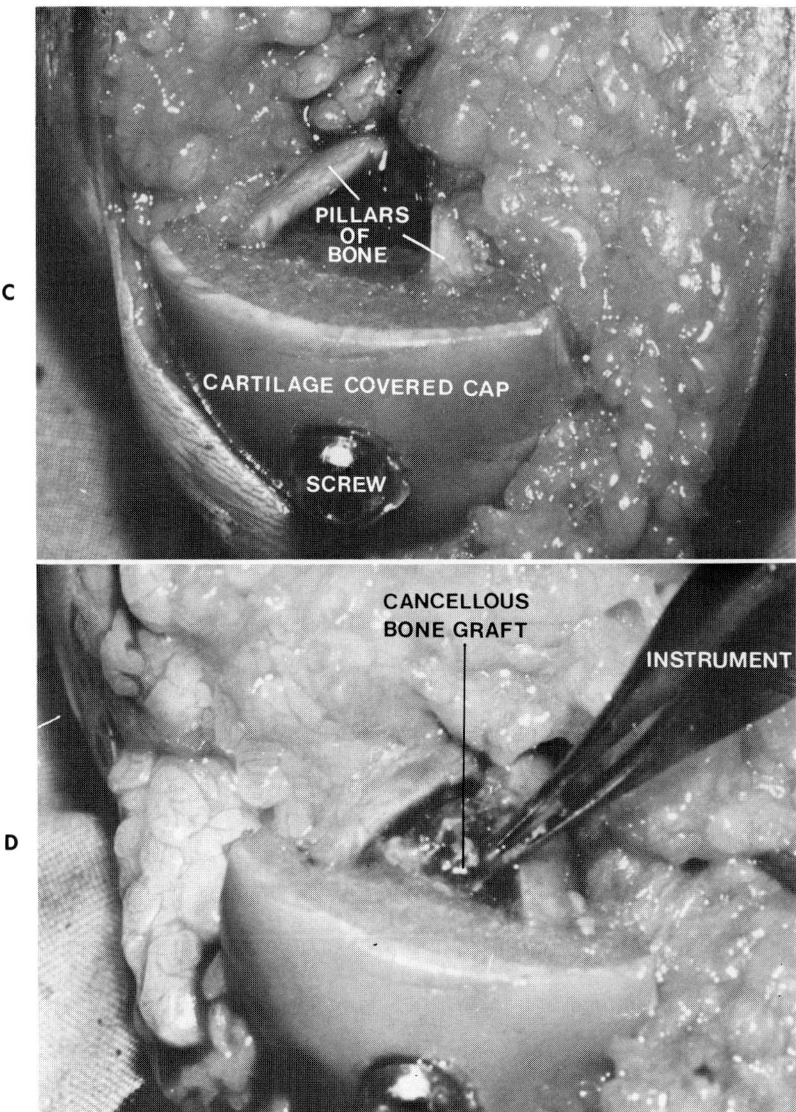

Fig. 41-9, cont'd. C, Tibia has been split and two pillars of bone separated. Cartilage covered cap has been attached and is held in place with single screw into center of shaft of tibia. **D,** Defect between capped pillars of tibia is now packed with autogenous cancellous bone graft.

nize that the success of this procedure depends, not only on the surgical technique, but also on the postoperative physical therapy training program, as well as on acceptance and use of a carefully designed prosthesis. These children should be maintained on a daily physical therapy program throughout growth. Just as the normal individual or the athlete requires constant conditioning to maintain maximum muscle strength and joint motion, so the limb-deficient child requires an ongoing training program.

Approximately 3 months after the stump-capping surgery, the conditioning, which is called for emphasis "end-bearing training," is commenced. The therapist teaches the patient to apply weight to the reconstructed stump. Initially, 2 or 3 kg of pressure are used and are gradually increased until the patient is able to take at least 50% of his body weight directly over the stump end. During this training an effort should be made to apply pressure to different surface areas of the stump so that the loading will ultimately be distributed over the entire stump end. This training is conducted in coordination with the other daily exercises necessary for rehabilitation. End-bearing training should be repeated at intervals throughout the day.

Immediately after the end-bearing training

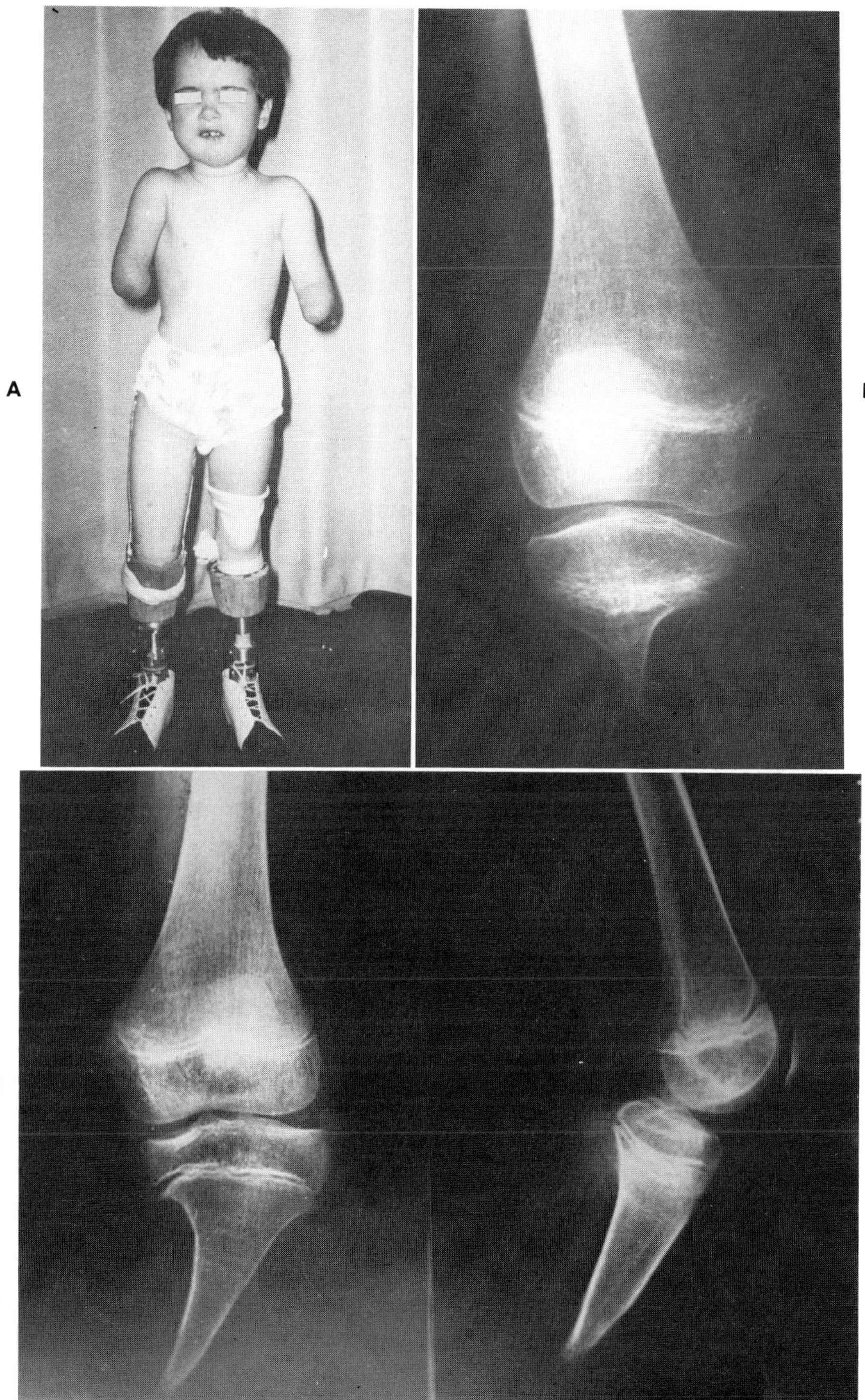

Fig. 41-10. A, At 26 months of age patient has been converted from stubbies to total-contact socket with supracondylar wedge suspension on left leg, and on right leg, because of ultrashort below-knee stump, she has been fitted with above-knee prosthesis with knee flexed at 90 degrees. Prostheses are unfinished at this stage. **B,** Prior to stump capping, right below-knee stump is very short. **C,** Prior to stump capping, left below-knee stump shows osseous overgrowth (spiking) and varus deformity, despite absence of fibula. At this point, painful bursa was clinically evident over area of osseous overgrowth.

Continued.

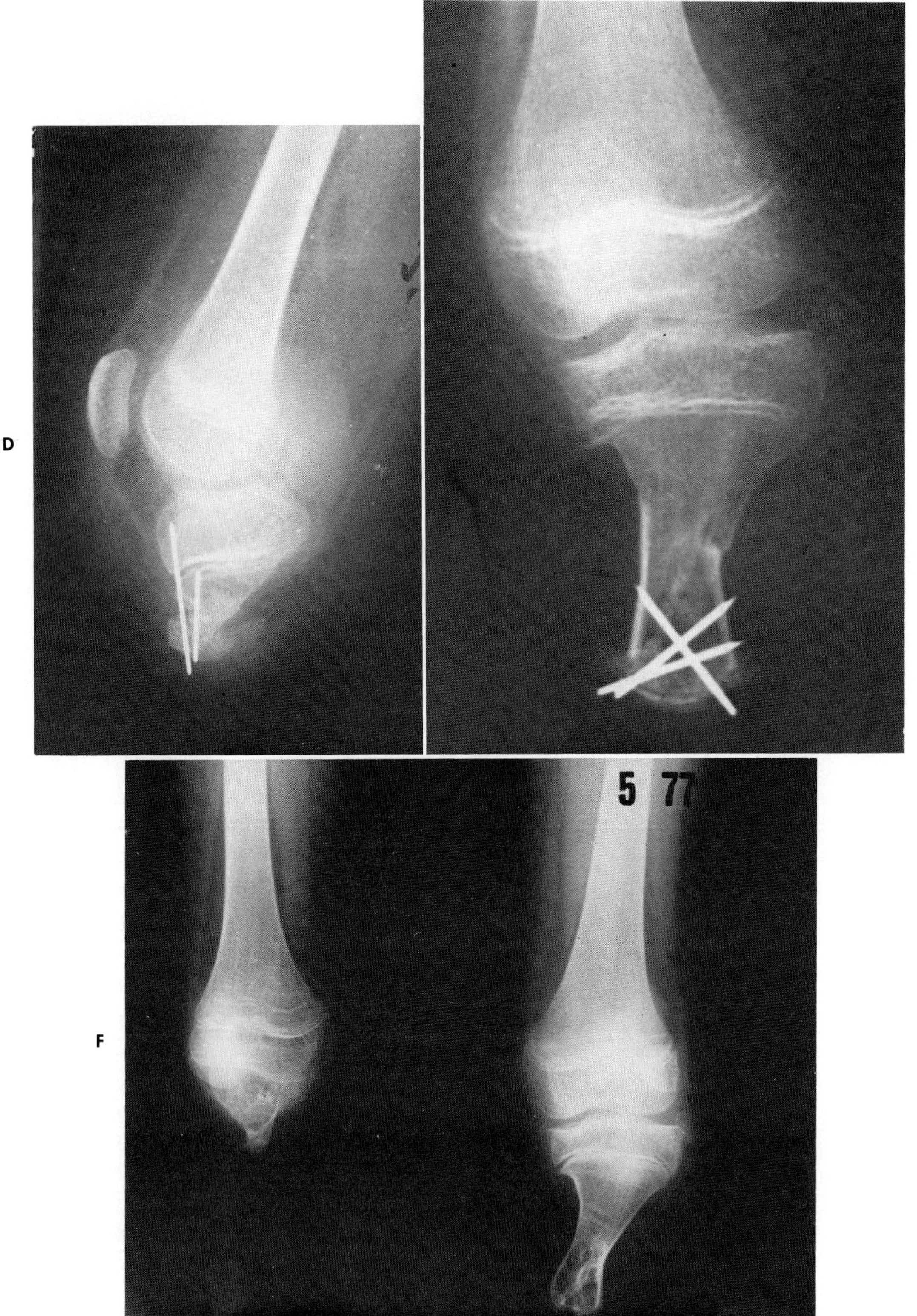

Fig. 41-10, cont'd. D, Roentgenogram of right below-knee stump 1 month after stump capping. **E,** Roentgenogram of left below-knee stump immediately after stump capping. **F,** Eleven months after stump capping, left cap is quite satisfactory. Right cap is beginning to absorb (6 months after surgical procedure).

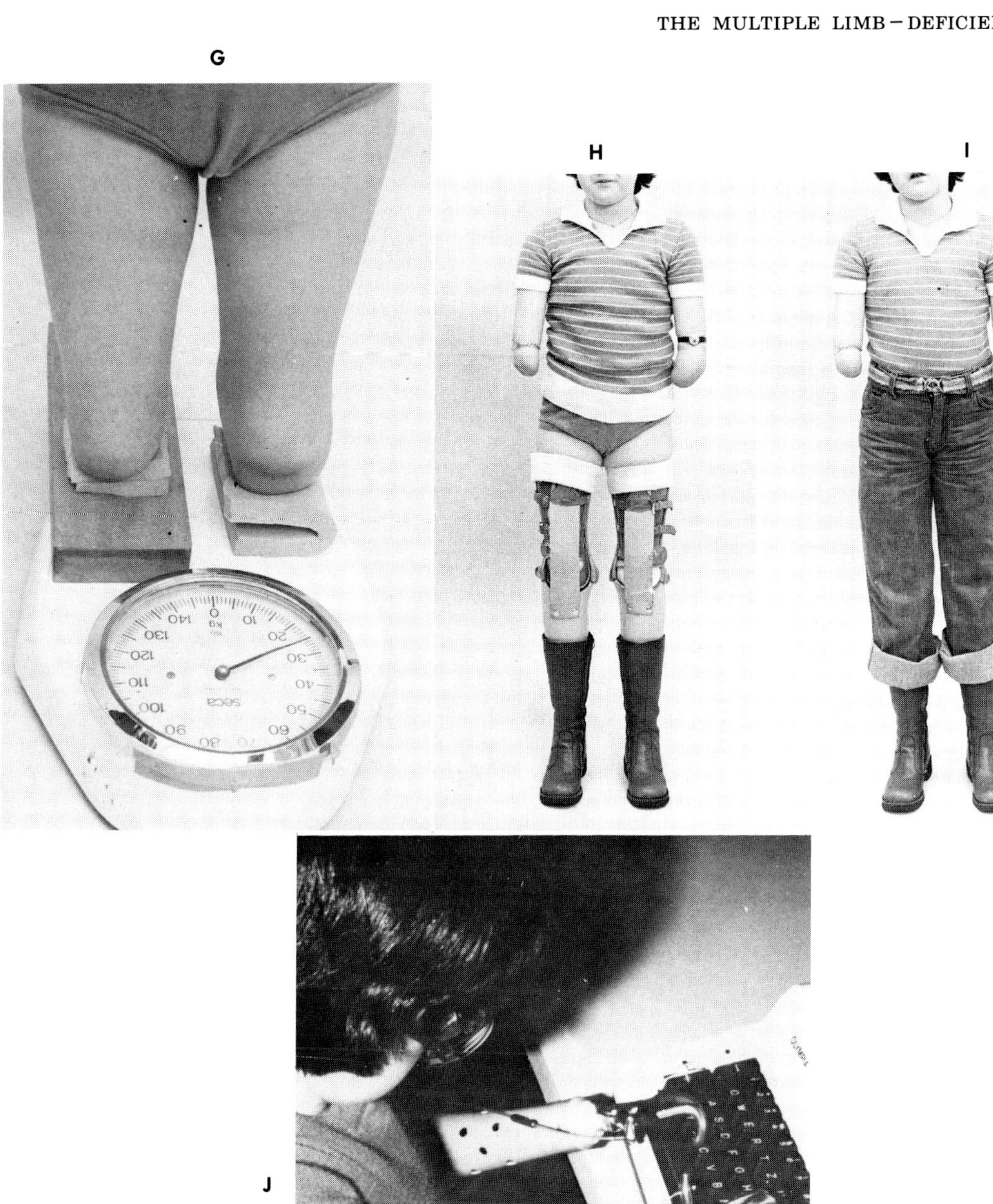

Fig. 41-10, cont'd. G, End-bearing training using scale to determine amount of pressure applied to stumps. End-bearing training must be continued throughout growth. **H,** Patient with new prostheses incorporating below-knee end-bearing on left leg. Absorption of graft on right leg negated beneficial effect of surgical procedure, and she is wearing again a right above-knee prosthesis with the knee flexed at 90 degrees with corset and side bars. She is fully ambulatory with these prostheses. **I,** Patient fully clothed wearing her new below-knee prosthesis on left leg and above-knee prosthesis with knee flexed 90 degrees on right leg, without arm prostheses. **J,** When arms are applied she uses them well and is even able to type.

session the therapist should also show the patient and the parent the technique of stretching the skin distally over the stump to prevent contracture or tightening of the skin over the reconstructed end. During this period of time the healing and conditioning of the stump should be evaluated and the decision made as to the time for prosthetic prescription and training. In the weight-bearing limbs the prosthesis should be designed to use the end-bearing capacity of the stump to ensure continued hypertrophy and tolerance.

Case report. The child in Fig. 41-10 was born on July 12, 1965, the first child of healthy parents with two normal siblings. There was no history of congenital limb deficiency in the family, nor were there other congenital anomalies. In the early pregnancy, however, the mother had had considerable illness and taken numerous medications. At the time of birth it was noted that the child had transverse deficiencies of all four limbs, with the forearm deficient in the upper third bilaterally and the leg similarly deficient in the upper third bilaterally, with aplasia of the fibula. Additionally the child had a micrognathia and dysplasia of the tongue. She was first seen in my outpatient clinic on May 2, 1966, and in August her first stubby prostheses were fitted to her lower limbs. In January of 1967, she was fitted with cable-controlled below-elbow prostheses and below-knee prostheses with a thigh corset, but no knee joints were prescribed. In 1968, she was fitted with a below-knee prosthesis for the left leg with supracondylar wedge suspension. On the right side, because of the extreme short below-knee stump, she was fitted with a bent-knee prosthesis, with the knee flexed at 90 degrees, and she walked independently with these prostheses. In June of 1969, she received two new below-elbow prostheses with Muenster sockets and Dorrance hooks, as well as two new lower limb prostheses. By December of 1970, osseous overgrowth of the left tibial stump was noted, and by October of 1972, this had increased even though she had received treatment of skin traction and "extension therapy" of the skin—manual stretching by the mother. New sockets were prescribed. In October of 1975, there was increased spiking at the distal end of the tibia, which was now being handled with liners in the plastic sockets of her prostheses. By June of 1976, she had a painful bursa about the area of spiking at the distal tibia of the left below-knee stump, and there was a varus deviation of the tibia despite the fact that the fibula was absent. In July of 1976, a stump-capping procedure of the left below-knee stump was carried out with a homologous cartilage bone transplant to the cap supplemented by autogenous cancellous bone to fill the gap between the two branches of the split tibia. In December of 1976, the same procedure was carried out on the right tibia. Postoperatively, end-bearing training was instituted, and the left side did well; however, the right showed reduction of the transplant and increased pain. It required revision in March of 1978. The left below-knee stump remained healthy. Presently, this patient is wearing an above-knee prosthesis on the right side with 90-degree knee flexion and below-knee prostheses on the left for 12 to 13 hours a day. She wears her forearm prostheses only part time; nonetheless, she is completely independent in all activities of daily living.

Angulation osteotomy of the humerus

An amputee with a long above-elbow deficiency can use a body-powered prosthesis quite effectively. With the conventional fitting, however, the important and useful function of active pronation and supination of the forearm is absent. This may be provided by passive rotation of the terminal device at the wrist, but must be preset by the patient. This is particularly difficult for the bilateral above-elbow amputee to accomplish. In addition, mediolateral positioning of the forearm segment and terminal device through humeral rotation is usually deficient in strength and range. Passive rotation through a turntable elbow unit or the use of an externally powered rotation unit has never been completely satisfactory.

Although most amputees with long or middle length stumps, have essentially normal shoulder function and strength, full abduction and, particularly, full shoulder rotation cannot be transmitted through the stump-socket interface to the terminal device with the conventional above-elbow fitting.

In an effort to provide the above-elbow amputee with a simpler and more effective prosthetic device that might help to provide these additional functions, I have developed a technique of angulation osteotomy of the humeral stump.[26] Following this osteotomy of the distal humerus, an open-socket prosthesis suspended only by two straps may be used.[35] In the long above-elbow amputee the dorsal end of the stump may be left exposed for tactile sensation. With this fitting, the artificial elbow joint is set somewhat proximal to the distal end. External locking hinges are used. In the middle length stump the distal angulated humeral segment is maintained by one or two straps. This strap suspension is easy for the bilateral amputee to apply himself. More important, however, is that it frees the shoulder for full abduction and elevation, as well as allows full internal and external rotation to be transmitted to the prosthesis. The flanges necessary for stability in the conventional prosthesis are eliminated, and rotational stability and motion are provided by the angulated distal end of the stump in the socket. When the forearm is in a moderately extended position, the humeral rotation can also transmit a useful amount of pronation and supination at the terminal device.

Although angulation osteotomy is used primarily for the long and middle length above-elbow stump, it has also been used in the very long below-knee stump. In this instance, it provides the amputee not only with improved suspension of the prosthesis, but also provides a partial end-bearing capacity. As with the stump-capping procedure, angulation osteotomy of the distal tibia and fibula or humerus, should be followed by daily training in end-bearing. This is mandatory for proper conditioning of the stump.

Surgical procedure. For planning of angulation osteotomy, the length of the remaining humeral segment should be carefully measured. The planned length of the distal osteotomy fragment will depend on the volume of the stump. In a long slender stump as little as 3 cm for the angulated distal fragment may be acceptable. To accomplish this, the osteotomy must be started 4 cm above the distal end of the stump. In a large, flabby stump, however, it is necessary to have at least 5 cm of bone in the angulated segment to provide adequate suspension for the socket. An anterior angulation of the distal end in the sagittal plane of from 70 to 90 degrees in the neutral-zero method of measurement is planned.

The incision should be planned to extend no further distally than the lower level of the osteotomy site. It is important to prevent any damage to the blood supply of the distal fragment. No stripping of the periosteum of this distal segment is carried out. An incision 5 to 7 cm long is made from the distal level of the planned osteotomy site proximally. The periosteum is incised longitudinally directly over the area from which the wedge of bone is to be removed, usually anteriorly. The

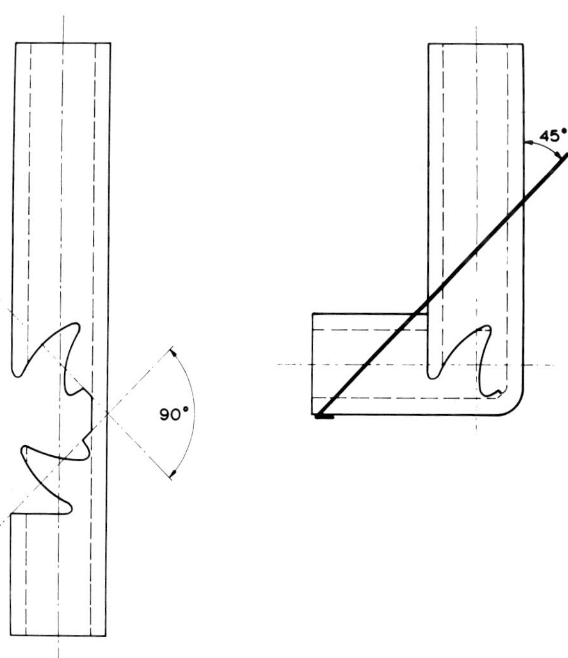

Fig. 41-11. Angulation osteotomy. **A,** Chosen osteotomy site is prepared by removal of trapezoidal wedge, using bone cutting forceps and rongeur. Using "interdigitating technique" irregular edges do not form trapezoidal fragment. **B,** When distal end is flexed, interdigitating areas provide for considerably more bony contact, and fixation with single Kirschner wire that crosses all four cortices should be carried out. Should posterior cortex fracture during bending maneuver, two Kirschner wires are necessary.

periosteum is carefully dissected from the area of wedge removal and further periosteal dissection carried only proximally to avoid denuding the distal fragment. Approximately three quarters of the thickness of the diameter of the bone is then removed in the shape of a trapezoid wedge. In the child, this can be most easily done with a bone-cutting forceps or rongeur. Proximally and distally the open cortex may be notched with a fine rongeur so that when the angulation osteotomy is closed, the notches will interdigitate to provide some stability and good bone apposition (Fig. 41-11).

The posterior cortex, supported by its intact periosteum, is now bent into the planned angulation. In the younger child this produces a fairly stable "green stick" fracturing, but maintains stability. The osteotomy is then fixed with a single Kirschner wire, which passes obliquely across the angulated bone at an angle of 45 degrees from the distal fragment through the proximal fragment, penetrating both cortices of each fragment. If, during the attempt to bend the posterior cortex, fracturing occurs and inherent stability is lost, a second Kirschner wire passed parallel to the first, but crossing the osteotomy, should provide the adequate fixation (Fig. 41-12). If there is any separation at the osteotomy site, the defect may be packed with cancellous bone from the removed wedge. The periosteum is then repaired. Suction drainage is placed, and the wound is closed in layers. A compression dressing is applied, but no

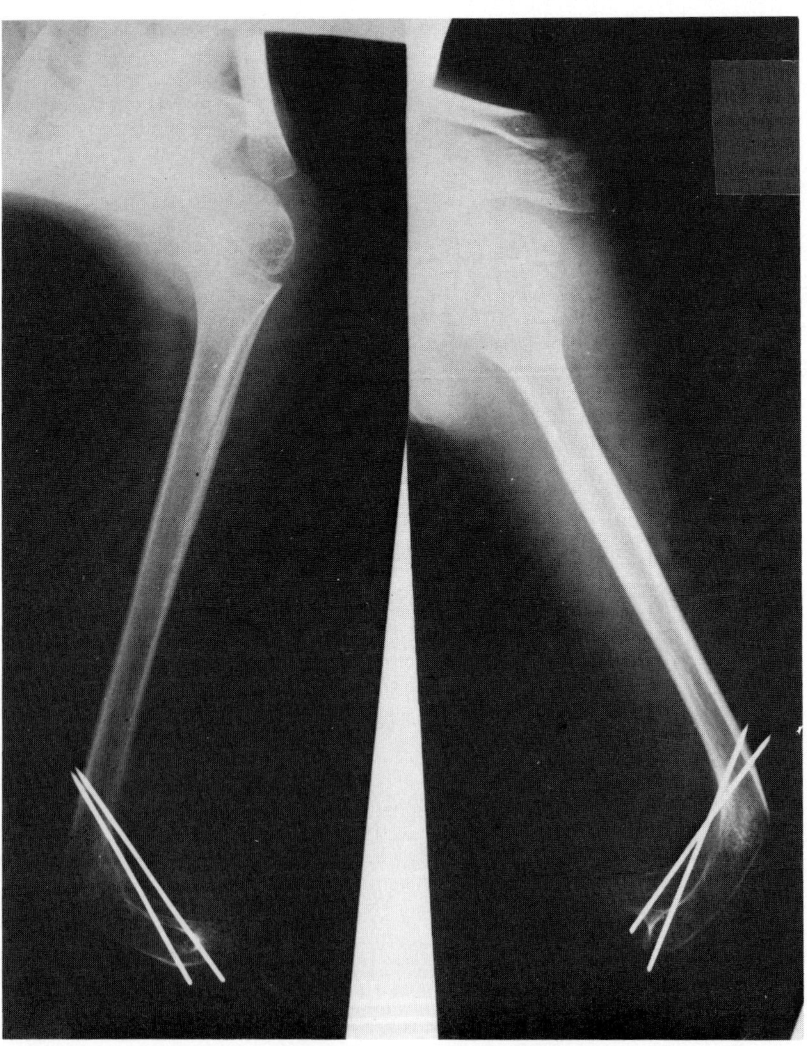

Fig. 41-12. Roentgenogram of angulation osteotomy. Osteotomy has been angulated approximately 60 degrees, and two Kirschner wires have been used for fixation. Kirschner wires should be pulled through posteriorly so as not to disrupt healing osteotomy when they are removed.

plaster of Paris cast is necessary. Suction tubes may be removed in 48 hours.

Patients with a shorter above-elbow stump may be treated by exposing the bone on its posterior side to carry out the posterior angulation osteotomy.

Postoperative care. At 6 to 8 weeks after angulation osteotomy the radiographs should demonstrate secure union. The Kirschner wires may be removed at this time. As with the stump-capping procedure, end-bearing training should be instituted as soon as bony healing is secure, in an effort to condition and prepare the stump for prosthetic use and over the long term to stimulate growth of bone both in size and length. Where angulation osteotomy has been used in the below-knee stump, it is particularly important to continue this training so that partial end bearing in the prosthesis can be used. In the humeral angulation osteotomy, the fitting with the new prosthesis

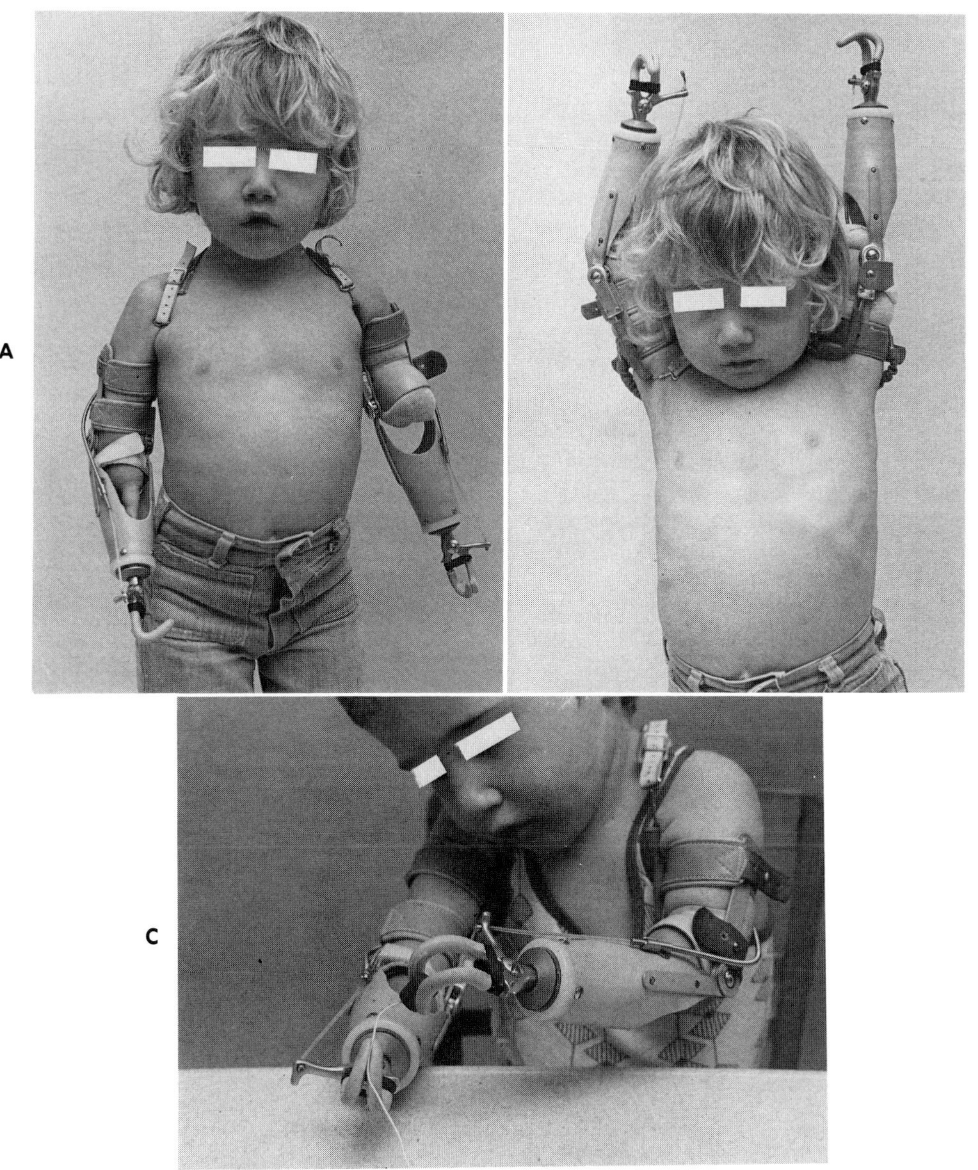

Fig. 41-13. A, Six-year-old patient, after humeral angulation osteotomy of long left above-elbow humeral stump, has been fitted with above-elbow prosthesis with "open splint construction," using outside locking elbow unit with closure straps, one anterior across upper humerus and second posterior across angulation osteotomy. **B,** This fitting provides for full mobilization of shoulder rather than restrictive fitting of conventional shoulder cap prosthesis for above-elbow amputee. **C,** Close-up shows frame construction with dual control cable.

may proceed at approximately 6 to 8 weeks after the operation (Fig. 41-13). In a young child it may be expected that the given angle will diminish approximately 1.3 to 1.5 degrees for every month of growth. However, a second or third angulation osteotomy during growth may be performed in preference to proximal revision of the amputation.

The Krukenberg procedure

In 1917, Hermann Krukenberg developed an operative procedure to convert a long forearm amputation stump into a pincer-like grasping organ with tactile sensation.[12] This operation has not received wide acceptance in the United States, probably due to cosmetic objections, but in Germany and elsewhere it is quite widely used.

It has been generally accepted that the prime indication for the Krukenberg procedure is the bilateral below-elbow amputee who is blind and absolutely requires tactile sensation for independence. Children with multimembral deficiencies, however, who have bilateral long or medium length below-elbow forearm stumps should also be considered for this procedure. I prefer to wait until the child is 10 years old before performing the procedure, since extensive training is required to gain the functional capacity needed. The younger child has difficulty in maintaining sufficient concentration and attention needed to satisfactorily work with the physical and occupational therapy training required.

Surgical procedure. In his original technique, Krukenberg used a simple U-shaped incision, bisecting the forearm with either one or two V-shaped flaps, based proximally, to cover the proximal portion of the cleft of the split forearm.[12] A large free skin graft was necessary to cover the grasping surface of the ulnar half of the forearm. To diminish bulk, some of the muscles of the distal forearm were excised. Bauer,[1] in 1947, described a similar incision but employed radical excision of all distal muscles, except brachioradialis, pronator teres, and supinator, to allow primary skin closure without grafting. Kreuz,[1] during and after World War II, performed approximately 700 Krukenberg operations. He did not excise muscle, believing that a better blood supply was thus preserved and a better grasping surface and proprioception created. Large skin grafts were, however, required on the grasping surface of the ulna.

In an attempt to combine the advantages of the Kreuz and Bauer modifications and avoid the necessity of excising muscles for closure, I use an incision with two L-shaped flaps rather than the simple bisecting U-shaped incision (Fig. 41-14).[29] In closure, the volar flap is advanced or rotated over the grasping surface of the ulna and the dorsal flap over that of the radius, so that the opposing tactile surfaces will be covered with skin having normal tactile sensation. Skin grafts are applied to the outer surfaces of the digits where sensation is less important. Interdigitating V flaps, based proximally, are used to cover the proximal web of the cleft. It is important that the surgeon review the anatomy of the cutaneous nerves of the forearm (Fig. 41-15), so that these are not transected in the incisions used for creating the flaps.

After developing the skin and fascial flaps, the forearm muscles are carefully dissected into radial and ulnar groups. The interosseous membrane is divided throughout its length along its ulnar periosteal attachment to avoid damage to the interosseous vessels and nerves (Fig. 41-16, *A*).

The musculature that will motor the forceps action of the reconstructed limb must be carefully dissected and preserved. The supinator will become the major adductor.[43] The pronator teres muscle is part abductor and part adductor. The brachioradialis will open the digits. After division

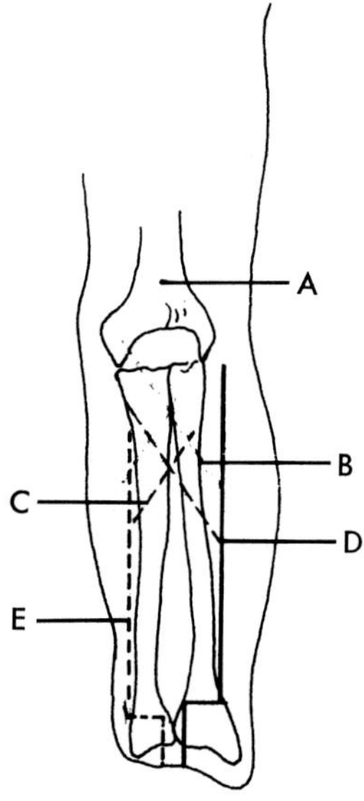

Fig. 41-14. Krukenberg procedure. *A*, Humerus. *B*, Radius. *C*, ulna. Cross dotted lines at antecubital fossa represent digitating V flaps that will cross at opening between radius and ulna. Solid line *D* represents L-shaped incision on volar aspect of radial side (it should end 4 to 5 cm distal to elbow), and line *E* represents opposing L-shaped incision on dorsum of ulnar side.

of the muscle groups, gentle separation of the radius and ulna is carried out to create an angle of 25 to 30 degrees. The distal fibers of the supinator must be carefully observed during this part of the procedure, since overstretching or tearing of its muscle fibers must be avoided.

If the radius is approximately 22 cm in length – an average normal for a 12- to 14-year-old – the length of the opening V of the digits will be approximately 12 cm and the opening span between the tips approximately 8 cm. Shorter stumps may have less opening, but useful function and power can be expected. In the very short stump, proximal transposition of the radial insertion of the pronator teres may be advisable to gain additional opening space and span.

When the dissection is completed and the radius and ulna spread to a maximum without damaging muscle, closure is carried out. The two L-shaped flaps are rotated so as to cover the grasping surfaces and sutured to the skin over the tips of each digit. The V flaps are sutured in an interdigitating fashion to cover the cleft between the separated radius and ulna. Skin defects will be present on the outer side of each forearm branch. These are covered with free full-thickness skin

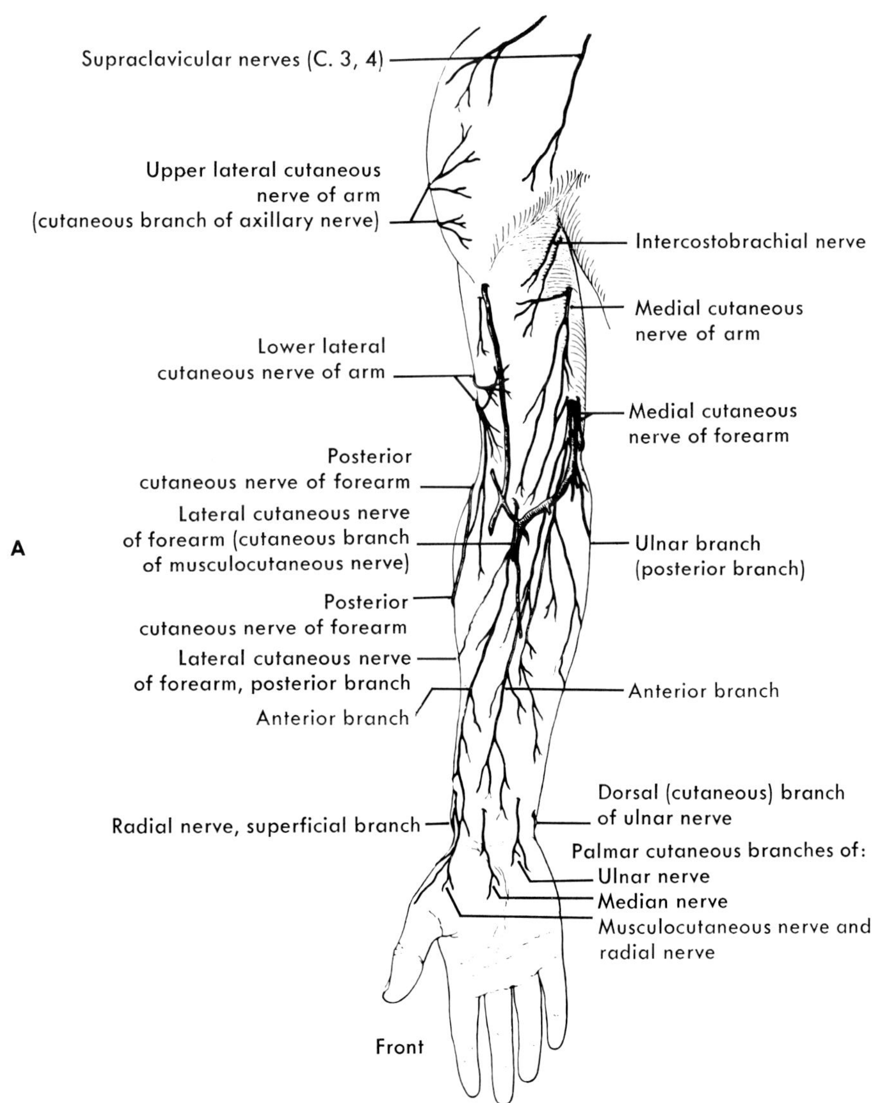

Fig. 41-15. A, Most important nerve for tactile sensation of grasping surface of ulna in Krukenberg stump is anterior branch of medial cutaneous nerve of forearm. L-shaped volar incision should be made sufficiently far lateralward that it will not cross this nerve. In all incisions, care must be taken to preserve these cutaneous nerves.

Continued.

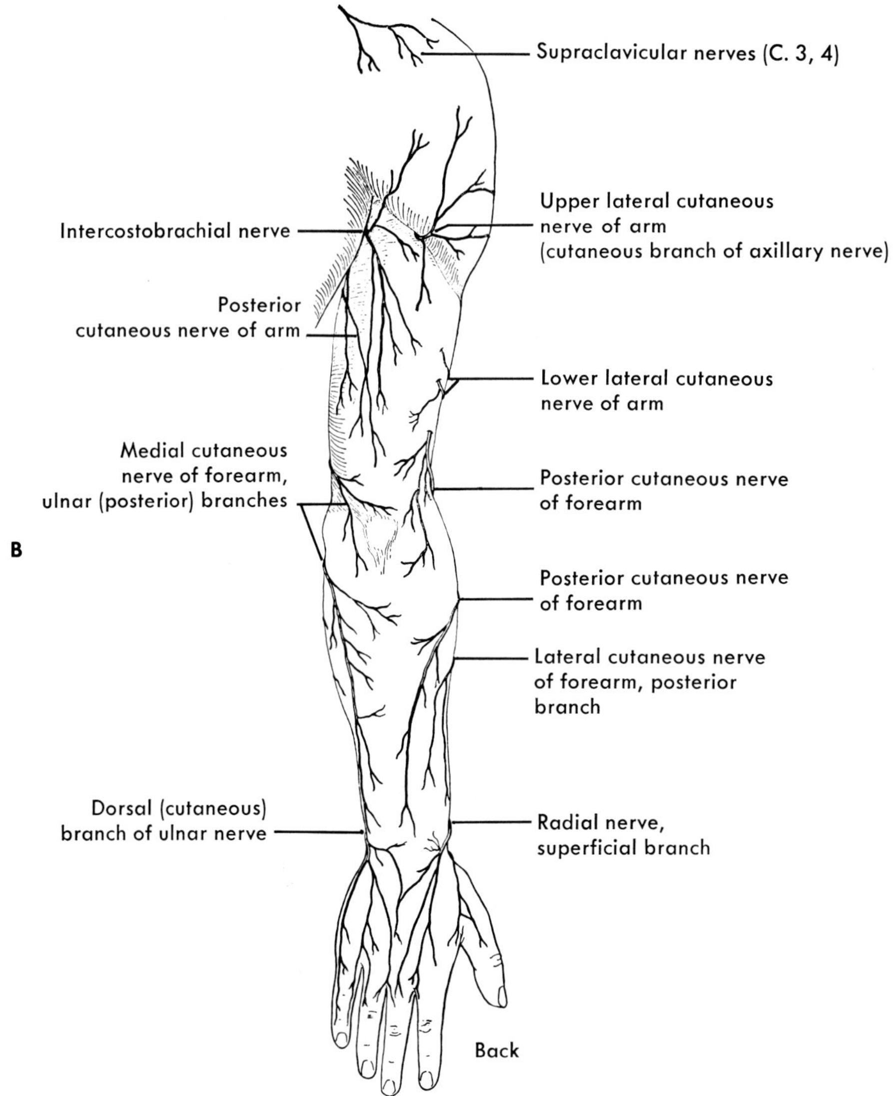

Fig. 41-15, cont'd. B, Most important nerve for grasping surface of radius is posterior cutaneous nerve of forearm. This nerve will not be damaged by incision described in **A.** Incision will parallel nerve and be slightly to radial side of ulna (posterior) branches of medial cutaneous nerve of forearm. (From Basmajian, J. V.: Grant's method of anatomy, ed. 9, Baltimore, 1975, The Williams & Wilkins Co.)

grafts taken from the groin. Suction drainage is placed beneath the V flaps in the cleft. Closure is completed with care to avoid undue tension (Fig. 41-16, *B* and *C*).

Following closure, the two branches are separated to a little less than maximum opening position and sterile dressings applied with a wedge of soft material to maintain the open position (Fig. 41-16, *D*).

Postoperative care. The suction drainage tubes are removed 2 days after the operation without disturbing the other dressing. All wounds are dressed at a minimum of 10 to 14 days after operation. It is advisable to thoroughly wet down the dressings so that they can be removed easily without damaging the skin grafts.

If healing is satisfactory, physical and occupational therapy may be started.[9] The voluntary actions to be exploited are pronation and supination. Pronation has been converted into an opening motion as the pronator teres, acting with the biceps and with the brachioradialis, abducts the radius away from the ulna, which is stabilized by the triceps. Supination has been converted to a closing action, since the supinator adducts the radius against the ulna.[43] During the training

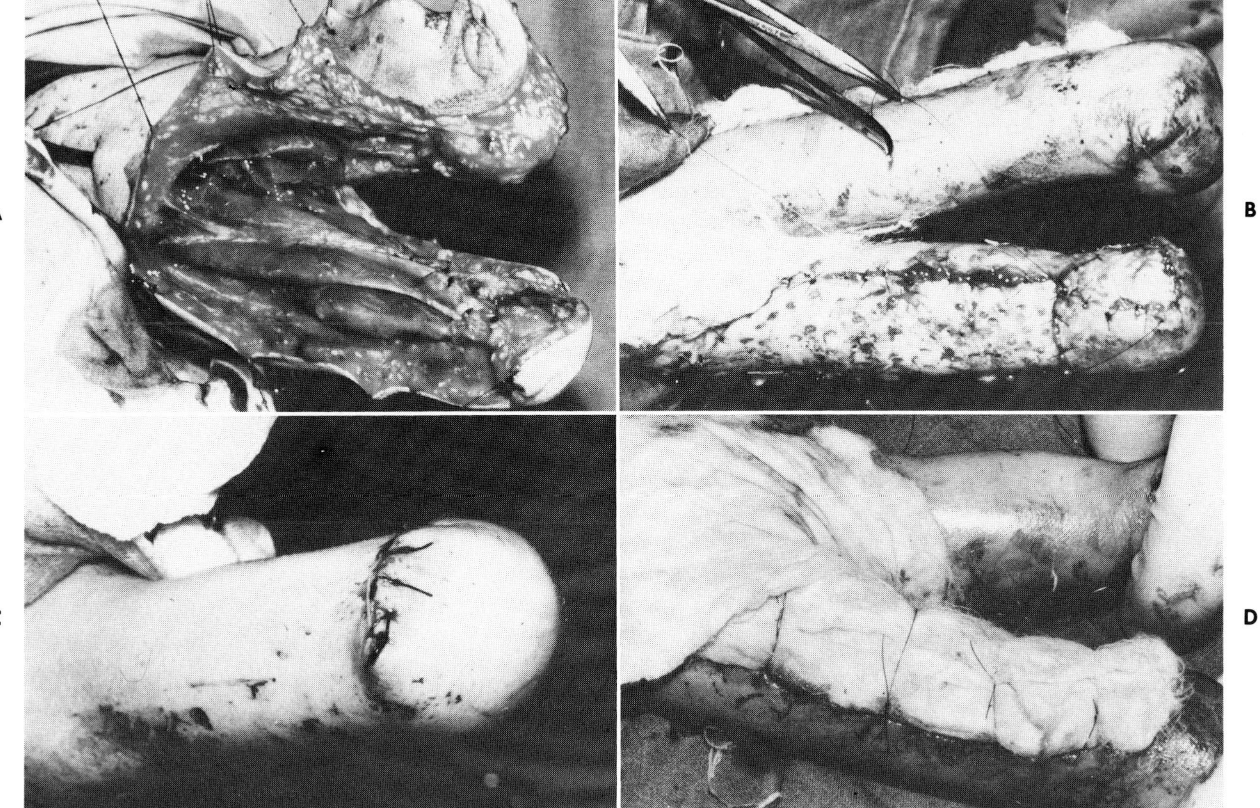

Fig. 41-16. Krukenberg technique. **A,** After developing skin and fascial flaps, forearm muscles are carefully dissected into radial and ulnar groups. Interosseous membrane is divided throughout its length along its ulnar periosteal attachment, avoiding damage to interosseous vessels and nerve. **B,** Two L-shaped flaps have been rotated so as to cover grasping surfaces, and sutured to skin over tips of each digit. Skin defects on outer side of each forearm branch are covered with free full-thickness skin grafts taken from groin. **C,** Close-up shows closure with tactile surface covered with sensate skin. **D,** Following closure, two branches are separated to maximum opening position, and sterile dressings applied. Wedge will be placed to maintain open position.

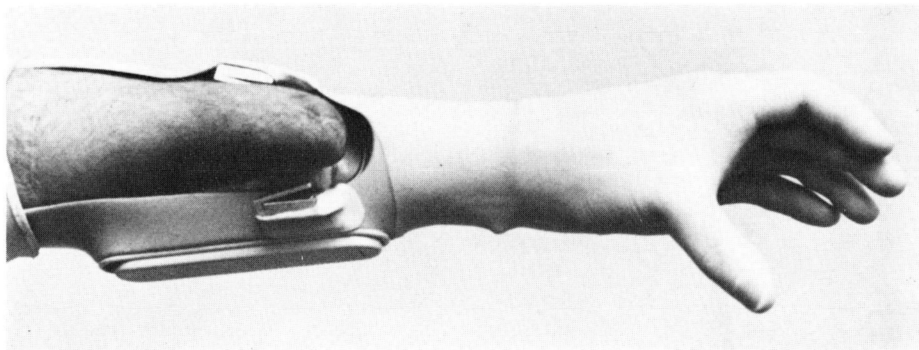

Fig. 41-17. Sunday hand. Prosthesis for Krukenberg patient emphasizes cosmesis over function. Here, powered electromechanical system with microswitches is used, completely self-contained, and fitted over Krukenberg stump.

period the patient must be taught to properly use and balance these muscles to gain this function.

Between training sessions the patient should be provided with a well-shaped wedge to maintain maximum opening and prevent contracture. For some period of each day, however, the wedge is removed and a circumferential bandage applied to maintain the fully closed position. In this way maximum mobility of the joint is maintained and the contractures prevented.

As the patient gains the primary function and strength in the forceps action of the stump, additional devices such as wedges, or clip ons, are fabricated to hold particular instruments for writing or eating. These assistive devices increase the versatility of the stump and allow the patient to perform specially needed tasks more easily.

In addition to these special devices, experience has shown that those patients who have good vision want, in addition to their Krukenberg stump, prostheses that will provide some function, but which are primarily desired for aesthetic reasons. These patients refer to the prostheses as their "Sunday hands." For this purpose a conventional body-powered prosthesis in which the socket is modified to accept the Krukenberg stump is usually prescribed. A powered electric system is also possible in which the microswitches are placed so as to activate terminal device opening by supination and closing by pronation (Fig. 41-17).

Case report. The child in Fig. 41-18 was born December 20, 1963, of healthy parents with two normal siblings. There was no history of drug ingestion, but there had been a threatened abortion in the third month. At the birth it was recognized that the child had bilateral complete carpal transverse deficiencies of both upper limbs. The child was first seen in March, 1965, at which time open-end prostheses were prescribed. He was admitted for training in the use of the prostheses but preferred the tactile contact with the stump, especially on the right side. In 1970, 10X Dorrance hooks were substituted for his earlier terminal devices and on June 15, 1978, a Krukenberg operation of the left upper limb was carried out. The decision to operate on the left side rather than the right was based on a subluxation of the proximal radius on the right side and a tendency to dysplasia in this limb. Postoperatively the boy became an excellent Krukenberg user and continues now to use an open-end prosthesis on the right side in association with his Krukenberg limb. He is completely independent in the activities of daily living. A "Sunday hand" was rejected by the patient for use in his social life.

Surgical considerations in the radial clubhand

The implication of radial clubhand as a component of multiple deficiencies is quite different from when it occurs as an isolated anomaly. In the child with multimembral anomalies in which longitudinal deficiency of the radius (radial clubhand) is present, consideration of the contraindications to surgery deserve more emphasis than do the indications. The position of uncorrected deformity in the bilateral case may have very significant functional advantages, which should not be sacrificed in attempts at cosmesis.

It has already been emphasized that in the infant and small child the shortened arm must be left exposed and not covered or concealed by clothing as parents often are wont to do, so that the child will develop maximum function of the fingers, elbow, and shoulder. During the day the hands and fingers should be free for play. Splints to maintain corrected position are used only at night, and the physical therapy program emphasizes maximum mobility of all joints.

In watching and assessing the developing function in these children the careful observer will note important compensatory functions that depend on the radial positioning of the hand. Many of these patients have limited elbow flexion, and radial abduction of the wrist is an important sub-

Fig. 41-18. Complete bilateral carpal transverse deficiency. **A,** Patient age 3½ years old has bilateral open-end sockets with voluntary opening terminal devices. He retains pronation and supination of forearm and tactile sensation from open-end prosthesis. Prosthetic training is underway at this age. **B,** Prosthetic training includes independent feeding. **C,** After Krukenberg procedure on left forearm, patient continues to wear right open-end prosthesis but uses Krukenberg arm for grasping with tactile sensation, as with cards shown. **D,** Patient uses Krukenberg arm to hold glass, with assistance from stump at open-end prosthesis. **E,** Special adaptive device for eating utensils. **F,** Lifting strength. Patient is excellent "Krukenberg-user" and is completely independent in activities of daily living.

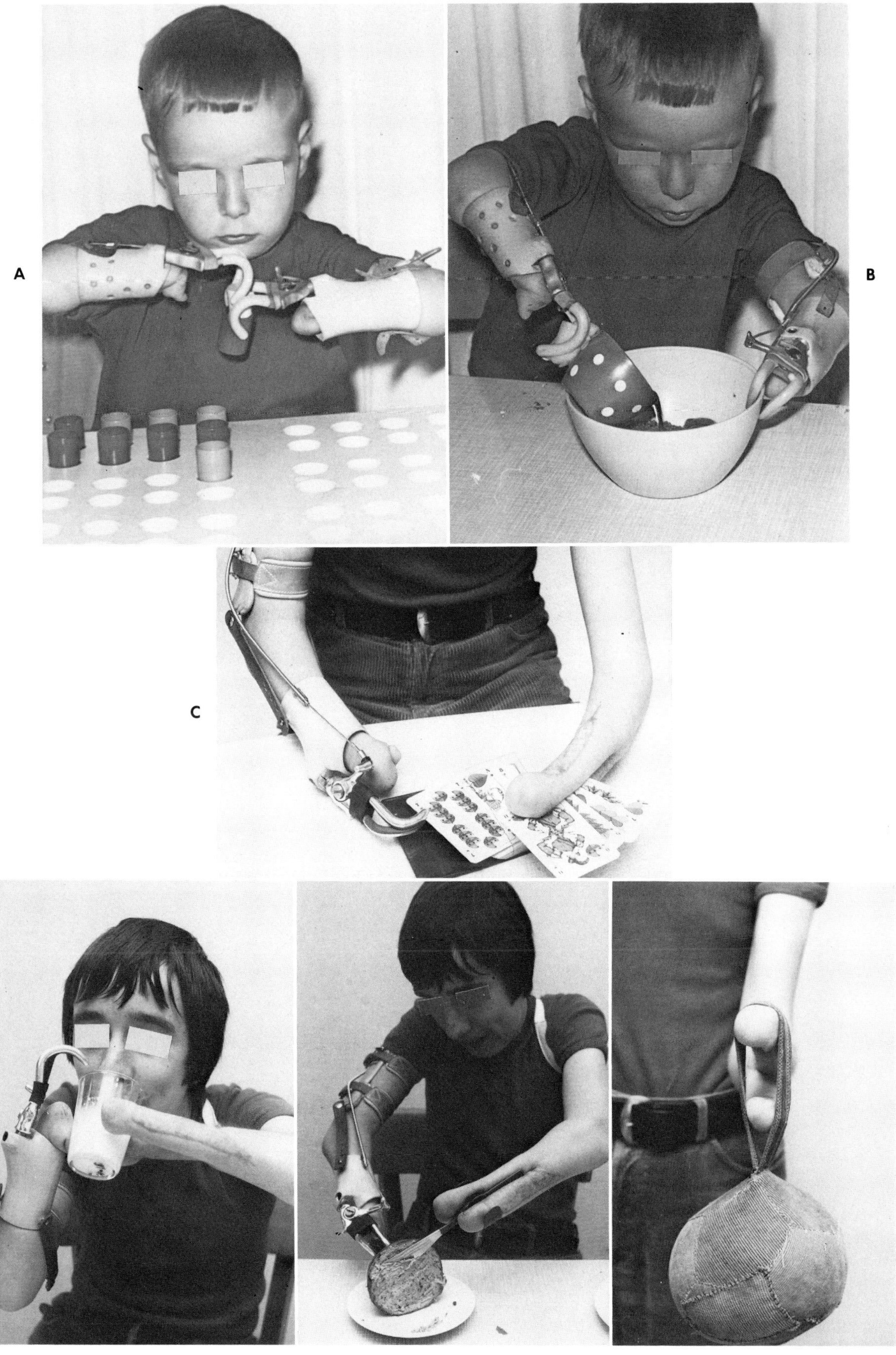

Fig. 41-18. For legend see opposite page.

stitution to bring the hand to the mouth or face. Radial abduction combined with volar flexion is often used for grasping. Hypermobility of the wrist and metacarpals substitute for lost pronation and supination (Fig. 41-19) and greatly enhance dexterity. In the radial clubhand the fifth finger is much more often used for fine pinch than is the index finger, when there is a hypoplastic or absent thumb, and may be more suitable for pollicization than the index in terms of useful function.

The range of motion of finger joints, particular-

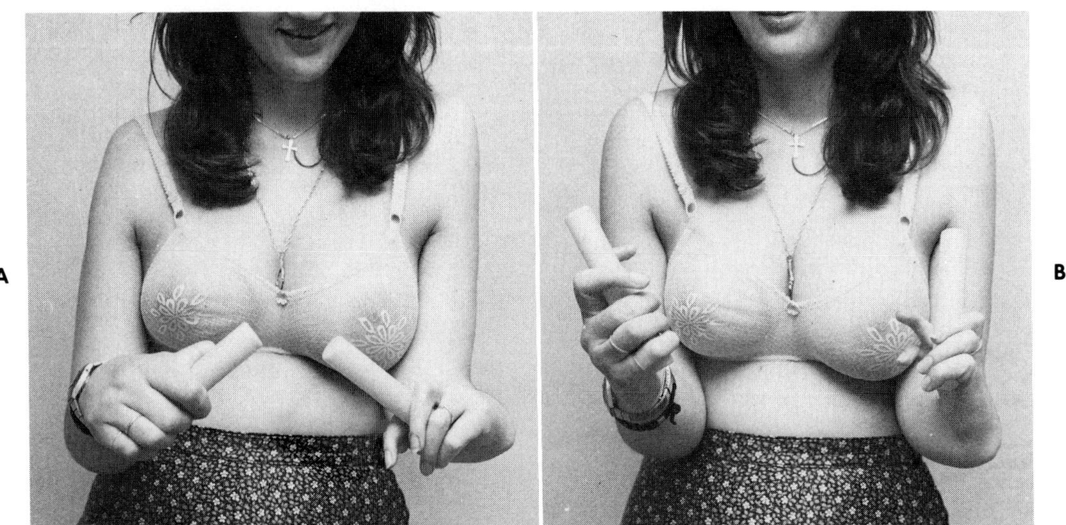

Fig. 41-19. Hypermobility of wrist and metacarpals in patient with radial deficiency permits compensatory function. **A,** Pronation. **B,** Supination.

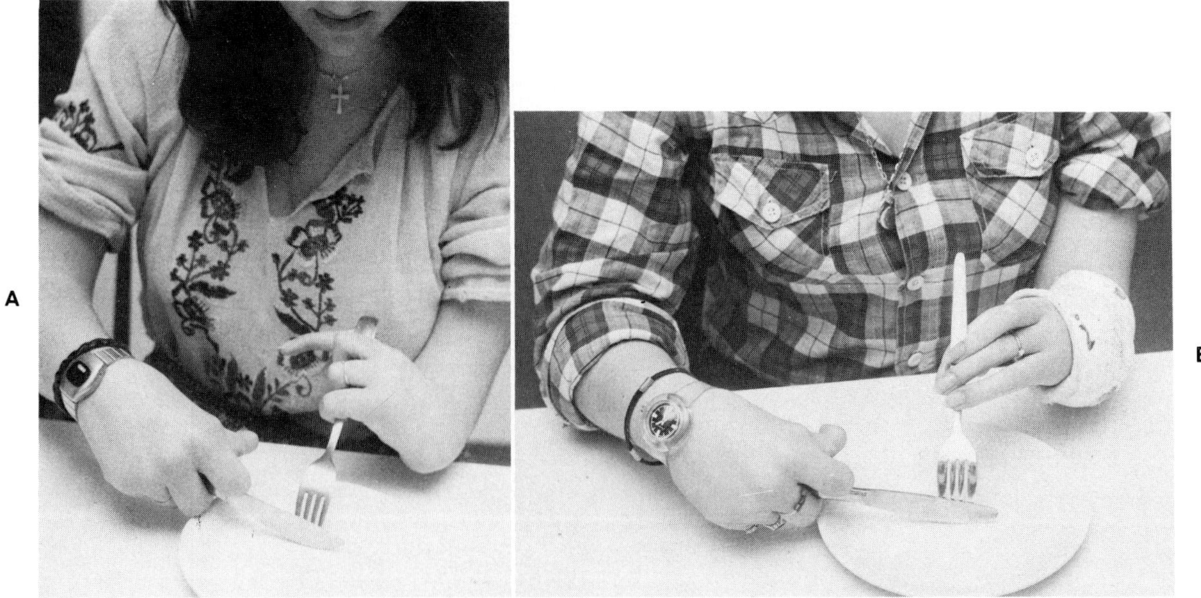

Fig. 41-20. Functional testing of radial clubhand prior to surgical intervention. **A,** Patient is tested with knife and fork. **B,** With cast applied in position of correction, patient is retested to be sure that no function will be lost. **C,** Preoperative roentgenogram shows radially deviated hand. **D,** Postoperative roentgenogram demonstrates centralized hand. **E,** Patient after centralization of left radial clubhand. Examination 2 years after operation showed same correction.

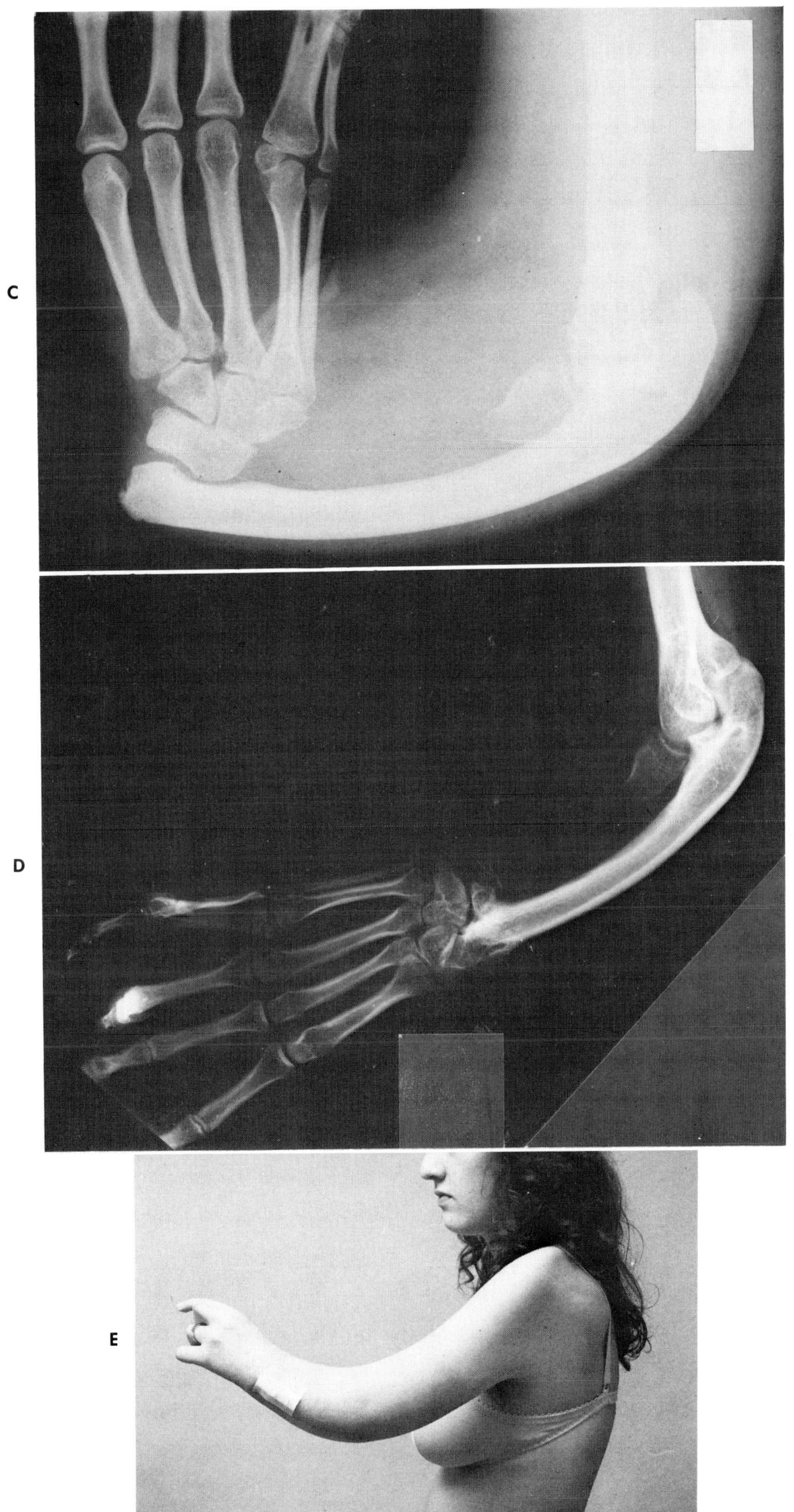

Fig. 41-20, cont'd. For legend see opposite page.

ly metacarpophalangeal joints, is important in assessing function. In many of these children the power of the hook created by radial deviation of the hand is the only power grasping action. They will develop fine grasp between the fingers, especially on the ulnar side.

These children must be carefully evaluated by both the surgeon and therapist before surgical treatment is planned to be sure that no important functions will be lost by centralization of the hand (Fig. 41-20). The contraindications should be recognized.[21,34,37,46] The most important is limited elbow flexion, which, with centralization of the hand, will prevent the individual from using it for any activity approaching the neck, throat, face, or mouth. It should be recognized that the radially deviated hand provides for lifting capacity with strength not available with weakened finger grasp. This function may be necessary in using a rail for stair climbing. Only when good function of all digits and the elbow joint is present should the centralization procedure be considered in the quadrimembral child. I recommend, in accordance with Witt, Cotta, and Jäger,[48] correcting the radial clubhand only after growth is completed. Centralization procedures in the young child are almost always followed by impairment of the distal growth plate of the ulna, which may result in further shortening and recurrent deformity.[34]

Surgical procedure (centralization of the hand). Where indicated, surgical correction of the radially deviated hand for centralization is carried out in two stages. The first, only for cases without the possibility of passive correction, is primarily a procedure in the form of a Z-plasty of the skin on the radial side of the wrist with soft tissue release.[37] After developing the skin flaps, the fascial contractures are released and tendons lengthened as necessary. This may be adequate to allow correction of the radial deviation, but in severe deformity it may be necessary to open the radial side of the wrist joint capsule. In this process care must be taken in the volar dissection to identify and protect the radially displaced median nerve. As the hand is deviated in an ulnar direction, care must be exercised to avoid stretching the nerve, which may, in fact limit the extent of correction at this first stage. With the desired correction attained, the flaps of the Z-plasty are reversed and the wound closed.

Schöllner[37] adds to the incision of the contracted radial structures the transposition of the tendon of the flexor carpi ulnaris to the dorsum of the carpus, together with the transposition of the tendon of the extensor carpi ulnaris into the carpus. The hand is positioned to avoid tension on skin sutures, and the correction is maintained in a plaster of Paris dressing. Postoperative therapy emphasizes function and motion of the fingers. In some instances, especially in patients with acutely angulated radial abduction who require the function of the clubhand position, this procedure is adequate to obtain enough correction to increase the range of movement, without losing this functional need. In other instances, this procedure is a preliminary release of the shortened radial structures to permit bony centralization of the hand on the ulna with a minimum of shortening of the bony elements.

The second stage is accomplished after the conclusion of growth and after thorough healing of the first stage, through an S-shaped dorsal incision beginning on the ulnar side of the distal forearm, curving around the styloid of the ulna, transversely crossing the proximal wrist, and then turning distally to the base of the second metacarpal. The transverse portion of the incision is superficial and the large dorsal veins and cutaneous nerves, as well as the extensor tendons, remain intact and protected. These structures are then elevated from the underlying ulna and dorsal carpal ligaments as an intact soft tissue bridge beneath which the procedure is completed.

The dorsal capsule is then elevated from the ulna and dissected distally to expose the carpus. The carpal bones are seldom normal. For the most part the carpal bones on the radial side of the wrist are extremely hypoplastic or absent. Frequently there are various degrees of synostosis of the carpal bones. The region of the lunate bone in the synostosis is excavated to form a bed for reception of the shortened ulna. The ulna is shortened sufficiently to obtain full correction of the clubhand. If the lunate and triquetral bones are separate, I propose to excavate both of them, carefully protecting their distal joints to prevent displacing them. These two bones together have a larger base and with it a better resistance against recurrent deformity than the lunate bone only (Fig. 41-21). The excellent mobility of the joints distal to these bones with regard to dorsiflexion and volar flexion will be preserved, and we should save mobility and function for the multimembral-deficient person as much as possible without increasing the risk of recurrent deformity. If there is insufficient shortening to permit centralization without excessive soft tissue tension, or if the lunate bone is too dysplastic, the lunate may be excised completely and the bed for the reception of the ulna excavated in the capitate bone or in the distal portion of the synostotic carpal block. Other techniques for correction of the radial clubhand have been described by Blauth[3,4] and by Schöllner[37] and are represented in Fig. 41-21.

As in the soft tissue release, reduction of the hand around the shortened ulna should be carried out gently and gradually and the tension on

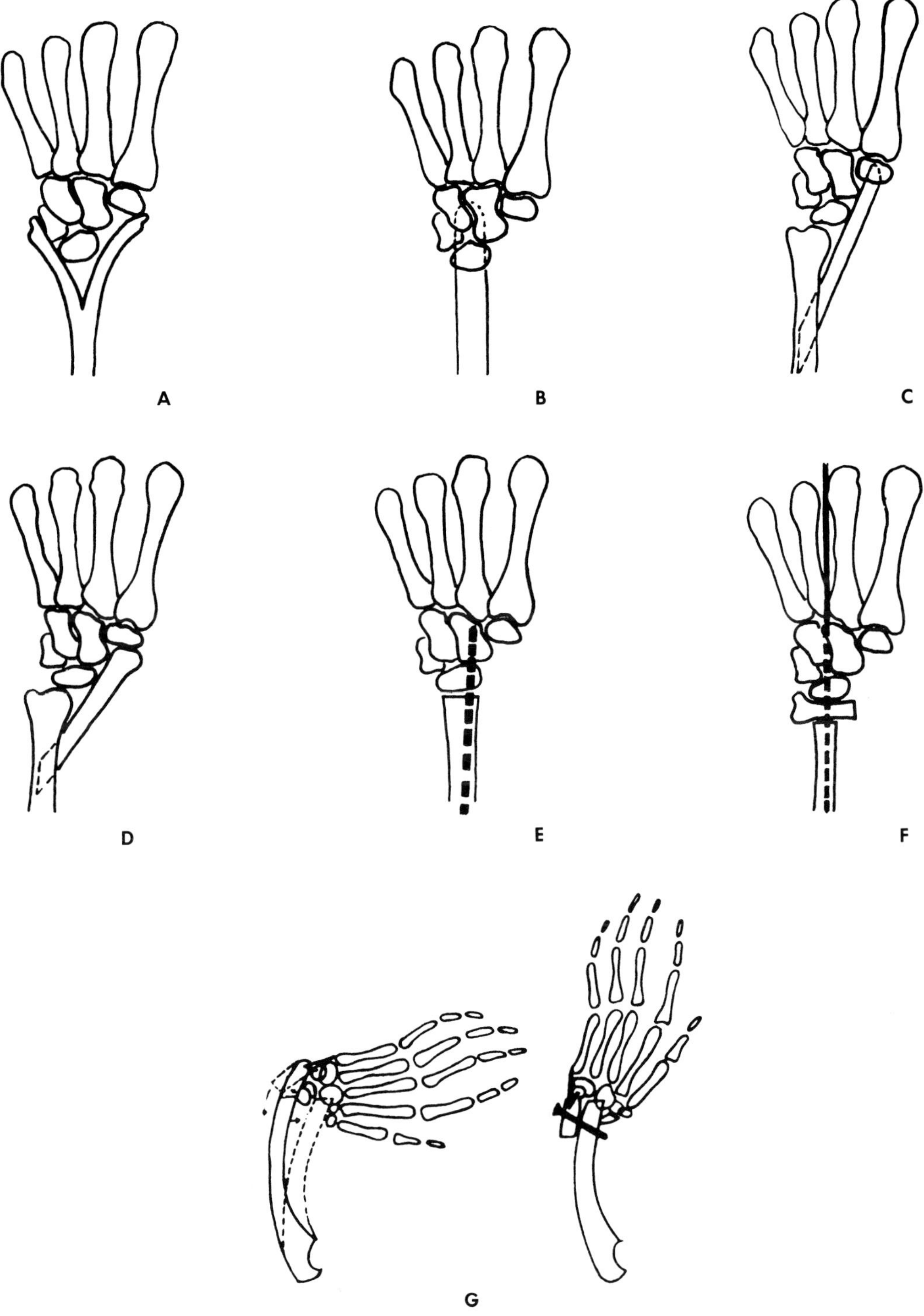

Fig. 41-21. Techniques of correcton of radial clubhand as described by Schöllner. **A,** Bardenheuer. **B,** Gocht. **C,** Albee. **D,** Starr. **E,** Stracker. **F,** Gardemin. **G,** Hepp. (From Schöllner, D.: Die Klumphand bei Radiusaplasie, Aktuelle Orthopädie, Stuttgart, 1972, Georg Thieme Verlag.)

nerves and vessels carefully observed. With correction obtained and centralization acceptable, fixation is accomplished by two crossed Kirschner wires. The shortening effected, which may be as much as 3 cm, will be more than compensated for by the relative lengthening provided by the length of the corrected hand.

Before the wound is closed, the tourniquet is released and circulation in hand and fingers observed. If circulation is satisfactory and bleeding controlled, repair of the wrist joint capsule is carried out. Suction drainage tubes are placed and the wound closed.

Immobilization is applied with sterile dressings and plaster of Paris, extending from above the elbow to the proximal interphalangeal joints of the fingers. The metacarpophalangeal joints are maintained in slight flexion.

Postoperative care. Suction drainage is removed at 48 hours. Plaster is changed and sutures removed at about 14 days postoperatively. Immobilization, however, after this procedure should be maintained a minimum of 3 months and, on occasion, up to 6 months to ensure stability. If immobilization is extended beyond 3 months, all finger joints should be freed, and physical therapy for finger motion should be instituted. When bony fusion of the ulna to the carpus is complete, the Kirschner wires may be removed and a full physical therapy program begun. Night splints maintaining full correction of the hand are employed for at least a year postoperatively.

Procedure with hypoplastic radius. For those patients in whom the radius is hypoplastic, rather than absent, with radial deviation of the hand, no attempt should be made to perform arthrodesis to the wrist. The procedure should be a release of the contracted structures on the radial side of the wrist, followed by elevation of a capsular flap and shortening by removal of a segment

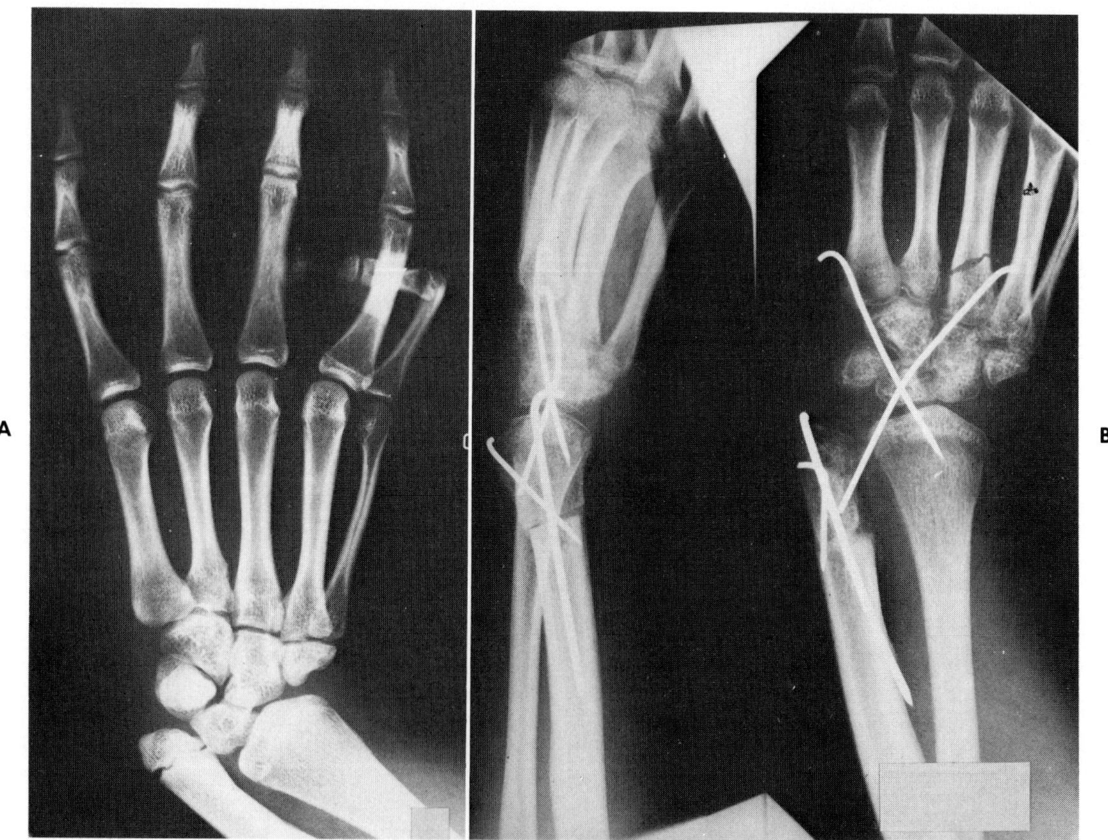

Fig. 41-22. Correction of radial deviation of hand in patient with hypoplastic radius. **A,** Roentgenogram shows radial deviation of hand with hypoplastic radius and ulna blocking correction. **B,** Wedge has been removed from ulnar side of carpus; ulna has been shortened and rotated. Fixation is with crossed Kirschner wires. Hand is centralized. **C,** Preoperatively, left hand is noted to be radially deviated approximately 70 degrees. **D,** Six months after surgery, centralization is excellent. **E,** Maximum dorsiflexion. **F,** Maximum volar flexion postoperatively. Examination 2 years after surgery shows same result.

of the ulna, preserving approximately 2 cm of its distal end. The ulna should be shortened to a level of about 1 mm proximal to the distal end of the radius. A wedge of bone with its base ulnarward and dorsalward is removed from the distal carpal row. When the wedge defect is closed, centralization and correction of the deformity is obtained (Fig. 41-22). As with the other procedures care must be taken not to place the neurovascular structures under tension. Circulation must be checked prior to internal fixation with crossed Kirschner wires. In this procedure an additional technical detail should be noted. In reducing the shortened ulna, the distal fragment should be externally rotated slightly so that the line of pull of extensor carpi ulnaris within its groove is partly changed to that of ulnar abductor. This tendon should be shortened proximal to the ulnar styloid process under sufficient tension, so that it prevents passive radial deviation of the wrist.

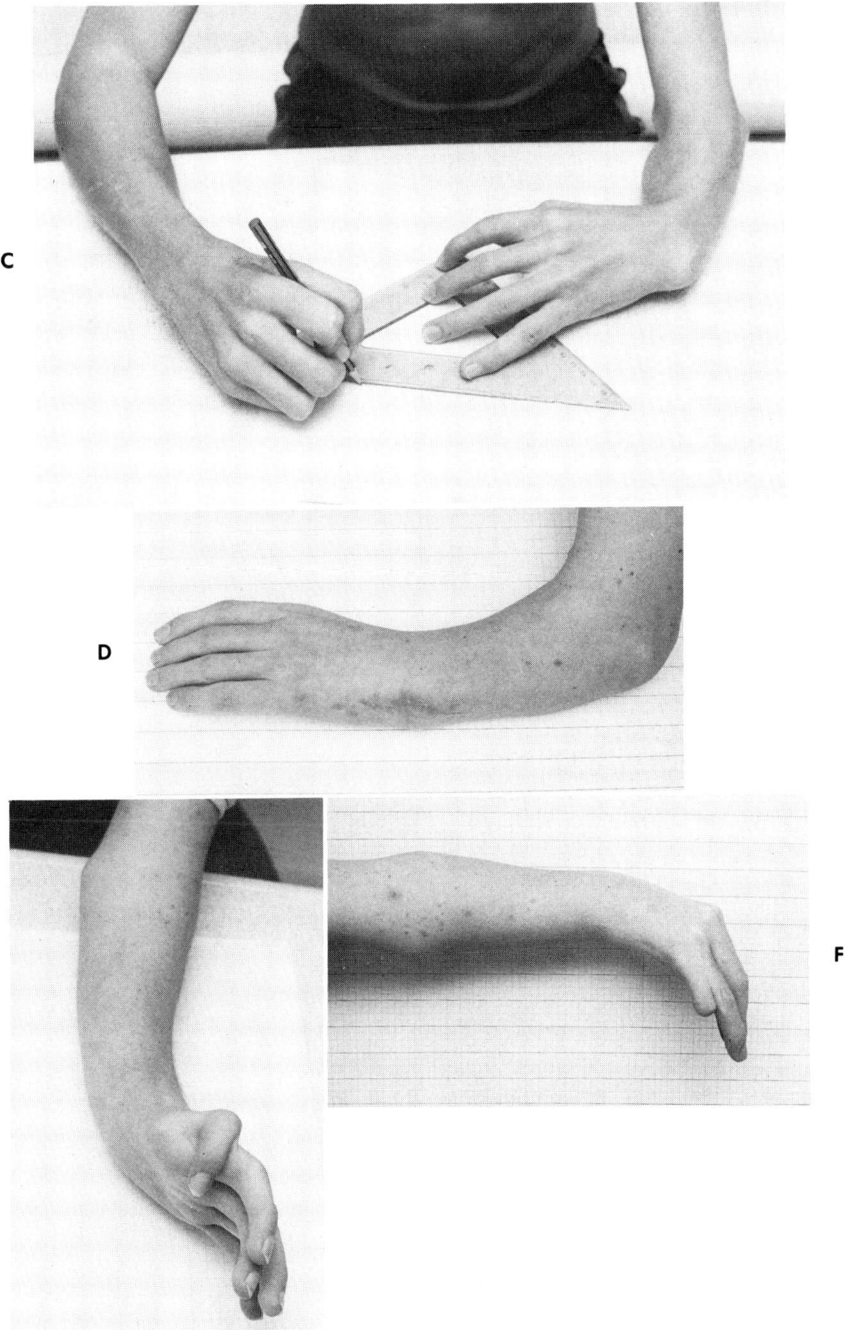

Fig. 41-22, cont'd. For legend see opposite page.

Immobilization and aftercare are similar to the procedure previously described.

CASE REPORTS

Retention of feet when hands are missing

Fig. 41-23 shows the first-born child of a 39-year-old mother. The child was born on June 15, 1971, by caesarean section with complete bilateral transverse deficiencies of the forearms, complete bilateral longitudinal deficiencies of the fibula, and with fifth metatarsophalangeal deficiencies also present. There were numerous lesser deformities, including some hypoplasia of the right femur, and, in particular, bowing of the tibiae bilaterally. She was first seen in the outpatient clinic in October of 1972 at age 16 months. Orthoprostheses were prescribed for the lower limbs, a thigh corset and knee joint on the right side, and more of an orthopaedic shoe on the left side. No upper limb prostheses were prescribed. By December of the same year, the child was beginning to take her first steps in a walker. She was not seen again until April of 1975, when it was recognized that she had a small rudimentary ulnar fragment present on the right. At this time upper limb prostheses were prescribed. In October, 1975, surgical intervention in the form of osteotomy of the tibia and fixation of a digital transplant from the great toe of this foot to the left ulnar fragment, to create a better below elbow stump, was carried out. New orthoprostheses were prescribed. Bilateral below-elbow cable-controlled prostheses were prescribed. Her parents would only consider functional hands and rejected the use of a hook. Between 1975 and 1977, the child was not seen. During this period she rejected her prostheses and resumed ambulation on her own feet but with gradual increasing deformities so that when she was again seen in October, 1977, she was independent in the activities of daily living using her forearm

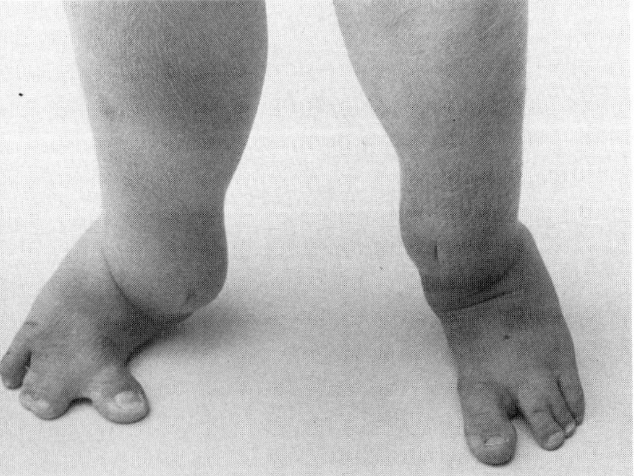

Fig. 41-23. A, Roentgenogram at first examination, October, 1972, reveals longitudinal deficiency of fibula bilaterally with some shortening of right femur and considerable shortening of right tibia. Knee joints and hip joints are intact. **B,** Lower limbs show classic anteromedial bowing with dimple of skin, absence of fifth ray with severe equinus and valgus deformity at ankle. **C,** Recidivism of deformities 2 years after osteotomy of right tibia. Child is wearing right orthoprosthesis and left orthopaedic shoe with leather thigh lacer. This combination equalizes her leg length, and she is independently ambulatory. **D,** After transplantation and fusion of phalanx of deviated digit to residual ulna in left limb, function is demonstrated. **E,** Child uses upper limb stumps for all activities of daily living, including tying her boots on. **F,** Functional hands are worn only part time, particularly when eating out in restaurant. **G,** Freedom of shoulders is demonstrated. Even with this freedom clumsiness of hand precluded full use during day.

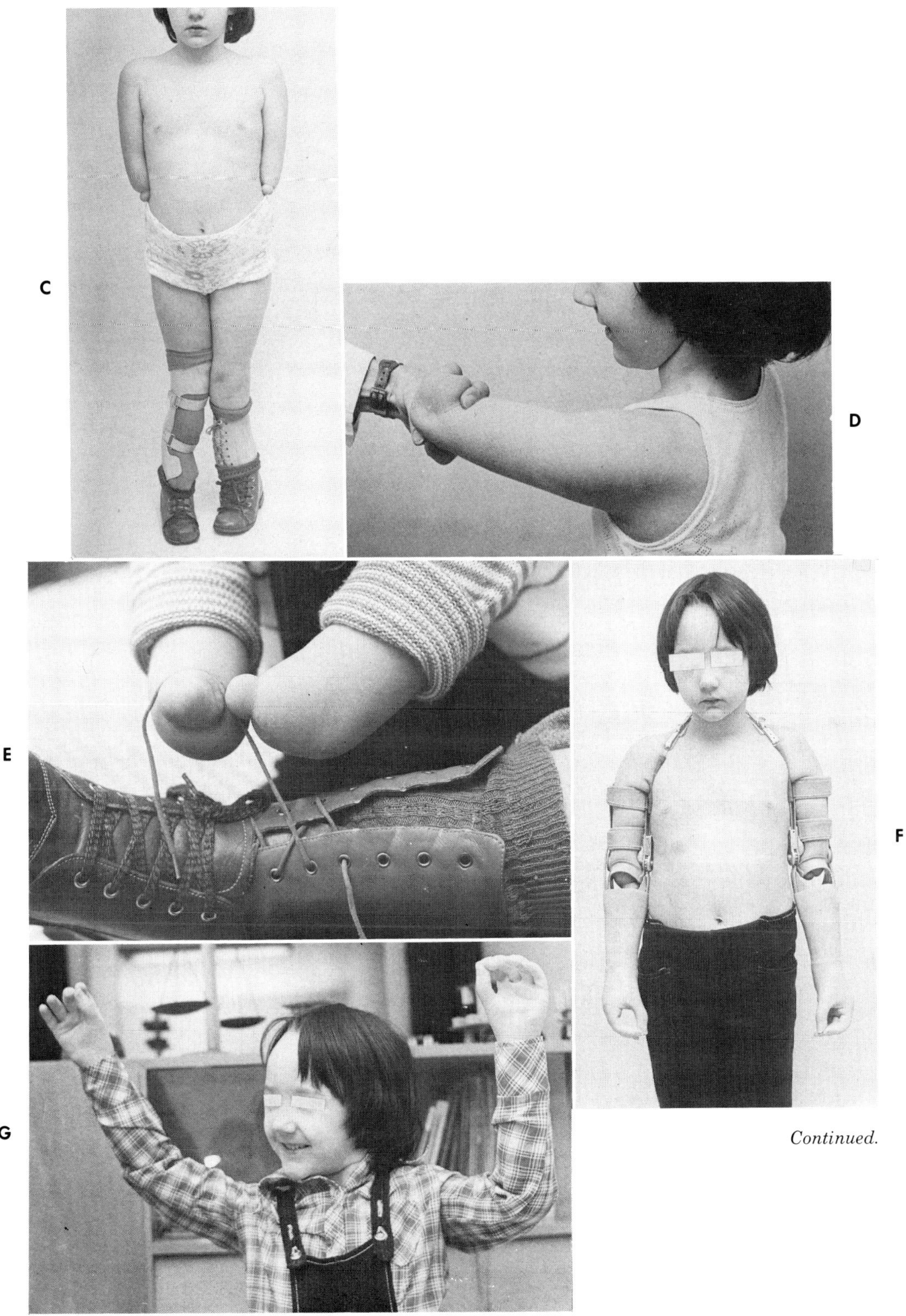

Continued.

Fig. 41-23, cont'd. For legend see opposite page.

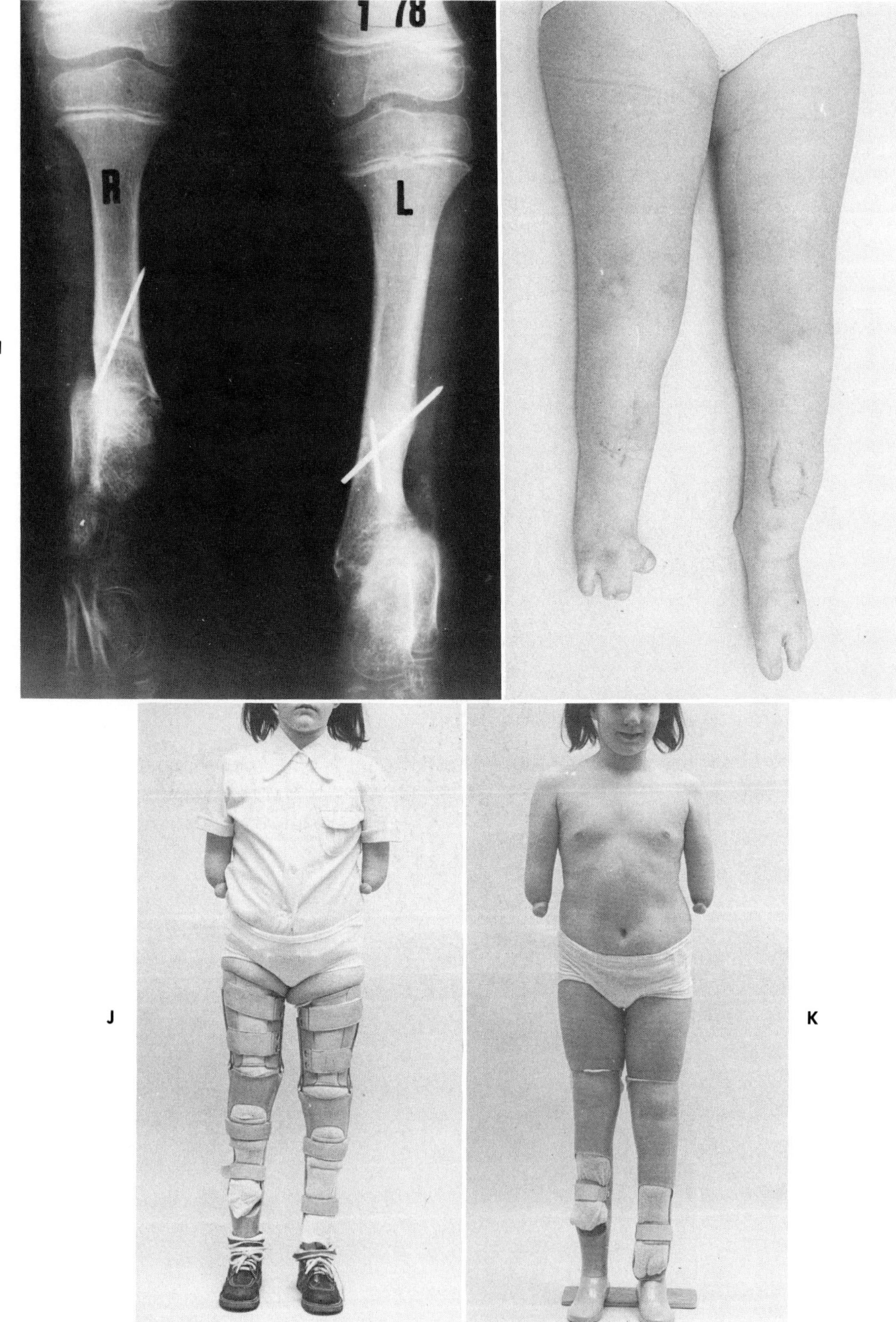

Fig. 41-23. cont'd. H, Roentgenograms after bilateral tibial osteotomy for correction of deformity. **I,** Realigned tibiae are now much more amenable to prosthetic restoration. Note that there is still difference of knee level due to shortening of right femur. **J,** Patient in orthoprostheses with knee joints and thigh corset for full active everyday wear. **K,** These can be replaced with PTS-type orthoprosthesis, which child prefers, particularly for beach and boating activities.

stumps, but not her prostheses. She did use her upper limb prostheses when she went to a restaurant. At this time Syme amputations for the lower limbs were considered, but after consultation with the parents, the decision was made against this and only further correction of the tibial deformity was carried out. In February of 1977, new lower limb orthoprostheses were prescribed (Fig. 41-23). The patient continues to use her forearm stumps for all activities at home but uses her arm prostheses at a restaurant. She is fully ambulatory on her lower limb orthoprostheses.

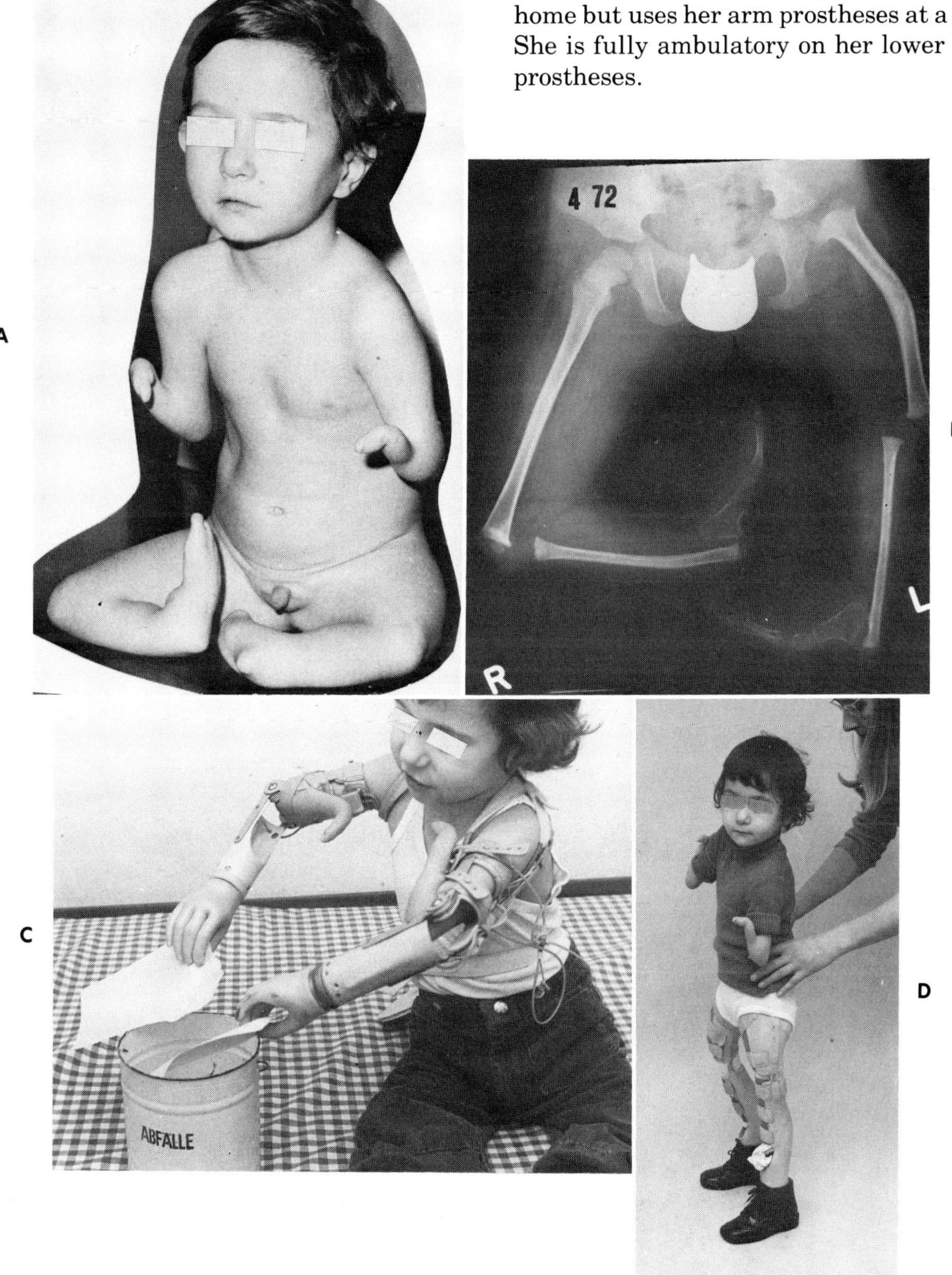

Fig. 41-24. A, This child was first seen in April, 1972, with bilateral upper and lower limb deficiencies. Upper limbs had longitudinal deficiencies of ulna, complete; carpus, partial; metacarpophalangeal, complete 2, 3, 4, and 5, with hypoplastic radius and humerus and flexion deformities at elbow. Lower limbs had bilateral longitudinal deficiencies of the tibia, complete; tarsal, partial; metatarsophalangeal 1 to 3, complete, with left coxa vara, bowing and hypoplasia of femur. **B,** Roentgenogram of lower limbs at initial visit. **C,** Pneumatic prostheses with outside elbow joints and functional hands. Child has developed independent function bilaterally. **D,** First lower limb prostheses or orthoprostheses with stiff knees and end bearing.

Continued.

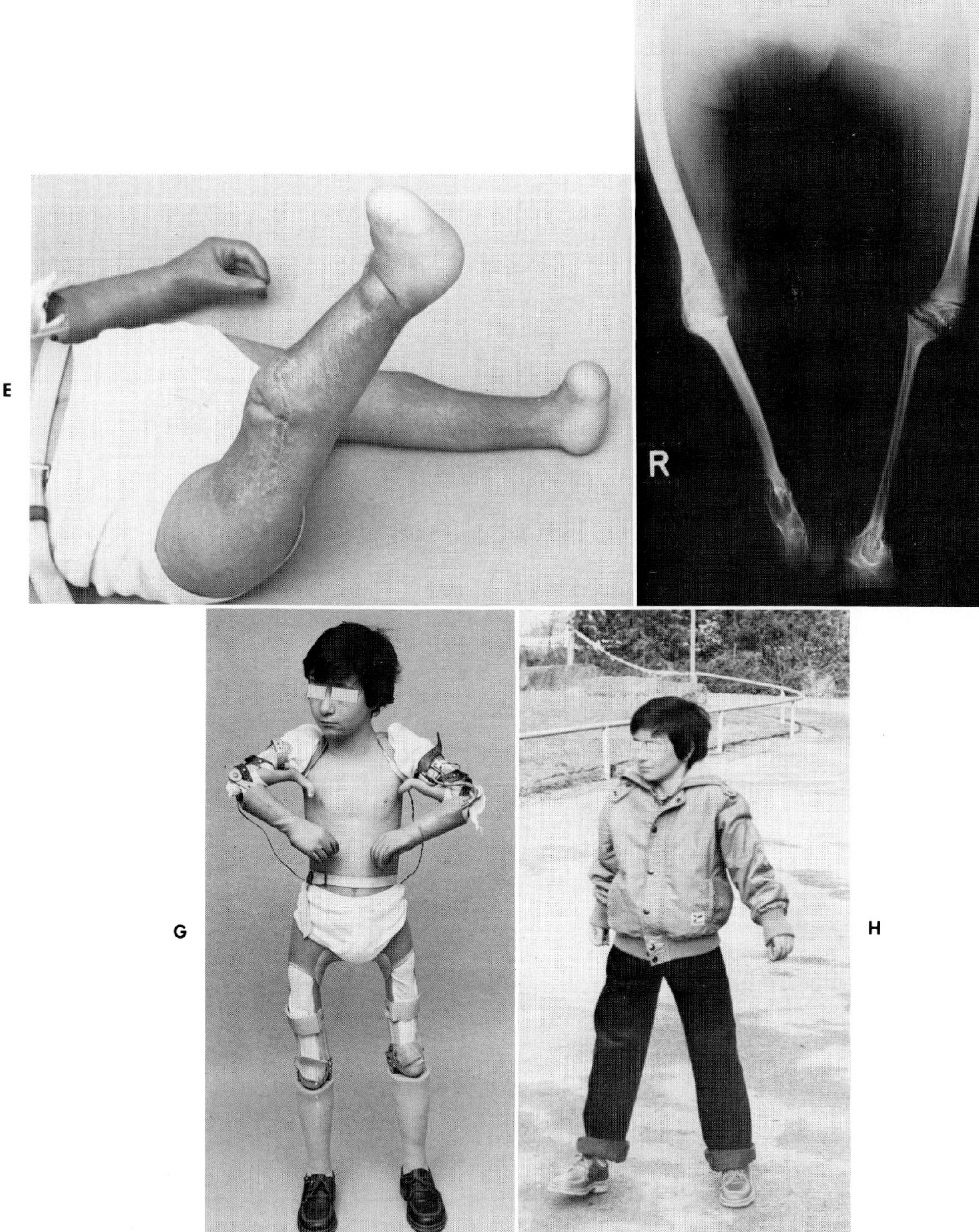

Fig. 41-24, cont'd. E, Following final surgical intervention, knees have been stiffened (fibulofemoral fusions), ankles have been stabilized, and partial foot amputations accomplished. **F,** Roentgenogram shows fusion of fibula to femur bilaterally as well as fusion of fibula to astragalus and partial foot amputation. **G,** Final prosthetic fitting demonstrates electric bilateral upper limb prostheses. Note that radius and digit have been left free for operation of microswitches, and outside elbow joints permit function of prosthetic hands without flexion deformity of elbow affecting this. Lower limbs have orthoprostheses with plastic sockets, and open window with Velcro strap suspension and end bearing. Artificial knee joints are fitted with Swiss locks, and articulated feet have been substituted for the SACH feet. **H,** Fully clothed, patient attends regular school, plays soccer, and, despite quadrimembral limb deficiencies, has normal personality.

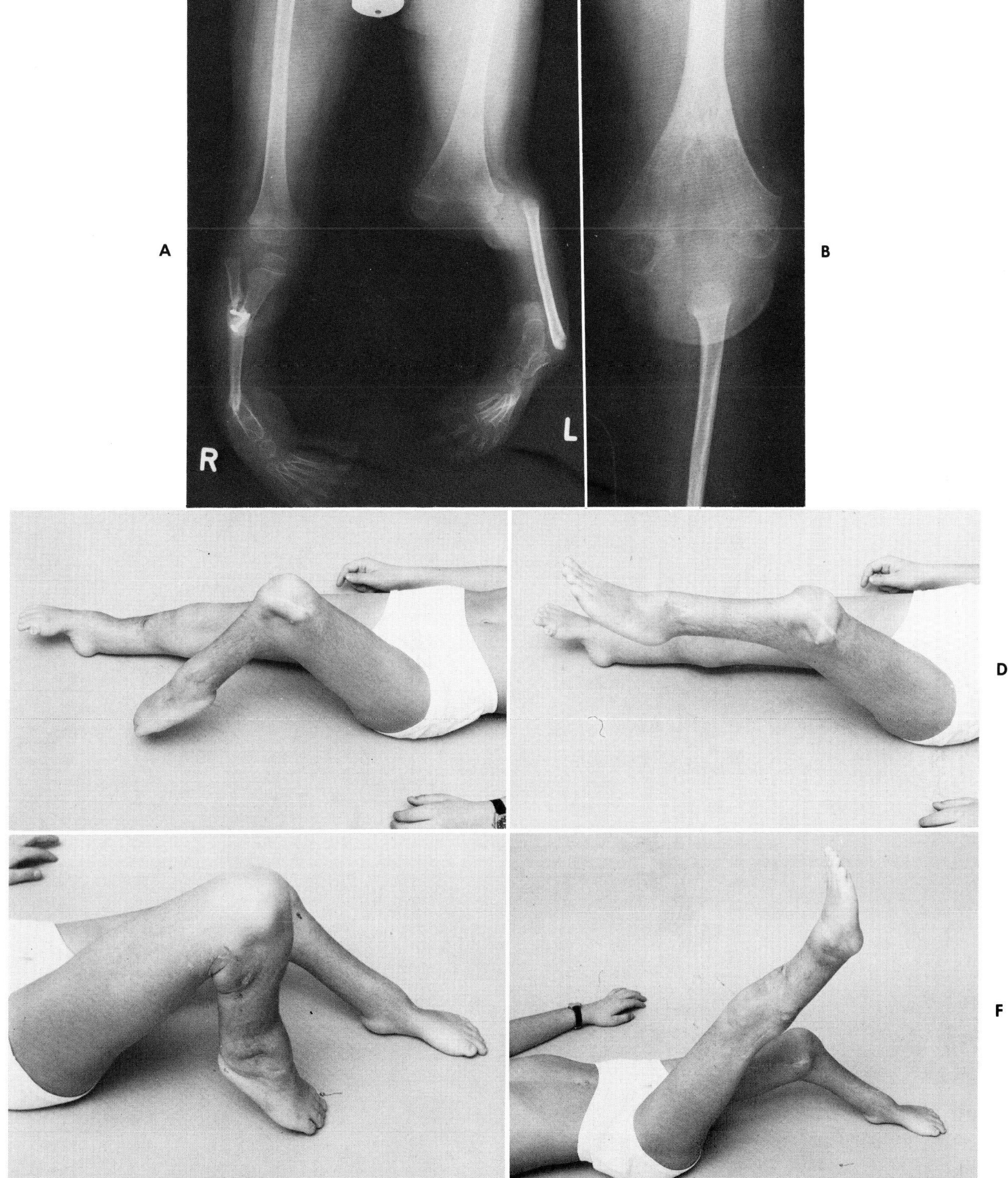

Fig. 41-25. Twin of patient in Fig. 41-24 was born with right partial deficiency of tibia and left complete deficiency of tibia. **A,** At time of first visit, April, 1972, roentgenogram shows prior effort at reconstruction on right leg with no reconstruction on left. Note that distal femoral epiphysis is bifid. **B,** After Brown procedure on left leg, centralization has been accomplished. **C,** Right synostosis between tibia and fibula has been redone. Left knee flexes to 90 degrees. **D,** Left knee lacks 20 degrees of extension. **E,** Right knee flexes to 110 degrees. **F,** Right knee has full extension.

Continued.

Reconstruction and prosthetic fittings for multiple limb deficiency

The child in Fig. 41-24 was born September 17, 1968, to healthy parents with a 3-year-old normal sibling. There was, however, a significant family history in that he was born with a twin who had limb dificiencies as well (Fig. 41-25). There was an additional history of the father's sister having given birth to twins who died at birth with unknown limb deficiencies. There was no history of unusual medication during the pregnancy.

At the time of birth, the infant was noted to have bilateral upper limb deficiencies, consisting of complete longitudinal deficiency of the ulna, partial carpal deficiency, and complete metacarpophalangeal deficiency 2 through 5. There was additionally hypoplasia of both the radius and humerus with a flexion deformity at the radiohumeral joint. The child had bilateral longitudinal deficiencies of the lower limbs consisting of complete tibia, partial tarsal, and complete metatarsophalangeal deficiences 1 through 3. The combination of complete ulna and tibia longitudinal deficiencies is extraordinary. There was also a left coxa vara with bowing and hypoplasia of the femur. The child's twin was born with bilateral lower limb deficiencies (Fig. 41-25).

The patient was first seen in April, 1972, at which time training in the activities of daily living was immediately instituted. Bilateral pneumatic upper limbs were prescribed for the child and reconstruction of the knees and feet undertaken. In August of 1972, he was fitted with his first lower limb prostheses. The initial fitting was temporary plaster of Paris sockets with SACH feet. These were replaced by orthoprostheses with stiff knees and SACH feet (Fig. 41-24, *D*). In December of 1972, the child was ambulatory. Meanwhile, his training with the upper limb prostheses was quite satisfactory, and he was able to feed himself as well as to play using the artificial limbs. Further efforts at recon-

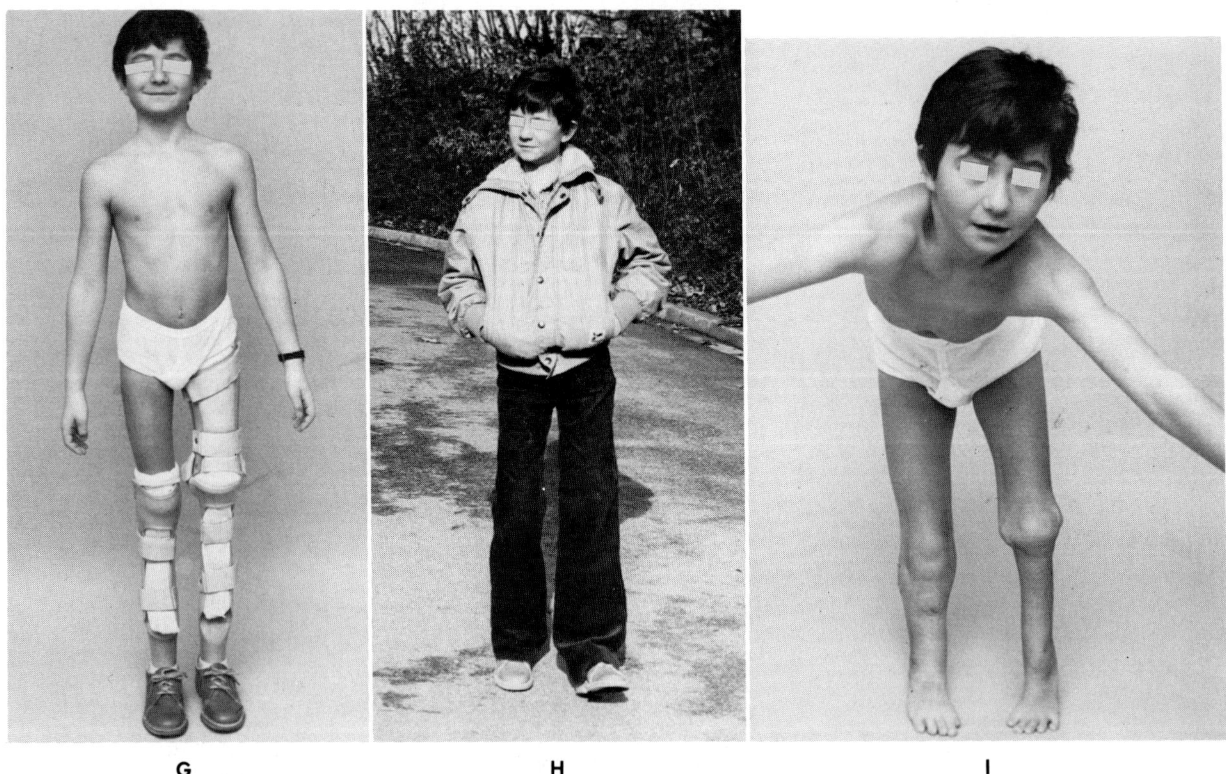

Fig. 41-25, cont'd. G, In March, 1979, patient has been fitted with his most recent prostheses. Right leg has PTS prosthesis with open socket and Velcro closures over tibia and foot. Left leg has been fitted with nonconventional technique, including open socket with Velcro straps for tibia and foot, outside knee joint with Swiss locks, and plastic thigh corset with Velcro closures. **H,** Patient wears his prostheses 12 to 14 hours a day, attends regular school, and is an entirely normal individual despite severe lower limb deficiencies. **I,** Patient can stand on feet without his prostheses.

struction concluded in June of 1977, with arthrodesis of both knees, partial foot amputation, and stabilization of the astragalus to the fibula bilaterally (Fig. 41-24, *E* and *F*). Knee disarticulation was contraindicated because of the hypoplasia of both femora and also to preserve his independence. Use of above-knee prostheses would have required the help of others to don them. Following this surgery, the child was fitted with new orthoprostheses. The prescription included plastic above-knee sockets with windows and Velcro suspension, knee joints with Swiss locks, and articulated feet. Again, he became ambulatory and independent in donning and doffing his four prostheses. New limbs were prescribed in February, 1979. The child is now fully ambulatory, wears his lower limbs full time, and is able to play soccer wearing them. He wears his upper limbs approximately 8 hours a day, attends regular school, and is independent in eating and drinking, but at home he removes the upper limbs for playing.

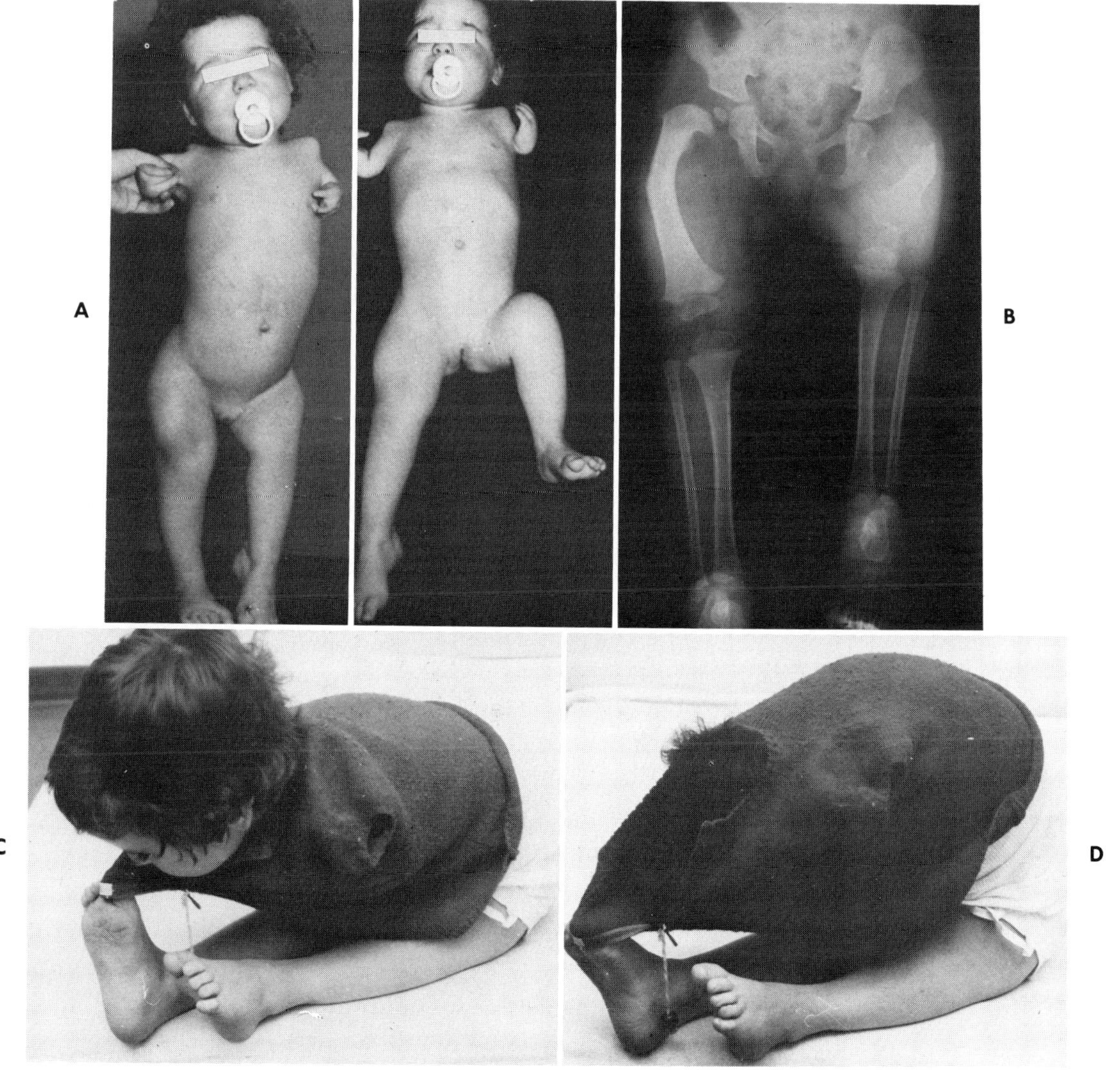

Fig. 41-26. A, Patient has bilateral upper limb phocomelia and bilateral lower limb deficiencies secondary to ingestion of thalidomide by mother. **B,** Roentgenogram of lower limbs shows coxa vara with bowing on right and left longitudinal deficiency of femur, partial (Aitken class A PFFD). **C,** In 1967, self-care training was undertaken in physical therapy and occupational therapy departments, emphasizing use of feet for prehension. **D,** Independence in dressing and undressing is taught. Note loops on undergarments at left hip region to assist in removal.

Continued.

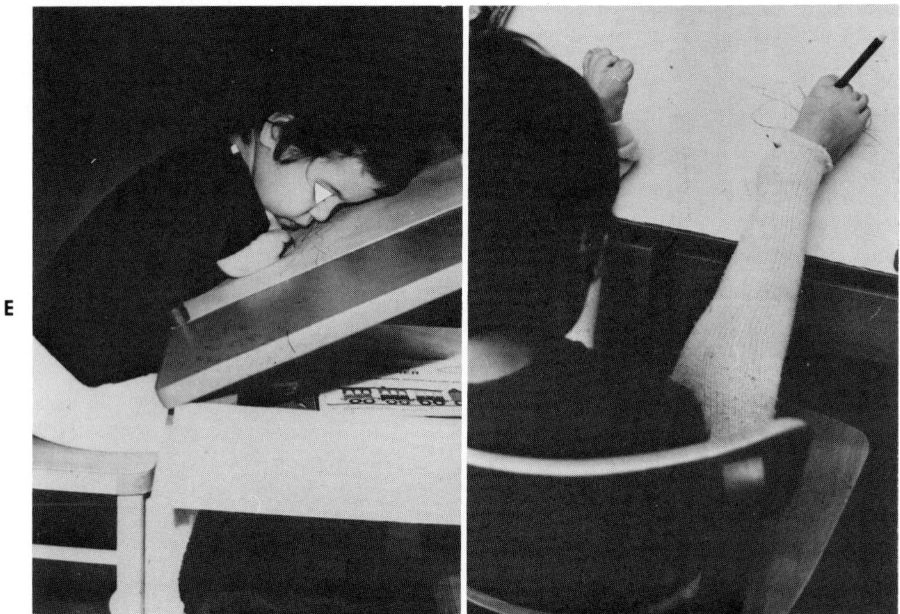

Fig. 41-26, cont'd. E, Child is able to use hypoplastic phocomelic hands for writing and drawing, but it is much easier for her to do this using her feet. **F,** PFFD with severe varus angulation is demonstrated here. **G,** First stage correction of severe varus following resection and fusion of subtrochanteric pseudarthrosis is demonstrated with internal fixation in place. **H,** After second-stage correction, better angle is achieved, and once again healing is solid with internal fixation. **I,** After removal of osteosynthesis hardware, Chiari osteotomy is fixed with Steinmann pin and distal transplantation of trochanter is fixed with single screw. Good coverage of femoral head has been attained.

Continued.

Hip reconstruction for PFFD with multimembral deficiency

The child in Fig. 41-26 was born on June 9, 1962, after a full-term pregnancy; the father and mother are both entirely normal as were three older siblings. There was no family history of limb deficiency or other congenital deformity. There was, however, a history of the mother having ingested thalidomide in the early pregnancy. The child was born with bilateral phocomelic upper limbs, consisting of hypoplastic rudimentary humeral segments synostosed with the ulna, longitudinal deficiency of the radius and complete metacarpophalangeal 1 and 2 deficiency, with hypoplasia of the remaining digits. The lower limbs showed left partial longitudinal deficiency of the femur (intermediate—the equivalent of an Aitken class A PFFD). On the right side there was a coxa vara with bowing. Other congenital anomalies included a mild scoliosis, strabismus, and a pyloric stenosis corrected by surgery on the second day of life. The child was first seen in September of 1962, at which time a physical therapy program was instituted as well as extension splinting of the lower limbs. In August of 1964, a valgus osteotomy of the right femur was carried out, and, in September, 1964, she was supplied with an extension orthosis for the left leg. In 1967, the child was admitted to the hospital for self-care training, especially in the technique of using the feet as well as the vestigial hands for activities of daily living. A full physical therapy program to maintain functional mobility of the spine was likewise undertaken. At this time a left upper limb prosthesis was prescribed. This was a ball bearing-supported elongation of the left upper limb with a pneumatic hook and a pneumatic wrist rotation unit operated by the left phocomelic hand (Fig. 41-5). By the following year the child had rejected the pneumatic prosthesis. In 1968, she was enrolled in a special preschool for the physically handicapped. In 1969, she was supplied with an orthoprosthesis for the left lower limb with a stiff knee and SACH foot (Fig. 41-4). In 1974, the left subtrochanteric pseudarthrosis was resected and the first stage of correction of the severe varus deformity undertaken, as well as correction of the severe hip flexion deformity. In 1975, the second stage for correction of the varus deformity was carried out and 6 weeks later the patient was fitted with a new orthoprosthesis. In 1976, the hardware

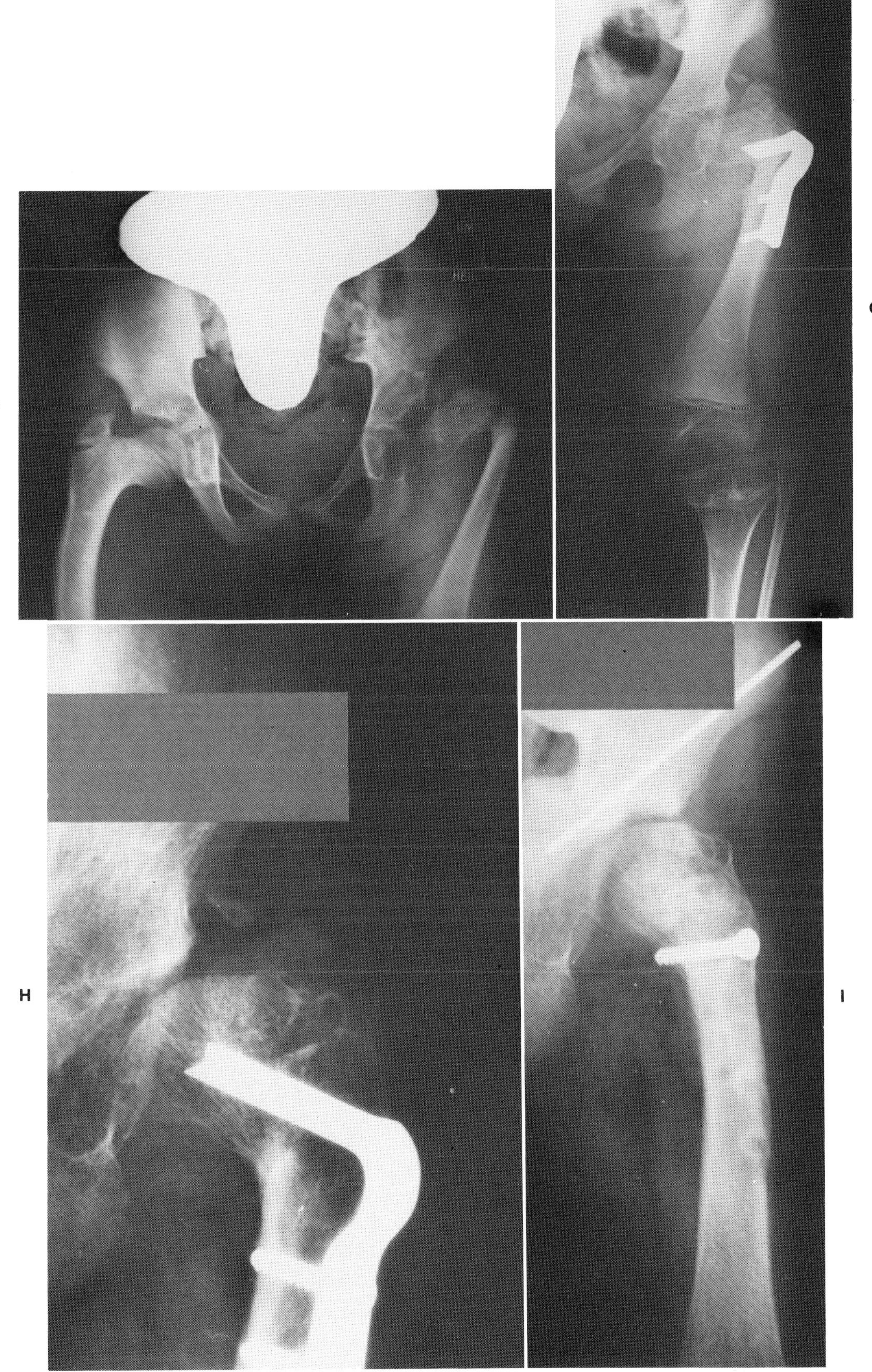

Fig. 41-26, cont'd. For legend see opposite page. *Continued.*

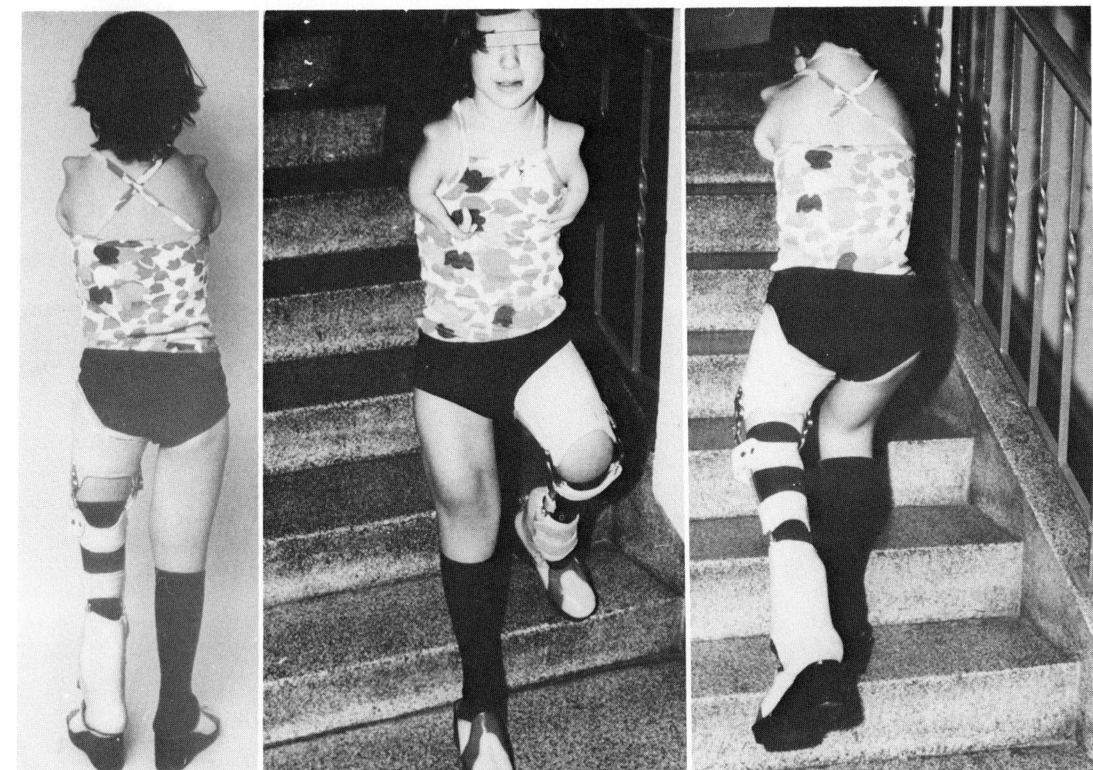

Fig. 41-26, cont'd. J, Child is fully ambulatory with her new orthoprosthesis and attends regular school in her own village. She has rejected pneumatic arm prescribed in childhood.

was removed and a Chiari osteotomy carried out to provide increased coverage of the femoral head. At this time the trochanter was also transplanted distally. After healing of this surgery a new orthoprosthesis was prescribed with a left thigh corset, free knee joint, and SACH foot. Presently, the child is fully and independently ambulatory, uses her toes as well as her vestigial hands for self-care, and attends school in her own village.

Reconstructive surgery in upper and lower limbs prior to prosthetic fitting

The child in Fig. 41-27 was born of healthy parents on May 15, 1961. The history, however, reveals that at approximately 6 weeks after her last menstrual period, the mother of the patient ingested thalidomide for a period of 3 days for surgery. The pregnancy was uneventful with a normal birth. The child had the following limb deficiencies: upper limbs showed bilateral hypoplasia of the radius with partial carpal absence and, on the right, partial absence metacarpophalangeal 1, whereas on the left, metacarpophangeal 1 was completely absent. In the lower limbs there was bilateral complete longitudinal deficiency of the tibia, with coxa vara of the femur on the right and longitudinal deficiency of the proximal femur on the left (Aitken class A) with subtrochanteric pseudarthrosis.

The patient was first seen in 1964, prior to which he had been fitted with stubby prostheses at the University of Tübingen. Shortly thereafter, centralization of the fibula under the femur and of astralgus under the fibula was carried out at Tübingen for stiffness on the right. In 1967, orthoprostheses as well as a night splint were provided, and he began a physical therapy and occupational therapy program. In 1968, the left index finger was pollicized.[3] In 1969, arthrodesis of the right knee was carried out, and, in 1970, new orthoprostheses were prescribed for the lower limbs. In 1971, pollicization of the right index finger was carried out in Heidelberg, and, in 1974, the left subtrochanteric pseudarthrosis was resected, and the varus deformity corrected, subsequent to which new prostheses were prescribed. In 1978, because of increasing flexion adduction deformity in the left knee, arthrodesis of this

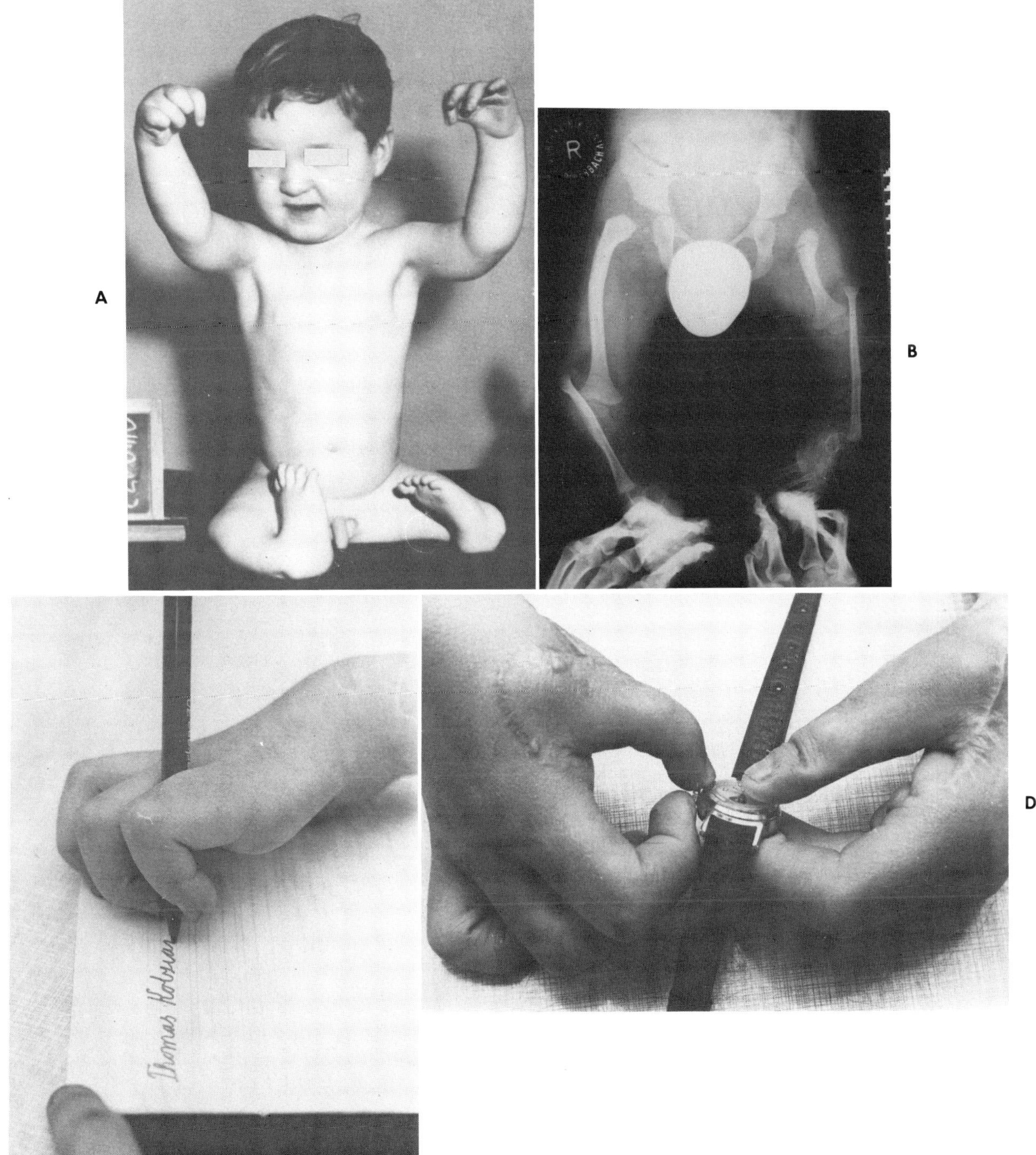

Fig. 41-27. A, Patient was born with longitudinal deficiency of tibia bilaterally and left longitudinal deficiency of proximal portion of femur, as well as associated deficiencies of first metacarpal ray. **B,** Roentgenograms demonstrate bilateral longitudinal deficiency of tibia as well as PFFD. **C,** Prior to reconstruction (pollicization), pencil is held by adduction of digits. **D,** After bilateral pollicizations, function is excellent.

Continued.

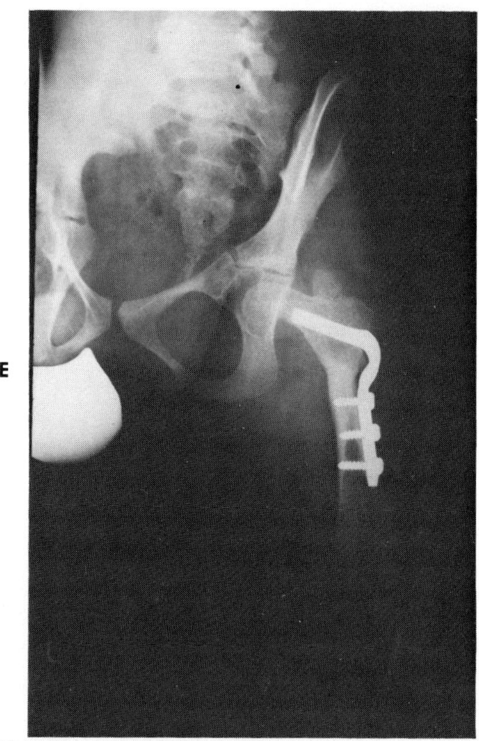

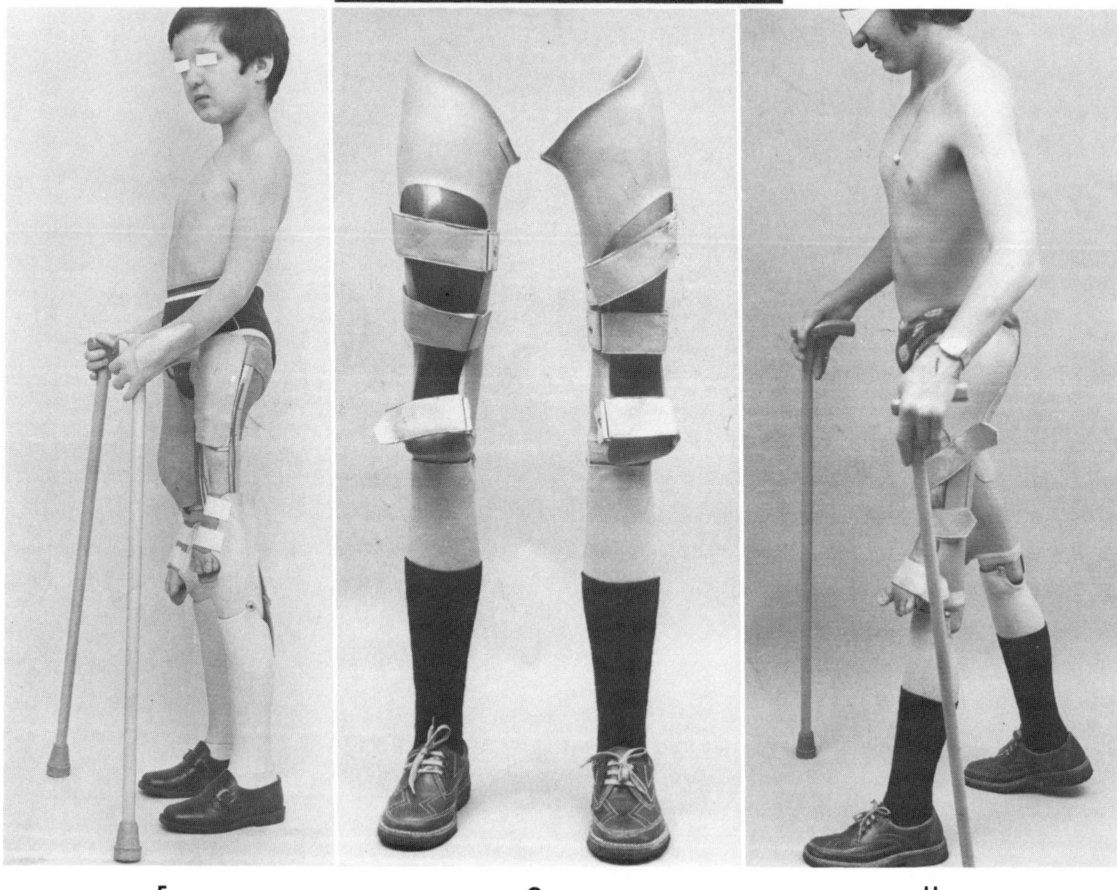

Fig. 41-27, cont'd. E, Roentgenogram shows left hip after reconstruction. **F,** Knees have been fused, and he is ready for prostheses. **G,** Orthoprostheses that were constructed for patient. **H,** Patient is ambulatory. Note use of pollicized digits to hold canes.

knee was carried out. New orthoprostheses were prescribed. In addition to all of his physical problems, this child has mental retardation and his schooling has been much delayed by these multiple surgical procedures. Nonetheless, as indicated in Fig. 41-27, he is independently ambulatory, and his pollicized index fingers function quite well as thumbs. This patient demonstrates the importance of reconstructive surgery in both the upper and lower limb prior to prosthetic fitting, but he demonstrates also the need for a better consideration of the child's psychic development if orthopaedic surgery and hospitalization are indicated.

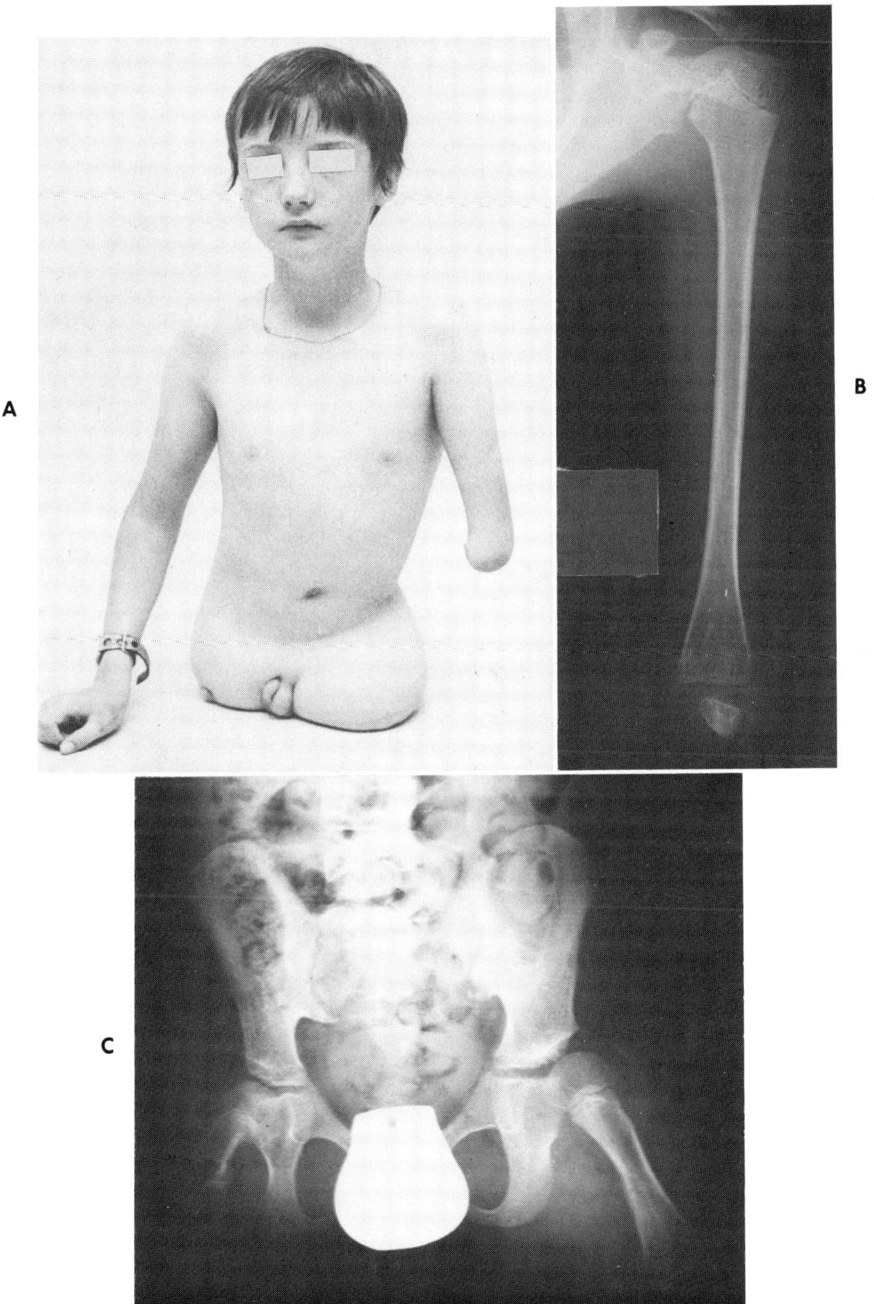

Fig. 41-28. Transverse deficiency of forearm, left upper third (very short ulnar fragment). Transverse deficiency of thigh, upper third bilateral (functional amelia). **A,** At age 11, patient has been trained in wheelchair. He is now ready for prosthetic limbs. **B,** Roentgenogram of left arm. Note very small ulnar fragment articulating with distal humerus. **C,** Roentgenogram of pelvis, showing very short remaining femoral segments.

Continued.

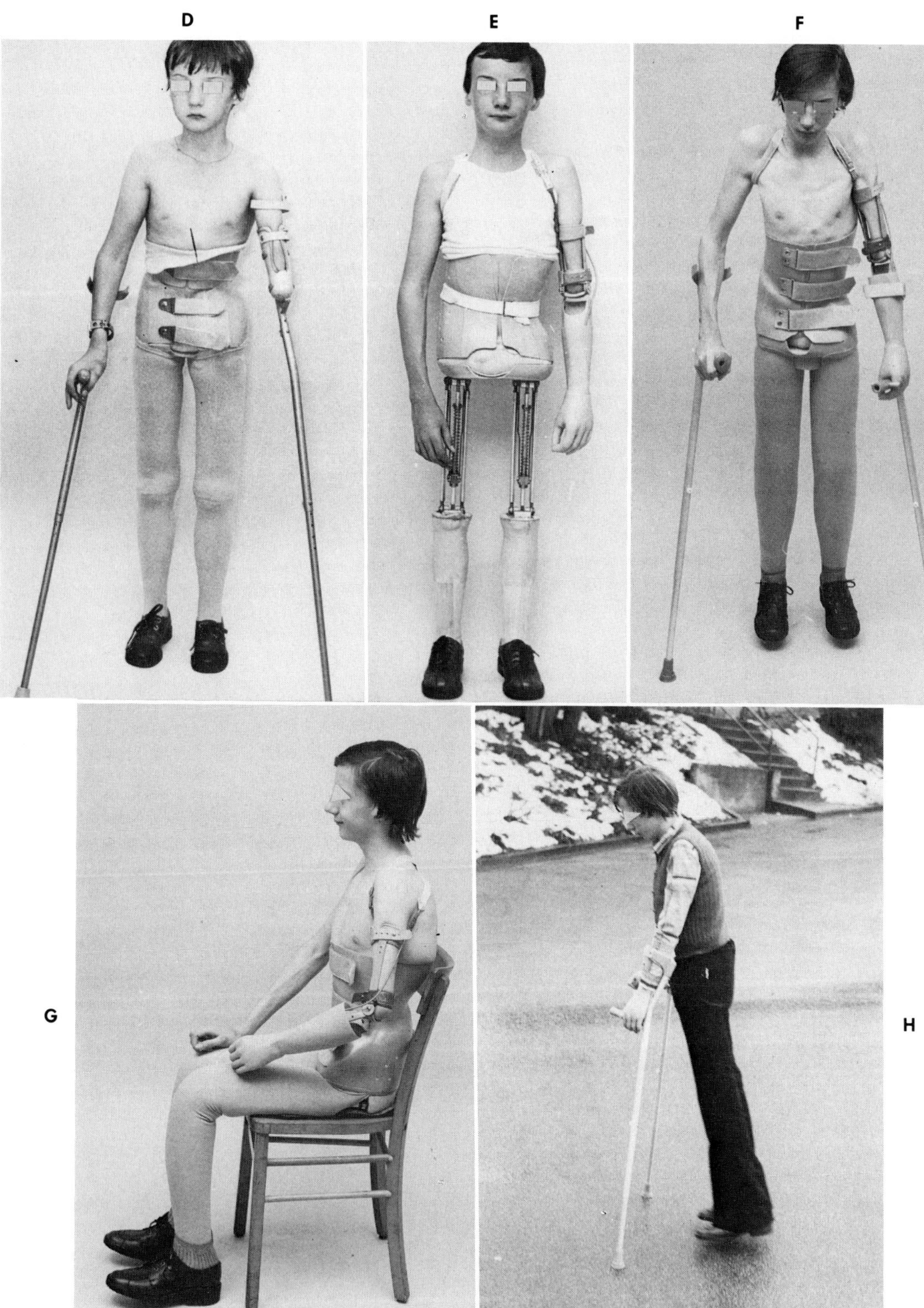

Fig. 41-28, cont'd. D, First prostheses. Plastic laminate pelvic bucket with parallellogram construction of hips and knees and SACH feet. Finished prostheses have foam covers. After 4 weeks of training, he was able to sit, stand, and walk with swing-through gait. **E,** Unfinished lower limb prostheses show parallellogram construction of knee and hip joints. Functional hand has been applied. **F** and **G,** With finished prostheses, patient demonstrates standing and sitting. **H,** Clothed, patient demonstrates swing-through gait. With his ability to sit and stand, as well as to ambulate independently, he has been permitted to attend regular school in his hometown, rather than special school for handicapped persons far away from home.

Hip disarticulation prostheses for bilateral lower limb deficiency

This child was born November 4, 1962 (Fig. 41-28). There was no family history of limb deficiencies and his two siblings were normal. There was no history of ingestion of any medication during the pregnancy.

The child was born with bilateral transverse lower limb deficiencies, thigh upper third, and a transverse deficiency of the forearm, proximal third (with a very short ulna segment remaining). He had other congenital anomalies.

The child was first evaluated in November, 1972, at which time he was using primarily a wheelchair but was able to get around on the floor using his hands. He was noted also to have a scoliosis. Bilateral lower limb prostheses were prescribed with automatic knee locks in the stance phase and automatic combined hip and knee flexion for sitting. A left above-elbow prosthesis was constructed with a crutch attached to the functional hand for ambulation. These prostheses were first applied July, 1973, and after 4 weeks of training he was able to ambulate on a level surface and, with considerable effort, even manage stairs. He was also able to sit and stand independently. Stairs were particularly important because without this ability, he would not be permitted to attend high school at home but would have to attend a special school. In 1974, his upper limb prosthesis was changed to a cable-controlled Hosmer outside locking elbow with a Dorrance 10X hook interchangeable with an Otto Bock hand. He was additionally supplied with a cosmetic forearm prosthesis for swimming. His lower limb socket had to be changed in 1976, again in 1978, and most recently in 1979, extending the socket somewhat proximally to act as a support for his progressive scoliosis. It was believed that because of his problems in ambulation with bilateral hip disarticulation-type prostheses that Harrington instrumentation should not be considered.

CONCLUSION

An effort has been made to document a philosophy for management of the multimembral-deficient child. Particular emphasis is placed on using all function in tactile areas, including vestigial digits on deficient upper limbs, in the early life of these children. Substitution patterns are discussed, especially the use of the foot for prehension by the armless child. Reconstructive procedures that have special benefits for the multimembral-deficient child as opposed to the unimembral-deficient child are discussed. Prosthetic solutions are presented for both upper and lower limb deficiencies. Stress is placed on the limitation of functional value and particularly on the excess of the weight of currently available externally powered upper limb devices. Finally, case studies are used to illustrate the complexity of the problems involved with the quadrimembral-deficient child. It is important to recognize that in no way could such a chapter as this cover all combinations of deficiencies and that this is an effort to present the problems in general with some particular solutions.

ACKNOWLEDGMENTS

I thank my co-workers, patients, and parents for their cooperation.

Special thanks I give to Dr. U. Banniza von Bazan and Dr. G. Suppelna for preliminary extracts of selected medical reports and for the preselection of photographs and x-ray films. I thank Mr. H. Brünler, head of our photography laboratory, for the photographs and x-ray reproductions, and last, but not least, Dr. Leon M. Kruger for his excellent help and great patience.

REFERENCES

1. Bauer, K. H.: Zum Problem der Ohnhänderversorgung und zur Frage der operativen Behandlung, insbesondere des Krukenberg-Armes, Verh. Dtsch. Orthop. Ges. **36**:51-53, 1949.
2. Biesalski, K.: Die Kunstglieder der Versuchs – und Lehrwerk – stätte des Oskar-Helene-Heims, Z. Orthop. **37**:174-278, 1917.
3. Blauth, W.: Erfahrungen in der operativen Behandlung von Klumphänden (Radius aplasien) Verh. Dtsch. Orthop. Ges. **54**:439-445, 1968.
4. Blauth, W., and Schneider-Sickert, F.: Handfehlbildungen – Atlas ihrer operativen Behandlung, Berlin, 1976, Springer Verlag.
5. Fischer: Z. Orthop. **37**:228-247, 1917.
6. Häefner, O.: Die pneumatisch bewegte prothese. Patentschrift des Patents der Bundesrepublik Deutschland, No. 828291, July 28, 1949.
7. Hepp, O.: Prothesen der oberen Extremität. In Hohmann, G., Hackenbrock, K., Lindemann, L., editors: Handbuch der Orthopädie, vol. 1, Stuttgart, 1957, Georg Thieme Verlag.
8. Hepp, O.: Die Häufung der angeborenen Defektmibildungen der oberen Extremitaten in der Bundesrepublik Deutschland, Med. Klin. **57**:419-426, 1962.
9. Heyne, S.: Ergotherapie bei blinden Ohnhändern mit Krukenberg-Plastik, Beschaftigungstherapie und Rehabilitation **17**(4):221-225, Dec., 1978.
10. Ķeyl, R.: Erfahrungen mit der Krukenberg-operation und deren Nachbehandlung, Verh. Dtsch. Orthop. Ges. **36**:61-64, 1949.
11. Kreuz, L.: Die Herrichtung des Unterarmstumpfes zum natürlichen Greifarm nach dem Verfahren von Krukenberg, Zentralbl. Chir. **37-38**:1170-1175, 1944.
12. Krukenberg, H.: Uber die plastihe Umwertung von Arm-

amputationstümpfen, Stuttgart, 1917, Ferdinand Enke Verlag.

13. Kuhn, G. G.: Kunstarmbau in GieSharztechnik, Stuttgart, 1968, Georg Thieme Verlag.
14. Lenz, W.: Diskussionsbemerkung von Privatdozent Dr. W. Lenz, Hamburg, zu dem Vortrag von R. A. Pfeiffer u. W. Kosenow: Zur Frage der oxogenen Entstehung schwerer Extremitaten-Missbildungen, Tagung der Rheinisch-Westfälischen Kinderärzte-vereinigung in Düsseldorf, am 19.11, 1961.
15. Lenz, W.: Missbildungen nach Medikamenteneinnahme während der Gravidität, Dtsch. Med. Wochenschr. **86:** 2555, 1961.
16. Lenz, W. and Knapp, K.: Die Thalidomid-Embryopathie, Dtsch. Med. Wschr. **87:**1232-1242, 1962. Lancet **1:**45, 1962.
17. Lindemann, K., and Marquardt, E.: Information on standard prostheses for armless children. Information on measures for habilitation of children with dysmelia, Heidelberg, 1963, Deutsche Vereinigung für die Rehabilitation Behinderter, pp. 52-55.
18. Marquardt, E.: Indications for an early treatment of children with dysmelia. Information on measures for habilitation of children with dysmelia. Heidelberg, 1963, Deutsche Vereinigung für die Rehabilitation Behinderter, pp. 56-57.
19. Marquardt, E.: Pneumatic arm prostheses for children. In Information on measures for habilitation of children with dysmelia, Heidelberg, 1963, Deutsche Vereinigung für die Rehabilitation Behinderter, pp. 34-41.
20. Marquardt, E.: Provision with active protheses of armless babies in the second year of life. In Information on measures for habilitation of children with dysmelia. Heidelberg, 1963, Deutsche Vereinigung für die Rehabilitation Behinderter, pp. 42-51.
21. Marquardt, E.: Einleitung der Diskussion über die Therapie der radialen Klumphand. In 1. Monographie über die Rehabilitation der Dysmeliekinder. Published by the Bundesminister für Gesundheitswesen, Bartmann, Frechen, 1965, pp. 48-51.
22. Marquardt, E.: The Heidelberg pneumatic arm prosthesis, J. Bone Joint Surg. **47B:**425-434, 1965.
23. Marquardt, E.: Erfahrungen mit pneumatischen prothesen, Verh. Dtsch. Orthop. Ges. **52:**346-352, 1966.
24. Marquardt, E.: The management of infants with malformation of the extremities. In Limb development and deformity: problems of evaluation and rehabilitation, Springfield, Ill., 1969, Charles C Thomas, Publisher, pp. 363-378.
25. Marquardt, E.: The total treatment of the limb deficient child. The Horowitz Lectures, 1968. Rehabilitation Monograph 44, 1969, Institute of Rehabilitation Medicine, New York University Medical Center.
26. Marquardt, E.: Steigerung der Effektivität von Oberarmprothesen nach Winkelosteotomie, Rehabilitation **11:** 244-248, 1972.
27. Marquardt, E.: Osteotomia katowa kikuta ramienia. In Tomaszewskiej, J., editor: Protesowanie typu czynnego po amputcjach w obrebie konczyn gornych. Warszawa-Poznan 1975, pp. 37-50.
28. Marquardt, E.: Plastische Operationen bei drohender Knochendurchspiessung am kindlichen Oberarmstumpf, Z. Orthop **114:**711-714, 1976.
29. Marquardt, E.: Die Krukenberg-Plastik, Originalmethode und Modifikationen für blinde Ohnhänder, Beschäftigungstherapie ünd Rehabil. **17**(4):221-225, Dec., 1978.
30. Marquardt, E., and Haefner, O.: Technical adequacy and practical application of the Heidelberg pneumatic prosthesis, New York, 1956, International Society for the Welfare of Cripples. In German: Archiv für orthopädische and Unfallchirurgie **48:**115-135, 1956.
31. Marquardt, E., and Roesler, H.: Prothesen und Prothesenversorgungen der oberen Extremität. In Witt, A. N., Rettig, H., Schlegel, F. K., Hackenbrock, M., and Hupfauer, W., editors: Orthopädie in praxis und Klinik, vol. 2. Stuttgart, 1981, Georg Thieme Verlag.
32. McBride, W. G.: Thalidomide and congenital abnormalities, Lancet **2:**1358, 1961.
33. McBride, W. G.: Thalidomide and congenital abnormalities, Med. J. Aust. **2:**689-693, 1963.
34. Neff, G., and Marquardt, E.: The radial club hand: the case for conservative therapy, Chirurgia Plastica **4:**279-287, 1979.
35. Neff, G., and Marquardt, E.: Angeborene Extremitätenmi bildungen. In Baumgartner, R.: Amputation und Prothesenversorgung beim Kind, Stuttgart, 1977, Ferdinand Enke Verlag.
36. Pfeiffer, R. A., and Kosenow, W.: Zur Frage einer exogenen Verursachung von schweren Extremitätenmissbildungen, Münchner Med. Wochenschr. **104:**68-74, 1962.
37. Schöllner, D.: Die Klumphand bei Radiusaplasie. Aktuelle Orthopädie, vol. 5, Stuttgart, 1972, Georg Thieme Verlag (extensive bibliography).
38. Simpson, D. C.: An externally powered prosthesis for the complete arm. The basic problems of prehension, movement, and control of artificial limbs, Proceedings of the Institution of Mechanical Engineers, vol. 183, Part 3J, 1968-1969, p. 11.
39. Simpson, D. C.: Eine Prothese für beidseitig armgeschädigte Dysmeliekinder, Orthop. Tech. **24:**363-364, 1972.
40. Spitzy, H., and Feldschareck: Die Versorgung beiderseits Armamputierter, Münchner Med. Wochenschr. **63:**1181-1186, 1916.
41. Steinruck. In Katthagen, A.: Versorgung von Hand und Armamputierten mit Werkprothesen, Verh. Dtsch. Orthop. Ges. **43:**193-200, 1955.
42. Swanson, A. B.: Silicone-rubber implants to control the overgrowth phenomenon in the juvenile amputee, Inter-Clin. Info. Bull. **11**(9):58, 1972.
43. von Volkmann, R.: Die Muskelfunktion im Krukenberg-Arm sowie einige operative Folgerungen, Verh. Dtsch. Orthop. Ges. **38:**293-297, 1951.
44. Wiedemann, H. R.: Hypo-und aplastische Fehlbildungen der Gliedmassen (Dysmelie-Syndrom), Med. Welt. **23:** 1863-1866, 1961.
45. Weil, S.: Die Heidelberger pneumatische Armprothese, Chirurg. **26:**351-354, 1955.
46. Witt, A. N., Cotta, H., and Jäger, M.: Die angeborenen Fehlbildungen der Hand, Stuttgart, 1966, Georg Thieme Verlag.

SUGGESTED READINGS

Boos, O.: Die Versorgung von Ohnhändern, Stuttgart, 1960, F. K. Schattauer Verlag.

Gocht, H.: Atiologie, Pathogenese und Therapie der Deformitäten im allgemeinen. In Hoffa, A.: Orthopädische Chirurgie, Stuttgart, 1925, Ferdinand Enke Verlag.

Hepp, O.: Information on measures for habilitation for children with dysmelia, Heidelberg, 1962 (German version), 1963 (English version), Deutsche Vereiningung für die Rehabilitation Behinderter e.V.

Jones, D., Barnes, J., and Lloyd-Roberts, G. C.: Congenital aplasia and dysplasia of the tibia with intact fibula: classification and management, J. Bone Joint Surg. **60B:**30-39, 1978.

Kallio, K. E.: Recent advances in Krukenberg's operation, Acta Chir. Scand. **97:**165, 1948.

Kessler, H. H.: Cineplasty, Springfield, Ill., 1947, Charles C Thomas, Publisher.

Kuhn, G. G: Neue technische Hilfen für schwer Körperbehinderte kinder. In Baumgartner, R.: Amputation und Prothesenversorgung beim Kind Stuttgart, 1977, Ferdinand Enke Verlag.

Lamb, D. W.: Radial club hand, J. Bone Joint Surg. **59A:**1-13, 1977.

Marquardt, E., and Neff, G.: The angulation osteotomy of above-elbow stumps, Clin. Orthop. **104:**232-238, 1974.

Nathan, P. A., and Nguyen, B. T.: The Krukenberg operation; a modified technique avoiding skin grafts, J. Hand Surg. **2**(2):127-130, 1977.

Sauerbruch, F.: Die willkürlich bewegbare künstliche Hand, eine Anleitung für Chirurgen and Techniker mit anatomischen Beiträgen von G. Ruge and W. Felix unter Mitwirkung von A.Stadler, Berlin, 1916, Julius Springer Verlag.

Swanson, A. B.: The Krukenberg procedure in the juvenile amputee, J. Bone Joint Surg. **46A:**1540, 1964.

Thomsen, W.: Diskussionsbeitrag zum Thema Krukenberg-Plastik, Verh. Dtsch. Orthop. Ges. **36:**60-61, 1949.

Willert, H. G., and Henkel, H. L.: Klinik und Pathologie der Dysmelie. Die Fehlbildungen an den oberen Extremitäten bei der Thalidomidembryopathie. Experimentelle Medizin, Pathologie und Klinik, Bd. 26, Berlin, 1969, Springer Verlag.

CHAPTER 42

Research in juvenile prosthetics

MADELYN M. LABORIEL
YOSHIO SETOGUCHI

Historically, the establishment of clinics specifically designed and staffed for child amputees occurred in the early 1950s. Clinicians who were aware of the unique needs of children with limb deficiencies or amputations believed that the care and management of these patients should be separated from the care provided to adult amputees. At that time, however, the only surgical techniques and prosthetic fittings available were those which had been developed for adult patients.

With the establishment of child amputee clinics, new management techniques and philosophies, together with new surgical techniques and prosthetic fittings, were developed specifically for children. Some centers, realizing the need for prosthetic research, developed their clinics for just such purposes. During the past 25 years, these centers have provided many new prosthetic devices and fitting techniques that are now considered "standard." The research has continued, and in the past 5 years, many new devices and techniques have been developed. To keep abreast of some of these developments, the major juvenile amputee research centers in the United States and Europe were recently contacted; this chapter is a summary of research activities as reported to us. We apologize if any researcher was inadvertently omitted.

The emphasis in research during the past 5 years has been in four major areas: (1) modular or endoskeletal prosthetic design, (2) body-powered components, (3) external power sources and component designs, and (4) sensory feedback studies. There has also been some interesting research in specialized devices, which will be discussed.

UPPER LIMB PROSTHESES

Modular systems

"Modular" has become one of the key words in prosthetics research in the past few years. It refers to a system of interchangeable components that can be easily assembled, permitting great flexibility in prosthetic design. With the modular system, prostheses can be tailored to the needs of an individual child or group of children without the prohibitive expenditure of time for a prosthetist.

Those who have had clinical experience with the child amputee know that the child cannot be viewed as a miniature adult, nor can children be regarded as a uniform group. The body proportions of an infant and toddler are quite distinct from those of the school and teen-aged child. The functional needs, too, are quite distinct. The activities of a 12-month-old infant who is crawling, beginning to walk, and clasping objects at his side, are different from those of a 24-month-old who is running, turning pages of a book, using crayons, and feeding himself with growing independence. Flexibility in prosthetic design and in the selection of components is imperative if the changing needs of a child are to be met. The modular system provides this flexibility.[10] Research using the modular concept is in progress at several locations.

One design for functional upper limb prostheses using the modular concept is being developed at the Child Amputee Prosthetics Project (CAPP), at the University of California, Los Angeles.[17] Standard functional upper limb prostheses are exoskeletal in design, with the structural support provided by an outer shell, which is hollow to the terminal device. The experimental design is endoskeletal. That is, the device is hollow in the socket area to accommodate the stump, but structural support is provided by an endoskeletal frame covered with a filler and cosmetic covering.

The prosthesis is lightweight, which encourages early acceptance and the rapid development of spontaneous use by the child. The soft, deformable filler provides a natural appearing contour and effective grip when the child clutches objects to the chest with the prosthesis. The cosmetic covering is capable of withstanding the rough treatment to which children subject their prostheses. As the prostheses are now designed, prosthetists are able to make repairs and adjustments easily, changing the length or combination of components in accordance with the child's growth or functional capabilities. The modular prosthesis is therefore good for the life of the socket.

Modular systems are also available for above-elbow and shoulder disarticulation deficits. CAPP has one such design. The German firm Otto Bock Orthopedic Industries, Inc., also has such a design with components that are commercially available in the United States. Research efforts are now focused on refinement of individual components.

Body-powered prostheses

CAPP terminal device. It is well established that 25% of all patients with congenital limb deficiencies have unilateral below-elbow deficiencies.[3] CAPP has designed and has in use a new terminal device designed expressly for children.[11] Unlike conventional terminal devices, this is not a miniaturization of adult designs but is distinctly different. It was developed as a result of clinical experience, which identified the special functional needs of the young child and the characteristics of the patient population. Fine manipulation of objects is carried out primarily by the unaffected limb and hand. The primary function of the prosthetic limb and terminal device is to provide a secure assistive grasp. The hook, designed primarily for fine manipulation by adults, becomes an inefficient tool for the young child to use because of the precise placement required to achieve a secure hold on an object.

The currently available CAPP terminal device (Fig. 42-1) consists of a lightweight plastic shell. The grasping surface is triangular with multiple "toothlike" compressible projections that provide maximum surface area and friction for secure grasp. This surface is opposed by a single aluminum opening lever, which is mounted on a shaft that also holds the spring. This design permits good grasp with maximum visibility. A control line passes centrally from the opening lever over a pulley within the shell and exits from the terminal device with straight-line pull.

Clinical testing of fifty-six patients in various centers throughout the United States has been encouraging. It was noted that surprisingly little

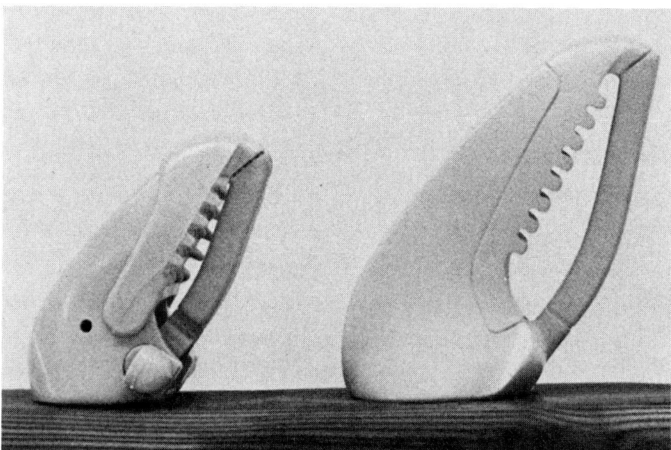

Fig. 42-1. CAPP terminal device. Left, size currently available. Right, design of experimental second size.

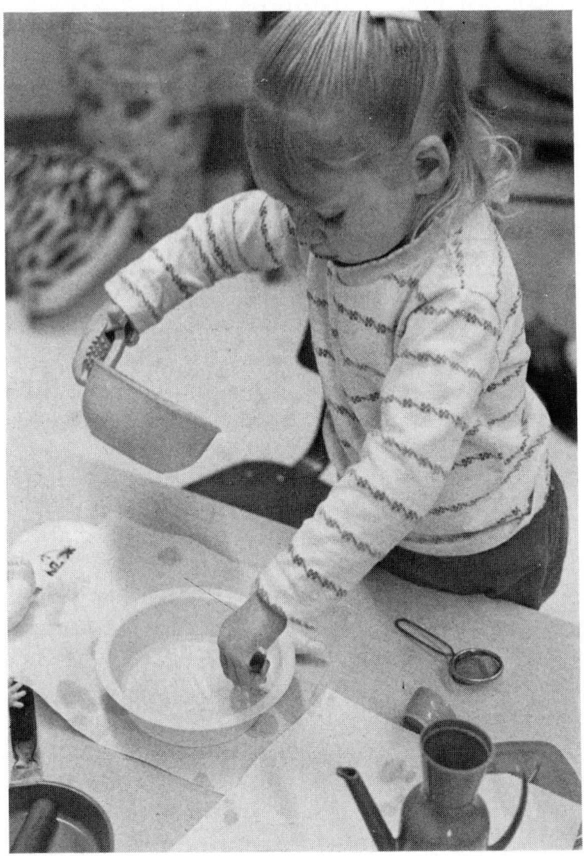

Fig. 42-2. Patient using CAPP terminal device. Note gripping, or frictional, surface.

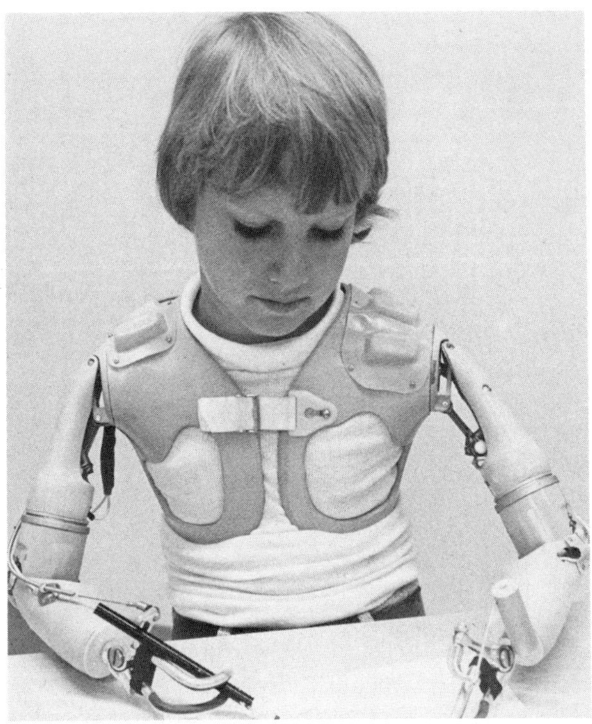

Fig. 42-3. Fitting of bilateral shoulder disarticulation prostheses with externally powered elbows.

pinch force (0.23 kg; 1/2 pound for children under age 3) was required for the child to obtain a secure hold on objects because of the broad, frictional, resilient gripping surface provided by the material used to make the cover. This cover also extended to the outer surface of the terminal device and was readily integrated into gross motor activities (Fig. 42-2). Placing objects into the terminal device presented no problem for young children, since they did not require precise positioning. The appearance was somewhat forbidding to some parents when seen in isolation, but was preferred to the hook by a substantial number of parents after being seen as a part of a complete prosthesis on a patient. Overall, the device appears to be clinically successful and plans for commercial manufacture are underway.

CAPP two-way shoulder joint. A two-way shoulder joint is under development that is designed to meet some of the needs of the child with a complete arm deficiency (amelia).[9] Among those needs is a joint that is sturdy and will provide easy and flexible positioning but that will be stable in the selected positions. The addition of a second plane of motion (abduction-adduction) contributes to the flexibility of choice of position and compensates for the torque and lateral forces that act on the humeral segment of the prosthesis by permitting "breakaway" into a second plane.

The new shoulder joint under development provides these movements in two planes and also provides improved cosmesis (Fig. 42-3). The joint is constructed of metal with a flesh-colored finish that requires no additional covering. Friction units for both planes have been designed to fit into the limited space provided, thereby avoiding as much bulk as possible.

Clinical testing of the joint has been successful. Children position the shoulder quite naturally by grasping and pulling the terminal device with the sound hand. A 2-year-old girl with little training has been observed to position the joint in such a way as to cause the prosthesis to match the position of her normal arm. She readily incorporated the abduction movement into her spontaneous use patterns. The cosmetic improvement was well-received by the patients and parents alike.

Frame shoulder socket. Fitting a shoulder disarticulation socket to a child is a difficult task,

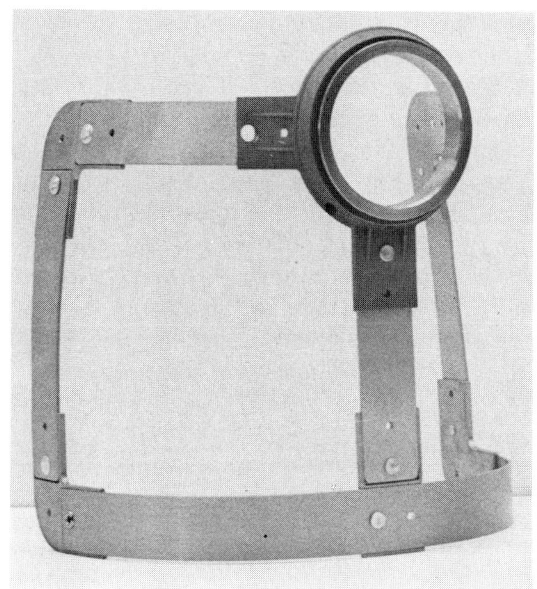

Fig. 42-4. CAPP frame socket.

a fact that is well known to clinicians. The chest contour of a child is not constant and is, in fact, quite malleable, so that a good cast is difficult to obtain when standard casting techniques are used. It is difficult to adequately distribute the forces and pressures that are exerted on the shoulder socket by the prosthesis, and sensitive pressure areas often develop. Standard shoulder disarticulation sockets cover half of the rib cage of the unilateral amputee and half of the torso of the bilateral amputee. A child whose total body surface is already decreased because of the absent limbs can ill afford this heavy covering of the torso. Under these conditions the problems of copious perspiration and temperature control take on major proportions.

Research is under way in several centers to design a "frame socket" that will help alleviate these problems. The Chailey Heritage Workshop in England[7] is experimenting with a carbon-fiber reinforced plastic (CFRP), which is very lightweight but has a high degree of stiffness and tensile strength. This material is being used instead of metal to make a strong frame that permits body temperature control with minimal addition of weight. Initial reports of clinical trials of this socket indicate excellent acceptance by the children.

A different approach to the frame socket design is found at CAPP. Design of the socket was based on a study of the patterns of the forces that act on the shoulder and socket when the prosthesis is in motion. It was postulated that if a satisfactory fit could be obtained to accommodate those forces, the result would be a combination of comfort and good function. This socket design is a prefabricated system of lightweight aluminum strips with a cosmetic finish that can be fitted directly on the patient by the prosthetist without any casting procedure (Fig. 42-4). The forces reflected from the prosthesis through the socket to the stump are distributed to areas of the torso that can receive them with comfort and provide stability.

Elimination of the casting procedure reduces the time normally required to make a shoulder socket by 75%, but this consideration is secondary to the improvement in accuracy of fit that can be obtained through the direct fitting of the frame socket to the patient. In addition to the superiority of the initial fitting, the socket can be easily adjusted when the growth of the child has changed his shape. An initial evaluation by clinical prosthetists of the fitting procecure has been successful. Clinical evaluation of the durability and comfort for the child ovver long periods of time should begin in the near future.

CAPP multiposition opposition post. Approximately 10% of congenital limb deficiencies are deficiencies of the hand.[3] The level of deficit varies from the presence of some digits to the absence of all but minimally mobile segments. The challenge to the clinician is to improve function by providing the ability to grasp independently with this partial hand without interfering with the child's other activities. Sophisticated hardware such as the wrist disarticulation prosthesis or the activated spatula result in a very high rejection rate. The loss of sensation and restriction of normal activities imposed by such devices are too high a price for the child to pay for minimal functional improvement.

In 1968, CAPP introduced the opposition post to prosthetic design.[15] The post is now a standard fitting in many clinics, but there are inadequacies in this design. Children often have difficulty in adjusting the grasp to accommodate objects of different size. Those children who have sufficiently long palmar segments can adjust anatomically. Others compensate by moving the post up and down the arm to change the paddle to the angle they desire. Many of the children only wear the post when it is useful for the task at hand, and then they remove it.

CAPP has now developed a multiposition opposition post (Fig. 42-5) to allow the child the option of changing the grasp capabilities from, for exam-

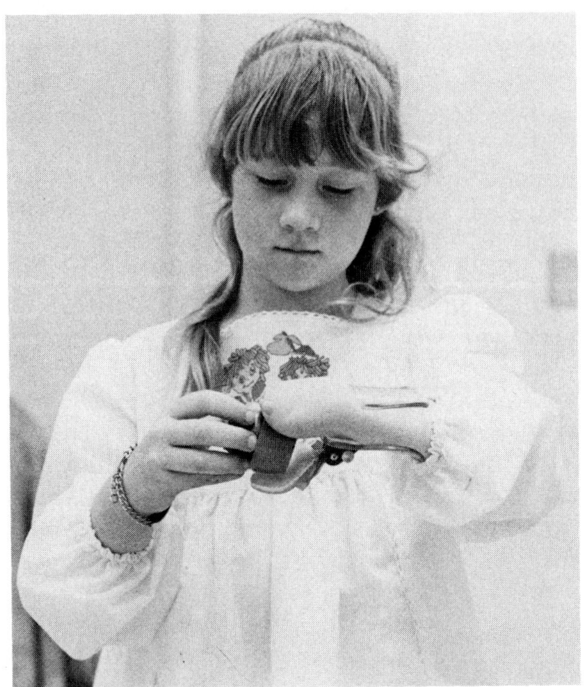

Fig. 42-5. CAPP multipositioned apposition post.

ple, sustained holding of a piece of paper to assisting in holding a hockey stick.

A strong hinge action joint has been designed that can be moved through multiple preselected position settings controlled by a simple push-button mechanism. A transparent plastic bracelet is attached to one end of the joint and a frictional surface grip paddle to the other end. The prosthetist, working with the child and the therapist, sets the angle of the paddle to accommodate the size range appropriate to the needs of the child. In general, the older child needs the capacity for fine manipulation, whereas the toddler needs a gross grasping capability. The design also features a mechanism for moving the paddle to a position flat against the forearm, completely out of the way. This feature eliminates the need to remove and reapply the post as activities change.

Externally powered prostheses

One of the major areas of research at present is in the use of external power to operate upper limb prostheses. Attempts to design powered prostheses have been made for over 20 years. The thalidomide episode from 1959 to 1961 led to the expenditure of considerable time and money for this purpose. During this period of time, several very ingenious designs were developed, using pneumatic or electric power sources. Early designs included the Heidelberg system, the coordinated arm developed at Grand Rapids, Michigan, pneumatic systems developed at New York University, and the coordinated systems from Roehampton, England. However, none of these units were used to any great degree outside of their own facilities. Although some clinical successes were originally reported, in almost all cases, the prostheses or their components were ultimately found to be less than ideal and the designs were never put into commercial production. In other cases, insufficient funds and/or lack of a manufacturer led to the discontinuance of a system under design.

Presently, only two manufacturers have commercially available powered components, not systems, although a third is in the process of marketing a powered hand terminal device.

Terminal devices. The first company to make a powered component commercially available was Otto Bock Orthopedic Industries, Inc., of Germany, which manufactured an electrically powered prosthetic hand. Unfortunately, the original hands did not come in sizes small enough for children under 12 to 13 years of age. Although the experience of fitting this terminal device has been different in different centers, in general, the greatest success rate has been in fitting unilateral below-elbow patients. At approximately the same time that the Otto Bock electrically powered hand was introduced, the Viennatone hand, which had been developed in Austria, was commercially marketed, but it had only limited success. Following the availability of these two powered hands, major research efforts (especially for adults) have been directed toward control systems and improvement in the packaging of the control systems, motors, and power sources.

Recognizing the lack of child-sized electronic devices, the Ontario Crippled Childrens Center (OCCC) in Toronto began in the mid 1960s to develop powered components for severely involved child amputees. Two devices from this research are presently available through Variety Village in Toronto. These devices are an electrically powered elbow and an electrically powered hand that comes in two sizes. These two items have been extensively field tested in the United States and Canada and are now being fitted to selected patients.

A third powered hand has been developed by Systemteknik AB in Sweden and is available for adults as well as for children as young as 2 years of age. The control of the hand is through two

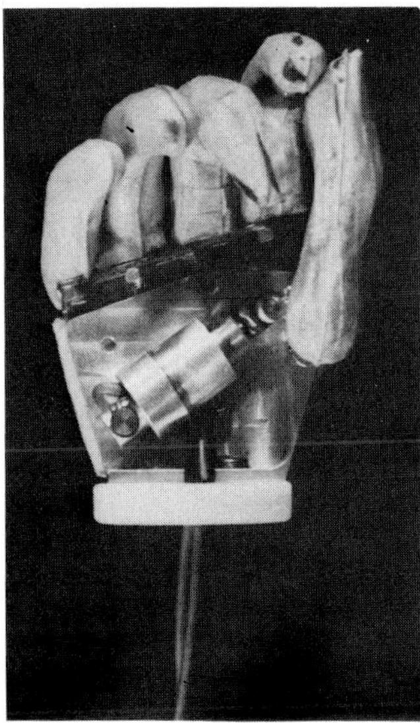

Fig. 42-6. Kenworthy externally powered hand. (Courtesy Orthopaedic Bio-Engineering Unit, Princess Margaret Rose Orthopaedic Hospital, Fairmilehead, Edinburgh, Scotland.)

myoelectric electrodes, which activate the motor that is installed in the hand. The adult myoelectric hand is more complex than the child size, providing adaptive grip, pronation and supination, and wrist flexion.

A powered hand that has good potential for children, but is still in the research stage, is being designed by Kenworthy (Fig. 42-6), in Scotland for use with the Edinburgh complete arm system.[5] The function of the hand grip is distinctive in that the thumb moves in a plane at a right angle to the plane of the fingers, facilitating the grasping of objects from tabletops and other flat surfaces without prepositioning the device. The mechanical design is simple, with emphasis placed on achieving durability and ease of repair. Stability of grip is provided through careful design of the relative positions of the index fingertip, long fingertip, and the thumb, which provide three-point contact. With the use of the proximal phalanx of the index finger, one can get a fourth point of contact. A conformable gripping surface is provided by the "power grip" system of Simpson,[13] which consists of a cloth-reinforced PVC skin filled with tiny glass beads. When the hand grips an object, the beads shift and pack, causing the surface to conform to the shape of the object and thereby increasing stability of the grip. Initial reactions to clinical testing have been favorable, with positive comments ranging from pleasure with the improved cosmesis to satisfaction with the ready use of normal feeding utensils.

Extended physiological proprioception system (EPP system). Simpson and Kenworthy have introduced an externally powered upper limb prosthesis with a new control system. The theoretical groundwork was laid in a paper by Simpson,[14] which explored the natural functioning of man's "hand-arm system."

Simpson observed that the extraordinary array of functions of the hand and upper arm appear to the careful observer to be almost automatic in the ease with which they are carried out, but are in fact extraordinarily difficult to duplicate with even the most intricate and sophisticated prosthetic machinery. The human hand and arm offer 3 positional DOF and 3 orientational ones in addition to many options of hand movements, all of which are apparently very easy to control. This is in notable contrast to, for example, the perceived complexities of driving a car, which involves only 2 DOF, but depends on visual feedback channels. Accident statistics alone attest to the complexities of this task.

The human hand and arm are not dependent on visual feedback, but apparently use a system of proprioceptive feedback to operate without the need for conscious control. It is known that joint angle receptors transmit data to the brain about the angle of each joint. This information alone is not sufficient to determine the position of the hand in space. Simpson, using a computer model, postulates the existence of some matrix of memory storage that carries data about the segment length between each joint. Simpson suggests that a "ready-made" biological system exists within the central nervous system for controlling position in space when given data about joint angles and interjoint lengths. The problem to the prosthetic designer, then, is to devise a control system that provides information to the human brain in the form in which it is most readily processed, which appears to be that of joint angles.

Simpson thus proposes a mechanism of control for the prosthetic arm that (1) matches the prosthetic interjoint lengths closely to those of the normal arm, and (2) makes each joint in the prosthetic arm correspond directly to an intact joint elsewhere in the body. Thus, for example, movement of a joint in the intact shoulder girdle could be designed to correspond directly to movement of the prosthetic elbow. This system has been called the "extended physiological proprioception (EPP) system."

The complete arm prosthesis designed by Simpson and Kenworthy[12] makes use of this approach.

A pneumatically powered system of "servoactivators" is controlled in the amelic patient by movements of the clavicles relative to the supporting harness. Each clavicle provides control movement for two functions by movement up or down, forward or back. Prehension is controlled by a waist belt device or by a digit if one is present.

The mechanism of the arm movements themselves depends on a complex gear train mechanism that permits arm movements to be considered as altering the position of the wrist with respect to the shoulder. Control of rotation of the hand in a horizontal axis in the plane of the arm has been included. Stabilization of the hand in the horizontal axis at a 90-degree angle to the arm is a feature that permits, for example, carrying a cup to the mouth without spilling. To date this system is being used in their facility with good success, although careful selection of patients and proper training is essential. A backup system is needed to ensure continued prosthetic use when the unit is broken.

INAIL myoelectric system. The INAIL project in Bologna, Italy, has designed both myoelectrically and switch-controlled upper limb prostheses for use by the older juvenile and adult patient.[8] Studies in that institution indicated the superiority of electrically over pneumatically powered components in grip strength, energy storage capacity, quantity of work between charges, and portability of the energy source. As a result of these studies electric power sources are used at the INAIL project.

The control systems are tailored to the needs of the individual patient so that maximum use is made of remaining stump function in movement of the prosthesis as a whole and in controlling its intrinsic movements. Controls are always built into the same side as the deficit. In choosing the appropriate control system, patients are divided into three groups: (1) transverse deficiencies, (2) phocomelia, and (3) amelia. Children with transverse deficiencies are fitted with a myoelectric system using the biceps and triceps muscles as signal sources. A simple locking Hosmer elbow is used. The stump itself is used for flexion and extension at the shoulder and for operation of the elbow lock.

Children with phocomelia usually have inadequate muscular development for myoelectric fitting, and therefore a system of microswitches or sensors are channeled through miniamplifiers, permitting operation of the limb through slight movements of the remnant appendage. In these prostheses, INAIL electric elbows are used with the now commercially available Otto Bock electric wrist flexors and electric hands.

Children with amelia are fitted with myoelectric controls using muscles that are active in forward, backward, and lifting motions of the shoulder. In addition, features have been included that permit operation of certain movements unilaterally or bilaterally through either myoelectric controls or microswitches.

Another total arm system is currently being evaluated in Hanover, Germany. It consists of an electromechanically powered shoulder joint, upper arm rotation unit, elbow joint, forearm supination and pronation, and hand (Otto Bock) components. By means of a special type of control, this arm permits the simultaneous performance of coordinated "flowing" movements of several joints. Control is obtained through use of a miniature potentiometer.

Sensory feedback systems. It has been apparent for some time that the conventional upper limb prostheses currently fitted are not widely accepted by the patients because the functional gains are limited. Although the prosthesis provides adequate and often even stronger prehension than that of the normal hand, and joint motion is satisfactorily reproduced, it cannot provide sensory feedback to the patient. Without the sensations of touch, pressure, and proprioception, the patient cannot recognize texture, shape, amount of force of grasp and pinch, or even the location of the prosthesis in space. The ability to recognize such factors is important for development of functional use of the hand. It is commonly accepted that the upper limb amputee wearing a prosthesis substitutes for the loss of normal sensory feedback by two means: (1) visual cues and (2) sensations received in the interfaces of socket-stump pressure and cable-harness skin pressure.

Much of the work in providing sensory feedback through the prosthesis itself has been done in the field of bioengineering. Unfortunately, little, if any, of the research has had clinical application. Almost all efforts to date have concentrated on feedback to the patient from the terminal device opening. Attempts to convey signals to the patient have included auditory signals, vibratory and other mechanical stimuli, and electrical stimulation. In the latter two methods, the skin of some part of the body, usually the amputation site, has been the receptor location. The advantage to electrical stimulation feedback is that the frequency, amplitude, and space interval information can be adjusted as desired. The primary objective has been to provide a feedback signal that is reliable and readily identifiable by the patient without being unpleasant or dangerous.

A recent attempt has been to combine surgery and electrical engineering techniques to provide a feedback system. Clippinger[2] developed a system whereby a stimulating electrode is implanted in the distal arm along the median nerve of below-elbow amputees. The transducer is located in the terminal device of the prosthesis. Stimulation varies in intensity in accordance with the amount of force exerted on an object by the terminal device. Because this is an invasive procedure, patient acceptance has been limited. Further research and development in this field is still needed.

LOWER LIMB PROSTHESES

As this chapter illustrates, the major research effort for juvenile amputees has been for those with upper limb deficiencies. The reasons for this are probably that (1) in the congenital limb deficiency population there are more upper than lower limb patients and (2) the success rate to date of upper limb acceptance has not been good. However, some research work is being done for the lower limb patients. As reported elsewhere in the book, Otto Bock has had a modular system for all levels of lower limb patients available for the past 10 years.

Polypropylene socket

An adjustable polypropylene socket has been developed for above-knee amputees.[4] All surgical amputees experience stump swelling and edema, which was conventionally treated with elastic bandaging until the stump size had stabilized. More recently, an intermediate fitting with an adjustable polypropylene socket has been used with great success.

The adjustable socket has also been of considerable help with fitting the juvenile cancer patient. Courses of chemotherapy cause significant changes in the shape and size of the stump, especially during the initial phases. The ability to vary the socket to fit the changing stump has averted prolonged periods of nonuse of the prosthesis.

The two-piece socket accommodates changes in the stump through adjustments of three Velcro straps that determine socket fit. The light weight of the modular design is particularly appropriate for those patients whose strength is often diminished by the side effects of chemotherapy.

The use of polypropylene has also led to the development of a lightweight, cosmetic, below-knee prosthesis. This concept has not yet been extensively tested on children.

CAPP foot

Children with lower limb amputations, particularly those with above-knee deficits, often experience instability while standing or walking on their prosthetic foot. Two factors contribute significantly to the instability of the conventional foot: instability at the point of heel strike and lack of accomodation to torsional forces. In the conventional foot, the reaction point is at the heel with compression at heel strike of either a heel cushion (SACH foot) or a rubber bumper (single-axis foot). This is the point of maximal instability. The amputee then shifts his weight forward until it is carried by the flat foot at midstance and then by the ball of the foot at toe-off. Toe-off becomes the period of maximum stability. The conventional foot does not accommodate to the torsional forces of walking on uneven ground, and most forces are simply transmitted upward to the stump. Some designers have created devices to be added to the conventional foot to deal with the problem like the STAR units and multiaxis ankle joints, but these represent significant additions of weight and expense and are not available in the smaller sizes required by children.

CAPP has designed a foot that addresses these problems within the foot itself (Fig. 42-7). At heel

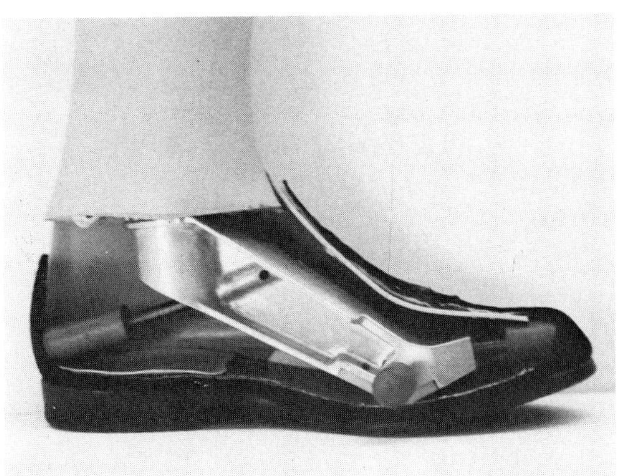

Fig. 42-7. CAPP artificial foot (still experimental).

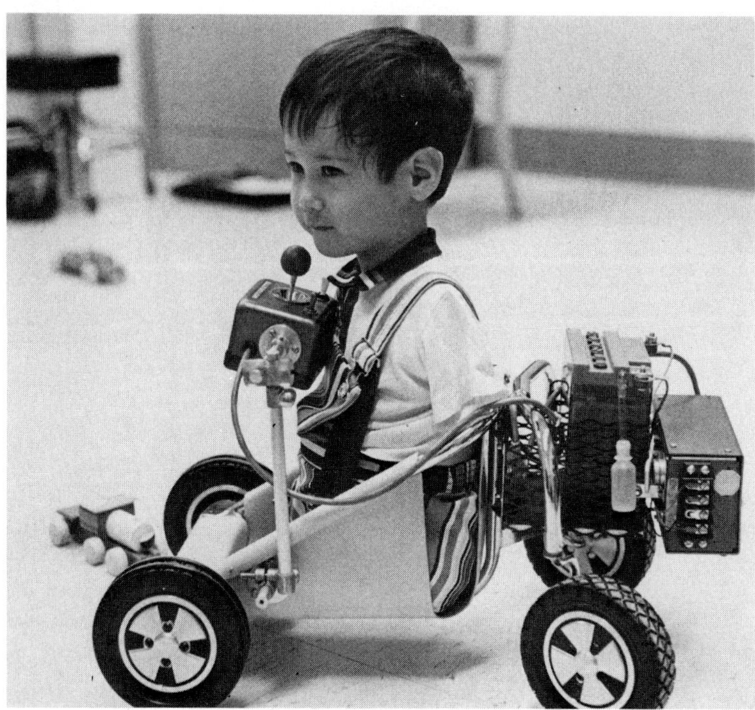

Fig. 42-8. CAPP infant electric cart.

strike, the heel flexshaft is deflected upward, and the weight of the amputee is immediately shifted to the ball of the foot. Stance phase stability is enhanced by this immediate shift to the position of maximum stability. In addition, when subjected to torsional forces, the flexshafts bend, and the foot shifts within the shoe. Any torsional forces generated by walking on uneven ground are dissipated by this shifting and are not transmitted to the stump. The stump, which is the "weak link" in the system, is protected and balance is greatly improved. This design also permits keying the foot to various shoe styles as well as making possible length adjustments for growth through three full shoe sizes.

Initial clinical trials have been satisfactory. Most patients adjust to the new action with no instruction and are pleased with the increase stability. Many children have shown greater confidence in their own abilities to walk as result of this device. This foot is still in the research design stage and is not commercially available.

Mobility systems

The multiple limb-deficient child is a challenge to the clinicians. Most children with less extensive limb deficiencies undergo a normal pattern of motor development, but the limbless child is limited in his ability to explore the environment and in his ability to move about and assert himself independently. Usually such an infant moves about by rolling on the floor and can manipulate objects only with his mouth. Independent sitting balance and upright ambulation are quite late in developing and assuming the upright position often does not occur until 4 or 5 years of age. This situation, in which the child must wait for the world to be brought to him, can have a stifling effect on his cognitive and social development.

Swivel walkers. Attempts have been made to achieve independent ambulation for the multiple limb-deficient patient using the swivel walker. In its simplest form, a swivel walker consists of a fitted pelvic socket to which are added two pylons with rocker-shaped footpieces. Movement is achieved by a combination of lateral rocking and alternate twisting of the trunk. One design by CAPP was reported in 1963[1] and found to be frustrating to the child because of the substantial output of energy required for relatively limited functional gain.

The OCCC developed a pylon arrangement designed mathematically to make maximally efficient use of the side-to-side oscillations in forward movement.[6] They reported good results in the

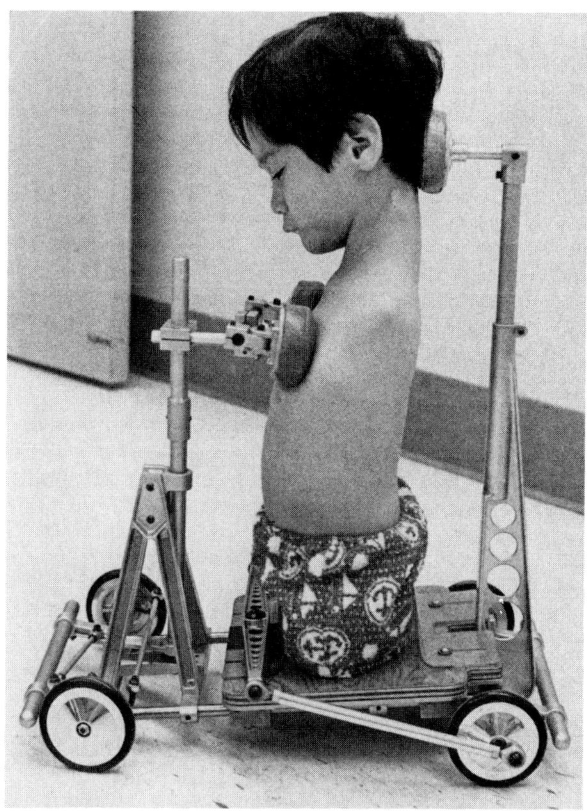

Fig. 42-9. CAPP shuffle cart.

young child with improved functional gain. Children averaged 120 steps per minute, with each step being approximately 7.5 cm (3 inches) when walking forward.

In the older child the main difficulty of the swivel walker becomes that of stability. The CG rises, and balance becomes quite precarious. In addition, it is quite difficult to achieve vertical lift. The edge of a rug or irregularities of the floor surface become serious obstacles to mobility.

CAPP electric cart. The need was recognized to provide the quadrimelic child with a safe means of independent mobility as early as possible. CAPP designed an electric cart to meet this need (Fig. 42-8).[16] The cart is controlled by a commercially available "joystick" control unit with slow speed. Initial clinical trials have been encouraging.

CAPP shuffle cart. The electric cart provides easy mobility but does not provide any outlet for the child's need to exercise. Too often the limbless child becomes inactive and passive and turns to food as a source of satisfaction. This, with the absence of exercise, leads to obesity, which even further decreases mobility. CAPP has therefore designed another cart primarily as an exerciser. This is known as the Shuffle Cart (Fig. 42-9). The Shuffle Cart is powered by pelvic rotation. The child sits on the platform stabilized by anterior and posterior supports and activates the cart with anterior pelvic tilt. This causes the platform to slide and the cart to move forward or backward, depending on the timing of the movement. Steering is accomplished by movements of the chest against the direction plate, which moves the front wheels. Despite some mechanical difficulties, those children who have used the Shuffle Cart have been enthusiastic about it.

REFERENCES

1. Blakeslee, B.: The limb deficient child, Los Angeles, 1963, University of California Press.
2. Clippinger, F. W.: A sensory feedback system for an upper-limb prosthesis, Bull. Prosthet. Res. **10**:247-258, 1974.
3. Compton, J.: Patient census at child amputee clinics—1975, Prosthetics and Orthotics Report, September, 1976, New York University Post-Graduate Medical School.
4. Irons, G. et al.: A lightweight above knee prosthesis with an adjustable socket, Orthot. Prosthet. **31**(1):3-15, 1977.
5. Kenworthy, G.: An artificial hand incorporating function and cosmesis, Biomed. Eng. **9**:559-562, 1974.
6. Motloch, W. M., and Elliott, J.: Fitting and training children with swivel walkers, Artif. Limbs **10**(2):24-38, 1966.
7. Ring, N. D., and Benford, J. M.: Carbon-fibre based harness for artificial arms, Biomed. Eng. **6**:17-21, 1971.
8. Schmidl, H.: The INAIL experience in fitting upper extremity dysmelia patients with myoelectric control, Orthop. Tech., 1977.
9. Setoguchi, Y.: The CAPP two-way shoulder joint, Inter-Clin. Info. Bull. **16**(1):1-8, 1974.
10. Setoguchi, Y.: Some non-standard prostheses for children, Orthot. Prosthet. **29**:11-18, 1975.
11. Shaperman, J.: The CAPP terminal device, Inter-Clin. Info. Bull. **14**(2):1-12, 1975.
12. Simpson, D. C.: Design of a complete arm prosthesis, Biomed. Eng. **8**:56-59, 1973.
13. Simpson, D. C., and Kenworthy, G.: Gripping surfaces for artificial hands, Hand **3**:12-14, 1973.
14. Simpson, D. C.: Choice of control system for the multimovement prosthesis: extended physiological proprioception (e.p.p.). In Herberts, P., editor: Control of upper extremity prostheses and orthoses, Springfield, Ill., 1974, Charles C Thomas, Publisher.
15. Sumida, C. et al.: An apposition post prosthesis for transcarpal deficiencies, Inter-Clin. Info. Bull. **8**(3):1-6, 1968.
16. Sumida, C. et al.: The CAPP electric cart, Artif. Limbs **15**(2):11-15, 1971.
17. Sumida, W., and Shaperman, J.: Clinical application of the infant modular below elbow prosthesis, Inter-Clin. Info. Bull. **13**(13):1-4, 1975.

Index

□Italicized numbers indicate illustrations, and t indicates a table.

C